D0890106

SEVENTH EDITION

CLINICAL PROCEDURES FOR MEDICAL ASSISTING

Kathryn A. Booth, RN-BSN, RMA (AMT), RPT, EFR, CPhT, MS
Total Care Programming, Inc.
Palm Coast, Florida

Leesa G. Whicker, BA, CMA (AAMA)
Central Piedmont Community College—Retired
Charlotte, North Carolina

Terri D. Wyman, CPC, CMRS, CMCS, AS
Baystate Wing Hospital
Palmer, Massachusetts

McGraw Hill

CLINICAL PROCEDURES FOR MEDICAL ASSISTING, SEVENTH EDITION

Published by McGraw-Hill Education, 2 Penn Plaza, New York, NY 10121. Copyright © 2021 by McGraw-Hill Education. All rights reserved. Printed in the United States of America. Previous editions © 2017, 2014, and 2011. No part of this publication may be reproduced or distributed in any form or by any means, or stored in a database or retrieval system, without the prior written consent of McGraw-Hill Education, including, but not limited to, in any network or other electronic storage or transmission, or broadcast for distance learning.

Some ancillaries, including electronic and print components, may not be available to customers outside the United States.

This book is printed on acid-free paper.

1 2 3 4 5 6 7 8 9 LWI 21 20

ISBN 978-1-260-47707-8 (bound edition)
MHID 1-260-47707-X (bound edition)
ISBN 978-1-260-47708-5 (loose-leaf edition)
MHID 1-260-47708-8 (loose-leaf edition)

Portfolio Manager: *William Lawrensen*
Product Developer: *Christine Scheid*
Marketing Manager: *Roxan Kinsey*
Content Project Managers: *Ann Courtney/Brent dela Cruz*
Buyer: *Sandra Ludovissy*
Designer: *David W. Hash*
Content Licensing Specialist: *Lori Hancock*
Cover Image: *Pefkos/Shutterstock*
Compositor: *SPi Global*

All credits appearing on page are considered to be an extension of the copyright page.

Library of Congress Control Number: 2019952528

mheducation.com/highered

Kathryn A. Booth, RN-BSN, RMA (AMT), RPT, EFR, CPhT, MS is a medical assistant (RMA) who started her career as a nurse (RN). She has a master's degree in education as well as certifications as a pharmacy technician and in phlebotomy and medical assisting. She is a certified emergency first responder and rescue scuba diver. Kathryn is an author, an educator, and a consultant for Total Care Programming, Inc. She has over 35 years of teaching, nursing, and healthcare experience that spans five states. As an educator, Kathy has been awarded the teacher of the year in three states where she taught various health sciences, including medical assisting in both a classroom and an online capacity. Kathy serves on the AMT Examinations, Qualifications, and Standards Committee and the Cardiac Credentialing International CRAT Exam Committee, as well as on the advisory board of two educational institutions. She stays current through volunteer employment and obtaining and maintaining certifications. Her goal is to develop up-to-date, dynamic healthcare educational materials to assist her and other educators and to promote healthcare professions especially medical assisting. Kathy values the medical assisting profession, recognizing that the diverse and dynamic professionals in it are essential to the future of our healthcare system.

Leesa G. Whicker, BA, CMA (AAMA) is a Certified Medical Assistant with a BA in art with a concentration in art history. She is an educator with more than 20 years of experience in the classroom. With 35 years of experience in the healthcare field as a medical assistant, a research specialist in molecular pathogenesis and infectious disease, and a medical assisting program director and instructor, she brought a broad background of knowledge and experience to the classroom. As a curriculum expert, she served on several committees, including the Writing Team for the Common Course Library for the North Carolina Community College System and the Curriculum Committee at Central Piedmont Community College. Leesa was among the first instructors to develop online courses at Central Piedmont Community College. She has presented Methods of Active and Collaborative Learning on the national level. She recently retired from Central Piedmont Community College in Charlotte, North Carolina. Though retired from teaching, she continues searching for novel and varied ways to reach the ever-changing learning styles of today's students.

Terri D. Wyman, AS, CPC, CMRS, CMCS has 35 years of experience in the healthcare field, first as a CMA specializing in hematology/oncology and homecare and then in the medical billing and coding field. At the suggestion of a coworker, she began her career in education as instructor and program director for both medical assisting and medical billing and coding programs for several technical schools in New England. Currently, Terri is the revenue management coordinator for the Baystate Health System's Eastern Region, where her love of teaching continues in the hospital setting. She is active with her local AAPC chapter and is on the National Advisory Board for the American Medical Billing Association (AMBA) and the executive advisory board for the Massachusetts Association of Patient Account Management. She provides continuing education opportunities for AMBA members by writing numerous billing and coding courses for them and speaking at their national conferences on medical coding and revenue management topics. In the rapidly changing world of healthcare billing and coding, she is excited to continue sharing the language of billing and coding with instructors, students, and career professionals. Terri sends special thanks to Dale for his unending support and to Francis Stein, MD, whose patience with a new medical assistant years ago showed her the joy of learning and education.

Brief Contents

Contents

CHAPTER 36

Patient Interview and History *465*

CHAPTER 37

Vital Signs and Measurements *487*

CHAPTER 38

Assisting with a General Physical Examination *508*

CHAPTER 44

Assisting with Minor Surgery 649

UNIT SEVEN

Assisting with Diagnostics

CHAPTER 45

Orientation to the Lab 676

CHAPTER 46

Microbiology and Disease 697

CHAPTER 47

Collecting, Processing, and Testing Urine and Stool Specimens *728*

CHAPTER 48

Collecting, Processing, and Testing Blood Specimens *757*

CHAPTER 49

Electrocardiography and Pulmonary Function Testing *793*

Procedures

*Indicates EHRClinic video

Digital Exercises and Activities

Administrative and Clinical Skills Videos

NEW! Application-Based Activities (ABAs) Including Practice Medical Office (PMO)

Find the complete list of of NEW! Application-Based Activities (ABAs) with the Instructor Resources on Connect.

A Closer Look

Medical assisting is a rock-solid career with a variety of essential tasks. These tasks are always expanding and changing as the healthcare environment changes. Learning these tasks and stacking them together can be a challenge. The seventh edition is updated to help students as well as instructors learn these ever-changing tasks and stay current in the healthcare environment. McGraw-Hill is committed to helping prepare students to succeed in their educational program and career by providing a complete and easy set of solutions for the educators of these programs. The following will give you a snapshot of some of the exciting solutions available with the seventh edition of *Medical Assisting: Clinical Procedures with Anatomy and Physiology* for your Medical Assisting course. Instructors across the country have told us how much preparation it takes to teach medical assisting. To help, we have added more detailed information on how to organize and utilize the many available practice features and activities, as well as a breakdown by Learning Outcomes for corresponding activities entitled the Comprehensive Asset Map, located in the Instructor Resources portion of Connect.

The Content—a Note from the Authors

The seventh edition of *Medical Assisting: Clinical Procedures with Anatomy and Physiology* has many exciting and noteworthy updates. With insightful feedback from our users and reviewers, our experienced author team set out to create a one-of-a-kind, dynamic, practical, realistic, *and* comprehensive set of tools for individuals preparing to become medical assistants as well as the instructors helping them to accomplish this task.

When you begin the book, you will find it is not just about rote memorization of concepts. *Medical Assisting* immerses you in the world of BWW Medical Associates, where you learn as you confront new workplace challenges in each chapter. All elements of the book—from the case studies in each chapter and the Soft Skills Success exercises to the EHRclinic screenshots and other visuals—immerse the student in a realistic learning environment. Case studies are built around a set of patients who regularly visit BWW Medical Associates, and you will get to know these patients as well as the employees of BWW Medical Associates as you move through the chapters and the accompanying EHR exercises.

Within this framework, we have worked to provide the most up-to-date information about all aspects of the medical assisting profession, with a focus on consistency, authenticity, and accuracy. Along with thousands of minor tweaks and updates, *Medical Assisting,* seventh edition, incorporates the following:

- **New!** Over 100 EHRclinic electronic health record exercises correlated to 34 chapters.
- **New!** A complete set of 23 EHRclinic exercises included with Chapter 12 Electronic Health Records that provides documentation of EHR proficiency and a "big picture" journey for the student.
- Dozens of BWW EHR documentation/progress note examples in both clinical and administrative chapters.

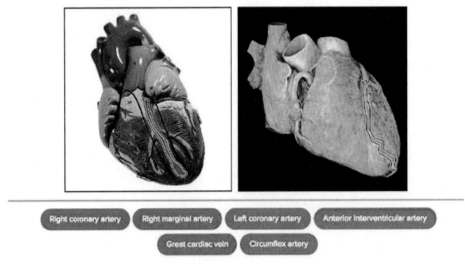

Coronary Circulation: Anterior View

Click on the name of each structure to reveal its location on the model and cadaver photos.

Right coronary artery　Right marginal artery　Left coronary artery　Anterior interventricular artery

Great cardiac vein　Circumflex artery

FIGURE FM-1 The new Practice Atlas.
©McGraw-Hill Education

- Soft Skills Success exercises located with the Chapter Review that test employability skills and link students to related modules in Practice Medical Office (PMO) and Application-Based Activities (ABAs).
- ⓥEHRclinic Over 30 ⓥEHRclinic screenshots throughout the text to showcase basic EHR skills in the context of the BWW Medical Associates.
- Case studies that are enhanced by the inclusion of more detailed clinical information and link to the new Soft Skills Success activities where applicable.
- Coding content focusing on ICD-10-CM, including detailed 1500 claim form instructions utilizing the 5010 updates to make the form compliant with ICD-10 requirements
- **New!** Thirteen math and dosage videos and questions located as assignments in Connect.
- Inclusion of content and terminology related to all of the current medical assisting standards to help ensure student certification success.
- Brand new level heading in all of the anatomy and physiology chapters titled "Diagnostic Exams and Test."
- **New! Medical Terminology Practice** feature with the anatomy and physiology chapters to bring further understanding of the power of the construction and deconstruction of medical terms, as well as corresponding practice questions in the Chapter Review.
- **New!** Corresponding practice of anatomy and physiology with **Practice Atlas** on Connect.

A more detailed list of chapter changes is covered in the next section.

Key Chapter-by-Chapter Changes

The following chapter-by-chapter list includes the essential changes and updates made to the book. A full list of changes is available in the transition guide provided in the Instructor Resources on Connect.

Chapter 1	The medical assistant as a patient navigator, scope of practice procedure, standard of care, and practice test provided by certification organizations. A new procedure titled Locate Your State's Legal Scope of Practice
Chapter 3	Professional use of personal electronic devices and social media, customer service as professionalism, cultural diversity with co-workers
Chapter 4	Introduction to Behavioral Health Issues, Substance Abuse, and Gender Identity and Sexuality and more detail about Roadblocks to Effective Communication
Chapter 5	POLST, Advance Medical Directive, DNR, and DNAR
Chapter 6	OPIM, transmission-based precautions, and OSHA education and training requirements for ambulatory care
Chapter 7	Computer Vision Syndrome, service dogs and comfort animals, visual relay services
Chapter 9	Mixing 10% bleach solution; key terms *anoscope, examination light, laryngeal mirror, nasal speculum, otoscope, penlight, reflex hammer*
Chapter 12	Meaningful Use, expanded coverage of shared data, general guidelines for using an EHR program, practice management systems, updated EHR content with new ⓥEHRclinic program
Chapter 14	Communicating with deaf, Uber, Lyft, and cell phone use
Chapter 15	Electronic media use, defined modeling versus return demonstration; sample e-newsletter, patient information form, and physician information figures added
Chapter 21	New Medical Terminology focus feature and "Diagnostic Exams and Tests" heading under Pathophysiology section
Chapter 22	Added melanin and modified burn and skin cancer sections, New Medical Terminology focus feature and "Diagnostic Exams and Tests" heading under Pathophysiology section
Chapter 23	New Medical Terminology focus feature and "Diagnostic Exams and Tests" heading under Pathophysiology section
Chapter 24	New Medical Terminology focus feature and "Diagnostic Exams and Tests" heading under Pathophysiology section
Chapter 25	Added *interatrial* and *interventricular* as related to the septum and additional information about capillaries; new Medical Terminology focus feature and "Diagnostic Exams and Tests" heading under Pathophysiology section
Chapter 26	New Medical Terminology focus feature and "Diagnostic Exams and Tests" heading under Pathophysiology section
Chapter 27	Removed HIV/AIDS section and revised Medical Terminology focus feature and "Diagnostic Exams and Tests" heading under Pathophysiology
Chapter 28	Added image of paranasal sinuses, new Medical Terminology focus feature and "Diagnostic Exams and Tests" heading under Pathophysiology section
Chapter 29	New Medical Terminology focus feature and "Diagnostic Exams and Tests" heading under Pathophysiology section
Chapter 30	New Medical Terminology focus feature and "Diagnostic Exams and Tests" heading under Pathophysiology section

Learning Outcomes, Key Terms, and Textbook Organization

Every learning outcome in *Medical Assisting,* seventh edition, is aligned with a level I heading. McGraw-Hill has made it even easier for students and instructors to find, learn, and review critical information. The chapter organization of the seventh edition is organized to promote learning based on what a medical assistant does in practice. The chapters build on one another to ensure student understanding of the many tasks they will be expected to perform. The chapters can be easily grouped together to create larger topics or units for the students to learn. For ease of understanding, content can be organized as follows:

- Unit One, Medical Assisting as a Career—Chapters 1, 3, 4, 5
- Unit Two, Safety and the Environment—Chapters 6, 7, 9
- Unit Three, Communication—Chapters 12, 14, 15
- Unit Four, Administrative Practices—Chapters 15 to 20
- Unit Five, Applied Anatomy and Physiology—Chapters 21 to 34
- Unit Six, Clinical Practices—Chapters 35 to 44
- Unit Seven, Assisting with Diagnostics—Chapters 45 to 50
- Unit Eight, Assisting in Therapeutics—Chapters 51 to 55
- Unit Nine, Medical Assisting Practice—Chapters 56 to 58

Key terms are called out at the beginning of each chapter and are set in bold throughout the text to further promote the mastery of learning outcomes.

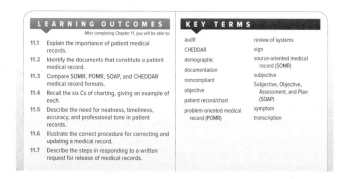

Content Correlations

Medical Assisting, seventh edition, also provides a correlation structure that will enhance its usefulness to both students and instructors. We have been careful to ensure that the text and supplements provide coverage of topics crucial to all of the following:

- CAAHEP (Commission on Accreditation of Allied Health Education Programs) Standards and Guidelines for Medical Assisting Education Programs

- ABHES (Accrediting Bureau of Health Education Schools) Competencies and Curriculum
- AAMA (American Association of Medical Assistants) CMA (Certified Medical Assistant) Occupational Analysis
- AMT (American Medical Technologists) RMA (Registered Medical Assistant) Task List
- AMT (American Medical Technologists) CMAS (Certified Medical Assistant Specialist) Competencies and Examination Specifications
- NHA (National Healthcareer Association) Certified Clinical Medical Assistant (CCMA)
- NHA (National Healthcareer Association) Certified Medical Administrative Assistant (CMAA)
- CMA (AAMA) Certification Examination Content Outline
- NCCT (National Center for Competency Testing) National Certified Medical Assistant (NCMA) Detailed Test Plan
- NAHP (National Association for Health Professionals) Nationally Registered Certified Medical Assistant (NRCMA) content outline
- NAHP (National Association for Health Professionals) Nationally Registered Certified Administrative Health Assistant (NRCAHA) content outline
- CAHIIM (Commission on Accreditation for Health Informatics and Information Management Education)
- SCANS Correlation

Correlations to these are included with the instructor resources located on Connect (see later pages for information about Connect™). In addition, CAAHEP requires that all medical assistants be proficient in the 71 entry-level areas of competence when they begin medical assisting work. ABHES requires proficiency in the competences and curriculum content at a minimum. The opening pages of each chapter provide a list of the areas of competence that are covered within the chapter.

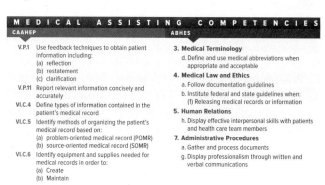

You will also find that each procedure is correlated to the ABHES and CAAHEP competencies within the workbook on the procedure sheets. These sheets can be easily pulled out of the workbook and placed in the student file to document proficiency.

Chapter Features

Each chapter opens with material that includes the Case Study, the learning outcomes, a list of key terms, the ABHES and CAAHEP medical assisting competencies covered in the chapter, and an introduction. Since the learning outcomes represent each of the level I headings in the chapter, they serve as the chapter outline. Chapters are organized into topics that move from the general to the specific. Updated color photographs, anatomical and technical drawings, tables, charts, and text features help educate the student about various aspects of medical assisting. The text features include the following:

- **Case Studies** are provided at the beginning of all chapters. They represent situations similar to those that the medical assistant may encounter in daily practice. The case studies include pictures of each of the patients who come to BWW Medical Associates for care (and, where applicable, matching *avatars* in the new ⍰EHRclinic and ABAs). Students are encouraged to consider the case study as they read each chapter. Case Study Questions in the end-of-chapter review check students' understanding and application of chapter content.

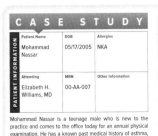

CASE STUDY		
PATIENT INFORMATION	**Patient Name** Mohammad Nassar	**DOB** 05/17/2005	**Allergies** NKA
	Attending Elizabeth H. Williams, MD	**MRN** 00-AA-007	**Other Information**

for his rescue inhaler in the last several days. His mother has brought him to the appointment, but Mohammad Nassar has asked that she remain in the reception area during his appointment. She does give you a list of Mohammad's current asthma medications and the previously completed new patient documents.

©David Sacks/Getty Images

Mohammad Nassar is a teenage male who is new to the practice and comes to the office today for an annual physical examination. He has a known past medical history of asthma, which has been relatively stable until recently. He states when he arrives that he has been experiencing an increasing need

Keep Mohammad Nassar (and his mother) in mind as you study this chapter. There will be questions at the end of the chapter based on the case study. The information in the chapter will help you answer these questions.

©David Sacks/Getty Images

CASE STUDY CRITICAL THINKING

Recall Mohammad from the case study at the beginning of the chapter. Now that you have completed the chapter, answer the following questions regarding his case.

1. As a new patient, which documents should be completed prior to Mohammad being seen by the

physician? What documents should he have brought with him, if available?

2. Your office uses a SOAP format for medical records. After Dr. Williams completes her exam, explain where each of the new documents or pieces of information obtained during Mohammad's exam will be filed using the SOAP format.

©David Sacks/Getty Images

- **Procedures** give step-by-step instructions on how to perform specific administrative or clinical tasks that a medical assistant will be required to perform. The procedures are referenced within the content when discussed and found in their entirety at the end of the chapter. In the workbook, the tearable procedure sheets mirror the exact procedures in the book and allow for easy practice and assessment. Critical procedures also can be studied in Clinical or Administrative skills video exercises on Connect, as well as new step-by-step videos of the procedures using the ⍰EHRclinic.

PROCEDURE 12-1 Creating a New Patient Record Using EHR Software

Procedure Goal: To create a new patient record using EHR software

OSHA Guidelines: This procedure does not involve exposure to blood, body fluids, or tissue.

Materials: Initial patient forms (patient information, advance directives, physician notes, referrals, and laboratory orders)

Method:

1. From the ⍰EHRclinic home screen, select "Tools" from the left side of the screen.

2. On this Administrative tools screen, under the Information Management window, click on the blue bar labeled "Manage practice data."

3. At the next screen, Information Management List, choose "Patient Information." At the top of the Patient Listing, click the "Add New Patient" button.

4. The patient's chart number will auto-populate on the

RATIONALE: *This is a legal record. The information must be entered completely and correctly.*

8. Any field marked with an * is a required field. For instance, the patient's address is a required field, as is the identification number. The insurance name field must be completed with the insurance company name. This field may also be used if the patient does not have insurance by entering "none" or used temporarily if the patient has insurance that is new to the practice that would be entered into the system. In any case, the insurance name field is required.

RATIONALE: *A required field is considered essential information by the practice, so the field cannot be skipped.*

9. Continue entering the information in each field, and use the scroll bar on the right-hand side of the screen to see all of the fields.

10. Inspect all information for accuracy. Once you are satisfied that all information is complete and accurate, click the "Add Patient" button to save the patient

- **Points on Practice** feature boxes provide guidelines on keeping the medical office running smoothly and efficiently.

- **Educating the Patient** feature boxes focus on ways to instruct patients about caring for themselves outside the medical office.

- **Caution: Handle with Care** feature boxes cover the precautions to be taken in certain situations or when performing certain tasks.

CAUTION: HANDLE WITH CARE

Maintaining Standards of Cleanliness in the Reception Area

Cleanliness is (and should be) one of a medical office's hallmarks. Not only is cleanliness required in the examination and testing rooms, it is also expected in the patient reception area. A messy patient reception area reflects badly on the practice. Patients may think, "If they don't care about this, what else do they not care about?" Maintaining standards of cleanliness helps ensure that the reception area is presentable and inviting at all times.

As a medical assistant, you may be involved—along with the physician, office manager, and other staff members—in setting the office's cleanliness standards. Standards are general guidelines. In addition to setting standards, you will need to specify the tasks required to meet each standard. You also may want to create a checklist of the tasks required to meet all of these standards. The following list outlines standards you may want to consider. Specific housekeeping tasks for meeting those standards are included in parentheses.

1. Keep everything in its place. (Complete a daily visual check for out-of-place items. Return all magazines to racks. Push chairs back into place.)

2. Dispose of all trash. (Empty trash cans. Pick up trash on the floor or on furniture.)

3. Prevent dust and dirt from accumulating on surfaces. (Wipe or dust furniture, lamps, and artificial plants. Polish doorknobs. Clean mirrors, wall hangings, and pictures.)

4. Spot-clean areas that become dirty. (Remove scuffmarks. Clean upholstery stains.)

5. Disinfect areas of the reception area if they have been exposed to body fluids. (Immediately clean and disinfect all soiled areas.)

6. Handle items with care. (Take precautions when carrying potentially messy or breakable items. Do not carry too much at once.)

After the standards have been established, type and post them in a prominent place for the office staff (but not the patients) to see. The cleaning activities checklist may be posted, but the person responsible for cleaning the office also should keep a copy. It is everyone's duty to keep the office looking clean and presentable.

A schedule of specific daily and weekly cleaning activities also should be posted. Less frequent housekeeping duties, such as laundering drapes, shampooing the carpet, and cleaning windows and blinds, can be noted in a tickler file so that they will be performed on a regular basis.

It is always a good idea to have a second staff member responsible for periodically working with the medical assistant on housekeeping responsibilities. That person also may be responsible for handling cleaning duties when the medical assistant is away from the office.

- **Pathophysiology** is featured in each of the chapters on anatomy and physiology. These sections provide students with details of the most common diseases and disorders of each body system and include information on the causes, common signs and symptoms, diagnostic exams and tests, treatment, and, where possible, the prevention of each disease.

PATHOPHYSIOLOGY   LO 23.11

Common Diseases and Disorders of the Skeletal System

Arthritis is a general term meaning "joint inflammation." Although there are more than 100 types of arthritis, we will discuss the two most common types: osteoarthritis and rheumatoid arthritis.

OSTEOARTHRITIS, also known as *degenerative joint disease (DJD),* is the most common type of joint disorder, affecting nearly everyone to some degree by the age of 70. DJD primarily affects the weight-bearing joints of the hips and knees, and the cartilage between the bones and the bones themselves begin to break down.

Causes. Research points to inflammatory processes or metabolic disorders as the etiology of DJD.

Signs and Symptoms. These include joint stiffness, aching, and pain, especially with weather changes. There is often fluid around the joint and grating noises with joint movement. The grating noise is usually caused by bone-on-bone contact.

Diagnostic Exams and Tests. X-rays of the affected joint are used to determine if osteoarthritis is present. Blood tests are

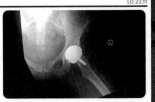

FIGURE 23-14 X-ray image of the Birmingham Hip Resurfacing prosthesis of the left hip.
©Total Care Programming, Inc.

Causes. RA is an autoimmune disease. The body's immune system attacks the synovium (lining) of the joints, triggering inflammation.

Signs and Symptoms. In this disease, immune system attacks cause edema (swelling), tenderness, and warmth in and around the joints. Tissue becomes granular and thick, eventually

Each chapter closes with a summary of the Learning Outcomes. The summary is followed by an end-of-chapter review with questions related to the case study, as well as 10 multiple-choice exam-style questions.

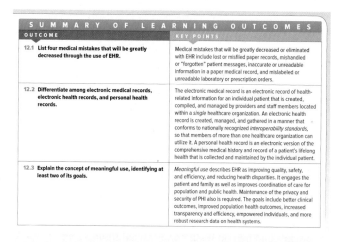

- **Medical Terminology** practice exercises have been added to all the anatomy and physiology chapters.

- **Soft Skills Success** practice scenarios emphasize employ-ability skills and critical thinking in complex situations. These new exercise features are included in most non-A&P chapters and are correlated to Practice Medical Office and Application-Based Activities where applicable.

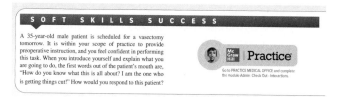

The book also includes a glossary and three appendices for use as reference tools. The glossary lists all the words presented as key terms in each chapter, along with a pronunciation guide and the definition of each term. The appendices present a list of common medical terminology, including prefixes, root words, and suffixes, as well as medical abbreviations and symbols. A Diseases and Disorders appendix provides a quick reference point for patient conditions that the student may encounter.

Digital Materials for *Medical Assisting*

For the seventh edition, we enhanced the integration between the textbook and our digital study materials and expanded our offerings to better cover all aspects of medical assisting. Links between the textbook and the key study resources are highlighted by eye-catching icons divided by resource type. Digital study resources with icons include BodyANIMAT3D, ⏻EHRclinic electronic health record exercises, and both Administrative and Clinical Skills videos. Real-life practice opportunities include Practice Medical Office and Application-Based Activities, with icons at the end of the chapter.

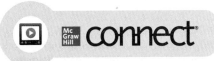

Go to CONNECT to see a video exercise about *Establishing and Conducting the Supply Inventory and Receiving Supplies.*

These different types of icons are then used to call out specific activities and exercises by name. For example, above you can see an icon for Connect skills videos (the resource) about Establishing and Conducting Supply Inventory and Receiving Supplies (the exercise name).

McGraw-Hill Connect® Medical Assisting

A number of our key resources for *Medical Assisting,* 7e—including BodyANIMAT3D activities, skills video exercises, and ⏻EHRclinic electronic health records exercises—are part of our Connect offering for Medical Assisting.

Here is more on what you can expect to find in Connect for *Medical Assisting,* 7e, specifically:

- NEW! ⏻EHRclinic Exercises
  - Over 101 *electronic health record actionable exercises* correlated to over 34 chapters of Booth *Medical Assisting,* 7th edition. These simulated exercises allow students to navigate the ⏻EHRclinic tool while learning the tasks of a Medical Assistant.
- NEW! ⏻EHRclinic *financial practice management exercises* designed to provide students with practical experience with electronic billing, charge capture, payment posting, and more.
- Pre- and Post-Tests
- End-of-Chapter Exercises
- Interactive Exercises
- Administrative and Clinical Skills Video Exercises*
- BodyANIMAT3D Exercises*
- ICD-10 Coding Exercises*
  - Utilizing scenarios developed by the authors, students can practice identifying and inputting the proper ICD-10 codes.

*in applicable chapters

- Medical Terminology Practice*
  - A refresher area for the body systems chapters with Word Part exercises on select terms as well as audio terms with associated spelling practice.
- NEW! Math and dosage videos with questions that reinforce basic math needed by Medical Assistant students.
- NEW! **Practice Atlas** exercises for all of the Anatomy and Physiology chapters. The Practice Atlas for Anatomy & Physiology is an interactive tool that pairs images of common anatomical models with stunning cadaver photography, which allows students to practice naming structures on both models and human bodies. Additional multiple choice questions for practice are available as assignments in Connect.
- A completely revised and updated Test Bank (also available through the Instructor Resources).

As part of Connect for *Medical Assisting,* we also offer SmartBook's adaptive reading experience, which is powered by LearnSmart, the most widely used adaptive learning resource.

For more information on Connect—the teaching and learning platform used with all McGraw-Hill Education products—and SmartBook, look for the section *Connect, Required=Results.*

Simulations and Games for Medical Assisting

⏻EHRclinic, McGraw-Hill's NEW electronic health record tool, allows for the look and feel of a real electronic health records system fully integrated with CONNECT. ⏻EHRclinic provides over 101 exercises directly correlated to 34 chapters of Booth *Medical Assisting,* 7e, with *Chapter 12 Electronic Health Records* being the most robust. These actionable exercises allow students to navigate the ⏻EHRclinic tool, providing practical experience using electronic health records while they learn the tasks of a medical assistant. These simulated exercises are assignable in Connect and are autograded. Chapter 12 includes 23 exercises that take the student through the paces of electronic health records including administrative functions and financial management. Completion of these exercises in total provides the basis for documenting electronic health record practical experience and gives the student "the big picture."

In **Practice Medical Office (PMO),** the student takes on the role of a new medical assistant in a 3D, immersive game focused on teaching the six key skills important to working in a medical office—professionalism, soft skills, office acumen, liability, medical knowledge, and privacy. **Practice Medical Office** features 12 engaging and challenging

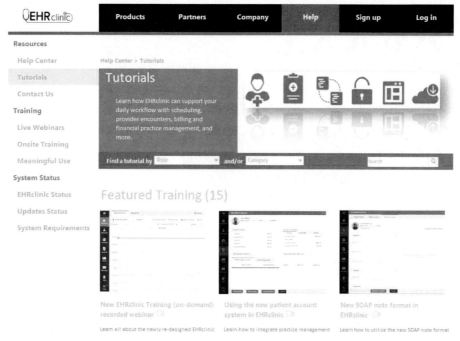

FIGURE FM-2 The new ◯EHR clinic

©McGraw-Hill Education

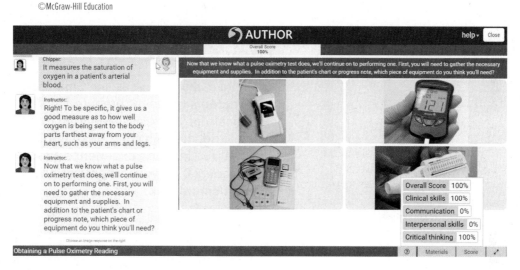

FIGURE FM-3 A new Application-Based Activity (ABA)

©McGraw-Hill Education

modules representing the functional areas of a medical practice: administrative check-in interactions, clinical interactions, and administrative check-out interactions. As the players progress through each module, they will be faced with realistic situations and learning events that will test their mastery of critical job readiness skills in a fun, engaging learning experience. The **PMO modules** will be found together with the **Application-Based Activities** described below.

For a demo of **Practice Medical Office,** please go to http://www.mhpractice.com/products/Practice_Medical_Office and click on "Play the Demo." An instructor's manual for PMO, correlated to ABHES and CAAHEP standards by learning event, is available in your Instructor Resources on Connect.

For the NEW **Application-Based Activities,** or **ABAs,** the student is immersed in a brief, microsimulation experience, with the ability to practice steps in key Procedures *outside* a lab and "virtually" with an instructor. Along with the **Procedure ABAs,** students will be able to practice real-life **Scenario ABAs** that call upon decision making and application of medical assisting knowledge. Depending on the **ABA,** students will be graded on Objectives such as Clinical Skills, Administrative Skills, Interpersonal Skills, Communication, and more, all of which are aligned with ABHES and CAAHEP standards in the instructor materials. Find a full list of the **ABAs,** as well as resources for how to incorporate in your course, in the Instructor Resources on Connect.

On Connect, both the **PMO modules** and the **ABAs** can be found within the "Add Assignment" menu, under "MH Practice Activity" (title at publication).

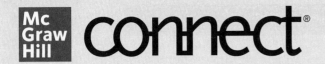

You're in the driver's seat.

Want to build your own course? No problem. Prefer to use our turnkey, prebuilt course? Easy. Want to make changes throughout the semester? Sure. And you'll save time with Connect's auto-grading too.

65%
Less Time Grading

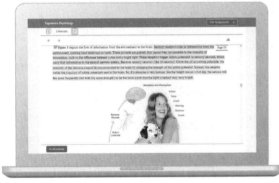

Laptop: McGraw-Hill; Woman/dog: George Doyle/Getty Images

They'll thank you for it.

Adaptive study resources like SmartBook® 2.0 help your students be better prepared in less time. You can transform your class time from dull definitions to dynamic debates. Find out more about the powerful personalized learning experience available in SmartBook 2.0 at **www.mheducation.com/highered/ connect/smartbook**

Make it simple, make it affordable.

Connect makes it easy with seamless integration using any of the major Learning Management Systems— Blackboard®, Canvas, and D2L, among others—to let you organize your course in one convenient location. Give your students access to digital materials at a discount with our inclusive access program. Ask your McGraw-Hill representative for more information.

Padlock: Jobalou/Getty Images

Solutions for your challenges.

A product isn't a solution. Real solutions are affordable, reliable, and come with training and ongoing support when you need it and how you want it. Our Customer Experience Group can also help you troubleshoot tech problems— although Connect's 99% uptime means you might not need to call them. See for yourself at **status. mheducation.com**

Checkmark: Jobalou/Getty Images

Effective, efficient studying.

Connect helps you be more productive with your study time and get better grades using tools like SmartBook 2.0, which highlights key concepts and creates a personalized study plan. Connect sets you up for success, so you walk into class with confidence and walk out with better grades.

Study anytime, anywhere.

Download the free ReadAnywhere app and access your online eBook or SmartBook 2.0 assignments when it's convenient, even if you're offline. And since the app automatically syncs with your eBook and SmartBook 2.0 assignments in Connect, all of your work is available every time you open it. Find out more at **www.mheducation.com/readanywhere**

"I really liked this app—it made it easy to study when you don't have your text-book in front of you."

- Jordan Cunningham, Eastern Washington University

No surprises.

The Connect Calendar and Reports tools keep you on track with the work you need to get done and your assignment scores. Life gets busy; Connect tools help you keep learning through it all.

Calendar: owattaphotos/Getty Images

Learning for everyone.

McGraw-Hill works directly with Accessibility Services Departments and faculty to meet the learning needs of all students. Please contact your Accessibility Services office and ask them to email accessibility@mheducation.com, or visit **www.mheducation.com/about/accessibility** for more information.

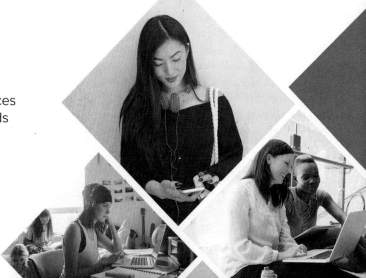

Additional Supplementary Materials

Student Workbook for Use with *Medical Assisting, 7e*—in print and full color (ISBN: 978-1-260-47702-3)

The *Student Workbook* provides an opportunity for the student to review and practice the material and skills presented in the textbook. The workbook is divided into parts and presented by chapter; the first part provides the following:

- Vocabulary review exercises, which test knowledge of key terms in the chapter
- Content review exercises, which test the student's knowledge of key concepts in the chapter
- Critical thinking exercises, which test the student's understanding of key concepts in the chapter
- Application exercises, which include figures and practice forms and test mastery of specific skills
- Case studies, which apply the chapter material to real-life situations or problems

Each section, Clinical and/or Administrative, contains the appropriate procedures, presented in the order in which they are shown in the student textbook. These have been revised for ease of use and include correlations to the ABHES and CAAHEP competencies mastered with the successful completion of each procedure. Accompanying Work Product Documentation (work/doc) provides blank forms for many of the procedures that require a specific type of document to complete the procedure. These documentation forms are used when completing many of the application activities as well as procedure competencies. Over 100 procedures as well as multiple application activities in the workbook include correlated work docs.

Pocket Guide for Use with *Medical Assisting, 7e* (ISBN: 978-1-260-47700-9)

The *Pocket Guide* is a quick and handy reference to use while working as a medical assistant or during training. It includes critical procedure steps, bulleted lists, and brief information all medical assistants should know. Information is sorted by Administrative, Clinical, Laboratory, and General content.

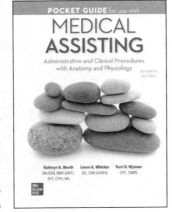

Instructor Resources

Medical Assisting also comes with the instructor resources you've come to expect, all of which can be found through the Instructor Resources section in Connect.

- An **Instructor's Manual** that contains everything to organize your course, complete with lecture outlines (with PowerPoint slide references), discussion points, learning activities, and case studies. Also included are the answer keys to the book and workbook.
- **Correlation Guides** map the standards of many accreditation bureaus, including the Accrediting Bureau of Health Education Schools (ABHES) Medical Assisting competencies and curriculum; the Commission on Accreditation of Allied Health Education Programs (CAAHEP) Standards and Guidelines for Medical Assisting Education Programs competencies; American Association of Medical Assistants (AAMA) Occupational Analysis; the Association of Medical Technologists (AMT) Registered Medical Assistant (RMA) Certified Exam Topics; the National Healthcareer Association (NHA) Medical Assisting Duty/Task List; the National Association for Health Professionals (NAHP) Nationally Registered Certified Medical Assistant (NRCMA) and Nationally Registered Certified Administrative Health Assistant (NRCAHA) content outlines; the Commission for Accreditation on Health Informatics and Information Management Education (CAHIIM); and the Secretary's Commission on Achieving Necessary Skills (SCANS) areas of competence, as well as others.
- **PowerPoint Presentations** have been fully updated to include the latest figures and content and to mirror the design of the book. Teaching notes offer suggestions—in addition to those in the Instructor's Manual—to keep your class running smoothly. We also have taken steps to make our PowerPoints more accessible, including adding alt tags for images and tables and ensuring that our slides are organized to be easily read by screen readers.
- A **Comprehensive Asset Map** breaks down all of the resources available through the book and Connect by chapter and by learning outcome to help you identify *what* you want to include in your course and *where* to find it.
- **New! Challenging Topics Asset Map** uses Heat Map data gathered from LearnSmart to determine the most challenging topics and Learning Objectives for students and then gives direction as to what resources and practice activities are available for those Learning Objectives, allowing the instructor to focus lectures or group chats on areas most needed.
- A **Transition Guide** to help users of earlier editions make the leap to this new edition, with thorough details outlined by the authors about changes big and small.

Test Builder in Connect

Available within Connect, Test Builder is a cloud-based tool that enables instructors to format tests that can be printed or administered within a LMS. Test Builder offers a modern, streamlined interface for easy content configuration that matches course needs, without requiring a download.

Test Builder allows you to:

- access all test bank content from a particular title.
- easily pinpoint the most relevant content through robust filtering options.
- manipulate the order of questions or scramble questions and/or answers.
- pin questions to a specific location within a test.
- determine your preferred treatment of algorithmic questions.
- choose the layout and spacing.
- add instructions and configure default settings.

Test Builder provides a secure interface for better protection of content and allows for just-in-time updates to flow directly into assessments.

Tegrity: Lectures 24/7

Tegrity in Connect is a tool that makes class time available 24/7 by automatically cap¬turing every lecture. With a simple one-click start-and-stop process, you capture all computer screens and corresponding audio in a format that is easy to search, frame by frame. Students can replay any part of any class with easy-to-use, browser-based viewing on a PC, Mac, iPod, or other mobile device.

Educators know that the more students can see, hear, and experience class resources, the better they learn. In fact, studies prove it. Tegrity's unique search feature helps students efficiently find what they need, when they need it, across an entire semester of class recordings. Help turn your students' study time into learning moments immediately supported by your lecture. With Tegrity, you also increase intent listening and class participation by easing students' concerns about note-taking. Using Tegrity in Connect will make it more likely you will see students' faces, not the tops of their heads.

Check out the Instructor Resources area on Connect for additional resources, including an image library, sample syllabi, printable procedure checklists and work documents, and more!

CASE STUDY

EMPLOYEE INFORMATION	Employee Name	Position	Credentials
	Sandro Peso	Student	In Training
	Supervisor	**Date of Hire**	**Other Information**
	Malik Katahri, CMM	10/11/2019	Assigned to Dr. Paul F. Buckwalter

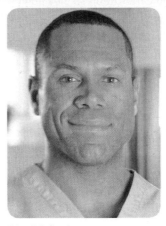
©Ryan McVay/Getty Images

Sandro Peso, a father of four in his mid-thirties, lost his job at a local factory. He is now a medical assistant-in-training and is currently working at BWW Medical Associates. He will be working in the administrative, clinical, and laboratory sections of the office. He wants to decide which area he likes best and where he might like to work when he finishes his training. It will not be long until he graduates and needs to take the test to become credentialed. He is nervous about the exam but really wants to do well to get the best job he can to help support his family.

Keep Sandro Peso in mind as you study this chapter. There will be questions at the end of the chapter based on the case study. The information in the chapter will help you answer these questions.

LEARNING OUTCOMES

After completing Chapter 1, you will be able to:

1.1 Recognize the duties and responsibilities of a medical assistant.

1.2 Distinguish various organizations related to the medical assisting profession.

1.3 Explain the need for and importance of the medical assistant credentials.

1.4 Identify the training needed to become a professional medical assistant.

1.5 Discuss professional development as it relates to medical assisting education.

KEY TERMS

accreditation
Accrediting Bureau of Health Education Schools (ABHES)
American Association of Medical Assistants (AAMA)
American Medical Technologists (AMT)
certification
Certified Medical Assistant (CMA)
Clinical Laboratory Improvement Amendments of 1988 (CLIA '88)
Commission on Accreditation of Allied Health Education Programs (CAAHEP)
continuing education
cross-training
Health Insurance Portability and Accountability Act (HIPAA)
licensed practitioner
multiskilled healthcare professional (MSHP)
Occupational Safety and Health Administration (OSHA)
patient navigator
professional development
Registered Medical Assistant (RMA)
registration
résumé
scope of practice
standard of care

V.C.12 Define patient navigator

V.C.13 Describe the role of the medical assistant as a patient navigator

X.C.1 Differentiate between scope of practice and standards of care for medical assistants

X.C.5 Discuss licensure and certification as they apply to healthcare providers

X.P.1 Locate a state's legal scope of practice for medical assistants

1. General Orientation

  a. Describe the current employment outlook for the medical assistant

  c. Describe and comprehend medical assistant credentialing requirements, the process to obtain the credential and the importance of credentialing

  d. List the general responsibilities and skills of the medical assistant

4. Medical Law and Ethics

  f. Comply with federal, state, and local health laws and regulations as they relate to healthcare settings

    (1) Define the scope of practice for the medical assistant within the state that the medical assistant is employed

    (2) Describe what procedures can and cannot be delegated to the medical assistant and by whom within various employment settings

10. Career Development

  b. Demonstrate professional behavior

  c. Explain what continuing education is and how it is acquired

▶ Introduction

Healthcare is changing at a rapid rate. Advanced technology, implementation of cost-effective medicine, and the aging population are all factors that have caused growth in the healthcare services industry. As the healthcare services industry expands, the US Department of Labor projects that medical assisting will grow 29% between 2012 and 2022, which is much faster than the average for all occupations. The growth in the number of physicians' group practices and other healthcare practices that use support personnel such as medical assistants will in turn continue to drive up demand for medical assistants. The multifunctional medical assistant is the perfect complement to the changing healthcare industry.

Medical assistants have the training to perform a variety of duties, which qualify them to fill many different job openings in the healthcare industry. This chapter provides an introduction to the medical assisting profession. It presents a general description of your future duties, credentials, and needed training. Some basic facts about professional associations, organizations, and development related to medical assisting also are discussed. All of this will help you understand the career of a medical assistant.

▶ Responsibilities of the Medical Assistant   LO 1.1

Your specific responsibilities as a medical assistant will depend on the type, location, and size of the facility, as well as its medical specialties. General tasks performed by most medical assistants include working and communicating with patients throughout the healthcare experience. In fact, medical assistants often perform the role of **patient navigator.** They help patients find their way through the sometimes complex healthcare system, helping them overcome any barriers they may encounter to help ensure that they get the diagnosis and treatment they need in a timely manner.

Medical assistants work in an administrative, clinical, and/or laboratory capacity. As an administrative medical assistant, you may handle the payroll for the office staff (or supervise a payroll service), obtain equipment and supplies, and serve as the link between the physician or other **licensed practitioner** and representatives of pharmaceutical and medical supply companies. As a clinical medical assistant, you will be the physician's or other licensed practitioner's right arm by maintaining an efficient office, assisting the practitioner during examinations, and keeping examination rooms in order. Note that a licensed practitioner in healthcare means an individual other than a physician who is licensed or otherwise authorized by the state to provide healthcare services. Your laboratory duties as a medical assistant may include performing basic laboratory tests and maintaining laboratory equipment. In small practices, you may handle all duties. In larger practices, you may specialize in a particular duty. As you grow in your profession, advanced duties may be required. The lists of duties in Table 1-1 are provided to help you better understand what you will be doing when you practice as a medical assistant.

TABLE 1-1   Daily Duties of Medical Assistants

Duty Type	Entry-Level Duties	Advanced Duties
General 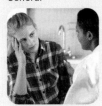 ©monkeybusinessimages/ iStockphoto/Getty Images	• Recognizing and responding effectively to verbal, nonverbal, and written communications • Explaining treatment procedures to patients • Providing patient education within scope of practice • Facilitating treatment for patients from diverse cultural backgrounds and for patients with hearing or vision impairments, or physical or mental disabilities • Acting as a patient navigator and advocate • Maintaining medical records	None
Administrative 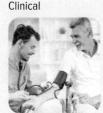 ©JGI/Daniel Grill/Blend Images/Getty Images	• Greeting patients • Handling correspondence • Scheduling appointments • Answering telephones • Creating and maintaining patient medical records • Handling billing, bookkeeping, and insurance processing • Performing medical transcription • Arranging for hospital admissions	• Developing and conducting public outreach programs to market the licensed practitioner's professional services • Negotiating leases of equipment and supply contracts • Negotiating nonrisk and risk managed care contracts • Managing business and professional insurance • Developing and maintaining fee schedules • Participating in practice analysis • Coordinating plans for practice enhancement, expansion, consolidation, and closure • Performing as a **HIPAA (Health Insurance Portability and Accountability Act)** compliance officer • Providing personnel supervision and employment practices • Providing information systems management
Clinical 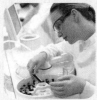 ©VGstockstudio/Shutterstock	• Assisting the licensed practitioner during examinations • Assisting with asepsis and infection control • Performing diagnostic tests, such as spirometry and ECGs • Giving injections, where allowed • Phlebotomy, including venipuncture and capillary puncture • Disposing of soiled or stained supplies • Performing first aid and cardiopulmonary resuscitation (CPR) • Preparing patients for examinations • Preparing and administering medications as directed by the licensed practitioner, and following state laws for invasive procedures • Recording vital signs and medical histories • Removing sutures or changing dressings on wounds • Sterilizing medical instruments • Instructing patients about medication and special diets, authorizing drug refills as directed by the licensed practitioner, and calling pharmacies to order prescriptions • Assisting with minor surgery • Teaching patients about special procedures before laboratory tests, surgery, X-rays, or ECGs	• Initiating an IV and administering IV medications with appropriate training and as permitted by state law • Reporting diagnostic study results • Assisting patients in the completion of advance directives and living wills • Assisting with clinical trials
Laboratory ©Adam Gault/AGE Fotostock	• Performing Clinical Laboratory Improvement Amendments (CLIA)–waived tests, such as a urine pregnancy test, on the premises • Collecting, preparing, and transmitting laboratory specimens • Teaching patients to collect specific specimens properly • Arranging laboratory services • Meeting safety standards (OSHA guidelines) and fire protection mandates	• Performing as an OSHA compliance officer • Performing moderately complex laboratory testing with appropriate training and certification

You also may choose to specialize in a specific area of healthcare. For example, podiatric medical assistants make castings of feet, expose and develop X-rays, and assist podiatrists in surgery. Ophthalmic medical assistants help ophthalmologists (doctors who provide eye care) by administering diagnostic tests, measuring and recording vision, testing the functioning of eyes and eye muscles, and performing other duties. A discussion of medical specialties is found in the chapter *Healthcare and the Healthcare Team.* For specific information about medical assistant duties within medical specialty practice, refer to the following chapters: *Assisting in Reproductive and Urinary Specialties, Assisting in Pediatrics, Assisting in Geriatrics, Assisting in Other Medical Specialties,* and *Assisting with Eye and Ear Care.*

▶ Medical Assisting Organizations   LO 1.2

Many organizations guide the profession of medical assisting. These include professional associations such as the American Association of Medical Assistants (AAMA), the American Medical Technologists (AMT), and National Healthcareer Association (NHA), as well as accrediting and registering organizations. As a future medical assistant, knowledge of these organizations will help you make critical decisions about your career.

Professional associations set high standards for quality and performance in a profession. They define the tasks and functions of an occupation, provide members with the opportunity to communicate and network with one another, as well as offer **continuing education.** Becoming a member of a professional association helps you achieve career goals and furthers the profession of medical assisting. Joining as a student is encouraged, and some associations even offer discounted rates to students for a specified amount of time after graduation.

American Association of Medical Assistants

The idea for a national association of medical assistants—later to be called the **American Association of Medical Assistants (AAMA)**—was suggested at the 1955 annual state convention of the Kansas Medical Assistants Society. The next year, at an American Medical Association (AMA) meeting, the AAMA was officially created. In 1978, the US Department of Health, Education, and Welfare declared medical assisting as an allied health profession.

AAMA's Purpose The AAMA works to raise standards of medical assisting to a more professional level. It is the only professional association devoted exclusively to the medical assisting profession. The AAMA provides the CMA (AAMA) credential.

AAMA Occupational Analysis In 1996, the AAMA formed a committee whose goal was to revise and update its standards for the **accreditation** of programs that teach medical assisting. The committee's findings were published in 1997 as the "AAMA Role Delineation Study: Occupational Analysis of the Medical Assistant Profession." In 2009, it was updated and named the "Occupational Analysis of the

CMA (AAMA)". In 2013, the study identified the 12 most frequently performed responsibilities of medical assistants. They are listed here in the order of most performed to least performed.

1. Abide by principles and laws related to confidentiality.
2. Adapt communications to an individual's understanding.
3. Demonstrate respect for individual diversity (culture, ethnicity, gender, race, religion, age, economic status).
4. Employ professional techniques during verbal, nonverbal, and text-based interactions.
5. Comply with risk management and safety procedures.
6. Interact with staff and patients to optimize workflow efficiency.
7. Maintain patient records.
8. Provide care within legal and ethical boundaries.
9. Practice standard precautions.
10. Document patient communication, observations, and clinical treatments.
11. Identify potential consequences of failing to operate within the scope of practice of a medical assistant.
12. Transmit information electronically.

Professional Support for CMAs (AAMA) When you become a member of the AAMA, you will have a large support group of active medical assistants. Membership benefits include:

- Professional publications, such as *CMA Today.*
- A large variety of educational opportunities, such as chapter-sponsored seminars and workshops about the latest administrative, clinical, and management topics.
- Group insurance.
- Legal information.
- Local, state, and national activities that include professional networking and multiple continuing education opportunities.
- Legislative monitoring to protect your right to practice as a medical assistant.
- Access to the website at http://www.aama-ntl.org.

American Medical Technologists (AMT)

American Medical Technologists (AMT) is a nonprofit certification agency and professional membership association representing over 45,000 individuals in allied healthcare. Established in 1939, AMT began a program to register medical assistants at accredited schools in the early 1970s. The AMT provides allied health professionals with professional certification services and membership programs to enhance their professional and personal growth. Upon certification, individuals automatically become members of AMT and start to receive benefits. You will read more about the benefits of joining a professional organization later in the chapter. The AMT provides many certifications, including the Registered Medical Assistant RMA (AMT) credential and the Certified Medical Assistant Specialist CMAS (AMT) credential.

Professional Support for RMA (AMT) and CMAS (AMT) The AMT offers many benefits. These include:

- Professional publications.
- Membership in the AMT Institute for Education.
- Group insurance programs—liability, health, and life.
- State chapter activities.
- Legal representation in health legislative matters.
- Annual meetings and educational seminars.
- Student membership.
- Access to the website at http://www.americanmedtech.org.

National Healthcareer Association (NHA)

The National Healthcareer Association (NHA) (http://www.nhanow.com) was established in 1989 as an information resource and network for today's active healthcare professionals. NHA provides certification and continuing education services for healthcare professionals and curriculum development for educational institutions. It offers a variety of certification exams, including Clinical Medical Assistant (CCMA), Medical Administrative Assistant (CMAA), Billing and Coding Specialist (CBCS), and Electronic Health Records Specialist (CEHRS).

Some of the NHA's programs and services include:

- Certification development and implementation.
- Continuing education curriculum development and implementation.
- Program development for unions, hospitals, and schools.
- Educational, career advancement, and networking services for members.
- Registry of certified professionals.

Healthcare educators working in their various fields of study develop the National Healthcare Association certification exams. The NHA is a member of the National Organization of Competency Assurance (NOCA).

Other Medical Assistant Organizations

Other organizations assist potential and current medical assisting professionals. These include the National Center for Competency Testing (NCCT) and the National Association for Health Professionals (NAHP).

The National Center for Competency Testing (NCCT) (https://www.ncctinc.com) is an independent agency that certifies the validity of competency and knowledge of the medical profession through examination. Medical assistants and medical office assistants receive the designation of National Certified Medical Assistant (NCMA) and National Certified Medical Office Assistant (NCMOA) after passing the certification examination. The NCCT avoids any allegiance to a specific organization or association.

The National Association for Health Professionals (NAHP) (http://www.nahpusa.com) offers multiple credentials for healthcare professionals. The organization, which has been in existence for 30 years, prides itself in making the process of obtaining a credential an accessible, affordable, and obtainable goal for individuals who wish to show commitment to their chosen profession. Having multiple credentials with one agency makes maintaining continuing education easier for practicing healthcare professionals. The NAHP offers many credentials, including the Nationally Registered Certified Medical Assistant (NRCMA), the Nationally Registered Certified Coding Specialist (NRCCS), and the Nationally Registered Certified Administrative Health Assistant (NRCAHA).

With the growth of the medical assisting field, new organizations have developed to serve professionals. For example, the American Medical Certification Association (AMCA), founded in 2010, provides certification for clinical and/or administrative medical assistants. The American Registry of Medical Assistants (ARMA) is also one of many national certifying organizations that certify/register medical assistants. Prospective medical assistants should be knowledgeable about the agency they will use to obtain their medical assistant credential.

▶ Medical Assistant Credentials   LO 1.3

Certification is confirmation by an organization that an individual is qualified to perform a job to professional standards. **Registration,** on the other hand, does not guarantee an individual's competence. Instead, registration is the granting of a title or license by a board that gives permission to practice in a chosen profession. Once credentialed, you earn the right to wear a pin that is obtained through the credentialing organization (Figure 1-1).

Medical assistant credentials such as certification and registration are not always required to practice as a medical assistant. However, employers today are aggressively recruiting medical assistants who are credentialed in their field. As discussed in the Medical Assisting Organizations, many credentials are available for medical assisting by various organizations. Small physician practices are being consolidated or merged into larger providers of healthcare, such as hospitals, to decrease operating expenses. Human resource directors of

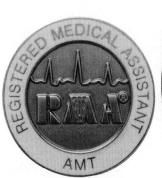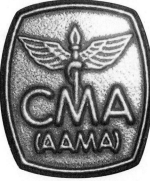

FIGURE 1-1   Wearing one of these pins indicates you have obtained a credential in medical assisting. Medical assistants registered by the American Medical Technologists must past the RMA exam to be certified and can wear the pin on the left. Members of the American Association of Medical Assistants who pass the CMA exam wear the pin on the right.
©Total Care Programming, Inc.

these larger organizations place great importance on professional credentials for their employees. Hiring credentialed medical assistants may lessen the likelihood of a legal challenge. Common administrative and clinical certifications are provided in Table 1-2.

State and Federal Regulations

Certain provisions of the **Occupational Safety and Health Administration (OSHA)** and the **Clinical Laboratory Improvement Amendments of 1988 (CLIA '88)** are making mandatory credentialing for medical assistants a logical step in the hiring process. OSHA and CLIA '88 regulate healthcare but presently do not require that medical assistants be credentialed. However, various components of these statutes can be met by demonstrating that medical assistants are certified. For example, some physician offices perform moderately complex laboratory testing onsite. The medical assistant can perform moderately complex tests if she or he has the appropriate training and skills.

AAMA Credential

The **Certified Medical Assistant (CMA)** credential is awarded by the Certifying Board of the AAMA. The AAMA's certification examination evaluates mastery of medical assisting competencies based on the Occupational Analysis of the CMA (AAMA), which is available at http://www.aama-ntl. org/resources/library/OA.pdf. The National Board of Medical Examiners (NBME) also provides technical assistance in developing the tests.

CMAs (AAMA) must recertify the credential every 5 years. To be recertified as a CMA (AAMA), 60 contact hours must be accumulated during the 5-year period: 10 in the administrative area, 10 in the clinical area, and 10 in the general area, with 30 additional hours in any of the three categories. In addition, 30 of these contact hours must be from an approved AAMA program. The AAMA also requires you to hold a current CPR card.

The recertification mandate requires you to learn about new medical developments through education courses or participation in an examination. Hundreds of continuing education courses are sponsored by local, state, and national AAMA

groups. The AAMA also offers self-study courses through its continuing education department.

Only students who have completed medical assisting programs accredited by CAAHEP and ABHES are eligible to take the certification examination. The AAMA offers the Candidate's Guide to the Certification Examination to help applicants prepare for the examination. This guide explains the test format and test-taking strategies. It also includes a sample examination with answers and information about study references. Some schools also have incorporated test preparation reviews into their programs.

The CMA (AAMA) examination is a computerized test that may be taken any time at a designated testing site in your area. You may search the Internet for an application and test review materials. Once you have successfully passed the CMA (AAMA) examination, you have earned the right to add that credential to your name, such as Miguel A. Perez, CMA (AAMA).

AMT Credentials

The American Medical Technologists (AMT) organization credentials medical assistants as **Registered Medical Assistants (RMA)** or Certified Medical Assistant Specialists (CMAS). Although this section focuses on the RMA credential, you can find more about the CMAS credential on the AMT website at https://www.americanmedtech.org/.

Requirements for the RMA (AMT) credential include:

- Graduation from a medical assistant program that is accredited by ABHES or CAAHEP or is accredited by a regional accrediting commission, by a national accrediting organization approved by the US Department of Education, or by a formal medical services training program of the US Armed Forces.
- Alternatively, employment in the medical assisting profession for a minimum of 5 years, no more than 2 years of which may have been as an instructor in the postsecondary medical assistant program.
- Passing the AMT examination for RMA (AMT) certification.

RMAs (AMT) must accumulate 30 contact hours for continuing education units (CEUs) every 3 years if they were

TABLE 1-2 Medical Assisting Credentials		
Type of Certification	**Certification Title**	**Certifying Organization**
Administrative and Clinical	Certified Medical Assistant (CMA)	AAMA
Administrative and Clinical	Registered Medical Assistant (RMA) AMT	AMT
Administrative and Clinical	National Certified Medical Assistant (NCMA)	NCCT
Administrative and Clinical	Nationally Registered Certified Medical Assistant (NRCMA)	NAHP
Clinical	Certified Clinical Medical Assistant (CCMA)	NHA
Administrative	Medical Administrative Assistant (CMAA)	NHA
Administrative	Certified Medical Assistant Specialist (CMAS)	AMT
Administrative	National Certified Medical Office Assistant (NCMOA)	NCCT
Administrative	Nationally Registered Certified Administrative Health Assistant (NRCAHA)	NAHP

certified after 2006. RMAs (AMT) who were certified before this date are expected to keep abreast of all the changes and practices in their field through educational programs, workshops, or seminars. However, there are no specific continuing education requirements. Once a medical assistant has passed the AMT exam, she has earned the right to add RMA (AMT) to her name: Kaylyn R. Haddix, RMA (AMT).

Credentialing Examinations

Credentialing examinations are rigorous. Participation in an accredited program will help you learn what you need to know. Each certification examination is based on a specific content outline created by the certifying organization. Most organizations provide their content outline as well as practice examinations for potential medical assistants to prepare. You should research the Internet to gain additional information regarding any of these certifications. See Procedure 1-1, Obtaining Certification/Registration Information Through the Internet.

▶ Training Programs   LO 1.4

With continuous changes in healthcare today, the role of the medical assistant has become dynamic and wide-ranging. These changes have expanded the expectations for medical assistants. The knowledge base of the modern medical assistant includes:

- Administrative and clinical skills.
- Patient insurance product knowledge (specific to the workers' geographic locations).
- Compliance with healthcare-regulating organizations.
- Exceptional customer service.
- Practice management.
- Current patient treatments and education.

The medical assisting profession requires a commitment to self-directed, lifelong learning. Healthcare is changing rapidly because of new technology, new healthcare delivery systems, and new approaches to facilitating cost-efficient, high-quality healthcare. A medical assistant who can adapt to change and is continually learning will be in high demand.

Formal programs in medical assisting are offered in a variety of educational settings, including vocational-technical high schools, postsecondary vocational schools, community and junior colleges, and 4-year colleges and universities. Vocational school programs usually last 9 months to 1 year and award a certificate or diploma. Community and junior college programs are usually 2-year associate's degree programs. Training can be obtained through traditional classroom as well as online settings.

An accredited medical assisting program is competency based; this means that standards are set by an accrediting body for skill and proficiency in administrative and clinical tasks. It is the educational institution's duty to ensure that medical assisting students learn all medical assisting competencies and that evidence is clearly documented for each student. Periodic evaluations are performed by the accrediting agencies to ensure the effectiveness of the program.

Program Accreditation

Accreditation is the process by which programs are officially authorized. The US Department of Education recognizes two national entities that accredit medical assisting educational programs:

- **Commission on Accreditation of Allied Health Education Programs (CAAHEP).** CAAHEP works directly with the Medical Assisting Educational Review Board (MAERB) of Medical Assistants Endowments to ensure that all accredited schools provide a competency-based education. CAAHEP accredits medical assisting programs in both public and private postsecondary institutions throughout the United States that prepare individuals for entry into the medical assisting profession.

- **Accrediting Bureau of Health Education Schools (ABHES).** ABHES accredits private postsecondary institutions and programs that prepare individuals for entry into the medical assisting profession.

Accredited programs must cover the following topics:

- Anatomy and physiology
- Medical terminology
- Medical law and ethics
- Psychology
- Oral and written communications
- Laboratory procedures
- Clinical and administrative procedures

High school students may prepare for these courses by studying mathematics, health, biology, office skills, bookkeeping, and information technology. You may obtain current information about accreditation standards for medical assisting programs from the AAMA.

Medical assisting programs also must include a practicum (externship) or work experience. This applied training is for a specified length of time in an ambulatory care setting, such as a physician's office, hospital, or other healthcare facility. Additionally, the AAMA lists its minimum standards for accredited programs. This list of standards ensures that all personnel—administrators and faculty alike—are qualified to perform their jobs. These standards also ensure that financial and physical resources are available at accredited programs.

Graduation from an accredited program helps your career in three ways. First, it shows that you have completed a program that meets nationally accepted standards. Second, it provides recognition of your education by professional peers. Third, it makes you eligible for registration or certification. Students who graduate from an CAAHEP- or ABHES-accredited medical assisting program are eligible to take the CMA (AAMA) or RMA (AMT) immediately.

Work Experience

Your practicum (externship) or work experience is mandatory in accredited schools. The length of your experience will vary, depending on your particular program, so familiarize yourself with the program requirements as soon as possible.

Because this is a required part of the program, no matter how good your grades are in class, if the work experience is not completed, you will not graduate from the program.

Your practicum (externship) or work experience is an extension of your classroom learning experience. You will apply skills learned in the classroom in an actual medical office or other healthcare facility. You also earn the right to include this applied training experience on your résumé under job experience, as long as you title it as "Medical Assistant Practicum, Externship, or Work Experience." The *Preparing for the World of Work* chapter will further explain your practical work experience.

▶ Professional Development   LO 1.5

Professional development refers to skills and knowledge attained for both personal development and career advancement. During your training, you should strive to improve your knowledge and skills. This will help you transition into your first job with ease. You also can gain valuable knowledge and skills through volunteering prior to or in addition to work experience obtained as a student.

Once you have entered the world of work as a medical assistant, you will want to continue to develop in your profession. You can do this through additional training, **cross-training,** and other forms of continuing education.

Volunteer Programs

Volunteering is a rewarding experience. Before you even begin a medical assisting program, you can gain experience in a healthcare profession through volunteer work. As a volunteer, you will get hands-on training and learn what it is like to assist patients who are ill, disabled, or frightened.

You may volunteer as an aide in a hospital, clinic, nursing home, or doctor's office, or as a typist or filing clerk in a medical office or medical record room. Some visiting nurse associations and hospices (homelike medical settings that provide medical care and emotional support to terminally ill patients and their families) also offer volunteer opportunities. These experiences may help you decide if you want to pursue a career as a medical assistant.

The American Red Cross also offers volunteer opportunities for student medical assistants. The Red Cross needs volunteers for its disaster relief programs locally, statewide, nationally, and abroad. As part of a disaster relief team at the site of a hurricane, tornado, storm, flood, earthquake, or fire, volunteers learn first-aid and emergency triage skills. Red Cross volunteers gain valuable work experience that may help them obtain a job.

Because volunteers are not paid, it is usually easy to find work opportunities. Just because you are not paid for volunteer work, however, does not mean the experience is not useful for meeting your career goals.

Include information about any volunteer work on your **résumé**—a document that summarizes your employment and educational history. Be sure to note specific duties, responsibilities, and skills you developed during the volunteer experience. Refer to the *Preparing for the World of Work* chapter for examples of résumés.

Multiskilled Healthcare Professionals

Many hospitals and healthcare practices are embracing the idea of a **multiskilled healthcare professional (MSHP).** An MSHP is a cross-trained team member who is able to handle many different duties.

Reducing Healthcare Costs By hiring multiskilled healthcare professionals, healthcare organizations can reduce personnel costs. MSHPs can perform the functions of two or more people, so they are cost-effective employees and are in high demand.

Expanding Your Career Opportunities Career opportunities are vast if you are self-motivated and willing to learn new skills. Following are some examples of positions for medical assistants with additional experience and certifications:

- Medical office manager
- Medical biller and coder
- Medical assisting instructor (with a specified amount of experience and education)
- ECG technician
- Sterilization technician
- Patient care technician

If you are multiskilled, you will have an advantage when job hunting. Employers are eager to hire multiskilled medical assistants and may even create positions for them.

You can gain multiskill training by showing initiative and a willingness to learn every aspect of the medical facility in which you are working. When you begin working in a medical facility, establish goals regarding your career path and discuss them with your immediate supervisor. Indicate to your supervisor that you would like cross-training in every aspect of the medical facility. Begin in the department in which you are currently working and branch out to other departments once you master the skills needed for your current position. This will demonstrate a commitment to your profession and a strong work ethic. Cross-training is a valuable marketing tool to include on your résumé.

Scope of Practice

Professional development includes knowing your **scope of practice** and working within it. Medical assistants are not "licensed" healthcare professionals, and most often work under a licensed healthcare provider, such as a nurse practitioner or physician. Licensed healthcare professionals may delegate certain duties to a medical assistant, providing he or she has had the appropriate training through an accredited medical assisting program or through on-the-job training provided by the medical facility or physician.

Questions often arise regarding the kinds of duties a medical assistant can perform. There is no universal answer to these questions. There is no single national definition of a medical assistant's scope of practice, so the medical assistant must research the state in which he or she works to learn about the scope of practice. You can find this information online by entering "medical assistant scope of practice" and the name of your state in any major search engine. See Procedure 1-2, Locating Your State's Legal Scope of Practice. In general, a medical assistant may not perform procedures for which he or she was not educated or trained. Examples of procedures medical assistants may not perform include administering intravenous medications (without advanced training), diagnosing patients or informing patients of a diagnosis, and giving any advice to a patient unless permitted by a facility's standard policies and procedures. The AAMA and AMT are good resources to assist you in your research. The AAMA Occupational Analysis is also a helpful reference source that identifies the procedures that medical assistants are educated to perform.

Do not confuse the terms *scope of practice* and *standard of care*. A medical assistant's scope of practice is the set of procedures that can be performed and the actions that can be taken under the terms of his or her professional license and training. **Standard of care** is a legal term that refers to the care that would ordinarily be provided by an average, prudent healthcare provider in a given situation.

Networking

Networking is building alliances—socially and professionally. It starts long before your job search. By attending professional association meetings, conferences, or other functions, medical assistants generate opportunities for employment and personal and professional growth. Networking, through continuing education conferences throughout your career, keeps the doors open to employment advancement.

PROCEDURE 1-1 Obtaining Certification/Registration Information Through the Internet   WORK // DOC

Procedure Goal: To obtain information from the Internet regarding professional credentialing

OSHA Guidelines: This procedure does not involve exposure to blood, body fluids, or tissue.

Materials: Computer with Internet access and printer

Method:

1. Open your Internet browser and use a search engine to search for the credential you would like to pursue—for example, Certified Medical Assistant or Registered Medical Assistant. If you are unsure of the credential you would like to pursue, you may just want to search for "Medical Assisting Credentials."

2. Select the site for the credential you are pursuing. Avoid sponsored links. These links are paid for and typically will not take you to the site of a credentialing organization.

   For example to navigate to the home page:

   - For the CMA (AAMA) credential, enter the site http://www.aama-ntl.org.

AMERICAN ASSOCIATION OF MEDICAL ASSISTANTS

   - For the RMA (AMT) or CMAS (AMT) credential, enter the site http://www.americanmedtech.org.

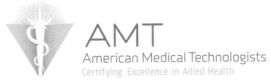
AMT American Medical Technologists
Certifying Excellence in Allied Health

   - For other selected credentials navigate to the selected organization.
     - National Association for Health Professionals (NAHP): http://nahpusa.com/
     - National Center for Competency Testing (NCCT): https://www.ncctinc.com/
     - National Healthcareer Association (NHA): http://www.nhanow.com/

3. Determine the steps you must take to obtain the selected credential. You will need to navigate to the information about the requirements for eligibility, certification standards, and the examination outline.

4. Print or write down the qualifications you must obtain.
   RATIONALE: *Maintaining a record of needed qualifications will be a reference as you pursue your chosen credential.*

5. Once you have met the qualifications, you will need to apply for the examination or certification. Download the application and the application instructions for the RMA (AMT) or the CMAS (AMT) or the candidate application and handbook for the CMA (AAMA).

6. To view or print these instructions, you may need to download Adobe Reader. You can click on a link to download Adobe Reader after you click on the "Apply Online" link for AMT or "Apply for the Exam" for AAMA.

7. Before or after you apply for the examination, you will need to prepare for the examination. Select the link "Study for the Exam" on the AAMA site or the "Prepare for Exam" link under the "Get Certified" drop-down menu on the AMT site.

8. Prepare for the exam by reviewing the content outline, obtaining additional study resources, or taking a practice exam online.

9. Print or save downloaded information in a file folder on your desktop labeled "Credentials" or another name you can recognize. To print, click the printer icon found at the bottom of the web page or click the printer icon in your browser.

Professionalism and Success

CASE STUDY

Employee Name	**Position**	**Credentials**
Kaylyn R. Haddix	Clinical Medical Assistant	RMA (AMT)
Supervisor	**Date of Hire**	**Other Information**
Malik Katahri, CMM	06/11/2018	Meeting with Malik at 1 P.M.

EMPLOYEE INFORMATION

Kaylyn R. Haddix does well with the "hands-on" skills and gets along fairly well with the other office personnel. However, Kaylyn has a problem with getting to work on time. She seems to show a pattern of poor planning, such as forgetting to set her alarm, losing her car keys, and neglecting to solve her various car problems when they first become apparent (brought on by skipped oil changes, worn tire treads, squeaky brakes, and a rusty muffler). The clinic suffers when

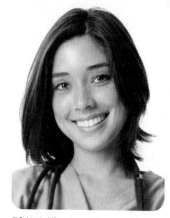

©Rubberball/Getty Images

Kaylyn is late because she is not ready to see the first patient upon arrival, causing patients to wait and disrupting the routines and schedules of other staff members. Following the third time she was late, Malik, the office manager, noted the problem in Kaylyn's record and informed Kaylyn that chronic tardiness could lead to termination. Although Kaylyn is sometimes afraid to ask questions, her performance is generally above average, so Malik is hoping that Kaylyn will improve.

Keep Kaylyn in mind as you study this chapter. There will be questions at the end of the chapter based on the case study. The information in the chapter will help you answer these questions.

LEARNING OUTCOMES

After completing Chapter 3, you will be able to:

3.1 Recognize the importance of professionalism in the medical assisting practice.

3.2 Explain the professional behaviors that should be exhibited by medical assistants.

3.3 Model strategies for success in medical assisting education and practice.

KEY TERMS

attitude
comprehension
constructive criticism
critical thinking
cultural diversity
empathy
hard skills
integrity
organization
patient advocacy

persistence
prioritize
problem solving
punctuality
self-confidence
soft skills
teamwork
time management
work ethic
work quality

V.A.1 Demonstrate:
(a) empathy

V.A.2 Demonstrate the principles of self-boundaries

V.A.3 Demonstrate respect for individual diversity including:
(a) gender
(b) race
(c) religion
(d) age
(e) economic status
(f) appearance

VII.A.1 Demonstrate professionalism when discussing patient's billing record

XI.P.2 Demonstrate appropriate responses to ethical issues

XI.A.1 Recognize the impact personal ethics and morals have on the delivery of healthcare

I.A.2 Incorporate critical thinking skills when performing patient care

5. Human Relations
b. Provide support for terminally ill patients
(1) Use empathy when communicating with terminally ill patients
c. Assist the patient in navigating issues and concerns that may arise (e.g., insurance policy information, medical bills, physician/provider orders)

10. Career Development
a. Perform the essential requirements for employment such as resume writing, effective interviewing, dressing professionally, time management, and following up appropriately
b. Demonstrate professional behavior

▶ Introduction

A profession is an occupation or a career based upon specialized educational training. Professionalism is behavior that exhibits the traits or features that correspond to the standards of that profession. Professional standards vary from occupation to occupation, and some vary within the same occupation, depending on the environment. And, of course, these standards go way beyond just personal appearance, although they do include this. Imagine the difference between the professional standards required of a commercial jet pilot who logs thousands of miles despite tough weather conditions and is responsible for the lives of 200-plus passengers at any given time versus those of a hobby pilot who likes to fly his Cessna solo for a few hours on sunny weekends. Will their uniforms or dress codes be different? Is punctuality equally important in both cases? Luckily, you will not need to worry too much about airplanes as a medical assistant, but this is just one example of how professional standards may differ in a particular industry.

As discussed in the *Introduction to Medical Assisting* chapter, standards for medical assisting education and the profession are developed by professional organizations, such as the American Association of Medical Assistants (AAMA), the American Medical Technologists (AMT), and the National Health Career Association (NHA). To be a professional medical assistant, not only do you need to know standards of the profession, but you also must be able to exhibit appropriate personal attributes and behaviors.

Success is a favorable or desired outcome. To achieve a favorable or desired outcome from your medical assisting education and in practice, you must follow the standards and exhibit the personal behaviors established by your school

and workplace. In this chapter, you will explore the professional behaviors required of a medical assistant in school and in practice, as well as the attributes and strategies needed for success in your education and career.

▶ Professionalism in Medical Assisting   LO 3.1

The mere fact that you are reading this book means you are embarking on the profession of medical assisting. To understand this profession, you should first understand what a profession consists of. A profession has two areas of competence (abilities):

1. **Hard skills**—specific technical and operational proficiencies
2. **Soft skills**—personal qualifications or behaviors that enhance an individual's interactions, job performance, and career prospects; these are sometimes called people skills (Figure 3-1)

Hard skills represent the minimum proficiencies necessary to do the job. Following are some examples of hard skills of medical assisting:

- Scheduling appointments
- Coding for insurance purposes
- Managing medical records
- Interviewing patients
- Taking vital signs
- Assisting a provider with patient examinations

These hard skills are the ones you will learn throughout this program, and your ability to perform them is readily observable. Your hard skills set is the first screen employers use to determine if you are qualified for the position.

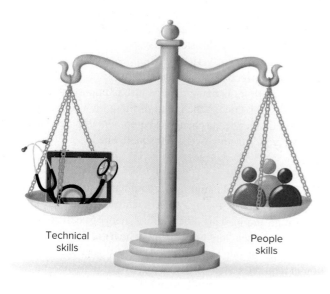

FIGURE 3-1 As a medical assistant, you need to have both technical skills (hard skills) and people skills (soft skills) and maintain a good balance between them.

Soft skills are less concrete and more difficult to observe and evaluate. These are the characteristics, attributes, or **attitudes** that people develop throughout their lives. Some examples are respect, dependability, and integrity. These personal attributes or qualities, which are sought after and significant for specific jobs, are also professional attributes or behaviors, and they tend to help define an individual's personality. Your professional behaviors together produce what is called a good **work ethic,** which is what employers seek.

A medical assisting credential and the technical skills associated with it are the reasons most graduates are hired. However, the lack of a specific soft skill or poor professional behavior is the reason for most terminations. Weakness in soft skills is also the major reason that some students do not successfully complete their medical assisting education. So knowing how to do something is important, but behaving professionally while practicing is essential.

Much of the medical assistant's role involves dealing with other people, whether this is a patient, a patient's family member, a coworker, an insurance agent, a pharmaceutical sales representative, a laboratory staff member, or anyone else with whom you may come in contact in the workplace. Because most professional behaviors and skills are about working with other people, it only makes sense that someone going into a profession that continually deals with people should possess these behaviors and skills to do a good job. As a student and in your medical assisting career, you will experience the ongoing assessment of your professional behaviors in the following environments:

- Classroom
- Student work experience
- Hiring process
- Workplace performance evaluation
- Promotion consideration

So no matter the circumstance, your professionalism contributes to your success and should always be on the top of your list of ongoing self-improvements. For example, what if a medical assistant did not know the proper instructions to give a patient regarding a diagnostic test? She was either too shy (lacked self-confidence) to ask or chose not to ask because of a lack of time or neglect. Consequently, she gave instructions based on what she thought might be appropriate (lacked knowledge). So it is highly probable that the patient would not be adequately prepared for the test. The results of this poor decision might be

- Difficulty in performing the test on the patient.
- Cancellation of the test, wasting time and resources.
- Repetition of the test, incurring increased costs that may not be reimbursed by insurance.
- Inaccurate test results, leading to incorrect diagnosis and treatment and a poor patient outcome.
- Potential litigation (lawsuit) against the medical practice.

The issue is not that the medical assistant did not know the correct instructions but that the medical assistant did not use the correct behaviors (communication, cooperation, knowledge, persistence, work quality) to obtain and give the correct instructions. Although this scenario may seem exaggerated, it has occurred. The importance of professional behaviors cannot be overemphasized.

▶ Professional Behaviors   LO 3.2

Certain behaviors distinguish medical assistants who behave professionally from those who just get by, as well as those who do not make it. Professional behaviors contribute to your overall success in life—as a medical assistant and as a human being on this planet. Let's explore essential medical assisting professional behaviors. As you read each of the following sections, take a moment to consider whether you exhibit this behavior or quality. When you have completed this section, review the sample self-evaluation document and Procedure 3-1, Self-Evaluation of Professional Behaviors, at the end of the chapter.

Comprehension

Comprehension is the ability to learn, retain, and process information. To function as a medical assistant, you must comprehend your role and responsibilities. This means not only to have information but also to be able to analyze that information, to know how to use it, and to retain it, no matter how infrequently you might use it. An example of comprehension is learning how to take a blood pressure, including the equipment needed, the steps in the procedure, what results to expect, how to record the results, and when to report a problem.

Persistence

Persistence is continuing in spite of difficulty—being determined and overcoming obstacles. Two other words for persistence are *perseverance* and *tenacity*. The slang is *stick-to-itiveness*. This attribute ensures that you will finish the job no matter how difficult, boring, annoying, or time-consuming it may be. One example that is not uncommon in the medical office is trying to reach a patient whose contact information is not up-to-date. The issue may be an abnormal laboratory report that requires follow-up or another vital matter. The practitioner must be able to count on you and know that you will follow through and make contact no matter how difficult it may be. The patient's well-being often depends on it.

Self-Confidence

Self-confidence means believing in oneself. It is a trait that puts people at ease. The patient, the licensed practitioner, and others are more comfortable when they feel that you know what you are doing. The self-assured medical assistant is generally the one whom the patient and the practitioner prefer to work with. However, some people are self-confident to excess, which is not a professional trait. Have you ever felt a test was easy, but when the score came back you did less than great? That is overconfidence. On the other hand, self-confidence is a professional trait that makes you desirable to be around. An overconfident person acts as if she knows everything; a self-confident person knows what she knows and what she doesn't know. Display your self-confidence by smiling, making eye contact, and remaining calm no matter what the situation.

Judgment

Judgment is evaluating a situation, reaching an appropriate conclusion, and acting accordingly. It is also referred to as **critical thinking** (Figure 3-2). Critical thinking is defined as purposeful decisions resulting from analysis and evaluation. You will examine the steps of critical thinking in the *Strategies for Success* section. Applying sound judgment in all situations—even when you are distracted, upset, or annoyed—is necessary as a medical assistant.

Knowledge

Knowledge is understanding gained through study and experience. Medical assisting is a profession that requires understanding theory (knowledge) and then applying psychomotor

skills or hands-on experience. You will acquire knowledge by learning the principles and then performing the procedures. Students who do not have an understanding of the procedure and only memorize the steps may have difficulty performing when equipment varies or if a procedure is done differently (yet correctly) at the externship site. Understanding "why" something is being done is just as important as knowing "how" it is done. When both of these knowledge sets are known and practiced, a change in equipment or procedure will not have you "starting over from square one."

Organization

Organization is planning and coordinating information and tasks in an orderly manner to efficiently complete a job in a given time frame. This attribute has many aspects, including time management and prioritizing, which will be discussed in more detail in the *Strategies for Success* section. Organization is required to know how to prioritize the issues and tasks while addressing them all in an efficient and timely manner. One example is prioritizing your work—deciding which are the most important tasks of the day and which are less important. On a day when everything seems to be "top priority," you must use your professional judgment, knowledge of office policies, and experience with providers and coworkers to determine what should be completed first, second, third, and so on.

Integrity

Integrity is adhering to the appropriate code of law and ethics and being honest and trustworthy. Ethics is a system of values that determines right or wrong behavior. Integrity involves relatively simple matters, such as not taking pens home from the workplace, to more complex matters, such as always being truthful with patients. It also deals with subjects that are punishable and illegal, such as taking cash, cheating on an exam, or falsifying a time card. Falsifying a time card is clearly dishonest, but knowingly extending breaks or lunches also demonstrates a lack of integrity. Knowing that a coworker or a classmate is doing something dishonest and your actions regarding that knowledge can demonstrate integrity or lack of integrity (Figure 3-3). If you do not report your facts or

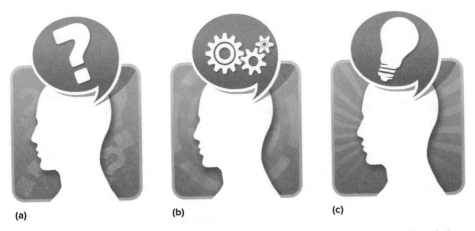

(a)   (b)   (c)

FIGURE 3-2   Using sound judgment through critical thinking requires (a) identifying a problem, (b) analyzing methods to solve it, and (c) determining an acceptable method to solve it.

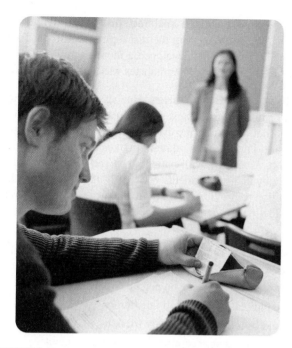

FIGURE 3-3 Being dishonest or not reporting something that you observe that is dishonest reduces your integrity and trustworthiness.
©Digital Vision

suspicion of the act, you could be considered an accomplice and subject to a penalty. Besides causing harm, once a person is involved in a dishonest act or is seen as lacking integrity, it is very difficult to regain the trust of others. The *Legal and Ethical Issues* chapter provides more details about standards of integrity that involve morals, laws, and ethics.

Growth

Growth is an ongoing effort to learn and improve. Being a professional brings with it an obligation to keep up with new standards, methods, procedures, and technologies in the field. Throughout this text and your medical assisting program, you will learn current practices. However, healthcare practices change frequently. For example, electronic health records (EHR) have replaced paper health records in many practices and facilities, and the standards for cardiopulmonary resuscitation (CPR) change frequently. Growth requires staying informed.

As discussed in the *Introduction to Medical Assisting* chapter, you should join one or more of the medical assisting professional organizations, such as AAMA, AMT, or NHA. Besides receiving the benefits, you are expected to earn a specific number of continuing education units (CEUs) within a specified time frame. These CEU offerings are credits given by the organization for participating in approved professional educational offerings. CEUs help you grow professionally and stay up-to-date with the latest information through taking seminars, reading articles, taking courses, and completing CEU modules, which may be accessed online, on a DVD or video stream, or in print.

Teamwork

Teamwork is working with others in the best interest of completing the job. The healthcare team, described in the *Healthcare and the Healthcare Team* chapter, is large and complex.

Like any team, its members must work together and cooperate with each other in order to increase the likelihood of achieving the goal. Also, studies show that in workplaces where staff members cooperate and help each other, job satisfaction and patient (client) satisfaction rates are higher than in those areas where cooperation is lacking.

In the healthcare practice, the overall goal should be providing good patient care, which is done through cooperation between team members. Everyone in the facility has an important job that depends on someone else. It is important to remember that the patient comes first and everyone is responsible for the care of that patient.

Another important aspect of teamwork and professionalism is the correct use of personal cell phones and other electronic devices while at work. Personal cell phones and other devices should never be used while you are working. Depending on the workplace policy, use of a personal cell phone or iPad may be allowed when you are on break, but otherwise you should place the device on mute or "airplane mode" and store it while you are working. In the same vein, although you may think of the computer you use at work as "yours," it belongs to your employer. Visiting social websites, such as Facebook, or checking personal e-mail or Twitter accounts should never be considered. Also, keep in mind that your work e-mail is not yours, either. Any e-mail you send from your work e-mail address reflects on your workplace and employer. Any sites you visit or e-mails you send may be tracked at any time by your employer. If you are tempted to send a "quick e-mail" to a friend or "quickly" check your Facebook account, remember, your employer and/or IT department has access to your work computer or network drive. Your employer will not ask you to work for him or her on your time; you should not be accessing personal websites and e-mail on work time.

Teamwork also requires coordination, which is the integration of activities. A typical patient may have three or more physician specialists, several prescriptions, home healthcare, routine blood work, physical therapy, hospital care, and outpatient procedures. This requires multiple appointments, one or more insurance plans, medical claims, and other processes. These processes require all the members of the team to work together for the benefit of the patient. Frequently, coordinating these patient care activities is the role of the medical assistant and requires cooperation and coordination with everyone involved. Team dynamics consist of:

- Assisting each other on a daily basis with the duties required.
- Avoiding interpersonal conflict with members of the team, and remaining professional at all times.
- Performing extra responsibilities without questioning or complaining.
- Being considerate of all other team members' duties and responsibilities.

Acceptance of Criticism

Acceptance of criticism is the willingness to consider feedback and suggestions to improve; it is taking responsibility for one's actions. In this context, let's focus on **constructive criticism,** which is counseling or advice that is intended to be useful

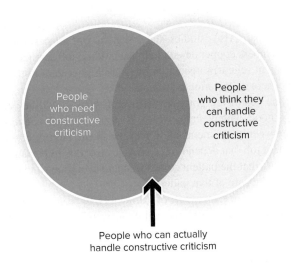

People who need constructive criticism

People who think they can handle constructive criticism

People who can actually handle constructive criticism

FIGURE 3-4 Accepting constructive criticism to improve your performance is essential to medical assisting practice. Get yourself inside the green zone.

with the goal of improving something. To grow and understand the areas in which you can improve, you must be able to accept constructive criticism (Figure 3-4). This may come from medical assisting educators, classmates, physicians, coworkers, or even patients. You will be evaluated throughout your education and workplace experience. Never expect a perfect evaluation because no one is perfect and improvements can always be made. Instead, be open to accepting criticism and suggestions, and offer your own thoughts on what you can do to improve. Do not be defensive or blame others. It is not about what your classmate or coworker does; it is about you.

Relations with Others

Relations with others—the ability to get along with those around you—involves treating everyone with respect and caring even when it is difficult. This sometimes includes **empathy,** feeling and understanding another's experience without having the experience yourself. In the healthcare environment, the medical assistant works with many patients who are experiencing great loss. It may be the loss of health or function or a terminal diagnosis. Or it may be a personal loss, such as the death of a spouse. As in any other workplace, coworkers also experience losses and unfortunate events. Sometimes medical assistants are very kind to patients but do not exhibit the same behaviors with coworkers. With coworkers, they may become involved in gossip and pettiness or display impatience and rudeness.

Caring is showing concern and appropriate attention, whereas enabling, or codependency, in this context is doing for others the things that they should be doing for themselves. When you enable, you become part of the disease process. For example, a young medical assistant learned this early in her career when she became attached to a 10-year-old juvenile diabetic patient. Every time the child came into the office, the MA gave her a stuffed animal or other gift. The patient started to have more and more problems, and the office visits became more frequent. An experienced medical assistant pointed out that the child was being rewarded for not managing her

illness. This exemplifies enabling. Instead of giving a gift (reward) for not managing the disease and becoming ill, the two medical assistants developed a more appropriate reward system for the patient if her diabetes was kept under control.

Professional Boundaries Having professional boundaries, or limitations, means always treating a patient as a client and not becoming involved in issues of his or her private life that do not directly relate to the healthcare. This is often difficult, especially with patients you see often and particularly enjoy and with patients you feel you may be able to help in addition to providing care in the medical office. Generally, the guidelines for maintaining professional boundaries are:

- Address the patient only by his or her last name unless first asking permission to use his or her first name (children are an exception).
- Avoid offering advice on personal matters.
- Use only tasteful, appropriate humor.
- Avoid becoming excessively friendly.
- Avoid giving or accepting money from a patient.
- Decline meeting a patient outside of the workplace unless you were acquainted prior to taking your position.

Cultural Diversity Have you heard the expression "it takes all kinds"? Professionalism involves understanding people who are different from you and respecting their right to be different. After all, from their point of view, you are the one who is different! Healthcare facilities serve patients from many countries who speak many languages. In addition, it is highly likely you will be working with people who are also from different cultures and belief systems. The variety of human social structures, belief systems, and strategies for adapting to situations in different parts of the world is referred to as **cultural diversity.** Showing respect to all individuals, regardless of culture, race, religion, age, gender, sexual orientation, physical challenges, special needs, lifestyle choices, or socioeconomic standing, impacts your relations with others (Figure 3-5). Being respectful does not mean that you have to agree with the lifestyles and beliefs of others. It means that

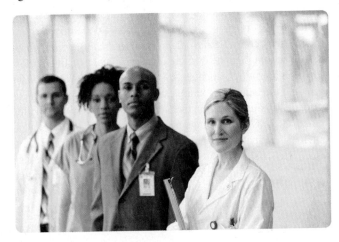

FIGURE 3-5 Respect and understanding for everyone is an essential professional behavior for the medical assistant.
©Terry Vine/Getty Images

you accept the idea that others have every right to be different from you and that as a medical assistant, you treat them appropriately. The following list gives some ideas that may help you understand and respect diversity.

- Increase your awareness of diversity. Communication with patients and coworkers will help you learn about individual similarities and differences.
- Increase your awareness of your own feelings. Everyone has biases. People tend to stereotype others, and this can lead to discrimination. Examine your own biases. Are they realistic?
- Look at individuals. As you learn about people as individuals, any group stereotypes you have often begin to break down.

Patient Advocacy As a medical assistant, you may be in a position to speak or act on behalf of the patient or the patient's family. This is called **patient advocacy.** Understanding your scope of practice, as well as being professional in your relations with others and being a good communicator, will help you be an effective advocate for the patient. Be sure you have all the facts before you act and include your supervisor or licensed practitioner as needed. Table 3-1 provides some examples of patient advocacy decisions.

Work Quality

Work quality means striving for excellence in doing the job and having pride in your performance. If you feel you need improvement in an area or would like to learn a new skill, consider taking a course, asking your supervisor or a coworker for help, or spending more time in that area. If you have an idea to improve a work process, make a suggestion. If you see something that is a potential risk, report it. Never say, "It is not my job." If it is not your job, simply state that you will get the person who can help and then get that person. Getting the job done is the focus. Being flexible is another part of work quality. If a staff member is absent or the schedule changes, the important thing is to get the job done. Again, do not worry about whose job it is as long as you are staying within your scope of practice.

Another way to look at this is to believe that patients are "customers" of the practice and, as such, deserve excellent customer service. Basically, this boils down to two things: The patient comes first and the patient is satisfied. When working with a patient, give him or her your undivided attention. Happy patients return to a practice and tell their friends about their experience. Be more than simply an employee; be part of building the practice. Keeping the following skills

TABLE 3-1	Examples of Patient Advocacy	
Circumstance	**Example**	**Suggested Action**
You have concern for the individual's safety.	You suspect an elderly patient is being abused.	Discuss with licensed practitioner; follow legal requirements and office protocols for reporting suspected elder abuse.
A complex situation requires your level of expertise.	A patient is having difficulty with an insurance claim.	Assist the patient as needed.
A potentially bad situation exists that your knowledge may help to avoid or resolve.	You are aware that a patient will not fill a prescription for an expensive drug because he cannot afford the insurance copay.	Inform the practitioner, who may be able to prescribe a generic version of the drug, or, with the practitioner's approval, contact the drug company to obtain free or reduced medications or contact a local pharmacy that provides low-cost medications if available.
Giving extra attention is likely to benefit the patient.	You are reviewing a 1-year-old patient's profile and notice that she is probably eligible for a nutritional program called WIC (Women, Infants, and Children).	Take the time to explain the program to the mother and provide the information for her to enroll.
The patient is capable of advocating for himself or herself.	The patient does not want to tell the provider that he does not understand why he needs a proposed procedure.	Encourage the patient to talk to the provider and assure him it is not unusual for patients to not fully understand the first time information is presented.
Anything that can be considered medical advice or a medical recommendation should be avoided.	The patient is asking your telephone advice regarding his symptoms.	Avoid saying anything that involves a potential diagnosis, such as "that sounds like the flu"; follow the office protocol for scheduling an appointment.
The action interferes with your job duties or presents a potential liability.	A patient asks you to keep an eye on her children during her exam.	Suggest the patient reschedule when she can arrange childcare; if needed, provide a contact number for a facility close to the office.
There are reasonable options.	A patient forgets to fill his monthly prescriptions and is consistently asking for an emergency refill. The office policy is that refills will be processed in 3 business days. He wants you to call and remind him each month.	Suggest to the patient that many pharmacies provide a monthly automatic refill or a monthly reminder.

sharp and using them consistently will lead to excellent customer service in the medical office.

- Using proper telephone techniques.
- Writing or responding to telephone messages.
- Explaining procedures to patients.
- Expediting insurance referral requests.
- Assisting with billing issues.
- Answering questions or finding answers to patient questions.
- Ensuring that patients are comfortable in your office.
- Creating a warm and reassuring environment.

Punctuality and Attendance

Being on time—**punctuality**—and coming to work every day that you are scheduled are essential for maintaining your job. Poor attendance is a frequent reason for termination. You are expected to be at your duty station or in your classroom, ready to work at the given time. Whether you are late or absent as a result of poor planning or an emergency, it still means that either your job is not getting done or you created additional work for your teammates. Patient care is impacted when you are not present. Recall Kaylyn in the chapter-opening case study, who is at risk for termination for frequent tardiness. Do not let this be you.

Professional Appearance

A medical professional always strives to maintain a neat appearance in the workplace, and personal cleanliness is an important part of this. Your appearance is the first impression you make on your patients, coworkers, and the providers you work with. Medical facilities are considered "conservative" work environments, and your appearance should reflect a conservative style. Listed here are a few professional guidelines to follow in the medical environment:

- Your approved uniform or other clothing should be clean, be pressed crisply, fit properly, and be in good repair.
- Your shoes should be comfortable, white, clean, and in good condition. Open-toed shoes should not be worn in the patient treatment areas to prevent injury or infection to yourself.
- Choose a hairstyle that is flattering and conservative. Hair should be clean and pulled back from your face and off your collar if it is long. Natural colors for hair are the most acceptable colors in a medical environment.
- Your nails should be kept at a short working length, no more than one-fourth of an inch, and of a natural color. Acrylic nails should not be worn, as they pose a risk for infection.
- Body odors, including the odor of smoke, are offensive. Even pleasant odors such as hairspray, perfumes, and lotions may trigger nausea or allergies in some patients and should be avoided.
- Jewelry should be kept to a minimum and in good taste. No more than one ring should be worn. Rings may tear through exam gloves. Ears can be pierced with one hole, and small

earrings are appropriate. Avoid dangling earrings, as patients (particularly pediatric patients) can tear these off.
- Visible tattoos, body piercings, and tongue piercings are not acceptable.

Communication

Effective communication involves careful listening, observing, speaking, and writing. Communication even involves good manners—being polite, tactful, and respectful. You must use good communication skills during every patient discussion and in every interaction you have with providers, other staff members, and other professionals with whom your practice does business.

Communication is giving and receiving accurate information. If a person is a poor communicator, it means that he or she cannot communicate or provide information that is accurate or understandable. Sometimes the patient leaves the office confused because he or she did not understand medical terms that were used and did not communicate that he or she did not understand. Sometimes the student leaves class confused because he or she did not understand the assignment and did not communicate to the instructor that he or she did not understand. In these scenarios, communication was poor from the sender because it was not understood. It was also poor from the receiver because lack of understanding was not communicated back to the sender. Effective communication is a two-way process, with a responsibility on both sides. It impacts every aspect of healthcare and is discussed in depth in the *Interpersonal Communication* chapter.

▶ Strategies for Success   LO 3.3

As you move toward and through your career as a medical assistant, you should be constantly improving your professional behaviors, as discussed earlier. As a medical assistant, you must practice specific strategies to ensure your success. These strategies include critical thinking and problem solving, time management and prioritizing, and stress management. The sections that follow will discuss these strategies, provide examples, and explain how to practice them.

Critical Thinking and Problem Solving

You will develop critical thinking skills over time as you apply your knowledge about and experience with human nature, medicine, and office skills to new situations. Critical thinking skills include quickly evaluating circumstances, solving problems, and taking action. For example, you must use critical thinking skills to assess how to react to emergency situations. If you see a patient suddenly pass out in the office reception area, you must immediately see that the patient receives first aid, notify a licensed professional, and alert the patient's family.

Critical thinking skills are used every day, and critical thinking relies on sound judgment. More specifically, critical thinking involves the ability to

- Analyze situations.
- Determine what aspects of a situation are most important.
- Reach conclusions that go beyond the obvious.

Critical thinking includes both factual problem identification and creative decision-making skills. It is the ability to see the whole picture and to reach reasonable conclusions based on the most important facts.

Problem solving can be broken down into a step-by-step approach (Figure 3-6):

- Identify the problem and define it clearly.
- Identify the potential effects of the problem.
- Clearly identify the objectives to be achieved.
- Identify as many potential solutions and strategies as possible.
- Analyze the potential solutions and strategies.
- Implement the strategy that appears to be the best solution.
- Evaluate the results and repeat the steps as needed.

Let's use the problem-solving steps to solve a patient problem. A patient approaches your desk and complains loudly that he does not have all day to wait for his provider to see him. His appointment was at 2:00 and the time is now 2:40. The patient is obviously angry about the delay. What should you do?

Step 1. Identify and define the problem: What is wrong with the patient?

The patient is angry because his provider did not see him promptly at his appointment time.

Step 2. Identify the potential effects of the problem: What effects might the patient's anger have?

The patient is disrupting the office; the practice may lose this client.

Step 3. Identify the objectives to be achieved: What is your goal for this situation?

Your goal is to end the disruption and calm the patient.

Step 4. Identify potential solutions and strategies: What can you do to end the disruption and calm the patient?

This is the step where you may be able to come up with more than one answer. For example, you may want to (a) inform your supervisor that the patient is causing a disruption, (b) ask the provider to speak with the patient, (c) tell the patient there is nothing you can do about it, or (d) explain the situation to the patient quietly and offer to reschedule the appointment. Remember that problem solving is not an exact science. You are attempting to come up with solutions so you can determine the one that will most effectively solve the problem.

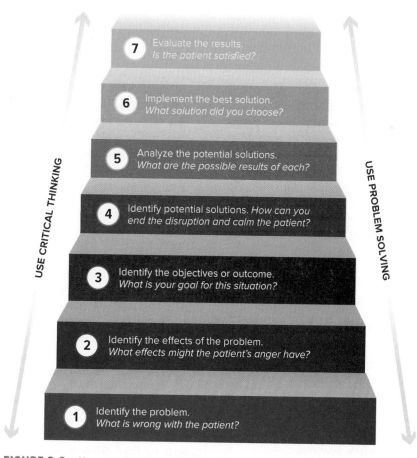

FIGURE 3-6 Use critical thinking and good judgment when following the steps of the problem-solving process.

Step 5. Analyze the potential solutions and strategies. What are the possible results from each solution?

For (a), you discover that the supervisor is busy in a room with another patient, and waiting for her to become available will allow the disruption to continue. For (b), you recall that the patient's provider expects the office staff to take care of this type of incident. For (c), you suspect that telling the patient you cannot do anything will not make him less angry. For (d), you think that talking quietly to the patient and offering to reschedule the appointment might work.

Step 6. Implement the best solution. What solution did you choose?

You explain that an emergency earlier in the day put the provider behind schedule and offer to reschedule the patient's appointment for a more convenient time. Of course, you will need to use your judgment to provide an explanation without violating the confidentiality of the patient who had the emergency earlier.

Step 7. Evaluate the results and repeat the steps as needed. How did it go? Is the patient satisfied and calmer now? If not, try a different strategy.

This step is important because learning from experience counts. If you chose to wait for the supervisor to become available to handle the situation and the patient stalked out of the office, saying he would not be back, you would hopefully do something different if faced with the same circumstance again. In this case, you explained the reason for the delay and offered to reschedule the patient, and he calmed down and decided to wait for his provider to see him. Often, individuals simply want to know that their concerns have been heard and understood.

Time Management and Prioritizing

Personal and professional time management skills are essential for medical assistants. **Time management** is controlling how you spend your time. People who use time management techniques routinely are the highest achievers in all walks of life, professionally and personally. Using these skills will help you function exceptionally well in the medical office, even under intense pressure. Even more importantly, you can say goodbye to the often intense stress of work overload. Setting goals and concentrating on results, not just being busy, are the main focus of time management.

Medical assistant students who are disorganized waste a great deal of time locating assignments and other materials before they get started on their work. Prepare in advance. Purchase a binder, notebook, or folders for storing your homework assignments; reminders about upcoming tests; your course syllabus; and other pertinent facts, such as your instructor's office hours and contact information and your classmates' information for study sessions. Obtain computer access with an Internet connection at home, through your school, or at the local library. Try these tips for organization:

- Study in a quiet area away from distractions.
- Find a study "buddy" who is just as committed to and focused on success as you are.

- Formal classroom courses require at least as much work time outside of class as inside it to prepare, so allow yourself enough preparation time.
- Budget your time between school and other responsibilities.
- Set aside study time by creating a study schedule.
- Set daily, weekly, or course-specific goals to accomplish the overall goal of completing your course.

The medical assistant must be organized. For example, the phone may be ringing at the same time a patient is trying to schedule a follow-up appointment, while a practitioner is inquiring about the results of a diagnostic report, and while a coworker is asking for information about a patient's immunizations. To be an effective medical assistant, you must be able to manage your time and **prioritize** effectively. When you decide on the order in which tasks should be completed based on things such as the task deadline and importance. Evaluate yourself, and use the following ideas to improve your ability to manage time and prioritize.

1. Have a plan for your day. Know what needs to be done. Set your daily goals and try to meet them.
2. Take advantage of your own productivity. That is, you may work better at a particular time of day. Choose to do the most difficult tasks when you are working at your best. Remember, everybody has sluggish times, so know when yours are—maybe right after lunch or near the end of the day. Plan accordingly.
3. Avoid distractions when you can. Of course, if your job is to answer the phone, then you must do so. But if someone is just chatting or your smartphone is constantly beeping to signal text messages, this probably means you are not accomplishing what needs to be done. Personal phone calls, text messages, tweets, or other communications are not supposed to occur during your working hours. However, business electronic communication is vital. Consider setting specific times during the day to look at business e-mail so you will not have constant interruptions.
4. Evaluate yourself on a daily basis. Consider whether you accomplished your daily goal, and come up with a plan to continue or do better the next day.

Stress and Burnout Professionals in the healthcare field, including medical assistants, may experience high levels of stress in their daily work environment. Stress can result from a feeling of being under pressure, or it can be a reaction to anger, frustration, or a change in your routine. Stress can increase your blood pressure, speed up your breathing and heart rate, and cause muscle tension. Stress also can cause you to behave or communicate ineffectively. For example, if you are feeling very pressured at work, you might snap at a coworker or patient, or you might forget to give the provider an important message.

Good or Bad Stress A certain amount of stress is normal. A little bit of stress—the kind that makes you feel excited or challenged by the task at hand—can motivate you to get things done and push you toward a higher level of productivity. For example, your supervisor may ask you to learn a new procedure. Learning something new, although stressful in itself, can be an exciting challenge and a welcome change of pace. Ongoing stress, however, can be overwhelming and affect you physically. For example, it can lower your resistance to colds and increase your risk for developing heart disease, diabetes, high blood pressure, ulcers, allergies, asthma, colitis, and cancer. It also can increase your risk for certain autoimmune diseases, which cause the body's immune system to attack normal tissue.

Some stress at work is inevitable. An important goal is to learn how to manage or reduce stress. Take into account your strengths and limitations, and be realistic about how much you can handle at work and in your life outside work. Pushing yourself a certain amount can be motivating. The *Points on Practice* box lists the potential causes of stress and ways to reduce stress.

Preventing Burnout Burnout is the end result of prolonged periods of stress without relief, an energy-depleting condition that will affect your health and career. Certain personality types are more prone to burnout than others. If you are a highly driven, perfectionist-type person, you will be more susceptible to burnout. Experts often refer to such a person as a characteristic Type A personality. A more relaxed, calm individual is considered a Type B person. Type B personalities are less prone to burnout but have the potential to suffer from it, especially if they work in healthcare.

According to some experts on stress, there are five stages of burnout:

1. *The honeymoon phase.* During the honeymoon phase, your job is wonderful. You have boundless energy and enthusiasm, and all things seem possible. You love the job and the job loves you. You believe it will satisfy all your needs and desires and solve all your problems. You are delighted with your job, your coworkers, and the organization.

2. *The awakening phase.* The awakening phase starts with the realization that your initial expectations were unrealistic. The job is not working out the way you thought it would. It does not satisfy all your needs, your coworkers and the organization are less than perfect, and rewards and recognition are scarce. As disillusionment and disappointment grow, you become confused. Something is wrong, but you cannot quite put your finger on it. Typically, you work harder to make your dreams come true. But working harder does not change anything, and you become increasingly tired, bored, and frustrated. You may question your competence and ability and start losing your self-confidence.

3. *The brownout phase.* As brownout begins, your early enthusiasm and energy give way to chronic fatigue and irritability. You become indecisive, and your productivity drops. Your work deteriorates. Coworkers and managers may even comment on it. You become increasingly frustrated and angry and project the blame for your difficulties onto others. You are cynical, detached, and openly critical of the organization, superiors, and coworkers. You are beset with depression, anxiety, and physical illness.

4. *The full-scale burnout phase.* Unless you interrupt the process or someone intervenes, brownout drifts remorselessly into full-scale burnout. Despair is the dominant feature of this final stage. It usually takes 3 to 4 years to get to this phase. You experience an overwhelming sense of failure and a devastating loss of self-esteem and self-confidence. You become depressed and feel lonely and empty. You talk about just quitting and getting away. You are exhausted physically and mentally and prone to physical and mental breakdowns.

5. *The phoenix phenomenon.* Just like a phoenix, you can arise from the burnout ashes. But this takes time. First, you need to rest and relax. Do not take work home. If you are like many people, the work will not get done, and you will only feel guilty for being lazy. Second, be realistic in your job expectations as well as your aspirations and goals. Third, create balance in your life. Invest more of yourself in family and other personal relationships, social activities, and hobbies. Spread yourself out so that your job does not have such an overpowering influence on your self-esteem and self-confidence.

Potential Causes of Stress

Sometimes stress can be difficult to measure. Just like varying thresholds for pain, different people can tolerate different amounts of stress. One person's stress may seem a lot worse than another's. For example, who can say that the stress you may be feeling over an upcoming exam is less nerve-wracking than the stress someone else may be feeling about paying off a large credit card balance? Stress can come in many forms from many directions, but here is a list of common potential causes.

- Death of a spouse or family member
- Divorce or separation
- Hospitalization (yours or a family member's) due to injury or illness
- Marriage or reconciliation from a separation
- Loss of a job or retirement
- Sexual problems
- A new baby
- Significant change in your financial status (for better or worse)
- Job change
- Children leaving or returning home
- Significant personal success, such as a promotion at work
- Moving or remodeling your home
- Problems at work, such as your boss's retirement, that may put your job at risk
- Substantial debt, such as a mortgage or overspending on credit cards

Tips for Reducing Stress

Managing your stress levels can benefit your overall well-being, both mentally and physically, at work and at home. The following is a list of helpful, doable tips for lowering stress.

- Maintain a healthy balance in your life among work, family, and leisure activities.
- Exercise regularly.
- Eat balanced, nutritious meals and healthful snacks.
- Avoid foods high in caffeine, salt, sugar, and fat.
- Get enough sleep.
- Allow time for yourself and plan time to relax.
- Rely on the support that family, friends, and coworkers have to offer. Do not be afraid to share your feelings.
- Try to be realistic about what you can and cannot do. Do not be afraid to admit that you cannot take on another responsibility.
- Try to set realistic goals for yourself. Remember, there are always choices, even when there appear to be none.
- Be organized. Good planning can help you manage your workload.
- Redirect excess energy constructively; clean your closet, work in the garden, volunteer, invite friends for dinner, or exercise.
- Change some of the things you have control over.
- Stay focused. Focus your full energy on one thing at a time and finish one project before starting another.
- Identify sources of conflict and try to resolve them.
- Learn and use relaxation techniques, such as deep breathing, meditation, or imagining yourself in a quiet, peaceful place. Choose what works for you.
- Maintain a healthy sense of humor, as laughter can help relieve stress. Joke with friends after work. See a funny movie.
- Try not to overreact. Ask yourself if a situation is really worth getting upset or worried about.
- Seek help from social or professional support groups, if necessary.

PROCEDURE 3-1 Self-Evaluation of Professional Behaviors WORK // DOC

Procedure Goal: To identify necessary professional behaviors and relate them to yourself in order to improve your performance as a medical assistant

OSHA Guidelines: This procedure does not involve exposure to blood, body fluids, or tissue.

Materials: Self-Evaluation Form (Procedure 3-1)

Method:

1. Read and review each professional behavior.
2. Rate yourself on each behavior, considering the level at which you exhibit them.
3. Identify at least one measure to improve yourself on each behavior, as needed.
4. Place the completed form in your portfolio and review it on an ongoing basis.
5. Reevaluate your professional behavior prior to your applied training experience (practicum).
6. Compare the two scores and identify any weaknesses.
7. Obtain feedback about your professional behaviors from your instructor, coworkers, classmates, practicum coordinator, or employer.

Behavior	Example(s)	Rate Yourself (5 = Best) 1	2	3	4	5	Improvements Needed
Integrity	Consistently honest; able to be trusted with the property of others; can be trusted with confidential information; completes tasks accurately						
Appearance	Clothing and uniform appropriate for circumstance; neat, clean, and well-kept appearance; good personal hygiene and grooming						
Teamwork	Places the success of the team above self-interest; does not undermine the team; helps and supports other team members; shows respect to all team members; remains flexible and open to change; communicates with others to help resolve problems						
Self-confidence	Demonstrates the ability to trust personal judgment; demonstrates an awareness of strengths and limitations; exercises good personal judgment						
Communication	Speaks clearly; writes legibly; listens actively; adjusts communication strategies to various situations						
Commitment to diversity	Consistently demonstrates respect for varied cultural backgrounds, ethnicities, religions, sexual orientations, social classes, abilities, political beliefs, and disabilities						
Punctuality and attendance	Arrives at class and work on the appointed day and time						
Acceptance of criticism	Listens when constructive criticism is given; does not become defensive with criticism; appreciates constructive criticism and incorporates suggestions into behavior as appropriate						
Organization	Coordinates more than one task at a time; keeps work area neat and orderly; anticipates future work; works efficiently and systematically						
Knowledge and comprehension	Learns new things easily; retains new information; associates theory with practice						

FIGURE Procedure 3-1   Self-evaluation of professional behaviors.

SUMMARY OF LEARNING OUTCOMES

OUTCOME	KEY POINTS
3.1 **Recognize the importance of professionalism in the medical assisting practice.**	Professionalism is behavior that exhibits the traits or features corresponding to the standards of that profession. Standards are developed by professional organizations and, in some states, by governmental entities. The skills are placed in two broad categories: hard skills and soft skills. Hard skills are specific technical and operational proficiencies. Soft skills are personal attributes or behaviors that enhance an individual. Professional behaviors are needed to function at a high level in medical assisting and produce a good work ethic.

Continued

OUTCOME	KEY POINTS
3.2 **Explain the professional behaviors that should be exhibited by medical assistants.**	Some essential professional behaviors include comprehension—learning, retaining, and processing information; persistence—continuing in spite of difficulty; self-confidence—believing in oneself; judgment—evaluating and determining an appropriate conclusion; organization—coordinating information and tasks in an orderly manner; integrity—adhering to law and ethics; growth—engaging in ongoing efforts to learn and improve; teamwork—working with others in the best interest of completing the job; acceptance of criticism—being willing to consider feedback and suggestions to improve; relations with others—getting along with all people in all circumstances; work quality—striving for excellence in doing the job; punctuality and attendance—showing up on appointed days and times; professional appearance—adhering to the standards and codes of dress; and communication—giving and receiving accurate information.
3.3 **Model strategies for success in medical assisting education and practice.**	Strategies for success as a medical assistant include cultivating your skills, such as critical thinking and problem solving, time management and prioritizing, stress management, and avoidance of burnout. Practicing effective strategies can assist you during your education and employment.

CASE STUDY CRITICAL THINKING

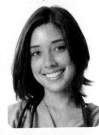

©Rubberball/Getty Images

Recall Kaylyn Haddix from the beginning of the chapter. Now that you have completed this chapter, answer the following questions regarding her case.

1. Why do you think Malik wants to meet with Kaylyn?
2. What professional behaviors does Kaylyn need to improve?
3. What strategies for success could Kaylyn use to prevent herself from losing her job?

EXAM PREPARATION QUESTIONS

1. (LO 3.1) The primary reason an employee is hired is usually associated with
   a. Hard skills
   b. Soft skills
   c. References
   d. Punctuality
   e. Cooperation

2. (LO 3.1) Which of the following is considered a soft skill?
   a. Communicating with a patient
   b. Measuring a patient's height
   c. Taking a telephone message
   d. Taking a patient's vital signs
   e. Scheduling an appointment

3. (LO 3.2) An indication that a person lacks integrity would be exhibited by
   a. Being rude to a coworker
   b. Coming into work late
   c. Ignoring the dress code
   d. Taking money from the cash drawer
   e. Gossiping

4. (LO 3.2) A significant part of critical thinking is
   a. Memorizing
   b. Analyzing
   c. Being tenacious
   d. Empathizing
   e. Criticizing

5. (LO 3.2) Adhering to the dress code and good personal hygiene demonstrates
   a. Persistence
   b. Growth
   c. Respect
   d. Knowledge
   e. Organization

6. (LO 3.2) If a medical assistant is not self-confident, this may lead to the patient feeling
   a. Confident
   b. Neglected
   c. Apprehensive
   d. Ignored
   e. Ill

7. (LO 3.2) An example of enabling, or codependency, would be
   a. Providing a wheelchair for a patient who is weak
   b. Helping a patient identify a community resource
   c. Scheduling a patient's next appointment
   d. Offering cookies to an obese patient
   e. Calling a taxi for a patient

8. (LO 3.2) Maintaining professional boundaries involves
   a. Showing a patient you care by being personal
   b. Being friendly but not excessively affectionate
   c. Avoiding any touch with the patient
   d. Babysitting for a patient
   e. Buying the patient lunch

9. (LO 3.3) Your coworker likes to talk about her kids and husband, usually right after lunch as you are returning to work and patients. What should you do?
   a. Talk with your coworker as much as you can because it is important to have good relationships at work
   b. Talk with your coworker because some personal discussions at work are OK anyway
   c. Consider telling your supervisor that your coworker talks too much and you find it disturbing
   d. Request that your supervisor ask your coworker to not talk to you so much because you cannot get your work done
   e. Realize that the time you speak with your coworker is preventing you from completing your goals, so politely explain this to your coworker

10. (LO 3.3) Once you have considered what the problem is and what effects it will have, what should you do next?
    a. Implement a solution
    b. Identify the problem
    c. Determine multiple solutions
    d. Determine the effects of the solution
    e. Evaluate your solution to determine if it works or worked

SOFT SKILLS SUCCESS

Learning the technical, or hard, skills required of a medical assistant is important. Why are the soft skills considered just as, if not more, important than these hard skills? Discuss at least four soft skills you will need as a medical assistant. At the end of each chapter, you will see an icon like the one below to direct you to the Practice Medical Office software where you can practice these important soft skills.

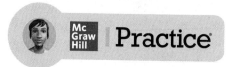

Go to PRACTICE MEDICAL OFFICE and complete the module Admin Check In: Interactions

Interpersonal Communication

CASE STUDY

PATIENT INFORMATION

Patient Name	DOB	Allergies
Cindy Chen	07/15/1993	NKA

Attending	MRN	Other Information
Alexis N. Whalen, MD	00-AA-001	History of depression

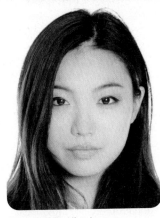

©excentric_01/iStock/Getty Images

Cindy Chen arrives at your office complaining of the inability to sleep and nervousness. She tested positive for HIV in 2014, although she has been asymptomatic on antiviral drugs. Currently, she lives with her aunt and is going to school to become a phlebotomist. During her interview, she says, "I'm just feeling so nervous. Do you have anything you can give me until I see the doctor?"

Keep Cindy Chen in mind as you study this chapter. There will be questions at the end of the chapter based on the case study. The information in the chapter will help you answer these questions.

LEARNING OUTCOMES

After completing Chapter 4, you will be able to:

4.1 Identify elements and types of communication.

4.2 Relate communication to human behavior and needs.

4.3 Categorize positive and negative communication.

4.4 Model ways to improve listening, interpersonal skills, and assertiveness skills.

4.5 Carry out therapeutic communication skills.

4.6 Use effective communication strategies with patients in special circumstances.

4.7 Carry out positive communication with coworkers and management.

KEY TERMS

active listening

aggressive

assertive

body language

boundaries

closed posture

conflict

feedback

hierarchy

homeostasis

hospice

interpersonal skills

open posture

passive listening

personal space

rapport

V.C.1   Identify styles and types of verbal communication

V.C.2   Identify types of nonverbal communication

V.C.3   Recognize barriers to communication

V.C.4   Identify techniques for overcoming communication barriers

V.C.5   Recognize the elements of oral communication using a sender-receiver process

V.C.14   Relate the following behaviors to professional communication:
(a) assertive
(b) aggressive
(c) passive

V.C.15   Differentiate between adaptive and nonadaptive coping mechanisms

V.C.17   Discuss the theories of:
(a) Maslow
(b) Erikson
(c) Kubler-Ross

V.P.1   Use feedback techniques to obtain patient information including:
(a) reflection
(b) restatement
(c) clarification

V.P.2   Respond to nonverbal communication

V.P.5   Coach patients appropriately considering:
(a) cultural diversity
(b) developmental life stage
(c) communication barriers

V.A.1   Demonstrate:
(a) empathy
(b) active listening
(c) nonverbal communication

V.A.3   Demonstrate respect for individual diversity including:
(a) gender
(b) race
(c) religion
(d) age
(e) economic status
(f) appearance

5. Human Relations

a. Respond appropriately to patients with abnormal behavior patterns

b. Provide support for terminally ill patients
(1) Use empathy when communicating with terminally ill patients
(2) Identify common stages that terminally ill patients experience
(3) List organizations and support groups that can assist patients and family members of patients experiencing terminal illnesses

c. Assist the patient in navigating issues and concerns that may arise (i.e., insurance policy information, medical bills, and physician/provider orders)

e. Analyze the effect of hereditary, cultural, and environmental influences on behavior

h. Display effective interpersonal skills with patients and healthcare team members

8. Clinical Procedures

j. Make adaptations for patients with special needs (psychological or physical limitations)

10. Career Development

b. Demonstrate professional behavior

▶ Introduction

Think about the last time you had a medical appointment. How well did the staff and practitioner communicate with you? Were you greeted pleasantly and invited to take a seat, or did someone thrust a clipboard at you and say, "Fill this out"? If you had a long wait in the reception area or examination room, did someone come in to explain the delay? Did you become frustrated and angry because nobody told you what was happening? The abilities to recognize human behaviors and to communicate effectively are vital to a medical assistant's success. This chapter takes a psychological approach to understanding human behavior and the challenges that influence therapeutic communication in a healthcare setting.

As the key communicator within the healthcare facility, the medical assistant must be able to communicate with each patient with professionalism and diplomacy. This includes patients from different cultures, socioeconomic backgrounds, educational levels, ages, and lifestyles. The medical assistant sets the tone for the communication circle and must be aware

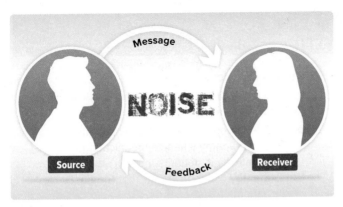

FIGURE 4-1 The process of communication involves an exchange of messages through verbal and nonverbal means.

of all the obstacles that can affect human communication. It is important that patients develop a good rapport and feel confident in the care they are receiving from your office. Developing strong communication skills in the medical office is just as important as mastering administrative and clinical tasks.

▶ Elements of Communication   LO 4.1

As you interact with patients and their families, you will be responsible for giving information and ensuring that the patient understands what you, the practitioner, and other staff members have communicated. You also will be responsible for receiving information from the patient. For example, patients will describe their symptoms. They also may discuss their feelings or ask questions about a treatment or procedure. In this case, it will be crucial that you understand exactly what the patient or his or her family member is stating or questioning so you can assist them efficiently and appropriately. The giving and receiving of information forms the communication circle.

The Communication Circle

The communication circle involves three elements: a message, a source, and a receiver. Messages are usually verbal, written, or nonverbal. (You will explore more about nonverbal messages later in this chapter.) The source sends the message and the receiver receives it. The communication circle is formed as the source sends a message to the receiver and the receiver responds (Figure 4-1).

Consider the following example, in which Miguel, BWW's clinical medical assistant, is speaking with Sylvia Gonzales, a patient who is having physical therapy for a back injury. Watch the communication circle at work.

Miguel: The physical therapist says you're making great progress and that you can start on some simple back exercises at home. I'd like to go over them with you. Then I'll give you a sheet that illustrates the exercises. How does that sound to you?

Sylvia Gonzales: I'm a little nervous about doing exercises. I still have some pain when I bend over.

Miguel: I understand. It's important, though, to start using those muscles again. Why don't you show me exactly where it hurts? Then we can go over proper body mechanics, such as bending down to pick something up and getting in and out of chairs, the car, and bed. Then we'll just start with one or two of the exercises and save the rest for next time, when you're feeling more ready.

Sylvia Gonzales: Okay, I will try, but I only feel up to doing a little bit today.

In this example, the medical assistant (the source) gives a verbal message about back exercises to the patient (the receiver). The patient responds by drawing attention to her pain and uneasiness about certain movements (feedback). The patient's response is also a message to the medical assistant, who responds in turn. The giving and receiving of information continues within the communication circle until the exchange is finished.

Feedback The receiver's response to the message is known as **feedback.** Feedback may be verbal or nonverbal evidence that the receiver got and understood the message. When you communicate information to a patient or ask a patient a question, always look for feedback. For example, if you calculate a pregnant patient's due date and tell her she's 12 weeks pregnant, look for a response. If she responds, "Oh, good, that means I'm out of danger of having a miscarriage," you may respond by saying that whereas most miscarriages occur in the first 12 weeks, some risk of miscarriage remains throughout the pregnancy. If she responds, "I thought I was 14 weeks pregnant," you need to clarify how you worked out your calculation and compare it with hers to uncover any discrepancy. Good communication in the medical office requires patient feedback at every step.

Noise Anything that changes the message in any way or interferes with the communication process can be referred to as noise. *Noise* refers not only to sounds, such as a siren or jackhammer on the street below the medical office suite, but also to room temperature and other types of physical comfort or discomfort, such as pain, or emotions, such as fear or sadness. If patients are feeling uncomfortable in a chilly or hot room, upset about their illness, or in great pain, they may not pay close attention to what you are saying. Conversely, if you are feeling upset about a personal problem outside work or if you are unwell or preoccupied with all the things you have on your to-do list, you may not communicate well.

As you deal with each patient, try to screen out or eliminate causes of noise. For example, before you start a conversation with a patient in an examination room, you might ask, "Are you too chilly or too warm? Is the temperature in here comfortable for you?" If there is construction going on outside the building, see if there is a less noisy inner room or office that you might use. If a patient seems nervous or upset, address those feelings before you launch into a factual discussion.

If you are feeling stressed or out of sorts, that feeling constitutes a type of noise. Try to take a "breather" between patients or a break from desk work—walk downstairs, get some fresh air, stretch your legs. Feeling dehydrated or hungry affects your communication efforts, too. Limit your caffeine and sugar intake. Drink plenty of water throughout the day. Eat a good breakfast and lunch and healthful snacks. Leave your personal problems at home.

▶ Human Behavior and Needs   LO 4.2

Medical assistants are exposed to many different personality types in addition to different illnesses. When you understand why a person is behaving in a certain way, you can adjust your communication style to adapt to that person. For example, as highly structured healthcare organizations and technological advances rapidly change the face of healthcare, many patients feel that healthcare is becoming impersonal, and consequently, they may become difficult. Every time you communicate with patients, you can counteract this perception by playing a humanistic role in the healthcare process. Being humanistic means that you work to help patients feel attended to and respected

as individuals, not just as descriptions in a chart. Remember to always treat each patient as an individual and not simply as the disease, condition, or problem that brought the patient to the office. The problem may be common to you, but it is new and often frightening for the patient. To humanize and improve communication, you should have an understanding of the developmental stages of the life cycle and Maslow's hierarchy of human needs.

Developmental Stages of the Life Cycle

Understanding the stages of human growth and development will enable you to enhance your communication skills, including patient education, with patients of all age groups, cultures, and religions. Human growth includes physical, psychological, and emotional growth. Many scientists and behaviorists have studied the developmental stages of human life and have developed guidelines to assist healthcare practitioners and staff in applying effective patient communication skills. Figure 4-2 is an example of a lifespan development model, created by Erik Erikson (1902–1994).

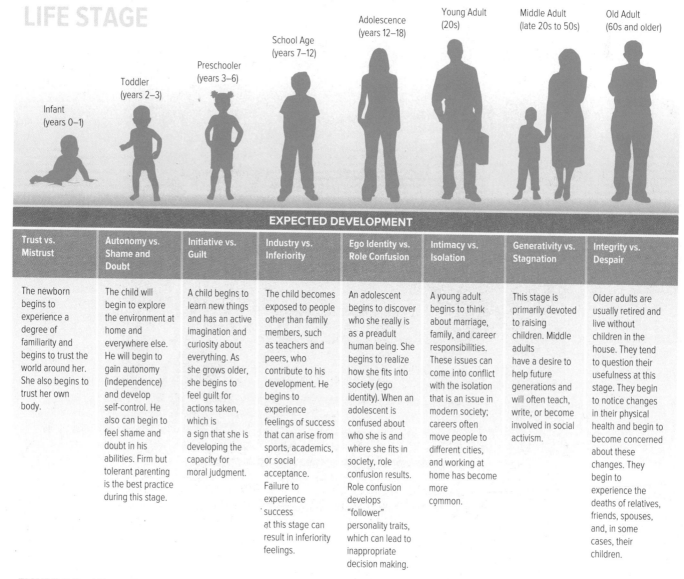

LIFE STAGE

Infant (years 0–1)	Toddler (years 2–3)	Preschooler (years 3–6)	School Age (years 7–12)	Adolescence (years 12–18)	Young Adult (20s)	Middle Adult (late 20s to 50s)	Old Adult (60s and older)

EXPECTED DEVELOPMENT

Trust vs. Mistrust	Autonomy vs. Shame and Doubt	Initiative vs. Guilt	Industry vs. Inferiority	Ego Identity vs. Role Confusion	Intimacy vs. Isolation	Generativity vs. Stagnation	Integrity vs. Despair
The newborn begins to experience a degree of familiarity and begins to trust the world around her. She also begins to trust her own body.	The child will begin to explore the environment at home and everywhere else. He will begin to gain autonomy (independence) and develop self-control. He also can begin to feel shame and doubt in his abilities. Firm but tolerant parenting is the best practice during this stage.	A child begins to learn new things and has an active imagination and curiosity about everything. As she grows older, she begins to feel guilt for actions taken, which is a sign that she is developing the capacity for moral judgment.	The child becomes exposed to people other than family members, such as teachers and peers, who contribute to his development. He begins to experience feelings of success that can arise from sports, academics, or social acceptance. Failure to experience success at this stage can result in inferiority feelings.	An adolescent begins to discover who she really is as a preadult human being. She begins to realize how she fits into society (ego identity). When an adolescent is confused about who she is and where she fits in society, role confusion results. Role confusion develops "follower" personality traits, which can lead to inappropriate decision making.	A young adult begins to think about marriage, family, and career responsibilities. These issues can come into conflict with the isolation that is an issue in modern society; careers often move people to different cities, and working at home has become more common.	This stage is primarily devoted to raising children. Middle adults have a desire to help future generations and will often teach, write, or become involved in social activism.	Older adults are usually retired and live without children in the house. They tend to question their usefulness at this stage. They begin to notice changes in their physical health and begin to become concerned about these changes. They begin to experience the deaths of relatives, friends, spouses, and, in some cases, their children.

FIGURE 4-2   Lifespan development. by Erik Erikson

Source: Erik Erikson (1902–1994).

Maslow's Hierarchy of Human Needs

Abraham Maslow, a well-known human behaviorist, developed a model of human behavior known as the **hierarchy** (classification) of needs (Figure 4-3). This hierarchy states that human beings are motivated by unsatisfied needs and that certain lower or base needs have to be satisfied before higher needs, such as self-actualization, are met. Maslow felt that people are basically trustworthy, self-protecting, and self-governing and that humans tend toward growth and love. He believed that humans are not violent by nature but are violent only when their needs are not being met. When thinking of Maslow's hierarchy, consider the basic needs as the base of the pyramid, which grows upward as each need is met. Essentially, as each need is met, a person is climbing toward the top of the pyramid.

Deficiency (Basic) Needs   According to Maslow, there are general types of needs—physiological, safety, love/belonging, and esteem—that must be satisfied before a person can act unselfishly. He called these deficiency (basic) needs.

Physiological Needs   Physiological needs are humans' very basic needs, such as air, water, food, sleep, and sex. When these needs are not satisfied, we may feel sickness, irritation, pain, and discomfort. These feelings motivate us to alleviate them as soon as possible to establish **homeostasis** (a state of balance, or equilibrium). Once our basic needs are met and our feelings are alleviated, we may think about other things.

Safety Needs   People have the need and desire to establish stability and consistency. These basic safety needs are security, shelter, and a safe environment.

Love/Belonging Needs   Humans have a desire to belong to groups: clubs, work groups, religious groups, families, and so on. We need to feel loved and accepted by others. Humans are like pack animals—we place great importance in belonging to society.

Esteem Needs   Humans like to feel that they are important and valuable to society. There are two types of self-esteem. The first results from competence, or mastery of a task, such as completing an educational program. The second is the attention and recognition that come from others.

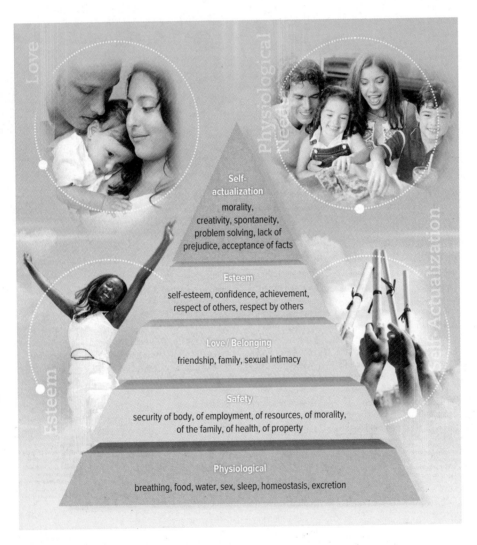

FIGURE 4-3   Maslow's hierarchy.

(top-left) ©Brand X Pictures/Getty Images, (top-right) ©BananaStock/age fotostock, (bottom-left) ©Gallo Images - Malcolm Dare/Getty Images, (bottom-right) ©baona/Getty Images

Self-Actualization Self-actualization is finding self-fulfillment and realizing one's potential. To reach this level, a person utilizes many tools to maximize potential, such as education, a fulfilling career, and a balanced personal life. Self-actualized people are generally comfortable with who they are and know their strengths and weaknesses.

Considering Patients' Needs When working and communicating with patients, remember this hierarchy of human needs and observe what need a patient is deficient in. For example, if an elderly patient has recently lost her husband, she may feel lonely and deficient in the love need. You may see homeless patients who are deficient in their physiological and safety needs. You may have a young girl as a patient who is overweight and has low self-esteem. On the other hand, you may have a high-level executive as a patient who has reached self-actualization. Each of these scenarios would require a communication style adjustment in order for you to effectively communicate with these patients.

▶ Types of Communication
LO 4.3

Each type of communication (verbal, nonverbal, or written) can be positive or negative. An effective communicator is familiar with these types of communication. This section focuses on verbal and nonverbal communication.

Positive Verbal Communication

In the medical office, communication that promotes patient comfort and well-being is essential. Treating patients brusquely or rudely is unacceptable in the healthcare setting. It is your responsibility to set the stage for positive communication.

When information—even bad news—is communicated with some positive aspect, patients are more likely to listen attentively and respond positively themselves. For example, you might explain to a patient who is about to get an injection, "This will sting, but only for a couple of seconds. When we are through, you are free to go." You would not just say, "This is going to hurt."

Other examples of positive communication are

- Being friendly, warm, and attentive ("It's good to see you again, Mrs. Armstrong. I know you're on your lunch hour, so let's get started right away.").
- Verbalizing concern for patients ("Are you comfortable?" "I understand it hurts when I do this; I'll be gentle." "This paperwork won't take long at all.").
- Encouraging patients to ask questions ("I hope I've explained the procedure well. Do you have any questions, or are there any parts you would like to go over again?").
- Asking patients to repeat your instructions to make sure they understand ("Will you explain to me how you plan to take your medicine?").
- Looking directly at patients when you speak to them.
- Smiling (naturally, not in a forced way).
- Speaking slowly and clearly, being sure to pronounce words correctly.
- Listening carefully.

Negative Verbal Communication

Most people do not purposely try to communicate negatively. Some people, however, may not realize that their communication style has a negative impact on others. Look for and ask for feedback to help you curb negative communication habits. Ask yourself, "Do the practitioners and my coworkers seem happy to speak with me? Are they open and responsive to me? Do patients seem at ease with me, or are they very quiet, turned off, or distant?" (Note that some patients may respond this way because of the way they feel, not because of the way you are communicating with them.) Here are some examples of negative communication (verbal and nonverbal):

- Mumbling.
- Speaking brusquely or sharply.
- Avoiding eye contact.
- Interrupting patients as they are speaking.
- Rushing through explanations or instructions.
- Treating patients impersonally.
- Making patients feel they are taking up too much of your time or asking too many questions.
- Forgetting common courtesies, such as saying please and thank you.
- Showing boredom.

A good way to avoid negative communication is to open your eyes and ears to others in service-oriented workplace settings.

The next time you buy something at a store, call a company for information over the phone, or eat at a restaurant, take note of the way the staff treat you. Do they answer your questions courteously? Do they give you the information you ask for? Do they make you feel welcome? What specifically makes their communication style positive or negative? You expect good customer service, and so do your patients, as discussed in the chapter *Professionalism and Success.* Remember, you can always improve your communication skills, and learning by observing others is a great start.

Nonverbal Communication

Whereas verbal communication is communication that is spoken, nonverbal communication, or **body language,** consists of facial expressions, eye contact, posture, touch, and attention to personal space. In many instances, people's body language conveys their true feelings, even when their words say otherwise. A patient might say, "I'm OK about that," but if she is sitting with her arms folded tightly across her chest and avoids looking at you, she may not mean what she says.

Facial Expression Your face is the most expressive part of your body. You often can tell whether someone has understood your message simply by his facial expression. For example, when you are explaining a procedure to a patient, look at his expression. Does he seem puzzled? Is his brow wrinkled? Does he look surprised? Facial expressions can give you clues about how to tailor your communication efforts. They also serve as a form of feedback. As stated previously, your facial expressions are just as important as your words. Remain open and interested in what the patient is saying. Never look bored or impatient with a patient.

Eye Contact Eye contact is an important part of positive communication. Look directly at patients when speaking to them. Looking away or down communicates that you are not interested in the person or that you are avoiding her for some reason. Be aware of cultural differences. For example, in some cultures, it is common to avoid eye contact out of respect for someone who is considered a superior. Thus, children may be taught not to look adults in the eye.

Posture The way you hold or move your head, arms, hands, and the rest of your body can project strong nonverbal messages. During communication, posture can usually be described as open or closed.

Open Posture A feeling of receptiveness and friendliness can be conveyed with an **open posture.** In this position, your arms lie comfortably at your sides or in your lap. You face the other person, and you may lean forward in your chair. This demonstrates that you are listening and are interested in what the other person has to say. Open posture is a form of positive communication.

Closed Posture A **closed posture** conveys the opposite of open posture—a feeling of not being totally receptive to what is being said. It also can signal that someone is angry or upset. A person in a closed posture may hold his arms rigidly or fold them across his chest.

He may lean back in his chair, away from the other person. He may turn away to avoid eye contact. He may even slouch—a kind of closed posture that can convey fatigue or lack of caring. Watch for patients with closed postures that may indicate tension or pain. Avoid closed postures yourself; they have a negative effect on your communication efforts.

Touch Touch is a powerful form of nonverbal communication. A touch on the arm or a hug can be a means of saying hello, sharing condolences, or expressing congratulations. Family background, culture, age, and gender all influence people's perception of touch. Some people may welcome a touch or think nothing of it. Others may view touching as an invasion of their privacy. In general, in the medical setting, a touch on the shoulder, forearm, or back of the hand to express interest or concern is acceptable.

Personal Space When communicating with others, it is important to be aware of the concept of personal space. **Personal space** is an area that surrounds an individual. By not intruding on patients' personal space, you show respect for their feelings of privacy. In most social situations, it is common for people to stand 4 to 12 feet away from each other. For personal conversation, you would typically stand between 1 and 4 feet away from a person. Some patients may feel uncomfortable and become anxious when you stand or sit close to them. Others prefer the reassurance of having people close to them when they speak. Watch patients carefully. If they lean back when you lean forward or if they fold their arms or turn their head away, you may be invading their personal space. If they lean or step toward you, they may be seeking to close up the personal space.

▶ Improving Your Communication Skills   LO 4.4

Sharpening your communication skills should be an ongoing effort and will help you become a more effective communicator. Among the skills involved in daily communication are listening skills, interpersonal skills, and assertiveness skills.

Listening Skills

Listening involves both hearing and interpreting a message. Listening requires you to pay close attention not only to what is being said but also to nonverbal cues communicated through body language.

Listening can be passive or active. **Passive listening** is simply hearing what someone has to say without the need for a reply. An example is listening to a news program on the radio; the communication is mainly one-way. **Active listening,** on the other hand, involves two-way communication. You are actively involved in the process, offering feedback or asking questions. As seen in Figure 4-4, active listening takes place, for example, when you interview a patient for her medical history. Active listening is an essential skill in the medical office.

Ways to improve your listening skills include:

- Prepare to listen. Position yourself at the same level (sitting, standing) as the person who is speaking and assume an open posture.
- Relax and listen attentively. Do not simply pretend to listen to what is being said.
- Maintain eye contact and appropriate personal space.
- Think before you respond.
- Provide feedback. Restate the speaker's message in your own words to show that you understand.
- If you do not understand something that was said, ask the person to repeat it.

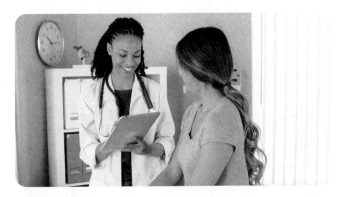

FIGURE 4-4 Active listening requires two-way communication and positive body language.
©Rocketclips, Inc./Shutterstock

Interpersonal Skills

When you interact with people, you use **interpersonal skills.** When you make a patient feel at ease by being warm and friendly, you are demonstrating good interpersonal skills. In addition to warmth and friendliness, valuable interpersonal skills include empathy, respect, genuineness, openness, consideration, and sensitivity.

Warmth and Friendliness

A friendly but professional approach, a pleasant greeting, and a smile get you off to a good start when communicating with patients. When your approach is sincere, patients will be more relaxed and open.

Empathy

The process of identifying with someone else's feelings is empathy. When you are empathetic, you are sensitive to the other person's feelings and problems. When you are sympathetic, you feel sorry *for* or feel pity *for* the person and his or her circumstances, but you don't really understand them. When you are empathetic, you are feeling *with* the person, putting yourself in his or her shoes. For example, if a patient is experiencing a migraine headache and you have never had one, you can still let her know you are trying to imagine, or relate to, her situation. In other words, you can acknowledge the severity of her pain and show support and care. If you were sympathetic to the patient's migraine, you would feel sorry that she did not feel well, but you would not try to put yourself in her shoes (or head) to understand how she is feeling.

Respect

Showing respect can mean using a title of courtesy such as "Mr." or "Mrs." when communicating with patients. It also can mean acknowledging a patient's wishes or choices without passing judgment.

Genuineness

Being genuine in your interactions with patients means that you refrain from "putting on an act" or just going through the motions of your job. Patients like to know that their healthcare providers are real people. In a medical setting, being genuine means caring for each patient on an individual basis, giving patients the full attention they deserve, and showing respect for them. Being genuine in your communication with patients encourages them to place trust in you and in what you say.

Openness

Openness means being willing to listen to and consider others' viewpoints and concerns and being receptive to their needs. An open individual is accepting of others and not biased for or against them.

Consideration and Sensitivity

You should always try to show consideration toward patients and act in a thoughtful, kind way. You must be sensitive to their individual concerns, fears, and needs.

Assertiveness Skills

As a professional, you need to be assertive—to be firm and to stand by your principles while still showing respect for others. Being assertive means trusting your instincts, feelings, and opinions (not in terms of diagnosing, which only the licensed practitioner can do, but in terms of basic communication with patients) and acting on them. For example, when you see that a patient looks uneasy, speak up. You might say, "You look concerned. How can I help you feel more comfortable?" versus asking the patient, "What is the matter with you?" Being assertive is different from being aggressive. When people are **aggressive,** they try to impose their position on others or try to manipulate them. Aggressive people are bossy and can be quarrelsome. They do not appear to take into consideration others' feelings, needs, thoughts, ideas, and opinions before they act or speak. To be **assertive,** you must be open, honest, and direct. Be aware of your body position: An open posture conveys the proper message. When you communicate, speak confidently and use "I" statements such as "I feel . . ." or "I think . . . ."

Developing your assertiveness skills increases your sense of self-worth and your confidence as a professional. Being assertive also will help you prevent conflicts or resolve them more peacefully and increase your leadership ability. People look up to and respect professionals who are assertive in the workplace. See Table 4-1 for a comparison of nonassertive, assertive, aggressive, and nonassertive aggressive behaviors.

TABLE 4-1 A Comparison of Nonassertive, Assertive, Aggressive, and Nonassertive Aggressive Behaviors				
	Nonassertive Behavior	**Assertive Behavior**	**Aggressive Behavior**	**Nonassertive Aggressive Behavior (NAG)**
Characteristics of the Behavior	Emotionally dishonest, indirect, self-denying; allows others to choose for self; does not achieve desired goal	Emotionally honest, direct, self-enhancing, expressive; chooses for self but not for others; may achieve goal	Emotionally honest, direct, self-enhancing, BUT at the expense of another; expressive; chooses for others; may achieve goal at expense of others	Emotionally dishonest, indirect, self-denying; chooses for others; may achieve goal at expense of others
Your Feelings	Hurt, anxious, possibly angry later	Confident, self-respecting	Righteous, superior, derogative at the time and possibly guilty later	Defiant, angry, self-denying; sometimes anxious, possibly guilty later
The Other Person's Feelings Toward You	Irritated, pity, lack of respect	Generally respected	Angry, resentful	Angry, resentful, irritated, disgusted
The Other Person's Feelings About Himself or Herself	Guilty or superior	Valued, respected	Hurt, embarrassed, defensive	Hurt, guilty or superior, humiliated

▶ Therapeutic Communication Skills LO 4.5

Therapeutic communication is the ability to communicate with patients in terms they can understand. At the same time, it helps patients to feel at ease with what you are saying. It is also the ability to communicate with other team members in technical terms that are appropriate in a healthcare setting. Therapeutic communication techniques can improve communication with patients. This communication must remain within your scope of practice, as discussed in the *Points on Practice* box. Therapeutic communication involves the following skills:

- *Being silent.* Silence allows the patient time to think without pressure.
- *Accepting.* This skill gives the patient an indication of reception. It shows that you have heard the patient and follow the patient's thought pattern. Some indicators of acceptance include nodding; saying, "Yes," "I follow what you said," and other such phrases; and open, positive body language.
- *Giving recognition.* Show patients that you are aware of them by stating their name in a greeting or by noticing positive changes. With this skill, you are recognizing the patient as a person and individual.
- *Offering self.* Make yourself available to the needs of the patient.
- *Giving a broad opening.* Allow the patient to take the initiative in introducing the topic. Ask open-ended questions such as "Is there something you'd like to talk about?" or "Where would you like to begin?"
- *Offering general leads.* Give the patient encouragement to continue by making comments such as "Go on" or "And then?"
- *Making observations.* Make your perceptions known to the patient. Say things like "You appear tense today" or "Are you uncomfortable when you . . . ?" By calling patients' attention to what is happening to them, you encourage them to notice it for themselves so that they can describe it to you.
- *Encouraging communication.* Ask patients to verbalize what they perceive. Make statements such as "Tell me when you feel anxious" or "What is happening?" Patients should feel free to describe their perceptions to you, and you must try to see things as they seem to the patients.
- *Mirroring.* Restate what the patient has said to demonstrate that you understand.

Some techniques that can be helpful in encouraging positive or therapeutic communication are listed here:

1. *Reflecting.* Encourage patients to think through and answer their own questions. By reflecting patients' questions or statements back to them, you are helping patients feel that their opinions about their health are of value. A reflecting dialogue may go like this:

   Patient: *"Do you think I should tell the doctor?"*

   Medical Assistant: *"Do you think you should?"*

2. *Focusing.* Focusing encourages the patient to stay on the topic. A focusing dialogue may go like this:

   Patient: *"My daughter told me I should come and see you for this leg. She always tells me what to do. I wish she was more understanding."*

   Medical Assistant: *"Tell me what happened to your leg."*

3. *Exploring.* Encourage patients to express themselves in more depth. Try to get as much detail as possible about a patient's complaint, but avoid probing and prying if the patient does not wish to discuss it.

   Patient: *"My knee hurts and so do the bottoms of my feet."*

   Medical Assistant: *"How much pain do you have? Are you able to walk?"*

4. *Clarifying.* Ask patients to explain themselves more clearly if they provide information that is vague or not meaningful.

   Patient: *"Every time I ride my bike, I feel kind of funny."*

   Medical Assistant: *"When you feel funny, what happens?"*

5. *Summarizing.* This skill involves organizing and summing up the important points of the discussion. It gives the patient an awareness of the progress made toward greater understanding.

   Patient: *"So what do you think?"*

   Medical Assistant: *"You said your shoulder hurts when you swim at about a level 8 out of 10 pain. It has been hurting for about 3 days and you do not know what started the pain, but you would like to find out what the problem is so you can swim again."*

POINTS ON PRACTICE
Communication and Scope of Practice

A medical assistant is a representative of the practice. However, patients may view you as a healthcare practitioner with medical decision-making ability. The physician or licensed practitioner will diagnose and prescribe treatment to a patient based on his or her examination and diagnostic test results. A medical assistant is not allowed to give his or her opinions on decisions made by the practitioner. Doing so puts a medical assistant in an "advising" position, which could cause legal complications for the practice. "Advising" is out of the scope of practice for a medical assistant and could be considered practicing medicine in most states, which is illegal.

Roadblocks to Therapeutic Communication

Often, people think they are communicating thoroughly, but they are not. Here are some roadblocks that can interfere with your communication style, making it ineffective or less effective than you would like.

- *Reassurance.* This type of communication indicates to the patient that there is no need for anxiety or worry. By doing this, you devalue the patient's feelings and give false hope if the outcome is not positive. The communication error here is a lack of understanding and empathy.

- *Approval.* This is usually done by overtly approving of a patient's behavior. This may lead the patient to strive for praise rather than progress.

- *Disapproval.* Overtly disapproving of a patient's behavior implies that you have the right to pass judgment on the patient's thoughts and actions. Find an alternate attitude when dealing with patients. Adopting a moralistic attitude may take your attention away from the patient's needs and instead direct it toward your own feelings.

- *Agreeing/disagreeing.* Overtly agreeing or disagreeing with thoughts, perceptions, and ideas of patients is not an effective way to communicate. When you agree with patients, they will have the perception that they are right because you agree with them or because you share their opinion. Opinions and conclusions should be the patient's, not yours. When disagreeing with patients, you become the opposition to them instead of their caregiver. Never place yourself in an argumentative situation regarding a patient's opinions.

- *Advising.* If you tell the patient what you think should be done, you place yourself outside your scope of practice. You cannot advise patients.

- *Probing.* This means discussing a topic that the patient has no desire to discuss.

- *Defending.* Protecting yourself, the institution, and others from verbal attack is classified as defending. If you become defensive, the patient may feel the need to discontinue communication.

- *Requesting an explanation.* This communication pattern involves asking patients to provide reasons for their behavior. Patients may not know why they behave in a certain manner. "Why" questions may have an intimidating effect on some patients.

- *Minimizing feelings.* Never judge or make light of a patient's discomfort. You need to be able to perceive what is taking place from the patient's point of view, not your own.

- *Making stereotyped comments.* This type of communication involves using meaningless clichés—such as "It's for your own good"—when communicating with patients. These types of comments are given in an automatic, mechanical way as a substitute for a more reasonable and thoughtful explanation.

Defense Mechanisms

When working with patients, it is important to observe their communication behaviors. Patients often develop unconscious defense mechanisms, or coping strategies, to protect themselves from anxiety, guilt, and shame. The following are some common defense mechanisms that a patient may display when communicating with the practitioner, medical assistant, or other healthcare team members. These mechanisms may be adaptive (have the ability to change or adjust) or nonadaptive (not have the ability to change or adjust).

- *Compensation:* Overemphasizing a trait to make up for a perceived or actual failing.

- *Denial:* An unconscious attempt to reject unacceptable feelings, needs, thoughts, wishes, or external reality factors.

- *Displacement:* The unconscious transfer of unacceptable thoughts, feelings, or desires from the self to a more acceptable external substitute.

- *Dissociation:* Disconnecting emotional significance from specific ideas or events.

- *Identification:* Mimicking the behavior of another to cope with feelings of inadequacy.

- *Introjection:* Adopting the unacceptable thoughts or feelings of others.

- *Projection:* Projecting onto another person one's own feelings, as if they had originated in the other person.

- *Rationalization:* Justifying unacceptable behavior, thoughts, and feelings into tolerable behaviors.

- *Regression:* Unconsciously returning to more infantile behaviors or thoughts.

- *Repression:* Putting unpleasant thoughts, feelings, or events out of one's mind.

- *Substitution:* Unconsciously replacing an unreachable or unacceptable goal with another, more acceptable one.

▶ Communicating in Special Circumstances   LO 4.6

If you make an effort to develop good interpersonal skills, most patients will not be difficult to communicate with. You will, however, encounter patients in special circumstances that can inhibit communication, such as when they are anxious or angry. Patients from different cultures may pose challenges to communication. Others may have some type of impairment or disability that makes communication difficult. Patients with terminal illnesses also may present communication difficulties. Learning about these patients' special needs and polishing your own communication skills will help you become an effective communicator in any number of situations.

The Anxious Patient

It is not uncommon for patients to be anxious in a medical office or other healthcare setting. This reaction is commonly known as the white-coat syndrome. In some cases, the anxiety even raises the patient's blood pressure. There can be many reasons for anxiety. A patient can become anxious because she is ill and does not know what is wrong with her—she may fear the worst. A patient may have recently been diagnosed with an illness that he knows nothing about, which may necessitate a severe lifestyle change. Fear of bad news or fear that some procedure is going to be painful can create anxiety. Regardless of what is causing it, anxiety can interfere with the communication process. For example, because of anxiety, a patient may not pay attention to what you are saying.

Some patients—particularly children—may be unable to verbalize their feelings of fear and anxiety. Watch for signs of anxiety, including a tense appearance, increased blood pressure and rates of breathing and pulse, sweaty palms, reported problems with sleep or appetite, irritability, and agitation. Procedure 4-1, at the end of this chapter, will help you communicate with anxious patients.

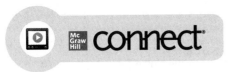

Go to CONNECT to see a video exercise about *Communicating with the Anxious Patient.*

The Angry Patient

In a medical setting, anger may occur for many reasons. It may be a mask for fear about an illness or the outcome of surgery. Anger may come from a patient's feeling of being treated unfairly or without compassion, or it may stem from a patient's resentment about being ill or injured. Anger also may be a reaction to frustration, rejection, disappointment, feelings of loss of control or self-esteem, or an invasion of privacy.

As a medical assistant, you will encounter angry patients and will need to help them express their anger constructively, for the sake of their health. At the same time, you must learn not to take expressions of anger personally; you may just be the unlucky target. The goal with angry patients is to help them refocus emotional energy toward solving the problem. Procedure 4-2, at the end of this chapter, will help you communicate with angry patients. Remember to document the facts of each encounter and its outcome in the patient's medical record (see the progress note example from Cindy Chen's chart).

Patients of Other Cultures

Our beliefs, attitudes, values, use of language, and world views are unique to us, but they also are shaped by our cultural background. Each culture and ethnic group has its own behaviors, traditions, and values. Rather than viewing these differences as communication barriers, strive to understand them (Figure 4-5). For example, many medical facilities are located in heavily populated ethnic locations, and it is important that the medical staff understand the differences among patient cultures. A medical assistant who is employed in a

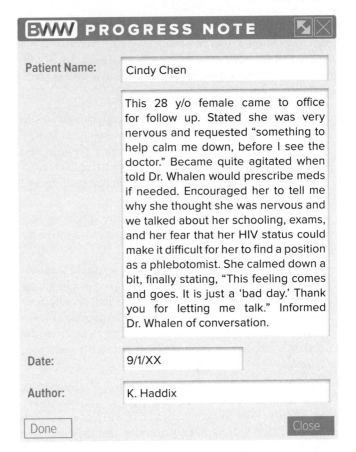

BWW PROGRESS NOTE

Patient Name: Cindy Chen

This 28 y/o female came to office for follow up. Stated she was very nervous and requested "something to help calm me down, before I see the doctor." Became quite agitated when told Dr. Whalen would prescribe meds if needed. Encouraged her to tell me why she thought she was nervous and we talked about her schooling, exams, and her fear that her HIV status could make it difficult for her to find a position as a phlebotomist. She calmed down a bit, finally stating, "This feeling comes and goes. It is just a 'bad day.' Thank you for letting me talk." Informed Dr. Whalen of conversation.

Date: 9/1/XX

Author: K. Haddix

Done   Close

medical facility in which the majority of patients are Latino should learn as much as possible about the specific Latin culture in that area in order to provide good customer service.

It is necessary to understand the difference between stereotyping and generalizing. *Stereotyping* is a negative statement about the specific traits of a group that is applied unfairly to an entire population. A *generalization* is a statement about common trends within a group, but it is understood that further investigation is needed to determine if the trend applies to an individual.

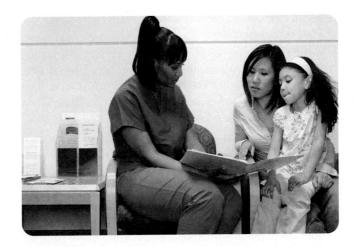

FIGURE 4-5 Knowing how to communicate across cultures is an essential skill of medical assistants.
©Image Source/Jupiterimages

Remember, the beliefs of other cultures are neither superior nor inferior to your own. They are simply different. Never allow yourself to make value judgments or to stereotype a patient, a culture, or an ethnic group. Each patient is an individual in her own right and deserves your respect and undivided attention.

Cultural Differences Patients' cultural backgrounds have an effect on their attitudes, perceptions, behaviors, and expectations toward health and illness. The following are examples of cultural differences. More information can be found online at the National Institutes of Health website, http://sis.nlm.nih.gov/outreach/multicultural.html.

- Many cultures believe that some illnesses are caused by a change in the "vital energy" or hot and cold forces in the body.
- Certain cultures may differ in the way they perceive and report symptoms. Some may express pain very emotionally because their culture may feel that suppressing pain is harmful. In contrast, people from other cultures may not admit that they are in pain, thinking that acknowledging pain is a sign of weakness.
- Patients of certain ethnic or cultural groups often consult other types of healers before seeing a doctor. They are likely to have different expectations of treatment from each.
- Patients from other cultures may be wary of certain treatments because these treatments are so different from what they are accustomed to. This is especially true of some of the medical procedures and interventions considered to be state-of-the-art, such as laser surgery or diabetes management.
- In some cultures, it may not be appropriate to suggest making a will for dying patients or patients with terminal illnesses; this is the cultural equivalent of wishing death on a patient.
- Some cultures do not look at those worthy of respect, such as healthcare workers, in the eye. If a patient does not look you in the eye when answering questions, it could be that in his culture he is not hiding anything but rather is showing you great respect.

Language Barriers Patients who cannot speak or understand English may have difficulty expressing their needs or feelings effectively. Although you may use a family member in certain circumstances, federal policies require healthcare providers who receive federal funds (that is, Medicare) to make interpretive services available to their patients with limited English. The interpreter should be a medically trained interpreter, especially for patients having surgery or if a consent form needs to be signed. If your medical office has a large number of non-English speakers, it is a good idea to have forms translated and available for use. Procedure 4-3, Communicating with the Assistance of an Interpreter, at the end of this chapter, will give you practice with this skill.

Limited Reading Skills You will find that some of your patients are functionally illiterate. They may try to hide this by saying, "I didn't bring my glasses with me" or "This is too much to read right now." Be polite, review the information

with them, and ask if they have any questions. Send the information home and have them further discuss it with a family member before requesting that they sign consent forms or forms that need to be signed before having surgery. Several vendors publish patient education materials on a specific readability level. It is recommended that patient education brochures not exceed fourth- to eighth-grade reading levels. Visual media can be provided through valid Internet resources that will improve communication as well.

Cultural Competence Your cultural competence relates to your ability to respond to the cultural and language needs of the patients you encounter. Consider the following techniques to improve your communication with patients of various cultures.

- If possible, learn and use a few phrases of greeting and introduction in the patient's native language. This conveys respect and demonstrates your willingness to learn about their culture.
- Use an interpreter whenever needed to assist with communication. Look at the patient, not the interpreter, during communication.
- Be aware of nonverbal communication and respond. For example, look for signs of pain such as a grimace.
- Avoid saying, "You must . . . ." Instead, teach patients their options and let them decide—for example, "Some people in this situation would . . . ."
- Always give the reason or purpose for a treatment or prescription.
- Make sure patients understand by having them explain it themselves.

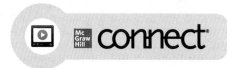

Go to CONNECT to see a video exercise about *Communicating Effectively with Patients from Other Cultures and Meeting Their Needs for Privacy.*

Terminally Ill Patients

Terminally ill patients are often under extreme stress and can be a challenge to treat. It is important that healthcare professionals respect the rights of terminal patients and treat them with dignity. It is also important that you communicate with the family and offer support and empathy as their loved one accepts her condition. You also should provide information on **hospice**, which is an area of medicine that works with terminally ill patients and their families. Hospice workers often go to the home of the terminally ill patient or work with patients in facilities. Hospice care is usually staffed with RNs and other healthcare providers who have specialized training in issues related to death and dying. They work with the family and patient in the beginning, assisting with medications, comfort care, and emotional support. If the patient dies at home, they may make arrangements with the funeral home and coroner.

Elisabeth Kübler-Ross, a world-renowned authority in the areas of death and dying, developed a model that describes the behavior patients will experience on learning their condition. This is called the stages of dying or stages of grief (Figure 4-6). This model is widely used in work with terminally ill patients.

Patients' Families and Friends

Family members or friends sometimes accompany a patient to the office. These individuals can provide important emotional support to the patient. Always ask patients if they want a family member or friend to accompany them to the examination room, however. Do not just assume their preference. Acknowledge family members and friends and communicate with them as you do with patients. They should be kept informed of the patient's progress, whenever possible, to avoid unnecessary anxiety on their part. You must always protect patient confidentiality, however. Too often, healthcare workers think that it is acceptable to discuss patient cases in detail with family members, even without the patient's consent.

AIDS and HIV-Positive Patients

Patients with acquired immunodeficiency syndrome (AIDS) and patients who have the human immunodeficiency virus (HIV), the virus that causes AIDS, may face social stigma or blame themselves. These patients often feel guilty, angry, and depressed.

To communicate effectively with these patients, you need accurate information about the disease and the risks involved. Take the initiative to educate yourself about AIDS and HIV. Patients will have many questions. Part of your role as a good communicator will be to answer as many questions as you can. If a patient asks a question you cannot answer, tell the patient's provider so he can respond quickly.

Remember, HIV is not transmitted through casual or common physical contact, such as brushing by a person in a crowded hall or shaking hands. It is transferred only through body fluids. Patients with AIDS and those who are HIV-positive need to know you are not afraid to be near them, to touch them, or to talk to them. Like any patient whose body is being ravaged by a serious illness, these patients need human contact (verbal and physical), and they need to be treated with dignity.

Patients with Behavioral Health Issues

When a patient has a behavioral or emotional health diagnosis, social stigma may be an issue. Behavioral health diagnoses include, but are not limited to, depression, attention deficit disorder with hyperactivity, dementia, and bipolar disorder.

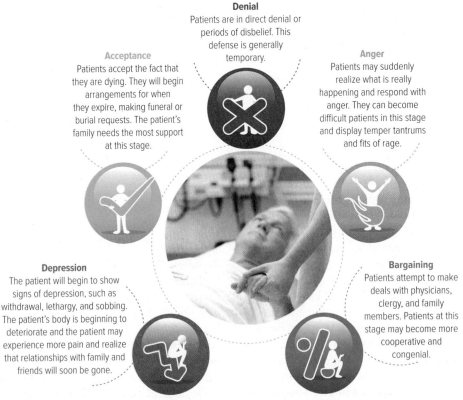

Kübler-Ross's stages of dying include five stages, which usually—but not always—progress in the following order:

Denial
Patients are in direct denial or periods of disbelief. This defense is generally temporary.

Acceptance
Patients accept the fact that they are dying. They will begin arrangements for when they expire, making funeral or burial requests. The patient's family needs the most support at this stage.

Anger
Patients may suddenly realize what is really happening and respond with anger. They can become difficult patients in this stage and display temper tantrums and fits of rage.

Depression
The patient will begin to show signs of depression, such as withdrawal, lethargy, and sobbing. The patient's body is beginning to deteriorate and the patient may experience more pain and realize that relationships with family and friends will soon be gone.

Bargaining
Patients attempt to make deals with physicians, clergy, and family members. Patients at this stage may become more cooperative and congenial.

Even though these stages have been generalized to dying, many experts have applied them to the grieving process as well. For example, after a stroke, a patient may go through the process of grieving his loss of body function.

FIGURE 4-6 Kübler-Ross's stages of dying.
©ERproductions Ltd/Blend Images LLC

In addition to dealing with the disorder itself and finding the correct treatment, these patients often feel they must try and hide their diagnosis because many in society feel they should be able to "fix themselves." Unlike cancer and other serious physical diagnoses, behavioral and emotional disorders are often not met with the same compassion as other medical illnesses. Treat patients with these illnesses with the same care, compassion, and discretion as you do any other patient.

Patients with Substance Abuse Issues

Alcohol, prescription drug, and illicit drug use and abuse are rampant in this country. If substance abuse has not affected you personally, it is very likely that it will one day. Patients may be in denial about their problem, or they may be seeking assistance with their own problem or even seeking assistance for a loved one. Substance abuse crosses all generations and all socioeconomic statuses. Many people with substance abuse issues are highly functional in their everyday lives and are embarrassed to admit there is a problem, to the point of denying that help is needed. Every office should have substance abuse hotline information available as well as that for local, state, and private agencies in your area capable of assisting patients (or even coworkers) fighting substance abuse issues. As with mental illnesses, substance abuse issues are also medical issues. Patients and their families deserve respect, compassion, and discretion during their ongoing recovery.

Gender Identity and Sexuality

According to the Human Rights Campaign survey on growing up LGBTQ (lesbian, gay, bisexual, transsexual, queer) in America, 42% of LGBTQ youth in America state they do not feel accepted by their community, and 26% feel they are not accepted by their families. Gender identity and sexuality are part of the human condition, and it is vital that patients be open and honest with their healthcare providers about their gender identity and their sexual practices. For this to occur, all members of the healthcare team must be respectful, sympathetic, and compassionate toward all patients so that they feel safe and comfortable talking about the intimate aspects of their lives. As always, address the patient as he or she prefers to be addressed, regardless of the sex listed on the record. When assisting the patient with disrobing, ask about the type of gown or drape that will make the patient most comfortable. Many people in the LGBTQ community feel judged by members of their own community. There should never be judgment of any kind in the medical community, only acceptance of everyone who enters seeking care.

▶ Communicating with Coworkers   LO 4.7

The quality of the communication you have with coworkers greatly influences the development of a positive or negative work climate and a team approach to patient care. In turn, the workplace atmosphere ultimately affects your communication with patients.

Positive Communication with Coworkers

In your interactions with coworkers, use the same skills and qualities that you use to communicate with patients. Have respect and empathy; be caring, thoughtful, and genuine; and use active listening skills. These skills will help you develop **rapport,** which is a harmonious, positive relationship, with your coworkers. Following are some rules for communication in the medical office.

- Use proper channels of communication. For example, if you are having problems getting along with a coworker, try first to work it out with her. Do not go over her head and complain to her supervisor. Your coworker may not have realized the effect of her behavior and may wish to correct it without involving her supervisor. If you go to the supervisor right away, working relationships can become even more strained.

- Have the proper attitude. You can avoid conflict and resolve most problems if you maintain a positive attitude. A friendly approach is much more effective than a hostile approach. Remember, many problems are simply the result of misinformation or lack of communication.

- Plan an appropriate time for communication. If you have something important to discuss, schedule a time to do so. For example, if you want to talk with the office manager about renewing the lease on a piece of office equipment, tell him you would like to discuss that topic and ask him to let you know a time that is convenient.

As an example of good communication with coworkers, consider this exchange between Kaylyn, a clinical medical assistant, and Miguel, her coworker at BWW Medical Associates. Note the way Kaylyn demonstrates assertiveness.

Kaylyn:	I know you spent a lot of time choosing the new toys for the reception area. I love the wooden safari animal puzzles.
Miguel:	Thanks. I think the children really enjoy themselves now.
Kaylyn:	I wanted to mention to you, though, that I'm concerned about the toy tea set with miniature cupcakes and sandwiches. Anything that's smaller than a golf ball is a choking hazard to infants and toddlers.
Miguel:	I don't think the little ones pay much attention to the tea set. It's mostly for older kids.
Kaylyn:	Yes, but I'm still afraid that a baby could put one of those pieces in his mouth. What if we put up a little shelf in the play area that is low enough for kids 4 years old or more to reach but high enough to be out of reach of the babies? We could put the tea set (and any other toys with small parts) on it in a clear plastic box.
Miguel:	I see your point. Sounds like a good idea to me.

Kaylyn started with a statement that acknowledged the coworker's situation and feelings. Then she stated her own opinion. When her coworker disagreed, she repeated her concern, describing what could happen if the situation remained unchanged. Then, she made a constructive suggestion for solving the problem without hurting the coworker's feelings. As you interact with coworkers, be sensitive to the timing of your conversations, the manner in which you present your ideas and thoughts, and your coworkers' feelings.

Communicating with Management

Positive or negative communication can affect the quality of your relationships with your supervisor or manager. For example, problems arise when communication about job responsibilities is unclear or when you feel that your supervisor does not trust or respect you, or vice versa. Consider these suggestions when communicating with your direct supervisor:

- Keep your supervisor informed. If the office copier is not working properly, talk to your supervisor about it before a breakdown occurs that will hold everyone up. If several patients express the same types of complaint about the examination rooms, make sure the right people are told. If the doctor asks you to call a patient and you reach the patient, tell the doctor.

- Ask questions. If you are unsure about an administrative task or the meaning of a medical term, for example, do not hesitate to ask your supervisor. It is better to ask a question before acting than to make a mistake. It is also better to ask than to risk annoying someone because you carried out a task or wrote a term incorrectly. Asking your supervisor or manager a question shows that you respect him or her professionally.

- Minimize interruptions. For example, before launching into a discussion, make sure your supervisor has time to talk. Opening with "Can I interrupt you for a moment or should I come back?" or "Do you have a minute to talk?" goes a long way toward establishing good communication. It is also better to go to your supervisor when you have several questions to ask rather than to interrupt her repeatedly.

- Show initiative. Any manager or supervisor will greatly appreciate this quality. For example, if you think you can come up with a more efficient way to get the office newsletter written and distributed, write out a plan and show it to your supervisor. He is likely to welcome any ideas that improve office efficiency or patient satisfaction.

Dealing with Conflict

Conflict, or friction, in the workplace can result from opposition of opinions or ideas or even from a difference in personalities. Conflict can arise when the lines of communication break down or when a misunderstanding occurs. Conflict also can result from preconceived notions about people or from lack of mutual respect or trust between a staff member and management. Whatever the cause, conflict is counterproductive to the efficiency of an office.

Following these suggestions can help prevent conflict in the office and improve communication among coworkers.

- Do not "feed into" other people's negative attitudes. For example, if a coworker is criticizing one of the doctors, change the subject or walk away.

- Try your best at all times to be personable and supportive of coworkers. For example, everyone has bad days. If a coworker is having a bad day, offer to pitch in and help or to run out and get her lunch if she is too busy to go out.

- Refrain from judging or stereotyping others (women are bad at math, men do not know how to communicate, and so on). Coworkers should show respect for one another and try to be tolerant and nonjudgmental.

- Do not gossip. You are there to work. Act professionally at all times.

- Do not jump to conclusions. For example, if you get a memo about a change in your schedule that disturbs you, take your concern to your supervisor. She may be able to be flexible on certain points. You do not know until you ask.

Setting Boundaries in the Healthcare Environment

As a medical assistant, your professional behavior is extremely important. In many instances, when dealing with patients, practitioners, and other staff members, you must set **boundaries,** whether physical or psychological. This will limit undesirable behavior.

If a patient, physician, or staff member is acting inappropriately toward you, you must take immediate action. Do not let the situation fester. You must act tactfully, assertively, and diplomatically. Let the aggressor know that his actions or language is inappropriate and that you are not obligated in any way to accept such behavior. If none of your efforts helps stop the unacceptable behavior, report the behavior to your immediate supervisor so she can assist you in identifying a solution. If the aggressor is your immediate supervisor, follow the office policy and procedure. Make yourself aware of policy and procedures ahead of time by reading the policy and procedure manual, which will be discussed in the *Practice Management* chapter.

PROCEDURE 4-1 Communicating with the Anxious Patient

Procedure Goal: To use communication and interpersonal skills to calm an anxious patient

OSHA Guidelines: This procedure does not involve exposure to blood, body fluids, or tissue.

Materials: Progress note

Method:

1. Identify signs of anxiety in the patient.
2. Acknowledge the patient's anxiety. (Ignoring a patient's anxiety often makes it worse.)
   RATIONALE: *Good therapeutic communication techniques can help reduce patient anxiety.*
3. Identify possible sources of anxiety, such as fear of a procedure or test result, along with supportive resources available to the patient, such as family members and friends.
   RATIONALE: *Understanding the source of anxiety in a patient and identifying the supportive resources available can help you communicate with the patient more effectively.*
4. Do what you can to alleviate the patient's physical discomfort. For example, find a calm, quiet place for the patient to wait, a comfortable chair, a drink of water, or access to the bathroom.
5. Allow ample personal space for conversation. Note: You would normally allow a 1- to 4-foot distance between yourself and the patient. Adjust this space as necessary.
6. Create a climate of warmth, acceptance, and trust.
   a. Recognize and control your own anxiety. Your air of calm can decrease the patient's anxiety.
   b. Provide reassurance by demonstrating genuine care, respect, and empathy.
   c. Act confidently and dependably, maintaining truthfulness and confidentiality at all times.
7. Using the appropriate communication skills, have the patient describe the experience that is causing anxiety, her thoughts about it, and her feelings. Proceeding in this order allows the patient to describe what is causing the anxiety and to clarify her thoughts and feelings about it.
   a. Maintain an open posture.
   b. Maintain eye contact, if culturally appropriate.
   c. Use active listening skills.
   d. Listen without interrupting.
   RATIONALE: *The use of open-ended questioning will result in more information about the patient's feelings of anxiety.*
8. Do not belittle the patient's thoughts and feelings. This can cause a breakdown in communication, increase anxiety, and make the patient feel isolated.
9. Be empathic to the patient's concerns.
10. Help the patient recognize and cope with the anxiety.
    a. Provide information to the patient. Patients are often fearful of the unknown.
    b. Suggest coping behaviors, such as deep breathing or other relaxation exercises.
    RATIONALE: *Helping them understand their disease or the procedure they are about to undergo will help decrease their anxiety.*
11. Notify the doctor of the patient's concerns.
    RATIONALE: *The patient's healthcare provider must be aware of all aspects of the patient's health, including anxiety, to allow for optimal patient care. Part of your job as a medical assistant is to act as a liaison between the patient and the practitioner.*
12. Document your encounter with the patient.

PROCEDURE 4-2 Communicating with the Angry Patient

Procedure Goal: To use communication and interpersonal skills to calm an angry patient

OSHA Guidelines: This procedure does not involve exposure to blood, body fluids, or tissue.

Materials: Progress note

Method:

1. Recognize anger and its causes. Anger is easy to recognize in most people, but it can be subtle in others. Patients who speak in a tense tone, are stubborn, or appear to ignore your attempts at communication may be angry.
2. Remain calm and continue to demonstrate genuineness and respect. Communicate that you respect and care about the patient's feelings.
3. Focus on the patient's physical and medical needs.
4. Maintain adequate personal space. Place yourself on the same level as the patient. If the patient is standing, encourage him to sit down. Maintain an open posture and eye contact but avoid staring.
   RATIONALE: *Open posture and eye contact show the patient you are receptive to listening. Staring at the patient may make the person angrier.*
5. Listen attentively and with an open mind to what the patient is saying. Avoid the feeling that you need to defend yourself or to give reasons the patient should not be angry.
   RATIONALE: *Most patients' anger will lessen if they know someone is really listening to them and showing an interest in their emotions and needs.*

6. Encourage patients to be specific in describing the cause of their anger, their thoughts about it, and their feelings. Be empathic and acknowledge the patient's feelings and perceptions. Follow through with any promises you make concerning correction of a problem, but avoid totally agreeing or disagreeing with the patient. State what you can and cannot do for the patient.

7. Present your point of view calmly and firmly to help the patient better understand the situation. If patients are receptive to your viewpoint, their perspective may change for the better.

8. Avoid a breakdown in communication. Allow the patient to voice anger. Trying to outtalk the patient or overexplain will only annoy and irritate him. If needed, suggest that the patient spend a few moments alone to gather his thoughts or to cool off before continuing any type of communication.

9. If you feel threatened by a patient's anger or if it looks as if the patient's anger may become violent, leave the room and seek assistance from one of the physicians or other members of the office staff.

10. Document any actual threats in the patient's chart.

PROCEDURE 4-3 Communicating with the Assistance of an Interpreter

WORK // DOC

Procedure Goal: To demonstrate techniques to effectively communicate with a non-English-speaking patient through an interpreter

OSHA Guidelines: This procedure does not involve exposure to blood, body fluids, or tissue.

Materials: Pen, forms, progress note, or computer and appropriate pictures and other visual aids if available

Method:

1. Identify the patient by name and ask if you pronounced the name correctly. Be sure to smile, even if you are feeling slightly awkward or unsure of yourself.
   RATIONALE: *A smile is a form of nonverbal communication that will help the patient feel more comfortable.*

2. Introduce yourself, with your title, to the patient and the interpreter.

3. Ask the interpreter to spell his full name and provide you with identification, such as his agency's identification or a business card. Retain his business card to file in the patient's medical record. If he does not have a business card, obtain contact information, which also will be filed in the patient's medical record.
   RATIONALE: *Healthcare facilities are required to provide an interpreter, and this information must be documented.*

4. Do not take it personally if the patient appears abrupt or even rude; this behavior may be considered appropriate in the patient's culture. For example, in some cultures, male patients may not deal with a female staff member, and that should be respected if possible. Ascertain from the interpreter if there is a problem.

5. Inquire of the interpreter if the patient speaks or understands any English and if there are any communication traditions or other customs that you should be aware of. For example, traditional Navajo people consider it rude to have direct eye contact.

6. Provide a quiet, comfortable area.

7. Speak directly to the patient and speak slowly if the patient has any understanding of English.
   RATIONALE: *Eye contact and other forms of nonverbal communication are important to convey and receive information.*

8. If forms are to be completed, instruct the interpreter to translate with appropriate intervals and give opportunities for the patient to ask questions to ensure understanding. For example, if the patient is providing general consent for treatment or permission to send information and receive payment directly from the insurance company, have one area translated at a time. Instruct the interpreter to ask if there are questions at each portion.

9. If the patient and interpreter are discussing an issue in depth or appear to be leaving you out of the conversation, ask the translator what is being said.

10. Provide the same information, services, and courtesies that you would to a native English speaker. If possible, provide written information in the patient's native language.

11. Document what you would ordinarily document; note on all forms that "translation was done by" and include the name, credential, and agency of the interpreter, as well as the date and time.

OUTCOME	KEY POINTS
4.1 **Identify elements and types of communication.**	The communication circle involves a message being sent, a source, and a receiver that responds. Feedback is the response to a message, and noise is anything that may interfere with or change the message.
4.2 **Relate communication to human behavior and needs.**	Understanding human behavior and needs, and their correlation with professional relationships is necessary to practicing as a medical assistant. Understanding the various stages of human life assists you in your communication skills with patients.
4.3 **Categorize positive and negative communication.**	Communication that promotes comfort and well-being is considered positive communication. Negative communication can be a turnoff. Medical assistants may not be aware of some of the signs of negative communication they display. Lack of eye contact with patients, except in specific cultures, or speaking sharply to a patient is considered negative communication. To help you avoid this type of communication, ask yourself, "Does this make me feel good?" or "Do I feel welcome?"
4.4 **Model ways to improve listening, interpersonal skills, and assertiveness skills.**	Listening and other interpersonal skills can be improved by becoming more involved in the communication process by offering feedback or asking questions of the patient. Assertive medical assistants trust their instincts. They respect their self-worth, while still making the patient feel comfortable and important. Aggressive medical assistants try to impose their positions through manipulation techniques.
4.5 **Carry out therapeutic communication skills.**	Therapeutic communication is the ability to communicate with patients in terms that they can understand and, at the same time, feel at ease and comfortable in what you are saying. Positive therapeutic skills can enhance communication. Be aware of negative therapeutic skills that can disrupt the communication. Recognize defense mechanisms in patients, and note whether the patient is using them to cope or is not able to cope.
4.6 **Use effective communication strategies with patients in special circumstances.**	Learning about the special needs of patients and polishing your communication skills will help you become an effective communicator. This will help you handle diversity in the workplace, handle anxious and annoyed patients, and deal with patients who have language barriers.
4.7 **Carry out positive communication with coworkers and management.**	The quality of communication you have with your coworkers and your supervisor greatly influences the development of a positive or negative work climate. Use proper channels of communication. Be open-minded. Keep supervisors informed of office problems as they arise, and show initiative in your work habits.

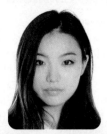

Recall Cindy Chen from the beginning of the chapter. Now that you have completed the chapter, answer the following questions regarding her case.

©excentric_01/iStock/Getty Images

1. Cindy Chen is nervous. What techniques could you use to improve your communication with her?
2. What should you do regarding Cindy Chen's HIV-positive health status?
3. How would you best answer Ms. Chen's question, "Do you have anything you can give me until I see the doctor?"
4. Ms. Chen becomes agitated when you answer her question. What should you do?

E X A M   P R E P A R A T I O N   Q U E S T I O N S

1. (LO 4.1) The main elements in the communication circle are
   a. A message (verbal and nonverbal), a source, and a receiver
   b. A message and a receiver
   c. A receiver, a response, a sender, and a source
   d. A source, feedback, and a receiver (verbal and nonverbal)
   e. A message, a receiver, and a response

2. (LO 4.7) Good relationships with coworkers would not include
   a. Professionalism
   b. Stress
   c. Cooperation
   d. Gossip
   e. Integrity

3. (LO 4.3) Which is an example of negative communication?
   a. Speaking sharply to the patient
   b. Listening carefully
   c. Being friendly and warm
   d. Looking directly at the patient
   e. Keeping quiet when appropriate

4. (LO 4.3) Which of the following is an example of positive communication?
   a. Treating patients impersonally
   b. Looking directly at patients when you speak to them
   c. Speaking brusquely or sharply
   d. Showing boredom
   e. Forgetting common courtesies, such as saying please and thank you

5. (LO 4.4) The ability to identify with someone else's feelings is called
   a. Sympathy
   b. Feedback
   c. Empathy
   d. Respect
   e. Assertiveness

6. (LO 4.3) Poor communication could lead to all of the following except
   a. Patient satisfaction
   b. Errors in billing
   c. Inefficient care
   d. Malpractice
   e. Anxiety

7. (LO 4.3) Personal space in a healthcare environment is approximately
   a. 7–18 feet
   b. 1–4 feet
   c. 3–6 feet
   d. 4–12 feet
   e. 3–10 feet

8. (LO 4.3) You want to convey an open posture while communicating with a patient. What should you do?
   a. Fold your arms and lean forward while looking into the patient's eyes
   b. Lean back gently while facing the patient
   c. Lean forward in your chair facing the patient
   d. Lean forward and avoid eye contact with the patient
   e. Extend your arms while leaning forward toward the patient

9. (LO 4.6) Your patient has been diagnosed with a terminal illness and makes the following comment: "If you could help me make it to my grandson's graduation next month before I get too sick, that would be perfect." Which of Kübler-Ross's stages of dying is this patient exhibiting?
   a. Denial
   b. Bargaining
   c. Depression
   d. Acceptance
   e. Anger

VIII.C.5 Differentiate between fraud and abuse

X.C.1 Differentiate between scope of practice and standards of care for medical assistants

X.C.2 Compare and contrast provider and medical assistant roles in terms of standard of care

X.C.3 Describe components of the Health Insurance Portability and Accountability Act (HIPAA)

X.C.4 Summarize the Patient Bill of Rights

X.C.5 Discuss licensure and certification as they apply to healthcare providers

X.C.6 Compare criminal and civil law as they apply to the practicing medical assistant

X.C.7 Define:
(a) negligence
(b) malpractice
(c) statute of limitations
(d) Good Samaritan Act(s)
(e) Uniform Anatomical Gift Act
(f) living will/advanced directives
(g) medical durable power of attorney
(h) Patient Self Determination Act (PSDA)
(i) risk management

X.C.8 Describe the following types of insurance:
(a) liability
(b) professional (malpractice)

X.C.10 Identify:
(b) Genetic Information Nondiscrimination Act of 2008 (GINA)

X.C.11 Describe the process in compliance reporting:
(c) conflicts of interest

X.C.13 Define the following medical legal terms:
(a) informed consent
(b) implied consent
(c) expressed consent
(d) patient incompetence
(e) emancipated minor
(f) mature minor
(g) *subpoena duces tecum*
(h) *respondeat superior*
(i) *res ipsa loquitur*
(j) *locum tenens*
(k) defendant-plaintiff
(l) deposition
(m) arbitration-mediation

X.P.2 Apply HIPAA rules in regard to:
(a) privacy
(b) release of information

X.P.6 Report an illegal activity in the healthcare setting following proper protocol

4. Medical Law and Ethics
b. Institute federal and state guidelines when:
   1) Releasing medical records or information
c. Follow established policies when initiating or terminating medical treatment
d. Distinguish between employer and personal liability coverage
e. Perform risk management procedures
f. Comply with federal, state, and local health laws and regulations as they apply to healthcare settings
h. Demonstrate compliance with HIPAA guidelines, the ADA Amendments Act, and the Health Information Technology for Economic and Clinical Health (HITECH) Act

Continued

CAAHEP	ABHES

XI.C.1   Define:
        (a) ethics
        (b) morals

XI.C.2   Differentiate between personal and professional ethics

XI.P.1   Develop a plan for separation of personal and professional ethics

XI.A.1   Recognize the impact personal ethics and morals have on the delivery of healthcare

▶ Introduction

Medical law plays an important role in medical facility procedures and the quality of patient care. Our modern society can be a litigious one, meaning people are inclined to sue when results or outcomes are not acceptable to them. This is particularly true with healthcare practitioners, healthcare facilities, and manufacturers of medical equipment and products. Patients, their relatives, and others expect favorable medical outcomes and often sue when these outcomes do not meet expectations. As a result, it is important for all medical professionals to understand medical law, ethics, and the Health Insurance Portability and Accountability Act (HIPAA), which began in 1996 and has expanded since that time.

As a medical assistant, having a basic knowledge of medical law and ethics can help you gain perspective in the following three areas:

1. *The rights, responsibilities, and concerns of healthcare consumers.* Healthcare professionals need to be concerned about how law and ethics impact their respective professions, and they must understand how legal and ethical issues affect patients. As medical technology advances and the use of computers increases, patients know more about their healthcare options and their rights as consumers, and more about the responsibilities of healthcare practitioners to their patients.

2. *The legal and ethical issues facing society, patients, and healthcare professionals as the world changes.* Every day new technologies emerge with solutions to biological and medical issues. These solutions often include social issues involving decisions about controversial topics such as reproductive rights, fetal stem cell research, and the confidentiality of sensitive medical records.

3. *The impact of rising costs on the laws and ethics of healthcare delivery.* Rising costs—of both healthcare insurance and medical treatment in general—can lead to questions concerning access to healthcare services and the allocation of medical treatment. For example, should everyone, regardless of age, race, or lifestyle, have the same access to scarce medical commodities such as transplant organs and very expensive medications?

Because medical treatment and decisions surrounding healthcare today have become so increasingly complex, it is important to be knowledgeable about, and aware of, the ethical issues and the laws that govern patient care. As a medical assistant and an important member of the healthcare team, always keep in mind that any health or financial information you obtain regarding a patient (past or present) is protected. It may be shared only with the patient's express permission, except in a few very specific instances, which will be discussed in this chapter.

▶ Laws and Ethics   LO 5.1

To understand medical law and ethics, it is helpful to know the difference between law and ethics. A **law** is defined as a rule of conduct or action prescribed or formally recognized as binding or enforced by a controlling authority, such as local, state, and federal governments. **Ethics** are standards of behavior based on concepts of right and wrong. Ethical behavior goes beyond the legal consideration in any given situation. *Moral values*—formed through the influence of family, culture, and society—serve as a basis for ethical conduct. Ethics will be discussed in further detail in section 5.7 of the chapter.

Classifications of Law

While a crime is any offense committed or omitted in violation of a public law, two types of law pertain to healthcare practitioners: criminal law and civil law. Whether the case is criminal or civil, there are always two sides, the plaintiff and the defendant. The party making the charge or claim is known as the *plaintiff*. The party against whom the charge or claim is made is the *defendant*.

Criminal Law **Criminal law** involves crimes against the state. When a state or federal law is violated, the government brings criminal charges against the alleged offender—for example, *Ohio v. John Doe*. Criminal laws prohibit such crimes as murder, arson, rape, and burglary. A criminal act may be classified as a felony or a misdemeanor. A **felony** is a crime punishable by death or by imprisonment in a state or federal prison for more than 1 year. Some examples of a felony include abuse (child, elder, or domestic violence), manslaughter, fraud, attempted murder, and practicing medicine without a license.

Misdemeanors are less serious crimes than felonies and are punishable by fines or imprisonment in a facility other than a federal prison for 1 year or less. Some examples of misdemeanors are thefts under a certain dollar amount, attempted burglary, and disturbing the peace.

Civil Law Civil law involves crimes against the person. Under civil law, a person can sue another person, a business, or the government. Court judgments in civil cases often require the payment of a sum of money to the injured party. Civil law includes a general category of law known as torts. A **tort** is broadly defined as a civil wrong committed against a person or property that causes physical injury or damage to someone's property or that deprives someone of his or her personal liberty and freedom. Torts may be intentional (willful) or unintentional (accidental).

Intentional Torts When one person intentionally harms another, the law allows the injured party to seek a remedy in a civil suit. The injured party can be financially compensated for any harm done by the person guilty of committing the tort. If the conduct is judged to be malicious, punitive damages also may be awarded. Examples of intentional torts include the following:

- **Assault** is the open threat of bodily harm to another, or acting in such a way as to put another in the "reasonable apprehension of bodily harm." In the medical office, if a patient were to feel threatened in any way, assault could be charged.
- **Battery** is an action that causes bodily harm to another. It is broadly defined as any bodily contact made without permission. In healthcare delivery, battery may be charged for any unauthorized touching of a patient, including such actions as suturing a wound, administering an injection, or performing a physical examination. For this reason, having a written record of a patient's informed consent is essential for all invasive medical procedures. Informed consent is discussed in section 5.2 of this chapter.
- **Defamation** is the act of damaging a person's reputation by making public statements that are both false and malicious. The full term for these actions is *defamation of character*. Defamation can take the form of slander and/or libel. *Slander* is speaking damaging words intended to negatively influence others against an individual in a manner that jeopardizes his or her reputation or means of livelihood. If a patient hears members of the staff speaking about him in an unprofessional manner or talking about his diagnosis with staff members who do not have a "need to know," it could be considered slanderous. *Libel* is publishing in print damaging words, pictures, or signed statements that will injure the reputation of another.
- False imprisonment is the intentional, unlawful restraint or confinement of one person by another. Preventing a patient from leaving the facility might be seen as false imprisonment.
- *Healthcare fraud* and *abuse* are closely related intentional torts. **Fraud** is an intentional deception or misrepresentation of services that an individual knows to be false and

that could result in an unauthorized reimbursement to a practice. An example of healthcare fraud would be billing for a procedure that is not performed. *Abuse* describes incidents or practices inconsistent with accepted and sound medical, business, or fiscal practices. Billing for unnecessary medical services is an example of healthcare abuse.

- Invasion of privacy is the interference with a person's right to keep personal matters private. Entering an exam room without knocking can be considered an invasion of privacy. The improper use of or a breach of confidentiality of medical records may be seen as an invasion of privacy.

Unintentional Torts The most common torts within the healthcare delivery system are those committed unintentionally. Unintentional torts are acts that are not intended to cause harm but are committed unreasonably or with a disregard for the consequences. In legal terms, such acts constitute negligence. **Negligence** is charged when a healthcare practitioner fails to exercise ordinary care and the patient is injured. Medical negligence is more commonly known as malpractice, which will be discussed in more detail later in section 5.3 of this chapter.

Contracts

A **contract** is a voluntary agreement between two parties in which specific promises are made for a consideration. The elements of a contract are important to healthcare practitioners because healthcare delivery takes place under various types of contracts. To be legally binding, four elements must be present in a contract:

1. *Agreement.* One party makes an offer and another party accepts it. Certain conditions pertain to the offer:
   - It can relate to the present or the future.
   - It must be communicated.
   - It must be made in good faith and not under duress or as a joke.
   - It must be clear enough to be understood by both parties.
   - It must define what both parties will do if the offer is accepted.

   For example, a physician offers a service to the public by obtaining a license to practice medicine and opening a business. Patients accept the physician's offer by scheduling appointments, submitting to physical examinations, and allowing the physician to prescribe or perform medical treatment. The contract is complete when the physician's fee is paid.

2. *Consideration.* Something of value is bargained for as part of the agreement. The physician's consideration is providing service; the patient's consideration is payment of the physician's fee.

3. *Legal subject matter.* Contracts are not valid and enforceable in court unless they are for legal services or purposes. For example, a contract entered into by a patient to pay for the services of a physician in private practice would be *void* (not legally enforceable) if the physician were not licensed to practice medicine. **Breach of contract** may be charged if either party fails to comply with the terms of a legally valid contract.

4. *Contractual capacity.* Parties who enter into the agreement must be capable of fully understanding all its terms and conditions. For example, a mentally incompetent individual or a person under the influence of drugs or alcohol cannot enter into a contract. In this context, *incompetent patients* are those who have mental conditions that make them incapable of understanding the concepts and meaning of a contract.

Types of Contracts The two main types of contracts are expressed contracts and implied contracts. An **expressed contract** is clearly stated in written or spoken words. A payment contract is an example of an expressed contract. **Implied contracts** are those in which the conduct of the parties, rather than expressed words, indicates acceptance and creates the contract. A patient who rolls up a sleeve and offers an arm for an injection is creating an implied contract.

Employment Contract Some medical practices—usually larger practices and hospitals—use employment contracts for their employees. This type of contract could include any or all of the following elements:

- A description of your duties and your employer's duties.
- Plans for handling major changes in job responsibilities.
- Salary, bonuses, and other forms of compensation.
- Benefits, such as vacation time, sick days, life insurance, and participation in pension plans.
- Grievance procedures.
- Exceptional situations under which the contract may be terminated by either you or your employer.
- Termination procedures and compensation.
- Special provisions, like job sharing, medical examinations, or liability coverage.

If you are offered an employment contract, study it closely. Consider any local laws that apply. It is wise to have a lawyer or business adviser review the contract prior to signing it.

▶ The Physician-Patient Contract LO 5.2

A physician has the right, after forming a contract or agreeing to accept a patient under his or her care, to make reasonable limitations (such as expecting the patient to follow through on the agreed-upon treatment plan) on the contractual relationship. The physician is under no legal obligations to treat patients who may wish to exceed those limitations (for example, expecting the physician to accept patient phone calls at home). Under the physician-patient contract, both parties have certain rights and responsibilities.

Physician Rights and Responsibilities

A physician has the right to:

- Set up a practice within the boundaries of his or her license to practice medicine.
- Set up an office where he or she chooses and to establish office hours.
- Specialize.

- Decide which services he or she will provide and how those services will be provided.

Within an implied contract, the physician is not expected, or bound, to:

- Treat every patient seeking care. A physician is free to use his or her discretion to form contracts within his or her practice, with one exception: If a physician is providing care to patients in a hospital emergency room or free clinic, then the physician must treat every patient who comes for treatment.
- Restore the patient to his or her original state of health.
- Make a correct diagnosis in every case.
- Guarantee the successful result of any treatment or operation. In fact, guarantees of "cures" may constitute fraud on the part of the physician.

Under an implied contract with the patient, the physician does have the responsibility (obligation) to:

- Use due care, skill, judgment, and diligence in treating patients, with the same care, skill, judgment, and diligence that peers of the same medical specialty use.
- Stay informed of the best (and current) methods of diagnosis and treatment.
- Perform to the best of his or her ability, whether or not he or she is to receive a fee.
- Furnish complete information and instructions to the patient about diagnoses, options, methods of treatment, and fees for services.

Medical Assistants and Liability All competent adults are liable (legally responsible) for their actions, in both their personal lives and their professional careers. As a medical assistant, it is important to know and understand your scope of practice within the state where you are working. As healthcare providers, medical assistants have general liability in the duties they perform, as well as toward the facility in which they work. By understanding the standard of care and the duty of care, you, as the office medical assistant, can function ethically and legally within the scope of practice for your profession. Medical assistants are held to the "reasonable person standard," which means to carry out your professional and interpersonal relationships without causing harm. This also means that you are held to a higher standard, both inside and *outside* of the office and both during and *outside* of office hours.

Patient Rights and Responsibilities

Each patient has the right to see the physician of the individual's choosing, although some managed care plans limit the physician choices to those who are "in-network." Patients also have the right to terminate a physician's services if they wish. Most states have adopted a version of the American Hospital Association's *Patient Care Partnership* (formerly called the Patient's Bill of Rights). The Patient Care Partnership is a list of standards that patients can expect in healthcare. The Joint Commission (TJC) requires hospitals to post a copy of these standards,

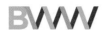

BWW Medical Associates, PC
305 Main Street, Port Snead YZ 12345-9876
Tel: 555-654-3210, Fax: 555-987-6543
Web: BWWAssociates.com

Paul F. Buckwalter, MD
Alexis N. Whalen, MD
Elizabeth H. Williams, MD

Patient Care Partnership
Understanding Expectations, Rights, and Responsibilities

Welcome to our medical practice. As our patient, you have the right to certain expectations, including

1. High-quality medical care.

2. A clean and safe environment for your medical care.

3. Informed involvement in your medical care.

4. Protection of your privacy.

5. Assistance obtaining referrals and appointments with outside providers.

6. Help with billing and insurance claim issues.

You will receive a brochure outlining the details of these rights for your records. If you have any questions, comments, concerns, or suggestions regarding the information within the brochure or regarding your care with us, please let us know. We are always interested in improving your patient care experience with us.

FIGURE 5-1   Example of a patient care partnership list.

and most managed care organizations require contracted physicians to post them. Figure 5-1 is an example of a typical patient care partnership list for a medical office. The brochure given to the patient would go into each point in more detail.

Patient Responsibilities Patients are also part of the medical team involved in their treatment. Under an implied contract, patients have the responsibility to:

- Follow any instructions given by the licensed practitioner and cooperate as much as possible.
- Give all relevant information to the licensed practitioner in order to reach a correct diagnosis. If a patient fails to inform a licensed practitioner of any medical conditions he or she has and an incorrect diagnosis is made, the licensed practitioner is not liable.
- Follow the licensed practitioner's orders for treatment.
- Pay the fees charged for services provided.

Consent means that the patient has given permission, either expressed or implied, for the licensed practitioner to examine him or her, to perform tests that aid in reaching a diagnosis, or to treat a known or found medical condition. *Expressed consent* is consent the patient gives in words. When the patient makes an appointment to be examined by a licensed practitioner, the patient has given *implied consent* to the examination and any (simple) diagnostic testing procedures needed for treatment.

Informed consent involves the patient's right to receive all information relative to his or her condition and to make a decision regarding treatment based upon that knowledge. The "doctrine of informed consent" is the legal basis for informed consent (or informed refusal of treatment) and is usually outlined in a state's medical practice acts. Informed consent implies that the patient understands:

- Proposed treatment modes.
- Why the treatment is necessary.
- The risks involved in the proposed treatment.
- Available alternative modes of treatment.
- The risks of alternative treatments.
- The risks involved if treatment is refused.

Adult patients who are of sound mind are usually able to give informed consent. Courts have ruled that emancipated minors (those under age 18, not living at home, and self-supporting) understand as a competent adult would and therefore are able to make decisions on their own. Mature minors—although defined differently by each state—are generally minors who, depending on their medical condition, are considered capable of making their own medical decisions and do not require a guardian's consent for certain procedures such as contraception, sexually transmitted infection (STI) treatment, and drug or alcohol addiction treatment. Keep in mind, however, that although mature minors may consent to treatment, they may not legally be allowed to enter into a financial contract for payment. The physician or business manager should make decisions regarding payment issues surrounding the treatment of mature minors.

Patients who cannot give informed consent include the following:

- **Minors** or persons under the age of majority, but excluding married minors.
- The mentally incompetent.
- Those who speak a foreign language—interpreters may be necessary.

Informed consent is a vital part of the practice of medicine. Physicians often are sued for negligence because of the failure to adequately inform patients of adverse surgical complications, drug reactions, and alternative treatment modes.

Terminating the Physician-Patient Contract

There are times when a physician feels it is necessary to terminate care of a patient. Terminating care is sometimes called withdrawing from a case and must be undertaken very carefully to avoid charges of abandonment. The following are some typical reasons a physician may choose to withdraw from a case:

- The patient refuses to follow the physician's instructions.

- The patient's family members complain incessantly to or about the physician.
- A personality conflict develops between the physician and the patient that cannot be reasonably resolved.
- The patient habitually does not pay for or fails to make satisfactory arrangements to pay for medical services. A physician may stop treatment of such a patient and end the physician-patient relationship only if adequate notice is given to the patient.
- The patient fails to keep scheduled appointments. To protect the physician from charges of abandonment, all missed and canceled appointments should be noted in the patient's chart.

A physician who terminates care of a patient must do so in a formal, legal manner, following these four steps:

1. Write a letter to the patient expressing the reason for withdrawing from the case and recommending that the patient seek medical care from another physician as soon as possible. Thirty days is the usual norm allowed for finding another physician. Figure 5-2 shows an example of a letter terminating patient care.

2. Send the letter by certified mail with a return receipt requested. This will provide evidence that the patient

BWW

BWW Medical Associates, PC
305 Main Street, Port Snead YZ 12345-9876
Tel: 555-654-3210, Fax: 555-987-6543
Web: BWWAssociates.com

Paul F. Buckwalter, MD
Alexis N. Whalen, MD
Elizabeth H. Williams, MD

December 12, 20XX

Jack Smallwood
20 Cedarview Court
Funton YZ 13254-0987

Dear Mr. Smallwood:

This letter is to inform you of my intent to discontinue providing medical care to you due to habitual and continued noncompliance with your treatment plan. My records indicate that you have missed several appointments and have not complied with ordered testing. In order to allow you sufficient time to establish yourself with another physician, this discontinuation will go into effect 30 days from the date of this letter. My office will be happy to forward your medical records to the physician of your choice.

If you require assistance in locating a new physician, please contact your insurance plan or the Port Snead Medical Society at 1-800-666-9898.

Sincerely,

Paul F. Buckwalter, MD

Paul F. Buckwalter, MD

FIGURE 5-2 Sample letter of withdrawal of medical care.

received the notification by providing a signature on the return receipt.

3. Place a copy of the letter (and the return receipt, when received) in the patient's medical record.

4. Summarize in the patient record the physician's reason for terminating care and the actions taken to inform the patient.

Just as a physician may choose to end the physician-patient contract, a patient also may choose to end this contract at any time. Often, the ending of the contract on the patient's part is much less formal; he may simply stop coming to appointments. If a patient suddenly stops coming to appointments, as a medical assistant, you should always attempt to reach the patient to ascertain the reason the patient has stopped coming to the office. If the patient expresses dissatisfaction with the care he has received, inform the physician as soon as possible and document the call in the patient's medical record. You will have a look at patient dissatisfaction and its connection with malpractice claims in section 5.3 of this chapter.

Standard of Care

As a medical assistant, you are expected to fulfill the standards of the medical assisting profession by practicing appropriate legal concepts for your profession. According to the AAMA, medical assistants should uphold legal concepts in the following ways:

- Maintain confidentiality.
- Practice within the scope of training and capabilities.
- Prepare and maintain medical records.
- Document accurately.
- Use appropriate guidelines when releasing information.
- Follow legal guidelines and maintain awareness of healthcare legislation and regulations.
- Maintain and dispose of regulated substances in compliance with government guidelines.
- Follow established risk management and safety procedures.
- Meet the requirements for professional credentialing.

Some state laws dictate what medical assistants may or may not do. For instance, in some states, it is illegal for medical assistants to give injections to patients. No states consider it legal for medical assistants to diagnose a condition, prescribe treatment, or allow a patient to believe that the medical assistant is a nurse. In addition to what is stated by law, you and the physician must establish your scope of practice—the procedures that are appropriate for you to perform while working under the physician's supervision. Once that scope of practice is agreed upon, you must continue to stay within that scope of practice unless the scope is updated or changed by mutual agreement. For instance, your scope of practice may change if laws change in your state or if you receive additional training, increasing your skill and/or credential level, which allows an increase in responsibilities for your position.

Closing a Medical Practice

Distressful economic circumstances may cause a medical practice to terminate and close its services to its patients. If this becomes necessary, make sure the medical staff and all physicians do the following:

- Comply with all HIPAA laws for maintaining confidentiality.
- Write letters to all patients informing them that your practice will be closing (Figure 5-3).
- Give patients an option of choosing another physician or make referrals. If the patient chooses another physician to take over his care, get written consent for his charts to be transferred to that physician properly.
- Keep all files in a secured location for the maximum amount of time files should be saved if contact with patients cannot be made. You will have to choose a vendor that stores files; make sure you choose a reputable vendor.
- Shred files if necessary; again, be sure to choose reputable vendors.
- Stay up-to-date on any HIPAA laws that will affect the practice.

▶ Preventing Malpractice Claims LO 5.3

Malpractice litigation not only adds to the cost of healthcare but also takes a psychological toll on both patients and healthcare practitioners. Both sides probably would agree that prevention is preferable to litigation. Healthcare practitioners who use reasonable care in preventing professional liability (malpractice) claims are less likely to be faced with defending themselves against these claims.

Risk management is the act or practice of controlling risk. This process includes identifying and tracking risk areas, developing risk improvement plans as part of risk handling, monitoring risks, and performing risk assessments to determine how risks have changed. Proper documentation, patient satisfaction, appropriate behavior, proper medical procedures, and safeguards against exposure assist with decreasing the risk of malpractice lawsuits brought against the medical facility, physicians, and their staff.

Medical Negligence

Malpractice claims are lawsuits by patients against physicians for errors in diagnosis or treatment. Medical *negligence* cases are those in which a person believes that a medical professional did not perform an essential action or performed an improper one, thus harming the patient.

The following are some examples of malpractice:

- *Postoperative complications.* For example, a patient starts to show signs of internal bleeding in the recovery room. The incision is reopened, and it is discovered that the surgeon did not complete closure (cauterization) of all the severed capillaries at the operation site.
- *Res ipsa loquitur.* This Latin term means "the thing speaks for itself" and refers to a case in which the doctor's fault is completely obvious—for example, a case in which a surgeon accidentally leaves a surgical instrument inside the patient.

The following are examples of medical negligence:

- *Abandonment.* A healthcare professional who stops care without providing an equally qualified substitute can be

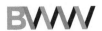

BWW Medical Associates, PC
305 Main Street, Port Snead YZ 12345-9876
Tel: 555-654-3210, Fax: 555-987-6543
Web: BWWAssociates.com

Paul F. Buckwalter, MD
Alexis N. Whalen, MD
Elizabeth H. Williams, MD

May 23, 20XX

Ms. Gisele Monahan
234 Cutter Lane
Port Snead, YZ 12345-6789

RE: Closing of Medical Practice

Dear Ms. Monahan:

I regret to inform you that our medical practice will be closing on July 30, 20XX. The practice has been purchased by the Vaughn Group, 2345 Williamsburg Court, Port Snead, YZ 12345-6789.

If you wish to use this group of medical practitioners, please sign the enclosed authorization to release medical records form so that your files may be forwarded to them promptly.

Should you choose another physician, please send me a written request with your signature, authorizing the release of your medical records to the physician of your choice. Should we not hear from you prior to the practice closing date, all records will be stored at the Vaughn Group location for retrieval at a future date.

It has been my pleasure to provide your medical care.

Sincerely,

Alexis N. Whalen, MD

Alexis N. Whalen, MD

Enc: Authorization to Release Information

FIGURE 5-3 Sample letter notifying patient of medical practice closure.

charged with **abandonment**. For example, a labor and delivery nurse is helping a woman in labor. The nurse's shift ends, but all the other nurses are busy and her replacement is late for work. Leaving the woman would constitute abandonment. A healthcare practitioner who intends to be away from her practice for an extended period of time may hire a ***locum tenens,*** literally "place holder." For example, a physician taking maternity leave may hire another qualified physician to temporarily take her place. The substitute physician will act as the practicing physician's agent; therefore, abandonment is not an issue.

- *Delayed treatment.* A patient shows symptoms of some illness or disorder, but the doctor decides, for whatever reason, to delay treatment. If the delay is the direct cause of patient harm, the patient may have a negligence case.

The following legal terms are sometimes used to classify medical negligence cases:

- *Malfeasance* refers to an unlawful act or misconduct.
- *Misfeasance* refers to a lawful act that is done incorrectly.
- *Nonfeasance* refers to failure to perform an act that is one's required duty or that is required by law.

Proving Medical Negligence In order for a patient to prove an injury was due to negligence, four legal elements must be satisfactorily proven. These four elements are often called the four Ds of negligence. They are:

1. *Duty.* Patients must show that a physician-patient relationship existed in which the physician owed the patient a duty.

2. *Derelict.* Patients must show that the physician failed to comply with the standards of the profession. For example, a gynecologist has routinely taken Pap smears of a patient and then, for whatever reason, does not do so. If the patient then shows evidence of cervical cancer, the physician could be said to have been derelict.

3. *Direct cause.* Patients must show that any damages were a direct cause of a physician's breach of duty. For example, if a patient fell on the sidewalk and damaged her cast, she could not prove that the cast was damaged because it was incorrectly or poorly applied by her physician. It would be clear that the damage to the cast resulted from the fall. If, however, the patient's leg healed incorrectly because of the way the cast had been applied, she might have a case.

4. *Damages.* Patients must prove that they suffered injury.

To go forward with a malpractice suit, a patient must be prepared to prove all four elements. If one or more of these elements cannot be proven, a legal case of medical negligence is unlikely.

Malpractice and Civil Law Malpractice (medical negligence) lawsuits are part of civil law, coming under the heading of torts. Recall that a tort is the intentional or unintentional breach of an obligation that causes harm or injury. A *breach of contract* is the failure of one of the parties to adhere to the terms of the contract.

In the case of medical care contracts, which are often implied contracts, either the provider or the patient can breach the contract. The provider can breach the contract by not maintaining patient confidentiality or by not providing adequate medical care (negligence). The patient can breach the contract by not showing up for appointments or by not following the physician's plan of care.

Settling Malpractice Suits Malpractice suits often require a trial in a court of law. Sometimes, however, they are settled through arbitration or mediation. *Arbitration* is a process in which the opposing sides choose a person or persons outside the court system, often with special knowledge in the field, to hear and decide the dispute. Arbitration is generally binding—that is, the parties agreeing to settle through arbitration must follow the solution arrived at by the arbitrator. Mediation is similar to arbitration in that the goal is to settle the case. The mediator does not judge the case but simply seeks a reasonable solution that both parties can agree upon. Mediation is generally nonbinding. (Your local or state medical society has information about the policy on arbitration or mediation for your state.) If injury, failure to provide reasonable care, or abandonment of the patient is proven to have occurred, the doctor must pay damages (a financial award) to the injured party.

If the physician you work with becomes involved in a lawsuit, you should be familiar with subpoenas and depositions. A *subpoena* is a written court order addressed to a specific person, requiring that person's presence in court on a specific date at a specific time. If you were directly involved in the patient case or have knowledge of the events that precipitated the lawsuit, you might be subpoenaed to provide testimony under penalty, known as *subpoena testificandum.* Another important term to know is *subpoena duces tecum,* which is a court order to produce specific, requested documents required at a certain place and time to enter into court records. If you are in charge of patient records at the practice, you will be required to locate, assemble, photocopy, and arrange for delivery of the requested records or be charged with contempt of court if you do not comply. Prior to appearing in court, a healthcare practitioner may be asked to give a deposition, either as a defendant or an expert witness. The **deposition** is a sworn statement regarding the facts of the case and is used to prepare the case for trial.

Law of Agency According to the law of agency, an employee is considered to be acting as a doctor's agent (on the doctor's behalf) while performing professional tasks. The Latin term *respondeat superior,* or "let the master answer," is sometimes used to refer to this relationship. For example, the medical assistant's word is as binding as if it were uttered by the doctor (so you should never promise a patient a cure). With the law of agency, the doctor is responsible, or *liable,* for the negligence of employees. A negligent employee, however, also may be sued directly because individuals are legally responsible for their own actions. So a patient can sue both the doctor and the involved employee for negligence. The employer, or the employer's insurance company, also can sue the employee. Most likely, in a case of negligence, the doctor would be sued (because you as an employee are acting on the doctor's behalf), and you are usually covered by the doctor's malpractice insurance. Some medical assistants (usually clinical MAs) choose to obtain malpractice insurance. Obtaining personal malpractice insurance is a professional decision that depends on the type of work or facility in which you are employed. The American Association of Medical Assistants (AAMA) offers medical assisting malpractice insurance through various insurance companies at reduced rates.

Courtroom Conduct Most healthcare providers will never have to appear in court, but should you be asked to appear, the following suggestions may prove helpful:

- Attend court proceedings as required. Failure to appear in court could result in charges of contempt of court or in the case being forfeited.
- Do not be late for scheduled hearings.
- Bring required documents to court and present them only when requested to do so.
- Before testifying, refresh your memory concerning all the facts observed about the matter in question, like dates, times, words spoken, and circumstances.

- Speak slowly, clearly, and professionally. Do not use medical terms. Do not lose your temper or attempt to be humorous.
- Answer all questions in a straightforward manner, even if the answers appear to help the opposing side.
- Answer only the question asked, no more and no less.
- Appear well groomed, and wear clean, conservative clothing.

Professional Liability Coverage Professional liability coverage, also known as malpractice insurance, is specialty coverage to protect the physician and staff against financial losses due to lawsuits filed against them by their clients or others. This coverage protects the physician if she is found to be negligent in her actions, and it protects the physician and her staff members if it is determined that any member is negligent in his or her actions. Though professional liability coverage likely covers you as a medical assistant, the employer's first responsibility is to the practice. For this reason, you may want to consider additional personal liability coverage. Personal coverage protects you in the event the employer's coverage does not extend to all aspects of your involvement in the case. Although professional liability coverage comes at an extremely high cost to the practice, personal coverage is affordable and covers you if you are no longer employed at the practice where the claim was made. Society in general, and patients in particular, have extremely high expectations of physicians and of the medical community. Malpractice lawsuits have become quite commonplace. You have likely seen billboards advertising lawyers who offer assistance to patients who are unhappy with the medical care they have received.

It is no surprise, then, that malpractice insurance can be one of the most expensive accounts payable for the office. Depending on the type of specialty and the area of the country in which the physician practices, costs for an internist can be as low as $3,500 per year in Minnesota (which has some of the lowest malpractice rates in the country) to a high of $48,000 annually (in 2014) in Florida, which has some of the highest rates in the country. OB/GYNs, who have some of the highest rates of any specialty, can expect to pay anywhere from $17,000 in Minnesota to $82,000 to $200,000 per year in Florida for coverage.

Reasons Patients Sue

The following reasons were researched by interviewing families and patients who have sued healthcare practitioners:

1. *Unrealistic expectations.* With modern advancements in medical technology, patients often expect perfection in medical outcomes. They may feel betrayed by the healthcare system when a medical outcome is not what was expected.
2. *Poor rapport and poor communication.* Patients usually do not sue healthcare practitioners whom they like and trust. Healthcare providers who do not return telephone calls or are otherwise unavailable to a patient's family members may be perceived as arrogant, cold, or uncaring. When such perceptions exist, patients and family members are more likely to sue if something goes wrong.

3. *Greed and our litigious society.* Financial gain is seldom the reason for medical malpractice, but in some cases, it may be an influencing factor. Malpractice attorneys sometimes make it very easy for patients to retain their services, such as with contingency arrangements.
4. *Poor quality of care.* Poor quality means that a patient is truly not receiving quality care. Poor quality in "perception" means that the patient believes he or she is not receiving quality care, even if it is not true. Either situation can lead to a malpractice lawsuit.

Statute of Limitations Statutes of limitations are laws that set the deadline or maximum period of time within which a lawsuit or claim may be filed. The most common length of time is 2 years. The deadlines may vary depending on the circumstances and the type of case or claim. The periods of time also vary from state to state and depend on whether the lawsuit or claim is filed in federal or state court. The lawsuit or claim is barred or disqualified if it is not filed before the statutory deadline. Under certain circumstances, a statute of limitations will be extended beyond its deadline. The following are examples for a civil claim for professional malpractice:

- *Medical:* 1 to 4 years from the act or occurrence of injury, or 6 months to 3 years from discovery; certain circumstances will extend the statute, including if the party is a minor, when a foreign object is involved, or in cases of fraud.
- *Legal:* 1 to 3 years from date of discovery, or a maximum of 2 to 5 years from the date of the wrongful act.

Four Cs of Medical Malpractice Prevention

1. *Caring.* As a healthcare professional, caring about your patients and colleagues is your most important asset. Showing patients that you care about them may result in an improvement in their medical condition and, if you are sincere, decreases the likelihood that patients will feel the need to sue if treatment has unsatisfactory results or if adverse events occur.
2. *Communication.* If you communicate in a professional manner and clearly ask for confirmation that you have been understood, you will earn respect and trust from your patients and other members of the allied health team.
3. *Competence.* Be competent in your skills and job knowledge by maintaining and updating your knowledge and skills frequently through continuing education.
4. *Charting.* Documentation is proof of competence. Make sure that all current reports and consultations have been reviewed by the physician and are evident in the chart. Chart every conversation or interaction you have with a patient.

How Effective Communication Can Help Prevent Lawsuits
Patients who see the medical office as a friendly place are generally less likely to sue. Physicians, medical assistants, and other medical office staff who have pleasant

personalities and are competent in their jobs will have less risk of being sued. Medical assistants can help by:

- Developing good listening skills and nonverbal communication techniques so that patients feel the time spent with them is not rushed.
- Setting aside a certain time during the day for returning patient phone calls.
- Checking to be sure that all patients or their authorized representatives sign informed consent forms (after all questions and concerns have been addressed) before they undergo medical or surgical procedures.
- Avoiding statements that could be construed as an admission of fault on the part of the physician or other medical staff.
- Using tact, good judgment, and professional ability in handling patients.
- Making every effort to reach an understanding about fees with the patient before treatment so that billing does not become a point of contention.

▶ Administrative Procedures and the Law

LO 5.4

Many of your administrative duties as a medical assistant are related to legal requirements and fall under the heading of risk management. When correct policies and procedures are followed, the risk of lawsuits decreases, but if a lawsuit is brought against the physician, the same policies and procedures will be the physician's best defense. Keep in mind that everything you do and do not do reflects not only on you but also on the physician and the practice. Always follow office policies and procedures, and follow your "best practices" at all times to do your part to avoid lawsuits.

Paperwork for insurance billing, patient consent forms for surgical procedures, and correspondence (such as a physician's letter of withdrawal from a case) must be handled correctly to meet legal standards. Documentation of appropriate and accurate entries in a patient's medical record not only provides proof of continuity of care but is legally important, should the physician ever require the record for a legal case involving the patient. You also may maintain the physician's appointment book—also considered a legal document—especially for tracking missed or canceled appointments. You will explore this aspect of medical assisting in the *Schedule Management* chapter.

In your role as a medical assistant, you also may be responsible for handling certain state reporting requirements. Items that must be reported include births; certain communicable diseases such as acquired immunodeficiency syndrome (AIDS) and STIs; drug abuse; suspected child abuse or abuse of the elderly; injuries caused by violence, such as knife and gunshot wounds; and deaths. Reports are sent to various state departments, depending on the content of the report. For example, suspected child and elder abuse cases are reported to the state department of social services. Addressing these state requirements is called the physician's public duty.

Phone calls also must be handled with an awareness of legal issues. For example, if the physician asks you to contact a patient by phone and you call the patient at work, you should not identify yourself or the physician by name to someone else without the patient's permission. You can say, for example, "Please tell Mrs. Arnot that her doctor's office is calling." If you do not take this precaution, the physician can be sued for invasion of privacy. You must abide by similar guidelines if you are responsible for making follow-up calls to a patient after a procedure or an office visit and when leaving messages on answering machines or on voicemail where someone other than the person you are attempting to reach may pick them up.

Documentation

Patient records often are used as evidence in professional medical liability cases, and improper documentation can contribute to the loss of a case. Physicians should keep records that clearly show exactly what treatment was performed and when it was done. It is important that physicians be able to demonstrate that nothing was neglected and that the care given fully met the standards demanded by law. One cliché to remember is "If it is not recorded, then it was not done." (On the same note, if it is recorded, it is assumed that it was done.) Pay attention to spelling in charts, and keep a medical dictionary handy if you are not sure of a spelling. Today's healthcare environment requires complete documentation of actions taken and actions not taken. Medical staff members should pay particular attention to the following situations.

Referrals Make sure the patient understands whether you will be making the appointment with the specialist, whether the specialty physician's staff will be calling to make the appointment with the patient, or whether the patient must call to set up the appointment. Document in the chart that the patient was referred, to whom, and how the appointment is to be made. If the date and time of the appointment are known, document this information also. Follow up with the specialist to verify that the appointment was kept. If a paper referral is necessary, make sure a hard copy is placed in the patient's chart. If the referral is made electronically, note the referral number in the patient's chart. Note whether reports of the consultation were received in your office, and document any further care the patient is to receive from the specialty physician.

Missed Appointments At the end of the day, a designated person in the medical office should document the charts of those patients who missed or canceled appointments without rescheduling. Charts should be dated and documented "No Call/No Show" or "Canceled/Not Rescheduled." The appointment book also is considered a legal document; make sure that all missed appointments are documented in the appointment book or within the electronic scheduling system. The treating physician should review these records and note whether follow-up is indicated.

Dismissals To avoid charges of abandonment, the physician must formally withdraw from a case. Be sure that a letter of withdrawal or dismissal has been filed in the patient's records (refer to Figure 5-2). All mailing confirmations should be filed in the record, such as the return receipt from certified mail.

All Other Patient Contact Patient records should include reports of all tests, procedures, and medications prescribed, including prescription refills. Make sure all necessary informed consent papers have been signed and filed in the chart. Make entries into the chart of all telephone conversations with the patient. Correct documentation requires the initials or signature of the person making the notation on the patient's chart as well as the date and time.

Medical Record Correction Errors made when making an entry in a medical record or errors discovered later can be corrected, but corrections must be made in a certain manner so that if the medical records are ever used in a medical malpractice lawsuit, it will not appear that they were falsified. So when deleting information, never black it out, never use correction fluid to cover it up, and never in any other way erase or obliterate the original wording. Draw a line through the original information so that it is still legible. Write or type in the correct information above or below the original line or in the margin. The *Medical Records and Documentation* chapter describes the proper procedure for correcting paper chart errors, and the *Electronic Health Records* chapter discusses the procedure for electronic health records.

Ownership of the Patient Record Patient medical records are considered the property of the owners of the facility where they were created. A physician in a private practice owns his or her charts or records, while records in a hospital or clinic belong to the facility. It is important to remember that although the facility in which the records were created owns the records, the patient owns the information they contain. Upon signing a release, patients may usually obtain access to or copies of their medical records, depending upon state law. Under HIPAA, patients who ask to see or copy their medical records must be accommodated with a few exceptions, such as with mental health records. If the physician decides it may be harmful to the patient to see the contents of the medical record and denies access, the physician is protected under the *doctrine of professional discretion.*

Retention and Storage of the Patient Record As a protection against legal litigation, records should be kept until the applicable statute of limitations period has elapsed, which is generally 7 years. In some cases, the medical records for minor patients must be kept for a specified length of time after they reach legal age. Some states have enacted statutes for the retention of medical records. Because the federal False Claims Act requires that financial records be kept for 10 years and medical records are often required to back up financial records, many legal experts suggest that medical records also should be kept for a minimum of 10 years. Most physicians retain records indefinitely to provide evidence in medical professional liability suits or for tax purposes. The medical record may provide the patient's medical history for future medical treatment. The chapter *Managing Medical Records* goes into more detail on this subject.

Credentialing *Credentialing* is used by various organizations, including insurance carriers, to ensure that healthcare providers are appropriately qualified to provide services and meet all the necessary requirements to do so. The qualifications are determined and approved by unbiased physician peer review groups. Specific criteria vary according to the physician or provider specialty and the provider's scope of practice. Physicians are broken into two types according to medical licensure—MD (medical doctor) or DO (doctor of osteopathy)—and then further broken down according to specialty.

As the office medical assistant, you may be responsible for credentialing any new providers joining the practice. In general, insurance companies require their doctors to hold and maintain the proper credentials. In order for a physician to participate with an insurance carrier such as Medicare, he must have the necessary professional credentials and go through the Medicare credentialing process, or he will not be allowed to bill Medicare for services provided to Medicare beneficiaries.

Medicare has three forms for credentialing:

1. Form 855B is used to establish or change a practice group number.

2. Form 855I is used to establish or reestablish a physician's individual number. In addition to completing this 29-page application, the physician also must provide his or her medical school diploma, individual national provider identifier (NPI), current license number, any board certifications for specialties, work history for at least 5 years, statement of any limitations, history of loss of licensure or felony convictions, history of loss or limitations of privileges or disciplinary actions, and outside verification of information provided.

3. Form 855R is used to link individual provider numbers to group practice numbers.

These forms are not complicated, but they are time-consuming. More information about Medicare's credentialing process can be found on the Centers for Medicare and Medicaid Services (CMS) website at http://www.cms.gov/. In addition to the paper-based forms, CMS has established the Internet-based Provider Enrollment Chain and Ownership System (PECOS). This system allows physicians, nonphysician practitioners, and provider and supplier organizations to enroll, make a change in their Medicare enrollment, view their Medicare enrollment information on file with Medicare, or check on the status of a Medicare enrollment application via the Internet. Regardless of the application method used, once the Medicare credential is received, many other insurance plans will follow suit with credentialing or linking so the provider also can bill them for services provided. If a separate credentialing process is required, it is generally much less complicated than that required by Medicare.

The Food and Drug Administration Regulatory Function

The Food and Drug Administration (FDA) requires that drug manufacturers perform clinical tests on new drugs before humans use these drugs. These tests include toxicity tests in laboratory animals, followed by clinical studies (frequently called clinical trials). Venipuncture is performed and blood is drawn from controlled groups of volunteers. See Figure 5-4. Some volunteers are patients; others are healthy subjects.

Clinical tests are designed to consider the ratio of benefits to the risk of adverse side effects. If the clinical tests prove that the drug is safe and effective, the FDA approves it for marketing. The manufacturer must continue to demonstrate the drug's safety and efficacy (therapeutic value) and must submit reports whenever it discovers unexpected adverse reactions. The FDA can withdraw a drug from the market at any time if evidence suggests that it is no longer safe or effective.

During the clinical trials, the pharmaceutical (drug) company studies all aspects of the pharmacology of the new drug. When the company seeks approval from the FDA, it must document the pharmacodynamics, pharmacokinetics, safety (how many and what kind of adverse effects), and efficacy of the drug. In addition, it must present data regarding the effective dose—the amount of drug given at one time.

After the FDA approves a drug, it continues its regulatory function to protect patients and consumers. These regulatory functions are discussed in detail in the *Principles of Pharmacology* chapter and include the following:

- Review of new indications proposals (applications from companies for new uses for a drug).
- Drug manufacturing—ensuring the proper identity, strength, purity, and quality of each drug.

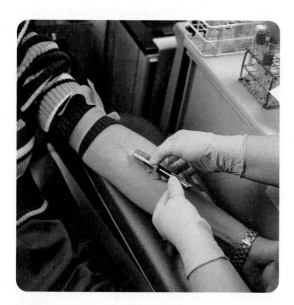

FIGURE 5-4   Blood tests provide baseline data on volunteers at the start of clinical drug trials.
©Liquidlibrary/Getty Images

- Over-the-counter (nonprescription) drugs—approving drugs for use without supervision by a healthcare practitioner.
- Prescription drugs—monitoring safety, use, and availability of drugs prescribed by healthcare practitioners.
- Pregnancy categories—risk categories established by the FDA based upon the degree to which available information has ruled out risk to the fetus or breastfed infant.
- Controlled substances—regulation of drugs or drug products that are potentially dangerous or addictive.
- The Comprehensive Drug Abuse Prevention and Control Act, also known as the Controlled Substances Act (CSA)—federal law established to strengthen regulation of potentially dangerous or addictive drugs by:
  - Creating the Drug Enforcement Administration (DEA).
  - Designating five schedules for drugs based on the degree of potential the substance has for abuse or nontherapeutic use.
  - Requiring doctors who administer, dispense, or prescribe any controlled substance to register with the DEA.

Legal Documents and the Patient

You need to be aware of several legal documents that are typically completed by a patient prior to major surgery or hospitalization or facing terminal illness. Advanced care planning documents including Physicians Orders for Life-Sustaining Treatment (POLST) forms, the advance medical directive, and the durable power of attorney. Additionally, you should be familiar with the uniform donor card. The Patient Self-Determination Act (PSDA), implemented in 1991, was designed to encourage patients and healthcare professionals to discuss end-of-life issues. According to the PSDA, certain healthcare facilities that are Medicare and Medicaid providers are required to ask each patient, age 18 or older, if he or she has an advance directive. Facilities also are required to inform patients of their policies regarding recognizing advance directives. They must discuss the patient's healthcare decision-making rights under state law regarding end-of-life issues. Contact your state's Public Health Department for additional information.

Advance Care Planning   Every adult capable of making his or her own decisions should plan, in advance, what actions medical professionals should take in the event of serious illness or injury. Advance care planning allows you to make your wishes known in the event you cannot speak for yourself. The process of advance care planning includes:

- Obtaining information about types of life-sustaining treatment.
- Choosing what types of treatment you want or do not want.
- Talking with family and loved ones about your wishes.
- Completing appropriate documents stating your wishes.

These documents include the Physician Orders for Life-Sustaining Treatment form, advance directives, durable power of attorney, and the living will.

Physician Orders for Life-Sustaining Treatment The **Physician Orders for Life-Sustaining Treatment (POLST) form** is a set of medical orders completed by a healthcare provider after a discussion with the patient regarding his or her desires for treatment. The POLST form is signed by the healthcare provider and serves as a set of portable treatment orders. The patient should keep the form with him or her at all times. According to the National POLST Paradigm, all but one state and the District of Columbia have or are developing POLST programs. The form has different names in different states. These include but are not limited to:

- MOLST: Medical Orders for Life-Sustaining Treatment
- MOST: Medical Orders for Scope of Treatment
- POST: Physician Orders for Scope of Treatment

The content of the medical orders varies from state to state but can include orders for the following medical interventions:

- Cardiopulmonary resuscitation (CPR)
- Intubation/airway management
- Artificial ventilation
- Blood transfusion
- Hospital transfer
- Antibiotics
- IV fluids
- Administration of artificial nutrition (feeding tube)
- Dialysis

Advance Medical Directive The advance medical directive is a legal document addressed to the patient's family and healthcare providers stating what type of treatment the patient wishes or does not wish to receive if she becomes terminally ill, unconscious, or permanently comatose (sometimes referred to as being in a persistent vegetative state). For example, an advance directive typically states whether a patient wishes to be put on life-sustaining equipment if she becomes permanently comatose. Some directives contain orders for medical personnel to refrain from starting CPR in the event a patient's heart stops. These orders are known as DNR (do not resuscitate) orders. The American Heart Association began using the term DNAR (do not attempt resuscitation) in 2005 in place of DNR. Additionally, some healthcare facilities use the term AND (allow natural death). Table 5-1 outlines the advantages and disadvantages of each of these terms. The directives are signed when the patient is mentally and physically competent to do so. They also must be signed by two witnesses. Advance medical directives are a means of helping families of terminally ill patients deal with the inevitable outcome of the illness. Having advance directives in place can lower the family's stress levels, as difficult decisions already have been made, and also may help limit unnecessary medical costs often occurred at the end of life.

Medical practices can help patients develop an advance medical directive, sometimes in conjunction with organizations that have resources for completing advance directives. The American Cancer Society (based in Atlanta, Georgia) is one such organization.

Your first impression might be that the POLST form and advance medical directives are the same. Though both honor a patient's right to receive or not to receive life-sustaining treatment, they are different in several ways. Advance medical directives go into effect only when the patient loses the capacity to make decisions. POLST forms are medical orders that go into effect as soon as they are signed. See Table 5-2.

Durable Power of Attorney Patients who have an advance medical directive are asked to name, in the second document, called a **durable power of attorney** (also known as a healthcare proxy), someone who will make decisions regarding medical care on their behalf if they are unable to do so. It is important that the person named in the durable power of attorney knows the patient's wishes ahead of time, so in the event that he is required to make medical decisions, he can be confident he is carrying out the patient's wishes. Durable power of attorney is not the same as a legal guardian. Legal guardianship is usually directed by a court, whereas a durable power of attorney is a legal document drawn up by an attorney without a court order.

The Uniform Donor Card In 1968, the Uniform Anatomical Gift Act was passed, setting forth guidelines for all states to follow in complying with a person's wish to

TABLE 5-1	Differences among Various Terms for Resuscitation Orders	
Medical Order	**Pros**	**Cons**
DNR (Do Not Resuscitate)	Widely known and understood	May give impression that resuscitation will succeed and patients and family members perceive they are choosing between life and death
DNAR (Do Not Attempt Resuscitation)	Language more clearly implies that resuscitation is attempted but may not result in recovery	Not widely used, may not be as familiar
AND (Allow Natural Death)	Language implies that patients and family understand that resuscitation attempts are unlikely to succeed and natural death is anticipated	Could be confused with the word *and;* should be accompanied by clarifying orders of what is and is not desired (pain control, fluids, etc.)

TABLE 5-2 Differences Between POLST and Advance Directives

	POLST Paradigm Form	Advance Directive
Type of Document	Medical Order	Legal Document
Who Completes the Document	Health care professional (which health care professional can sign varies by state)	Individual
Who Should Have One	Any seriously ill or frail individual (regardless of age) whose health care professional wouldn't be surprised if he or she died within the year	All competent adults
What Document Communicates	Specific medical orders	General treatment wishes
Can This Document Appoint a Surrogate Decision-Maker?	No	Yes
Surrogate Decision-Maker Role	Can engage in discussion and update or void form if patient lacks capacity	Cannot complete
Can Emergency Personnel Follow This Document?	Yes	No
Ease in Locating / Portability	Patient has original; a copy is in patient's medical record. A copy may be in a state registry (if state has one).	No set location. Individuals must make sure surrogates have most recent version.
Periodic Review	Health care professional responsibilities for reviewing with patient or surrogate	Patient is responsible for periodically reviewing.

Table 1 from "POLST: Advance Care Planning for the Seriously Ill," http://polst.org. Copyright © by National POLST Paradigm. All rights reserved. Used with permission.

make a gift of one or more organs (or the whole body) upon death. An anatomical gift is typically designated for medical research, organ transplants, or placement in a tissue bank. The uniform donor card is a legal document that states one's wish to make such a gift. People often carry the uniform donor card in their wallets. Many medical practices offer the service of helping their patients obtain and complete a uniform donor card. In some states, the Department of Motor Vehicles makes the process simple by asking you at the time you renew your driver's license if you would like to be an organ donor, with a card being issued to you at that time and a notation made on the driver's license that you are an organ donor. The patient's family should be aware of this wish to be an organ donor so that it is carried out upon the patient's death.

▶ Federal Legislation Affecting Healthcare

LO 5.5

Congress has passed legislation intended to improve the quality of healthcare in the United States, reduce fraud, and ensure that insurance providers will not discriminate against patients. The most significant healthcare laws passed in recent years are the Health Care Quality Improvement Act of 1986, the False Claims Act, the Genetic Information Nondiscrimination Act of 2008, and the Health Insurance Portability and Accountability Act of 1996. In addition, Occupational Safety and Health Administration regulations are vital to the practice of healthcare and the safety of its practitioners, and these, too, are reviewed and often updated by the administration.

Health Care Quality Improvement Act of 1986

The Health Care Quality Improvement Act of 1986 (HCQIA) is a federal statute passed to improve the quality of medical care nationwide. Congress created HCQIA after discovering an increasing occurrence of medical malpractice and a need to improve the quality of medical care. The act requires professional peer review in certain cases, limits damages to professional reviewers, and protects from liability those who provide information to professional review bodies. One of the most important provisions of the HCQIA was the establishment of the National Practitioner Data Bank, designed to improve the quality of medical care nationwide by encouraging effective professional peer review of physicians. Information that must be reported to the National Practitioner Data Bank includes medical malpractice payments, adverse licensure actions, adverse clinical privilege actions, and adverse professional membership actions. This data bank is a resource to assist state licensing boards, hospitals, and other healthcare entities in investigating the qualifications of physicians and other healthcare practitioners.

False Claims Act

The False Claims Act is a federal law that allows individuals to bring civil actions on behalf of the US government for false claims made to the federal government, under a provision of the law call *qui tam* (from Latin, meaning to bring an action for the king and for one's self). The law was enacted because of the rising cost of healthcare, fraud, and abuse within the healthcare industry. As a result, laws have been passed to control three types of illegal conduct:

1. *False billing claims.* Fraudulently billing for services not performed is prohibited.
2. *Kickbacks.* Giving financial incentives to a healthcare provider for referring patients or for recommending services or products is prohibited under the federal Anti-Kickback Law and by state laws.
3. *Self-referrals.* Referring patients to any service or facility where the healthcare provider has financial interests is prohibited by the Federal Ethics in Patient Referral Act and other federal and state laws.

Violations of laws against healthcare fraud and abuse can result in imprisonment and fines, the loss of professional licensure, the loss of healthcare facility staff privileges, and exclusion from participating in federal healthcare programs such as Medicare and Medicaid.

Genetic Information Nondiscrimination Act of 2008

The Genetic Information Nondiscrimination Act of 2008 (GINA) was enacted by Congress to protect the rights of individuals from discrimination based on their genetic information. Protected genetic information includes the following:

- An individual's genetic test information.
- Genetic test information of an individual's family member.
- Information about a disease or disorder that has occurred in an individual's family member.

This act prohibits insurance carriers and employers from using genetic information as a basis for denying insurance coverage or employment. Title I of GINA states that insurance carriers may not use genetic information to determine an individual's eligibility, coverage, underwriting, or premium cost. Health insurers may not require individuals to have genetic testing in order to obtain insurance coverage. Insurers also may not use previous genetic testing results to determine enrollment or coverage. Title II of GINA states that employers also are restricted from requiring genetic testing or using previous genetic testing results to determine eligibility for employment.

Occupational Safety and Health Administration

The Occupational Safety and Health Administration (OSHA), a division of the US Department of Labor, enforces federal laws to protect healthcare workers from health hazards on the job. Medical personnel may accidentally contract a dangerous or even fatal disease by coming into contact with the body fluids of a patient contaminated with a virus. Medical assistants also may be exposed to toxic substances in the office. OSHA regulations describe the precautions a medical office must take with clothing, housekeeping, recordkeeping, and training to minimize the risk of disease or injury.

Some of the most important OSHA regulations are those for controlling workers' exposure to infectious disease. These regulations are set forth in the OSHA Bloodborne Pathogens Protection Standard of 1991. A pathogen is any microorganism that causes disease. Microorganisms are microscopic living bodies, such as viruses or bacteria, that may be present in a patient's blood or other body fluids (saliva or semen). Of particular concern to medical workers are the human immunodeficiency virus (HIV), which causes AIDS, and the hepatitis B virus (HBV). AIDS damages the body's immune system and thus its ability to fight disease. HBV is a highly contagious disease that causes inflammation of the liver and may cause liver failure.

OSHA requires that medical professionals in medical practices follow what are called Standard Precautions. These were developed by the Centers for Disease Control and Prevention (CDC) to prevent medical professionals from exposing themselves and others to bloodborne pathogens. Exposure can occur, for example, through skin that has been broken from a needle puncture or other wound and through mucous membranes, such as those in the nose and throat. If these areas come into contact with a patient's (or coworker's) blood or body fluids, a virus could be transferred from one person to another. The chapter *Infection Control Fundamentals* discusses OSHA and Standard Precautions in more detail.

Health Insurance Portability and Accountability Act

On August 21, 1996, the US Congress passed the Health Insurance Portability and Accountability Act (HIPAA). The primary goals of the act were to improve the portability and continuity of healthcare coverage in group and individual markets; to combat waste, fraud, and abuse in healthcare insurance and healthcare delivery; to promote the use of medical savings accounts; to improve access to long-term care services and coverage; and to simplify the administration of health insurance.

The primary purposes of HIPAA are to:

- Improve the efficiency and effectiveness of healthcare delivery by creating a national framework for health privacy protection that builds on efforts by states, health systems, individual organizations, and individuals.
- Protect and enhance the rights of patients by providing them access to their health information and controlling the inappropriate use or disclosure of that information.
- Improve the quality of healthcare by restoring trust in the healthcare system among consumers, healthcare professionals, and the multitude of organizations and individuals committed to the delivery of care.

HIPAA is divided into two main sections of law: Title I, which addresses healthcare portability, and Title II, which covers the prevention of healthcare fraud and abuse, administrative simplification, and medical liability reform. Although in this text you will study Titles I and II in more detail, you also should be aware of three other titles included in HIPAA regulations: Title III—tax-related health provisions governing medical savings accounts; Title IV—application and enforcement of group health insurance requirements; and Title V—revenue offset governing tax deductions for employers providing company-owned life insurance premiums.

Title I: Healthcare Portability The issue of portability deals with protecting healthcare coverage for employees who change jobs, allowing them to carry their existing plans with them to new jobs. HIPAA provides the following protections for employees and their families:

- Increases workers' ability to get healthcare coverage when starting a new job.
- Reduces workers' probability of losing existing healthcare coverage.
- Helps workers maintain continuous healthcare coverage when changing jobs.
- Helps workers purchase health insurance on their own if they lose coverage under an employer's group plan and have no other healthcare coverage available.

The specific protections of this title include the following:

- Limits the use of exclusions for preexisting conditions.
- Prohibits group plans from discriminating by denying coverage or charging extra for coverage based on an individual's or a family member's past or present poor health.
- Guarantees certain small employers, as well as certain individuals who lose job-related coverage, the right to purchase health insurance.
- Guarantees, in most cases, that employers or individuals who purchase health insurance can renew the coverage regardless of any health conditions of individuals covered under the insurance policy.

Title II: Prevention of Healthcare Fraud and Abuse, Administrative Simplification, and Medical Liability

Reform The HIPAA Standards for Privacy of Individually Identifiable Health Information (IIHI) provided the first comprehensive federal protection for the privacy of both IIHI and personal, or protected, health information. The *HIPAA Privacy Rule* is designed to provide strong privacy protections that do not interfere with patient access to healthcare or the quality of healthcare delivery. The privacy rule is intended to:

- Give patients more control over their health information.
- Set boundaries on the use and release of healthcare records.
- Establish appropriate safeguards that healthcare providers and others must achieve to protect the privacy of health information.
- Hold violators accountable, with civil and criminal penalties that can be imposed if they violate patients' privacy rights.
- Strike a balance when public responsibility supports disclosure of some forms of data—for example, to protect public health.

Before the HIPAA Privacy Rule, the personal information transferred among healthcare providers and third-party payers fell under a patchwork of federal and state laws. This meant that unless forbidden by state or local law, IIHI could be distributed, for reasons that had nothing to do with a patient's medical treatment or healthcare reimbursement, to other agencies. For example, patient information held by a health plan could be passed on to a lender, who could then deny the patient's application for a home mortgage or a credit card; or it could be given to an employer, who could use it in personnel decisions—all without patient knowledge or consent. HIPAA stopped that.

Individually identifiable health information includes:

- Patient name, address, phone numbers, and e-mail address.
- Patient dates (birth, death, admission, discharge, etc.).
- Social Security number.
- Medical record numbers.
- Health plan beneficiary numbers.
- Account numbers.
- Certificate or license numbers.
- Vehicle identifiers and serial numbers, including license plate numbers.
- Device identifiers and serial numbers.
- Web universal resource locators (URLs) and Internet protocol (IP) addresses.

The core of the HIPAA Privacy Rule is the protection, use, and disclosure of *protected health information (PHI)*. Protected health information means individually identifiable health information that is transmitted or maintained by electronic or other media, such as computer storage devices. The Privacy Rule protects all PHI held or transmitted by a covered entity, which includes healthcare providers, health plans, and healthcare clearinghouses. Other covered entities include employers, life insurers, schools or universities, and public health authorities. PHI can come in any form or medium, such as electronic, paper, or oral, including verbal communications among staff members, patients, and other providers. The Privacy Rule covers the following PHI:

- The past, present, or future physical or mental health or condition of an individual.
- Healthcare that is provided to an individual.
- Billing or payments made for healthcare provided.

Information that is not individually identifiable or is unable to be tied to the identity of a particular patient is not subject to the Privacy Rule.

Use and *disclosure* are the two fundamental concepts in the HIPAA Privacy Rule. It is important to understand the differences between these terms. *Use* limits the sharing of information within a covered entity. Performing any of the following actions to PHI by employees or other members of an organization's workforce means the information is being used:

- Sharing
- Employing
- Applying
- Utilizing
- Examining
- Analyzing

Disclosure restricts the sharing of information outside the entity holding the information. Performing any of the following actions so that information is transmitted outside the entity constitutes disclosure:

- Releasing
- Transferring
- Providing access to
- Divulging in any manner

Managing and Storing Patient Information Because of HIPAA, medical facilities have undergone many changes to the way they manage and store patient information. Many facilities now contract with consultants that specialize in HIPAA, and large facilities, such as hospitals, often employ a compliance officer. Patients must be given the opportunity to read the office privacy practices and receive a copy of them, signing an acknowledgment that they have received them. Should the patient refuse to sign the acknowledgment, the refusal should be documented in the medical record to prove *due diligence* and a "good faith effort" by the office to provide the patient with the privacy practices. The Privacy Rule requires the provider to perform activities including:

- Notifying patients of their privacy rights and how their information is used.
- Adopting and implementing privacy procedures for its practice, hospital, or plan.
- Training employees so that they understand the privacy procedures.
- Designating an individual responsible for seeing that the privacy procedures are adopted and followed.
- Securing patient records containing IIHI so that they are not readily available to those who do not need them.

Patient Notification Since the HIPAA Privacy Rule's effective date, medical facilities have made major changes in how they inform patients of their HIPAA compliance. You may have noticed, as a patient yourself, the forms and information packets that are now provided by your healthcare providers. The first step in informing patients of HIPAA compliance is the communication of patient rights, conveyed through a document called Notice of Privacy Practices (NPP). This notice must:

- Be written in plain, simple language.
- Include a header that reads, "This notice describes how medical information about you may be used and disclosed and how you can get access to this information. Please review carefully."
- Describe the covered entity's uses and disclosures of PHI.
- Describe an individual's rights under the Privacy Rule.
- Describe the covered entity's duties.
- Describe how to register complaints concerning suspected privacy violations.
- Specify a point of contact.
- Specify an effective date.
- State that the entity reserves the right to change its privacy practices.

See Figure 5-5 for an example of a HIPAA Notice of Privacy Practices. Procedure 5-1, found at the end of this chapter, outlines the steps in obtaining a signature for receipt of the NPP.

In addition to the office obligations under HIPAA, remember, it also has given patients an increased understanding about their right to privacy regarding their health information. These rights include the following:

- The right to access, copy, and inspect their healthcare information.
- The right to request an amendment to their healthcare information.
- The right to obtain an accounting of certain disclosures of their healthcare information.
- The right to alternate means of receiving communications from providers.
- The right to complain about alleged violations of the regulations and the provider's own information policies.

Figure 5-6 gives an example of a typical privacy violation complaint form, which the office should keep on hand in case a patient feels his privacy rights have been violated. As the medical assistant, you may need to help the patient complete this form. Procedure 5-2, at the end of this chapter, provides practice in assisting with this form.

Sharing Patient Information When sharing patient information, HIPAA will allow the provider to use healthcare information for *treatment, payment, and operations (TPO)*:

- *Treatment.* Providers are allowed to share information in order to provide care to patients.
- *Payment.* Providers are allowed to share information in order to receive payment for the treatment provided.
- *Operations.* Providers are allowed to share information to conduct normal business activities, such as quality improvement.

If the use of patient information does not fall under TPO, then written authorization must be obtained before sharing information with anyone (Figure 5-7). Some of the core elements of an authorization form are:

- Specific and meaningful descriptions of the authorized information.
- Persons authorized to use or disclose protected health information.
- Purpose of the requested information.
- Statement of the patient's right to revoke the authorization.
- Signature of the patient and date signed.

Procedure 5-3, at the end of the chapter, outlines the steps to be taken to obtain an authorization to release PHI.

HIPAA Security Rule In February 2003, the final regulations were issued regarding the administrative, physical, and technical safeguards to protect the confidentiality, integrity, and availability of health information covered by HIPAA.

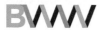

BWW Medical Associates, PC
305 Main Street, Port Snead YZ 12345-9876
Tel: 555-654-3210, Fax: 555-987-6543
Web: BWWAssociates.com

Paul F. Buckwalter, MD
Alexis N. Whalen, MD
Elizabeth H. Williams, MD

Notice of Privacy Practices

I understand that BWW Medical Associates, PC creates and maintains medical records describing my health history, symptoms, examinations, test results, diagnoses, treatments, and plans for my future care and/or treatment. I further understand that this information may be used for any of the following:

1. Plan and document my care and treatment
2. Communicate with health professionals involved in my care and treatment
3. Verify insurance coverage for planned procedures and/or treatments for the applicable diagnoses
4. Application of any medical or surgical procedures and diagnoses (codes) to my medical insurance claim forms as application for payment of services rendered
5. Assessment of quality of care and utilization review of the healthcare professionals providing my care

Additionally, it has been explained to me that

1. A complete description of the use and disclosure of this information is included in the *Notice of Information of Privacy Practices,* which has been provided to me.
2. I have had a right to review this information prior to signing this consent.
3. BWW Medical Associates, PC has the right to change this notice and their practices.
4. Any revision of this notice will be mailed to me at the address I provided to them prior to its implementation.
5. I may object to the use of my health information for specific purposes.
6. I may request restrictions as to the manner my information may be used or disclosed in order to carry out treatment, payment, or health information.
7. I understand that it is not required that my requested restrictions be honored.
8. I may revoke this consent in writing, except for those disclosures which may have taken place prior to the receipt of my revocation.

At the time of the document signing, I request the following restrictions to disclosure or use of my health information: _____

_____

_____   _____
Printed Name of Patient or Legal Guardian   Signature of Parent or Legal Guardian

_____   _____
Printed Name of Witness/Title   Signature of Witness/Title

Date: _____

FIGURE 5-5   Example of a Notice of Privacy Practices and acknowledgment.

The *Security Rule* specifies how patient information is protected on computer networks, the Internet, disks, and other storage media and extranets. However, the rapidly increasing computer use in healthcare has created new dangers for confidentiality breaches. The Security Rule mandates that:

- A security officer must be assigned the responsibility for the medical facility's security.
- All staff, including management, must receive security awareness training.
- Medical facilities must implement audit controls to record and examine staff who have logged into information systems that contain PHI.

- Organizations must limit physical access to medical facilities that contain electronic PHI.
- Organizations must conduct risk analyses to determine information security risks and vulnerabilities.
- Organizations must establish policies and procedures that allow access to electronic PHI on a need-to-know basis.

Computers are not the only concern regarding workplace security. The facility layout can pose a possible violation if not designed correctly. All facilities must take measures to reduce the identity of patient information. Some examples of facility design that can help reduce a confidentiality breach include the security of patient medical records (including

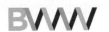

BWW Medical Associates, PC
305 Main Street, Port Snead YZ 12345-9876
Tel: 555-654-3210, Fax: 555-987-6543
Web: BWWAssociates.com

Paul F. Buckwalter, MD
Alexis N. Whalen, MD
Elizabeth H. Williams, MD

Privacy Violation Complaint

As per our Privacy Policies and Procedures, we are providing this form for individuals who feel they have a complaint regarding how their protected health information was handled by our office. You have the right to make a complaint and we may take no retaliatory actions against you because of it. We will respond to this complaint within 30 days of its receipt.

Patient Name: _____

Address: _____

DOB: _____ Date of Complaint: _____

Phone: Home _____ Cell _____ Work _____

Best time to reach you: _____

Reason for the complaint (please be as specific as possible, attaching additional documentation as necessary): _____

_____

_____

_____

_____

_____   _____
Signature   Date

Office Use Only

Received by: _____ Date _____

Follow-up Started on (date): _____

FIGURE 5-6   Sample of a Privacy Violation Complaint form.

charts), the reception area, the clinical station (or patient care area), and the location of fax machines.

- *Chart security.* When paper health records are used, patient charts and the information contained within them can be kept confidential by following these rules:

  1. Charts that contain a patient's name or other identifiers cannot be in view at the front reception area or nurse's station. Some offices have placed charts in plain jackets to prevent information from being seen.

  2. Charts must be stored out of view of a public area to prevent unauthorized individuals from seeing them.

  3. Charts should be placed on the filing shelves without the patient name showing.

  4. Charts should be locked when not in use. Many facilities have purchased filing equipment that can be locked and unlocked without limiting the availability of patient information.

  5. Every staff member who uses patient information must be logged and a confidentiality statement signed. Signatures of staff should be on file with the office.

- *Reception area security.* To be compliant with security rules, the following steps should be taken to secure the reception area:

  1. Log off or lock your computer or terminal, shutting off the monitor, when leaving your terminal or computer.

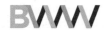

BWW Medical Associates, PC
305 Main Street, Port Snead YZ 12345-9876
Tel: 555-654-3210, Fax: 555-987-6543
Web: BWWAssociates.com

Paul F. Buckwalter, MD
Alexis N. Whalen, MD
Elizabeth H. Williams, MD

Authorization to Release Health Information

I, _____ , residing at

_____ and DOB of

_____ , give permission to (name of practice) _____

to release to _____ of BWW Medical Associates, PC the

following information: _____

_____

_____

Reason for the Request: _____

_____

Signature of Patient or Legal Guardian _____

Printed Name of Patient or Legal Guardian _____

If Guardian, Relationship to Patient _____

This authorization will expire on _____

YOU MAY REFUSE TO SIGN THIS AUTHORIZATION. You may revoke this authorization at any time by notifying BWW Medical Associates, PC in writing. Revocation will have no effect on actions taken prior to receipt of any revocation. Any disclosure of information carries the potential for unauthorized redisclosure and the information may not be protected by federal confidentiality rules.

FIGURE 5-7 An example of an Authorization to Release Health Information form.

2. The computer must be placed in an area where patients and unauthorized personnel cannot see the screen.

3. Many facilities are purchasing flat screen monitors to prevent visibility of the screen.

4. Patient sign-in sheets may be used but must not include the reason or nature of the patient visit. Likewise, patient names may be called out as long as no reference to the reason for the visit is made.

5. Call centers and reception area phone conversations must be kept confidential. Many offices put the administrative office behind sliding glass windows to allow for privacy when on the phone with other patients or offices, so that people in the reception area cannot hear phone conversations.

- *Patient care area security.* All healthcare personnel should follow these guidelines to protect PHI in patient care areas:

1. Log off or lock computer terminals, turning off the monitor, when leaving the computer station.

2. When placing charts in exam room racks or shelves, the name of the patient or other identifiers must be concealed from view.

3. When discussing a patient with the physician or another staff member, make sure your voice is lowered and that all doors to the exam rooms are

closed. Avoid discussing patient conditions in heavy-traffic areas.

4. When discussing a condition with a patient, make sure that you are in a private room or area where no one else can hear you.

5. Avoid discussing patients in lunchrooms, hallways, or any other place in a medical facility where someone can overhear you.

- *Fax security.* As a vital link among healthcare providers, insurance plans, and others, much information is exchanged over the fax machine in a medical office, particularly if the office is paper-based and does not have access to electronic communication. Private health information can be exchanged via faxes sent to covered entities, but PHI still must be safeguarded as much as possible by taking the following precautions:

1. Use a fax cover page. State clearly on the fax cover sheet that confidential and protected health information is included. Further state that the information included is to be protected and must not be shared or disclosed without the appropriate authorizations from the patient.

2. Keep the fax machine in an area that is not accessible by individuals who are not authorized to view PHI.

3. Faxes received containing PHI must be stored promptly in a protected, secure area.

4. Always confirm the accuracy of fax numbers to minimize the possibility of faxes being sent to the wrong person. Call recipients to confirm the fax was received.

5. Program the fax machine to print a confirmation for all faxes sent, and staple the confirmation sheet to each document sent.

6. Train all staff members to understand the importance of safeguarding PHI sent or received via fax.

- *Copier security.* Medical assistants should follow these guidelines to protect PHI at the copier:

1. Do not leave confidential documents anywhere on or near the copier where others can read the information.

2. Shred copies containing PHI when no longer needed—do not discard copies in a trash container.

3. If a paper jam occurs, after removing the paper causing the jam, shred it if PHI is contained within the document.

- *Printer security.* To maintain the confidentiality of printed materials, follow these guidelines:

1. Do not print confidential material on a printer shared by other departments or in an area where others can read the material.

2. Do not leave the printer unattended while printing confidential material.

3. Before leaving the printing area, make sure all data storage media containing confidential information and all printed material have been collected.

4. Be certain that the print job is sent to the correct printer location.

5. Shred any discarded printouts—do not throw them in a trash container.

Violations and Penalties Each staff member is responsible for adhering to HIPAA privacy and security regulations to ensure that PHI is secure and confidential. If PHI is abused or confidentiality is breached, the medical facility can incur substantial penalties or even the incarceration of staff. Violations of HIPAA law can result in both civil and criminal penalties.

- *Civil penalties* for HIPAA privacy violations can be up to $100 for each offense, with an annual cap of $25,000 for repeated violations of the same requirement.

- *Criminal penalties* for the knowing, wrongful misuse of individually identifiable health information can result in penalties ranging from $50,000 to $250,000 in fines and between 1 and 10 years in prison.

Administrative Simplification The main key to the set of rules established for HIPAA administrative simplification is standardizing patient information throughout the healthcare system with a set of transaction standards and code sets. The codes and formats used for the exchange of medical data are referred to as *electronic transaction records.* Regulated transaction information receives a transaction set identifier. For example, a healthcare claim would receive an identifier of ASC X12N 837 version 5010—a standard transaction code given to any facility that submits an electronic healthcare claim to an insurance company.

Standardized code sets are used for encoding data elements. The following books are used for the standardized code sets for all healthcare facilities:

- *ICD-10-CM.* This book is used to identify diseases and conditions.
- *CPT 4.* This book is used to identify physician services or procedures.
- *HCPCS.* This book is used to identify health-related services and procedures, such as pharmaceuticals or hearing and vision services, that are not included in the CPT manual.

▶ Confidentiality Issues and Mandatory Disclosure   LO 5.6

Related to law, ethics, and quality care is the issue of when a healthcare worker, including a medical assistant, can disclose information and when it must be kept confidential. The incidents that doctors are legally required to report to the state were outlined earlier in the chapter. A doctor can be charged with criminal action for not following state and federal laws.

Ethics and professional judgment are always important. Consider the question of whether to contact the partners of a patient who has a sexually transmitted infection (STI) and whether to keep the patient's name from those people. The law says that the physician must instruct patients on how to notify possibly affected third parties and give them referrals to get the proper assistance. If the patient refuses to inform involved outside parties, then the doctor's office may offer to

CAUTION: HANDLE WITH CARE

Notifying Those at Risk for Sexually Transmitted Infection

Few things are more difficult for a patient with an STI than telling current and former partners about the diagnosis. In fact, some patients elect not to do so. When patients refuse to alert their partners, the medical office can offer to make those contacts. Often that responsibility lies with the medical assistant.

You are most likely to encounter such a situation if you are a medical assistant working in a family practice, an OB/GYN practice, or a clinic. So becoming familiar with all facets of the situation—from ensuring patient confidentiality to handling potentially difficult confrontations—will help you best serve the patient.

The first step is to get the appropriate information from the patient who has contracted the STI. Because the patient may be sensitive about revealing former and current partners, help him feel more comfortable. First, spend some time talking about the STI. How much does the patient know about it? Educate him about implications, including the probable short- and long-term effects of the infection. Explain how the STI is transmitted. Alert the patient as to precautions to take so he will not continue to transmit the infection to others. Help the patient understand why it is important for people who may have contracted the infection from him to be told they may have it.

Then, offer to contact the patient's former and current partners. Fully explain each step in the notification process, assuring the patient that his name will not be revealed under any circumstances. Answer any questions and address any concerns about the notification process. If the patient is still reluctant to provide information, give him some time to think about it away from the office and follow up with a phone call.

Once the patient agrees to reveal names, write down the names and other information, preferably phone numbers. To make sure you have correct information, read it back to the patient, spelling each person's name in turn and reciting the phone number or address. Write down the phonetic pronunciations of any difficult names. Tell the patient when you will make the notifications.

You now are ready to contact these individuals. Professionals who work with STI patients recommend the following guidelines for contacting current and former partners to alert them about potential exposure to an STI. Note that these guidelines are applicable only to STIs other than AIDS. Determine how you will contact each individual: in writing, in person, or by phone.

1. If you use US mail, mark the outside of the addressed envelope "Personal." On a note inside, simply ask the person to call you at the medical office. Do not put the topic of the call in writing.

2. If you make the contact in person, ask where you can talk privately. Even if the person appears to be alone, others still may be able to overhear the conversation.

3. If you use the phone, identify yourself and your office and ask for the specific individual. Do not reveal the nature of your call to anyone but that person. If pressed, tell the person who answers the phone that you are calling regarding a personal matter.

Once on the phone or alone with the person, confirm that you are talking to the correct person. Mention that you wish to talk about a highly personal matter and ask if it is a good time to continue the discussion. If not, arrange for a more appropriate time. Inform the individual that she has come in contact with someone who has an STI and recommend that she visit a doctor's office or clinic to be tested for the infection.

Be prepared for a variety of reactions, from surprise to anger. Respond calmly and coolly. Expect to respond to questions and statements such as

- Who gave you my name?
- Do I have the disease?
- Am I really at risk? I haven't had intercourse recently (or) I've only had intercourse with my spouse.
- I feel fine. I just went to my doctor recently.

Let the person know that you cannot reveal the name of the partner because the information is strictly confidential. Assure the person that you will not reveal her name to anyone, either. Explain that exposure to the disease does not mean a person has contracted it. Encourage the person to get tested to know for sure.

Tell the person that she is still at risk, even if she hasn't had intercourse recently or has had it only with a spouse. Let the person know that someone with whom she came in close contact at some point has contracted the disease. Even if the person says, "I feel fine," she still may have the infection. Again, stress the importance of getting tested.

Provide your name and phone number for contact about further questions. Recommend local offices and clinics for testing and provide phone numbers. If the person will come to your office, offer to make the appointment.

Finally, document the results of your call. Log in the original patient's file the date that you completed notification. Include any pertinent details about the notification. Alert the patient when all people on the list have been notified.

---

notify current and former partners. The *Caution: Handle with Care* section addresses this issue.

In general, the patient's ethical right to confidentiality and privacy is protected by law. Only the patient can waive the right to confidentiality. A physician cannot publicize a patient case in journal articles or invite other health professionals to observe a case without the patient's written consent. Most states also prohibit a doctor from testifying in court about a patient without the patient's approval. When a patient sues a physician, however, the patient automatically gives up the right to confidentiality.

The following are six principles for preventing improper release of information from the medical office.

1. When in doubt about whether to release information, it is better not to release it.

2. It is the patient's right, not the physician's, to keep patient information confidential. If the patient wants to disclose the information, it is unethical for the physician not to do so.

3. All patients should be treated with the same degree of confidentiality, whatever the healthcare professional's personal opinion of the patient might be.

4. You should be aware of all applicable laws and of the regulations of agencies such as public health departments.

5. When it is necessary to break confidentiality and when there is a conflict between ethics and confidentiality, discuss it with the patient. If the law does not dictate what to do in the situation, the attending physician should make the judgment based on the urgency of the situation and any danger that might be posed to the patient or others.

6. Get written approval from the patient before releasing information. For common situations, the patient should sign a standard release-of-records form.

The AMA has several standard forms for authorization of disclosure and includes disclosure clauses in many other forms. For example, the consent-to-surgery form includes a clause about consenting to picture taking and observation during the surgery. When using a standard form, cross out anything that does not apply in that situation. Medical practices often develop their own customized forms.

▶ Ethics   LO 5.7

Medical ethics is a vital part of medical practice, and following an ethical code is an important part of your job. Ethics deals with general principles of right and wrong, as opposed to requirements of law. A professional is expected to act in ways that reflect society's ideas of right and wrong, even if such behavior is not enforced by law. Often, however, the law is based on ethical considerations.

Bioethics: Social Issues

Bioethics deals with issues that arise related to medical advances. For many people, bioethical issues are particularly sensitive and highly personal issues. This may be true for you on a personal level as well. Remember that, as a medical assistant, you must remain nonjudgmental at all times regarding patient healthcare dilemmas and decisions. Here are three examples of bioethical issues.

1. A treatment for Parkinson's disease was developed that uses fetal tissue. Some women, upon learning about this treatment, might get pregnant just to have an abortion and sell the fetal tissue. Is this ethical?

2. If a couple cannot have a baby because of a medical condition of the mother, using a surrogate mother is an option some couples choose. The surrogate mother is artificially inseminated with the sperm of the husband and carries the baby to term. The couple then raises the child. Ethically speaking, who is the real mother, the woman who bears the child or the woman who raises the child? If the surrogate mother wants to keep the baby after it is born, does she have a right to do so?

3. When a liver transplant is needed by both a famous patient who has had a history of alcohol abuse and a woman who is a recipient of public assistance, what criteria are considered when determining who receives the organ? Who makes the decision? Ethically, treating physicians should not make the decision of allocating limited medical resources. Such decisions should consider only the likelihood of benefit, the urgency of need, and the amount of resources required for successful treatment. Nonmedical criteria such as ability to pay, age, social worth, perceived obstacles to treatment, patient's contribution to illness, or the past use of resources should not be considered.

Practicing appropriate professional ethics has a positive impact on your reputation and the success of your employer's business. As a result, many medical organizations have created guidelines for the acceptable and preferred manners and behaviors, or etiquette, of medical assistants and physicians.

The principles of medical ethics have developed over time. The Hippocratic oath, in which medical students pledge to practice medicine ethically, was developed in ancient Greece (see http://www.nlm.nih.gov/hmd/greek/greek_oath.html). It is still used today and is one of the original bases of modern medical ethics. Hippocrates, the 4th-century B.C. Greek physician commonly called the "father of medicine," is traditionally considered the author of this oath, but its authorship is actually unknown.

Among the promises of the Hippocratic oath are to use the form of treatment believed to be best for the patient, to refrain from harmful actions, and to keep a patient's private information confidential.

The AMA defines ethical behavior for doctors in *Code of Medical Ethics: Current Opinions with Annotations* (Use of 174 words from the American Medical Association's *Code of Medical Ethics: Current Opinions and Annotations,* found within the 2015 CPT *Professional Edition.* © American Medical Association [1995–2015]. All rights reserved.) Medical assistants as well as doctors need to be aware of these principles, some of which are included in italics here and explained as follows:

A physician shall be dedicated to providing competent medical service with compassion and respect for human dignity.

This means that medical professionals will respect all aspects of the patient as a person, including intellect and emotions. The doctor must decide what treatment would result in the best, most dignified quality of life for the patient and must respect a patient's choice to forgo treatment.

A physician shall deal honestly with patients and colleagues and strive to expose those physicians deficient in character or competence or who engage in fraud or deception.

Medical professionals, including medical assistants, should respect colleagues, but they also must respect and protect the profession and public welfare enough to report colleagues who are breaking the law, acting unethically, or unable to perform competently. Dilemmas may arise where one suspects, but is not able to prove, for instance, that a coworker has a substance abuse problem or another problem that is affecting performance. Ignoring such a situation in medical practice could cost someone's life as well as lead to lawsuits.

In terms of billing, a doctor should bill only for direct services, not for indirect ones such as referrals. The doctor also should not bill for services that do not really pertain to the practice of medicine, such as dispensing drugs.

It is also unethical for the doctor to influence the patient about where to fill prescriptions or obtain other medical services when the doctor has a personal financial interest in any of the choices. For example, it can be considered a conflict of interest if a physician has ownership in a surgical center and refers patients to the center without disclosing this financial interest to the patient.

A physician shall respect the law and also recognize a responsibility to seek changes in requirements that are contrary to the patient's best interests.

Several legal or employer requirements have come under scrutiny as being contrary to a patient's best interests. Among them are discharging patients from the hospital after a certain time limit for certain procedures, which may be too soon for many patients. Insurance company payment policies sometimes have been criticized as unfair. So have health maintenance organization (HMO) financial policies that conflict with a doctor's treatment preference.

A physician shall respect the rights of patients, of colleagues, and of other health professionals and shall safeguard patient confidences within the constraints of law.

As previously mentioned, the Patient Care Partnership: Understanding Expectations, Rights and Responsibilities, originally established by the American Hospital Association in 1973 and revised in 1992, lists ethical principles protecting the patient. Some states have even passed this code of ethics into law. Among a patient's rights are the right to information about alternative treatments, the right to refuse to participate in research projects, and the right to privacy.

A physician shall continue to study; apply and advance scientific knowledge; make relevant information available to patients, colleagues, and the public; obtain consultation; and use the talents of other health professionals when indicated.

Keeping up with the latest advancements in medicine is crucial for providing high-quality, ethical care. Most states require doctors to accumulate continuing education units to maintain a license to practice. These units are earned by means of educational activities such as courses and scientific meetings. As discussed in the *Introduction to Medical Assisting* chapter, medical assistants who are certified by the AAMA or AMT have similar requirements by the sponsoring certification board to earn CEUs to maintain their credentialed status.

A physician shall, in the provision of appropriate patient care, except in emergencies, be free to choose whom to serve, with whom to associate, and the environment in which to provide medical services.

Ethically, doctors can set their hours, decide what kind of medicine to practice and where, decide whom to accept as a patient, and take time off as long as a qualified substitute performs their duties. Doctors may decline to accept new patients because of a full workload. In an emergency, however, a doctor is ethically obligated to care for a patient, even if the patient is not of the doctor's choosing. The doctor should not abandon that patient until another physician is available.

A physician shall recognize a responsibility to participate in activities contributing to an improved community.

This ethical obligation also holds true for the allied health professions. In addition to knowing the physician's codes of ethics, medical assistants should follow the code of ethics for their certifying body, be it the AAMA or the AMT. See the *Points on Practice* box for the AAMA's Code of Ethics and Figure 5-8 for the AMT's Standards of Practice.

POINTS ON PRACTICE
Medical Assisting Code of Ethics

The Medical Assisting Code of Ethics of the AAMA sets forth principles of ethical and moral conduct as they relate to the medical profession and the particular practice of medical assisting.

Members of the AAMA dedicated to the conscientious pursuit of their profession, and thus desiring to merit the high regard of the entire medical profession and the respect of the general public which they serve, do pledge themselves to strive always to:

A. Render service with full respect for the dignity of humanity.

B. Respect confidential information obtained through employment unless legally authorized or required by responsible performance of duty to divulge such information.

C. Uphold the honor and high principles of the profession and accept its disciplines.

D. Seek to continually improve the knowledge and skills of medical assistants for the benefit of patients and professional colleagues.

E. Participate in additional service activities aimed toward improving the health and well-being of the community.

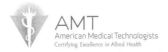

AMT Standards of Practice

The American Medical Technologists is dedicated to encouraging, establishing and maintaining the highest standards, traditions, and principles of the disciplines which constitute the allied health professions of the certification agency and the Registry.

Members of the Registry and all individuals certified by AMT recognize their professional and ethical responsibilities, not only to their patients, but also to society, to other health care professionals, and to themselves.

The AMT Board of Directors has adopted the following Standards of Practice which define the essence of competent, honorable and ethical behavior for an AMT-certified allied health care professional. Reported violations of these Standards will be referred to the Judiciary Committee and may result in revocation of the individual's certification or other disciplinary sanctions.

I.   While engaged in the Arts and Sciences that constitute the practice of their profession, AMT professionals shall be dedicated to the provision of competent and compassionate service and shall always meet or exceed the applicable standard of care.

II.   The AMT professional shall place the health and welfare of the patient above all else.

III.   When performing clinical duties and procedures, the AMT professional shall act within the lawful limits of any applicable scope of practice, and when so required shall act under and in accordance with appropriate supervision by an attending physician, dentist, or other licensed practitioner.

IV.   The AMT professional shall always respect the rights of patients and of fellow health care providers, shall comply with all applicable laws and regulations governing the privacy and confidentiality of protected healthcare information, and shall safeguard patient confidences unless legally authorized or compelled to divulge protected healthcare information to an authorized individual, law enforcement officer, or other legal or governmental entity.

V.   AMT professionals shall strive to increase their technical knowledge, shall continue to learn, and shall continue to apply and share scientific advances in their fields of professional specialization.

VI.   The AMT professional shall respect the law and pledges to avoid dishonest, unethical or illegal practices, breaches of fiduciary duty, or abuses of the position of trust into which the professional has been placed as a certified healthcare professional.

VII.   AMT professionals understand that they shall not make or offer a diagnosis or dispense medical advice unless they are duly licensed practitioners or unless specifically authorized to do so by an attending licensed practitioner acting in accordance with applicable law.

VIII.   The AMT professional shall observe and value the judgment of the attending physician, dentist, or other attending licensed practitioner, provided that so doing does not clearly constitute a violation of law or pose an immediate threat to the welfare of the patient.

IX.   AMT professionals recognize that they are responsible for any personal wrongdoing, and that they have an obligation to report to the proper authorities any knowledge of professional abuse or unlawful behavior by any party involved in the patient's diagnosis, care and treatment.

X.   The AMT professional pledges to uphold personal honor and integrity and to cooperate in protecting and advancing, by every lawful means, the interests of the American Medical Technologists and its Members.

(Revised by the AMT Board of Directors July 7, 2013)

10700 W. Higgins Road, Suite 150 | Rosemont, Illinois 60018 | (847) 823-5169 | www.americanmedtech.org

FIGURE 5-8   AMT Standards of Practice.

▶ Legal Medical Practice Models LO 5.8

There are five basic types of medical practice:

- Sole proprietorship
- Partnership
- Group practice
- Professional corporation
- Clinics

Laws governing the types of practice vary, but medical office personnel should be aware of the laws that apply to their employers' practice management models.

Sole Proprietorship

This type of practice is often referred to as a "solo practice." In this type of practice, a physician practicing alone assumes all the benefits for and liabilities of the business. Sole proprietorship practice management is no longer a popular option, as a result of the increased expenses and decreased insurance reimbursements. So more physicians are joining group practices or professional corporations.

Partnership

When two or more physicians decide to practice together, they may form a partnership based on a legal contract that specifies the rights, obligations, and responsibilities of each partner. One advantage of partnerships is sharing the workload, expenses, profits, and assets. A disadvantage is that each partner has equal liability for acts of misconduct, losses, and deficits of the practice, unless specified otherwise in the contract.

Group Practice

Group practice is a medical practice model in which three or more licensed physicians share the collective income, expenses, facilities, equipment, records, and personnel for the practice. Physicians in group practice may be engaged in the same specialty, calling themselves, for example, Associates in Cardiology, or several physicians may offer similar specialties, such as OB/GYN and pediatrics.

Professional Corporations

A corporation is a body formed and authorized by state law to act as a single entity. Physicians who form corporations are shareholders and employees of the organization. Forming a corporation has financial and tax advantages, and the fringe benefits for employees may be greater than in a sole proprietorship or partnership.

In forming a corporation, the incorporators and owners have limited liability in lawsuits. Some medical practices are managed by for-profit corporations that are formed by outside business interests or subsidiary corporations organized by hospitals. Physicians are hired as salaried employees with bonus options. The management corporation provides the facility, office personnel, employee benefits, human resource services, and operating expenses.

Clinics

Patients can be admitted to clinics for special circumstances and research. In many cases, clinics are hard to distinguish from large medical facilities.

Clinics are broad in their range of specialties and subspecialties, and many have sophisticated medical equipment and renowned medical practitioners. Clinics may be housed inside of a hospital or be free-standing. Urgent care centers, also known as walk-in clinics, exist so that patients have the option of being seen without an appointment.

In-store clinics are becoming more prevalent. Housed in large major chain stores and sometimes in chain pharmacies, they offer minor medical services such as flu shots, other vaccinations, and eye exams.

Employment Law

Many medical assistants find themselves promoted into supervisory and managerial positions. Knowledge of employment and labor laws such as those involving civil rights, sexual harassment, employment of persons with disabilities, fair labor standards, and family medical leave are important to all employees but particularly so for those who oversee other employees. Labor and employment laws are covered in detail in the *Practice Management* chapter.

PROCEDURE 5-1 Obtaining Signature for Notice of Privacy Practices and Acknowledgment `WORK // DOC`

Procedure Goal: To follow HIPAA guidelines and obtain the patient's signature that he or she has received and understands the office privacy policies

OSHA Guidelines: This procedure does not involve exposure to blood, body fluids, or tissue.

Materials: Preprinted Notice of Privacy Practices and Acknowledgment (see Figure 5-5), pens, and a copy machine

Method:

1. Explain to the patient the office privacy policy regarding protected health information.

   RATIONALE: *Some patients understand the spoken word more easily than the written word.*

2. Ask the patient to read the policy carefully and to feel free to ask any questions he may have regarding the policy. Answer any questions that arise.

   RATIONALE: *Patients must have a thorough understanding in order to acknowledge receipt of the privacy policy.*

3. When the patient's questions have been answered, witness the patient (or guardian) sign and print his name. Note any restrictions placed on the document.

   RATIONALE: *Restrictions must be noted so inadvertent release of information does not occur.*

4. Print your name and sign the document as witness, including your title.

5. Date the document when all signatures have been completed.

6. Make a copy of the document to file in the patient medical record and give the original to the patient.
RATIONALE: *It is important that copies of all signed documents are in the patient's record in case of any legal proceedings that arise.*

PROCEDURE 5-2 Completing a Privacy Violation Complaint Form

WORK // DOC

Procedure Goal: To assist the patient in completing a Privacy Violation Complaint form if she feels her PHI has been compromised

OSHA Guidelines: This procedure does not involve exposure to blood, body fluids, or tissue.

Materials: Privacy Violation Complaint form (see Figure 5-6), pens, private room to complete form, and a copy machine

Method:

1. Explain to the patient that all formal complaints must be made in writing.
   RATIONALE: *This provides legal documentation in case it is ever needed in court.*

2. Ask the patient if she feels assistance will be needed completing the form. If not, the patient may complete the form on her own. Answer any questions she may have regarding completion of the form.

3. When the patient completes the form, read it carefully, making sure it is complete and legible and the information regarding the breach of privacy is clear.
   RATIONALE: *In order to address the alleged breach, a thorough understanding of the complaint is needed.*

4. If the patient requires that any copies be made of documentation backing the claim, make the copies, returning any originals to the patient.

5. Make sure the patient signs and dates the complaint.

6. As the person receiving the complaint, sign the document as indicated and date it.

7. Explain to the patient that the office will respond to the complaint within 30 days of today's receipt.

8. Make a copy of the document for the patient and keep the original for the office files.
   RATIONALE: *Copies of all legal documents must be kept on file.*

PROCEDURE 5-3 Obtaining Authorization to Release Health Information

WORK // DOC

Procedure Goal: To follow HIPAA guidelines when obtaining the patient's protected health information without violating confidentiality regulations

OSHA Guidelines: This procedure does not involve exposure to blood, body fluids, or tissue.

Materials: Preprinted Authorization to Release Health Information form (see Figure 5-7), pens, and a copy machine

Method:

1. Explain to the patient the need for the requested medical information.
   RATIONALE: *In order for the consent to be valid, the patient must understand the need for the release of information.*

2. Obtain the name and address of the practice to which the authorization is to be mailed.

3. Fill in the patient's name, address, and DOB as required.

4. Enter the physician's or practitioner's name from your practice who is requesting the PHI.

5. Enter the information that is being requested.
   RATIONALE: *Only the required information may be requested and released to the practice.*

6. Complete the reason for request, explaining why the patient is requesting the information be sent to your office.
   RATIONALE: *To comply with HIPAA guidelines, a reason for the record release is necessary.*

7. Enter an expiration date for the authorization, giving a reasonable amount of time for the request to be fulfilled.

8. Prior to signing the release, go over with the patient the information contained within the release, answering any questions that arise. Be sure the patient understands the request may be withdrawn (in writing) at any time.

9. Witness the patient (or guardian) signature and date; if necessary, be sure the guardian relationship area is completed.

10. Sign and date the document as witness, including your title.

11. Make a copy of the document to file in the patient medical record and, if requested, give a copy to the patient.

RATIONALE: *The release is a legal document and must be kept with the patient medical record.*

12. Make a notation in the medical record of the document signing, and note the date the authorization is mailed.

RATIONALE: *If the records are not received in a timely manner, the office will need to be contacted.*

SUMMARY OF LEARNING OUTCOMES

OUTCOME	KEY POINTS
5.1 Differentiate between laws and ethics.	A law is a rule of conduct or action prescribed or formally recognized as binding or enforced by local, state, or federal government. Ethics are standards of behavior or concepts of right or wrong beyond what the legal consideration is in any given situation.
5.2 Identify the responsibilities of the patient and physician in a physician-patient contract, including the components for informed consent that must be understood by the patient.	Physician responsibilities in a physician-patient contract include using due care, skill, judgment, and diligence in treating the patient; staying informed of the current diagnosis and treatment; performing to the best of the physician's ability; and providing complete information and instructions to the patient. Regarding informed consent, the physician must provide the following information: proposed treatment modes; why the treatment is necessary; risks of the proposed treatment; alternative treatments available; risks of the alternatives; and the risks if all treatment is refused. Patient responsibilities in a physician-patient contract include following instructions given by the provider and cooperating as much as possible; giving relevant information to the provider; following physician instructions for treatment; and paying fees for services provided.
5.3 Describe the four elements of negligence that must be satisfied in order to prove malpractice, and explain the four Cs of malpractice prevention.	The four elements of negligence are duty—it must be proven that a physician-patient relationship exists; derelict—it must be proven that the physician failed to comply with standards of the profession; direct cause—it must be proven that any damages were directly caused by the physician's breach of duty; and damages—it must be proven that the patient suffered an injury. The four Cs of medical malpractice prevention are caring—the most important asset; communication—which earns respect and trust; competence—which proves abilities by maintaining and updating knowledge; and charting—which documents all aspects of patient interaction.
5.4 Relate the term *credentialing,* and explain the importance of the FDA and DEA to administrative procedures performed by medical assistants.	The term *credentialing* refers to the approval process a healthcare provider must go through to be allowed to bill Medicare and other insurance carriers for providing medical services to patients under their insurance plans. Often, the medical assistant is in charge of submitting the required paperwork and documentation for the provider to gain this approval. The Food and Drug Administration (FDA) approves drugs for use on humans. It also regulates whether drugs are prescription-based or accessible OTC. The Drug Enforcement Agency (DEA) is responsible for controlling and overseeing the prescribing of controlled substances. Physicians must obtain and renew their license with the DEA in order to prescribe controlled substances.

OUTCOME	KEY POINTS
5.5 **Summarize the purpose of the following federal healthcare regulations: HCQIA, False Claims Act, OSHA, and HIPAA.**	Congress enacted HCQIA in 1996 because it found that there was an increasing occurrence of medical malpractice and a need to improve the quality of medical care. The False Claims Act allows individuals to bring civil *qui tam* actions on behalf of the US government for false claims made to the federal government. OSHA enforces federal laws to protect healthcare workers from health hazards on the job. Title I of HIPAA was created so that employees could still have access to health insurance coverage when leaving employment for any reason. Title II was created to protect patients' individually identifiable personal information as well as their personal health information. It also allows patients access to their medical information on request and allows them to limit the sharing of that information. Additionally, patients on written request must be allowed to see a record of how their PHI has been shared and with whom.
5.6 **Identify the six principles for preventing improper release of information from the medical office.**	The six rules for preventing improper release of information include the following: (1) When in doubt about whether to release information, it is better not to release it. (2) It is the patient's right, not the physician's, to keep patient information confidential. (3) All patients should be treated with the same degree of confidentiality. (4) Be aware of all applicable laws and of the regulations of agencies involved with confidentiality. (5) When it is necessary to break confidentiality and when there is a conflict between ethics and confidentiality, discuss it with the patient. The physician may need to make the final decision. (6) Get written approval from the patient before releasing information.
5.7 **Discuss the importance of ethics in the medical office.**	Ethics reflects the general principles of right and wrong. A professional, particularly a medical professional, is expected to follow especially high ethical standards.
5.8 **Explain the differences among the practice management models.**	There are five basic types of practice management models: (1) sole proprietorship (one physician), (2) partnership (two or more physicians), (3) group practice (three or more physicians), (4) professional corporation (a body formed and authorized by state law to act as a single entity; physicians are stakeholders and employees of the organization), and (5) clinics.

CASE STUDY CRITICAL THINKING

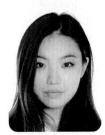

©Ryan McVay/Getty Images

Recall Cindy Chen from the beginning of the chapter. Now that you have completed the chapter, answer the following questions regarding her case.

1. How will you respond to the extern's concerns?
2. Once Cindy becomes a phlebotomist, how should the information regarding her HIV-positive status be handled? Will the situation change if she develops AIDS?

1. (LO 5.1) A standard of behavior with a concept of right and wrong beyond the legal considerations is called
   a. Civil law
   b. Moral values
   c. Medical ethics
   d. Etiquette
   e. Ethics

2. (LO 5.1) The two types of law that pertain to healthcare professionals are
   a. Contract law and agency law
   b. Civil law and criminal law
   c. Civil law and medical law
   d. Litigation and malpractice
   e. Contract law and medical negligence

3. (LO 5.2) The physician's responsibility within the physician-patient contract includes all of the following *except*
   a. Setting up a practice within the boundaries of his or her license to practice medicine
   b. Setting up an office where he or she chooses and establishes office hours
   c. Determining whether to specialize
   d. Deciding which services to provide and how those services will be provided
   e. Treating every patient seeking care

4. (LO 5.3) Cases in which a person believes that a medical professional did not perform an essential action or performed an improper one, thus harming the patient, may result in
   a. Charges of slander
   b. Charges of medical negligence
   c. Charges of abandonment
   d. Charges of defamation
   e. Charges of fraud

5. (LO 5.3) Under the _____, words uttered to a patient by the medical assistant can be said to be the responsibility of the employer-physician.
   a. Law of agency
   b. Employee contract
   c. Civil law
   d. Criminal law
   e. Ethical considerations

6. (LO 5.4) The process used by various organizations, including insurance carriers, to ensure that healthcare providers are appropriately qualified to provide services and meet all the necessary requirements to do so is called

   a. Arbitration
   b. *Qui tam*
   c. Credentialing
   d. Subpoena
   e. Tort

7. (LO 5.5) Which of the federal acts was passed by Congress to improve the quality of medical care nationwide?
   a. HIPAA Title I
   b. HIPAA Title II
   c. OSHA
   d. HCQIA
   e. False Claims Act

8. (LO 5.6) Incidents and diseases, although normally considered confidential, that must be reported to federal, state, or local agencies come under the heading of
   a. Medical ethics
   b. HIPAA security rule
   c. STIs and AIDS
   d. Mandatory disclosure
   e. Civil law

9. (LO 5.7) Issues relating to medical advances come under the heading of
   a. Ethics
   b. Bioethics
   c. Religious freedoms
   d. Misfeasance
   e. Malfeasance

10. (LO 5.8) Which practice model provides the most legal protection for the physicians who form the practice?
    a. Sole proprietorship
    b. Partnership
    c. Group practice
    d. Professional corporation
    e. Clinics

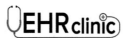

Go to CONNECT to complete the EHRclinic exercises: 5.01 Add an Acknowledgement of Receipt of NPP to a Patient's EHR and 5.02 Add an Authorization to Release Health Information to a Patient's EHR.

You are a medical assistant at the family practice office of Dr. Janice Parrish. Elizabeth James and her daughter Anne have been patients at the practice for 10 years. Anne is 20 years old. Elizabeth is in the office for a blood pressure check. While you are taking her blood pressure, she tells you that Anne was in to see Dr. Parrish last week. She also says that she thinks Anne has been acting strangely and asks you if her daughter is pregnant. How would you respond to Elizabeth? What can you legally tell Elizabeth about her daughter?

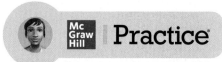

Go to PRACTICE MEDICAL OFFICE and complete the module Admin Check In: Privacy and Liability.

Infection Control Fundamentals

6

CASE STUDY

PATIENT INFORMATION	Patient Name	DOB	Allergies
	Shenya Jones	11/03/1985	Cinnamon, peanuts
	Attending	**MRN**	**Other Information**
	Elizabeth Williams, MD	00-AA-002	Wound C&S sent to Laboratory Services

Shenya Jones arrives at the office with a swelling and a red pustule on her face. She states the problem started 2 days ago as a small pimple near her nose. It became irritated, then became extremely swollen and painful overnight. This morning, there was yellow drainage at the site and the swelling has increased. The area of drainage is approximately 1 cm in diameter. The upper lip, side of the face, and nose are all

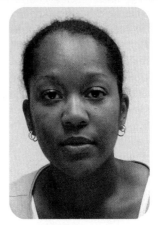
©McGraw-Hill Education

swollen. She rates the pain in her face as 7 out of 10. The physician thinks the condition may be impetigo or methicillin-resistant *Staphylococcus aureus* (MRSA), a type of skin infection that is resistant to the common antibiotics used to treat it. Dr. Williams will culture the wound to find out what type of microorganisms are present and what specific antibiotics could be used to treat the infection.

Keep Shenya Jones in mind as you study this chapter. There will be questions at the end of the chapter based on the case study. The information in the chapter will help you answer these questions.

LEARNING OUTCOMES

After completing Chapter 6, you will be able to:

6.1 Identify Occupational Safety and Health Administration (OSHA)'s role in protecting healthcare workers.

6.2 Illustrate the cycle of infection and how to break it.

6.3 Summarize the Bloodborne Pathogens Standard and universal precautions as described by OSHA.

6.4 Describe how transmission-based precautions supplement standard precautions.

6.5 Summarize OSHA's education and training requirements for ambulatory care settings.

KEY TERMS

alcohol-based hand disinfectants (AHD)

asepsis

carrier

endogenous infection

engineered safety devices

exogenous infection

fomite

general duty clause

healthcare-associated infections (HAI)

other potentially infectious materials (OPIM)

pathogen

reservoir host

standard precautions

susceptible host

transmission-based precautions

vector

work practice controls

III.C.2 Describe the infection cycle including:
  (a) the infectious agent
  (b) reservoir
  (c) susceptible host
  (d) means of transmission
  (e) portals of entry
  (f) portals of exit

III.C.3 Define the following as practiced within an ambulatory care setting:
  (a) medical asepsis

III.C.4 Identify methods of controlling the growth of microorganisms.

III.C.5 Define the principles of standard precautions.

III.C.6 Define personal protective equipment (PPE) for:
  (a) all body fluids, secretions, and excretions
  (b) blood
  (c) non-intact skin
  (d) mucous membranes

III.C.7 Identify Centers for Disease Control (CDC) regulations that impact healthcare practices

III.P.1 Participate in bloodborne pathogen training

III.P.2 Select appropriate barrier/personal protective equipment (PPE)

III.P.3 Perform handwashing

III.P.10 Demonstrate proper disposal of biohazardous material:
  (a) sharps
  (b) regulated wastes

III.A.1 Recognize the implications for failure to comply with the Centers for Disease Control (CDC) regulations in healthcare settings

XII.C.1 Identify:
  (b) symbols
  (c) labels

4. Medical Law and Ethics
  f. Comply with federal, state, and local health laws and regulations as they relate to healthcare settings

8. Clinical Procedures
  a. Practice standard precautions and perform disinfection/sterilization techniques

9. Medical Laboratory Procedures
  c. Dispose of biohazardous materials

▶ Introduction

From whooping cough in California to Ebola in West Africa, it is hard to open a newspaper or newsfeed without reading about an outbreak of disease. Despite all the medical advances of the modern world, humans continue to contract infectious diseases. As a medical assistant, you play an important role in stopping the spread of infections. In this chapter, you will be introduced to the fundamentals of infection control, including OSHA's role in protecting healthcare workers, the cycle of infection, OSHA Bloodborne Pathogens Standard, standard precautions, transmission-based precautions, and OSHA-required education and training for healthcare workers.

▶ Occupational Safety and Health Administration

LO 6.1

The Occupational Safety and Health Administration's (OSHA) mission is to "assure safe and healthful working conditions for working men and women by setting and enforcing standards and by providing training, outreach, education and assistance." Healthcare workers face safety challenges specific to caring for the sick and injured. For this reason, the Centers for Disease Control and Prevention (CDC) works closely with OSHA to ensure that these workers have documented best practices to follow. The CDC makes recommendations and guidelines regarding specific health and safety practices, and

OSHA makes and enforces regulations based on these recommendations and guidelines. Copies of these guidelines can be obtained from many sources, including local OSHA offices; the CDC in Atlanta, Georgia; many industrial organizations throughout the country; and the Internet.

If a specific standard exists, its guidelines must be followed; however, if no specific standard has been developed, the **general duty clause** takes effect. This clause requires an employer to maintain a workplace free from hazards that are recognized as likely to cause death or serious injury. For example, all employers are expected to ensure that all exits are clear of obstacles and unlocked when the building is occupied. If an employer blocks a fire exit, a fire breaks out, and employees are injured because they are unable to safely leave the building, the employer has violated the general duty clause.

Employer Responsibilities

Employers have a legal responsibility to provide a safe working environment. In order to fulfill this responsibility, employers must:

- Ensure that the workplace is free from serious recognized hazards and comply with Occupational Safety and Health Administration rules and regulations.
- Inspect workplace conditions, confirming they conform to OSHA standards.
- Provide safe and properly maintained equipment.
- Maintain operating procedures and communicate new and updated procedures to employees.
- Provide accessible safety training to all workers.

Employee Responsibilities

Healthcare workers must follow regulations related to workplace safety, including chemical exposure, fire safety, electrical safety, and ergonomics and physical safety (see the chapter *Safety and Patient Reception*). In order to protect yourself, your coworkers, and your patients, you must follow the procedures, guidelines, and regulations outlined in your facility's infection control plan. Before you can understand the elements of an infection control plan, you first must understand how infections are transmitted.

▶ The Cycle of Infection   LO 6.2

As a medical assistant, your role in helping to create and maintain a safe and healthy environment for both patients and employees is key. This role includes understanding how infections occur and are transmitted in the population and practicing all necessary infection control precautions. To understand how infections are spread, you need to understand the cycle of infection.

Five elements make up the cycle of infection (Figure 6-1). These five parts all must be present for infection to occur:

1. Reservoir host
2. Means of exit
3. Means of transmission
4. Means of entrance
5. Susceptible host

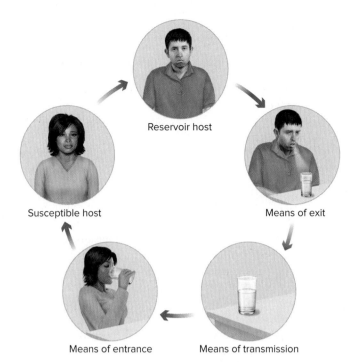

FIGURE 6-1 The cycle of infection must be broken at some point to prevent the spread of disease caused by pathogens.

Reservoir Host

The infection cycle begins when the **pathogen** invades the reservoir host. The **reservoir host** is an animal, insect, or human whose body is capable of sustaining the growth of a pathogen. Many pathogens require a reservoir host to provide nutrition and a place to multiply.

The presence of the pathogen in the reservoir host may cause an infection in the host. At times, however, the host avoids full infection. A human **carrier** is a reservoir host who is unaware of the presence of the pathogen and so spreads the disease. The carrier exhibits no symptoms of infection. A human host also may have a subclinical case, which is a manifestation of the infection that is so slight that it is unnoticeable. The host experiences only some of the symptoms of the infection or milder symptoms than in a full case. A wide range of diseases can be manifested subclinically.

An infection in the reservoir host may be either endogenous or exogenous. An **endogenous infection** is one in which an abnormality or a malfunction in routine body processes has caused normally beneficial or harmless microorganisms to become pathogenic. A bladder infection caused by *Escherichia coli* bacteria (commonly known as *E. coli*) is an endogenous infection. *E. coli* are beneficial bacteria normally found in the intestinal tract, but when introduced into the bladder via the urethra, *E. coli* can cause a bladder infection. An **exogenous infection** is one that is caused by the introduction of a pathogen from outside the body. A wound infection that occurs as the result of a healthcare worker transferring staph bacteria from her hands to a surgical site is an example of an exogenous infection.

Means of Exit

The next step in the cycle of infection is the pathogen's exiting from the reservoir host. Common routes of exit include:

- Through the nose, mouth, eyes, or ears.
- In feces or urine.
- In semen, vaginal fluid, or other discharge through the reproductive tract.
- In blood or blood products from open wounds.

Means of Transmission

To reproduce after it has exited from the reservoir host, the pathogen must spread to another host by some means of transmission, either direct or indirect. Direct transmission occurs when the pathogen moves immediately from one host to another (through contact with the infected person or with the discharges of the infected person, such as saliva or blood).

Indirect transmission is possible only if the pathogen is capable of existing independently of the reservoir host. In this case, the pathogen survives until a new host encounters it and the pathogen takes up residence in that new host.

Airborne Transmission Pathogens can be transmitted to a new host through the air. For example, microorganisms may enter the respiratory tract of a new host by inhalation. Respiratory diseases such as influenza, or flu, are often transmitted this way.

Pathogens may be inhaled from a variety of sources, such as soil particles or secretion droplets from a sneeze or cough. When people inhale contaminated soil particles, fungal diseases may be contracted. If contaminated droplets are inhaled, diseases including influenza, chickenpox, and tuberculosis may be contracted. Because pathogens can spread relatively rapidly through airborne transmission, they may cause large epidemics among susceptible people. See the feature *Caution: Handle with Care* for more information on respiratory hygiene and cough etiquette.

Bloodborne Transmission Pathogens also can enter a new host through contact with blood or blood products. Bloodborne pathogens may be transmitted in a variety of ways:

- Indirectly—when pathogens are transferred through blood transfusions, needlestick injuries, or improperly sterilized dental equipment.
- Directly—when the contaminated blood of one person comes into contact with another person's broken skin or mucous membrane, or when a pregnant woman transmits a disease to her fetus across the placenta.

Transmission During Pregnancy or Birth If a mother becomes infected during her pregnancy, she can pass on pathogens to the fetus. An infection may be transmitted while the fetus is in the mother's uterus, which may result in damage to the fetus. This transmission is a form of bloodborne transmission.

Some bloodborne infections that produce only mild symptoms in the mother may be devastating to the fetus (for example, rubella). Other infections, such as herpes, gonorrhea, syphilis, or streptococcal infections, may infect the baby during passage through the birth canal. An infection that is present in a child at the time of birth is said to be congenital.

Foodborne Transmission A new host may be exposed to pathogens by ingesting contaminated food or liquids. Food can become contaminated when it is handled by an infected person who has poor hygiene habits, such as a customer at a self-service salad bar who did not wash his hands. The amount of contamination needed in a food to make someone ill varies. People who produce less stomach acid may become infected with a smaller dose of pathogens than those with higher acid production because stomach acid kills many microorganisms. An example of a pathogen transmitted by ingestion is a strain of *E. coli,* which can cause severe food poisoning.

Vector-Borne Transmission A living organism that carries microorganisms from an infected person to another person is known as a **vector.** The most common carriers are insects such as fleas, flies, mosquitoes, and ticks.

- Fleas carry the organism responsible for plague. Though the number of cases in the United States is very low, plague has been identified as a possible bioterrorism agent.

CAUTION: HANDLE WITH CARE

Respiratory Hygiene and Cough Etiquette

With the recent increase in widespread respiratory disease outbreaks such as severe acute respiratory syndrome (SARS) and H1N1 influenza, the CDC identified the need to establish a set of guidelines to protect patients and their families in the healthcare setting. These guidelines include:

- Educating healthcare workers, patients, and their families about cough etiquette.
- Posting cough etiquette signs.
- Posting signs reminding patients to report flu symptoms.

- Controlling the source of transmission by covering coughs with a tissue and properly disposing of the tissue.
- Coughing or sneezing into your elbow or sleeve if no tissue is available.
- Using proper hand hygiene consistently.
- Separating patients with respiratory infections so they are at least 3 feet away from other patients in waiting areas or asking them to wear a mask.

- Common houseflies carry pathogens from garbage and feces on their bodies and feet. When they land on food, they mechanically transfer these microorganisms to the food.
- Mosquitoes are carriers of several diseases of importance in the United States. They carry the organisms responsible for West Nile virus, Zika virus, and malaria.
- Ticks carry the microorganisms responsible for Lyme disease and Rocky Mountain spotted fever.

Transmission by Touching Direct or indirect contact through touch is another method of transmitting infection. Direct transmission occurs through contact with an infected person's mucous membranes. Sexually transmitted infections are spread through the direct contact of one mucous membrane with another (in the penis, vagina, urethra, mouth, or anus) during sexual activity.

Indirect transmission occurs through contact with **fomites.** A fomite is any inanimate reservoir of pathogenic microorganisms. Examples of fomites include drinking glasses, door-knobs, shopping cart handles, pencils, and almost any surface or object that can temporarily hold microorganisms. So any object that can be contaminated by an infected person and then can transmit the infective agent to a susceptible host is considered a fomite.

Means of Entrance

Just as the pathogen needs a means of exit from the reservoir host, it also needs a means of entrance into the new host. Pathogens can enter a new host through any cavity lined with mucous membrane, such as the mouth, nose, throat, vagina, or rectum. They also can enter through the ears, eyes, intestinal tract, urinary tract, reproductive tract, or breaks in the skin. Most pathogens can take advantage of any means of exit and entry. For example, the droplets from an infected child's sneeze can land on a toy in a common play area. The next child to pick up the toy can transfer the infected droplets to her own nose, spreading the infection.

Susceptible Host

A final requirement must be met for the infection cycle to remain intact. The person into whom the pathogen has been transmitted must be an individual who has little or no immunity to infection by that organism. This individual is called a **susceptible host.**

Susceptibility is determined by a variety of factors—some related to the host, some to the pathogen, and some to the environment. Factors related to the host include the following:

- Age
- Genetic predisposition to certain illnesses
- Nutritional status
- Other disease processes
- Stress levels
- Hygiene habits
- General health

Factors related to the pathogen include the number and concentration of pathogens, the strength (virulence) of the pathogen, and the point of entry. Environmental factors, such as the host's living conditions and exposure to hazardous substances, also affect susceptibility.

Once a new host has been infected, the cycle can continue. This host becomes the reservoir host and eventually transmits the pathogen to yet another host.

Environmental Factors in Disease Transmission

The climate, food, water, animals, insects, and people in a community may greatly influence the types and courses of infection that exist there. In a highly dense population, the infection rate may be higher than in a low-density population because pathogens spread more quickly from person to person when people are in closer proximity. Proximity is one reason for the increase in respiratory disease during seasons when people are indoors for long periods.

Animals also can play a role in infection, as infections related to pathogens are found in domestic and wild animals. Unpasteurized milk from an infected cow may cause disease. Some pathogens can infect both animals and people. Butchers, hunters, and people in occupations dealing with animals may be at greater risk than other individuals for infection by those pathogens.

The environment affects the incidence of diseases carried by insects. Whether a potentially disease-carrying insect is in a certain area depends on whether that area has the appropriate climate and environment the insect needs to live. For instance, ticks may carry Rocky Mountain spotted fever or Lyme disease.

Economic and political factors also influence the pattern of infection transmission. They help determine the cleanliness of an area, the availability of medical care, and people's knowledge about preventing infection. Other factors that influence infection transmission include the availability of transportation, urbanization, population growth rates, and sexual behavior.

Breaking the Cycle

The principles of **asepsis** must be applied to break the cycle of infection and its spread. Asepsis is the condition in which pathogens are absent or controlled. For example, killing all microorganisms by sterilizing a suture removal kit and reducing the number of microorganisms on your hands by thoroughly washing them are types of aseptic practice. In medical settings, where many people are hosts to pathogens and many others are susceptible, asepsis can break the cycle by preventing the transmission of pathogens.

Specific measures to help break the cycle of infection include:

- Maintaining strict housekeeping standards to reduce the number of pathogens present.
- Adhering to government guidelines to protect against diseases caused by pathogens.
- Educating patients in hygiene, health promotion, and disease prevention.

Hand Hygiene

Transmission by touching is the most common means of transmitting pathogens. The single most important aseptic procedure for a medical assistant is proper hand hygiene. The two most common methods of hand hygiene in the medical office are handwashing with plain or antimicrobial soap and water and hand disinfection with alcohol-based hand disinfectants (AHD). Consistent hand hygiene using appropriate methods protects the patient, your coworkers, and you from healthcare-associated infections.

Handwashing Aseptic handwashing removes accumulated dirt and microorganisms that could cause infection under the right conditions. Procedure 6-1 describes how to perform aseptic handwashing. In most cases, plain soap and water are adequate. There is some evidence that overuse of antimicrobial soap leads to antibiotic-resistant pathogens. For this reason, only use antimicrobial soap after assisting with exams and procedures where body fluids are present.

Alcohol-Based Hand Disinfectants An alternative to handwashing is the use of **alcohol-based hand disinfectants (AHD).** These are gels, foams, or liquids that have an alcohol content of 60% to 95%. AHD are the preferred method of routine decontamination and may be safely used in most situations; however, conditions in which they should not be used include:

- When hands are visibly dirty or contaminated.
- Before and after eating.
- After using the bathroom.
- If you suspect you have come in contact with spore-forming bacteria.

A number of factors can affect the effectiveness of AHD:

- The type of alcohol used.
- The concentration of alcohol.
- Whether the hands are wet when the product is applied.
- The contact time.
- The amount used.

If your hands feel dry before the recommended amount of time has passed, you most likely did not use enough. You should reapply the AHD using a larger amount. Procedure 6-2 describes the proper use of an alcohol-based hand disinfectant.

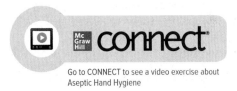

Go to CONNECT to see a video exercise about Aseptic Hand Hygiene

Fingernail Length Fingernails are a haven for pathogens. There is ample documentation that a large number of bacteria and some types of yeast can be cultured from underneath and around the nail, especially right next to the border of the skin and the nail. The CDC recommends that natural nail length be less than 1/4 inch.

Nail Polish and Artificial Nails The use of nail polish and artificial nails is discouraged in healthcare workers, as

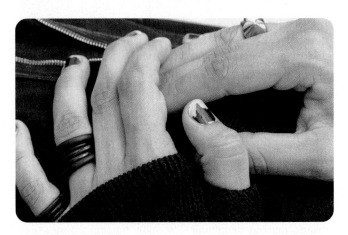

FIGURE 6-2 Chipped nail polish should not be worn by healthcare workers because it has a much higher bacteria count than natural, unpolished nails.
©Medioimages/Photodisc/Getty Images

there is enough evidence that nail polish and artificial nails harbor pathogens. Although freshly applied nail polish has not been shown to contain increased numbers of bacteria more research is needed, and polish that is chipped has a much higher bacteria count than natural, unpolished, or freshly polished nails (Figure 6-2). Healthcare workers who wear artificial nails or extensions have more gram-negative bacteria on their fingers than healthcare workers with natural nails. These increases are seen both before and after handwashing. The CDC recommends that healthcare workers not wear artificial nails or extensions when working with high-risk patients. The World Health Organization (WHO) recommends that healthcare workers not wear artificial nails when working with any patients.

▶ OSHA Bloodborne Pathogens Standard and Universal Precautions LO 6.3

You must know the laws that require basic practices of infection control, also called infection prevention, in a medical office and how to apply these laws in your office. Federal regulations related to infection control and asepsis were developed by the Department of Labor's Occupational Safety and Health Administration and described in the OSHA Bloodborne Pathogens Standard of 1991. OSHA enforces these laws, but it is the responsibility of a qualified medical office professional to make sure the laws are being followed correctly. These laws protect healthcare workers from health hazards on the job, particularly from accidentally acquiring infections. They also help protect patients and any other people who come into the medical office.

OSHA Bloodborne Pathogens Standard

To ensure that biohazardous materials do not endanger people or the environment, laws set forth in the OSHA Bloodborne Pathogens Standard of 1991 dictate how you must handle infectious or potentially infectious waste generated during medical or surgical procedures. According to these rules, any potentially infectious waste materials must be appropriately discarded or held for processing in biohazardous waste containers. These wastes include the following:

- Blood products.
- Body fluids.
- Human tissues.
- Cultures.
- Vaccines (special preparations administered to produce immunity).
- Table paper, linen, towels, and gauze containing body fluids.
- Used scalpels, needles, sutures with needles attached, and other sharp instruments (known as sharps).
- Specula.
- Inoculating loops.
- Used gloves, disposable instruments, cotton swabs, and disposable applicators.

Many medical offices use only disposable paper gowns, drapes, coverings, and towels. Some offices, however, use cloth linens, which must be laundered. Certain rules apply to the laundering of cloth linens that are soiled with potentially infectious materials.

Medical offices use outside, licensed waste management services approved by the Environmental Protection Agency (EPA) to dispose of medical waste. A waste management service can provide instructions for preparing items before they are taken away.

The disposition and handling of contaminated sharps are of special concern because these instruments can easily puncture the skin and expose you to extremely dangerous viruses. Used sharps must never be bent, broken, recapped, or otherwise tampered with. After use, place them in a rigid, leakproof, puncture-resistant biohazardous waste container for sharps. Procedure 6-3 demonstrates the correct method for using a biohazardous sharps container. Disposable and reusable sharps are kept in separate containers. Metal basins containing disinfectant are often used to store reusable sharps until they can be processed. The outside waste management company may supply containers for the disposable items, sterilize them on its premises, and discard them in the city trash dump or incinerate them. See the *Caution: Handle with Care* section for a discussion of the guidelines you must follow when disposing of biohazardous waste and potentially infectious laundry waste.

CAUTION: HANDLE WITH CARE

Proper Use of Biohazardous Waste Containers and Handling of Infectious Laundry Waste

Biohazardous waste containers are available in a variety of designs. Frequently, more than one design is used in the clinical setting. These containers often are provided by outside sterilization and waste management companies. Examples of biohazardous waste containers include:

- Bags or containers that are red or have a biohazardous waste label (for any material contaminated with blood or body fluids, such as used dressings or gloves).
- Boxes with biohazardous waste labels (sometimes lined with red bags and used for disposable gowns, examination table covers, and similar items that may be contaminated with blood or body fluids).
- Rigid, leakproof, and puncture-proof sharps containers that are red or have a biohazardous waste label (for lancets, needles, and other sharp objects).

Every biohazardous waste container has a lid that you must replace immediately after use. In addition, you may not overfill the container, and you must replace it when it is two-thirds full. All biohazardous waste containers must have a fluorescent orange or orange-red label with the biohazard symbol and the word *BIOHAZARD* in a contrasting color (Figure 6-3). Red bags or red containers may be substituted for containers with biohazardous waste labels.

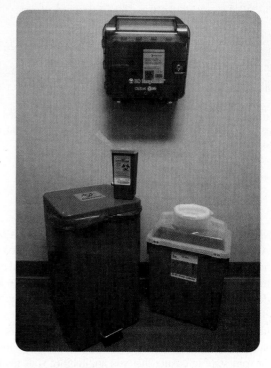

FIGURE 6-3 All biohazardous sharps containers must be rigid, leakproof, and labeled with the biohazard symbol.

©McGraw-Hill Education/David Moyer, photographer

You must follow these guidelines when handling biohazardous waste:

- Always wear gloves.
- Place biohazardous waste in the appropriate biohazardous waste container immediately or as soon as possible.
- Keep biohazardous waste containers close to the place where the waste material is generated.
- Keep the containers closed when not in use, close them before removing them from the area of use, and keep them upright to avoid any spills.
- If outside contamination of the primary container occurs, place that container in a secondary container to prevent leakage during handling, processing, storage, and transport.
- Drop—do not push—intact contaminated needles into the biohazardous waste container for sharps (Figure 6-4).
- To avoid accidental puncture wounds, never break off, recap, reuse, or handle needles after use.

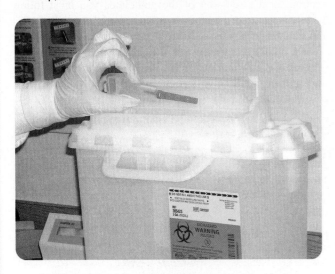

FIGURE 6-4 A sharps disposal container is a receptacle for used needles, lancets, specimen slides, transfer pipettes, and other disposable pointed or edged instruments, supplies, and equipment.
©Leesa Whicker

- If there is a danger of biohazardous waste puncturing the primary container, place that container in a secondary container.
- Do not open, empty, or clean reusable sharps containers by hand.
- When they are two-thirds full, discard disposable sharps containers in large biohazardous waste containers.

Spills of hazardous chemicals or biohazardous materials can happen anywhere in the office. Immediately clean up spills or splashes of potentially contaminated material. Depending on the material, you may need to use special hazardous waste control products. Be sure to dry the area if appropriate or clearly indicate that the area is still wet. When cleaning up spills, take the following measures:

- Place material in a biohazardous waste bag.
- Ensure that the bag is leakproof on the sides and bottom and can be closed tightly.
- Place the plastic bag in a cardboard box also marked with the biohazard symbol.

The outside waste management agency will pick up the box for incineration before disposing of it in a public landfill. Procedure 6-4 demonstrates the proper disposing of biohazardous waste.

Potentially infectious laundry waste also must be handled in a specific manner. OSHA has issued these regulations for handling this type of waste:

- Place contaminated laundry in a red laundry bag that is marked with the biohazard symbol or recognizable to facility employees as contaminated material to be handled using standard precautions.
- Pack any laundry to be transported so that it does not leak in transit.
- Have the laundry washed in a designated area onsite or at a professional laundry facility.

Any laundry service the medical office uses should abide by all OSHA regulations. For example, anyone handling laundry must wear gloves and handle contaminated materials as little as possible.

OSHA's laws for hazardous waste disposal, as well as other OSHA regulations about measures to prevent the spread of infection, provide a margin of safety, ensuring that medical facilities meet at least the minimal criteria for asepsis. These laws include requirements for training personnel, keeping records, housekeeping, wearing protective gear, and other measures.

Although federal laws exist, individual states have some discretion in applying them. You should become familiar with the laws in your state to ensure that you are helping your medical office comply. Any outside cleaning service used by the office also should be made aware of these standards. Penalties for failing to comply with regulations can be severe (see Table 6-1).

To be in compliance with the Bloodborne Pathogens Standard, an employer must meet these requirements:

- A written OSHA Exposure Control Plan must be created and updated annually or whenever procedures that require exposure to potentially contaminated material are added or changed. The plan must be available to all employees and to authorized OSHA authorities.
- Training must be provided to all employees describing the documentation mandated by the standard. This documentation includes the symptoms, methods of transmission, and epidemiology of infectious diseases caused by bloodborne pathogens. Employees also must be instructed in the use of personal protective equipment (PPE), universal precautions, and engineering controls designed to prevent exposure. Procedures to follow in the event of exposure or emergency situations also must be part of the training.

TABLE 6-1 Infectious Waste Disposal: Penalties for Not Following Regulations, as Set Forth by OSHA

Type of Violation	Characteristics of Violation	Penalties for Violation
Other than serious violation	Direct relationship to job safety and health but would probably not result in death or serious physical harm	Fine of up to $13,260 (discretionary)
Serious violation	Substantial probability that death or serious physical harm could result; employer knew, or should have known, of the hazard	Fine of up to $13,260 (mandatory)
Willful violation	Violation committed intentionally and knowingly	Fine of up to $132,598 with a $9,472 minimum; if violation resulted in death of employee, additional fine and/ or up to 6 months' imprisonment
Repeated violation	Substantially similar (but not the same) violation found upon re-inspection; not applicable if initial citation is under contest	Fine of up to $132,598
Failure to correct prior violation	Initial violation not corrected	Fine of up to $13,260 for each day the violation continues past the date it was supposed to stop

New employee training is required before the worker can perform a task that might pose a risk of occupational exposure and then on a yearly basis. Additional training is required when a new task or procedure is introduced that may change the employees' occupational exposure risk.

- The employer must make the hepatitis B vaccine available at no charge to all employees who are at risk for occupational exposure. Employees must either receive the vaccination or decline it in writing. The employer must maintain documentation of vaccinations and refusals. Employees who initially decline the vaccine are free to reverse their decision at any point during their employment.

Universal Precautions

OSHA requires medical professionals to follow specific "universal blood and body fluid precautions" as set forth by the Department of Health and Human Services' Centers for Disease Control and Prevention. These universal precautions prevent healthcare workers from exposing themselves and others to infections. Following universal precautions means assuming that all blood, body fluids, and **other potentially infectious materials (OPIM)** are infected with bloodborne pathogens. Universal precautions apply to the following:

- Blood and blood products
- Human tissue
- Semen and vaginal secretions
- Saliva from dental procedures
- Cerebrospinal, synovial, pleural, peritoneal, pericardial, and amniotic fluids, which bathe various internal structures in the body
- Other body fluids, if visibly contaminated with blood or of questionable origin in the body
- Any unfixed human tissue

Breast milk, although not on the list of fluids covered by universal precautions, is generally treated as such because it has been shown that mothers can pass along the human immunodeficiency virus (HIV) to their infants through breast milk.

Healthcare facilities now use **standard precautions,** which are a combination of universal precautions and rules to reduce the risk of disease transmission by means of moist body substances (known as Body Substance Isolation [BSI] guidelines). Standard precautions apply to the following:

- Blood
- All body fluids, secretions, and excretions except sweat
- Nonintact skin
- Mucous membranes

Standard precautions are used in healthcare facilities for the care of all patients. All body fluids, except sweat, are included whether or not they are known to be infectious. For this reason, standard precautions are an important measure for preventing the transmission of disease in the healthcare setting.

As mentioned earlier, some types of pathogens can be transmitted when the host's infected blood comes in contact with another person's skin. Skin that has been broken from a needle puncture or other wound and mucous membranes, such as those lining the nose and throat, are the areas that need the most protection. If a patient's (or coworker's) blood or body fluids come in contact with such areas, pathogens can be transferred from the patient's body to that of the medical worker.

OSHA outlines the routine safeguards to take when performing each medical procedure or task, depending on that task's level of risk. The degree of risk is determined by how much exposure to potentially infectious substances you are likely to encounter. When a procedure is explained, particular icons will be used to represent each of the OSHA guidelines. Figure 6-5 shows these icons.

OSHA requires that each employer keep a list of job classifications in which an employee working in that job has a potential for exposure to bloodborne pathogens. These tasks can be sorted in the following categories.

1. Category I tasks are those that expose a worker to blood, body fluids, or tissues or tasks that have a chance of spills or splashes. These tasks always require specific protective measures.

2. Category II tasks do not usually involve risk of exposure. Because they may involve exposure in certain situations, however, OSHA requires that precautions be taken.

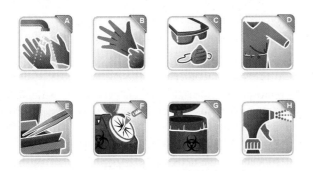

FIGURE 6-5 These icons will appear at the beginning of each Procedure to let you know which OSHA guidelines you should follow. They represent (A) handwashing, (B) gloves, (C) mask and protective eyewear or face shield, (D) laboratory coat or gown, (E) reusable sharps container, (F) sharps disposal, (G) biohazardous waste container, and (H) disinfection.

3. Category III tasks do not require any special protection. These tasks, such as taking a patient's blood pressure, involve no exposure to blood, body fluids, or tissues. (Observe patients for open wounds before you touch them to perform such tasks.)

Category I Tasks A Category I task you might perform is assisting with a minor surgical procedure in the office, such as the removal of a cyst. This procedure requires that you wash your hands before and after the procedure and that you wear protective gloves, a mask and protective eyewear or a face shield, and protective clothing. After the procedure, you must follow the guidelines for dealing with disposable and nondisposable sharps equipment and decontaminating work surfaces.

Category II Tasks A Category II task you might perform is giving mouth-to-mouth resuscitation to a patient. Because blood is usually not visible in such situations, the task is not classified as Category I. Gloves are still recommended, however, although you may not have time to get them in an emergency. Because you will be exposed to saliva in such a procedure, OSHA recommends using disposable airway equipment and resuscitation bags (shown in Figure 6-6), which medical offices are required to supply.

OSHA recommends taking these precautions to decrease the risk of transmitting infectious diseases through mouth-to-mouth resuscitation. Of particular concern to healthcare workers are HIV, which causes AIDS, and the hepatitis B virus (HBV).

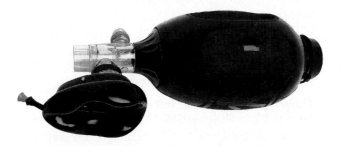

FIGURE 6-6 Resuscitation bags are used when a person requires mouth-to-mouth resuscitation. You must use one of these bags or another barrier device when performing mouth-to-mouth resuscitation.
©Stockbyte/Getty Images

AIDS damages the body's ability to fight disease and is ultimately fatal in most instances. Hepatitis B is a highly contagious and potentially fatal disease that causes inflammation of the liver and sometimes liver failure. Healthcare workers become infected with these viruses at work every year. Hepatitis B infection occurs far more frequently on the job than does HIV infection.

Category III Tasks A Category III procedure you may perform is giving a patient medicated nose drops. This task involves tilting the patient's head and holding the dropper above the patient's nostril. Although you must perform aseptic handwashing before and after the procedure, there are no other protective requirements. Some Category III tasks require no precautions. Examples of these tasks are instructing a patient in how to use a heating pad and how to take care of a cast for a broken leg.

Written Exposure Plan

In order to reduce the risk of bloodborne pathogen exposure, OSHA requires that every medical facility have a written exposure control plan (ECP). Employees who are at risk of bloodborne exposure must have access to the ECP. This plan must be reviewed with new employees at the onset of employment and with all employees on an annual basis. A written copy of the plan must be made available if an employee requests it. The ECP must include the following:

- Determination of employee exposure.
- Implementation of exposure control methods, including universal precautions, engineering and work practice controls, personal protective equipment, and housekeeping.
- Hepatitis B vaccination.
- Postexposure evaluation and follow-up.
- Communication of hazards to employees and hazard training.
- Recordkeeping.
- Procedures for evaluating circumstances surrounding exposure incidents.

Exposure Incidents

The OSHA Bloodborne Pathogens Standard also specifies what to do in case of an exposure incident. An exposure incident is one in which a worker, despite all precautions, has reason to believe that he has come in contact with a substance that may transmit infection. Contact may occur when a medical worker accidentally sticks himself with a used needle. A puncture exposure incident is the most common kind of exposure.

The basic rules covering exposure incidents apply to all serious infections, such as HBV and HIV. The rules covering HBV also include vaccination.

When an exposure incident occurs, the physician or employer must be notified immediately. This prompt action is extremely important because quick and proper treatment can help prevent the development of many diseases, such as hepatitis B. Timely action also can prevent the worker from exposing other people to a potentially acquired infection. Reporting the incident helps to prevent the same type of accident from happening again.

After such an exposure, the employer must offer the exposed employee a free medical evaluation. The employer must refer the employee to a licensed healthcare provider who can counsel the employee about what happened as well as about how to prevent the spread of any potential infection. The healthcare provider also takes a blood sample and prescribes appropriate treatment. If the employee does not want to participate in the medical evaluation and treatment, he has the right to refuse it. If this occurs, the employee's refusal should be documented.

If an employee who has not received the HBV vaccination and is not known to be immune is exposed to any infected person, especially someone who is HBV-positive or at high risk, it is recommended that the employee be tested for HBV and receive the vaccination if necessary. This vaccination may prevent infection. When the source person's HBV status is unknown and the person does not wish to be tested, the employee should be tested. If the source person agrees to be tested, the law requires that the employee be informed of the test results. The employee may agree to give blood but not to be tested. In such a case, the blood sample must be kept for 90 days in case the employee later develops symptoms of HBV or HIV infection and decides to be tested then.

The healthcare provider who performs the postexposure evaluation must give the employer a written report stating whether HBV vaccination was recommended and received and that the employee was informed of the results of any blood tests. Any additional information must be kept confidential.

Other OSHA Requirements

OSHA also requires that all healthcare workers who have occupational exposure to blood or other potentially infectious materials have the opportunity to receive the HBV vaccine, free of charge, as needed throughout employment. Within 10 days of a medical worker's starting a job, the doctor or employer is required to offer the worker the opportunity to receive this vaccination. The vaccine is recommended for all healthcare workers *unless*:

- They have received it in the past;
- A blood test shows them to be immune to the virus; and/or
- There are medical reasons for which the vaccine is contraindicated.

In most cases, the employee is permitted to decline the vaccination if she signs a form accepting all the conditions. (A few employers require HBV vaccination as a condition for employment.) Even if the healthcare worker declines the vaccination when beginning employment, she still has the opportunity to receive the free vaccine and any necessary booster shots throughout her employment.

Needlestick Safety and Prevention Act In response to the Needlestick Safety and Prevention Act, which was signed into law in November 2000, OSHA revised the Bloodborne Pathogens Standard. The additional provisions to the standard are:

- Healthcare employers must evaluate new safety-engineered control devices on an annual basis and implement the use of devices that reasonably reduce the risk of needlestick injuries.
- Healthcare facilities must maintain a detailed log of sharps injuries incurred from contaminated sharps.
- Healthcare employers must solicit input from employees involved in direct patient care to identify, evaluate, and

implement engineering and **work practice controls** (controlling injuries by altering the way a task is performed).

In an effort to reduce needlestick injuries, the National Institute for Occupational Safety and Health (NIOSH) has specific recommendations for employers and employees regarding **engineered safety devices,** devices specifically designed to isolate or remove the hazard, and work practice controls. NIOSH recommendations for employers include the following:

Engineering Controls

- Eliminate the use of needles where safe and effective alternatives are available.
- Implement the use of engineered safety devices and evaluate their use on a regular basis.

Needlestick Prevention Programs

- Analyze sharps injuries to identify hazard trends in the workplace.
- Ensure employees are properly trained in the proper use and disposal of sharps.
- Adapt work practices that involve sharps to make them safer.
- Make safety awareness in the workplace a priority.
- Have established procedures for reporting all needlestick injuries.
- Evaluate prevention procedures and provide feedback to employees.

NIOSH recommendations for employees include the following:

- Avoid using needles if a safe alternative exists.
- Participate in choosing engineered safety devices.
- Use the engineered safety devices provided by your employer.
- Do not recap needles if possible.
- Before beginning a procedure, make sure you have a means of safe sharps disposal close by and ready for use.
- Dispose of used needles promptly and appropriately.
- Promptly report all sharps-related injuries.
- Advise your employer if you see sharps hazards in the workplace.
- Participate in bloodborne pathogen training.

▶ Transmission-Based Precautions LO 6.4

In addition to strict adherence to standard precautions, there may be situations that require an additional level of precaution you must take in order to protect yourself, the facility staff, and other patients from exposure to infectious disease. For this reason, the CDC has developed guidelines known as **transmission-based precautions.** These guidelines are meant as a supplement to standard precautions when caring for patients with suspected or confirmed infection.

Transmission-based precautions include three categories:

- Contact precautions
- Droplet precautions
- Airborne precautions

Contact Precautions

Contact transmission is transmission by touching and is the most common means of spreading infectious diseases. The two subgroups of contact transmission are direct and indirect. As you learned in section 6.2 of the chapter, direct contact involves the spread of microorganisms from person to person by touching without an intermediate object. Microorganisms are spread indirectly by touching contaminated surfaces and objects.

Applying Contact Precautions You must use contact precautions with patients who have any of the following conditions or diseases:

- Stool incontinence/severe, uncontrolled diarrhea
- Draining wounds
- Uncontrolled secretions
- Decubitus ulcers (pressure sores)
- Ostomy tubes
- Generalized rash

   Contact precautions include:

- Washing your hands before and after touching the patient.
- Wearing gloves.
- Wearing a gown if considerable contact is expected.
- Washing hands after removing gloves.
- Disinfecting the exam room with EPA-registered disinfectant.

Droplet Precautions

Transmission of microorganisms by contact with secretions from the nose, throat, airways, lungs, and digestive tract is known as droplet contact. Droplets from coughs and sneezes can carry up to 3 feet from the source (Figure 6-7). Follow droplet precautions when assisting with patients suspected of having influenza, pertussis (whooping cough), mumps, respiratory syncytial virus, norovirus, and *Neisseria meningitidis* (a bacterium that causes meningitis).

Applying Droplet Precautions Patients suspected of being infected with a pathogen transmitted by droplets should be placed in an exam room as quickly as possible. If you do not have an open exam room, ask the patient to put on a face mask and place the patient as far away from other patients as possible. When caring for a patient with influenza or other droplet-transmitted infection, put on a mask before entering the room. If the patient is coughing or sneezing uncontrollably and substantial spraying of respiratory droplets is expected, you also should wear gloves, a gown, and goggles or a face shield. Wash your hands before and after touching the patient or contacting respiratory secretions. Ask the patient to wear a mask when leaving the exam room, and instruct her in respiratory hygiene and cough etiquette. Always clean and disinfect the exam room before allowing the next patient to enter.

Airborne Precautions

Some microorganisms are able to float in the air for substantial distances. For this reason, special airborne precautions must be taken if a patient is suspected of being infected with any known pathogen capable of being transmitted through the airborne route. The most common pathogens transmitted by the airborne route include tuberculosis, measles, chickenpox, and, in some cases, herpes zoster (shingles).

Applying Airborne Precautions Because airborne pathogens float in the air, anyone in the vicinity of an infected patient can easily be exposed. For this reason, it is important to isolate the patient as soon as possible. Have the patient enter through a different entrance than other patients, avoiding the reception area. Place the patient in a special airborne infection isolation room (AIIR), if one is available. If this type of room is not available, you should give the patient a face mask, close the door to the exam room, instruct the patient to keep the mask on, and change it if it becomes wet. The healthcare practitioner treating the patient will most likely transfer the patient to a facility equipped with special isolation rooms and fit-tested respirators. While caring for a patient with a suspected airborne pathogen, be sure to perform hand hygiene before and after patient contact and wear a mask, gloves, and a gown. Have the patient wear a mask at all times. After the patient leaves the room, keep the room empty for at least an hour, depending on the ventilation rate of the room. If you must enter the room before the prescribed time, you must use respiratory protection.

▶ OSHA-Required Education and Training

LO 6.5

In order for healthcare personnel to adhere to infection control policies and procedures, they must be properly trained. This training must be comprehensive and ongoing, and the trainers must have documented and demonstrated competency related to the task. Employers are required to provide infection control training at the onset of employment and then on a regular basis (usually yearly) or when a policy or procedure changes or there is a change in circumstances, such as an outbreak of influenza. Training should include the scientific rationale for infection control procedures. Understanding the rationale helps healthcare workers perform the procedures correctly and alter them safely

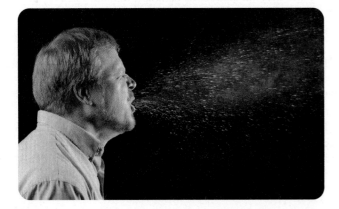

FIGURE 6-7 Uncovered coughs and sneezes can spread droplets for several feet.

Source: CDC/James Gathany

to specific situations when necessary. Anyone working in a healthcare facility who could be reasonably expected to come in contact with an infectious agent must be trained. This includes any contract worker from an outside agency, such as students participating in onsite training, housekeeping personnel, and equipment maintenance personnel who repair and maintain clinical equipment. This training must include but is not limited to the following:

- Proper PPE selection and use.
- Job-specific infection prevention.

Improvement in adherence to infection control procedures and subsequent reduction in **healthcare-associated infections (HAI)** has been documented. Research shows that periodic assessment and feedback regarding healthcare workers' adherence to infection control practices in addition to education result in better adherence to those practices. Reduction in the transmission of infectious disease requires that not only healthcare workers understand how to break the chain of infection but also patients and their families. Patients and family members should be given information on standard precautions, respiratory hygiene, cough etiquette, and the importance of vaccination.

PROCEDURE 6-1 Aseptic Handwashing

Procedure Goal: To remove dirt and microorganisms from under the fingernails and from the surface of the skin, hair follicles, and oil glands of the hands

OSHA Guidelines: This procedure does not involve exposure to blood, body fluids, or tissues.

Materials: Liquid soap, disposable brush or nail cleaner, and paper towels

Method:

1. Remove all jewelry (plain wedding bands may be left on and scrubbed).

2. Turn on the faucets using a paper towel, and adjust the water temperature to moderately warm. (Sinks with knee-operated faucet controls prevent contact of the surface with the hands.)

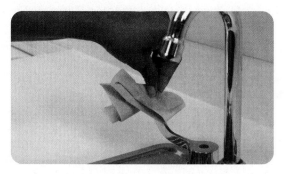

FIGURE Procedure 6-1 Step 2   Using a paper towel to turn on the faucet reduces the possibility of cross contamination.
©McGraw-Hill Education

3. Wet your hands and apply the recommended amount of liquid soap. Use a clean, dry paper towel to activate soap pump. Liquid soap, especially when dispensed automatically or with a foot pump, is preferable to bar soap. **RATIONALE:** *There is less available area for dirt to accumulate on a liquid soap dispenser than on bar soap,*

and there is a smaller chance of dropping the soap dispenser into the sink or onto the floor.

4. Work the soap into a lather, making sure that all surface areas of both hands are lathered. Rub vigorously in a circular motion for 2 minutes. Keep your hands lower than your forearms so that dirty water flows into the sink instead of back onto your arms. Your fingertips should be pointing down. Interlace your fingers to clean between them, and use the palm of one hand to clean the back of the other. It is important that you wash every surface of your hands. **RATIONALE:** *Microorganisms are found on every surface of the hand and, if not washed away, can be transferred to the patient.*

5. Use a single-use disposable nailbrush or plastic, single-use nail cleaner under running water to dislodge dirt around your nails and cuticles. **RATIONALE:** *Microorganisms under the nails are not directly subjected to the running water and must be dislodged so that they can be washed away.*

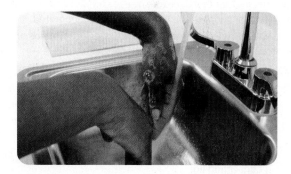

FIGURE Procedure 6-1 Step 6   Keep your hands lower than your forearms and avoid touching the sink when rinsing after an aseptic handwash.
©McGraw-Hill Education

6. Rinse your hands well, keeping your hands lower than your forearms and not touching the sink or faucets.

7. With the water still running, dry your hands thoroughly with clean, dry paper towels.

8. Turn off the faucets using a clean, dry paper towel. Discard the towels.

PROCEDURE 6-2 Using an Alcohol-Based Hand Disinfectant

Procedure Goal: To use an alcohol-based hand-cleansing substance to reduce pathogens on the hand surfaces and prevent recontamination

OSHA Guidelines: This procedure does not involve exposure to blood, body fluids, or tissue.

Materials: 60% to 95% alcohol-based foam, gel, or liquid rub

Method:

1. Remove all jewelry (plain wedding bands may be left on).
2. Pump the recommended amount of AHD onto the palm of the hand.
   RATIONALE: *You must use enough AHD to cover all surfaces of the hands, and there must be enough so that it does not dry too quickly.*

3. Rub the hands together vigorously, ensuring the alcohol comes in contact with all surfaces, including backs of hands, between fingers, and fingernails.
   RATIONALE: *Microorganisms are found on every surface of the hand and, if not exposed to the AHD, can be transferred to the patient.*

4. Continue to rub the solution in a rotary fashion until it is evaporated and the hands are dry (10–15 seconds). Do not wave hands to hasten drying.
   RATIONALE: *Once they evaporate, AHDs have no effect on pathogens.*

PROCEDURE 6-3 Using a Biohazardous Sharps Container

Procedure Goal: To ensure safe use of a sharps disposal unit

OSHA Guidelines:

Materials: Approved sharps container and gloves

Method:

1. Wash your hands and put on gloves.
2. Ensure that biohazardous waste containers are close to the place where the waste material is generated.
   RATIONALE: *To avoid accidental puncture wounds or exposure to biohazardous waste*
3. Hold the article by the unpointed, or blunt, end.
4. Drop the object directly into an approved container. (If you are using an evacuation system, do not unscrew the needle. Drop the entire system with the needle attached and the safety device engaged into the receptacle.) The container should be puncture-proof, with rigid sides and a tight-fitting lid.
   RATIONALE: *To avoid needlestick injuries*

5. Place sharps in an appropriate biohazardous waste container immediately or as soon as possible.
6. Keep containers closed when not in use. Close them before removing them from the area or use, and keep them upright to avoid spills.
7. Place the container in a secondary container if the outside of the primary container becomes contaminated.
8. Drop—do not push—intact contaminated needles into the biohazardous waste container for sharps.
   RATIONALE: *To avoid accidental puncture wounds*
9. Never break off, recap, reuse, or handle needles after use.
   RATIONALE: *To avoid accidental puncture wounds*
10. Do not open, empty, or clean sharps containers.
11. Discard sharps containers that are two-thirds full in large biohazardous waste containers. Depending on your office's procedures, the container and its contents may be sterilized before further disposal, or they may be collected by an authorized waste management agency.
12. Remove the gloves and wash your hands.

PROCEDURE 6-4 Disposing of Biohazardous Waste

Procedure Goal: To correctly dispose of contaminated waste products, including sharps and contaminated cleaning and paper products

OSHA Guidelines:

Materials: Biohazardous waste containers, gloves, and waste materials

Method:

1. Wash your hands and put on gloves.
2. Carefully deposit the biohazardous materials in a properly marked biohazardous waste container. A standard biohazardous waste container has an inner plastic liner (either red or orange and marked with the biohazard symbol) and a puncture-proof outer shell (also marked with the biohazard symbol).

3. Never "dump" the contents of one biohazardous waste container into another.
   RATIONALE: *Doing so puts you at risk of exposure to biohazardous materials.*
4. If the container is full, secure the inner liner and place it in the appropriate area for biohazardous waste.
   RATIONALE: *Biohazardous waste must be held in an area separate from regular waste and trash.*
5. Remove the gloves and wash your hands.

SUMMARY OF LEARNING OUTCOMES

OUTCOME	KEY POINTS
6.1 Identify Occupational Safety and Health Administration (OSHA)'s role in protecting healthcare workers.	The US Department of Labor created OSHA to protect the employees' safety in the workplace. Through the creation and enforcement of standards such as the Bloodborne Pathogens Standard, Hazard Communication, and the Needlestick Safety and Prevention Act, OSHA serves to protect healthcare workers from hazards.
6.2 Illustrate the cycle of infection and how to break it.	In order for an infection to occur, these five elements must be in place: a reservoir host, a means of exit, a means of transmission, a means of entrance, and a susceptible host. The most effective means of breaking the cycle of infection is by using aseptic techniques. These include maintaining strict housekeeping standards; adhering to government health guidelines; and educating patients in hygiene, health promotion, and disease prevention.
6.3 Summarize the Bloodborne Pathogens Standard and universal precautions as described by OSHA.	Laws set forth in the OSHA Bloodborne Pathogens Standard of 1991 dictate how you must handle infectious or potentially infectious waste generated during medical or surgical procedures. According to these rules, any potentially infectious waste materials must be discarded or held for processing in biohazardous waste containers.
6.4 Describe how transmission-based precautions supplement standard precautions.	Transmission-based precautions are meant to supplement standard precautions by adding an additional level of precautions. These include contact precautions, droplet precautions, and airborne precautions.
6.5 Summarize OSHA's education and training requirements for ambulatory care settings.	All ambulatory care settings must train employees and contract workers in the proper selection and use of PPE and job-specific infection prevention. This training must be done when the worker is hired and on a regular basis after that. In addition, patients and their families should be given information about preventing the spread of infection.

CASE STUDY CRITICAL THINKING

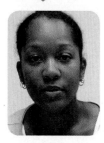

©McGraw-Hill Education

Recall Shenya Jones from the beginning of the chapter. Now that you have completed the chapter, answer the following questions regarding her case.

1. What aseptic technique practices would be most important with this patient?
2. Whom do these aseptic technique practices protect?
3. Why is it important that Dr. Williams do a wound culture?

1. (LO 6.1) The general duty clause requires
   a. That every employee perform every duty in the office
   b. An employer to maintain a safe workplace
   c. That each employee follow OSHA regulations
   d. That safety plan duties be well defined
   e. That healthcare workers not wear artificial nails when working with any patients

2. (LO 6.2) A bladder infection caused by *Escherichia coli* would be considered what type of infection?
   a. Vector-borne
   b. Exogenous
   c. Opportunistic
   d. Endogenous
   e. Foodborne

3. (LO 6.4) The guidelines set forth by the CDC that are meant to supplement standard precautions are known as
   a. Transmission-based precautions
   b. Training guidelines
   c. Respiratory hygiene
   d. OSHA supplemental procedures
   e. NIOSH recommendations

4. (LO 6.4) Droplet precautions pertain to someone who has which of the following?
   a. Ostomy tube
   b. Stool incontinence
   c. Draining wound
   d. Generalized rash
   e. Influenza infection

5. (LO 6.2) Which of the following is the *most* common means of transmitting pathogens?
   a. Ingesting food
   b. Sneezing
   c. Coughing
   d. Sexual contact
   e. Touching

6. (LO 6.2) Which of the following would be considered a fomite?
   a. Mosquito
   b. Pencil
   c. Sneeze
   d. *E. coli*
   e. Mucus

7. (LO 6.5) OSHA requires that all workers have initial training in PPE selection and
   a. Respirator use
   b. Job-specific infection prevention
   c. Sharps control
   d. Microbiology
   e. Equipment handling

8. (LO 6.3) Exposure to which of the following would be considered an exposure incident?
   a. Influenza
   b. Mumps
   c. HPV
   d. HIV
   e. Scabies

9. (LO 6.3) Which of the following would be considered a Category II task?
   a. Performing oral surgery
   b. Performing CPR
   c. Taking vital signs
   d. Measuring height
   e. Controlling bleeding

10. (LO 6.3) Means of controlling injuries by altering the way a task is performed is known as
    a. Universal precautions
    b. Engineering controls
    c. Personal protection
    d. Work practice controls
    e. Safety plan controls

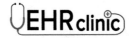

Go to CONNECT to complete the EHRclinic exercise: 6.01
Add a Note to a Patient's EHR.

You are a new graduate of a medical assisting program and have just been hired by an internal medicine practice with seven practitioners. This is a very busy office, and you are excited to be working in the clinical area. Because you are new to the practice, you will shadow with Mary Benton, RMA. This morning is particularly busy, and you have seen several patients with suspected influenza. After the morning patient session, Mary approaches you and says that you could save time by not washing your hands so much. She tells you that if you are wearing gloves, you don't have to wash your hands after you take them off. How do you respond to Mary, and what action should you take?

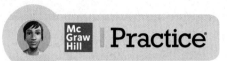

Go to PRACTICE MEDICAL OFFICE and complete the module Admin Check In: Office Operations.

Safety and Patient Reception

CASE STUDY

Patient Name	DOB	Allergies
Peter Smith	03/28/1946	NKA

Attending	MRN	Other Information
Paul F. Buckwalter, MD	00-AA-003	Mrs. Smith requests to speak privately with MD.

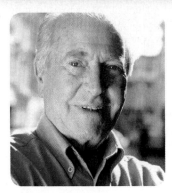

©Image Source/Getty Images

Peter Smith has mild Type 2 diabetes. When he called to schedule today's appointment, he stated that he was feeling very anxious and fatigued and that he was having difficulty eating and sleeping. He arrives at the reception desk today, appearing "flat" in affect. After he signs in, his wife whispers to you, "I want to talk with the doctor about him, before he sees the doctor." Once Peter Smith sits down, you notice him lean over and try to pick up a magazine from a table. His chair tips onto two legs while he continues to try to reach the magazine.

Keep Peter Smith in mind as you study the chapter. There will be questions at the end of the chapter based on the case study. The information in the chapter will help you answer these questions.

LEARNING OUTCOMES

After completing Chapter 7, you will be able to:

7.1 Describe the components of a medical office safety plan.

7.2 Summarize OSHA's Hazard Communication Standard.

7.3 Describe basic safety precautions you should take to reduce electrical hazards.

7.4 Illustrate the necessary steps in a comprehensive fire safety plan.

7.5 Summarize proper methods for handling and storing chemicals used in a medical office.

7.6 Explain the principles of good ergonomic practice and physical safety in the medical office.

7.7 Articulate the cause of most injuries to medical office workers and the four body areas where they occur.

7.8 List the design items to be considered when setting up an office reception area.

7.9 Summarize the housekeeping tasks required to keep the reception area neat and clean.

7.10 Relate how the Americans with Disabilities and Older American Acts have helped to make physical access to the medical office easier for all patients.

7.11 Describe the functions of the front office staff, including patient registration and accepting payments from patients.

7.12 Implement policies and procedures for opening and closing the office.

Americans with Disabilities Act (ADA)

color family

contagious

ergonomics

Globally Harmonized System of Classification and Labeling of Chemicals (GHS)

Hazard Communication Standard (HCS)

hazard label

infectious waste

Older Americans Act of 1965

reception

Safety Data Sheets (SDS)

MEDICAL ASSISTING COMPETENCIES

CAAHEP

X.C.4 Summarize the Patient Bill of Rights

XII.C.1 Identify:
(a) safety signs
(b) symbols
(c) labels

XII.C.2 Identify safety techniques that can be used in responding to accidental exposure to:
(a) blood
(b) other body fluids
(c) needle sticks
(d) chemicals

XII.C.3 Discuss fire safety issues in an ambulatory healthcare environment

XII.C.4 Describe fundamental principles for evacuation of a healthcare setting

XII.C.5 Describe the purpose of Safety Data Sheets (SDS) in a healthcare setting

XII.C.6 Discuss protocols for disposal of biological chemical materials

XII.C.7 Identify principles of:
(a) body mechanics
(b) ergonomics

XII.P.1 Comply with:
(a) safety signs
(b) symbols
(c) labels

XII.P.2 Demonstrate proper use of:
(a) eyewash equipment
(b) fire extinguishers
(c) sharps disposal containers

XII.P.3 Use proper body mechanics

XII.P.5 Evaluate the work environment to identify unsafe working conditions

XII.A.2 Demonstrate self-awareness in responding to an emergency situation

ABHES

4. Medical Law and Ethics

b. Institute federal and state guidelines when:
1. releasing medical records or information

f. Comply with federal, state, and local health laws and regulations as they relate to healthcare settings

h. Demonstrate compliance with HIPAA guidelines, the ADA Amendments Act, and the Health Information Technology for Economic and Clinical Health (HITECH) Act

5. Psychology of Human Relations

c. Assist the patient in navigating issues and concerns that may arise (e.g., insurance policy information, medical bills, and physician/provider orders)

8. Clinical Procedures

a. Practice standard precautions and perform disinfection/sterilization techniques

g. Recognize and respond to medical office emergencies

j. Make adaptations for patients with special needs (psychological or physical limitations)

9. Medical Laboratory Procedures

c. Dispose of biohazardous materials

▶ Introduction

In general, the medical office is divided into two broad, functional categories: The "back office" is the clinical area where patient care takes place, and the "front office," including the reception area, is where business and nonclinical tasks take place. Whether you are working in the clinical area or the administrative area, safety should be foremost in your mind. Patients and staff members can fall or cut themselves and be exposed to numerous safety hazards. As a medical assistant, you have

be moved. Lock the wheels of the wheelchair. Remove the wheelchair footrests if possible. Have the patient help as much as possible. If a transfer device is available, use it. Transfer devices include gait belts, sliding boards, pivot discs, and sling-type transfer equipment.

- Adjust your seat to the correct position to prevent back strain.
- If you are using a computer, take frequent breaks to reduce eyestrain and hand cramping.

Your employer has the responsibility to provide a safe work environment, including equipment designed to reduce injury and workstations that adjust to the worker. Many employers offer training seminars for reducing work-related injuries. It is your responsibility to follow safe practice when using equipment or performing tasks where there is a possibility of work-related injury.

Physical Safety

There are many ways to ensure physical safety in the medical office. You must understand and apply all the appropriate safeguards. Because accidents can happen, however, post emergency numbers in multiple locations throughout the office. Once each quarter, make sure the numbers are accurate and up-to-date.

Some safeguards come under the heading of common sense, meaning their application requires no special knowledge. These include:

- Walk, do not run, in the office.
- Prevent falls by wiping or mopping up spills immediately.
- Clear the floor of dropped objects.
- If the floor is carpeted, make sure there are no snags or tears that could cause someone to trip and fall.
- Spilled medications, chemicals, and other substances pose a threat to young children, who may ingest anything they find on the floor. Destroy and dispose of medications that are accidentally dropped on the floor.
- Be careful when carrying objects through the facility, especially when approaching blind corners.
- Close all cabinets, closet doors, desks, and worktable drawers.
- Routinely inspect the furniture in the exam room and reception area. Make sure there are no rough edges or sharp corners on the examining table, countertop, chairs, or other furniture.
- Electrical cords and medical and office equipment cables should run along the walls and be taped or fastened down securely.
- Never use damaged equipment or supplies, such as cracked or chipped glassware.

If you are asked to work in the laboratory, being aware of the laboratory environment will help you protect your health and well-being. Other safeguards to practice in the laboratory include:

- Do not eat or drink in the laboratory, and do not store food there. Never use laboratory supplies, such as beakers or flasks, for eating or drinking.

- Do not put anything in your mouth while working in the laboratory. (Some people have a habit of chewing on the end of their pencils, for example.)
- Do not apply makeup or lip balm or insert contact lenses in the laboratory.
- Familiarize yourself with the location of the first-aid kit. If you are responsible for the kit in your area, check it weekly to make sure it is adequately stocked with supplies and that expiration dates on medications have not passed. (See Figure 7-7).
- Familiarize yourself with the location and operation of the emergency eyewash and shower stations.

Additionally, in your efforts to promote safe practice in the laboratory, always wear appropriate protective gear and clothing. Use heat-resistant mitts or gloves to prevent burns. Wear sturdy, low-heeled, closed-toe shoes with rubber soles to prevent injury if you drop or spill something and to avoid slipping. Do not wear dangling jewelry or loose clothing that could get caught in laboratory equipment. Keep hair pulled back or covered for the same reason.

When you work with laboratory equipment, always follow manufacturers' guidelines. For example, wait for centrifuges to stop spinning before you open them.

Many laboratory materials and supplies require special handling and precautions, which include:

- Do not attempt to grasp bottles, jars, or other containers if your hands or the containers are wet.
- Close containers immediately after use.
- Clean up spills immediately.
- Clean up broken glass with a broom. Do not handle the debris. If the material is biohazardous, use tongs or forceps to pick up the glass. Package the pieces in a sturdy container with a label identifying the contents.

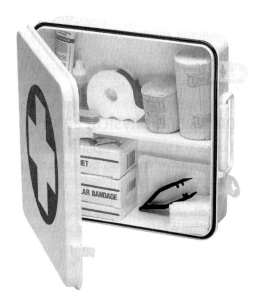

FIGURE 7-7 First-aid kit.
©Comstock/Alamy Stock Photo

▶ Preventing Injury in the Front Office

LO 7.7

In addition to taking care of patients, medical assistants also must be aware of their environment in the medical office and how it affects their ability to perform the job effectively.

The medical office environment's many work functions require many physical tasks. Examples are using the computer, carrying and unpacking boxes, filling copy machine trays, and helping patients with impairments. The associated movements are often performed using repetitive motions, such as typing, lifting, bending, stooping, and sitting. The most common office-related injuries are those occurring to office workers, including medical assistants, who spend much of their workday seated at a computer station. Common injuries or conditions involve the forearm, wrist, hand, and back. Table 7-1 contains ergonomic excerpts from an OSHA computer station checklist to use in prevention of these common injuries.

The ideal medical office environment is an efficient, safe, and caring place for patients, visitors, and staff. You will find the *Caution: Handle with Care* feature helpful in preventing carpal tunnel syndrome (CTS), as well as identifying the symptoms and treatments for CTS, should it occur.

TABLE 7-1 OSHA Computer Workstations Checklist
1. Head and neck to be upright or in line with the torso (not bent down or back).
2. Head, neck, and trunk to face forward (not twisted).
3. Trunk to be perpendicular to floor (may lean back into backrest but not forward).
4. Shoulders and upper arms to be in line with the torso, generally about perpendicular to the floor and relaxed (not elevated or stretched forward).
5. Upper arms and elbows to be close to the body (not extended outward).
6. Forearms, wrists, and hands to be straight and in line (forearm at about 90 degrees to the upper arm).
7. Wrists and hands to be straight (not bent up or down or sideways toward the little finger).
8. Thighs to be parallel to the floor and lower legs to be perpendicular to floor (thighs may be slightly elevated above knees).
9. Feet rest flat on the floor or are supported by a stable footrest.
10. Backrest provides support for your lower back (lumbar area).
11. Seat width and depth accommodate the specific user (seat pan not too big or small).
12. Seat front does not press against the back of your knees and lower legs (seat pan not too long).
13. Seat has cushioning and is rounded with a "waterfall" front (no sharp edge).
14. Armrests, if used, support both forearms while you perform computer tasks, and they do not interfere with movement.
15. Keyboard/input device platform(s) is stable and large enough to hold a keyboard and an input device.
16. Input device (mouse or trackball) is located right next to your keyboard so it can be operated without reaching.
17. Input device is easy to activate, and the shape and size fits your hand (not too big or small).
18. Wrists and hands do not rest on sharp or hard edges.
19. Top of the screen is at or below eye level so you can read it without bending your head or neck down or back.
20. User with bifocals or trifocals can read the screen without bending the head or neck backward.
21. Monitor distance allows you to read the screen without leaning your head, neck, or trunk forward or backward.
22. Monitor position is directly in front of you so you don't have to twist your head or neck.
23. Glare (for example, from windows or lights) is not reflected on your screen, which can cause you to assume an awkward posture to clearly see information on your screen.
24. Thighs have sufficient clearance space between the top of the thighs and your computer table/keyboard platform (thighs are not trapped).
25. Legs and feet have sufficient clearance space under the work surface so you are able to get close enough to the keyboard/input device.
26. Document holder, if provided, is stable and large enough to hold documents.
27. Document holder, if provided, is placed at about the same height and distance as the monitor screen so there is little head movement or need to refocus when you look from the document to the screen.
28. Wrist/palm rest, if provided, is padded and free of sharp or square edges that push on your wrists.
29. Wrist/palm rest, if provided, allows you to keep your forearms, wrists, and hands straight and in line when using the keyboard/input device.
30. Telephone can be used with your head upright (not bent) and your shoulders relaxed (not elevated) if you do computer tasks at the same time.
31. Workstation and equipment have sufficient adjustability so you are in a safe working posture and can make occasional changes in posture while performing computer tasks.
32. Computer workstation, components, and accessories are maintained in serviceable condition and function properly.
33. Computer tasks are organized in a way that allows you to vary tasks with other work activities, or to take microbreaks or recovery pauses while at the computer workstation.

Source: http://www.osha.gov/SLTC/etools/computerworkstations/checklist.html (2012).

Carpal Tunnel Syndrome

As the number of computers used in the home and workplace has escalated in recent years, the number of cases of carpal tunnel syndrome also has risen dramatically. Carpal tunnel syndrome is a hand disorder often associated with computer use. The term for this condition comes from the name for a canal (the carpal tunnel) located in the wrist. Several tendons pass through this tunnel, allowing the hand to open and close.

Carpal tunnel syndrome results from repetitive motion, such as keyboarding, for hours at a time. This motion may cause swelling to develop around the tendons and carpal tunnel. The swelling compresses the nerve. The people most likely to develop this disorder are workers whose jobs require them to perform repetitive hand and finger motions.

Symptoms

The symptoms associated with carpal tunnel syndrome include:

- Tingling or burning in the hands or fingers.
- Weakness or numbness in the hands or fingers.
- Hands that go to sleep frequently.
- Difficulty opening or closing the hands.
- Pain that stems from the wrist and travels up the arm.

Tips for Prevention

If you use a keyboard for extended periods, you should practice proper techniques, as outlined in the following bullets, to prevent carpal tunnel syndrome (Figure 7-8).

- While seated, hold your arms relaxed at your sides. Make sure your keyboard is positioned slightly higher than your elbows. As you input, keep your elbows at your sides and relax your shoulders.
- Use only your fingers to press keys and do not use more pressure than necessary. Use a wrist rest and keep your wrists relaxed and straight.
- When you need to strike difficult-to-reach keys, move your whole hand rather than stretching your fingers.

When you need to press two keys at the same time, such as "Control" and "F1," use two hands.

- Try to break up long periods of keyboard work with other tasks that do not require computer use.

Tips for Relieving Symptoms

If you have carpal tunnel syndrome symptoms, try these suggestions for relief:

- Elevate your arms.
- Wear a splint on the hand and forearm.
- Discuss your symptoms with a physician, who may prescribe medication.

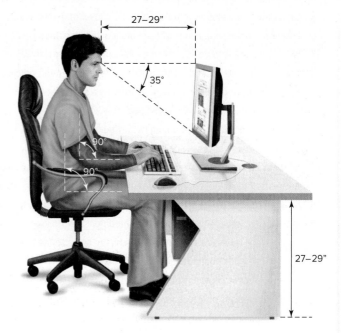

FIGURE 7-8 Maintaining proper posture and hand position helps avoid straining of the neck, back, arms, and eyes when using a computer.

In addition to carpal tunnel syndrome, long-term use of computers, tablets, and cell phones can cause a disorder known as computer vision syndrome. The *Caution: Handle with Care* feature will help you recognize and prevent the symptoms of computer vision syndrome.

Special Safety Precautions Some patients, such as children and people with disabilities, may be particularly susceptible to accidents in your office. You need to take special precautions to ensure their safety.

Children Follow these precautions when assisting children:

- Keep sharp instruments out of the reach of children.
- Store toxic items in high cabinets.

- Keep all medications and objects out of the reach of young children because children are likely to pick up items and put them in their mouths and could choke or be poisoned.
- Keep children's toys and books in the reception area or exam room picked up and stored safely when not in use.
- Toys should be washable and made of safe materials.
- Sanitize toys that children put in their mouths daily; sanitize other toys weekly.
- If well children and sick children use the same reception area or exam room, sanitize and disinfect toys after sick children play with them.
- Periodically check toys for sharp edges that might cause cuts.
- Ensure toys do not have small parts or pieces that could cause choking if swallowed.

Computer Vision Syndrome

Continued and long-term use of computers, tablets, and cell phones has resulted in computer vision syndrome, sometimes called digital eye strain. Symptoms increase as screen time increases. According to the American Optometric Association, symptoms usually decrease once work on digital screens ends; however, some will experience long-lasting symptoms.

Symptoms

The symptoms associated with computer vision syndrome include:

- Eyestrain
- Headaches
- Blurred vision
- Dry eyes
- Neck and shoulder strain

Tips for Prevention

If you use a computer monitor, tablet, or cell phone for long periods of time, you should follow the 20-20-20 rule.

Spend 20 seconds every 20 minutes to look at something at least 20 feet away.

Tips for Relieving Symptoms

If you have symptoms of computer vision syndrome, it is important that you see an eyecare professional. You also should take the following steps when using a computer or other device with a screen.

- Locate computer screen so that it is approximately 28 inches from your eyes and you are looking slightly downward.
- Avoid glare by using antiglare screens and using lower wattage bulbs in desk lamps and overhead lighting.
- Take frequent rest breaks. Use the 20-20-20 rule.
- Blink frequently to keep the outer eye moist.

Patients with Physical Disabilities Patients with disabilities are more likely than other patients to fall. Some patients may use walkers or canes for support, whereas others may simply be unsteady on their feet. Follow these recommendations when assisting patients with physical disabilities:

- Provide assistance as needed with disrobing prior to an exam or redressing afterward.
- Never leave severely disabled patients alone in an exam room. Check office policies for guidelines regarding appropriate chaperones for patients with disabilities.

In addition, keep in mind that patients with vision impairments may have difficulty seeing obstacles, stairs, and other potential hazards. Safe flooring and handrails in the reception area, bathroom, hallways, and exam room help ensure the safety of patients with impaired mobility or vision.

▶ Design of the Reception Area   LO 7.8

The word **reception** means the place or event where one is greeted. In the medical office, reception describes the area where the patient enters the practice, informs the staff of his or her presence by "signing in," receives a greeting, and waits to be seen. Avoid using the term *waiting room* because waiting is only one function and the term does not have a positive association. Although the practice manager is usually responsible for the office design, awareness of the aspects that affect the design is valuable knowledge for any medical assistant. The primary consideration in the design is the type of practice. For example, the furnishings, colors, and patient flow patterns of a pediatric office will differ from those of an internal medicine office.

Size and Schedule

After identifying the type of practice, size is the next factor. Knowledge of the number of practitioners and the number of patients anticipated daily is important. Knowing when individual physicians plan to utilize the space is equally important. For example, one surgeon in the practice may have office hours on Mondays, Wednesdays, and Fridays and perform surgeries on Tuesdays and Thursdays. Another surgeon may perform surgeries in the morning and see patients in the afternoon. These differences in physician scheduling allow better utilization of space and relative ease in planning for the reception size. Other offices may have staggered hours in which one physician will see patients between 7:00 a.m. and 3:00 p.m. and another physician in the practice will see patients from 11:00 a.m. to 7:00 p.m. This is challenging because more space is needed during the 4 overlap hours than the remainder of the day. Dealing with overlapping office hours and other time and space issues is often part of the medical assistant's role.

Utilization of Space

Utilization of space differs by type of practice. For example, an orthopedic office or geriatric office where a significant number of patients will need room for wheelchairs and walkers requires more open space for mobility and devices than does a cardiologist's office. There may be the false assumption that pediatric offices need a smaller reception area because the patients are smaller, but this is incorrect for a few reasons. First, a caregiver always accompanies the pediatric patient. Second, children require play space. Third, pediatric offices may need separate "well child" and "sick child" areas in an attempt to avoid cross-contamination from sick to well patients.

Overcrowding in a reception area is undesirable for patient comfort and for the potential of disease transmission. The reception area, which allows the patient to sit while waiting to be seen, is usually separated from the functional areas of the practice by a high counter and a sliding window (Figure 7-9). These areas should be HIPAA-compliant so the patient at the counter cannot overhear staff talking to or about other patients and cannot view an open computer screen or paper record.

Décor

Colors and fabrics are the primary elements that make up a room's décor. Colors can be used throughout the room—on walls, furniture, carpeting, and other items. Fabrics are used primarily on furniture and draperies.

When using several colors, it is important to decorate in color families to avoid a jarring, unprofessional look. A **color family** is a group of colors that work well together. In general, colors fall within two basic areas: cool and warm. Using all cool colors—such as white, blue, and mauve—creates a more harmonious impression in the reception area than mixing cool colors with warm ones such as red, orange, and hot pink. When choosing the color family, consider the mood you want to create, as studies demonstrate that the use of color affects mood. For example,

- Red increases heart rate and blood pressure.
- Blue causes the body to produce calming chemicals.
- Green is easy on the eyes and relaxing.
- Light browns are warm and inviting.
- Black and dark browns are associated with power and depression.
- White is related to cleanliness and purity.

Traditionally, the pediatric office incorporates primary colors for a lively atmosphere (although the use of red should be limited). Obstetric offices are often decorated in pastels; geriatric offices often use soft colors in beige tones.

Other offices tend to use popular decorator color palettes such as earth tones and jewel tones (Figure 7-10). Colors also may reflect the cultural preferences of the dominant patient population. You also might want to consider the effect of color when choosing your scrubs or other office attire.

Fabrics, too, add to the atmosphere in the room. Heavy fabrics such as velvet or brocade are more formal, whereas lightweight or sheer fabrics create a soft, delicate appearance. Patterns on fabrics or wallpaper can immediately change the mood of the room. No matter what the design, fabrics should be easy to clean and maintain.

Many medical offices are carpeted for greater appeal and improved noise reduction. Carpeting, available in a variety of colors and patterns, also provides a comfortable cushion when people walk through the office. Carpeting should be easy to clean and durable enough to handle a large volume of patient traffic. Scatter rugs, which can cause injuries if someone slips on or trips over them, should be avoided.

Furnishings

Chairs should be comfortable but have a straight back to allow the patient to get up easily, especially in obstetric, geriatric, and orthopedic offices. Many attractive stain-resistant cloth fabrics are available for medical use. Choose chairs and tables with rounded—not sharp—corners to avoid injuries.

Arranging Furniture The furniture arrangement can make the office seem comfortable or uncomfortable. If furniture is too close together, patients do not have sufficient space to move around easily or to stretch their legs. They may feel cramped. To ensure that patients have adequate room, a good rule of thumb is to allow 12 square feet of space per person. By this measurement, a 120-square-foot room (10 feet by 12 feet) can accommodate 10 people comfortably.

The furniture arrangement should allow maximum floor space. Patients should be able to stretch out their legs when seated and to walk around the reception area if they wish. Placing chairs against the wall usually produces the greatest amount of floor area. Additional seating in the middle

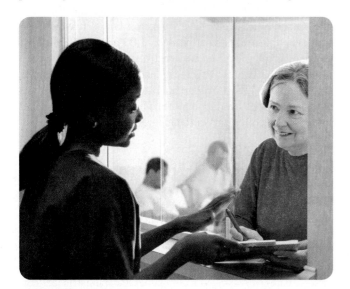

FIGURE 7-9 The receptionist's desk and window are part of every patient reception area and allow for privacy during patient check-in.
©Thinkstock Images/Getty Images

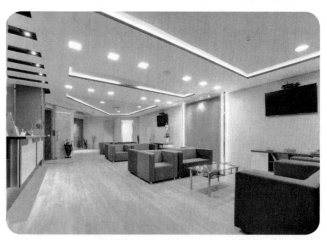

FIGURE 7-10 Decorator colors and furniture groupings make for a comfortable reception area.
©Eviled/Shutterstock

of the room can be placed back-to-back to conserve space. Seats should be grouped so that families or friends can sit together. Remember to reserve room for patients in wheelchairs and to allow enough space for wheelchairs with extended leg supports. Also, keep in mind that some patients value their privacy; placing single chairs or small groups of chairs in corners of the room offers patients some measure of privacy, if needed.

Specialty Items Accessories or specialty items can make the reception area more comfortable and inviting. The following are additional items to be considered when selecting or modifying medical office furnishings:

- Artificial plants and floral arrangements are preferred due to allergies, poisons, and the potential for microbes associated with living plants; these should be kept dust-free.
- Aquariums are popular and soothing but require upkeep. Some offices employ a service to care for the aquarium; others have virtual aquariums.
- Heavy objects such as large aquariums should be built into a wall if possible or securely fastened and stabilized to avoid injury. Likewise, large pictures, shelving, and bookcases should be securely fastened to walls.
- Toys and toy pieces should be easily and frequently disinfected and be larger than would fit into a small child's mouth. Balls and other throwing toys are dangerous in the medical environment.

Although specialty pieces can enhance the room's décor, they should be kept to a minimum. Too many pieces can create a cluttered look. Try to select specialty items that will be pleasing or helpful to patients. A clock is one example. Another useful item is a coat rack, which helps prevent clutter by providing a place for coats, umbrellas, and briefcases. Avoid accessories such as scented candles or potpourri that may be offensive to some people or cause allergic reactions.

Other Considerations

Lighting Most medical offices use fairly bright lighting in the reception area, allowing patients to see their surroundings easily. Subdued lighting, like that sometimes used in restaurants, could be hazardous, as it may cause patients to trip over or bump into hard-to-see objects. In addition, bright lighting is essential for reading—a common activity in the patient reception area. Bright lighting also conveys an impression of cleanliness. Be aware, however, that extremely bright light can be harsh on the eyes and create an annoying glare.

Room Temperature Patients will be uncomfortable if the reception area is too hot or too cold. In an uncomfortable setting, waiting time can seem much longer than it really is, so maintaining an average, comfortable temperature is important.

To ensure a comfortable versus an uncomfortable temperature, keep the thermostat at a temperature that feels comfortable to you and to the office staff. You might periodically survey patients to see if they are comfortable and adjust the setting accordingly. Many elderly people feel cold because of lowered metabolisms. You may want to increase the temperature setting

for a geriatric practice or if the office sees a large number of elderly patients. The room temperature in the reception area may be a bit cooler than in the examination rooms, where patients may be required to disrobe.

Music Many medical offices pipe soothing background music through speakers to the reception area as well as elsewhere in the office. Because the music is meant to calm patients, it should be chosen accordingly. Classical music, light jazz, and soft rock are appropriate choices, whereas heavy metal and rap music are not. Some offices use prepared compact discs. Others tune in to an "easy listening" local (or satellite) radio station.

Educational/Entertainment Materials

Practice-appropriate educational and entertainment materials are more likely to be read by patients if the materials are placed on tables close to the seating. While wall and countertop racks are appropriate and conserve space, keep some materials on tables for easier access by the elderly and differently abled (Figure 7-11). Magazines, newspapers, and other reading material also may be present. The publications should be relatively current and reflect the interests and languages of the populations served. Materials should be neatly arranged, tasteful, and not torn or dirty. Avoid tabloids. Some large-print editions should be available for elderly and other sight-impaired patients.

Magazines and Books Choosing the right mix of reading material to interest all patients is a challenge. You probably have been in offices that have wonderful selections and in an

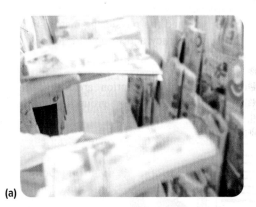

(a)

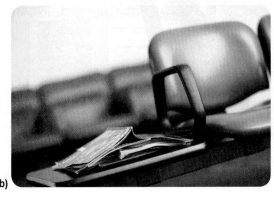

(b)

FIGURE 7-11 (a) Magazine racks save space, but do not forget to have (b) some reading material on tables for elderly or differently abled patients.
(a) ©Indeed/Getty Images, (b) ©Fuse/Getty Images

Maintaining Standards of Cleanliness in the Reception Area

Cleanliness is (and should be) one of a medical office's hallmarks. Not only is cleanliness required in the examination and testing rooms, it is also expected in the patient reception area. A messy patient reception area reflects badly on the practice. Patients may think, "If they don't care about this, what else do they not care about?" Maintaining standards of cleanliness helps ensure that the reception area is presentable and inviting at all times.

As a medical assistant, you may be involved—along with the physician, office manager, and other staff members—in setting the office's cleanliness standards. Standards are general guidelines. In addition to setting standards, you will need to specify the tasks required to meet each standard. You also may want to create a checklist of the tasks required to meet all of these standards.

The following list outlines standards you may want to consider. Specific housekeeping tasks for meeting those standards are included in parentheses.

1. Keep everything in its place. (Complete a daily visual check for out-of-place items. Return all magazines to racks. Push chairs back into place.)

2. Dispose of all trash. (Empty trash cans. Pick up trash on the floor or on furniture.)

3. Prevent dust and dirt from accumulating on surfaces. (Wipe or dust furniture, lamps, and artificial plants. Polish doorknobs. Clean mirrors, wall hangings, and pictures.)

4. Spot-clean areas that become dirty. (Remove scuffmarks. Clean upholstery stains.)

5. Disinfect areas of the reception area if they have been exposed to body fluids. (Immediately clean and disinfect all soiled areas.)

6. Handle items with care. (Take precautions when carrying potentially messy or breakable items. Do not carry too much at once.)

After the standards have been established, type and post them in a prominent place for the office staff (but not the patients) to see. The cleaning activities checklist may be posted, but the person responsible for cleaning the office also should keep a copy. It is everyone's duty to keep the office looking clean and presentable.

A schedule of specific daily and weekly cleaning activities also should be posted. Less frequent housekeeping duties, such as laundering drapes, shampooing the carpet, and cleaning windows and blinds, can be noted in a tickler file so that they will be performed on a regular basis.

It is always a good idea to have a second staff member responsible for periodically working with the medical assistant on housekeeping responsibilities. That person also may be responsible for handling cleaning duties when the medical assistant is away from the office.

waste, is waste that can be dangerous to those who handle it or to the environment. Infectious waste includes human waste, human tissue, and body fluids such as blood and urine. It also includes any potentially hazardous waste generated in the treatment of patients, such as needles, scalpels, cultures of human cells, and dressings.

Although infectious waste is not commonly generated in the patient reception area, it can happen—for example, when a patient vomits or bleeds on the rug or on furniture. If that situation should occur, you must clean up the waste promptly. Remember, infectious waste must be handled in accordance with federal law and following OSHA guidelines. Your office may choose to purchase commercially prepared hazardous waste kits for use in cleaning up spills. After cleaning infectious waste from the patient reception area, deposit it in a biohazard container. Disinfect the site to eliminate possible contamination of other patients. Refer to the chapter *Infection Control Fundamentals* to review OSHA guidelines and standard precautions.

▶ Office Access for All   LO 7.10

The path patients must take to get from the parking area or street to the office and then back out again is called the office access. Some offices have easier access than others, but ease of access is important to your patients, particularly those who are older or differently abled (see Figure 7-13).

Parking Arrangements

Although some patients walk to the medical office or take public transportation, the majority of patients will probably travel by their personal vehicles. Patients who drive to the office need a place to park.

The office can offer either on-street parking or a parking lot or parking garage. On-street parking requires patients to fend for

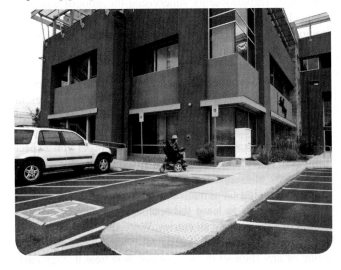

FIGURE 7-13   All patients should have access to ample parking and easy access to the office.

©McGraw-Hill Education/David Moyer, photographer

themselves. They may have to put money into parking meters, and parking spaces may be difficult to find. Both the money required and the potential problems in finding parking spots limit the ease with which patients can gain access to the office.

On the other hand, a free parking lot or parking garage improves office access. Parking lots and garages should be well lit for safety. The number of spaces needed depends on the number of patients scheduled for a specified time period and the average amount of time they spend in the facility. If patients generally spend an hour at the facility and 10 patients are scheduled per hour, then you will need no fewer than 10 parking spaces. Keep in mind that you will need to account for patients who spend more time in the office, and you will need a parking space for each staff member. Periodically reevaluate the office's parking needs because they may change over time. All offices also must provide handicapped parking spaces for patients. Visit http://www.adaptiveaccess.com/handicap_parking.php for more information on handicapped parking. You will read more about patients with special needs later in the chapter.

Entrances

The entrance to the office should be clearly marked so that patients can find the office easily. The name of the practice and of the physician(s) should be on the door or beside the door. Just outside the doorway should be a doormat to help control the amount of dirt tracked into the office. If the office door opens directly to the outside, people inside will feel a sudden change in temperature each time the door is opened in hot or cold weather. A foyer or double-door arrangement helps minimize the weather's effects by keeping the office at a consistent, comfortable temperature. All doorways must be wide enough to accommodate patients using wheelchairs and walkers. Hallways should be well lit and without obstructions.

Safety and Security

Safety and security are important concerns in any public building, and they are especially important for a medical office. To ensure both patient and staff safety, including protection from hazardous wiring or poorly lit hallways, there are guidelines for businesses, some of which pertain to the patient reception area. The medical office also must be secure from burglary.

Building Exits Make sure you and the office staff members are familiar with *all* building exits. As you learned earlier in the chapter, it may be necessary to leave the office quickly, as during a fire, flood, or other emergency. Refer to the instructions in *Emergency Action Plans and Drills,* discussed earlier, for more information about office exits and evacuating the office.

Security Systems No matter where the medical office is located, a security alarm system is a wise investment, even if security personnel patrol the office building. A security alarm system offers valuable protection for the confidential patient information housed in a medical office. After the alarm system is installed, all office staff members should thoroughly familiarize themselves with it. They should be able to arm and disarm it easily and know what to do if it is accidentally activated. Each staff member should have her or his own individually assigned security access code. This number is required to authorize locking or unlocking the system. Like a credit card, bank, or other security PIN (personal identification number), it should never be shared.

Considerations for Patients with Special Needs

Some patients who come into the medical office will have disabilities; that is, they were born with or have acquired a condition that limits or changes their abilities. A more positive way to refer to these patients who are differently abled is the use of the term *special needs*. For example, people who are paralyzed from the waist down have special needs; so do people who are visually impaired. This does not mean that these people cannot perform the same tasks that other people can; they may simply need special accommodations to do so. With some forethought and planning, the office can appropriately accommodate special needs patients. Ensuring wheelchair access through doors and hallways, as mentioned earlier, is just one way. Using ramps instead of steps, as shown in Figure 7-14, allows easier access not only for wheelchair users but also for others who have limited mobility. Allowing additional space in the reception area for wheelchairs, walkers, crutches, and service dogs accommodates several types of special needs patients. Procedure 7-4, found at the end of the chapter, explains how to organize the patient reception area to meet the special needs of patients who are physically challenged. For more information on meeting the needs of the differently abled, visit the Adaptive Access website at http://www.adaptiveaccess.com/index.php.

Americans with Disabilities Act Individuals with special needs are often singled out for their differences and are sometimes discriminated against. For example, if a company building does not have access ramps for wheelchairs, workers in wheelchairs cannot qualify for jobs there. This would

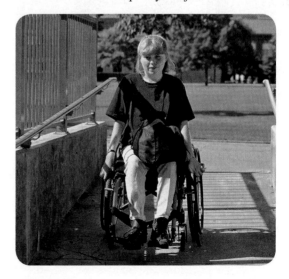

FIGURE 7-14 Ramps allow people using wheelchairs and other assistive devices easier access to the office.
©Patrick Clark/Getty Images

violate the **Americans with Disabilities Act (ADA),** which prevents discrimination based solely on a person's physical or mental disability.

Passed in 1990, this federal act is sometimes referred to as the civil rights act for people with disabilities because it forbids discrimination based on physical or mental disabilities. The intent of the ADA is to provide equal access and reasonable accommodation in several important areas, including employment, facilities, sports, and education. The two sections involving medical practices are employment (discussed in the *Practice Management* chapter) and facilities. The following are required and reasonable facility accommodations:

- Handicapped parking
- Wheelchair ramps
- Wheelchair-accessible doors, halls, and bathrooms
- Handrails in halls and bathrooms
- Handicapped bathrooms including toilets, sinks, and room for a wheelchair to turn
- Braille elevator floor indicators
- Large-print patient forms
- Devices to communicate with the hearing impaired, as discussed in the *Telephone Techniques* chapter

Service Animals A service animal, as defined by the Americans with Disabilities Act, is any dog that is individually trained to do work or perform tasks for the benefit of an individual with a disability, including a physical, sensory, psychiatric, intellectual, or other mental disability (Figure 7-15) The tasks a service dog may perform include but are not limited to the following:

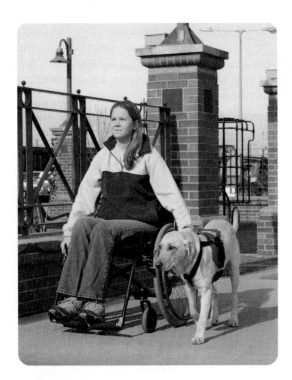

FIGURE 7-15 Service animals should not be disturbed or distracted when working.
©Digital Vision/Getty Images

- Guiding a person with a visual impairment
- Pulling a wheelchair
- Picking up dropped items
- Alerting a person if his blood sugar is high or low
- Reminding a person to take her medications

Service animals wear a special vest that identifies them and they should have a certification. In addition to service animals, you may encounter emotional support animals, also known as comfort animals. These are most often dogs but also may be cats, rabbits, or other animals. Emotional support animals provide comfort to individuals with anxiety, depression, phobias, and other emotional disabilities. In contrast to service animals, emotional support animals are not required to have special task-specific training, and there is no ADA requirement to allow them in workplaces, medical facilities, or other public places.

Vision and Hearing Impairments Although they should, there are still many offices that do not make special accommodations for patients with vision or hearing impairments. As a medical assistant, you can do your part in the office by posting prominent signs in the reception area with information that patients need to know. A staff member should offer to assist patients with hearing or vision impairments as needed from the reception area to the examination room when it is their turn to see the doctor.

Patients who are hearing impaired may request the presence of a certified sign language interpreter to assist in communicating with the medical staff. If requested, federal law requires that the office provide and pay for this interpreter.

It is also helpful, but not required by law, to provide hearing-impaired patients with an alternative communication device for communicating by telephone. This device might be a telecommunications device for the deaf (TDD). This specially designed telephone, formerly called a TTY (teletypewriter), looks similar to a laptop computer with a cradle for the receiver of a traditional telephone. The receiver is placed in the cradle and the hearing-impaired patient can then type the communication on the keyboard. The message can be received by another TDD or relayed through a specialty relay service.

Another type of telecommunications relay service available to hearing-impaired individuals is Video Relay System (VRS). This service allows individuals who use American Sign Language to use a telephone to communicate with others through a communications assistant (CA). The CA and the VRS user can see each other and communicate through signed conversation. The CA can relay the conversation to the other party more quickly and smoothly. You will read more about telecommunications relay services in more detail in the *Telephone Techniques* chapter.

Preparing the Reception Area for a Child with Autism In a medical office, you will most likely have patients who have an autism spectrum disorder (ASD). Individuals with ASD have difficulty with communication and social interactions. Children with ASD are often affected by changes in routine or schedule and new environments and may have severe reactions to sensory overload from loud noises or bright lights. For this reason, patients with ASD may need special accommodations when visiting a medical facility. As a medical assistant, you can make the visit to the healthcare facility easier by:

- Scheduling the appointment first thing in the morning or last in the afternoon.
- Reducing the number of other patients and staff the patient encounters.
- Keeping the lights in the reception area low.
- Turning the volume of music down or off in the room where a patient with ASD is located.
- Taking the patient to the exam room as soon as possible.
- Alerting the healthcare practitioner that the patient is ready.
- Using visual aids and stories to explain procedures.

Older Americans Act of 1965 The fastest-growing segment of the American population is the elderly. Like those who are differently abled, many elderly people face discrimination. One reason for the discrimination may be that with age come medical conditions and disorders that create physical limitations.

Congress passed the **Older Americans Act of 1965** to eliminate discrimination against the elderly. Among other benefits, the act guarantees elderly citizens the best possible healthcare regardless of ability to pay, an adequate retirement income, and protection against abuse, neglect, and exploitation.

What does the Older Americans Act mean for the medical office reception area? If the practice serves elderly patients, the office staff must be sensitive to their special needs. The patient reception area should be as comfortable as possible for patients with arthritis, failing eyesight, and other common ailments of the elderly. Make sure there are a few straight-backed chairs located near the front door and near the examination rooms. These chairs are easier to get into and out of than soft sofas and offer greater back support than low chairs or couches with sinking cushions. In addition, arms on chairs provide support when sitting and standing for patients who are unsteady.

Place reading materials within easy reach of the chairs so that elderly patients do not have to get up from their chairs for them. Have large-print books and magazines available, if possible, for patients with poor eyesight. You also might offer magnifying glasses for patients who like to use them. In addition, make sure that the print on all office signs is large and easy to read. As stated earlier, the patient reception area and restrooms should be well lit to help everyone, including elderly patients, see more clearly.

Special Situations Patients in a medical practice are usually a diverse group of people. Their interests, needs, and medical conditions can have an impact on the design of the reception area.

Patients from Diverse Cultural Backgrounds
The United States has long been called a melting pot because of its mixture of people and cultures. Each culture lends its own special qualities, and together the cultures combine to create a unique blend of people called Americans.

You may work in a neighborhood that has a distinct culture or one in which many cultures are represented. To help patients feel comfortable, make the reception area reflect aspects of the local cultural backgrounds whenever possible. This effort will help patients feel more welcome.

Suppose, for example, that the medical office where you work serves many Latino patients. Posting signs in Spanish and English acknowledges the fact that both languages are spoken in that neighborhood. Providing reading materials, such as newspapers and magazines, in a second language—for both adults and children—is another way to show respect and interest. Decorating the office for Spanish holidays in addition to American ones demonstrates that you care about what is important to patients. Displaying artwork created by local artists and artisans is another idea.

Patients Who Are Highly Contagious Patients may have to come into the physician's office when they are highly contagious. This fact is a concern for all patients, but it is especially critical for patients who are immunocompromised. The immune system of an immunocompromised patient is not functioning at a normal level. Because these patients do not have the normal ability to fight off disease, they are at greater risk than the average person for becoming sick. Patients undergoing chemotherapy and patients with AIDS, for example, have compromised immune systems. Follow transmission-based precautions when dealing with any patient who is highly contagious.

▶ Functions of the Reception Staff LO 7.11

The person who works at the *front desk* is commonly called the receptionist. The receptionist's main function is to greet people, register them, give them direction, and answer the phone. In the past, people have taken the receptionist for granted, but truly, the receptionist is one of the most important people in the practice. Just as the reception area décor gives the patient his first impression of the office itself, it is the receptionist who gives the first impression of the office staff and sets the perception of the care the patient will receive from the medical staff. The multiple tasks the receptionist is responsible for provides the very basis for the patient's medical care and for the overall positive impression you wish to convey to your patients. It is her attitude and communication skills that create this positive (or negative) first impression. This staff member, who is frequently an administrative medical assistant, should immediately acknowledge and greet the arriving patient with a smile and pleasant voice. If the receptionist is on the phone, looking up at the patient with a smile and head nod is appropriate to acknowledge the patient and let him know she will be with him shortly. This small gesture will convey that the office staff is attentive and put the patient at ease from the start of the appointment.

Patient Registration and HIPAA
Patient registration is often referred to as patient check-in or sign-in. In many offices, upon arrival, patients are asked to "sign in" to notify staff that they are there. Two commonly used forms of check-in or sign-in are the paper version and

the digital or electronic version. Both may include the arrival time, the appointment time, and the practitioner's name. As you read in section 5.5, under HIPAA, personal health information (PHI) is considered private and confidential; however, the rules do state that sign-in sheets are allowable, as long as the reason for the visit is not included on the sign-in sheet. If the physician specialty is of a confidential nature (such as psychology or drug treatment), it is suggested that sign-in sheets not be used—by the very nature of seeing the practitioner, an "assumption" about the nature of the visit can be made.

If an electronic sign-in is utilized, two methods are approved:

- Providing a digital pad (similar to electronic debit or charge).
- Use of a computer in the reception area for patients to input information.

Once the patient has signed in, the receptionist will provide him or her with appropriate forms. Returning patients may receive a copy of their information to update. Some offices will interview the patient, line-by-line, and input this information directly into the system. This method is usually more time-consuming than having the patient provide hard copy and then inputting directly from the form. Regardless of which method is used, the information given should be reviewed with the patient.

New patients receive a complete new patient registration packet that includes:

- Demographic/insurance coverage form.
- Authorizations for release of information to insurance carriers, assignment of benefits, and financial responsibility.
- Notice of Privacy Practices.
- Health history.
- Information regarding the payment and other policies of the practice.

The forms must be completed and signed. The patient's or insured party's insurance card and a picture identifier, such as a driver's license, are copied or scanned. The picture identifier is one method to help reduce healthcare fraud by preventing a friend or family member who may not have health insurance from "borrowing" another's insurance card. The ID should be checked every time the patient comes into the office. You will explore medical identity theft in more detail a bit later in this section. From the demographic and health information provided by the patient, the medical assistant initiates a medical record or electronic health record. The record may be totally electronic or a combination of electronic health record and hard-copy financial information or electronic financial information and paper health record. The components of the medical record are covered in the *Medical Records and Documentation* and *Electronic Health Records* chapters. When all forms are completed and signed, the appropriate clinical staff member is notified that the patient is ready to be seen.

Payment

Another reception responsibility is collecting the patient's insurance copayment, which is usually done prior to the visit. The amount of the copayment, if applicable, is usually shown on the patient's insurance card. Depending on the office, acceptable payment methods are cash, check, debit cards, and charge cards. Third-party checks should never be accepted, and any personal checks should be written for the exact amount. Cash and checks are kept in a cash drawer that is locked when the reception desk is unmanned. In some offices, the patient will return to the reception area after the visit and may make any payments due at that time. All financial transactions will be discussed in depth in the chapter *Patient Collections and Financial Management*. Follow-up and referral appointments are often also scheduled at the front desk. Once all patient transactions are completed, the receptionist should extend a pleasant farewell to all patients.

Observation and Updates

Another function of the front desk staff is to be observant. As discussed earlier, some patients should not sit in the main reception area. These include patients who are:

- Having chest pain (adults).
- Experiencing shortness of breath.
- Bleeding.
- Feeling faint (syncope), dizzy, light-headed.
- Vomiting.
- Experiencing an undiagnosed or contagious rash.

If a patient complains of any of these symptoms or if you notice a change in a patient's status, immediately notify a member of the clinical staff, who will determine where to place the patient. If you are concerned about the condition of any patient, do not hesitate to ask the clinical staff for advice.

As mentioned in section 7.6 of this chapter, the receptionist (or any office staff member) should address spills, trash, and any potential hazards—such as frayed cords, broken furniture, or tears in rugs—as quickly as possible. If the reception area becomes overcrowded, "traffic control" is required. Ensure chairs are not occupied with personal items and determine if there is room in treatment areas. Keeping patients updated if appointments are running late is another important function of the front office staff. If the wait time is significant, giving patients the option of rescheduling their appointments shows respect for the patient's time.

The Identity Theft Prevention Program

In many instances, HIPAA and medical identity theft go hand in hand. The person in the practice with the dual responsibility is generally the privacy or compliance officer. A three-pronged approach for the medical office's prevention program is recommended:

1. Prevention—implementing sound electronic and other security systems maintaining HIPAA compliance.
2. Detection—staff training on what to look for and electronic "red flagging" such as automatic on-screen identification of a difference in date of birth.
3. Mitigation—ensuring medical records of the perpetrator and the authentic patient are not co-mingled; the medical assistant should know what to look for in suspicious behaviors and both how to report such behaviors and how to find out if suspicious behavior by the patient has been previously reported.

▶ Opening and Closing the Office   LO 7.12

You are learning that efficiency in the medical office is a result of good organization and adherence to office policies and procedures. These policies include establishing set procedures for opening and closing the facility. This is generally the responsibility of the staff member in the reception area. Following a set routine and using specially designed check sheets ensure no process is overlooked. Some offices perform specific tasks when opening the office, such as restocking supplies, and other offices perform these tasks at closing. Let's take a general look at both of these procedures.

Beginning the Day

The person opening the office arrives approximately 30 minutes prior to the scheduled time for office operations to begin. Safety is a consideration. Be aware of the activity outside the office door such as persons in the parking area, elevators, or hallways. If you feel uncomfortable, notify the facility's security or await the arrival of another staff member. Laboratory specimens, such as blood, obtained by staff for delivery to reference laboratories are often placed in a special container on the office door or in the vicinity. Upon arrival in the morning, ensure the specimens were picked up from the previous day. Do not completely turn your back while unlocking the door. Once inside, deactivate the security system.

The first priority is accessing the answering service or answering machine to determine if any staff member may have called in with an emergency, patients have canceled appointments, patients need a same-day appointment, or hospitals reported patients seen during the night. Convey this vital information to the correct staff member as soon as possible. Other tasks may be to turn on a fax machine or coffee machine. Some offices divide the responsibility for the administrative areas and the clinical areas. Table 7-2 provides a general guideline for opening the medical office.

Ending the Day

Table 7-3 includes typical duties for ending the day efficiently, which is just as important as beginning the day

TABLE 7-2	Daily Checklist for Opening the Office						
Daily Checklist for Opening BWW Medical Associates, PC					W/E_____		
	M	T	W	Th		F	S
1. Security system is disarmed.							
2. Voicemail/answering service messages are retrieved.							
3. Messages are routed and ready for callback.							
4. Computers are turned on.							
5. Appointments and insurance rosters are checked.							
6. If needed, charts are pulled and paperwork is attached.							
7. Equipment is working properly.							
8. Rooms are supplied and ready.							
9. Refrigerator temperature is checked.							
10. Emergency supplies, including O$_2$, are checked.							
11. Reception area is in order and patient education material is available.							
12. Lab specimens from the day before were picked up.							

TABLE 7-3	Daily Checklist for Closing the Office						
Daily Checklist for Closing BWW Medical Associates, PC					W/E_____		
	M	T	W	Th		F	S
1. Computers are logged off and shut down.							
2. Contaminated supplies/equipment are properly disposed of or tagged for cleaning/sterilization.							
3. Areas are restocked.							
4. If needed, patient charts are pulled/reviewed for next day and all test results are available.							
5. Laboratory specimens are in pickup receptacle.							
6. All office equipment is turned off (including kitchen).							
7. Reception area is neat and organized.							
8. Calls are forwarded to voicemail/answering machine.							
9. Medical records are secured.							
10. All doors and windows are locked.							
11. Security system is armed.							

During a Splash or Splatter Emergency

9. Help the victim to the eyewash station.

10. Activate the system.

11. If the eyewash is a plumbed unit, have the victim lean into the eyewash, keeping her eyes continuously open. You may have to don gloves and gown and assist the victim by holding her eye or eyes open.

12. Continuously flush the eyes for at least 15 minutes or the length of time recommended on the SDS, if applicable.

13. Alert the physician or EMS.
    RATIONALE: *So that the victim receives prompt and appropriate postexposure care*

PROCEDURE 7-3 Creating a Pediatric Reception Area

Procedure Goal: To create an appropriate environment for children in the patient reception area of a medical (pediatric) practice

OSHA Guidelines: This procedure does not involve exposure to blood, body fluids, or tissue.

Materials: Children's books and magazines, games, toys, nontoxic crayons and coloring books, television and DVD player, children's DVDs, child- and adult-size chairs, child-size table, bookshelf, boxes or shelves, decorative wall hangings, or educational posters (optional)

Method:

1. Place all adult-size chairs against the wall. Position some of the child-size chairs along the wall with the adult chairs.

2. Place the remainder of the child-size chairs in small groupings throughout the room. In addition, put several chairs with the child-size table.

3. Put the books, magazines, crayons, and coloring books on the bookshelf in one corner of the room near a grouping of chairs.

4. Choose toys and games carefully. Avoid toys that encourage active play, such as balls, or toys that require a large area. Make sure that all toys meet safety guidelines. Watch for loose or small (smaller than a golf ball) parts. Toys also should be easy to clean.
   RATIONALE: *Helps ensure safety in the patient reception area*

5. Place the activities for older children near one grouping of chairs and the games and toys for younger children near another grouping. Keep the toys and games in a toy box or on shelves designated for them. Consider labeling or color-coding boxes and shelves and the games and toys that belong there to encourage children to return the games and toys to the appropriate storage area.

6. Place the television and DVD player on a high shelf, if possible, or attach them to the wall near the ceiling. Keep children's DVDs behind the reception desk and periodically change the video in the DVD player.
   RATIONALE: *Doing so helps ensure safety in the patient reception area, as DVDs and video equipment are easily damaged or destroyed by young patients. Young patients also may be harmed in trying to reach the equipment.*

7. To make the room more cheerful, decorate it with wall hangings or posters.

PROCEDURE 7-4 Creating a Reception Area Accessible to Patients with Special Needs

Procedure Goal: To arrange elements in the reception area to accommodate patients with special needs

OSHA Guidelines: This procedure does not involve exposure to blood, body fluids, or tissue.

Materials: Ramps (if needed), doorway floor coverings, chairs, bars or rails, adjustable-height tables, magazine rack, television/DVD player, large-type and Braille magazines

Method:

1. Arrange chairs to create gaps that allow substantial space along walls and near other chair groupings for wheelchairs. Keep the arrangement flexible so that chairs can be removed to allow room for additional wheelchairs if needed.
   RATIONALE: *To meet all the requirements of the Americans with Disabilities Act*

2. Remove any obstacles that may interfere with the space needed for a wheelchair to swivel around completely. Also, remove scatter rugs or any carpeting that is not attached to the floor. Such carpeting can cause patients to trip and creates difficulties for wheelchair traffic.
   RATIONALE: *Helps ensure safety in the patient reception area*

3. Position coffee tables at a height and location accessible to people in wheelchairs.

4. Place office reading materials, such as magazines, at a height accessible to people in wheelchairs (for example, on tables or in racks attached midway up the wall).

5. Locate the television and DVD within full view of patients sitting on chairs and in wheelchairs so that they do not have to strain their necks to watch.

6. For patients who have a vision impairment, include large-type and Braille reading materials.

7. For patients who have difficulty walking, make sure bars or rails are attached securely to walls 34 to 38 inches above the floor, to accommodate requirements set forth in the Americans with Disabilities Act. Make sure the bars are sturdy enough to provide balance for patients who need it. Bars are most important in entrances and hallways, as well as in the bathroom. Consider placing a bar near the receptionist's window for added support as patients check in.
   RATIONALE: *To meet all the requirements of the Americans with Disabilities Act*

8. Eliminate sills of metal or wood along the floor in doorways. Otherwise, create a smoother travel surface for wheelchairs and pedestrians with a thin rubber covering to provide a graduated slope. Be sure that the covering is attached properly and meets safety standards.
   RATIONALE: *Helps ensure safety in the patient reception area*

9. Make sure the office has ramp access.
   RATIONALE: *To meet all the requirements of the Americans with Disabilities Act*

10. Solicit feedback from patients with physical disabilities about the accessibility of the patient reception area. Encourage ideas for improvements. Address any additional needs.
    RATIONALE: *Doing so lets patients know that their comfort and well-being are important to you.*

PROCEDURE 7-5 Opening and Closing the Medical Office WORK // DOC

Procedure Goal: To ensure readiness and to receive and care for patients in an efficient, organized, and safe manner

OSHA Guidelines: This procedure does not involve exposure to blood, body fluids, or tissue.

Materials: Checklist for opening and closing the office (Tables 7-2 and 7-3 may be used as samples), pen, telephone, and pad of paper

Method:

1. Using Table 7-2, Daily Checklist for Opening the Office, as a guide, simulate the functions of opening the office. Enter the week ending date.
   RATIONALE: *Using a checklist ensures no task is inadvertently skipped.*

Daily Checklist for Opening BWW Medical Associates, PC	W/E _____					
	M	T	W	Th	F	S
1. Security system is disarmed.						
2. Voicemail/answering service messages are retrieved.						
3. Messages are routed and ready for callback.						
4. Computers are turned on.						
5. Appointments and insurance rosters are checked.						
6. If needed, charts are pulled and paperwork is attached.						
7. Equipment is working properly.						
8. Rooms are supplied and ready.						
9. Refrigerator temperature is checked.						
10. Emergency supplies, including O_2, are checked.						
11. Reception area is in order and patient education material is available.						
12. Lab specimens from the day before were picked up.						

FIGURE Procedure 7-5 Step 1   Use a daily checklist when opening the office.

a. Begin by disarming the security system.
b. Telephone the answering service to pick up messages or set the office answering machine or voicemail system to answer calls. Document any messages and notify the appropriate person of the call.
c. Conduct each task on the form, placing your initials in the column for the correct day of the week.
   RATIONALE: *It is important to know who performed each task in case questions arise.*

2. Using Table 7-3, Daily Checklist for Closing the Office, as a guide, simulate the functions of closing the office. Enter the week ending date.

Daily Checklist for Closing BWW Medical Associates, PC	W/E _____					
	M	T	W	Th	F	S
1. Computers are logged off and shut down.						
2. Contaminated supplies/equipment are properly disposed of or tagged for cleaning/sterilization.						
3. Areas are restocked.						
4. If needed, patient charts are pulled/reviewed for next day, and all test results are available.						
5. Laboratory specimens are in pickup receptacle.						
6. All office equipment is turned off (including kitchen).						
7. Reception area is neat and organized.						
8. Calls are forwarded to voicemail/answering machine.						
9. Medical records are secured.						
10. All doors and windows are locked.						
11. Security system is armed.						

FIGURE Procedure 7-5 Step 2   Use a daily checklist to close the office.

a. Begin with logging out and turning off the computers.
b. Use the telephone to turn on the answering machine/voicemail or notify the answering service that the office is closing.
c. Conduct each task on the form, placing your initials in the column for the correct day of the week.
   RATIONALE: *It is important to know who performed each task in case questions arise.*

OUTCOME	KEY POINTS
7.1 **Describe the components of a medical office safety plan.**	The medical office safety plan should include OSHA's Hazard Communication Standard; electrical, fire, and chemical safety; emergency action plans; bloodborne pathogen exposure plans; PPE; and needlestick prevention plans.
7.2 **Summarize OSHA's Hazard Communication Standard.**	The US Department of Labor created OSHA to protect the employees' safety in the workplace. Through the creation and enforcement of standards such as the Bloodborne Pathogens Standard, Hazard Communication Standard, and the Needlestick Safety and Prevention Act, OSHA serves to protect healthcare workers from hazards.
7.3 **Describe basic safety precautions you should take to reduce electrical hazards.**	To reduce electrical hazards in the medical office, you should avoid using extension cords, repair or replace damaged cords, avoid overloading circuits, ensure that all plugs are grounded, dry your hands before using electrical devices, and keep electrical devices away from sinks or other sources of water.
7.4 **Illustrate the necessary steps in a comprehensive fire safety plan.**	A comprehensive fire safety plan must include fire prevention strategies, actions to take in the event of a fire, building evacuation routes and plans, fire drills, and local emergency contacts.
7.5 **Summarize proper methods for handling and storing chemicals used in a medical office.**	When using chemicals in the medical office, you should always wear protective gear, carry the container with both hands, work in a well-ventilated area, never combine chemicals unless it is specifically required in the test procedures, always add acid to other substances if the procedure requires that you combine chemicals, and properly clean up spills immediately.
7.6 **Explain the principles of good ergonomic practice and physical safety in the medical office.**	In order to protect yourself from work-related musculoskeletal disorders at work, you must follow the principles of good body mechanics. Your physical safety at work depends on understanding and applying appropriate workplace safeguards, including never running in an office, taking care when carrying objects through the facility, closing cabinets and drawers, and following appropriate safety procedures in the lab.
7.7 **Articulate the cause of most injuries to medical office workers and the four body areas where they occur.**	Most office-related injuries are those associated with repetitive motions, such as typing, lifting, bending, stooping, and sitting. Common injuries or conditions involve the forearm, wrist, hand, and back.
7.8 **List the design items to be considered when setting up an office reception area.**	The size of the space you have to work with and the schedule of the physicians seeing patients must be considered first. Utilize the space to give as much room and privacy as possible. The décor should include a color family to suit the practice type. Furnishings should be comfortable but easy to get in and out of and easy to clean. Lighting should be appropriately bright to avoid accidental falls. Accessories such as wall hangings, aquariums, coat racks, and magazine racks should complement the décor but not make the room feel cluttered. Current magazines and other reading materials on multiple topics should be available to entertain and inform the patients. TV and/or informational DVDs also may be played. If the practice sees children, special accommodations to entertain them also must be made.

OUTCOME	KEY POINTS
7.9 **Summarize the housekeeping tasks required to keep the reception area neat and clean.**	Housekeeping tasks for the reception area include overseeing the professional cleaning staff (if one is employed), keeping everything in its place, disposing of trash, preventing visible dust and dirt on surfaces, spot-cleaning areas that become soiled, disinfecting areas exposed to body fluids, and handling items with care. OSHA guidelines should be followed in all aspects of keeping the office neat and clean. Standards of office cleanliness should be created and posted for all staff to see.
7.10 **Relate how the Americans with Disabilities and Older American Acts have helped to make physical access to the medical office easier for all patients.**	The Americans with Disabilities Act and the Older Americans Act both prevent discrimination based solely on a person's physical or mental disability or his or her age. Both of these acts mandate accessibility for the differently abled, including, but not limited to, adequate parking for vehicles with and carrying assistive devices such as wheelchairs, ramps instead of stairs, wider doorways and hallways, well-lit areas throughout the office, large-print instructions, and Braille markings for elevators and other instructions.
7.11 **Describe the functions of the front office staff, including patient registration and accepting payments from patients.**	The front office staff greet people, register them, give them direction, observe and report when patients should be transferred quickly to the clinical area, and answer the phone. They also may accept payment for patient visits.
7.12 **Implement policies and procedures for opening and closing the office.**	Maintaining specific policies and procedures for opening and closing the office ensures the necessary tasks are completed daily in a uniform manner. This results in an efficient and prepared medical office each day.

CASE STUDY CRITICAL THINKING

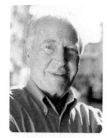

©Image Source/Getty Images

Recall Peter Smith from the beginning of the chapter. Now that you have completed the chapter, answer the following questions regarding his case.

1. How should you respond to Mrs. Smith's request that she be allowed to speak with Dr. Buckwalter privately?
2. Summarize your role as the "first person" Peter Smith (and all patients) sees as he enters the office.
3. What action should you take to prevent Peter Smith and possibly other patients from falling while trying to reach the magazines on the table?

EXAM PREPARATION QUESTIONS

1. (LO 7.8) When designing the reception area for a medical practice, the first consideration should be the
   a. Color
   b. Furnishings
   c. Patient education material
   d. Type of practice
   e. Music

2. (LO 7.2) Which of the following are the sheets that must accompany every hazardous chemical?
   a. GHS
   b. HCS
   c. SDS
   d. OSHA
   e. ADA

3. (LO 7.9) Which federal agency produces guidelines for maintaining office cleanliness and the SDS for cleaning solutions?
   a. HIPAA
   b. ADA
   c. OSHA
   d. FDA
   e. DEA

4. (LO 7.10) A violation of the ADA might be not permitting
   a. Smoking
   b. Pharmacy refills
   c. Charge cards
   d. Service animals
   e. Beverages in the reception area

5. (LO 7.2) OSHA requires that every facility keep a master list of hazardous chemicals in the facility. This is part of
   a. Global System of Hazardous Chemicals
   b. Hazmat Standard
   c. DOT Safety Rule
   d. Chemical Convention Rule
   e. Hazard Communication Standard

6. (LO 7.7) Which injury may be caused by repetitive motions using a computer?
   a. Eye strain
   b. Scoliosis
   c. Arthritis
   d. Whiplash
   e. CTS

7. (LO 7.4) PASS is an acronym for a system outlining the proper use of which of the following?
   a. Fire extinguisher
   b. Chemical hood
   c. Gas-fed open flame
   d. Alcohol-based hand disinfectant
   e. Evacuation plan

8. (LO 7.2) Which of the following requires that all employees receive workplace hazard training?
   a. Standard precautions
   b. Emergency action plans
   c. Needlestick prevention regulations
   d. Hazard Communication Standard
   e. Bloodborne Pathogens Standard

9. (LO 7.11) When the physician is running very late, the receptionist should
   a. Inform patients they will be seen soon
   b. Offer refreshments while the patients are waiting
   c. Cancel appointments
   d. Provide patients with the option to reschedule appointments
   e. Avoid eye contact with waiting patients

10. (LO 7.6) The study of the way people work is known as
   a. Economics
   b. Kinesiology
   c. Ergonomics
   d. Posturing
   e. Accommodation

SOFT SKILLS SUCCESS

You are working in the front office of a medical facility. The office is very busy; the reception area is full of patients waiting to be seen, and you are currently on the phone when a man walks in and says he has to see the doctor immediately. You notice that the man is about 60 years old and appears very pale, is sweating, and is clutching his chest. What action should you take?

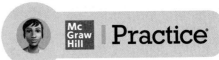

Go to PRACTICE MEDICAL OFFICE and complete the module Admin Check In: Work Task Proficiencies.

Examination and Treatment Areas

CASE STUDY

<table>
<tr><td rowspan="4" style="writing-mode:vertical">PATIENT INFORMATION</td><td>**Patient Name**</td><td>**DOB**</td><td>**Allergies**</td></tr>
<tr><td>Shenya Jones</td><td>11/03/1985</td><td>Peanuts and cinnamon</td></tr>
<tr><td>**Attending**</td><td>**MRN**</td><td>**Other Information**</td></tr>
<tr><td>Elizabeth H. Williams, MD</td><td>00-AA-002</td><td>CA-MRSA. Patient information brochure given to patient.</td></tr>
</table>

Shenya Jones arrives at the office with swelling and a red pustule on her face. She states that the problem started 2 days ago as a small pimple near her nose. It became irritated, and then extremely swollen and painful overnight. This morning, she noticed yellow drainage at the lesion site, and the swelling has increased. The area of drainage

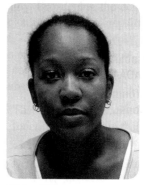
©McGraw-Hill Education

is approximately 1 cm in diameter. Her upper lip, side of the face, and nose are all swollen. The examination and treatment areas need to be prepared before you bring her to the back office.

Keep Shenya in mind as you study this chapter. There will be questions at the end of the chapter based on the case study. The information in the chapter will help you answer these questions.

LEARNING OUTCOMES

After completing Chapter 9, you will be able to:

9.1 Describe the layout and features of a typical examination room.

9.2 Differentiate between sanitization and disinfection.

9.3 List steps to prevent the spread of infection in the exam and treatment rooms.

9.4 Describe the importance of temperature, lighting, and ventilation in the exam room.

9.5 Identify instruments and supplies used in a general physical exam, and tell how to arrange and prepare them.

KEY TERMS

accessibility

ADA Amendments Act of 2008 (ADAAA)

anoscope

consumable

disinfection

examination light

fixative

general physical examination

laryngeal mirror

lubricant

nasal speculum

occult blood

otoscope

penlight

reflex hammer

sanitization

spores

sterilization

Refrigerator Temperature Control

Health inspectors visit medical facilities periodically to check that health and safety standards are being upheld. One of the first things they check is the temperature of refrigerators. To prevent spoilage or deterioration of testing kits, blood specimens, and other stored materials, the laboratory refrigerator temperature should be maintained between 36°F and 46°F (2°C and 8°C). Keep a thermometer in the refrigerator to monitor the temperature. See Figure 9-5.

Similar guidelines apply to the refrigerator in the employee area. Food spoils quickly in a refrigerator if the temperature is not low enough. The temperature of the food refrigerator should be maintained between 32°F and 40°F (0°C and 4.4°C). In addition to monitoring the temperature, make sure food is not stored in the refrigerator too long. All food containers, including brown bags containing lunches, should be dated and thrown out when their freshness has expired. You can prevent bacteria growth by wiping up food spills immediately and cleaning the interior and exterior of the refrigerator routinely.

Follow office procedures for the routine cleaning of both laboratory and food refrigerators and for the proper temperature maintenance of refrigerated contents while the refrigerator interiors are cleaned. Specimens, for example, must be kept at a specific temperature at all times. For documentation purposes, keep a log of dates when the laboratory refrigerator is cleaned.

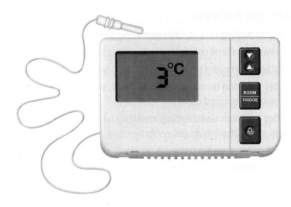

FIGURE 9-5 A temperature monitor is used to maintain a temperature within the refrigerator that prevents spoilage and deterioration of laboratory and food items.

for testing. These specimens must be handled and stored properly because they have the potential to be biohazards. Exposure that can spread disease may occur through the following routes:

- Inhalation (breathing)
- Ingestion (swallowing)
- Transcutaneous absorption (absorption through a cut or crack in the skin)

Occupational Safety and Health Administration (OSHA) regulations require storing biohazardous materials separately from food and beverages. Do not place food and beverages in refrigerators, freezers, or cabinets where blood or other potentially infectious materials are present or put specimens in a refrigerator otherwise used to store food and beverages.

It is dangerous to put food or beverages in the laboratory refrigerator for several reasons. If a biohazardous substance is not clearly labeled and you are in a hurry, you might accidentally ingest it. There is always the possibility that containers of biohazardous substances might leak or spill or that residue from the hazardous material might not have been thoroughly cleaned from the outside of containers. This residue could contaminate food or beverages.

OSHA regulations also require that a warning label containing the biohazard symbol be clearly and securely posted on the outside of refrigerators, freezers, and cabinets where biohazardous materials are stored. The government also recommends keeping the laboratory refrigerator and the refrigerator for the employees' personal use in separate rooms.

These measures help prevent employees from accidentally putting food and beverages in the wrong place.

OSHA regulations prohibit medical personnel from doing any of the following activities in a room where potentially infectious materials are present:

- Eating
- Drinking
- Smoking
- Chewing gum
- Applying cosmetics
- Handling contact lenses
- Putting pencils or pens in your mouth
- Rubbing eyes

These work practice controls, like all OSHA regulations, represent safeguards to protect workers against the health hazards of bloodborne pathogens.

Testing kit and specimen storage often involves refrigeration as a means of preservation. Adequate preservation requires maintaining careful temperature control in a refrigerator. Read the *Caution: Handle with Care:* Refrigerator Temperature Control section for more information on preventing spoilage by controlling refrigerator temperature.

Putting the Room in Order

After ensuring that the examining table is clean, all surfaces are properly disinfected, and all necessary items are stored, take time to straighten the exam room and put things in order. A neatly arranged room boosts patient confidence and supports the impression of a well-run office. It also contributes to the physical safety of patients and staff. Tasks include the following:

- Putting the rolling stool in its place
- Pushing in the examining-table step
- Returning supplies to containers
- Securing sample medications and solutions, prescription pads if used, and other items that may have been left in the room

▶ Room Temperature, Lighting, and Ventilation LO 9.4

No patient wants to sit in an unkempt exam room. Nor do patients feel comfortable in a cold, dimly lit, or stuffy room. Adjusting the temperature, lighting, and ventilation is part of keeping the exam room in good order and fit for use.

Room Temperature
Because patients may be wearing only a thin paper gown or drape while in the exam room, you must be sure the exam room is warm enough. Set the thermostat to maintain the temperature between 70°F and 72°F, and make sure there are no drafts from windows or doors. Patients often feel anxious while waiting for the physician; a warm room can help them relax.

Lighting
Good lighting is required to make accurate diagnoses, to correctly carry out medical procedures, and to read orders and instructions. A well-lit room also helps prevent accidents. Adjust room lights and blinds or drapes as necessary in preparation for an exam. If there is an exam lamp with a movable arm, be sure the arm is positioned appropriately. Replace all burned-out lightbulbs as soon as possible.

Ventilation
The air in the exam area should smell fresh and clean. Periodically, you may have to deal with offensive odors from urine, vomitus, body odors, or laboratory chemicals. First you must eliminate the source of the odor, especially if the source is potentially infectious or toxic. Then you can take steps to remove the odor.

Some exam rooms have a ventilation system with an odor-absorbing filter. If the rooms in your office do not, you may be able to turn on a high-speed blower to vent room air to the outside. In some cases, an open window and a fan may be sufficient to freshen the air. Remember to check the room temperature after using fresh-air approaches to odor control.

If necessary, you can temporarily mask unpleasant odors with a room deodorizer or spray. Some sprays also help kill germs. Be careful that the room deodorizer you choose does not have a strong odor.

▶ Medical Instruments and Supplies LO 9.5

Physicians require various instruments and supplies to perform an exam or procedure. Instruments are tools or implements physicians use for particular purposes. Disposable instruments are often referred to as supplies. You must maintain all instruments and supplies needed in the exam room. This responsibility involves the following three tasks:

- Ordering and stocking all supplies needed for exams and treatment procedures.
- Keeping the instruments sanitized, disinfected, or sterilized (as appropriate) and in working order.
- Ensuring all instruments and supplies are placed where the physician can easily reach them.

Instruments Used in a General Physical Exam
Many of the instruments physicians use are made of reusable fine-grade stainless steel. Some of these instruments may have disposable parts. Physicians also use a number of disposable instruments, such as curettes and needles, because these instruments are both convenient and sanitary. Place any such items contaminated with blood or other body fluids in appropriate biohazardous waste containers.

These commonly used instruments are shown in Figure 9-6:

- An **anoscope** is used to open the anus for an exam. Although not always used for the general physical examination, a stool specimen is usually obtained in order to check for blood.
- An **examination light** provides an additional source of light during the exam. It is usually on a flexible arm to permit light to be directed to the area being examined.
- A **laryngeal mirror** reflects the inside of the mouth and throat for exam purposes.
- A **nasal speculum** is used to enlarge the opening of the nose to permit viewing. This type of speculum may consist of a reusable handle with a disposable speculum tip, or it may be a disposable one-piece unit.
- An *ophthalmoscope* is a lighted instrument used to examine the inner structures of the eye.
- An **otoscope** is used to examine the ear canal and the tympanic membrane. The otoscope consists of a light source, a magnifying lens, and an ear speculum. An otoscope also may be used to examine the nostrils and the anterior sinuses. Like a nasal speculum, an otoscope may have disposable tips.
- A **penlight** is a small flashlight used when additional light is necessary in a small area. It also may be used to check pupil response in the eye.
- A **reflex hammer**—used to check a patient's reflexes—has a hard rubber triangular head.
- A *sphygmomanometer,* or blood pressure cuff, is a piece of equipment used to measure blood pressure.
- A *stethoscope* is used to listen to body sounds. It is described in more detail in the *Vital Signs and Measurements* chapter.

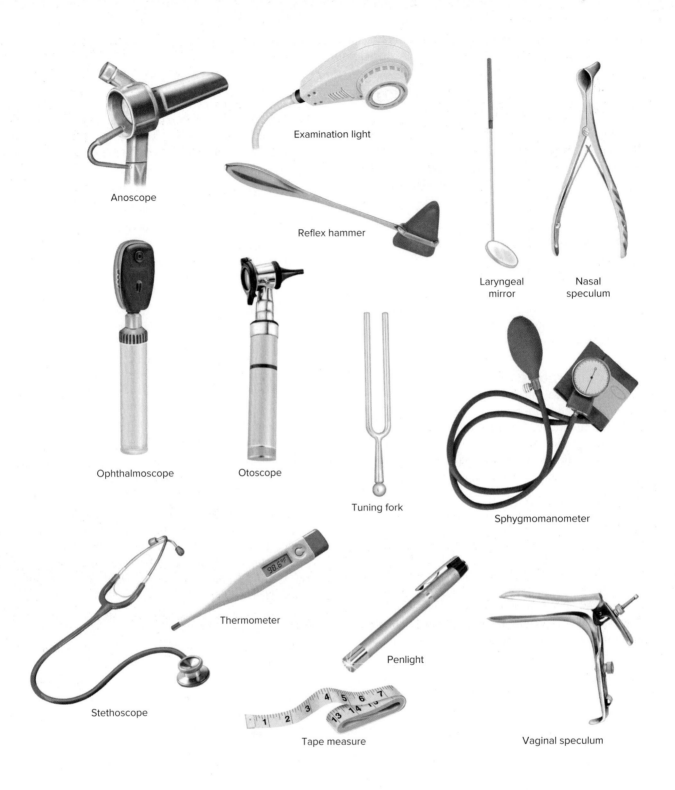

FIGURE 9-6 These instruments may be used in a general physical exam.

- A *tape measure* is a long, narrow strip of fabric, marked off in inches and sometimes in centimeters, used to measure size or development of an area or part of the body.
- A *thermometer* is used to measure body temperature.
- A *tuning fork* tests patients' hearing.
- A *vaginal speculum* is used to enlarge the vagina to make the vagina and the cervix accessible for visual exam and specimen collection. This instrument is used only for

a female when an examination and testing of the female reproductive system are done.

Inspecting and Maintaining Instruments Prior to the exam, make sure all instruments are sanitized, disinfected, or sterilized (as appropriate) and in good working order. For example, test the otoscope and ophthalmoscope to make sure the lights work. Place all rechargeable batteries in a battery charger when the instruments are not in use.

Medical instruments are expensive and are designed to work in precise ways. Read the manufacturers' directions so you are familiar with the care and maintenance of various instruments. Routinely check instruments for chipping and rusting, and report to the physician any instruments that need repair or replacement.

Arranging Instruments The physician must be able to find and reach instruments easily during an exam. You can assist by placing instruments in the same place for every exam or by arranging them in the order the physician will use them.

Physicians usually begin a general physical exam by examining the patient's head and face and working down the body. They may want instruments placed in that order. Other physicians may have individual preferences about how they want instruments arranged. In any case, make certain you know each physician's preferences. Figure 9-7 shows a typical arrangement of instruments.

With the exception of the stethoscope, which most physicians carry with them, instruments are kept in one of three places during an exam:

- Mounted on the wall (sphygmomanometer, some otoscopes and ophthalmoscopes)
- Set out on the countertop (penlight, reflex hammer, tape measure, tuning fork, thermometer, some otoscopes and ophthalmoscopes)
- Set on a clean (or sterile, if appropriate) towel or tray (anoscope, laryngeal mirror, nasal speculum, vaginal speculum)

Preparing Instruments You must prepare some instruments before they can be used. For example, you may need to warm a vaginal speculum by holding it under warm water just prior to the exam. You might warm the mirrored end of the laryngeal mirror with warm water to reduce fogging when the physician is using it. You also can spray it with a special spray that prevents fogging. Any time you will be handling instruments, you must first wash your hands. If the instruments are sterile, you also must wear sterile gloves.

Cleaning Instruments After the exam, put used instruments in a container and take them to the cleaning area. Always handle instruments carefully because mishandling can alter their precision. Dispose of supplies in the appropriate containers, and use approved procedures for sanitizing, disinfecting, and sterilizing reusable instruments and equipment. Refer to Table 9-3 for general guidelines on cleaning instruments.

Supplies for a General Physical Exam

Supplies for a general physical exam may be either disposable or consumable.

Disposable supplies are items that are used once and discarded. These include the following:

- Cervical scraper (a plastic or wooden scraper used to obtain samples of cervical secretions used for female exams only)
- Cytobrush or broom (specialized collection devices often used in conjunction with a cervical scraper to obtain cervical secretions)

TABLE 9-3	General Guidelines for Cleaning Instruments	
Process	**Guidelines***	**Instruments**
Sanitization	• Use detergent, or as indicated by the manufacturer. • Applies to instruments that do not touch the patient or that touch only intact skin • Disinfect these instruments after sanitization if they have come in contact with blood or other body fluids.	• Ophthalmoscope • Otoscope • Penlight • Reflex hammer • Sphygmomanometer • Stethoscope • Tape measure • Tuning fork
Disinfection	• Use only EPA-approved chemical or a 10% bleach solution to kill infectious agents outside the body. • Applies to instruments that touch intact mucous membranes but do not penetrate the patient's body surfaces	• Laryngeal mirror • Nasal speculum
Sterilization	• Use an autoclave or approved method to kill all microorganisms. • Applies to instruments that penetrate the skin or contact normally sterile areas of the body	• Anoscope • Curette • Needle (reusable) • Syringe (reusable) • Vaginal speculum

*Keep in mind, these guidelines are general. Each office may have its own methods and schedule for cleaning instruments, depending on the office's specialty.

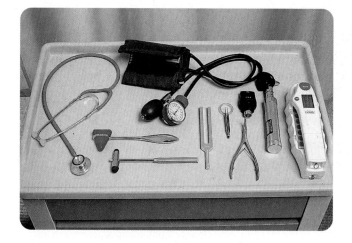

FIGURE 9-7 Arrange the instruments for a general physical exam so that they are convenient for the doctor.
©David Kelly Crow

- Cotton balls
- Cotton-tipped applicators
- Curettes
- Disposable needles
- Disposable syringes
- Gauze, dressings, and bandages
- Glass slides

- Gloves, both sterile and exam (nonsterile) types
- Paper tissues
- Prepared paper slides used to test the stool for the presence of **occult blood** (blood not visible to the naked eye)
- Specimen containers
- Tongue depressors

Consumable supplies are items that can be emptied or used up in an exam. These items include the following:

- **Fixative** (a chemical spray used for preserving a specimen obtained from the body for pathologic exam)
- Isopropyl alcohol (for cleansing skin)
- Lubricant

As they do with instruments, physicians may have a preferred arrangement of supplies for the general physical exam. Figure 9-8 shows typical types and arrangement of supplies. Certain supplies, such as needles, medications, and prescription blanks, if used, should be kept in a locked cabinet away from patient access.

Storing Supplies You can use the cabinets and drawers in the exam room to store nonperishable supplies. Store every item in its own place so you can find it quickly. Consider color-coding or labeling drawers and cabinets so you can easily locate items. Store supplies that come in various sizes, such as bandages, according to size and routinely straighten and clean the insides of all exam room cabinets and drawers.

Restocking Supplies To be sure you have a sufficient quantity of items on hand, order new supplies well in advance

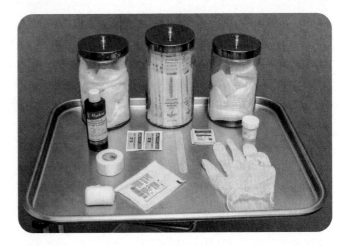

FIGURE 9-8 These supplies may be used in a general physical exam.
©McGraw-Hill Education/Aaron Roeth, photographer

of needing them. A good guideline to follow is to order a new supply when the first half of a box, tube, or bottle has been used up. A recordkeeping system will help you determine which supplies you need to restock most frequently and how long it takes for new supplies to arrive. Keep track of the following information in order to develop such a system:

- The types of supplies your office uses.
- The quantities of each type of supply used in a given amount of time, such as a month.
- The frequency with which you must reorder particular supplies.
- The names of various suppliers, along with the amount of time it takes to receive your orders.

PROCEDURE 9-1 Performing Sanitization with an Ultrasonic Cleaner

Procedure Goal: To decontaminate items safely and effectively using an ultrasonic cleaner

OSHA Guidelines:

Materials: Ultrasonic cleaner, contaminated items and instruments, ultrasonic cleaning fluid, and manufacturer's directions

Method:
1. Review the manufacturer's directions for safe operation of the ultrasonic cleaner.
2. Fill the container of the ultrasonic cleaner with water. Look for the fill line on the machine. In some cases, you may use distilled water.
3. Add the directed amount of ultrasonic cleaning fluid. Typically, only a small amount of fluid is used. Check the directions.

4. Plug in and turn on the ultrasonic cleaner. Some cleaners require a warm-up period. Check the instructions.
5. Separate instruments and equipment made of different metals.
   RATIONALE: *Different metals may fuse together during the cleaning process, making them useless.*
6. Separate instruments with sharp points.
   RATIONALE: *To avoid injury*
7. Open hinges on instruments and equipment.
   RATIONALE: *Contaminated materials can become trapped between two surfaces.*
8. Place instruments and equipment in the ultrasonic cleaner, but do not overfill.
9. Close the lid, turn on the machine or timer, and wait for the cycle to be completed.
10. Rinse each instrument or piece of equipment in cool, running water and then distilled or demineralized water as policy dictates.
    RATIONALE: *Ultrasonic cleaning fluid may cause damage to instruments or equipment.*
11. Dry each instrument or piece of equipment.

12. Prepare each item for storage or further disinfection or sterilization.
13. Replace ultrasonic cleaning solution according to office policy and manufacturers' guidelines.

RATIONALE: *Cleaning solution can be used for several cleaning baths but must be replaced as needed to maintain effectiveness.*

PROCEDURE 9-2 Guidelines for Disinfecting Exam Room Surfaces

Procedure Goal: To reduce the risk of exposure to potentially infectious microorganisms in the exam room

OSHA Guidelines:

Materials: Utility gloves, disinfectant (10% bleach solution or EPA-approved disinfecting product), paper towels, dustpan and brush, tongs, forceps, and a clean sponge or heavy rag

Method:
1. Wash your hands and don utility gloves.
2. Remove any visible soil from exam room surfaces with disposable paper towels or a rag.
   RATIONALE: *Removing visible soil first allows for better penetration of the disinfectant.*
3. Thoroughly wipe all surfaces with the disinfectant.

4. In the event of an accident involving a broken glass container, use tongs, a dustpan and brush, or forceps to pick up shattered glass, which may be contaminated.
   RATIONALE: *Using your fingers to pick up broken glass puts you at risk for exposure to bloodborne pathogens.*
5. Remove and replace protective coverings, such as plastic wrap or aluminum foil, on equipment if the equipment or the coverings have become contaminated. After removing the coverings, disinfect the equipment and allow it to air-dry. (Follow office procedures for the routine changing of protective coverings.)
6. When you finish cleaning, dispose of the paper towels or rags in a biohazardous waste receptacle. (This step is especially important if you are cleaning surfaces contaminated with blood, other body fluids, or tissue.)
7. Remove the gloves and wash your hands.
8. If you keep a container of 10% bleach solution on hand for disinfection purposes, replace the solution daily to ensure its disinfecting potency.

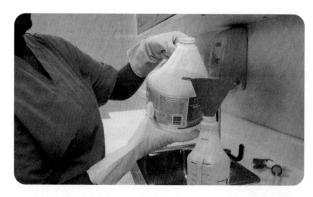

FIGURE Procedure 9-2 Step 8 Replace the bleach solution each day to ensure its disinfecting potency.
©McGraw-Hill Education

FIGURE Procedure 9-2 Step 4 Because broken glass may be contaminated, never pick it up directly with your hands. Use a brush and dustpan, tongs, or forceps to clean it up.
©Cliff Moore

OUTCOME	KEY POINTS
9.1 **Describe the layout and features of a typical examination room.**	A typical examination room is about 8 × 12 feet, large enough to accommodate the physician, the patient, and one assistant. Instruments and equipment in the room should be easily accessible.
9.2 **Differentiate between sanitization and disinfection.**	Sanitization is the scrubbing of instruments and equipment with special brushes and detergent to remove blood, mucus, and other contaminants or media where pathogens can grow. Disinfection uses special cleaning products applied to instruments and equipment to reduce or eliminate infectious organisms.
9.3 **List steps to prevent the spread of infection in the exam and treatment rooms.**	Steps involved in preventing the spread of infection in the examination room include covering the examination table with a paper cover and changing the cover between each patient. It is also important to disinfect all surfaces that come in contact with blood or other body fluids after each patient and at the beginning and end of the day.
9.4 **Describe the importance of temperature, lighting, and ventilation in the exam room.**	A comfortably warm, well-lit, and properly ventilated room will help the patient feel comfortable and more relaxed during the examination.
9.5 **Identify instruments and supplies used in a general physical exam, and tell how to arrange and prepare them.**	A variety of instruments and supplies are used in a general physical examination. To ensure the examination room always has the necessary instruments and supplies, the medical assistant should order and stock all supplies needed for examinations and treatment procedures; keep the instruments sanitized, disinfected, or sterilized and in working order; and place all instruments and supplies where the physician can easily reach them.

CASE STUDY CRITICAL THINKING

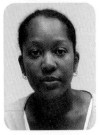

©McGraw-Hill Education

Recall Shenya Jones from the beginning of the chapter. Now that you have completed the chapter, answer the following questions regarding her case.

1. How should you prepare the exam room before Shenya Jones is brought back into the room?

2. Shenya Jones is diagnosed with community-acquired MRSA (a highly contagious microorganism). What measures should you take to ensure there is no transfer of infection?

3. After Shenya Jones has her examination, you will need to use an ultrasonic cleaner for sanitization. Describe how you would proceed and what source you would use if you had questions about the cleaner you are using.

1. (LO 9.1) Door-opening hardware required by the ADA can be grasped with one hand and
   a. Can be locked securely
   b. Is marked with reflective tape
   c. Does not require twisting the wrist to open
   d. Does not catch completely
   e. Opens automatically

2. (LO 9.5) Which of the following is a disposable supply?
   a. Glass slides
   b. Lubricant
   c. Fixative
   d. Isopropyl alcohol
   e. Nasal speculum

3. (LO 9.2) Which of the following may be sanitized and reused without further disinfection or sterilization?
   a. Curette
   b. Otoscope
   c. Laryngeal mirror
   d. Anoscope
   e. Vaginal speculum

4. (LO 9.1) Which of the following would you be *least* likely to find in an examination room?
   a. High-intensity lamp
   b. Medications
   c. Biohazardous sharps container
   d. Rolling stool
   e. Metal wastebasket with lid

5. (LO 9.2) Which disinfectant would *least* likely be corrosive or require ventilation when in use?
   a. Alcohol
   b. Bleach
   c. Hydrogen peroxide
   d. Formaldehyde
   e. Iodine

6. (LO 9.3) In which of the following situations would alcohol-based hand cleaner most likely be acceptable for use?
   a. After cleaning up a blood spill
   b. After changing the paper on the exam table
   c. After assisting with suturing
   d. After your break
   e. After helping a patient in the restroom

7. (LO 9.3) How often should you discard a 10% bleach solution?
   a. Monthly
   b. Weekly
   c. Daily
   d. Hourly
   e. Bleach solution is stable; do not discard it.

8. (LO 9.4) A patient vomits in exam room 2. Which of the following would be your best course of action?
   a. Immediately call the housekeeping department to clean it up.
   b. Spray the room with deodorizer and leave it empty for at least 15 minutes.
   c. Clean up the vomit and then open the window or spray a room deodorizer.
   d. Clean up the vomit, then turn off the ventilation system so the odor does not permeate the entire office.
   e. Turn on the ventilation system and spray deodorizer.

9. (LO 9.5) What instrument is used to look inside the ear?
   a. Ophthalmoscope
   b. Anoscope
   c. Nasal speculum
   d. Vaginal speculum
   e. Otoscope

10. (LO 9.5) Which of the following consumable supplies is used to preserve a specimen obtained during an exam?
    a. Lubricant
    b. Alcohol
    c. Hydrogen peroxide
    d. Fixative
    e. Bleach

Recall Shenya from the case study at the beginning of the chapter. Dr. Williams has finished seeing Shenya and asks you to help her with a patient having a mole removal in the procedure room. Dr. Williams is on a tight schedule because she needs to get to the hospital to see another patient. You know that the room in which Shenya was seen previously still needs to be disinfected and restocked, so you ask Michelle, another medical assistant in the office, to clean the room for you. You explain that Dr. Williams has asked you to assist with a mole removal. Michelle tells you that she does not want to clean the room because Shenya has MRSA and she doesn't want to get it. She also states that because the room is your responsibility, she doesn't think that she should have to clean the room. How should you respond to Michelle?

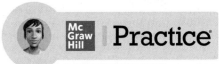

Go to PRACTICE MEDICAL OFFICE and complete the module Clinical: Office Operations.

Electronic Health Records

CASE STUDY

PATIENT TO PATIENT

Patient Name	DOB	Allergies
Ken Washington	12/01/1958	Sulfa

Attending	MRN	Other information
Paul F. Buckwalter, MD	00-AA-008	Takes OTC Excedrin® for headaches

Ken Washington arrives for a routine visit. Although he has not been diagnosed with hypertension, Ken has a strong family history of hypertension. He is concerned about this history and mentions today that he has had occasional weakness in his left arm and he feels that he has had an increase in headaches recently, which are readily

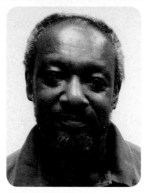

©McGraw-Hill Education

addressed by OTC Excedrin®. While you are checking him in, you notice him looking at the computer monitor on your desk. The monitor is displaying the screen saver for the new EHR program recently installed at the office. He asks, "What is EHR?"

Keep Ken Washington in mind as you study the chapter. There will be questions at the end of the chapter based on the case study. The information in the chapter will help you answer these questions.

LEARNING OUTCOMES

After completing Chapter 12, you will be able to:

12.1 List four medical mistakes that will be greatly decreased through the use of EHR.

12.2 Differentiate among electronic medical records, electronic health records, and personal health records.

12.3 Explain the concept of meaningful use, identifying at least two of its goals.

12.4 Contrast the advantages and disadvantages of electronic health records.

12.5 Illustrate the steps in creating a new patient record and checking in and rooming a patient using EHR software.

12.6 Describe some of the capabilities of EHR software programs.

12.7 Explain how you might alleviate a patient's security fears surrounding the use of EHR.

KEY TERMS

customized
electronic health record (EHR)
electronic medical record (EMR)
face page
face sheet

HITECH Act
meaningful use
personal health record (PHR)
practice management system

MEDICAL ASSISTING COMPETENCIES

CAAHEP

VI.C.8	Differentiate between electronic medical records (EMR) and a practice management system
VI.C.12	Explain meaningful use as is applies to EMR
VI.P.1	Manage appointment schedule using established priorities
VI.P.3	Create a patient's medical record
VI.P.4	Organize a patient's medical record
VI.P.6	Utilize an EMR
VI.P.7	Input patient data utilizing a practice management system
X.C.3	Describe components of the Health Information Portability and Accountability Act (HIPAA)
X.C.10	Identify: (a) Health Information Technology for Economic and Clinical Health (HITECH) Act
X.P.3	Document patient care accurately in the medical record
X.A.2	Protect the integrity of the medical record

ABHES

4. **Medical Law and Ethics**
   f. Comply with federal, state, and local health laws and regulations as they relate to healthcare settings
      (3) Comply with meaningful use regulations
5. **Human Relations**
   h. Display effective interpersonal skills with patients and healthcare team members
7. **Administrative Procedures**
   a. Gather and process documents
   b. Navigate electronic health records systems and practice management software.
   e. Apply scheduling principles
   g. Display professionalism through written and verbal communications
   h. Perform basic computer skills
10. **Career Development**
   b. Demonstrate professional behavior

▶ Introduction

Has your primary care physician (PCP) ever referred you to a specialist, and in the specialist's office, you spent the first 15 minutes filling out a medical history form so the medical staff had "the same medical history" that they have on file at your PCP's office? Have you ever been asked about any medication allergies or your surgical history, and you just could not remember the name of the new drug you developed an allergy to or the year you had your appendix removed? Now, imagine that before you even arrive at the office, the medical staff already has that information at their fingertips, thanks to their new electronic health record (EHR) system. All you need to do is review the information with the specialist to verify that everything is correct to the best of your knowledge. Welcome to the world of electronic health records (EHR).

▶ A Brief History of Electronic Medical Records   LO 12.1

In the early 1990s, it became apparent that paper medical records could no longer meet patients' or healthcare providers' needs. The increasing need for coordination of care (consider how many physicians you see), rising healthcare costs (17.8% of the U.S. gross national product as of 2015), and the rather alarming increase in medical errors fueled this realization. Medical errors as the cause of patient death in the United States is on the rise. Depending on the statistics given and the method used to calculate these statistics, medical errors are somewhere between the third and eighth leading cause of death for hospitalized patients. Most of these errors can be traced to communication problems, including:

- Lost or misfiled paper records.
- Mishandled or "forgotten" patient messages.
- Inaccurate or unreadable information in a paper medical record.
- Mislabeled or unreadable laboratory or prescription orders.

President George W. Bush signed an executive order in August 2006 to promote the overall efficiency and quality of healthcare in America. The base goal was for most Americans to have access to electronic health records by 2014. In most areas of the country, particularly in urban areas, this goal has been met, and electronic medical records are now the rule rather than the exception. The overall goal of this order was to decrease medical errors through record legibility and record uniformity, and to increase information available among patients, medical providers, and the insurance carriers who pay for that care. Meeting this overall goal would help to control the rising cost of healthcare to both the patient and the insurance carriers, including government-funded programs such as Medicare and Medicaid. Although implementation can be expensive, the electronic record (see Figure 12-1) is

have access to the "track records" of licensed practitioners to allow them to choose the best provider for their needs and get answers to questions such as these: Where is the best facility for treating breast cancer or leukemia? Who is most successful in helping patients and families with alcohol and substance abuse issues? Where is the most research being done on current health issues facing single parents or adult caregivers of elderly parents? All of these questions can be answered through the sharing of electronic health information. By sharing information with patients regarding their risk factors, illness, and treatment options, practitioners are engaging patients in medical decisions. Patients who are engaged partners in their care are more likely to adhere to the agreed-upon care plan when they understand the reasoning behind what they are being asked to do. Likewise, when caregivers listen to their patients, the results are more positive for the patient experience, regardless of the ultimate treatment outcome.

The government initiative through the Centers for Medicare and Medicaid Services (CMS) had completed Stage 1 of the EHR implementation, which focused on data capture and sharing of information, as well as Stage 2, which focused on advanced clinical reporting processes. Stage 3 was implemented in March 2017 and, at this writing, is ongoing. It focuses on improved clinical outcomes through the use of EHR programs, known as CEHRT (certified EHR technology). Stage 3 uses the following criteria for this focus:

- Improving quality, safety, and efficiency, leading to improved health outcomes.
- Decision support for national high-priority conditions.
- Patient access to self-management tools.
- Access to comprehensive patient data through patient-centered health information exchange (HIE).
- Improving population health.

As Stage 3 for the EHR initiative is still in process at this time, users and participants of EHR programs are in continual contact with CMS and its subsidiaries to obtain and meet the continually updating standards for this program. Although there are no longer incentives for using EHR programs, for hospitals and larger practices, there are financial penalties for not utilizing and reporting on an approved EHR program. Figure 12-2 shows a typical "dashboard" in an EHR program allowing providers to track their progress in meeting the attestation measures required during each reporting period.

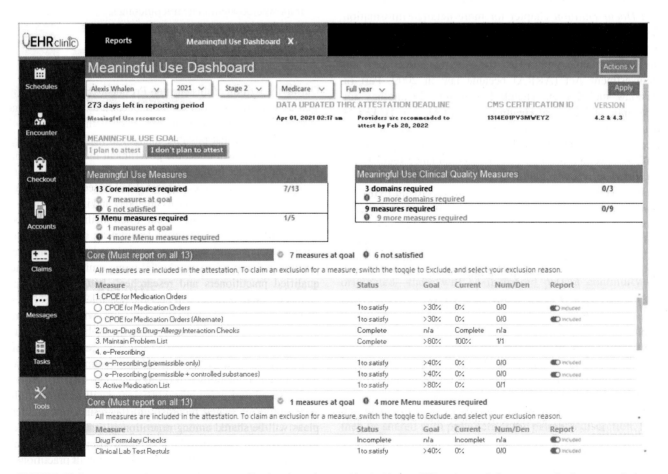

FIGURE 12-2 A meaningful use reporting system like that shown here resides inside your EHR system and allows you to check your practice's progress toward achieving the stages of meaningful use.

Advantages and Disadvantages of EHR Programs

LO 12.4

The government and proponents of EHR programs talk about all the advantages, but there are those who are reluctant to implement EHR. Let's take a look at the pros and cons of EHR programs.

Advantages of EHR Programs

Some of the advantages of EHR programs are:

- Fewer lost medical records (charts do not require pulling or refiling).
- Eliminated (or reduced) transcription costs.
- Increased readability/legibility of charts.
- Ease of chart access for multiple users.
- Chart availability outside of office hours.
- Increased access to patient education materials.
- Decreased duplication of test orders.
- More efficient transfer of records.
- More efficient billing processes using electronic billing methods.
- Greatly decreased storage needs.

In addition to these advantages, a fully functioning EHR program presents other advantages. If a practitioner is at home and needs to access a patient's record, he can access the EHR program from any computer (using his secure access code and password) at any time, review or update the file, and save it to the central computer. See Figure 12-3.

Computerized records also can be used in teleconferences, where people in different locations can look at the same record on their computer screens at the same time. Computer access to patient records is also helpful for healthcare providers with satellite offices in different cities or different parts of a city, and access may be used by a practitioner who is covering a practice while the patient's usual provider is out of town.

Disadvantages of EHR Programs

Cost is the primary reason most providers give for not implementing electronic records in their offices. Although costs for some practice management and EHR programs have come down, for smaller practices, the initial outlay to establish a new system, which also may require new computers to accommodate the system requirements, is simply too steep. Remember too, once a system is implemented, there are yearly maintenance and support costs that also must be factored in. Some practices do not have the initial financial outlay available, nor do they feel the time needed to recoup the initial cost to implement the program justifies the initial (and ongoing) cost of the system. Aside from financial concerns, other reasons for not implementing electronic health records include:

- Staff training requirements.
- Possible need for a full-time or part-time IT staff member.
- Possible damage to the system and to software and/or required upgrades.
- Existing programs that do not fit the needs of the practice.

Working with an Electronic Health Record

LO 12.5

By now, you are beginning to understand some of the EHR advantages. As a medical assistant concerned with patient care and patient confidentiality, you also should understand that the basic rules for working with a medical record do not change when that record is electronic instead of paper. The way you work with the record may change, but the way you treat a record does not. You may refer back to the chapter *Written and Electronic Communication* regarding the basic rules of working with a patient medical record.

General Guidelines for Using an EHR Program

As a medical assistant working with electronic records, you should keep the following in mind:

- Become familiar with the software and hardware used at your facility. Make sure you are not focused on the computer when you are with a patient. Becoming comfortable with the system you are using will help you to focus on the patient. If necessary, take notes and enter them into the computer when the patient is not present until you become comfortable.
- Retrieve the patient record carefully, just as you would with a paper record. Make sure you have identified the patient with at least two identifiers such as the name, date of birth, and/or medical record number.

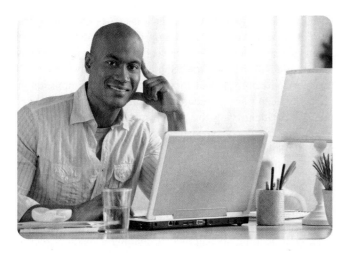

FIGURE 12-3 Electronic health records and a laptop computer with Internet access provide practitioners with easy record access no matter where they are.
©JGI/Blend Images LLC

- Keep your password information secure. Change your password on a regular basis or as directed by the healthcare facility.
- Secure the computer that maintains the electronic records, and keep a backup of electronic files.
- Check your entries carefully before hitting the enter button. An EHR is a legal document just like a paper chart. What is written in the chart occurred, and what is omitted from the chart did not occur.

In addition to these guidelines, many medical record software programs use abbreviations in medical records that may or may not be used in a paper record. Common abbreviations in EHR programs include:

PX for physical exam

SX for symptoms

RX for therapy, treatment, and/or prescriptions

DX for diagnosis

Additionally, because EHR programs are able to incorporate multimedia, graphs are commonly used to track ongoing results such as BP readings, weight, recurring lab results (such as cholesterol or blood sugar), or even photos with measurements to track skin lesions. Be sure you learn and understand how to update the multimedia documents as well as how to work with the standard patient record format.

Another positive in many EHR programs is the ability to enter alerts into a patient's record to remind the practitioner if the patient is due for periodic testing such as a mammogram or colonoscopy. They also can be set up to alert the healthcare provider to abnormal test results, so that the patient can be contacted or counseled. More sophisticated programs can even document health trends, provide voice recognition, and convert notes to complete sentences.

Patient Records and Tracking Using EHR Software

Keep in mind that even though EHR programs eventually will be required to communicate with each other and they are similar in many ways, there will be differences. With practice and time, you will become an expert in your office's EHR program. All programs will have a template that will require completion for each new patient. Included in that template will be *required fields,* such as the patient's full name, date of birth, address, next of kin, gender, and insurance information (Figure 12-4). This information is sometimes part of a **face page,** also known as a **face sheet,** which provides an overview, or "snapshot," of patient demographic information in an EHR system. However, the way you complete these fields will vary with each software package. Procedure 12-1 at the end of this chapter outlines the basic procedure for creating a new patient record using an EHR program.

In addition to allowing you to create patient records, the EHR program allows patients to be tracked and basic information to be recorded when they arrive at the medical facility and are screened. Procedure 12-2, found at the end of this chapter, outlines basic steps to check in and room a patient using an EHR program.

Correcting an Electronic Health Record

As you learned in chapter 11, when correcting a paper medical record, you neatly draw a line through the error and make the correction as close to the original entry as possible. Obviously, once information is saved in an electronic format, a line cannot be drawn through it. In fact, because electronic medical records are legal documents, once information has been saved, it cannot be changed in any way (which is why you want to double-check your work prior to clicking "save"). When an error or omission is found in an electronic record, an addendum to the omitted or incorrect information is made as soon as possible once the error or omission is noted. If an error is noted in a previous entry, many programs allow a note to be inserted at the original entry, telling the user to look at a further entry in the record for the corrected information.

▶ Other Functions of EHR Programs LO 12.6

In addition to the obvious advantages of electronic health records, all interoperable EHR programs have numerous other capabilities. When EHR programs have numerous capabilities, in addition to creating and storing medical records, they are often referred to as **practice management systems.** Let's look at some of the common options for practice management and EHR programs.

Tickler Files

As stated earlier, many electronic health record programs have the capability to act as tickler files (files that need periodic attention). For example, they can alert staff members about patients who are due for yearly checkups and patients who require follow-up care. Some hospitals have begun to use electronically scanned images of patient thumbprints or photos to keep track of records. This also assists with patient security by identifying the patient at the time of each visit, which can cut down on insurance fraud. This system saves time and helps maintain patient record security. (Review the *Office Equipment and Supplies* chapter for more information on computer use in the medical practice.)

Specialty Specific

Once you become accustomed to reading a medical record and documenting in it, you will begin to notice there are similarities in many of the records within any specific specialty. Cardiologists use certain terms such as *cardiomegaly, congestive heart failure, echocardiogram,* and *hypertension*

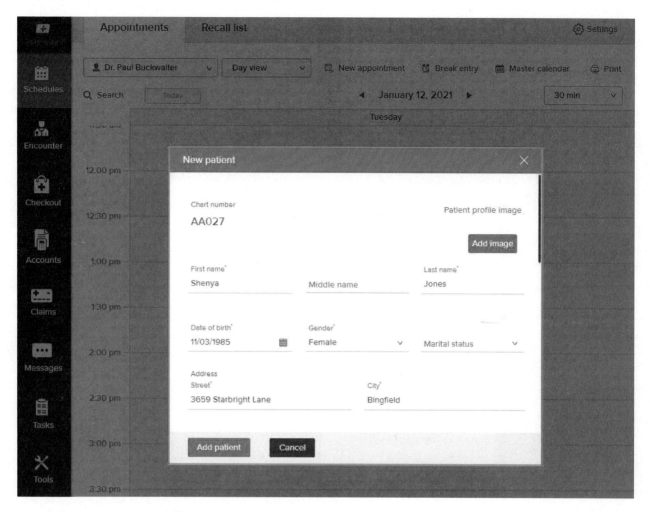

FIGURE 12-4 Screen shot from ⵔEHRclinic showing Shenya Jones being added. Note the black scroll bar on the right will be used to move through the screen and insert the required patient information.

©McGraw-Hill Education

in many of their medical records. On the other hand, an OB/GYN would seldom use those terms, but you would see terms and abbreviations such as *LMP, gravida, para,* and *C-section* in these records. Similarly, when dictating or documenting a physical exam or writing up an operative summary, physicians, like all of us, are creatures of habit and frequently use the same phrases time and time again. Recognizing this, EHR software programs may be **customized** to suit a specific specialty and style of a physician's office. Often, templates or "checkoffs" are available, so with a few simple clicks of the mouse, the physician may add entire sentences or phrases, instead of typing the same information repetitively—saving time and cutting down on errors.

Electronic Schedulers

When working with a paper appointment book, only one user at a time may make appointments. If a staff member is using the appointment book and a patient calls about an appointment, the patient on the phone must wait for the appointment

book to be free before she can be assisted. Ever forget the date of an appointment? In a traditional paper book, the scheduler must go page by page in order to find the forgotten appointment—inefficient at best! Electronic schedulers (Figure 12-5) have several advantages over the traditional appointment book. Multiple users may use them at any time. Depending on the software package you are using, if you need to find a patient's appointment, you can search by the patient's name or even look up the patient's record and the date of the next appointment in the record. In addition to these tasks, electronic schedulers can keep a list of patients who want an earlier appointment if one becomes available and allow you to search for appointments by time frame or appointment type needed (such as a complete physical or a BP check).

One disadvantage of electronic schedulers is the fact that if the computer is down, appointments cannot be made and the day's schedule is not accessible. So it is always a good idea to print out a copy of each day's schedule at

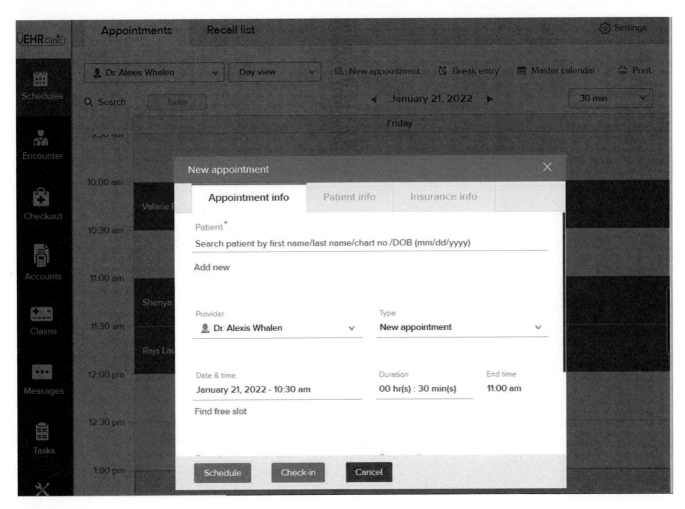

FIGURE 12-5 An electronic scheduler program has many advantages over paper scheduling.
©McGraw-Hill Education

the beginning of the day. Some offices also keep a backup appointment book handy in case of power failure. Some EHR scheduler programs also include appointment reminder and confirmation programs to automatically remind patients of their appointments. These programs then give patients the option to either confirm attendance or change the appointment by phone or online. Procedure 12-3, at the end of the chapter, outlines the steps in creating an electronic scheduler appointment matrix. Procedure 12-4 outlines the (generic) process for booking a patient appointment using an electronic scheduler.

Eligibility Verification and Referral Management

It is always wise—before performing any procedure—to verify the patient's insurance coverage. Many practice management programs make this process easier by assisting with online insurance verification. In addition to verifying coverage, most programs also allow for capturing the patient's demographic information at the same time.

Many managed care programs require the patient's PCP to provide any specialist with a referral before the specialist can

see the patient and before most procedures can be performed. Most EHR software programs not only allow the physicians to readily share information about the patient via the software package but also allow for electronic transmission of referrals among the PCP, the specialist, and the insurance plan involved. In addition, the number of visits allowed by the referral, the time frame involved, and the number of visits left on any given day can be tracked within the patient's medical record.

Billing and Coding Software

Many practice management systems and EHR programs include billing and coding software, allowing for electronic coding of medical records and electronic claims submission to insurance carriers. Depending on the software program being used, the procedure and diagnosis codes may be automatically chosen by the software program based on the medical record or may be coded and inserted manually by the office medical coder (Figure 12-6). Alerts to the system may be added, so if a charge does not match a diagnosis code, a flag is produced. An example would be a patient is seen for a skin

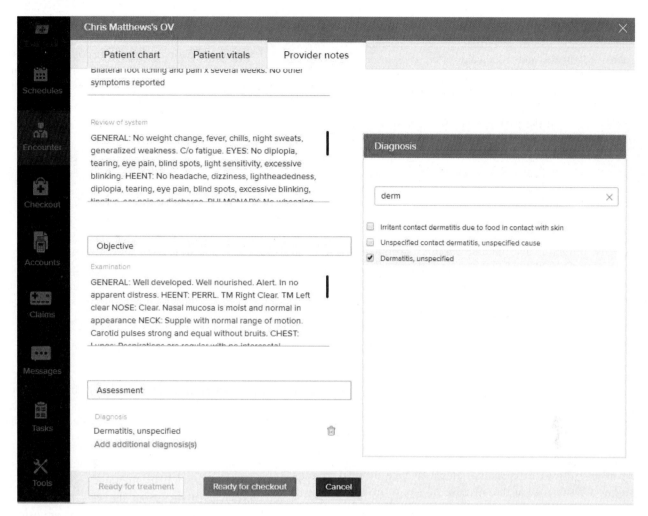

FIGURE 12-6 ◡EHRclinic screen shot of office visit details for Chris Matthews, including the addition of a new diagnosis.
©McGraw-Hill Education

biopsy, but the only diagnosis for the visit is hypertension. Because hypertension is not a reason to do a skin biopsy, an alert would appear stating the diagnosis does not meet medical necessity guidelines. Even if an electronic coding program is being used, an experienced coder should perform random internal coding audits several times a year to ensure that coding is being performed correctly. Once coding is completed, the electronic claim is submitted to the insurance carrier.

Once the insurance carrier has paid the claim, most programs also include a patient billing component so the administrative staff can produce a billing statement for the patient. This statement lists the total amount of the charges, the amount paid by the insurance plan, deductibles, and the copayment or coinsurance balance due from the patient. You will learn more about medical billing and coding in the chapters covering these subjects later in this text.

Report Generators

Most EHR programs also include a report generator, also known as a report writer. This part of the EHR program extracts information from one or more of the patient files and presents that information in a specific format to be used for other purposes. Multiple files are accessed that meet certain conditions. Reports can be used for things such as research or billing and accounting. Report formats may be preset, or you can create your own report to reuse when needed. The types of reports that may be produced include:

- Patient demographics (name, address, phone, marital status, insurance information, etc.).

- Office accounts receivable (A/R) and accounts payable (A/P).

- Office statistics (including the number of individual procedures done during a specified time frame).

- Revenue generated by specific procedures.

- Other tracking mechanisms to assist the office business manager in tracking both profitable and nonprofitable procedures for the practice.

- Patient and insurance carrier aging reports (reports of unpaid invoices arranged according to how long ago the invoices were generated) to see who is or who is not paying the office claims and statements promptly.

Electronic Prescriptions

To encourage the use of electronic prescribing and EHR programs, Medicare and Medicaid offered e-prescribing incentives, and now virtually all EHR programs include prescription writers. These programs allow entry of prescriptions, which may be transmitted directly to the pharmacy or printed and given to the patient. Lists of the most common medications (and dosages) prescribed by the physician also may be kept in the program. Because the program communicates with the patient's individual medical record, any allergies can cause a flag for an ordered prescription; possible medication interactions will do the same.

Ancillary Order Integration

Many EHR programs also include ancillary programs for labs, X-rays, and other diagnostic and therapeutic services. Orders can be submitted to the lab or ancillary office electronically at the time the patient appointment is made. Once testing is complete, the results of the test(s) are transmitted back to the office as soon as they are available, allowing for immediate upload to the patient's medical record. This greatly cuts down on patient and physician wait time for results. Additionally, results may be faxed, scanned, or e-mailed as necessary.

Patient Access

Most patients today are technically quite savvy. In fact, many prefer most communication to occur through electronic means instead of spending telephone time on hold or waiting for someone at the office to be free to make an appointment or provide routine information. Recognizing this, many EHR packages and offices provide patient portals so that a patient can access routine information and perform routine tasks, such as making an appointment, accessing a child's immunization record, or even paying a balance on his account online.

▶ Security and Confidentiality and EHR LO 12.7

When medical records are kept electronically, it is essential that the facility have policies in place to ensure the security and confidentiality of records. As already discussed, all users of the EHR program will have individual access codes and passwords. The access code will allow each user access to only the areas of the record to which the user is entitled, based on his or her job description. Additionally, these access codes insert a date and time stamp within the medical record, including the user's initials, so that office administration and the patient (if requested) may know who is accessing each medical record.

The office also should have a written procedure in place to document when someone requests information from the patient file, if the patient has given permission to release that information, and when it was released. When requested by the patient, this listing must be provided as part of the HIPAA privacy and security act. Protecting the confidentiality of patient records in computer files is the greatest concern of electronic health records. Electronic health records should be kept just as secure as paper records are kept.

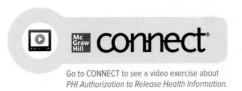

Go to CONNECT to see a video exercise about *PHI Authorization to Release Health Information.*

Remember, too, that whether you are documenting by hand or electronically, accuracy is always important. Careful key entry is essential to maintaining accurate electronic health files to protect both the patient and the medical office. In addition, processes must be in place to back up electronic files on a regular basis to avoid accidental data loss.

Reassuring Others About EHR Confidentiality and Security

As the office medical assistant, it often will be part of your job to reassure patients and other staff members that the office EHR program and the information it contains are confidential and secure. There are several ways you can do this.

- Be knowledgeable about all the confidentiality and security aspects of the office EHR program.
- Never display negativity about the new program, even when things don't go exactly right when you are using it. Remember, there is a learning curve with every new process. Remain patient and interested in the process.
- Suggest the office create a pamphlet or flyer for the patients regarding the office EHR program, and assist in preparing the document.
- When working in the program, show the patient his own medical record and how information is entered, maintained, and saved, including the backup process. Explain the security systems that are in place in easy-to-understand terms to reassure the patient that his medical information is accurate, safe, and secure.
- Explain the office access process to the patients, including the fact that they may view the list of people or companies (such as insurance carriers) that have accessed their information, when the access took place, and why.

Overall, the benefits of electronic health records far outweigh the drawbacks, and because the federal government stepped in to mandate the conversion to EHR, change was inevitable. As the office medical assistant, always be willing to learn any new process, including EHR; assist others with their learning process; and help the patients understand that EHR has only improved the healthcare they receive from your office.

PROCEDURE 12-1 Creating a New Patient Record Using EHR Software

Procedure Goal: To create a new patient record using EHR software

OSHA Guidelines: This procedure does not involve exposure to blood, body fluids, or tissue.

Materials: Initial patient forms (patient information, advance directives, physician notes, referrals, and laboratory orders)

Method:

1. From the)EHRclinic home screen, select "Tools" from the left side of the screen.

2. On this Administrative tools screen, under the Information Management window, click on the blue bar labeled "Manage practice data."

3. At the next screen, Information Management List, choose "Patient Information." At the top of the Patient Listing, click the "Add New Patient" button.

4. The patient's chart number will auto-populate on the new patient screen.

5. If a patient photo is available, select the "Add image" button to upload the image.

6. Using the patient registration form completed by the patient, carefully enter information in each field for this new patient.

7. Some fields, such as *gender* and *marital status,* are completed using a drop-down box obtained by clicking the arrow to the right of the field.

RATIONALE: *This is a legal record. The information must be entered completely and correctly.*

8. Any field marked with an * is a required field. For instance, the patient's address is a required field, as is the identification number. The insurance name field must be completed with the insurance company name. This field may also be used if the patient does not have insurance by entering "none" or used temporarily if the patient has insurance that is new to the practice that must be entered into the system. In any case, the insurance name field is required.
   RATIONALE: *A required field is considered essential information by the practice, so the field cannot be skipped.*

9. Continue entering the information in each field, and use the scroll bar on the right-hand side of the screen to see all of the fields.

10. Inspect all information for accuracy. Once you are satisfied that all information is complete and accurate, click the "Add Patient" button to save the patient information.
    RATIONALE: *This information will become part of the patient's permanent medical record. Proofread all information and verify accuracy before saving.*

11. At the confirmation box, which gives the patient's name and assigned chart or medical record number, click "OK."
    RATIONALE: *The confirmation must be "okayed" or the patient's record will not be saved.*

PROCEDURE 12-2 Checking in and Rooming a Patient Using an Electronic Health Record

Procedure Goal: To follow standard procedures for checking in and rooming a patient using an electronic health record

OSHA Guidelines: This procedure does not involve exposure to blood, body fluids, or tissue.

Materials: Access to the patient's EHR and other pertinent information or documents containing the patient's vital signs and measurements

Method:

1. Using)EHRclinic at the home screen, select "Schedules" from the menu on the left side of the screen.

2. From the provider drop-down, choose the provider the patient is to see and verify that the default date is today's date.
   RATIONALE: *To locate the correct patient, the correct provider and the date of service must be chosen.*

3. Scroll through the schedule to locate the desired patient, and double-click the entry to open the appointment information.

4. On the open patient appointment screen, click the "Check In" button at the bottom of the screen.
   RATIONALE: *If the patient is not checked in to the practice, no information can be added to the medical record.*

5. Complete the additional information related to the patient's appointment on the next screen. This includes auto, employment, or other accident. The default answer for each question is "No." Should the visit be related to one of these accident types, change the default answer to "Yes." Scroll down the entire field and enter any additional information related to the patient's appointment, including the "Date of current illness, injury,

pregnancy"; "Hospitalization dates related to current services"; "Dates patient unable to work in current occupation"; and "Name of the referring provider or other source," if applicable. Once this screen is completed, double-check the accuracy of all your entries, then click the "Check In" button once again. At the confirmation screen, click "Okay."

RATIONALE: *All information must be complete and accurate and the patient is now confirmed as checked in for the visit.*

6. Returning to the menu on the left side of the screen, choose, "Encounter." Locate the patient in the checked-in patient list and click the patient's name once to open the encounter.

7. Complete the patient's vital signs and measurements by either keying the information or using the drop-down menus when available. Enter the height and weight, and the BMI will *auto-populate*. Enter all information available, including the BP, arm examined, patient position, pulse, respiration, pain scale, temperature, temperature type, head circumference, and SpO$_2$ saturation. If any of these readings are not taken, leave the respective field blank.

8. Verify all readings taken are recorded and accurate. Click the "Ready for provider" button. At the confirmation screen, which states, "[patient name] is moved to provider encounter list," click "Okay" to complete the patient check-in process.

RATIONALE: *Without the acknowledgment at the confirmation screen, the check-in process is not complete and the provider will not be notified that the patient is ready to be seen.*

PROCEDURE 12-3 Creating an Appointment Matrix for an Electronic Scheduling System

Procedure Goal: Using an electronic scheduling system to indicate the days and times when the office is not scheduling appointments

OSHA Guidelines: This procedure does not involve exposure to blood, body fluids, or tissue.

Materials: Electronic scheduling program; physician schedule of meetings, conferences, vacations, and other times of unavailability, including staff meetings and hours when patients are not seen

Method:

1. Using ⊖EHRclinic at the home screen, select "Schedules" from the task choices down the left side of the screen.

2. Select the provider for whom the matrix is being created from the provider drop-down field, and then choose "Break Entry" from the top of the screen.

3. Choose the date required for the schedule update or the start date for a repetitive break. For example, the provider may be out of the office for a day or have a staff meeting once a week or month.

4. Verify the time chosen to start the break, then enter the length of time for the break and whether it is to occur in the a.m. or p.m.

5. If this is a repeated break, such as lunch time, choose the repetition required, and then, from the drop-down list, select a reason for the break, such as "lunch."

6. If a further description is desired, you may key a free text description in the description field.

7. Verify that all the information is correct, then click the "Break entry" button.

RATIONALE: *The reason that the time will not be used for patients will appear in the schedule for future reference.*

PROCEDURE 12-4 Scheduling a Patient Appointment Using an Electronic Scheduler

Procedure Goal: Utilizing a matrix to book patient appointments, applying the correct amount of time for each appointment

OSHA Guidelines: This procedure does not involve exposure to blood, body fluids, or tissue.

Materials: Electronic scheduler and template outlining time frames for patient appointment types

Method:

1. Establish the type of appointment required by the patients, particularly noting if the appointment is for a new patient or an established patient.

RATIONALE: *In general, new patient appointments take longer time frames than do existing patient appointments.*

2. If needed, consult the office template for the amount of time required for the patient appointment. Keep in mind the reason for the appointment, as that may affect timing.

RATIONALE: *If a patient is required to be fasting, for example, the appointment should be made earlier in the day and not in the afternoon.*

3. When possible, schedule appointments earlier in the day first, and then move to later time frames. Do ask if the patient has a preferred time frame and, if possible, honor the request.

4. From the ⓊEHRclinic home screen, choose "Schedules" from the task choices listed down the left side of the screen.

5. Select the provider required from the drop-down list at the top of the screen.

6. Click "New appointment." In the Patient field, type the first few letters of the patient's first or last name to locate an existing patient or click "Add New."
RATIONALE: *This allows you to enter the name of a new patient, or once you enter a few letters of an existing patient, choose the correct patient from the drop-down list.*

7. Verify the correct provider for this appointment is listed, or select the correct provider. Select the appointment type, either "New appointment" or "Follow up," using the drop-down arrow to the right of the field.
RATIONALE: *The visit type is required to give the provider an idea of the type of visit scheduled.*

8. Creating the appointment may be done in two ways: using the *Calendar* or using the *Find free slot* option.
   a. Using the *Calendar* option, select the date and time for the visit by clicking the current date and opening the calendar. Choose the date requested and then the start time. Click "a.m." to change the designation to p.m., if required and then click "Done."

   Returning to the Appointment screen, enter the duration required for the appointment

   If repeated appointments are required, choose the repetition type required and the end date for the repetitions.

   b. Using the *Find free slot* option, click the "Find free slot" button.

   Use the From and To calendars at the top of the window to choose the desired date range.

   Choose the appointment duration to change the default duration time, if required.

   From the list produced, choose the requested time slot and click "Select."

   If repeated appointments are required, use the repetition type required and the end date for the repetitions.
   RATIONALE: *This makes it easier to complete multiple appointments for a patient at one time.*

9. Enter the reason for the appointment, verify that all information is correct, and click "Schedule."

SUMMARY OF LEARNING OUTCOMES

OUTCOME	KEY POINTS
12.1 List four medical mistakes that will be greatly decreased through the use of EHR.	Medical mistakes that will be greatly decreased or eliminated with EHR include lost or misfiled paper records, mishandled or "forgotten" patient messages, inaccurate or unreadable information in a paper medical record, and mislabeled or unreadable laboratory or prescription orders.
12.2 Differentiate among electronic medical records, electronic health records, and personal health records.	The electronic medical record is an electronic record of health-related information for an individual patient that is created, compiled, and managed by providers and staff members located within a *single* healthcare organization. An electronic health record is created, managed, and gathered in a manner that conforms to nationally recognized *interoperability standards,* so that members of more than one healthcare organization can utilize it. A personal health record is an electronic version of the comprehensive medical history and record of a patient's lifelong health that is collected and maintained by the individual patient.
12.3 Explain the concept of meaningful use, identifying at least two of its goals.	*Meaningful use* describes EHR as improving quality, safety, and efficiency, and reducing health disparities. It engages the patient and family as well as improves coordination of care for population and public health. Maintenance of the privacy and security of PHI also is required. The goals include better clinical outcomes, improved population health outcomes, increased transparency and efficiency, empowered individuals, and more robust research data on health systems.

OUTCOME	KEY POINTS
12.4 **Contrast the advantages and disadvantages of electronic health records.**	Advantages of EHR include fewer lost medical records, elimination of transcription costs, increased readability/legibility of charts, ease of chart access for multiple users, chart availability outside of office hours, increased access to patient education materials, decreased duplication of medical tests, more efficient records transfer, more efficient billing processes using electronic billing methods, and decreased need for storage space. Disadvantages include cost, need for training, possible need for F/T or P/T IT personnel, and need for computer hardware/software upgrades or changes.
12.5 **Illustrate the steps in creating a new patient record and checking in and rooming a patient using EHR software.**	The same rules apply for EHR as for paper-based medical records when initiating or documenting in a patient's electronic health record. Follow the basic steps in Procedure 12-1 for setting up a new patient EHR and Procedure 12-2 for checking in and rooming a patient using an electronic health record.
12.6 **Describe some of the capabilities of EHR software programs.**	Aside from housing patient electronic health records, many EHR programs also can perform the following functions: tickler files, specialty-specific software, electronic scheduler, eligibility verification and referral management, billing and coding capabilities, report generation, electronic prescriptions and ancillary order integration, and a patient access portal.
12.7 **Explain how you might alleviate a patient's security fears surrounding the use of EHR.**	Be knowledgeable on all aspects of the office EHR program, and never display a negative attitude about it. Assist in preparing written information for the patients regarding the EHR program, including how the patient's medical information will remain confidential and secure. When the patient is in the office, offer to show the patient his EHR, and explain how information is added, entered, maintained, and kept secure. Understand and be able to explain the backup process for the EHR program. Understand the office access policy as it pertains to HIPAA, and explain it to the patients.

CASE STUDY CRITICAL THINKING

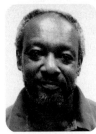

©McGraw-Hill Education

Recall Ken Washington from the case study at the beginning of the chapter. Now that you have completed the chapter, answer the following questions regarding his case.

1. How will you explain the benefits of using electronic health records to Ken Washington?

2. The screen Ken Washington has seen displays only the screen saver for the new EHR program. What precautions should be taken to ensure that patients do not see another patient's information on the computer monitor?

3. The practice you work for wants to review all of the patients who have similar problems as Ken Washington. What function of the EHR program would you use, and what problems would you search for?

1. (LO 12.1) What is the number one patient-related issue to (hopefully) be decreased by the use of EHR programs?
   a. Charting errors
   b. Lost records
   c. Illegible handwriting
   d. Deaths due to medical errors
   e. Decreased risk of falls/injuries for inpatients

2. (LO 12.2) Patient electronic health information created in a format meeting *interoperability standards* is defined as being in a(n)_____ format.
   a. EMR
   b. EHR
   c. PHR
   d. EMR or EHR
   e. None of these

3. (LO 12.2) An individual's lifelong health record is a(n)
   a. EMR
   b. EHR
   c. PHR
   d. Any of these
   e. None of these

4. (LO 12.3) What is the ultimate goal of EHR implementation and meaningful use?
   a. Ability to read practitioner notes
   b. Replacement of transcriptionists
   c. Selling of more practice management systems
   d. Better patient care
   e. Better care of at-risk populations

5. (LO 12.3) Part of meaningful use is to empower patients and families. How is that to happen?
   a. Patients should be given reading material.
   b. Providers should make sure patients understand all their options.
   c. Patients should be given websites to look up information.
   d. Patients should be given material, and providers should make sure patients understand all of their options.
   e. All of these

6. (LO 12.5) Many EHR programs use the term _____ for a correction made to an electronic health record.
   a. Deletion
   b. Error
   c. Addendum
   d. Omission
   e. Correction

7. (LO 12.6) Which of the following functions of the EHR program will be most helpful to the administration when reviewing the financial health of the practice?
   a. Report generator
   b. Tickler file
   c. Billing/coding
   d. Electronic scheduler
   e. Specialty-specific programs

8. (LO 12.6) Which of the functions of the EHR program would be most helpful to the staff member who schedules appointments for patients with specialists?
   a. Billing coding
   b. Specialty-specific programs
   c. Ancillary order integration
   d. Electronic prescriptions
   e. Insurance verification

9. (LO 12.7) Which item maintains each user's ability to work in certain areas of a patient's electronic health record?
   a. Password
   b. Access code
   c. Confidentiality
   d. HIPAA
   e. None of these

10. (LO 12.7) Which of the following will *not* reassure patients about the privacy and security of the office EHR system?
    a. Showing the patient how information is entered in his medical record
    b. Being knowledgeable about the security of the office EHR system
    c. Sharing "computer frustrations" with the patient
    d. Explaining how the backup system for the EHR program works
    e. Assisting in the creation of a pamphlet for the patients regarding the new office EHR system

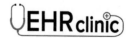

Go to CONNECT to complete the EHRclinic exercises for maintaining Electronic Health Records. See the Table of Contents for a complete list of exercises.

Recall Ken Washington from the case study at the beginning of the chapter.

1. You have just assured Ken Washington that his medical information will be safe on the office's new EHR system. As he is checking out, the administrative assistant, who had been looking up something in his record for the physician, leaves her station momentarily just as Ken walks by. He sees his record up on the screen and is upset. What should you say to Ken?

2. As a follow-up to the incident that occurred with Ken Washington, you have been asked to create a poster for the lounge to help remind the providers and staff of policies related to the use of the new EHR. What things should you include in the poster?

Go to PRACTICE MEDICAL OFFICE and complete the module Admin Check Out: Privacy and Liability.

Telephone Techniques

CASE STUDY

Employee Name	Position	Credentials
Reagan Patrick	Medical Assistant Extern	Student
Supervisor	**Date of Hire**	**Other Information**
Malik Katahri	Externship Start: 04/07/2019	Honors student. Puts a lot of pressure on herself.

Reagan Patrick has been selected by Malik Katahri and his team as their MA extern for this semester. BWW was Reagan's first choice; although excited to be working with this office, she also feels a lot of pressure to be "perfect" during this experience. She has been with them for a few days, and today she will be helping Miguel Perez, the administrative MA, with the phones and front office duties. Reagan feels

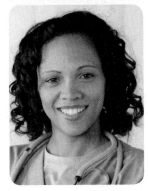
©Terry Vine/Blend Images LLC

she is ready but knows from the little time she has been in the office that as soon as they take the phones off the automated answering system, she is going to have to be at the top of her game as the voice of BWW Medical Associates. As the phone rings for the first time, she takes a deep breath; puts a smile on her face; and, answering on the third ring, says, "Good morning, BWW Medical Associates, this is Reagan. How may I help you?" and her morning begins.

Keep Reagan Patrick in mind as you study this chapter. There will be questions at the end of the chapter based on the case study. The information in the chapter will help you answer these questions.

LEARNING OUTCOMES

After completing Chapter 14, you will be able to:

14.1 Explain the purpose of the telecommunications equipment commonly found in the medical office.

14.2 Relate the five Cs of effective communication to telephone communication skills.

14.3 Define the following terms involved in making a good impression on the telephone: *telephone etiquette, pitch, pronunciation, enunciation,* and *tone.*

14.4 Describe how to appropriately handle the different types of calls coming into the medical practice.

14.5 Summarize the purpose of the office routing list with regard to call screening.

14.6 Carry out the procedure for taking a complete telephone message.

14.7 Outline the preparation required prior to making outgoing calls and the skills used in making the phone call.

KEY TERMS

automated voice response unit

enunciation

etiquette

interactive pager

pitch

pronunciation

telecommunications device for the deaf (TDD)

telephone triage

video relay services (VRS)

V.P.1   Use feedback techniques to obtain patient information, including:
     (c)   clarification

V.P.6   Demonstrate professional telephone techniques

V.P.7   Document telephone messages accurately

V.A.1   Demonstrate:
     (a)   empathy
     (b)   active listening

X.P.3   Document patient care accurately in the medical record

4. **Medical Law and Ethics**
   a. Follow documentation guidelines
   b. Institute federal and state guidelines when:
     (1) releasing medical records or information
   f. Comply with federal, state, and local health laws and regulations as they relate to healthcare settings
     (2) Describe what procedures can and cannot be delegated to the medical assistant and by whom within various employment settings

5. **Human Relations**
   h. Display effective interpersonal skills with patients and health care team members

7. **Administrative Procedures**
   g. Display professionalism through written and verbal communications

10. **Career Development**
   b. Demonstrate professional behavior

▶ Introduction

Most offices have policies and procedures for routing calls that come into the office. You will learn which types of calls you may handle and which should be directed to clinical medical personnel or the practitioner. You will learn to triage (prioritize) calls so that emergencies are handled correctly. Of equal importance, you will learn how to take a complete telephone message, how to be prepared when placing calls, how to leave effective and HIPAA-compliant messages for patients, and how to handle difficult telephone calls, including those from angry patients with complaints and from callers who will not identify themselves.

Finally, in addition to using the telephone correctly, you will learn how other communication devices are used in the medical office, including setting up and using automated telephone menu equipment, voicemail, answering services and machines, TDDs, cell phones, and pagers.

▶ Telecommunications Equipment   LO 14.1

When thinking about telecommunications equipment in the medical office, the first item that naturally comes to mind is the office telephone system. In addition to the office telephone line(s), you also will explore how cell phones, pagers (beepers), answering machines, voicemail, and answering services play vital roles in the medical office's management.

Telephone System

The telephone is one of the most important pieces of communication equipment in the medical practice. It is not only the primary instrument patients use to communicate with the office but also the primary means of communication among providers, hospitals, laboratories, and other businesses important to the practice.

Advances in technology and the advent of the Internet are dramatically changing voice communications. Technologies such as voice over Internet protocol (VoIP), also known as Internet voice, allow the integration of voice and data communication through the computer and Internet service. This means that medical practices have the option of using the computer for Internet access and telephone conversations.

Multiline Phones

Few practices can function with just one or two telephone lines. Most modern medical offices have a telephone system that includes several telephones and multiple lines for incoming or outgoing calls, an intercom system, and the ability to transfer calls, leave voicemail, and put calls on hold (Figure 14-1). The larger the practice, the greater the demand on the phone system. Larger practices often need complex communications systems to handle all their needs.

Call Routing

The telephone system can be set up so that all incoming calls ring on all the telephones in the office, but the more common setup is that one or more "main phones" receive all calls. The receptionist then routes calls to the appropriate telephone extensions.

The **automated voice response unit** is quickly becoming a popular alternative to the traditional phone system, which requires someone to answer each call. An automated menu

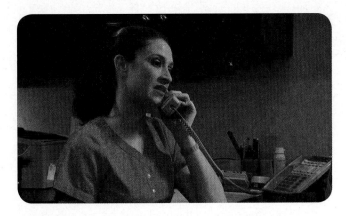

FIGURE 14-1 Most modern medical offices have multiline phones that are capable of multiple functions.
©McGraw-Hill Education

system answers calls for the office, separating requests into categories so that the appropriate staff member can deal with each call efficiently. Using an automated system saves time for office personnel because someone does not have to answer each call and then route it manually to the appropriate person or department. This allows the front office staff to complete other work without interruption.

Patients who reach an automated system hear a recorded message identifying the business. The message gives the caller a list of options from which to choose. Keep in mind that the first instruction the caller should hear is that if the call relates to a medical emergency, the caller should hang up and dial 911. After that, the caller will select an option by pressing the corresponding button on the telephone or by speaking the number of the option. The following are typical options that callers hear.

"Press or say 1 for appointments."

"Press or say 2 for prescription renewals."

"Press or say 3 for the clinical staff and triage nurse."

"Press or say 4 for the billing department."

"Press zero or say 'operator' to speak with an administrative medical assistant."

The last option is of utmost importance so that the patient never feels lost in the system or unable to reach a "live person." Once a caller has chosen an option, the call is automatically routed to the chosen department. If no one is immediately available to answer the call, the caller may leave a message on the voicemail system, which should ask the patient to leave her name, the date and time of the call, and a brief message including a phone number she may be reached. For the voicemail portion of the automated system to be considered "successful" by the patients and other callers, it is imperative that the office staff check the system frequently (at least every hour) and return calls promptly.

Although using an automated voice response unit is efficient for the office staff, its purchase and use must be approved by the office manager and the practitioners before it is implemented. Some practitioners maintain that handling the call of the patient, as the customer and the reason for the practice, is of utmost importance above all other office tasks. If that is the belief of the practitioner, he may be hard-pressed

to feel anything other than a "live person" should be the first voice a patient hears when calling the office. Even when an automated system is in the office, always use the system per office protocol, making no changes without speaking to the office manager and licensed practitioners beforehand.

Other Automated Telephone Options

In addition to using automated voice response systems, many practices use an automated system to place routine reminder calls to patients. Medical assistants spend a great deal of time on the telephone calling patients to remind them of appointments, calling patients about no-shows, and leaving other types of messages.

Keeping in mind that although some licensed practitioners believe that someone should always answer the phone, many other practitioners feel that they can make better use of staff time and ultimately save the practice some money by automating as much of the phone system as possible. A good automated system can offer much more than financial benefits. In addition to reminding patients of upcoming appointments, it can allow them to leave messages for staff. Some systems also can conduct patient surveys and give patients their test results through a privacy mechanism (usually a patient password). Many systems also can assist in managing referrals and authorizations from the managed care organizations requiring them and can assist with preventive care by giving direct access to nurses or medical assistants for minor problems and concerns via the automated routing system.

Voicemail and the Office Phone

As mentioned earlier, an automated menu often includes voicemail. If the office is closed or the person the patient is calling is on the phone or away from her desk, voicemail answers the call, and the caller can leave a message. The advantage of a voicemail system is that the caller never receives a busy signal. Another advantage is that voicemail is a secure system, in that each person on a voicemail system has a unique password to retrieve only her messages.

Answering Machine

If the office phone system does not include voicemail, many offices use a telephone answering machine to answer calls after office hours, on weekends and holidays, and when the office is closed for any reason. A typical recorded message announces that the office is closed and states the usual business hours. In addition, the message must always indicate how the caller can reach the covering provider in the case of an emergency.

Answering Service

Instead of, or in addition to, an answering machine, many medical offices use an answering service. Unlike answering machines, answering services provide people who answer the telephone. They take messages and communicate them to the physician on call, who is responsible for handling emergencies that occur when the office is closed at night or on weekends or holidays. Upon receiving a message from the answering service, the provider returns the patient's call and decides on the course of action.

Answering services can be used in a number of ways. The medical office may use an answering machine to record calls of a routine nature and give the number of the answering service to call in emergencies. Alternatively, the answering service may have a direct connection to the provider's office, picking up calls after a certain number of rings day or night or during specific hours. This ensures that calls do not get missed if the office is very busy and the staff cannot get to the phone.

Some answering services specialize in medical practices. These medical specialty services ask the medical practice to give specific directives for the triage of calls. Although most answering services provide satisfactory, sometimes even outstanding, service, it is good practice to check up on the service every so often by calling it during its coverage hours. This quality check ensures that the service meets office standards and expectations. Always ask any service for references before signing a contract for service.

Cell Phones—Personal and Business Use

Cell phones today are as common as people wearing shoes. In fact, cell phone use is so widespread that many people no longer have a land line. Instead, they depend solely on their cell phones, not only for calls but also for texting, directions, and many online applications (apps) for information and communication. Practitioners, medical practice employees, and patients may all be carrying their own cell phones into the medical office. With all that technology available at a button's touch, cell phone etiquette is a key concern. Generally, it is appropriate to turn off all personal cell phones while inside a medical office. In fact, it is not unusual for offices to have signs posted requesting that cell phones be shut off when entering the office or at least when patients are in the treatment areas. The patients should be shown the same consideration by the practitioners and medical staff. Cell phone calls from outside the practice are usually an interruption in the communication among the practitioners, the staff, and the patient, who, as the *customer* of the practice, should have your full attention. More important, personal cell phone use should be avoided within the office, as it can interfere with other electronic equipment.

However, cell phones play an important part in the business functioning of the medical office. Licensed practitioners may use a cell phone to respond quickly to a message from staff or a hospital. Office staff may use personal cell phones in an emergency when traditional phone systems fail. Some medical practices even issue a cell phone to key employees who conduct business for the practice outside the office. In addition, patients may use their cell phones to call for a ride to take them to their next destination after an appointment. If your medical office allows staff and patient cell phone use, make sure it is clearly noted in which areas cell phone use is permitted and, for employees, when personal cell phones may be used. In most offices, personal cell phones may be used only during break times; at other times, they must be turned off or left in vibrate mode.

Pagers (Beepers)

Physicians and other medical personnel often need to be reached when they are out of the office, so in addition to a cell phone, many also carry pagers (also known as beepers). Pagers are small electronic devices that give users a signal to indicate that someone is trying to reach them. Although generally considered outdated technology, pagers are still used in some places, particularly in rural areas, where cell phone signals are not as reliable.

Technology of Paging Like a cell phone, each paging device is assigned a telephone number. When the number is called, the pager picks up the signal and beeps, buzzes, or vibrates to indicate a call has been made. Most pagers have a window that displays either the caller's telephone number or a short message so that the receiver can return the call. Pagers also can store the telephone number so that the receiver can return several calls without having to write down the numbers.

Calling a Pager Many telephone messages can wait until the practitioner returns to the office or calls in for messages. When a message needs to be delivered immediately and a cell phone is not an option, paging is an efficient response. A list of pager (and cell phone) numbers for each practitioner in the practice should be kept in a prominent place in the office, such as by the main telephone or switchboard. Make sure you know where these numbers are kept. The paging process is as simple as making a telephone call.

1. Look up the telephone number for the pager of the practitioner you need to contact.
2. Dial the telephone number for the pager.
3. You will hear the telephone ringing and the call picked up. Listen for a high-pitched tone, which signals the connection between the telephone and the pager.
4. To operate most pagers, dial the telephone number you wish the practitioner to call, followed by the pound sign (#). (Some pager services have an operator and work much like an answering service. Give the operator a message, and the operator will contact the practitioner.)
5. Listen for a beep or a series of beeps signaling that the page has been transmitted. Then hang up the phone. The practitioner should call the number at his earliest convenience.

Interactive pagers (I-pagers) are designed for two-way communication. The individual is paged in much the same way as with the traditional pager. The pager can be set on "Audio" or "Vibrate" to alert the carrier that a message is coming in. However, the interactive pager screen displays a printed message and allows the provider to respond by way of a mini-keyboard.

The user can respond to the printed page by typing a return message, which is relayed back to the office in real time. The office computer and the user enter into a conversation much like with e-mail, texting or an Internet chat room. Many problems can be handled quickly and efficiently in this manner. Additionally, because the I-pager can function silently, the provider can communicate with her office while in a restaurant without disturbing others or compromising patient confidentiality.

Each interactive pager has its own wireless Internet address. The user types in the receiving party's e-mail address and creates a message on a monitor screen. The interactive pager indicates on the screen when the message has been sent, received, or read. I-pagers can communicate with other I-pagers as well, and they have broadcast capability, meaning the sender can send to more than one receiver at a time. For this reason, I-pagers can be very helpful for practices with multiple practitioners, especially in areas where cell phone service is not always reliable.

I-pagers also can send messages to traditional telephones. The message is typed into the pager, and the system "calls" the telephone number. When the telephone is answered, an electronic voice reads the message to the individual who has answered.

Communicating with Deaf Patients

In conjunction with the Americans with Disabilities Act (ADA) and more importantly in the interest of optimal patient care, it may be necessary for your office to provide assistance in communicating with patients who are severely hearing impaired or deaf. In face-to-face interactions, as in the office setting, many patients are adept at reading lips and/or using American Sign Language (ASL). The question is, how will the office staff and providers respond to allow an equally proficient means of communication on the healthcare end? In the office, if the patient cannot bring someone with her to act as an interpreter, an ASL interpreter may need to be provided. Interpreters may be located (with sufficient notice: several days to several weeks may be necessary) through individual state websites or through through organizations that provide services, such as www.languagesunlimited.com/American-Sign-Language or www.deafservicesunlimited.com. As part of ADA, the practice will be providing this service and will be responsible for any charges related to the interpreting services, not the patient.

The options available for communicating with deaf and hard-of-hearing patients also exist by phone and video service. You may have heard of, or even had experience with, a specially designed phone known as a **TDD** or **telecommunications device for the deaf,** which allows deaf individuals to communicate via telephone using a specialized keyboard that transmits information through another TDD or through a specialty relay service. Today, technological advancements are rapidly replacing TDD with **video relay services** or **VRS**.

VRS, sometimes also known as video interpreting services, is currently the preferred and most common type of telecommunication used by the deaf community. It allows those with hearing disabilities who utilize American Sign Language (ASL) to communicate via telephone using video equipment instead of typed text. The video equipment links the deaf user with an ASL interpreter/VRS operator known as a communication assistant (see Figure 14-2). The patient and assistant can then conduct an ASL conversation using the video monitors. At the patient's request, the communication assistant

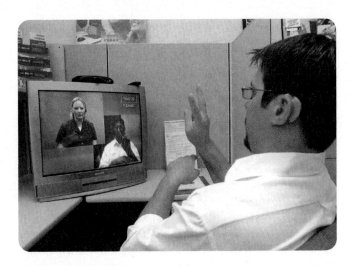

FIGURE 14-2 Video relay services (VRS) allow communication using American Sign Language.

©Lindy Keast Rodman/AP Images

then calls the office and acts as translator between the hearing impaired patient and the office personnel. The office also can "call" the patient by contacting the patient's VRS provider and requesting their assistance. Procedure 14-1, at the end of the chapter, outlines the procedure for using a VRS. More information on communicating with the deaf community may be found at the National Association of the Deaf on its website, https://www.nad.org. Information on VRS services may be found at https://www.fcc.gov/consumers/guides/video-relay-services, as well as at numerous other websites.

▶ Effective Telephone Communication
LO 14.2

When you answer the telephone, you may be someone's first contact with the practice. The impression you leave can be either positive or negative. Your job is to ensure that it is positive.

Good telephone management leaves callers with a positive impression of you, the practitioners, and the practice. Poor telephone management can result in negative feelings, misunderstandings, and an overall unfavorable impression. The image you present over the phone should convey the message that the staff is caring, attentive, and helpful. Showing concern for each patient's welfare is a quality that patients rate highly when evaluating healthcare professionals. In addition, you must sound professional and knowledgeable when handling telephone calls. Using proper telephone management skills will help keep patients informed and ensure their satisfaction with the medical practice.

Communication Skills

Excellent communication skills are important in telephone management because they help project a positive image and thus satisfy the patient's needs and expectations. Individuals who are adept at effective communication employ many of the same communication skills when communicating over the phone as they use when communicating in person. These skills include:

- Displaying tact and sensitivity.
- Showing empathy.
- Giving respect.
- Appearing genuine.
- Displaying openness and friendliness.
- Refraining from passing judgment or stereotyping others.
- Being supportive.
- Asking for clarification and feedback.
- Using paraphrasing to ensure that you understand what others are saying.
- Being receptive to each patient's needs.
- Knowing when to speak and when to listen.
- Exhibiting a willingness to consider other viewpoints and concerns.

As a medical assistant, in addition to using your *active listening* skills (refer to the *Interpersonal Communication* chapter), you also should apply the five Cs of communication. Doing so will allow you to be as effective when using the telephone as you are when having a face-to-face conversation with someone. Get to know and use the five Cs of effective communication in all forms of communication:

- *Completeness:* The message must contain all necessary information.
- *Clarity:* The message must be legible and free from ambiguity.
- *Conciseness:* The message must be brief and direct.
- *Courtesy:* The message must be respectful and considerate of others.
- *Cohesiveness:* The message must be organized and logical.

Guidelines for Using the Telephone Effectively

The following guidelines will help you use the telephone effectively and professionally.

- Answer the phone promptly, by the second or third ring.
- Hold the telephone to your ear, or use a headset to hold the earpiece securely against your ear. Do not cradle the telephone with your shoulder; doing so can cause muscle strain.
- Hold the mouthpiece about an inch away from your mouth and leave one hand free to write with.
- When answering the phone, greet the caller first with the practice name, then with your name. If accepting a call routed by an automated answering system or forwarded to you by someone else, always identify yourself by name.
- Acknowledge the caller. Demonstrate your willingness to assist the caller by asking, "Ms. Jones, how may I help you?"
- Be courteous, calm, and pleasant no matter how hurried you are.

- Identify the nature of the call and devote your full attention to the caller. Do not attempt to multitask while on the phone.
- At the end of the call, allow the caller to hang up first to be sure any questions have been answered. Always say good-bye and use the caller's name.

Following HIPAA Guidelines

As you learned in the *Legal and Ethical Issues* chapter, HIPAA is the law concerned with the privacy and confidentiality of patient information, including information communicated via the telephone. Healthcare providers are allowed to disclose patient information for the purpose of treatment, payment, and health care operations (known as TPO) only. Any use of this information outside of these reasons requires a written authorization from the patient, except in emergency situations or in cases of information required by government agencies for compliance issues. As a general rule, patient information should not be revealed over the phone unless you are speaking directly to the patient or have written consent from the patient to speak to another person about his condition. Always follow your office policy and procedures manual with regard to disclosing patient information. It is also important to note that cell phones are not considered secure methods of communication, so texting should not be used if the message contains any patient PHI.

It is equally important to maintain patient confidentiality regarding patient appointments or their presence in the office. In the same way that you would not share patient information with anyone outside the office, you should never reveal to anyone, whether in person or on the telephone, that a patient has an appointment, is in the office, or is being treated by a member of the healthcare team. It is solely up to the patient to reveal that information.

▶ Telephone Etiquette

LO 14.3

Proper telephone **etiquette** means handling all calls politely and professionally using good manners. Confidence in your role of providing quality patient care includes the ability to communicate effectively not only in person but also on the telephone. Your professionalism and caring attitude must come through the phone to the caller.

Your Telephone Voice

Customer service is critical when using the telephone. After all, your voice is representing the medical office. You must present your message effectively and professionally. Because you cannot rely on body language or facial expressions to help you communicate over the telephone, it is important to make the most of your telephone voice. Use the following tips to make your voice pleasant and effective.

- Speak directly into the receiver. Otherwise, your voice will be difficult to understand.
- Smile. The resulting "smile" in your voice will convey your friendliness and willingness to help (Figure 14-3).
- Visualize the caller and speak directly to that person.
- Convey a friendly and respectful interest in the caller.

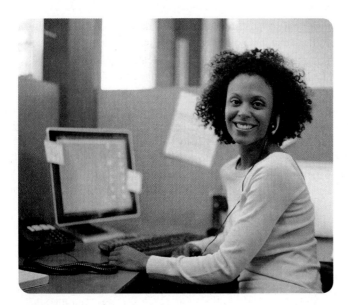

FIGURE 14-3 Smiling comes over the phone, making patients feel you want to help them.
©Thomas Barwick/Getty Images

- Be helpful and alert.
- Use language that is nontechnical and easy to understand. Never use slang.
- Speak at a natural pace, not too quickly or too slowly.
- Use a normal conversational tone.
- Try to vary your pitch while you are talking. **Pitch** is the high or low level of your speech. Varying the pitch of your voice allows you to emphasize words and makes your voice more pleasant to listen to.
- Make the caller feel important.

Pronunciation Proper **pronunciation** (saying words correctly) is one of the most important telephone skills. If you are unsure how to pronounce the name of the person on the phone, ask him to repeat it for you. This demonstrates respect for the person and shows him that he has your undivided attention. When clarifying the spelling of a name, verify letters that sound alike by repeating the letter and including a word that begins with that letter. Examples include D as in dog, V as in Victor, and M as in Mary.

Enunciation The term **enunciation** (clear and distinct speaking) means the opposite of *mumbling*. Good enunciation helps the person you are speaking to understand you, which is especially important when you are trying to convey medical information.

Speaking clearly over the telephone is very important because the speaker cannot be seen. Correct interpretation of the message is determined by hearing the words precisely. Activities such as chewing gum, eating, or propping the phone between the ear and shoulder hinder proper enunciation. Many offices today provide the medical assistant and/or the receptionist with a wireless headset. This hands-free device eliminates the need to hold the phone between your ear and shoulder, reducing office-related neck, back, and shoulder

pain. The wireless headset allows you to speak with the patient and multitask if it is related to the reason for the patient's phone call, such as booking an appointment or accessing her electronic health record. Because each patient deserves your undivided attention, you should not perform tasks unrelated to the caller. While using a wireless headset, always keep patient confidentiality in mind. Anything you say can be heard by people within listening range. As a general rule, do not walk around the office while on the phone with a patient unless an emergency demands that you do so. See Figure 14-4.

Tone Because you are not face-to-face with the caller, the most important measurements of good telephone communication are voice quality and tone. Always speak with a positive and respectful tone.

Making a Good Impression
In a sense, your telephone duties include public relations skills. How you handle telephone calls will have an impact on the medical practice's public image.

Exhibiting Courtesy Show common courtesy by projecting an attitude of helpfulness. Always use the person's name during the conversation and apologize for any errors or delays. When ending the conversation, be sure to ask the caller if there is anything else you can do for him and thank him before hanging up.

Giving Undivided Attention Do not try to answer the telephone while continuing to carry out another task. Before answering the phone, complete any conversations occurring in the office or excuse yourself while you answer the phone. Once you make sure that the call is not for an emergency, ask the caller if you may either put her on hold for a moment or call her back shortly. By interrupting the patient in the office briefly and giving the caller the option as to how she would like her call handled, both patients receive the undivided attention they deserve.

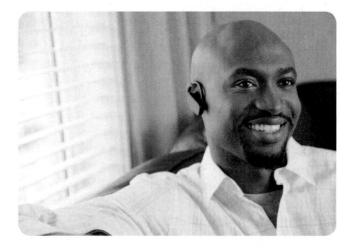

FIGURE 14-4 A wireless device, such as this one, allows you to move around the office, however, always keep patient confidentiality in mind when doing so.
©Kate Kunz/Glow Images

Putting a Call on Hold Although you should try not to put a caller on hold, there will be times when it is unavoidable. Calls may come in on another line, or a situation in the office may prevent you from devoting your full attention to the caller. Sometimes you may have to check a file or ask someone else in the office a question on behalf of the caller. Before putting a call on hold, however, always let the caller state the reason for the call. This step is essential so that you do not inadvertently put an emergency call on hold. Never answer the phone, "Dr. Buckwalter's office, please hold," and immediately put the call on hold. You must ask permission to put the caller on hold and wait for the response.

Your medical office may have a standard procedure for placing a call on hold. Typically, you will ask the caller the purpose of the call, state why you need to place the call on hold, and explain how long you expect the wait to be. Ask the caller if she would like to hold or if she would prefer you to return her call. If she requests a return call, ask her if there is a time that is best for the return call. If she decides to wait on hold and if you cannot end the task at hand quickly, return to the caller every 2 to 3 minutes, asking her if she wishes to remain on hold. An excessive wait on hold makes people feel they have been forgotten or are unimportant. Checking in with them and giving options minimizes these negative thoughts and feelings.

If you know you can return to the line shortly, put the caller on hold and complete your current task or call. If you need to answer a second call, get the second caller's name and telephone number, and unless this call includes an emergency situation, put the call on hold until you have completed the first call. You can then return to the second call. If possible, ask a coworker to assist with the second call, minimizing wait time for both callers.

Returning Patient Calls Some people do not like to hold and will request that you call them back. Obtain the caller's name and phone number, taking the time to repeat both to avoid errors. Return the call in a reasonable amount of time or as close as possible to the time requested by the caller, and give the patient your undivided attention. Be sure to apologize for the inconvenience and thank the caller for her patience.

Remembering Patient Names When patients are recognized by name, they are more likely to have positive feelings about the practice. Using a caller's name during a conversation makes the caller feel important. If you do not recognize a patient's name, it is better to ask, "Has it been some time since you've been in the office?" rather than to ask if the patient has been to the practice before.

Checking for Understanding When communicating by telephone, you do not have visual signals to convey the caller's feelings and level of understanding of the information you are discussing. If a call is long or complicated, summarize what was said to be sure that both you and the caller understand the information. Ask if the caller has any questions about what you have discussed. You may even want to have the caller repeat any instructions to make sure she

understands. If a situation requires a lengthy conversation, it might be best to have the patient come in to the office or to follow up the phone call with a written summary of the discussion. Do not forget to document the call in the patient's medical record.

Communicating with Empathy Whenever information is conveyed over the telephone, feelings also are communicated. When dealing with a caller who is nervous, upset, or angry, try to show empathy (an understanding of the other person's feelings). Communicating with empathy helps the caller feel more positive about the conversation and the medical office.

Ending the Conversation It is not useful to let a conversation run on if you can effectively complete the call sooner. Before hanging up, however, take a few seconds to complete the call so that the caller feels properly cared for and satisfied. You can complete the call by summarizing the important points of the conversation and thanking the caller. Let the caller hang up first.

Occasionally, you will encounter a patient who simply will not hang up. Often these patients are merely lonely, and your friendliness and helpfulness ease their loneliness. In this case, you may find that you must politely but firmly explain that another patient (or a member of the medical team) needs your assistance and you must complete the call. When you put the receiver down, never slam it—even if the caller has already hung up. Remember, all your actions reflect the medical practice's professional image. Patients in the reception area may see (and hear) you when you are talking on the telephone.

▶ Types of Incoming Calls LO 14.4

In dealing with incoming telephone calls, you will encounter a variety of questions and requests from numerous people. Many incoming calls are from patients. You also will receive calls from various people, including attorneys, healthcare providers, pharmaceutical sales representatives, and other salespeople.

Calls from Patients

Patients call the medical office for a variety of reasons, including rescheduling appointments and requesting prescription renewals. If you will be discussing clinical matters over the telephone, it is a good idea to pull the patient's chart. If the office uses EHR technology, this may be as simple as accessing the medical record on the computer screen. If paper records are used, you may need to ask the caller to hold for a moment while you retrieve the record. The information in the chart will often enable you to address any problems quickly. Pulling the chart also allows you to document the conversation immediately.

Always keep in mind that the practice is legally responsible for your actions, including relaying information to patients over the telephone. The office policy manual typically specifies what you may and may not discuss with patients. If you are uncertain about giving particular information to a patient, it is best to discuss the situation with the patient's practitioner or have the practitioner return the patient's call.

Appointment Scheduling Follow office procedures for making or changing appointment times over the telephone. Ask the patient to provide his name, a telephone number where he can be reached during the day, and the reason for the visit. Repeat the information back to the patient to verify all information before ending the call. (Scheduling appointments is discussed in the *Schedule Management* chapter.)

Billing Inquiries If a patient calls about a billing problem, you will need to pull the patient's billing information and possibly the medical record. With this information, you can compare the charges with the actual services performed.

If a patient claims to have been overcharged, check to see if the correct fee was charged. If you find that an error was made, apologize and tell the patient the office will send a corrected statement. Ask the patient to wait for the new statement before sending payment. If, in fact, the proper fee was charged, it may be helpful to speak to the provider before responding to the patient; she may be able to tell you if there were special circumstances regarding the visit or charge in question. Allowing the patient to pay the bill in installments is usually an acceptable option. The details on arranging for payment plans are discussed in the *Patient Collections and Financial Management* chapter.

Many offices use billing services instead of taking care of the insurance submission and monthly patient billing in the office. In that case, the patient may have called the billing service about charges and has now been referred to the office to dispute either the performance of a procedure or its cost. In this case, you may not have access to information about individual charges and may need to refer the patient to the office manager. Be aware that the patient may be upset about the bill and now is being referred to yet another person. Listen patiently to the patient, and take notes regarding the complaint, remaining tactful and understanding about his concerns and possible frustration because obtaining an answer does not appear to be a simple process. No matter what your office policy is, if a patient is dissatisfied, document all appropriate comments and relay the information to the patient's practitioner and/or the office manager. If a bill has not been paid, ask if there are special circumstances affecting the patient's ability to pay. Figure 14-5 gives an example of appropriate documentation of such a call.

Requests for Laboratory or Radiology Reports

If a patient calls the office requesting the results of a test, obtain the patient's chart to see if the report has been received. If it has not, suggest that the patient call back in a day or two. If the need for the result is urgent, you may call the laboratory or radiology office to obtain the results over the phone.

In some offices, you may be authorized to give laboratory results by telephone if they are normal, or negative, so the patient does not have to wait for results to be mailed or for a return phone call from the practitioner. Make a note on

the patient's chart if you provide any information about test results. If a test result is abnormal, the provider will usually wish to speak with the patient. In such a case, tell the patient that the office has received the results and that the provider will call as soon as possible. Then place the patient's chart and the telephone message on the provider's desk. See Figure 14-6 for a chart note example of such a telephone call.

Questions About Medications One of the most common calls from patients involves questions about medications. A patient may ask about using a current prescription or may want to renew an existing one.

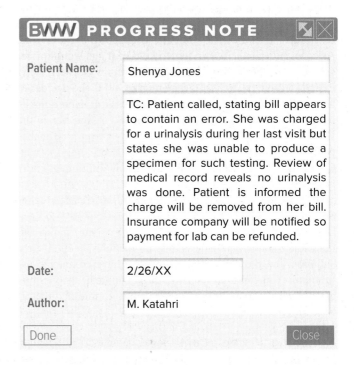

BWW PROGRESS NOTE

Patient Name:	Shenya Jones
	TC: Patient called, stating bill appears to contain an error. She was charged for a urinalysis during her last visit but states she was unable to produce a specimen for such testing. Review of medical record reveals no urinalysis was done. Patient is informed the charge will be removed from her bill. Insurance company will be notified so payment for lab can be refunded.
Date:	2/26/XX
Author:	M. Katahri

Done   Close

FIGURE 14-5 Medical record documentation of a patient telephone call.

BWW PROGRESS NOTE

Patient Name:	Sylvia Gonzales
	TC: Patient called inquiring about FBS result performed 5/10/XX. Reading of 130 given to patient. Per Dr. Whalen, patient is to remain on current insulin dosage.
Date:	5/12/XX
Author:	M. Perez

Done   Close

FIGURE 14-6 Typical chart note documenting patient receipt of lab results by phone.

Prescription Renewals Calls for prescription renewals may come from the patient's pharmacy or from the patient. A pharmacist usually calls to check before dispensing refills if more than a year has passed since the original prescription was written. If the prescriber has indicated in the patient's medical record that renewals are approved, you may authorize the pharmacy to renew a prescription. In any other case, only the prescriber may authorize renewals. If the prescriber authorizes a renewal, you may be asked to phone it in to the patient's pharmacy. Procedure 14-2 at the end of this chapter outlines the instructions for renewing a prescription by telephone. All renewals must be documented in the patient's medical record, with the date and the initials of the person authorizing the renewal. See Figure 14-7.

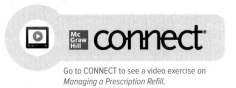

Go to CONNECT to see a video exercise on
Managing a Prescription Refill.

Old Prescriptions Patients may call to ask if they can use a medication that was prescribed for a previous condition. In these instances, recommend that the patient come in for an appointment. Explain why the medication should not be used: It may be old and no longer effective, the current problem may not be the same as the previous one, the medication may not be helpful, and using the medication may mask the symptoms of the current problem, making a diagnosis (and so identifying the proper treatment) more difficult.

If the patient does not want to make an appointment, relay the information to the patient's practitioner, as he or she will probably want to speak with the patient. Again, briefly document the conversation in the patient medical record.

Progress Reports Practitioners often ask patients to call the office to let them know how a prescribed treatment is working. If a patient has a satisfactory progress report, it is not usually necessary that the patient speak to the practitioner. It is important, however, that the medical assistant relay the information to the practitioner and log the call in the patient's medical record immediately. You also may be responsible for making routine follow-up calls to patients to verify that they are following treatment instructions. See Figure 14-8 for an example of a patient's progress report made by telephone. Figure 14-9 shows a patient phone call recorded using)EHRclinic).

Requests for Advice Sometimes patients call the office about problems or symptoms they are having. Although a patient may ask you for your medical opinion, as a medical assistant, you are not licensed to give medical advice of any kind. Explain that you are not trained to make a diagnosis or licensed to prescribe medication. Stress that the patient must see the licensed practitioner. Listen attentively to the patient. If the patient is in distress, try to schedule an appointment that day or as soon as possible.

If the patient cannot come in to the office, assure her that the practitioner will return the call or that you will call back after discussing the problem with the practitioner. Write down the patient's symptoms completely, accurately, and immediately. In many instances, the practitioner may be able to suggest simple emergency relief measures that you can relay to the patient. Occasionally, a patient will want to speak only with the practitioner, not other staff members. You must honor this request.

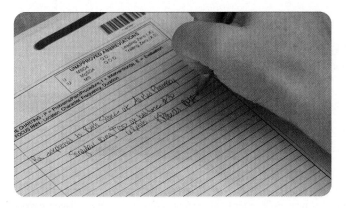

FIGURE 14-7 Documenting a prescription refill.
©McGraw-Hill Education

BWW PROGRESS NOTE

Patient Name:	Mohammad Nassar
	TC: Mohammad called in today to report that the addition of Flovent® to his medication regime is having a positive effect. He has used his rescue inhaler x2 in 3 days. Next appt in one week for recheck.
Date:	5/28/XX
Author:	K. Haddix

Done   Close

FIGURE 14-8 Patient progress note called in by telephone and documented in the medical record.

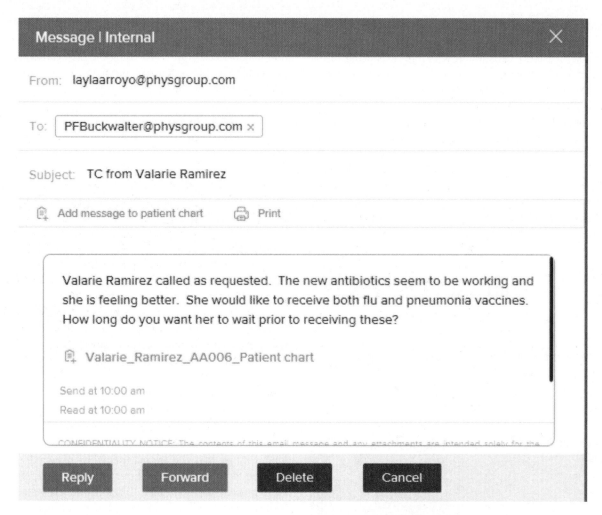

FIGURE 14-9 Telephone message from Valarie Ramirez to Dr. Buckwalter documented using ⊍EHRclinic®.
©McGraw-Hill Education

In some cases, the healthcare provider may feel that a patient's symptoms warrant immediate attention and will insist on seeing the patient before prescribing any treatment. If the patient refuses to come to the office, note the reason on the chart and suggest a visit to the emergency room or to a nearby medical office or urgent care center. As discussed in the *Legal and Ethical Issues* chapter, it is important to document such conversations completely in the patient's chart, including the refusal of treatment. It is always appropriate and professional to offer to take a message to have the patient's provider return the call. Figure 14-10 gives an example of such documentation.

Complaints Even when an office provides the highest-quality care, complaints still occur. When a patient calls with a complaint, such as a medication that does not appear to be working, it is important to listen carefully, without interrupting. Take careful notes of all the details, and read them back to the caller to ensure that you have written them down correctly. Let the caller know the person to whose attention you will bring the complaint and, if possible, when to expect a response.

Always apologize to the caller for any inconvenience the problem may have caused, even if the problem occurred through no fault of the office. Make sure the proper person receives the information about the complaint.

Sometimes a patient who calls with a complaint is angry. Responding to this type of call can be difficult and uncomfortable. Your first priority is to stay calm and try to pacify the caller. Follow these guidelines when dealing with an angry caller.

- Listen carefully and acknowledge the patient's anger. By understanding the problem, you will be better able to work toward a solution.
- Remain calm and speak gently and kindly. Do not act superior or talk down to the patient. Do not interrupt the patient. Do not return the anger or blame.
- Let the patient know that you will do your best to correct the problem. This message will convey that you care.
- Take careful notes and be sure to document the call.
- Do not become defensive.
- Never make promises you cannot keep.

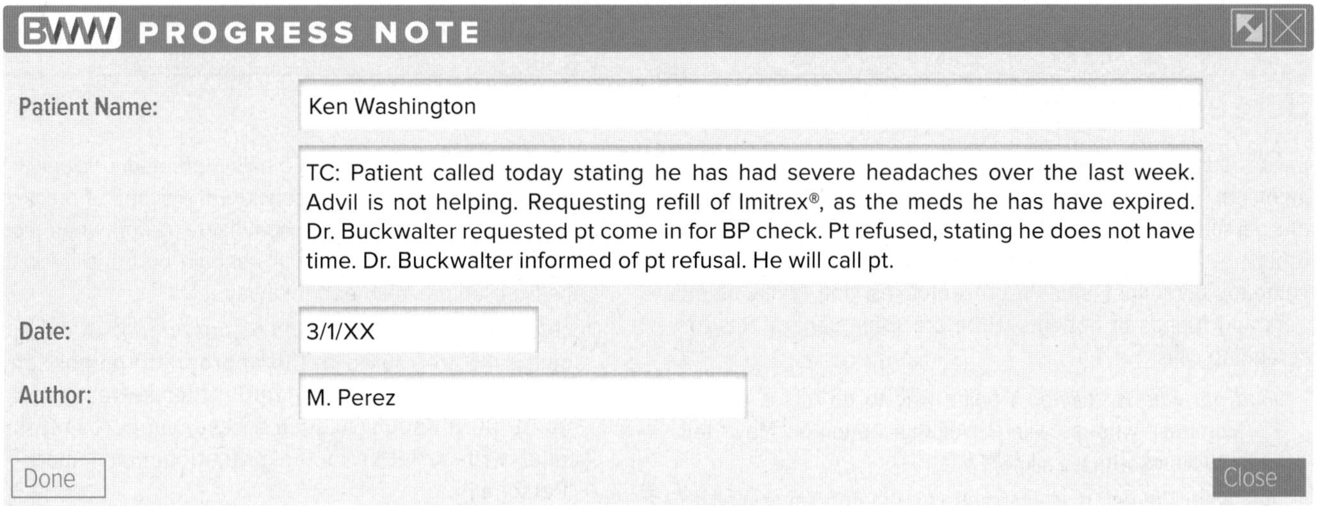

Patient Name:	Ken Washington

TC: Patient called today stating he has had severe headaches over the last week. Advil is not helping. Requesting refill of Imitrex®, as the meds he has have expired. Dr. Buckwalter requested pt come in for BP check. Pt refused, stating he does not have time. Dr. Buckwalter informed of pt refusal. He will call pt.

Date:	3/1/XX
Author:	M. Perez

Done | Close

FIGURE 14-10 Chart note documenting patient refusal of a treatment request.

- Follow up promptly on the problem.
- Any time a staff member has a difficult time with a patient, it is important to inform the patient's practitioner or the office manager, even when the situation is resolved. Always inform the practitioner and/or your supervisor immediately if an angry patient threatens legal action against the office.

Other Calls

Besides calls from patients, a medical office receives many other types of calls. For example, family members and friends of practitioners may call providers at the office. However, the use of the office telephone is never appropriate for personal calls. Always follow office policies and procedures when handling these calls.

Remember, a patient's information is confidential. As discussed previously, HIPAA requires medical providers to obtain authorization from the patient before any information can be disclosed. This is usually in the form of a written, patient-signed authorization indicating what type of information may be given out and to whom. The following are guidelines for managing calls from attorneys, other practitioners, and salespeople.

Attorneys Refer to the procedures listed in the office policies and procedures manual regarding how to handle calls from attorneys. Follow the office guidelines closely, and ask the practitioner or practice manager how to proceed if you receive a call that does not fall within the guidelines. Remember, never release any patient information to an outside caller unless the patient's provider has asked you to do so.

Other Healthcare Providers Patients at your practice may be referred to surgeons, specialists, and other licensed practitioners for consultations. Consequently, you may receive calls from those providers or from their offices. Route those calls to the appropriate practitioner if the caller requests that you do so. Always remember to ask if the call is about a medical emergency. Also keep in mind that you may not give out any patient information—even to another healthcare provider—unless you have a written, signed release from the patient. The exception to this rule is information requested by practitioners to whom you have referred the patient for care. Because of the referral, there is a contract involved for continuity of care. You may release medical information specific to the care that the practitioner has been asked to provide.

Salespeople As a medical assistant, you will probably be the contact for salespeople, unless the office policy manual states that another staff member should handle this duty. On the telephone, ask the salesperson to send you information about any new products or equipment. Pharmaceutical sales representatives may want to meet with the prescribing practitioners. Forward such messages to the providers with a request to let you know when to schedule the appointment. Many prescribing practitioners see pharmaceutical sales representatives on certain days at specific times. Sometimes they limit the number of representatives they will see in one day or one week. Make sure you know your office policy and each prescriber's preferences.

Conference Calls Periodically, providers may need to have a conference call with several individuals. For example, the physician, the nurse, and the medical assistant may need to talk with the insurance company representative at the same time. Telephone conferencing is an ideal setup in this case. All of today's telephone equipment has features for establishing and joining conference calls. In addition, offices with computerized systems now frequently use Internet-based programs, such as Go to Meeting, to allow conferencing among many participants.

Screening Incoming Calls

Each medical office has its own policy about how to screen incoming calls before transferring them to the appropriate person. Calls come not only from patients but also from other physicians, hospital personnel, pharmacists, insurance company personnel, sales representatives, and family members and friends of patients. Here are some general tips for screening calls.

Find out who is calling. A polite way to do this is to say, "May I ask who is calling?" Another option is "May I tell Dr. Williams who is calling?"

Ask what the call is in reference to. When a caller asks to speak with the practitioner, you should ask the purpose of the call. Depending on the answer, you may determine that you or someone else in the office can handle the situation without disturbing the practitioner. The response may be as simple as solving a billing problem or clarifying instructions. Remember to consider the scope of practice for each member of the healthcare team when you transfer a call. Emergency calls should be transferred to the licensed practitioner right away.

Decide whether the call should be put through. Although most calls are routed to the appropriate person, any callers who refuse to identify themselves should not be put through. In such a case, suggest that the caller write a letter to the practitioner and mark it "Personal."

Determine what to do if the matter is personal. The practitioner may ask you to take a message in these instances. Inform the caller that the practitioner will return the call as soon as possible.

▶ Managing Incoming Calls
LO 14.5

Screening Calls

Even if your office uses an automated answering unit, it is likely that part of your responsibility as the office medical assistant will be screening calls. Screening involves deciding which calls should be put through immediately and which calls are better handled by taking a message and allowing a callback at a more convenient time. The *Points on Practice: Screening Incoming Calls* describes some guidelines for screening calls. The procedure will remain basically the same, whether the calls come directly to you as you answer the phone or are directed to you by a telephone answering system.

Routing Calls

Incoming phone calls can generally be separated into three distinct groups: calls dealing mainly with administrative issues; emergency calls that require immediate action by the practitioner; and calls relating to clinical issues that require the attention of the physician, physician assistant, nurse practitioner, office nurse, or clinical medical assistant. Procedure 14-3, at the end of this chapter, will provide the outline for you to practice screening and routing calls.

Calls Requiring the Practitioner's Attention Certain calls will require the practitioner's personal attention:

- Emergency calls that include serious or life-threatening medical conditions, such as severe bleeding, a reaction to a drug, injuries, poisoning, suicide attempts, loss of consciousness, severe burns, or whatever your medical office deems an emergency; Table 14-1 lists symptoms and conditions that require immediate help.
- Calls from other providers.

- Patient requests to discuss test results, particularly abnormal results.
- Reports from patients concerning unsatisfactory progress.
- Requests for prescription renewals (unless previously authorized in the patient's chart).
- Personal calls.

Many practitioners have a set time, such as a half hour in the late morning or at the end of the day, for returning non-emergency patient calls. If a patient prefers to discuss symptoms with his provider, you may tell the patient to expect a phone call from the provider within this set time. If the practitioner does not have a set time for returning phone calls, do not make a commitment as to the time of the return phone call.

In many practices, some of these calls may be handled by others on the staff, such as a nurse practitioner or physician assistant. For example, a nurse practitioner may be able to order a renewal of a regular prescription, provide advice for the care of a sprain, or answer well-baby questions or questions about the side effects of a drug.

Calls Handled by the Medical Assistant The most common calls to a medical office involve administrative and clinical issues. Depending on the practice, the office manager or someone in the billing department may handle some administrative calls. The calls handled by the medical assistant may include:

- Appointments (scheduling, rescheduling, canceling)
- Questions concerning office policies, fees, and hours
- Billing inquiries
- Insurance questions
- Other administrative questions
- X-ray and laboratory reports

- Allergic reactions to foods or insect stings

- Broken bones: Symptoms include being unable to move or bear weight on the injured body part; the injured part is very painful or looks misshapen

- Chemical or foreign objects in the eye

- Choking

- Drowning

- Electrical shock

- Fires, severe burns, or injuries from explosions

- Heart attack: Symptoms include chest pain or pressure; pain radiating from the chest to the arm, shoulder, neck, jaw, back, or stomach; nausea or vomiting; sweating; weakness; shortness of breath; pale or gray skin color

- Heatstroke (sunstroke): Symptoms include confusion or loss of consciousness; flushed skin that is hot and may be moist or dry; strong, rapid pulse

- Human bites or any deep animal bites

- Hypothermia (drop in body temperature during prolonged exposure to cold): Symptoms include becoming increasingly clumsy, unreasonable, irritable, confused, and sleepy; slurred speech; slipping into a coma with slow, weak breathing and heartbeat

- Injuries to the head, neck, or back

- Lack of breathing (apnea) or difficulty breathing (dyspnea)

- Poisoning

- Pressure or pain in the abdomen that will not go away

- Severe bleeding

- Severe vomiting or bloody stools

- Shock: Symptoms include paleness; feeling faint and sweaty; weak, rapid pulse; cold, moist skin; confusion or drowsiness

- Snake bites

- Stroke: Symptoms include seizures, severe headache, slurred speech, and sudden inability or difficulty in moving a body part or one side of the body

- Unconsciousness

- Vehicle collisions

*If someone calls the office on behalf of a patient who is experiencing any of these symptoms or conditions, you may instruct the caller to dial 911 to request an ambulance. Procedure 14-4 at the end of the chapter describes the steps for handling emergency calls. If in the office, the physician should be called to the telephone immediately to offer assistance.

- Reports from hospitals regarding a patient's progress
- Reports from patients concerning their progress
- Requests for referrals to other providers
- Requests for prescription renewals, where prior approval for refills is noted in the chart
- Complaints from patients about administrative matters

The Routing List Each medical office has a standard policy that documents how incoming telephone calls are to be routed and handled. A routing list, such as the one shown in Figure 14-11, specifies who is responsible for the various types of calls in the office and how the calls are to be handled. For example, the routing list indicates which calls should be put through to the practitioners immediately and which ones can be returned later.

The routing list may simply identify the general title of the person responsible for handling a call. When more than one person in the office have the same title, however, the name of the individual who has that responsibility should be specified.

Telephone Triage

Depending on individual state regulations and on individual preference, some practitioners delegate part of the clinical decision making that is done over the telephone to other experienced staff members. In these instances, **telephone triage** is used to decide what action to take. The word *triage* refers to the screening and sorting of emergency incidents. Performing triage correctly is an important skill.

Using Triage Guidelines Proper office staff training is vital in providing safe, sound, and cost-effective medical care over the telephone. An increasing number of medical practices are preparing guidelines for the telephone staff to follow when patients call the office with specific medical problems or questions.

Guidelines are often written for common questions, such as how to deal with sniffles and fevers during cold and flu season or how to make a child with chickenpox more comfortable. Members of the telephone staff must realize, however, that their responsibility is to determine whether a caller needs additional medical care. They cannot diagnose or treat the patient's problem.

Office guidelines outline the specific information the telephone staff must obtain from the patient. In general, this information is the same type as that obtained during an office visit and should include the patient's age, the patient's symptoms, when the problem began, and the patient's level of anxiety about the problem.

Categorizing Problems and Providing Patient Education After the patient information is obtained, the guidelines help the staff categorize the problem according to severity. The medical assistant then decides whether the problem can be handled safely with advice over the telephone, the patient needs to come in to the office, or the problem requires immediate attention at an emergency room. For instance, if a caller is having chest pains, you would be performing a type of triage by instructing her to go to the emergency room immediately, preferably by ambulance.

If a problem is deemed appropriate for telephone management, the guidelines may include recommendations for nonprescription treatment that may relieve symptoms and anxiety. This information falls under the category of patient

	Route to doctor immediately	Take message for doctor	Route to nurse or assistant
Emergencies: bleeding, drug/allergic reaction, difficulty breathing, injury, pain, poisoning, shock, unconsciousness, incoherence or hysteria	X		
Calls from other physicians	If possible		
Patient progress report		X	
Patient request for laboratory report		X (if abnormal)	Kaylyn (if normal)
Patient questions re medication		X	
Patient questions re billing or insurance			Miguel
Patient complaints			Kaylyn
Appointments			Kaylyn
Prescription renewals or refills		X	
Office business			Miguel
Personal business		X	
Salespeople			Miguel

FIGURE 14-11 A routing list identifies the staff member responsible for each type of incoming call.

education. Advise the caller that recommendations are based on the symptoms and are not a diagnosis. Remember, only the licensed practitioner is authorized to make a diagnosis and prescribe medication. Ask the caller to repeat any instructions you give, and tell the patient to call back within a specified time if symptoms do not improve or worsen. Be sure to document in the medical record the critical elements of the conversation that relate to the patient's health status.

▶ Taking Complete and Accurate Phone Messages   LO 14.6

Always have paper or a telephone message pad (Figure 14-12) and pen near the telephone so that you are prepared to write down messages. Proper documentation protects the provider if the caller takes legal action. A record of telephone calls also should be included in a patient's file or electronic health record as part of a complete medical history. Because of their importance as part of the patient's legal health record, messages should never be taken on pieces of scrap paper, which are easily misplaced or accidentally discarded.

Documenting Calls
Documenting telephone calls is essential in a medical office, and several options are available to help medical assistants take a complete message every time. You can use the previously mentioned telephone message pads, a manual telephone log book, or an electronic (computerized) telephone log. Again, remember that many calls (for example, those concerning al problems or referrals) and the

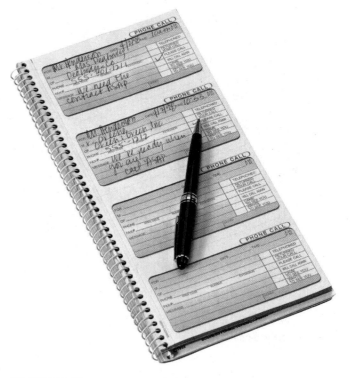

FIGURE 14-12 Using a telephone message pad ensures that no important information is omitted when the message form is filled out completely.
©Lawrence Manning/Getty Images

actions or decisions they lead to must be documented in patients' charts. Every entry into a patient's chart is considered a legal document, so the information must be accurate and legible.

Telephone Message Pads You can use preprinted telephone message pads, which often come in brightly colored paper, to record the following information:

- Date and time of the call.
- Name of the person for whom you took the message.
- Caller's name, or the patient's name if different from the caller.
- Caller's telephone number (always include the area code and extension, if any).
- A description or an action to be taken, including comments such as "Urgent," "Please call back," "Wants to see you," "Will call back," or "Returned your call".
- The complete message, such as "Dr. Stephenson wants to reschedule the committee meeting".
- Name or initials of the person taking the call.

Figure 14-13 shows an example of a completed preprinted telephone message.

The Manual Telephone Log Some medical offices use spiral-bound, perforated message books with carbonless forms to record messages (refer to Figure 14-12). The top copy, or original, of each message is given to

the appropriate person, and a copy is kept in the book for future reference in the event that the original is misplaced or accidentally destroyed.

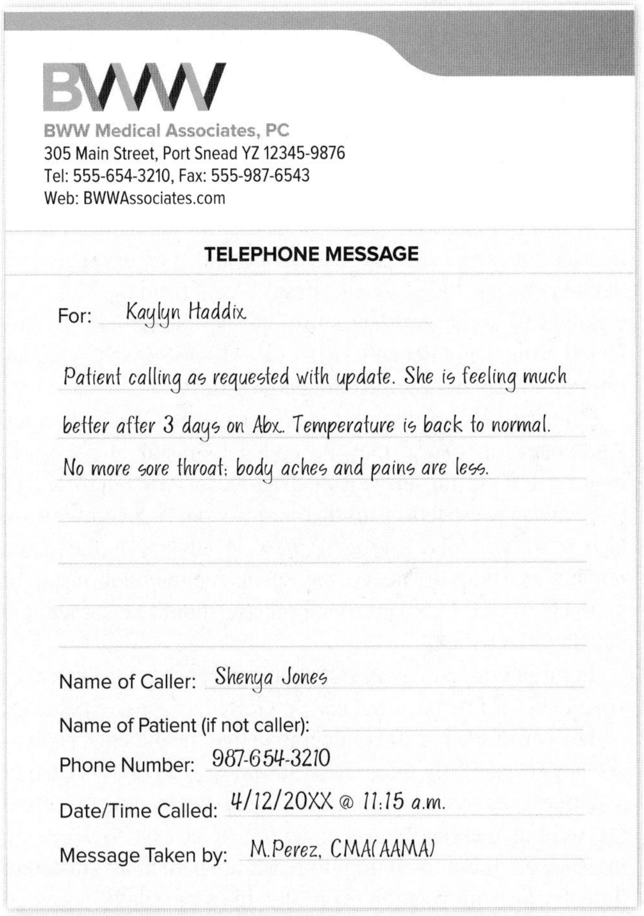

Electronic Telephone Messaging Offices that use practice management software programs often include electronic messaging systems, which allow the telephone messages to be transmitted directly to the intended recipient's computer. These messages may be input directly into the system while on the phone with the caller instead of using the traditional message pad or telephone log. Regardless of the method used, the information to be obtained from the caller remains the same and must be complete.

Tips for Ensuring Accurate Messages The following suggestions will help you provide accurate documentation for incoming messages:

- Always have a pen and paper on hand. If an electronic system is used, keep the software minimized on your computer screen so you can access it quickly.
- Jot down notes as the information is given.
- Verify information, especially the spelling of patient or caller names and the correct spelling of medications.
- Obtain the patient's full name and date of birth if pulling the chart is necessary, in case there are two patients with the same name.
- Verify the correct callback number.
- When taking a phone message, never make a commitment on behalf of the intended recipient by saying, "I'll have him call you." A more appropriate response would be "I will give your message to Dr. Buckwalter."

Maintaining Patient Confidentiality

Even if you are not using a wireless headset, when you are on the phone with a patient discussing confidential information, be aware of the people around you and the volume of your voice when verifying such information. If necessary, move to a private office for such conversations so that patient confidentiality will not be inadvertently breached. When leaving paper patient messages for a practitioner containing confidential information, insert the message into a folder marked "Confidential" so it cannot readily be seen by others. If using an electronic system, each user will access the system using his or her confidential password to access all messages, allowing for maintenance of confidentiality.

▶ Placing Outgoing Calls   LO 14.7

You often will be required to place outgoing calls on behalf of the medical office. You may need to return calls, obtain information, provide patient education, pick up messages from the answering service or voicemail, or arrange patient consultations with other physicians. If you are making a long-distance call, it is important to determine the time zone

BWW
BWW Medical Associates, PC
305 Main Street, Port Snead YZ 12345-9876
Tel: 555-654-3210, Fax: 555-987-6543
Web: BWWAssociates.com

TELEPHONE MESSAGE

For: Kaylyn Haddix

Patient calling as requested with update. She is feeling much better after 3 days on Abx. Temperature is back to normal. No more sore throat; body aches and pains are less.

Name of Caller: Shenya Jones
Name of Patient (if not caller):
Phone Number: 987-654-3210
Date/Time Called: 4/12/20XX @ 11:15 a.m.
Message Taken by: M.Perez, CMA(AAMA)

FIGURE 14-13 It is important that messages be filled out as completely as possible.

and the time of day in the location you are calling before you place the call. Time zones can be determined by checking the front of the phone book, going online, or speaking with a telephone operator. For information on time zones, go to http://www.time.gov.

Locating Telephone Numbers

The medical office should have at least one telephone directory, or telephone book, for the local calling area and perhaps additional directories for surrounding areas. Use these books, an Internet phone directory such as http://www.anywho.com/ (by AT&T), the company website, or directory assistance to locate telephone numbers for outside calls. The office also may have a card file, a list, or an electronic record of commonly used telephone numbers, or these numbers may be listed in the office policies and procedures manual. If you are calling a patient, the telephone number should be in the patient's chart.

If you need to find a long-distance telephone number, many offices use the directory assistance service. You can reach this service by dialing 1-[area code]-555-1212. You also can search the Internet for free "411" services. Use directory assistance only when you have exhausted other options, however, because most long-distance carriers charge a fee each time you use the service. If you are required to call out of the country, you will need to use an international dialing code. These codes, as well as area codes and long-distance numbers, can be located through the Internet and through directory assistance. Two websites that are helpful for finding information on area codes are http://www.lincmad.com/areacodemap.html and http://www.nanpa.com.

Applying Your Telephone Skills

You can apply the telephone skills you use for answering incoming calls when placing outgoing calls. Here are additional tips for handling outgoing calls:

- Plan before you call. Have all the information you need in front of you. Plan what you will say and decide what questions to ask so you will not have to call back for additional information.
- Double-check the telephone number. If in doubt, look it up in the telephone directory. If you do dial a wrong number, be sure to apologize for the mistake.
- Allow enough time, at least a minute or about eight rings, for someone to answer the telephone. When calling patients who are elderly or physically disabled, allow additional time.
- Identify yourself. After reaching the person to whom you placed the call, give your name and state that you are calling on behalf of the doctor or practice.
- Ask if you have called at a convenient time and whether the person has time to talk with you. If it is not a good time, ask when you should call back.

- Be ready to speak as soon as the person you called answers the telephone. Do not waste the person's time while you collect your thoughts.
- If you are calling to give information, ask if the person has a pencil or pen and piece of paper available. Do not begin with dates, times, or instructions until the person is ready to write down the information.

Reaching Voicemail or an Answering Machine

On occasion, it is important to leave a message on a patient's answering machine or voicemail. It is now required by HIPAA that you use these pieces of equipment correctly and confidentially to guard the patient's private medical information. The goal in calling a patient's home is to speak directly to the patient or to leave a message with enough information to get the patient to call back. It is unlawful to disclose confidential patient information to anyone but the patient. HIPAA requires that you *never* leave any information if you are unsure of the phone number dialed. As a medical assistant, you cannot ensure that only the intended patient will receive any message left on an answering machine or voicemail. To guard the patient's privacy, *state only the following information:*

- The name of the individual for whom the message is intended.
- The date and time of the call.
- The name of your office or practice (see caution below).
- Your name as the contact person in the office (see caution below).
- The phone number of your office or practice.
- The hours the office is open for a return call.

A word of caution: Leave the name of the practice only if it does not reveal the purpose of the call. For instance, you would not state, "Please call Tiffany Heath from the STI." An example of an appropriate substitute is "Please call Tiffany Heath from Dr. Greene's office at 413-788-0001, Monday through Friday between 8 a.m. and 5 p.m."

Alternatively, when patients sign the Office Privacy Agreement, a release may be added inquiring if messages may be left on an answering machine or voicemail and if there are any restrictions to that permission. A second release also may be added asking if there is anyone at the home number to whom the office may speak and the relationship of that person to the patient. Each release should be signed and dated by the patient.

Improper or careless use of a patient's answering system or voicemail (or fax machine) can be viewed as abusive behavior in the eyes of the law. It is imperative that the patient's right to privacy be carefully guarded at all times. If in doubt whether a patient's privacy might be violated by leaving a verbal (or written message) on a machine, it is best to leave no message at all but to attempt to reach the patient at a different time. Further information regarding this topic can be accessed on the HIPAA website, https://www.hhs.gov/hipaa.

Retrieving Messages from the Answering System or Service

If callers are allowed to leave messages on an answering machine or voicemail system, the medical assistant is usually responsible for retrieving these messages at the start of each day and, if the office closes for a lunch break, to check for messages after this break as well. Never use the speakerphone setting when retrieving messages from an answering machine, as a patient may leave personal information in a message that might be heard by others in the office. This could be considered a breach of patient confidentiality.

When an answering service is used, it is a good idea to call the service to retrieve messages at a set time (or multiple times, if the service or system is employed during office hours) each day. In doing so, you ensure that messages are not missed. When calling the service to retrieve messages, as when taking any message, verify the information for correctness and completeness before ending the call. Procedure 14-5, at the end of this chapter, describes how to do this.

Arranging Conference Calls

It may be necessary for you to schedule conference calls with patients, hospital personnel, or other practitioners to discuss tests or surgical results. When dealing with several people, suggest several time slots in case someone is not available at a particular time. Also keep in mind the various time zones in the country. Make sure that all the conference call participants are given the proper time in their time zone to expect the call. As mentioned earlier in this chapter, the office phone system will likely have an option allowing you to set up a conference call.

Additionally, there are services that provide "call-in conferencing." The host will provide a number and the time for you or your physician to call in as a participant, or your office may host the call. All of the participants are given a code and are asked to identify themselves as they call into the system. The service will ask for an e-mail address to confirm the information, time, date, and passcodes that will be given to each individual. More information on free conference calling services can be found online. Two such services can be found at https://www.freeconference.com and https://www.freeconferencecalling.com.

PROCEDURE 14-1 Using a Video Relay Service with an American Sign Language Interpreter

Procedure Goal: To properly communicate with the hearing-impaired patient using a VRS

OSHA Guidelines: This procedure does not involve exposure to blood, body fluids, or tissue.

Materials: Telephone, patient chart for documentation, and a pen or EHR program as available

Method:

Answering a Call from a VRS

1. The communication assistant (interpreter) will explain that she is acting as an interpreter for the patient using a video relay service.
   RATIONALE: *It is important to understand that the caller is acting as an interpreter for the patient at the other end of the relay service.*

2. Allow the interpreter to explain the nature of the call as provided to her by the patient.

3. Once the initial introduction has been made, if there are any questions, relay them to the interpreter/assistant.
   RATIONALE: *The assistant will then use ASL (American Sign Language) via the video hookup to the patient to relay the question(s) to the patient.*

4. Be patient while waiting for the interpretation to occur. The assistant will then relay any response from the patient.
   RATIONALE: *Remember that the assistant is acting as interpreter for both you and the patient and she must*

understand both sides of the conversation for effective communication.

5. Once the conversation is completed and all questions from both sides have been answered, the call may be completed as usual.

6. Prior to hanging up with the relay service assistant, be sure to obtain the relay service name and contact information so that the same service may be utilized should you need to contact the patient in the future. Document this information in the patient's record for use in the future.
   RATIONALE: *This allows for continuity of care utilizing the service with which the patient has developed a relationship.*

Making a Call with a VRS

1. Using the previously saved information, call the VRS company known to the patient.

2. When the call is answered, state the reason for the call, giving the office information and the name of the patient to whom you wish to speak.
   RATIONALE: *It is important the interpreter knows who is calling the patient/client and the reason for the call.*

3. Give a concise statement to the communication assistant regarding the reason for the call so that the information may be relayed to the patient when the phone is answered.

RATIONALE: *This gives the interpreter a basic understanding of the reason for the call that can be used as an introductory statement for the patient.*

4. Once the patient answers the phone, the introductory information will be given to the patient by the assistant using ASL via the video relay. You will remain on the line during this translation.

5. Should the patient have any questions or comments, the assistant will relay this information to you via the telephone. Your responses will again be sent to the patient via the video portion of the relay until all parties are satisfied.

RATIONALE: *Remember to wait patiently while the assistant translates information back and forth to be sure all communication is clear to both the patient and the office staff involved.*

6. As with all calls, be sure to inform the patient at the end of the call that should any questions or problems arise at a later time, they should contact the office with any questions or issues.
   RATIONALE: *The patient must always know the office is there to serve his needs.*

PROCEDURE 14-2 Renewing a Prescription by Telephone

WORK // DOC

Procedure Goal: To ensure a complete and accurate prescription is received by the patient

OSHA Guidelines: This procedure does not involve exposure to blood, body fluids, or tissue.

Materials: Telephone, appropriate phone numbers, message pad, or prescription refill request form, pen, and patient chart or progress note with prescription order

Method:

1. Take the message from the call or the message system. For the prescription to be complete, you must obtain the patient's name, date of birth, phone number, pharmacy name and/or phone number, medication, and dosage.

2. Follow your facility policy regarding prescription renewals. Typically, the prescription is usually called into the pharmacy the day it is requested. An example policy may be posted at the facility and may state, "Nonemergency prescription refill requests must be made during regular business hours. Please allow 24 hours for processing."

3. Communicate the policy to the patient. You should know the policy and the time when the refills will be reviewed. For example, you might state, "Dr. Williams will review the prescription between patients and it will be telephoned within 1 hour to the pharmacy. I will call you back if there is a problem."
   RATIONALE: *Letting the patient know the policy demonstrates good communication skills and will result in fewer misunderstandings as to when the prescription will be available for pickup.*

4. Obtain the patient's chart or reference the electronic chart to verify you have the correct patient and that the patient is currently taking the medication. Check the patient's list of medications, which is usually part of the chart.

5. Give the prescription refill request and the chart to the physician or prescriber. Do not give a prescription refill request to the licensed practitioner without the chart or chart access information. Wait for an authorization from the practitioner before you proceed.
   RATIONALE: *All prescription refills must be authorized by the prescribing practitioner.*

6. Once the practitioner authorizes the prescription, prepare to call the pharmacy with the renewal information. Be certain to have the practitioner order, the patient's chart, and the refill request in front of you when you make the call. The request should include the name of the drug, the drug dosage, the frequency and mode of administration, the number of refills authorized, and the pharmacy's name and phone number. Note: You cannot call in Schedule II or III medications; these are medications that have the greatest possibility of abuse. Renewals can be called in for Schedule IV and V medications.

7. Telephone the pharmacy. Identify yourself by name, the practice name, and the practitioner's name.
   RATIONALE: *Only an identified representative from a medical practice can authorize a prescription refill.*

8. State the purpose of the call (example: "This is Miguel Perez from BWW Medical Associates. I am calling to request a prescription refill for a patient.").

9. Identify the patient. Include the patient's name, date of birth, address, and phone number.
   RATIONALE: *It is essential that the correct drug be prescribed for the correct patient according to the physician's order.*

10. Identify the drug (spelling the name when necessary), the dosage, the frequency and mode of administration, and any other special instructions or changes for administration (such as "take at bedtime").
    RATIONALE: *Accuracy and complete information are essential for medication administration.*

11. State the number of refills authorized.

12. If leaving a message on a pharmacy voicemail system set up for prescribers, state your name, the name of the doctor you represent, and your phone number before you hang up.

    RATIONALE: *If the pharmacist has any questions, she must be able to reach the prescriber.*

13. Document the prescription renewal in the chart after the medication has been called in to the pharmacy. Include the date, the time, the name of the pharmacy, and the person taking your call. Also include the medication, dose, amount, directions, and number of refills. Sign your first initial, last name, and title. In an EHR, your credentials may be on file. Refer to the Progress Note.

BWW PROGRESS NOTE

Patient Name: Shenya Jones

Rx telephoned to Beth Stone at Noname Pharmacy: Zyrtec 10 mg, one tablet daily at bedtime, #30, 6 refills

Date: 05/03/XX

Author: M.A. Perez

Done   Close

PROCEDURE 14-3 Screening and Routing Telephone Calls

WORK // DOC

Procedure Goal: To properly screen incoming telephone calls

OSHA Guidelines: This procedure does not involve exposure to blood, body fluids, or tissue.

Materials: Telephone, telephone message sheet, pen or pencil, appointment book or computerized scheduling software (computer), and office routing list

Method:
Use the office routing list to route calls appropriately.

1. Make sure all of the materials are within reach of the telephone equipment.

2. Answer the telephone promptly within two to three rings.

3. Identify the medical office and identify yourself. Make sure you know office procedure for answering the phone in your facility even if a telephone answering system is employed to route calls to you—for example, "BWW Medical Associates, this is Malik. How may I help you?"

4. If the caller does not identify himself, ask him to do so and the number he is calling from, and write down this information. Find out the reason for the call. Is it an emergency? (Refer to Table 14-1.) If so, follow office policy.

RATIONALE: *As soon as you make certain a call is an emergency, it is important for the patient's welfare that you follow the office protocol for these situations.*

5. If you can handle the call, take care of the query. Listen carefully to what the caller has to say, paying particular attention to tone and feeling.

    RATIONALE: *If the caller's query is within your scope of practice and job description, it is up to you to take care of the patient's problem or request as quickly and professionally as possible.*

6. If this is a call that needs to be transferred to someone (per the routing list), tell the caller to whom and to what number you will be transferring the call. Make sure you write down the caller's name and phone number in case the call is accidentally dropped. If the other staff member does not answer promptly or is on another line, ask the caller if he would like to be transferred to the staff member's voicemail (if available) or would like to leave a message. See Figure 14-11.

7. If you need to take a message, make sure you repeat the information that is given to you, especially the name of the person and his phone number. Take a complete message.

    RATIONALE: *If the message is not complete, the person receiving it may not take the appropriate action or the patient may end up needlessly being directed to multiple people.*

PROCEDURE 14-4 Handling Emergency Calls

WORK // DOC

Procedure Goal: To determine whether a telephone call involves a medical emergency and to learn the steps to take if it is an emergency call

OSHA Guidelines: This procedure does not involve exposure to blood, body fluids, or tissue.

Materials: Office guidelines for handling emergency calls; list of symptoms and conditions requiring immediate medical attention; telephone numbers of area emergency rooms, poison control centers, and ambulance transport services; and telephone message sheets or a telephone message log

Method:

1. When someone calls the office regarding a potential emergency, remain calm.

    RATIONALE: *This attitude will help calm the caller and enable you to gather necessary information in the most efficient manner.*

2. Obtain the following information, taking accurate notes:

    a. The caller's name.

    b. The caller's telephone number and the address from which the call is being made.

    RATIONALE: *It may be necessary for you to put the call on hold or to hang up so you can call for medical assistance. Before you do so, however, be sure to read the information back to the caller to ensure that you have written it down correctly. If you deem the call a medical emergency, ask another medical assistant to dial 911 and give the information you have written down.*

    c. The caller's relationship to the patient (if it is not the patient who is calling).

    d. The patient's name (if the patient is not the caller).

    e. The patient's age.

    f. A complete description of the patient's symptoms.

    g. If the call is about an accident, a description of how the accident or injury occurred and any other pertinent information.

    h. A description of how the patient is reacting to the situation.

    i. Treatment that has been administered.

3. Read back the details of the medical problem to verify them.

    RATIONALE: *Details are necessary to determine whether or not an emergency exists and the steps you need to take next.*

4. If necessary, refer to the list of symptoms and conditions that require immediate medical attention to determine if the situation is indeed a medical emergency.

If the Situation Is a Medical Emergency

1. Put the call through to the patient's provider immediately, or handle the situation according to the established office procedures.

    RATIONALE: *Medical emergencies take precedence over all other matters.*

2. If the provider is not in the office, follow established office procedures. These may involve one or more of the following:

    a. Transferring the call to the nurse practitioner or other medical personnel, as appropriate.

    b. Instructing the caller (if not the patient) to hang up and dial 911 to request an ambulance for the patient.

    c. Instructing the patient to be driven to the nearest emergency room.

    d. Instructing the caller to telephone the nearest poison control center for advice and supplying the caller with its telephone number.

    e. Paging the doctor.

If the Situation Is Not a Medical Emergency

1. Handle the call according to established office procedures.

2. If you are in doubt about whether the situation is a medical emergency, treat it as an emergency. You must always alert the patient's provider immediately about an emergency call, even if the patient declines to speak with the doctor.

    RATIONALE: *It is better to be overly cautious than to let an emergency go untreated. The doctor should be the one to decide how to handle these situations.*

PROCEDURE 14-5 Retrieving Messages from an Answering Service or System

WORK // DOC

Procedure Goal: To follow standard procedures for retrieving messages from an answering service or system

OSHA Guidelines: This procedure does not involve exposure to blood, body fluids, or tissue.

Materials: Telephone message sheets, pen or pencil, manual telephone log, or electronic telephone log and writing instrument if needed

Method:

1. Set a regular schedule for calling the answering service (system) to retrieve messages.

    RATIONALE: *A regular schedule ensures the procedure will not be forgotten and calls will not be missed.*

2. Call at the regularly scheduled time(s) to see if there are any messages.

3. If calling a service, identify yourself and state that you are calling to obtain messages for the practice.

    RATIONALE: *Most services have a list of people at the office who are allowed to pick up messages.*

4. If calling an answering system, when the call is answered, you will enter the passcode for the office.

    RATIONALE: *The passcode is given only to staff members allowed to retrieve messages.*

5. For each message, write down all pertinent information on the telephone message pad or telephone log, or key it into the electronic telephone log. Be sure to include the caller's name and telephone number, time of call, message or description of the problem, and action taken, if any.

    RATIONALE: *Always take a complete message for the convenience of the caller and the person receiving the message.*

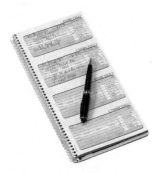

FIGURE Procedure 14-5 Step 5   Write down all pertinent information to take a complete message.
©Lawrence Manning/Getty Images

6. If calling an answering service, repeat the information, confirming you have the correct spelling of all names and the complete, correct information.
   RATIONALE: *This step ensures you have the information correct.*

7. If calling an answering system, be sure you listen carefully and replay messages if necessary to get complete information given within each message.
   RATIONALE: *This step ensures you have complete and correct information.*

8. When you have retrieved all messages, route them according to office policy.

SUMMARY OF LEARNING OUTCOMES

OUTCOME	KEY POINTS
14.1 Explain the purpose of the telecommunications equipment commonly found in the medical office.	Telecommunications equipment found in the medical office includes multiline phones for incoming and outgoing calls, which may include voicemail for picking up messages; an automated voice response unit to route calls automatically to the correct person or department using a series of prompts, answered by the caller; an answering machine or answering service to pick up calls and messages when the office is extremely busy or after business hours; and cell phones and/or pagers to reach medical staff when they are not in the office. Additionally, a VRS (or other communication assisting device) may be used in the office—for communication with deaf patients.
14.2 Relate the five Cs of effective communication to telephone communication skills.	The five Cs of effective communication are important in all types of communication, and the telephone is no exception. All forms of communication are more easily understood using these principles: completeness of the message, clarity of the message, conciseness of the information, courtesy when delivering the message, and cohesiveness (logic and organization) of the message.
14.3 Define the following terms involved in making a good impression on the telephone: *telephone etiquette, pitch, pronunciation, enunciation,* and *tone.*	Telephone etiquette means to handle all calls professionally and politely using good manners. Pitch is the high or low level of your voice, projecting interest in what you are saying. Pronunciation is saying words correctly, and enunciation is saying them clearly. Tone projects how you are feeling; in the office, your tone should always be positive and respectful.
14.4 Describe how to appropriately handle the different types of calls coming into the medical practice.	The medical assistant may receive calls from patients, attorneys, and others. Always refer to the office policies and procedures manual regarding how to handle incoming calls appropriately. Remember, always be courteous to the caller.
14.5 Summarize the purpose of the office routing list with regard to call screening.	Screening calls categorizes the importance of the call in regard to how quickly the patient's problem or question needs to be handled. The routing list is a guideline for the entire staff to recognize which types of calls should go to each member of the medical staff, following office protocol as to the duties and scope of practice for each team member.

OUTCOME	KEY POINTS
14.6 **Carry out the procedure for taking a complete telephone message.**	In addition to complete information from the caller regarding what the call is about, each complete telephone message should contain the following information: date and time of the call; name of the person for whom the message was taken; the caller's name and name of the patient (if different from the caller); the caller's telephone number with area code; a description or action to be taken; a complete and concise message; and the name or initials of the person taking the message.
14.7 **Outline the preparation required prior to making outgoing calls and the skills used in making the phone call.**	Prior to placing an outgoing call, be sure to have all necessary information in front of you, including the name of the person to be reached and the correct phone number. Dial the number carefully, identifying yourself when the phone is answered and asking for the person you need to reach. As always, use the five Cs of communication to complete the exchange.

CASE STUDY CRITICAL THINKING

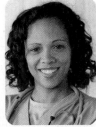

©Terry Vine/Blend Images LLC

Recall Reagan Patrick from the case study at the beginning of the chapter. Now that you have completed the chapter, answer the following questions regarding her case.

1. The first phone call is easy—a routine appointment for next week, which Reagan books without a problem. The next caller states he must speak with Dr. Buckwalter immediately. How should Reagan handle this call?

2. The next caller is Nancy Evans. Reagan remembers from her appointment earlier this week that Mrs. Evans has possible early-onset dementia. Mrs. Evans states she has not seen Dr. Williams in several months and wants to know why she does not "care about her anymore." While Reagan is trying to speak with Mrs. Evans, another line rings. How should Reagan handle Mrs. Evans and the ringing phone?

EXAM PREPARATION QUESTIONS

1. (LO 14.1) Which of the following is *not* a common function of many of today's multiline phones?
   a. Transfer options
   b. Hold
   c. Voicemail
   d. Intercom
   e. Voice recognition

2. (LO 14.1) What is the main reason pagers are not used as often in medical offices?
   a. Physicians hate carrying them.
   b. Improved healthcare means fewer "emergencies."
   c. Cell phones are being used more often.
   d. It is becoming harder to find signals for pagers.
   e. E-mail is used more often.

3. (LO 14.2) Which of the following is *not* one of the five Cs of effective communication?
   a. Compassion
   b. Clarity
   c. Conciseness
   d. Cohesiveness
   e. Completeness

4. (LO 14.2) Which of the following is an appropriate statement for answering the office telephone?
   a. "Doctor's office, Jayden speaking."
   b. "Jayden here, this is BWW Medical Associates."
   c. "BWW Medical Associates, Jayden. Hold please."
   d. "BWW Medical Associates; this is Jayden. How may I help you?"
   e. All of these

5. (LO 14.3) Speaking clearly and distinctly is called
   a. Tone
   b. Enunciation
   c. Etiquette
   d. Pronunciation
   e. Clarity

6. (LO 14.4) Which of the following is *not* a common reason patients call the office?
   a. Appointment requests
   b. Billing inquiries
   c. Seeking lab or X-ray reports
   d. Compliments to the medical staff
   e. All of these

7. (LO 14.5) Deciding how emergent a patient's problem is and how it may best be handled is a procedure known as
   a. Screening
   b. Routing
   c. Triage
   d. Paging
   e. Etiquette

8. (LO 14.5) _____ is being done when a call is transferred to an appropriate person based on the caller's request.
   a. Screening
   b. Routing
   c. Triage
   d. Paging
   e. Etiquette

9. (LO 14.6) Taking an effective message involves which of the following items?
   a. Date and time of call
   b. Whom the call is for
   c. Name and phone number of caller
   d. Message and action to be taken
   e. All of these and more

10. (LO 14.7) When placing a call to a patient with medical information, if you reach the patient's answering machine, what should you do?
   a. Leave a complete message; it is the patient's private answering machine.
   b. Leave your name, the name of the practice, and your phone number so the patient can call back.
   c. Leave your name and phone number, stating there is a medical issue that requires discussion.
   d. Leave the practice name only if the reason for the call is not easily identifiable, your name, and your phone number; if unsure, try calling back at another time.
   e. Leave your name and number with no message.

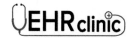

Go to CONNECT to complete the EHR exercises: 14.01 Create an Electronic Telephone Encounter, 14.02 Create an Urgent Electronic Telephone Encounter, and 14.03 Complete a Prescription Refill Request.

SOFT SKILLS SUCCESS

Recall Reagan Patrick from the case study at the beginning of the chapter.

1. Reagan is on the phone with Nancy Evans, who is obviously confused about when she last saw her physician. What type of soft skills should be used with this patient?

2. Later, while on break, another employee who heard about the phone call from Mrs. Evans started laughing about the "crazy woman" who did not remember coming

in to the office a couple of days ago. How should Reagan (or you) respond to such a comment?

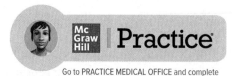

Go to PRACTICE MEDICAL OFFICE and complete the module Admin Check In: Office Operations.

Patient Education

CASE STUDY

	Patient Name	DOB	Allergies
PATIENT INFORMATION	Sylvia Gonzales	09/01/1968	Penicillin
	Attending	**MRN**	**Other Information**
	Alexis N. Whalen, MD	00-AA-004	04/22/XX: FBS - 152 mg/dL, A1C - 6.7% 06/18/XX: GTT - 232 mg/dL, A1C - 6.9%

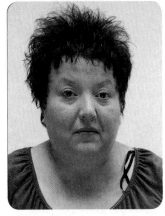

©McGraw-Hill Education

Sylvia Gonzales, a female in her early fifties, is at the office for a 3-month return check for newly diagnosed Type 2 diabetes. She appears overweight and is snacking on a bag of potato chips and chocolate milk when you take her into the exam room. She states, "I was hungry; I missed my breakfast, but I have been taking the medication the doctor game me for my 'sugar.'" She wants me to have a special 'sugar test' this time." Her medication list includes Januvia, 100 mg daily, a medication to help lower her blood sugar.

Keep Sylvia Gonzales in mind as you study the chapter. There will be questions at the end of the chapter based on the case study. The information in the chapter will help you answer these questions.

LEARNING OUTCOMES

After completing Chapter 15, you will be able to:

15.1 Identify the benefits of patient education and the medical assistant's role in providing education.

15.2 Describe factors that affect learning and teaching.

15.3 Implement teaching techniques.

15.4 Choose reliable patient education materials used in the medical office.

15.5 Explain how patient education can be used to promote good health habits.

15.6 Describe the types of information that should be included in the patient information packet.

15.7 Describe the benefits and special considerations of patient education prior to surgery.

KEY TERMS

consumer education
factual teaching
modeling
participatory teaching

philosophy
return demonstration
screening
sensory teaching

V.C.6   Define coaching a patient as it relates to:
- (a) health maintenance
- (b) disease prevention
- (c) compliance with treatment plan
- (d) community resources

V.C.8   Discuss applications of electronic technology in professional communication

V.P.4   Coach patients regarding:
- (a) office policies
- (b) health maintenance
- (c) disease prevention
- (d) treatment plan

V.P.9   Develop a current list of community resources related to patients' healthcare needs

V.P.10   Facilitate referrals to community resources in the role of a patient navigator

VI.P.6   Utilize an EMR

X.C.3   Describe components of the Health Information Portability and Accountability Act (HIPAA)

X.P.3   Document patient care accurately in the medical record

X.P.4   Apply the Patient's Bill of Rights as it relates to:
- (a) choice of treatment
- (b) consent for treatment
- (c) refusal of treatment

2. Anatomy and Physiology
- d. Apply a system of diet and nutrition
  - (2) Educate patients regarding proper diet and nutrition guidelines

4. Medical Law and Ethics
- f. Comply with federal, state, and local health laws and regulations as they relate to healthcare settings
  - (1) Define scope of practice for the medical assistant within the state where employed

5. Human Relations
- h. Display effective interpersonal skills with patients and health care team members

7. Administrative Procedures
- b. Navigate electronic health records systems and practice management software
- g. Display professionalism through written and verbal communications

8. Clinical Procedures
- h. Teach self-examination, disease management, and health promotion
- i. Identify community resources and Complementary and Alternative Medicine practices (CAM)
- j. Make adaptations for patients with special needs (psychological or physical limitations)

10. Career Development
- b. Demonstrate professional behavior

▶ Introduction

Health education should be a lifelong pursuit for all of us. The ultimate goal of all medical professionals is to encourage and teach healthy habits and behaviors to all patients. People first have to understand what is good for them, and then they have to make a decision to follow that advice. In patient education, the medical assistant shares health information and encourages patients to make good health decisions. To be a credible patient educator, you should make good personal health decisions because patients watch medical personnel to see if they "practice what they preach."

In this chapter, you will learn about patient education. Understanding your role and scope of practice related to patient education is necessary. Then you will develop skills in recognizing and overcoming roadblocks to education. You will become more comfortable with teaching and demonstrating procedures to others. Most importantly, you will begin to recognize the incredible responsibility of the medical assistant to correctly lead others to their highest level of health.

▶ The Educated Patient   LO 15.1

Patient education is an essential process in the medical office. It encourages patients to take an active role in their medical care. It results in better compliance with treatment programs. When patients are suffering from illness, disease, or injury, education can often help them regain their health and independence more quickly. Simply put, patient education helps patients become healthy and stay healthy. Educated patients are more likely to comply with instructions if they understand the "why" behind the instructions. Also, educated patients are more likely to be satisfied clients of the practice.

Patients benefit from education, but the medical office benefits as well. Preoperative instruction to surgical patients, for example, lessens the chance that procedures will have to be rescheduled because surgical guidelines were not followed. Educated patients also will be less likely to call the office with questions. Thus, the office staff will have to spend less time on the telephone.

Patient Education and Scope of Practice

A medical assistant must be competent and knowledgeable before he or she can provide patient education. If a licensed practitioner asks you to perform education, the content of that education must be approved by that practitioner. You must understand the content in order to teach it, but you should not go beyond the content you have been asked to teach. In addition, while performing education, you must not make any judgments or answer any questions that require diagnosis, assessment, or evaluation.

Patient education takes many forms and includes a variety of techniques. It can be as simple as answering a question that comes up during a routine visit, or it can be detailed instruction regarding a procedure such as wound care. In some cases, it may involve printed materials. In others, the patient may be asked to participate by responding correctly to instructions. As a medical assistant, the amount and type of patient education you provide will be decided by your place of employment and scope of practice. See *Caution: Handle with Care: Patient Education and Scope of Practice.* Even if you are not providing the education, you should be aware of the patient's educational needs and ability to understand. In addition, being a role model by practicing good health behaviors helps you and the patients who may be watching you.

▶ Learning and Teaching LO 15.2

To provide patient education, it is necessary to understand the process of learning. Learning is the acquiring of new knowledge, behaviors, or skills, which also are known as the *domains of learning.* Knowledge, the cognitive domain, includes the factual or practical understanding of a subject and the ability to recall it. Behavior, the affective domain, is how one approaches learning. It includes feelings, values, appreciation, enthusiasms, motivations, and attitudes. Skills, the psychomotor domain, include physical movement, coordination, and use of motor skills to complete a task. See Figure 15-1.

To better understand these domains, let's use the example of our patient, Sylvia Gonzales, who just found out she is diabetic. For her to be able to manage her diabetes and have the best outcome for her health, she will need to learn through all three of the domains.

- *Cognitive (knowledge):* Sylvia will need to understand the basic information about diabetes, including the effects of diet, exercise, and treatments. The information can come in many formats, as discussed later in this chapter.
- *Affective (behaviors):* Sylvia must have the desire or be motivated to make a change in order to improve her health. Once she appreciates the need, is motivated, and has a positive attitude, she will then be able to make the change.

This is part of the learning process. If she does not have the desire to learn about diabetes or is not motivated to improve her health, she will not make any change. Being aware of a patient's level of motivation and encouraging the patient are important parts of the teaching process.

- *Psychomotor (skills):* Once Sylvia has the basic knowledge and correct behavior, she will be able to learn and perform the skills necessary to improve her condition and keep her diabetes under control. This may include eating better foods, increasing exercise, and taking any medications that are prescribed.

For learning to occur, all three domains of learning must be considered during the teaching process. The patient, Sylvia, must be provided the information, she must be motivated and have a desire to learn the information, and then she must perform the skills, doing what is necessary to improve her condition.

▶ Teaching Techniques LO 15.3

Patient education can take many forms. Any instructions—verbal, written, or demonstrative—that you give to patients are types of patient education. When providing education, three types of teaching can occur: factual, sensory, and participatory. These three types of teaching correspond to the three domains of learning.

The combination of these teaching methods gives the patient an overall understanding because it encourages learning through all three of the domains of learning.

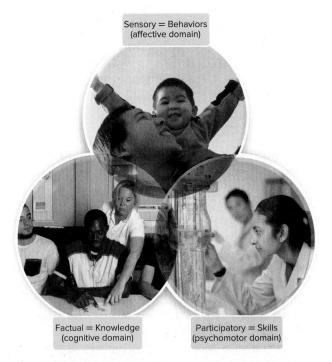

Sensory = Behaviors
(affective domain)

Factual = Knowledge
(cognitive domain)

Participatory = Skills
(psychomotor domain)

FIGURE 15-1 Learning occurs through three domains: cognitive, affective, and psychomotor. Teaching is accomplished by factual, sensory, and participatory techniques.

(top) ©Purestock/SuperStock; (left) ©franky242/Alamy Stock Photo; (right) ©ERproductions LTD/Blend Images LLC

Factual Teaching (Cognitive Domain)

Factual teaching provides detailed information about a subject. For example, when preparing a patient for surgery, you should tell the patient what will happen during the surgery, when it will happen, and why the procedure is necessary. Factual information provided to a patient before surgery also can include restrictions on diet or activity that may be necessary both before and after surgery. Factual information is usually supported with written materials so that the patient can refer to the information as needed at a later date.

Sensory Teaching (Affective Domain)

Sensory teaching provides patients with a description of the physical sensations they may have as part of the learning or the procedure involved. This learning relates to how the person is affected—that is, the affective domain. For example, prior to surgery, you might need to explain how much pain or what other sensations, such as numbness or tingling, the patient may feel. All five senses may be involved: feeling, seeing, hearing, tasting, and smelling.

Participatory Teaching (Psychomotor Domain)

Participatory teaching includes demonstrations of techniques that may be necessary to show that something has been learned. For example, as part of preoperative teaching, aspects of postoperative care include cleaning the wound, changing the dressing, and applying ice packs. A newly diagnosed diabetic might need to be taught how to check his blood sugar. During this phase of teaching, you need to first describe the technique to the patient and then demonstrate it. By demonstrating the procedure, you are **modeling** it for the patient, or showing the patient exactly what to do. Then you should ask the patient to perform the same procedure while you watch. This practice is called **return demonstration.** The return demonstration has two purposes. First, it allows you to be sure the patient fully understands the procedure. Second, by actually performing the procedure, the patient uses motor skills and engages the psychomotor domain. Physically performing the procedure helps cement the steps in the patient's mind.

Verifying Patient Understanding

The key to the success of any educational process is verifying that patients have actually understood the information. A good way to check for understanding is to have patients explain in their own words what they have learned. This is a form of feedback. In addition, have them engage in return demonstrations.

Cultural and Educational Barriers

Some practices serve patients who cannot read well or who do not speak or understand English. It may be necessary to create educational materials written in very simple terms that present information through pictures and charts. The information also may need to be translated into one or more languages. Patients must understand the office's policies and procedures as well as any other educational information provided.

One-on-one explanations may be required for these patients. However, printed materials should still be given to these patients to take home for reference. Family members or friends may be able to read the materials for them, reinforcing what they learned in the office. When demonstrating a procedure to patients, keep in mind any physical limitations they have and adjust the procedure accordingly. Make sure patients understand the instructions by asking them to perform the procedure for you.

It is important to match the learning materials to the patient's needs and to his or her level of understanding. Consider the patient's cultural background, age, medical condition, emotional state, learning style, educational background, disabilities, religious background, and readiness to learn when providing new materials. Review the *Points on Practice: Respecting Patients' Cultural Beliefs*. Keep in mind that patients can refuse treatment and information. If they do, notify the doctor and document the event in the patient's chart.

▶ Patient Education Materials LO 15.4

Patient education materials inform patients and enable and encourage them to become involved in their own medical care. Most formal types of patient education involve some printed information. They also may include visual materials, such as the medical practice's website, podcasts, DVDs, and other Internet sites.

Printed Materials

Printed educational materials come in a variety of formats. They can be as simple as a single sheet of paper, or they can be several sheets folded or stapled together to form a booklet.

Brochures, Booklets, and Fact Sheets Many medical offices have materials available that explain procedures performed in the medical office or give information about specific

---

POINTS ON PRACTICE
Respecting Patients' Cultural Beliefs

Patients come from many diverse cultures and have different beliefs about the causes and treatments of illness. These differences may affect their treatment expectations, as well as their willingness to follow medical directions. Consider these simple steps when giving instructions to patients of diverse cultures:

- Speak clearly at a steady pace.
- Request or provide a translator as needed.
- Ask for and look for feedback from the patient, indicating that she understands and intends to follow the patient instructions.
- Ask the patient if there is any reason that she will not be able to follow the instructions.
- Address any concerns indicated by the patient, notifying the doctor if the concerns mean that the patient is not likely to follow the instructions.

diseases and medical conditions. For example, women who have had a cesarean section delivery may be given a fact sheet describing simple exercises they can do in bed to help regain strength in the abdominal muscles. Many educational aids are prepared by pharmaceutical or other healthcare companies and are provided free of charge to medical offices. Others may be written by the licensed practitioner or members of the office staff. You may be asked to help prepare some of these materials.

Electronic health record systems provide the ability to create or import informational materials for patients. Once electronic patient instructions are created, education is provided to the patient and documented in the patient's chart. See Figures 15-2 and 15-3 as well as Procedure 15-1, Creating Electronic Patient Instructions, at the end of this chapter.

Whenever written materials of any kind are given to a patient, it must be noted in the patient's chart. Be sure to document exactly which brochure or leaflet was distributed. Using electronic health records, you can create and document patient receipt of pertinent information quickly and easily.

Educational Newsletters A popular patient education tool is the medical office newsletter. Newsletters contain timely, practical healthcare tips. Regular newsletters also can offer updates on office policies, information about new diagnostic tests or equipment, and news about the office staff. Newsletters are often written by the doctor or office staff. Some publishing companies and medical groups also offer newsletters that can be customized to a particular practice, using the Internet or software programs such as Microsoft® Publisher. See Figure 15-4.

Community-Assistance Directory Patients often require the assistance of health-related organizations within the community. For example, an elderly patient may need the services of a visiting nurse or a Meals on Wheels food program. Other patients may need the services of a day-care center, speech therapist, or weight clinic.

There are many community resources available in your local area that provide needed services to patients. The medical assistant should be aware of these resources and be able to navigate patients to them. The first step is to develop a community resource library by gathering a listing of local agencies. You will need the correct name, address, web address, phone number, contact person, and directions for submitting a referral for each resource listed. It may take some research on your part to locate and organize this information. Contact the community

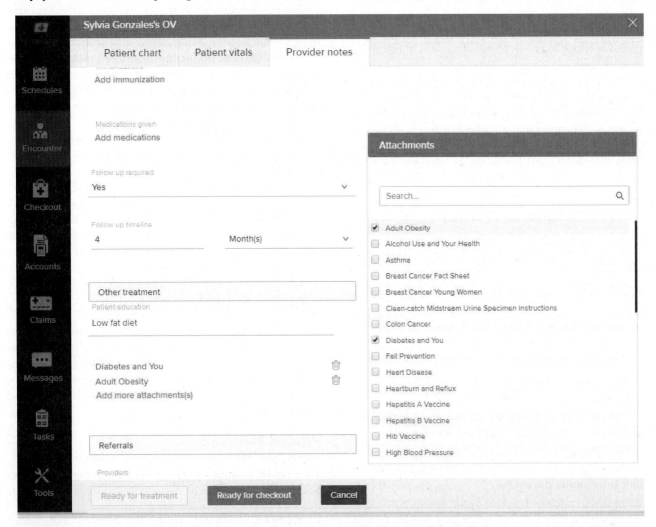

FIGURE 15-2 Patient education and materials are provided to the patient, then attached to the patient's EHR as shown in this screen from ◡EHRclinic.
©McGraw-Hill Education

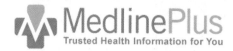
MedlinePlus
Trusted Health Information for You

Search MedlinePlus [GO]

About MedlinePlus Site Map FAQs Contact Us

Health Topics   **Drugs & Supplements**   **Videos & Tools**   **Español**

Home → Health Topics → Diabetes Type 2

Diabetes Type 2
Also called: Type 2 Diabetes

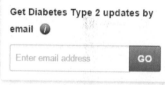

On this page

Basics
- Summary
- Start Here
- Latest News
- Diagnosis/Symptoms
- Treatment
- Prevention/Screening

Learn More
- Alternative Therapy
- Nutrition
- Coping
- Disease Management
- Specific Conditions
- Related Issues

Multimedia & Tools
- Health Check Tools
- Videos

Research
- Financial Issues
- Clinical Trials
- Genetics
- Research
- Journal Articles

Reference Shelf
- Dictionaries/Glossaries
- Directories
- Organizations
- Newsletters/Print Publications
- Law and Policy
- Statistics

For You
- Men
- Women
- Seniors
- Patient Handouts

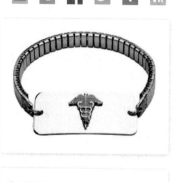

Get Diabetes Type 2 updates by email ⓘ

Enter email address [GO]

Summary

Diabetes means your blood glucose, or blood sugar, levels are too high. With type 2 diabetes, the more common type, your body does not make or use insulin well. Insulin is a hormone that helps glucose get into your cells to give them energy. Without insulin, too much glucose stays in your blood. Over time, high blood glucose can lead to serious problems with your heart, eyes, kidneys, nerves, and gums and teeth.

You have a higher risk of type 2 diabetes if you are older, obese, have a family history of diabetes, or do not exercise. Having prediabetes also increases your risk. Prediabetes means that your blood sugar is higher than normal but not high enough to be called diabetes.

The symptoms of type 2 diabetes appear slowly. Some people do not notice symptoms at all. The symptoms can include

- Being very thirsty
- Urinating often

MEDICAL ENCYCLOPEDIA

A1c test

Diabetes - what to ask your doctor - type 2

Diabetes type 2 - meal planning

Giving an insulin injection

High blood sugar

Type 2 diabetes

Type 2 diabetes - self-care

Related Health Topics

Blood Sugar

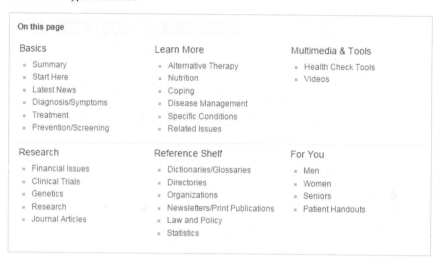

FIGURE 15-3   MedlinePlus is an excellent source of credible patient education materials.
Source: U.S. National Library of Medicine; ©Stockbyte/Getty Images

resources and request information such as brochures, newsletters, and referral applications. See Procedure 15-2, Identifying Community Resources, at the end of this chapter. Type up an inventory sheet or spreadsheet of your resources, and make sure that all appropriate departments have a copy. A filing drawer can be used to organize and maintain the informational material regarding each resource. A complete and up-to-date community resources directory prepared by the office that is accessible to staff and patients is a valuable aid for referring patients to appropriate agencies. A medical assistant provides good customer service if he is able help the patient navigate her health care using this directory. Assisting patients to navigate their health care helps to improve patient health and well-being.

Visual Materials

Many patients are better able to comprehend complicated medical information when it is presented in a visual format. When using visual educational materials, it is useful to provide corresponding written materials that patients can keep for reference, when needed.

BWW Wire

Our e-newsletter is your guide to current health news, practitioner-written articles, and upcoming events for BWW Medical Associates.

BWW Staff Profile

New Year, New Electronic Health Records for All!

Over the past year, the staff of BWW prepared for the transition to a new electronic health record system. On January 1, 2015, all of our pre-existing files were officially integrated with our new Practice Fusion® EHR, and we have started primarily using electronic health records. We are excited to be able to continue to offer you the very best possible care utilizing this new system. We hope you will be patient with us as our staff get accustomed to using the new system. By January 2016, we are planning to have a patient portal system that will allow you—the patient—to access your medical records from the comfort of your home computer and to more easily request the release of your records to specialists and other providers.

Crunch Camp Challenge

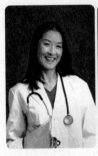

Ring in the New Year with the BWW staff as we challenge ourselves to eat healthier and exercise more. In the reception area, you'll be able to see a graph of our progress as we compete for the title of Crunch Challenge Champion and a new Vitamix blender.

Right now, Miguel is in the lead. With his marathon training regimen, he is logging an impressive number of exercise hours. Newcomer Marissa, however, is dominating the healthy eating component of the competition with her impressively varied and nutritious diet. You can log your own hours on our Crunch Camp app or at BWWAssociates.com to see if your can beat your favorite member of the BWW staff and win yourself a Vitamix blender.

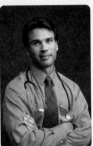

Meet Marissa T. Wang, NP and Andrew V. Utkin, PA

Starting in the New Year, BWW is happy to welcome Mrs. Wang and Mr. Utkin to our practice. Marissa started her career as a healthcare provider in the inner city, where she was a trauma nurse, before she decided to volunteer her time for a year with Doctors without Borders. She met her husband, a pharmacist, in south Sudan. Mrs. Wang just became a Nurse Practitioner, and she and her husband are expecting their first child this summer. Andrew will be splitting his time between BWW and a local non-profit clinic. Born to Ukrainian parents, Andrew spent his formative years abroad before moving to the United States for high school. He decided to enter the medical field after seeing the effects of war and the shortage of quality public healthcare.

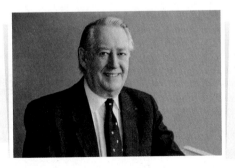

Happy Anniversary, Dr. Buckwalter

For the past 30 years, ever since he founded BWW Medical Associates, Dr. Buckwalter has called Port Snead his home. By founding his practice, Dr. Buckwalter brought quality medical care to this underserved waterfront community. A leading citizen, Dr. Buckwalter is known for his active involvement in local government and his Scottish Terrier Jamie. Dr. Buckwalter will be retiring from practice at the end of 2015; however, we plan to make his last year one to remember!

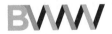
BWW Medical Associates, PC
305 Main Street, Port Snead YZ 12345-9876, Tel: 555-654-3210, Fax: 555-987-6543, Web: BWWAssociates.com

FIGURE 15-4 Practice newsletters are a great tool for patient education. They also keep patients up-to-date on practice events and advances.

©Stockbyte/Getty Images; ©Stockbyte/Getty Images; ©Corbis/VCG/Getty Images

Online Health Information The Internet is a widely used source of medical information. There are many reputable patient education websites for research. Websites should be checked for credibility before using them or referring your patients to them. See Procedure 15-3, Locating Credible Patient Education Information on the Internet, at the end of this chapter. Developing a list of reputable sites to suggest to patients as part of patient education as well as to use to create custom patient education materials is a must. After you have established the list, check the websites about every 6 months to be sure they are still active.

Streaming Videos or DVDs Streaming videos and DVDs are often used to educate patients about a variety of topics and to instruct them in self-care techniques. The use of a streaming video or DVD is especially effective when teaching about complex subjects and procedures. Examples of helpful streaming videos or DVDs used in patient education include those on breast self-examination, dressing change, prostate self-examination, and infant care.

Seminars and Classes Many physicians conduct or arrange educational seminars or classes for their patients. For example, an obstetrician might offer classes in childbirth preparation for patients and their partners. Other seminars and classes may be conducted depending on the type of medical practice.

Libraries and Patient Resource Rooms Most public libraries have an assortment of books, magazines, and electronic media or databases pertaining to health and medical topics. Hospitals may provide patient resource rooms, which include a variety of educational materials—such as books, brochures, electronic media, and DVDs—for public use. Some hospitals provide patient education materials on demand through televisions in patient rooms. A medical librarian is a healthcare team member and, if available, a good contact to assist you with obtaining and providing patient education materials.

Associations Thousands of health organizations and associations can be contacted for information about preventive healthcare and virtually every known disease or disorder. Table 15-1 provides a sample list of patient resource organizations. Search the Internet to obtain the latest contact information for each organization.

Once you are comfortable with the types of learning and teaching as well as the educational materials available, you should be ready to start patient teaching. Begin by creating a patient education plan. This plan includes identifying the education needs of the patient, creating an outline, collecting resources for teaching, carrying out the teaching, and then evaluating the effectiveness. Keep in mind that education is an ongoing process. However, the patient education plan gives you a place to start. See Procedure 15-4, Developing a Patient Education Plan, at the end of this chapter.

TABLE 15-1 Patient Resource Organizations	
Organization	**Web Address**
Academy of Nutrition and Dietetics	http://www.eatright.org
Alzheimer's & Related Dementias Education & Referral Center	http://www.nia.nih.gov/alzheimers
American Academy of Pediatrics	http://www.aap.org
American Cancer Society	http://www.cancer.org
American Diabetes Association	http://www.diabetes.org
American Heart Association	http://www.heart.org
American Lung Association	http://www.lung.org
Arthritis Foundation	http://www.arthritis.org
Asthma and Allergy Foundation of America	http://www.aafa.org
Centers for Disease Control and Prevention, U.S. Department of Health and Human Services	http://www.cdc.gov
National AIDS Hotline	http://www.thebody.com
National Health Information Center	http://www.health.gov/nhic
National Kidney Foundation	http://www.kidney.org
National Organization for Rare Disorders	http://www.rarediseases.org
President's Council on Sports, Fitness & Nutrition	http://www.fitness.gov
Substance Abuse and Mental Health Services Administration	http://www.samhsa.gov

▶ Promoting Health and Wellness Through Education   LO 15.5

Maintaining or improving your health is the best way to protect yourself against disease and illness. It is also part of being a good role model in your position as a medical assistant. **Consumer education** is geared toward the average person. It is provided in clear, everyday (nonmedical) language to help Americans become more aware of the importance of good health.

There are many ways to achieve good health. You can develop healthy habits, take steps to protect yourself from injury, and take preventive measures to decrease the risk of disease or illness. Patient education in the medical office should help patients achieve these goals.

Healthy Habits
Patient education can be used to promote good health habits by teaching patients the importance of:

- Good nutrition, including limiting fat intake and eating an adequate amount of fruits, vegetables, and fiber.
- Regular exercise.
- Adequate rest (7 to 8 hours of sleep a night).
- Avoiding tobacco and drug use.
- Limiting alcohol consumption.

- Safe-sex practices.
- A balanced lifestyle of work and leisure activities (moderation).
- Safety practices.

Whenever possible, these guidelines should be recommended to patients of all ages. Good health should be a top priority in life. Although it is best to adopt healthy behavior before illness develops, remind patients that it is never too late to work toward improving their health.

Protection from Injury

Many accidents happen because people fail to see potential risks and do not develop plans of action. Following safety measures at home, at work, at play, and while traveling can help prevent injury. A discussion of ways to avoid accidents and injury should be part of the educational process. See *Educating the Patient*: Tips for Preventing Injury to help patients avoid injury at home and at work.

Another essential aspect of educating patients about injury prevention is teaching them about the proper use of medications. A prescription includes specific instructions for taking the medication. Emphasize to the patient that these instructions must be followed exactly. In addition, the patient must not change the dosage or mix medications of any kind without first checking with the physician. Patients who do not adhere to these rules run the risk of potentially dangerous side effects. Tell patients to report to the physician any unusual reactions experienced when taking medications. Patients also must be cautioned to never share their medications with anyone else, no matter how tempting it may be to "help" a family member or friend.

When providing a patient with a new prescription, always ask the patient if he has told the doctor about all the medications he is already taking, including herbs, vitamins, and over-the-counter (OTC) medications. If the patient tells you that he has not, immediately inform the physician before the patient leaves the office. Some medications taken together or with certain foods can interfere with how well the drug works or cause side effects or adverse reactions. The physician needs to know about all drugs as well as herbal preparations and OTC medications the patient is taking.

EDUCATING THE PATIENT

Tips for Preventing Injury

To avoid accidents and injury, teach patients to use common sense and follow these guidelines.

At Home

- Install smoke detectors, carbon monoxide detectors, and fire extinguishers.
- Keep all medicines, chemicals, and household cleaning solutions out of the reach of children or adults with cognitive deficits.
- Purchase products in childproof containers. Lock or attach childproof latches to all cabinets, medicine chests, and drawers that contain poisonous items.
- Keep chemicals in their original containers, and store them out of reach of children and adults with cognitive deficits.
- Install adequate lighting in rooms and hallways.
- Install railings on stairs.
- Use nonskid backing on rugs to help prevent falls, or remove rugs altogether.
- Stay with young children and anyone prone to falls when they are in the bathroom.
- Do not rely on bath seats or rings as a safety device for babies and children.
- Set the water temperature on the water heater at 120°F.
- Never use appliances in the bathtub or near a sink filled with water.
- Practice good kitchen safety: Store knives and kitchen tools properly. Unplug small appliances when not in use. Wipe up spills immediately.

- When cooking, turn all handles of pots and pans inward, toward the cooking surface, to avoid spills and burns.
- Use twist-ties to shorten long electrical cords and speaker wires, or secure them with electrical tape. Avoid plugging too many electrical appliances into the same outlet.
- Exercise caution when using electrical appliances. Use outlet covers when outlets are not in use.
- To reach high places, use proper equipment, such as stepladders, not chairs.
- Use child safety gates at the top of stairwells.

At Work

- Use appropriate safety equipment and protective gear, as required.
- Lift heavy objects properly: Bend at the knees, not at the waist. As you straighten your legs, bring the object close to your body quickly. That way, strong leg muscles do the lifting, not weaker back muscles.
- Never attempt to move furniture on your own. Request that a member of the office building maintenance staff be engaged to do so.
- Use surge protectors on computer and other electronic equipment to prevent overloading outlets.
- Make sure hallways, entrance areas, work areas, offices, and parking lots are well lit.
- If your job involves desk work, practice proper posture when sitting. Do not sit for long periods of time. Get up and stretch, or walk down the hall and back.

Preventive Measures

Preventive healthcare is an area in which patient education plays a vital role. Patients need to know that they can decrease their chances of getting or living with certain illnesses and diseases and improve their quality of life by taking preventive measures and avoiding certain behaviors. Preventive techniques can be described on three levels: *health-promoting behaviors, screening,* and *rehabilitation.* (See Figure 15-5.)

Health-Promoting Behaviors The first level of disease and illness prevention is to form habits that lower the risk of illness or injury. Examples of these healthy habits were discussed earlier. Health-promoting behaviors also include understanding the symptoms and warning signs of disease. When these signs are recognized early in the disease process, the disease often can be treated more easily and sometimes even avoided altogether.

Screening The second level of disease prevention is screening. **Screening** involves the diagnostic testing of a patient who is typically free of symptoms. Screening allows early diagnosis and treatment of certain diseases. Examples of screening tests include colonoscopy, mammography and Pap smear for women, and prostate examination for men.

Regular screening examinations are necessary to health maintenance. Although the requirements differ according to the age and condition of the patient, screenings examinations usually include routine blood work, urinalysis, electrocardiogram (ECG), and a physical examination (PE).

Rehabilitation The third level of disease prevention involves the rehabilitation and management of an existing illness. At this level, the disease process remains stable, but the body will probably not heal any further. The objective is to maintain functionality and avoid further disability. Examples of this level of prevention include stroke rehabilitation programs, cardiac rehabilitation, and pain management for conditions such as arthritis.

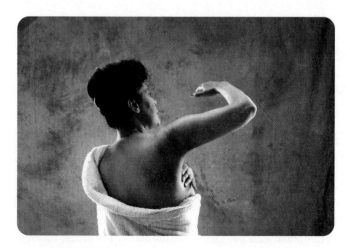

FIGURE 15-5 A breast self-exam is one example of a health-promoting behavior and is especially important when a family history of breast cancer is present.

Source: Bill Branson/National Cancer Institute

▶ The Patient Information Packet LO 15.6

When patients come to the medical practice, they need to learn not only about health and medical issues but also about the medical office itself. The patient information packet explains the medical practice and its policies. Unlike most other patient education materials, the patient information packet deals mainly with administrative matters rather than medical issues.

The patient information packet may be as simple as a one-page brochure or pamphlet. It may be a multipage brochure or a folder with multiple-page inserts. In many practices, the patient information packet is available online or through the EHR system for review or printing. See Figure 15-6.

Benefits of the Information Packet

The patient information packet is a simple, effective, and inexpensive way to improve the relationship between the office and the patients. It provides important information about the practice and the office staff. This information helps patients feel more comfortable with the qualifications of the healthcare professionals involved in their care. The packet may help clarify the roles that each office staff member has in patient care.

The information packet also informs patients of office policies and procedures. Patients will learn the doctor's office hours, how to schedule appointments, the office's payment policies, and other administrative details. This information helps limit misunderstandings about these procedures.

The patient information packet also benefits the office staff. It is both an excellent marketing tool and an aid to running the office more smoothly. Providing patients with a prepared information packet saves staff time by answering a number of potential patient inquiries. The information packet is also a good way to acquaint new office staff members with office policies.

Contents of the Information Packet

Regardless of the material the information packet contains, it must be written in clear language so that patients are able to read and understand it. All materials should be written at a sixth-grade reading level to accommodate the greatest number of patients. Information should not be presented in a technical medical style. Because you may be responsible for developing portions of the information packet, you should be familiar with the contents of a typical packet.

Introduction to the Office A brief introduction welcomes the patient to the office. It may be helpful to summarize the office's philosophy of patient care. The office's **philosophy** means the system of values and principles the office has adopted in its everyday practices.

Physician's Qualifications The packet commonly includes information about the physician's professional qualifications, including where he received his medical degree and any medical specialties. It usually lists his credentials, such as board certification, and membership in professional associations. For a group practice, the information packet may contain

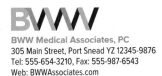

BWW Medical Associates, PC
305 Main Street, Port Snead YZ 12345-9876
Tel: 555-654-3210, Fax: 555-987-6543
Web: BWWAssociates.com

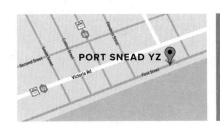

NEW PATIENT INFORMATION PACKET

PATIENT NAME: _____

DATE & TIME OF APPOINTMENT: _____

PHYSICIAN NAME: _____

Welcome to BWW Medical Associates, PC. Thank you for choosing us to assist in your healthcare needs.
We have included the following information in this packet:

☐ Letter of Introduction

☐ Map to provide directions to our clinic

☐ Description of our practice, staff, and office policies

Below you will find a checklist of information to complete prior to your appointment in our office.
Please fill out the entire packet and bring it in with you on your initial visit or complete it online at
www.BWWAssociates.com prior to your appointment.

☐ Medical history forms

☐ Patient information sheet

☐ An authorization for release of medical information

☐ HIPAA forms

☐ Please bring all medications that you are currently taking to this appointment

☐ Please bring your insurance card(s) and a photo ID so we may make copies for your chart

☐ Please bring all radiology procedures on a CD or film to your appointment
   (CTs, PET Scan, MRIs, X-rays, etc.)

It is our desire to make your visit to BWW Medical Associates, PC as pleasant as possible.
Should you have any questions, please do not hesitate to contact us at 555-654-3210 or by e-mail at
patientrelations@bwwassociates.com.

FIGURE 15-6   Every clinic should have its own patient information packet for new patient orientation.

a paragraph or a page for each physician. It also may include the qualifications of physician assistants or nurse practitioners who work in the physician's office. See Figure 15-7.

Description of the Practice The information packet should include a brief description of the practice, particularly if it is a specialty practice. Explaining the types of examinations or procedures that are commonly performed in the office as well as a list of any special services the office provides, such as physical examinations for employment, workers' compensation cases, or other occupational services, would be helpful. Be sure to make medical terms and specialties clear by avoiding the use of acronyms. Spell out everything the first time the reference is made and place the appropriate initials in parentheses.

Introduction to the Office Staff Many patients are not familiar with the qualifications and duties of the various members of the office staff. It is a good idea, therefore, to identify the staff positions according to their responsibilities and duties. Patients need to understand that some duties commonly thought to be a nurse's responsibilities may also be

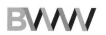

BWW Medical Associates, PC
305 Main Street, Port Snead YZ 12345-9876
Tel: 555-654-3210, Fax: 555-987-6543
Web: BWWAssociates.com

Alexis N. Whalen, MD

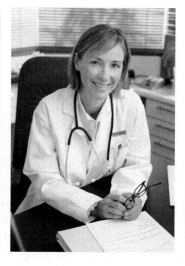

Dr. Whalen's Qualifications:

- Former Staff Pediatrician at Seattle Children's Hospital

- Board Certified OB/GYN and Pediatrician

- Residency in Family Medicine: Loyola University Chicago, Stritch School of Medicine, Chicago, IL

- Fellowship in Obstetrics & Gynecology: Stanford University, Stanford, CA

- Fellowship in Pediatrics: Seattle Children's Hospital, Seattle, WA

Dr. Whalen is a recognized expert in pediatric medicine, obstetrics, and gynecology.

Raised in Topeka, KS, Dr. Whalen completed her undergraduate studies at The University of Kansas, where she graduated first in her biochemistry class while also majoring in opera performance.

After graduation, she spent two years touring with an off-Broadway opera troop before starting medical school at Loyola University Chicago, where she went on to complete her residency in Family Medicine. During her residency, Dr. Whalen's talents for pediatrics, obstetrics, and gynecology shone, allowing her to acquire two competitive fellowships at the top research centers of Stanford and Seattle Children's Hospital.

A very well-received research study on Pediatric Cardiomyopathy earned Dr. Whalen a spot as a staff pediatrician at Seattle Children's Hospital.

While Dr. Whalen enjoyed the hustle and bustle of working at a major research hospital and the mild climate of Seattle, she and her husband decided to move back to his hometown of Port Snead five years ago.

Dr. Whalen enjoys long waterfront walks with her border collie Scout and her twin daughters Leslie and Lenore.

FIGURE 15-7 Healthcare personnel are the face of any medical practice. Providing patients with credentialing information as well as some personal information will help put new patients at ease.
©Chris Ryan/AGE Fotostock

performed by a medical assistant. It may be helpful to include the professional credentials and licenses of key staff members.

Office Hours This section should list the days and hours the office is open, including holidays. In addition, patients need to know what to do if an emergency occurs outside regular office hours. Patients should know what number to call first (for example, the answering service, 911, or the hospital emergency room) and what to do next. Include the telephone number and address of the emergency room at the hospital

with which the doctor is affiliated. Assure patients that the doctor or a physician partner can be reached at all times through the answering service. Some practices have multiple offices, and the physicians rotate from office to office on a regular schedule. List all office addresses and phone numbers, along with directions to all office sites.

Appointment Scheduling This section of the packet should explain the procedure for scheduling and canceling appointments. You might suggest that patients can benefit by scheduling routine checkups and visits as far in advance as possible. Also note if certain times of the day are reserved for sudden or unexpected office visits.

In this section, encourage patients to be on time for appointments. Explain the problems that result from late or broken appointments. If the office charges a fee for breaking an appointment without advance notice, mention it here. Be careful to address these sensitive areas with a positive, non-threatening tone. The office's written material should simply state the office policies and the problems that can result when the policies are not followed.

Communication Policy Providing the office's communication policies in the information packet can help save time for the office staff. Explain which procedures can be handled over the telephone and through e-mail and which cannot. Explain procedures such as calling in for prescription renewals or laboratory test results. If the physician returns patients' calls at a certain time of day, mention that policy in this section. Some practices bill patients for telephone calls in which medical advice is given but not for follow-up calls. For example, if a parent of a child who was vomiting uncontrollably called the physician to get immediate medical advice, the call might be billed. If the physician called to inform a patient of test results, however, the call would not be billed. It is important that patients know about these policies, particularly because many insurance plans do not cover charges for medical advice given over the phone, so the patient will be responsible for these charges.

Some offices (particularly pediatric offices) schedule a certain time of the day for patients (or parents and guardians) to call the physician for answers to their questions. This type of policy benefits both the office and the patients. The patients (or parents) have the assurance that they can speak with the physician about their concerns, and the office is spared interruptions during other times of the day.

Payment Policies Inform patients of the office's policies regarding payment and billing. State whether payment is expected at the time of a visit or whether the patient can be billed. List accepted forms of payment (for example, cash, personal checks, and credit cards). It is not common practice to mention specific fees in an information packet.

Insurance Policies List the major insurance carriers accepted by your office, or state that "most major insurance plans are accepted." Advise patients to bring proof of insurance coverage and a picture ID if this is their first visit to the office. A copy of this ID should be made and inserted in the patient's medical chart. State whether the office submits insurance claim forms directly to the insurance company or whether the patient has this responsibility. Generally, there is no charge for submission of the first insurance claim form; however, if the office charges for submission of secondary insurance forms, this should be stated. Outline the practice's policy for handling Medicare coverage, including whether the office accepts assignment on Medicare claims. If the office does not submit insurance claims directly, explain that the staff will help patients fill out insurance forms when necessary

and will provide the appropriate paperwork (usually a super-bill) containing dates of service and procedure and diagnosis codes for attachment to the claim form.

Patient Confidentiality Statement The information packet must include a copy of the office privacy policy. Complete information regarding the privacy policy and HIPAA regulations can be found in the *Legal and Ethical Issues* chapter. An important first step of HIPAA compliance is informing the patient of his or her rights. These rights are communicated through the Notice of Privacy Practices (NPP) (discussed in the *Legal and Ethical Issues* chapter), which must adhere to certain specifications.

The information packet also must state that no information from patient files will be released without a signed authorization from the patient. Each patient who receives a copy of the privacy notice must sign a document stating that he received the privacy notice and had the opportunity to have his questions about the notice answered. This document should remain in the patient's medical file.

Other Information The patient information packet may include the practice's policy on referrals. It may provide information about access to available community health resources or agencies. It also may include special instructions for common office procedures (for example, whether the patient needs to fast before a procedure or to avoid certain foods).

Distributing the Information Packet

For the information packet to be effective, you must make sure that new patients receive and read it. One way is to hand the packet to new patients at the time of their first office visit and briefly review the contents with them. Explain that they can find answers to many questions in the packet. Encourage patients to take the packet home, read the information, and keep it handy for future reference. However, you must be sure to obtain the signed documentation that the patient has received and read the privacy notice for the office files.

In many cases, the physician's office maintains a website where patients can view the information packet, make an appointment to see the physician, and get a map or directions to the office. The website also may allow patients to complete patient registration and consent for treatment forms online or download the forms, complete them by hand, and bring them to the office on the day of their appointment (Figure 15-8). Patients without Internet access may request to receive this information by mail, or they may be asked to arrive early for their appointment to complete the necessary forms.

▸ Patient Education Prior to Surgery

LO 15.7

When a patient undergoes a surgical procedure, patient education is vital to a successful outcome. Although exact instructions vary according to the procedure, their purpose is to prepare the patient for the procedure and to aid the patient during the recovery period.

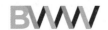

BWW Medical Associates, PC
305 Main Street, Port Snead YZ 12345-9876
Tel: 555-654-3210, Fax: 555-987-6543
Web: BWWAssociates.com

Paul F. Buckwalter, MD
Alexis N. Whalen, MD
Elizabeth H. Williams, MD

Consent for Treatment

I voluntarily give my permission to the healthcare providers of BWW Medical Associates, PC and such assistants and other healthcare providers as they may deem necessary to provide medical services to me. I understand that by signing this form, I am authorizing them to treat me for as long as I seek care from BWW Medical Associates, PC or until I withdraw my consent in writing.

_____
Signature of Patient or Guardian

_____
Date

_____
Printed Name of Patient or Guardian

_____
Relationship to Patient

Statement of Financial Responsibility/Assignment of Benefits

I acknowledge that I am legally responsible for all charges in connection with the medical care and treatment provided by BWW Medical Associates, PC and Associates. I assign and authorize payments to BWW Medical Associates, PC. I understand my insurance carrier may not approve or reimburse my medical services in full due to usual and customary rates, benefit exclusions, coverage limits, lack of authorization, or medical necessity. I understand I am responsible for fees not paid in full, co-payments, and policy deductibles and co-insurance except where my liability is limited by contract or State or Federal law.

_____
Signature of Patient or Guardian

_____
Date

_____
Printed Name of Patient or Guardian

_____
Relationship to Patient

A duplicate or faxed copy of this form is considered the same as the original document.

FIGURE 15-8   Sample patient consent for treatment form.

Providing Patient Education

Patients must receive information from the licensed practitioner (*not* the medical assistant) about the need for surgery and its nature. Educating and preparing patients for surgery may be your responsibility. You should provide support and explanations to patients. You must verify that they understand any information they have been given by other members of the healthcare team. Preoperative instruction may include discussion of postoperative care issues, such as temporary dietary restrictions or surgical wound care.

Determining whether patients have all the information they need before surgery is essential from both educational and legal standpoints. All patients who are undergoing a surgical procedure must first sign an informed consent form. This legal document provides specific information about the surgical procedure, including its purpose, the possible risks, and the expected outcome. The medical assistant may be asked to witness the patient's signature on this form. The signed informed consent form, along with documentation of all preoperative instructions, must be put in the patient's chart. (See Figure 15-9.)

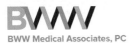

BWW Medical Associates, PC
305 Main Street, Port Snead YZ 12345-9876
Tel: 555-654-3210, Fax: 555-987-6543
Web: BWWAssociates.com

Paul F. Buckwalter, MD
Alexis N. Whalen, MD
Elizabeth H. Williams, MD

Patient Surgical Consent Form

Your surgeon for this procedure is: _____

I hereby authorize and request the surgeon, along with any assistants he/she feels are necessary, to perform upon me the following operation(s):

_____

I understand that the nature and purpose of the above mentioned procedure(s) is/are to:

_____

_____

I also authorize the surgeon to do any therapeutic procedure or investigation that in his/her judgment may be advisable for my well-being.

The nature of the planned operation has been thoroughly explained to me by my surgeon and I have decided to proceed with this form of therapy over other alternative methods. The risks, benefits, and alternatives, including doing nothing, have been explained to me. I understand that the practice of medicine and surgery is not an exact science and I acknowledge that no guarantees have been made about the results of the operation or procedure planned. Furthermore, the risks and complications inherent in the operation have been explained to me and I accept these.

I further give permission to have such anesthetics administered to me as the surgeon or the anesthetist deems necessary or advisable.

Pictures may be taken of the treatment site for record purposes. I understand that these photographs/videos will be the property of the attending physician.

☐ I DO agree to allow these pictures to be used for publication or teaching purposes.
☐ I DO NOT agree to allow these pictures to be used for publication or teaching purposes.

If I agree, I understand that my name and identity will be kept confidential and protected.

I agree to keep the office of the surgeon informed of my postoperative progress and I agree to cooperate with instructions given for my postoperative care.

Patient or Legal Guardian (Signature) _____
Patient or Legal Guardian (Please Print) _____
Surgeon as Witness (Signature) _____
Surgeon as Witness (Please Print) _____
Date _____
  Year   Month   Day

I hereby acknowledge receiving a copy of the postoperative instructions, which have been reviewed with me. I understand the advice and restrictions given and agree to abide by them. I will notify my doctor immediately if any unusual bleeding, respiratory problems, or acute pain occurs after my discharge from this surgical facility.

Patient (Signature) _____   Witness (Signature) _____
Patient (Please Print) _____   Witness (Please Print) _____
Date _____
  Year   Month   Day

FIGURE 15-9 Sample patient surgical consent form.

Preoperative Education

Preoperative education increases patients' overall satisfaction with their care. It helps reduce patient anxiety and fear, use of pain medication, complications following surgery, and recovery time. Letting the patient know what to expect during the surgery and afterward allows the patient to emotionally educate himself about the surgical procedure. The use of effective teaching techniques is essential to ensure patient understanding. Make sure the patient has a patient instruction sheet and can repeat the expectations back to you.

It may be difficult for a patient to visualize exactly what will take place in some surgical procedures. For example, think of arthroscopy of the knee. When told that the doctor will insert a viewing instrument into the knee, patients probably have no idea of the size of this scope. As a result, they may be particularly fearful of the procedure. An anatomical model, diagram, or photo is

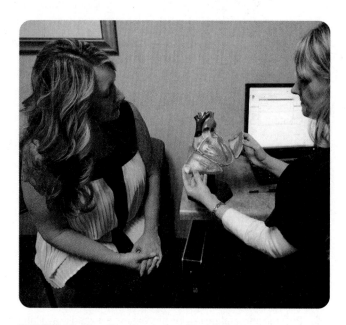

FIGURE 15-10 An anatomical model can help patients visualize what will happen during surgery.

©McGraw-Hill Education/David Moyer, photographer

useful to show exactly what will happen and ease patients' fears. For example, an anatomical model may help a patient who is having a surgery related to her heart see how the surgical procedure will help correct her problem. (See Figure 15-10.)

Helping Relieve Patient Anxiety

When you provide preoperative education, be aware that the fear and anxiety of patients who are about to undergo a surgical procedure can adversely affect the learning process. Consequently, allow extra time for repetition and reinforcement of material.

Always consider your choice of words carefully, stressing the positive rather than the negative whenever possible. Involving family members in the educational process is often beneficial, particularly if the patient is especially apprehensive about the surgery. Provide patients with contact information in case they have additional questions after they leave. Present your instructions and explanations in straightforward language that they can understand. Remember to be reassuring but to not promise a specific result for which the physician may be held liable if the expected result is not the actual result. Remember to verify that they understand everything. This also will help to reduce their anxiety level. Procedure 15-5, at the end of this chapter, will guide you through the process of outpatient surgery teaching.

PROCEDURE 15-1 Creating Electronic Patient Instructions

Procedure Goal: To create and administer patient instructions electronically

OSHA Guidelines: This procedure does not involve exposure to blood, body fluids, or tissue.

Materials: ⊍EHRclinic or another electronic health records software program that includes a patient instructions feature

Method:

1. Search the ⊍EHRclinic to find the button or icon to create patient instructions. (Check the "Help" button or review the training manual.)

2. Determine if you will need to write your own or can select from a previously created list of patient instructions. Select the correct button to proceed.

3. From the home screen of the ⊍EHRclinic, select "Tools" from the menu on the left side of the screen. On this Administrative tools screen, under the information management window, click on the blue bar labeled "Manage practice data."

4. Select "Patient education" and review the list to determine if the instructions needed for your patient are available. If not, you will need to create new instructions by using the "Add new attachment" feature.

5. Within a web browser, you can create new instructions by navigating to a credible Internet site, such as MedlinePlus, for patient instruction. If available on the site, select the "printer friendly" version. Highlight the information you want to use from the website, place your cursor at the beginning of the text, and, with your left mouse button depressed, drag the cursor to the end of the instruction page. Right-click on any highlighted area and choose Copy. Click in the patient instruction window or in the word processing program and, using the keypad, press the [Ctrl] and [V] keys.
RATIONALE: *All patient instructions must be accurate and credible.*

6. Identify and credit the web location where you obtain the data if they are copyrighted. Close the web page and return to the ⊍EHRclinic.

7. Import instructions by selecting "Add new attachment" under Patient education in the Information management section of the Administrative tools menu of ⊍EHRclinic.

8. Key the title and description of the instructions you just created. Then click the "Browse" button and navigate to the location of the instructions. Click "Choose."

9. Select "Add attachment," then scroll to the bottom of the list of instructions to ensure your instructions are available.

10. The instructions are provided to the patient and recorded in the ⊍EHRclinic to become a permanent part of the patient record.

PROCEDURE 15-2 Identifying Community Resources

Procedure Goal: To create a list of useful community resources for patient referrals

OSHA Guidelines: This procedure does not involve exposure to blood, body fluids, or tissue.

Materials: Computer with Internet access, phone directory, printer

Method:

1. Determine the needs of your medical office and formulate a list of the types of community resources that may be needed. The specific needs of your patients will help you formulate your list. Being able to help patients find outside assistance when necessary is the goal.

2. Use the Internet and/or phone directory to research the names, addresses, web addresses, and phone numbers of local resources such as state and federal agencies, home healthcare agencies, long-term nursing facilities, mental health agencies, and local charities. Locate local agencies such as Meals on Wheels; Alcoholics Anonymous; shelters for abused individuals; hospice care; Easter Seals; Women, Infants, and Children (WIC); and support groups for grief, obesity, and various diseases.

3. Contact each resource and request information such as business cards and brochures. Some agencies may send a representative to meet with you regarding their services. If patients can access information easily, they are more likely to take advantage of the services available to them.

4. Compile a list of community resources with the proper name, address, phone number, e-mail address, web address, and contact name. Include any information that may be helpful to the office.

5. Update and add to the information often, at least every 6 months, because outdated information will only frustrate you and your patients, creating even more anxiety.

6. Post the information in a location where it is readily available both in the office and on the practice's website, if available. Maintain an electronic record for easy reference.

7. Navigate patients to community resources when necessary.

PROCEDURE 15-3 Locating Credible Patient Education Information on the Internet

Procedure Goal: To determine the credibility of patient education information on the Internet

OSHA Guidelines: This procedure does not involve exposure to blood, body fluids, or tissue.

Materials: Computer with Internet access

Method:

1. Open your Internet browser and locate a search engine. Search engines vary in the way they search, so you may want to use more than one search engine for different results.

2. Search the topic. Be specific when entering the search term. For example, if you want to know about the proper diet for high cholesterol, you should type "high cholesterol diet." For different or more medical sites, try using different terms; instead of "high cholesterol," try "hyperlipidemia."

3. Select a site from the list of results and evaluate the source.

   a. Click the "About us" link to find out who developed the site. Sites should have an active link available to contact the webmaster and verify the source.

   b. Sites developed by professional organizations, educational institutions, or a branch of the federal government are generally better than those developed by an individual or a commercial company.

   RATIONALE: *These sites have less bias, and in most cases, their information can be reproduced for patient education use.*

4. Review the "About us" page to determine the quality of the information.

   a. Review the mission statement or other detailed information about the developer.

   b. Look for information about the writers or authors of the site. Make sure they are medical professionals.

5. Check the content of the site.

   a. Avoid sites that have sensational writing or make claims that are too good to be true.

   b. Make sure the language of the information is at a level that you can understand. Avoid sites that use lots of technical jargon for patient instruction.

6. Make sure the information is current by checking the copyright or by checking with the contact information on the site. Medical information changes frequently, so check the date and avoid information over 5 years old.

7. Avoid websites that are potentially biased. For example, if the site is written by a pharmaceutical company, the site will only present information about the medication manufactured by that company. There may be alternative medications. Sites written by individuals are interesting but may be biased as well.

8. Protect your privacy. If the sites require you to register, review their privacy policy. They may be able to share your or your patient's information with other companies.

9. Once you have evaluated the site and decide to use it, you may want to have your supervisor or licensed practitioner review and approve the information you will be providing to the patient.

PROCEDURE 15-4 Developing a Patient Education Plan

Procedure Goal: To create and implement a patient teaching plan

OSHA Guidelines: This procedure does not involve exposure to blood, body fluids, or tissue.

Materials: Pen, paper, various educational aids (such as instructional pamphlets, brochures, or EHR), and/or visual aids (such as posters and electronic media)

Method:

1. Identify the patient's educational needs in order to provide instruction at the patient's point of need. Consider the following:
   a. The patient's current knowledge.
   b. Any misconceptions the patient may have.
   c. Any obstacles to learning (loss of hearing or vision, limitations of mobility, language barriers, and so on).
   d. The patient's willingness and readiness to learn (motivation).
   e. How the patient will use the information.
   RATIONALE: Knowing what the patient already knows and understanding any special learning needs will help you tailor the instruction to the specific patient.

2. Using the various educational aids available, develop and outline a plan that addresses all the patient's needs. Include the following areas in the outline:
   a. What you want to accomplish (your goal).
   b. How you plan to accomplish it.
   c. How you will determine if the teaching was successful.
   RATIONALE: Developing an educational plan before providing the education ensures that all patient needs will be addressed.

3. Write the plan. Try to make the information interesting for the patient.

4. Before carrying out the plan, share it with the licensed practitioner to get approval and suggestions for improvement as well as to stay within your scope of practice.

5. Perform the instruction. Be sure to use more than one teaching method. For instance, if written material is being given, be sure to explain or demonstrate the material instead of simply telling the patient to read the educational materials.

6. Document the teaching in the patient's chart.
   RATIONALE: All patient education must be documented in the patient's medical chart for continuity of care and as a legal record.

7. Revise your plan as necessary to make it even more effective. To be an effective teacher, you must evaluate the methods you use.

PROCEDURE 15-5 Outpatient Surgery Teaching [WORK // DOC]

Procedure Goal: To inform a preoperative patient of the necessary guidelines to follow prior to surgery

OSHA Guidelines: This procedure does not involve exposure to blood, body fluids, or tissue.

Materials: Patient chart or progress note, surgical guidelines

Method:

1. Review the patient's chart to determine the type of surgery to be performed, and then ask the patient what procedure is being performed.
   RATIONALE: This confirms the patient's choice, knowledge, and understanding of the procedure including alternative treatments, the patient's right to refuse, and the patient's consent for the procedure.

2. Tell the patient that you will be providing both verbal and written instructions that should be followed prior to surgery.

3. Inform the patient about policies regarding makeup, jewelry, contact lenses, wigs, dentures, and so on.

4. Tell the patient to leave money and valuables at home.

5. If applicable, suggest appropriate clothing for the patient to wear for postoperative ease and comfort.

6. Explain the need for someone to drive the patient home following an outpatient surgical procedure.
   RATIONALE: Driving after even simple surgery can be very dangerous. Surgery can be canceled if a patient does not identify a responsible driver before surgery occurs.

7. Tell the patient the correct time to arrive at the office, surgery center, or hospital for the procedure.

8. Inform the patient of dietary restrictions. Be sure to use specific, clear instructions about what may or may not be ingested and at what time the patient must abstain from eating or drinking. Also explain these points:
   a. The reasons for the dietary restrictions.
   b. The possible consequences of not following the dietary restrictions.
   RATIONALE: Surgery can be canceled if the patient has not followed dietary instructions.

9. Ask patients who smoke to refrain from or reduce cigarette smoking during at least the 8 hours prior to the procedure. Explain to the patient that reducing smoking improves the level of oxygen in the blood during surgery.

10. Suggest that the patient shower or bathe the morning of the procedure or the evening before.

11. Instruct the patient about medications to take or avoid before surgery. For example, patients may need to stop taking a daily aspirin or vitamin E before surgery to reduce the risk of bleeding.

    RATIONALE: *Surgery can be canceled if the patient has not followed medication instructions.*

12. If necessary, clarify any information about which the patient is unclear.

13. Provide written surgical guidelines and suggest that the patient call the office if additional questions arise.

    RATIONALE: *Patients may not understand or remember verbal instructions. Written instructions can be taken home and reviewed again.*

14. Document the instructions in the patient's chart for continuity of care and as a legal record. Refer to the Progress Note.

    RATIONALE: *All patient education must be documented in the patient's medical chart for continuity of care and as a legal record.*

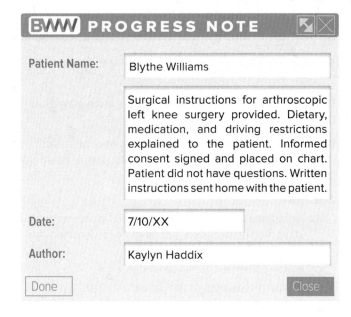

BWW PROGRESS NOTE

Patient Name: Blythe Williams

Surgical instructions for arthroscopic left knee surgery provided. Dietary, medication, and driving restrictions explained to the patient. Informed consent signed and placed on chart. Patient did not have questions. Written instructions sent home with the patient.

Date: 7/10/XX

Author: Kaylyn Haddix

Done   Close

SUMMARY OF LEARNING OUTCOMES

OUTCOME	KEY POINTS
15.1 Identify the benefits of patient education and the medical assistant's role in providing education.	Patients benefit from patient education because it can help them regain their health and independence more quickly. The medical office also benefits because patients will be less likely to call the office with questions, and therefore, the office staff can spend less time on the telephone. Educated patients take a more active role in their medical care.
15.2 Describe factors that affect learning and teaching.	Learning occurs in three domains: knowledge, behaviors, and skills. The patient must be able to recall the information, have the right attitude and be motivated to learn, and then implement the skills needed to demonstrate that the knowledge is retained.
15.3 Implement teaching techniques.	Teaching methods and formats are adjusted for the best possible result, depending on patient need and level of understanding. The best possible education plan comes from knowing your patient and his needs and abilities, as well as the goal of the instruction. Always assess your instruction at its completion and revise the plan as needed.
15.4 Choose reliable patient education materials used in the medical office.	The types of patient education materials in medical offices include brochures, booklets, fact sheets, newsletters, DVDs, Internet sites, and community-assistance directories. Using already completed print or electronic patient instruction sheets, ensuring that Internet sources are credible, and obtaining assistance from other healthcare team members are all methods of ensuring reliability of educational materials.
15.5 Explain how patient education can be used to promote good health habits.	Patient education promotes good health by teaching patients the importance of developing healthy habits such as eating properly and exercising regularly.

OUTCOME	KEY POINTS
15.6 Describe the types of information that should be included in the patient information packet.	The contents of the patient's information packet should include an introduction to the medical office, the physician's qualifications, a description of the practice, an introduction to the staff, office hours, appointment scheduling, telephone policies, payment and insurance policies, a confidentiality statement, and other pertinent information.
15.7 Describe the benefits and special considerations of patient education prior to surgery.	Educating patients prior to surgery is vital to a successful outcome. Patients should learn proper procedures before surgery and sign a surgical consent.

CASE STUDY CRITICAL THINKING

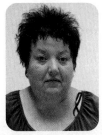

©McGraw-Hill Education

Recall Sylvia Gonzales from the case study at the beginning of the chapter. Now that you have completed the chapter, answer the following questions regarding her case.

1. What might be important to consider when creating an educational plan for Sylvia?
2. What factors could block effective patient education?
3. Why are good listening skills an important part of teaching?
4. What do you consider behaviors that indicate you are "talking down" or behaving inappropriately to a patient?
5. How can you personally be a better patient educator for Sylvia?

EXAM PREPARATION QUESTIONS

1. (LO 15.6) A benefit of the patient information packet is that it
   a. Promotes better compliance with treatment programs
   b. Helps patients feel more comfortable with the qualifications of the healthcare professionals who are caring for them
   c. Can answer a treatment question that may come up during an office visit
   d. Encourages patients to help themselves achieve better health
   e. Ensures patient compliance

2. (LO 15.3) Which of the following types of teaching gives patients a description of the physical sensations they may have during the procedure?
   a. Factual
   b. Sensory
   c. Participatory
   d. Modeling
   e. Media

3. (LO 15.4) Which of the following is the *most* difficult way to create electronic patient instructions?
   a. Type the instructions directly into a new document
   b. Import the instructions from the Internet
   c. Use previously created instructions
   d. Print the instructions directly from the Internet
   e. Use preprinted instructions

4. (LO 15.1) Which of the following is the *least* likely patient benefit of patient education?
   a. Patients are less likely to call the office.
   b. Patients take a more active role in their medical care.
   c. Office staff are not interrupted as often by patient phone calls.
   d. Patients will not need as much medication.
   e. Patients are more likely to understand instructions.

5. (LO 15.2) Which of the following is an example of the psychomotor learning domain?
   a. The patient is willing to read the brochure.
   b. The patient performs his own blood glucose test.
   c. The medical assistant tells the patient how she is going to feel during a procedure.
   d. The medical assistant provides the patient with a patient information package.
   e. The patient searches the Internet for information about his condition.

6. (LO 15.4) When checking an Internet site for credibility, which of the following is *least* likely to be necessary?
   a. Use caution if the site uses a sensational writing style.
   b. Look for the author of the information you plan to use.
   c. Check the date of the document you plan to use.
   d. Click links on the site to make sure they are not broken and are kept up-to-date.
   e. Ensure that the site is listed on at least two search engines.

7. (LO 15.6) Which of the following would *least* likely be in the patient information packet?
   a. Office policies and hours
   b. Patient instruction sheet regarding common tests done at the practice
   c. Patient instruction sheet about healthy living
   d. List of the physicians with their qualifications
   e. Patient confidentiality statement

8. (LO 15.7) What visual tool is especially helpful when performing preoperative education?
   a. Anatomical model
   b. Printed information sheet
   c. Line drawing
   d. Class or seminar
   e. Sensory teaching

9. (LO 15.5) Which of the following is a healthy habit that should be part of patient teaching?
   a. Getting adequate rest (4 to 5 hours of sleep a night)
   b. Limiting fruits, vegetables, and fiber
   c. Using tobacco in moderation
   d. Balancing lifestyle of work and leisure activities (moderation)
   e. Exercising about 15 minutes per day

10. (LO 15.5) Your patient has a history of cardiovascular disease. Which of the following is *least* likely a screening procedure that would be done?
   a. Blood work
   b. Colonoscopy
   c. Chest X-ray
   d. ECG
   e. Cardiac rehabilitation

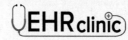

Go to CONNECT to complete the EHRclinic exercises: 15.01 Document Administration of Patient Education and 15.02 Document Administration of Pre- and Post-Operative Instructions.

SOFT SKILLS SUCCESS

A 35-year-old male patient is scheduled for a vasectomy tomorrow. It is within your scope of practice to provide preoperative instruction, and you feel confident in performing this task. When you introduce yourself and explain what you are going to do, the first words out of the patient's mouth are, "How do you know what this is all about? I am the one who is getting things cut!" How would you respond to this patient?

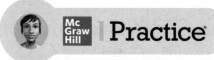

Go to PRACTICE MEDICAL OFFICE and complete the module Admin Check Out: Interactions.

21

Organization of the Body

CASE STUDY

Patient Name	DOB	Allergies
John Miller	12/05/1954	Bee Stings

Attending	MRN	Other information
Paul F. Buckwalter, MD	00-AA-005	Ordered: CXR-AP and Lateral Views

John Miller arrives at the clinic complaining of his shoes not fitting and feeling like he cannot take a deep breath. During the patient interview, he also states he is having intermittent pain in his chest. He has not taken his blood pressure medication for 2 weeks because he ran out of the medication and there were no refills left on his prescription.

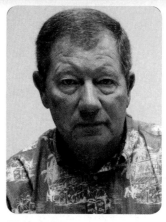

©McGraw-Hill Education

He is hoping to get this medication renewed. The licensed practitioner wants to evaluate his congestive heart failure and orders a chest X-ray. You know from your study of anatomy that the X-ray will provide an image of the structures in the thoracic cavity.

Keep John Miller in mind as you study this chapter. There will be questions at the end of the chapter based on the case study. The information in the chapter will help you answer these questions.

LEARNING OUTCOMES

After completing Chapter 21, you will be able to:

21.1 Explain the importance of understanding both anatomy and physiology when studying the body.

21.2 Illustrate body organization from simple to more complex levels.

21.3 Describe the locations and characteristics of the four main tissue types.

21.4 Describe the body organ systems, their general functions, and the major organs contained in each.

21.5 Use medical and anatomical terminology correctly.

21.6 Explain anatomical position and its relationship to other anatomical positions.

21.7 Identify the body cavities and the organs contained in each.

21.8 Relate a basic understanding of chemistry to its importance in studying the body.

21.9 Name the parts of a cell and their functions.

21.10 Summarize how substances move across a cell membrane.

21.11 Distinguish the stages of cell division.

21.12 Explain the uses of these genetic techniques: the polymerase chain reaction and DNA fingerprinting.

21.13 Describe the different patterns of inheritance and common genetic disorders.

21.14 Describe the causes, signs and symptoms, diagnosis, and treatments of various genetic diseases and disorders.

▶ Introduction

The human body is complex in its structure and function. Think of your own body for a moment. If you were to choose just one body part—say, your eyes—consider everything about how they look, how they function, how they are connected to the rest of your face, and how your skull supports them. Consider what happens to your eyes when you smile, cry, or glimpse bright sunlight. What about when a misguided insect or piece of dirt makes its way into them and you have to rub one eye with your finger and end up scratching it accidentally, causing temporarily blurred vision.

Of course, the eyes are just one example. You have your entire body to deal with. This chapter provides an overview of the human body. It introduces you to the way the body is organized from the chemical level all the way up to the organ system level. You will learn important terminology used to describe body positions and parts. You also will explore how diseases develop at the genetic and organism levels. This knowledge will help you function successfully as a medical assistant.

▶ The Study of the Body   LO 21.1

Anatomy is the scientific term for the study of body structure. For example, the heart may be described as a hollow, cone-shaped organ that is an average of 14 centimeters long and 9 centimeters wide. Understanding anatomy allows us to understand the normal positions of body structures and how to describe these positions precisely and correctly. **Physiology** is the term for the study of the function of the body's organs. For example, the physiology of the heart can be described by saying that the heart pumps blood into blood vessels to transport nutrients throughout the body. Anatomy and physiology are commonly studied together because they are intimately related. For example, the anatomy of the heart (a hollow, muscular organ) allows it to do its function (pump blood into tubular blood vessels). If the heart were not hollow, it could not allow blood to flow into it. If the heart were not muscular, it could not pump blood.

Knowledge of anatomy and physiology will help you grasp the meaning of diagnosis and procedure codes and help you understand the clinical procedures you will perform and assist with as a medical assistant. Understanding anatomy and physiology also can make it easier to see how and why certain diseases develop. Diseases develop in the body when homeostasis—the relative consistency of the body's internal environment—is not maintained. Body conditions that must remain within a stable range include body temperature, blood pressure, and the concentration of various chemicals within the blood. Individual cells also must maintain homeostasis. For example, if chemicals within a cell change the deoxyribonucleic acid (DNA), or genetic makeup of the cell, that cell can become cancerous.

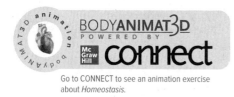

Go to CONNECT to see an animation exercise about *Homeostasis.*

Structural Organization of the Body

LO 21.2

The body's structure can be divided into different levels of organization. The chemical level is the simplest level—the billions of atoms and molecules in the body. Atoms are the simplest units of all **matter,** anything that takes up space and has weight, and many are essential to life. The four most common atoms in the human body are carbon, hydrogen, oxygen, and nitrogen. **Molecules** are made up of atoms that bond together. Proteins and carbohydrates are examples of molecules that consist of hundreds of atoms.

Molecules join together to form **organelles,** which can be thought of as cell parts. Organelles combine to form cells such as leukocytes (white blood cells), erythrocytes (red blood cells), neurons (nerve cells), and adipocytes (fat cells). **Cells** are considered to be the smallest living units in the body. When similar types of cells organize together, they form **tissues.** Two or more tissue types combine to form **organs,** and organs arrange to form **organ systems.** Finally, organ systems combine to form an **organism.** Figure 21-1 illustrates the organization of the body's organ systems.

Major Tissue Types

LO 21.3

Tissues are groups of cells that have similar structures and functions. The four major tissue types in the body are epithelial, connective, muscle, and nervous tissue. These are explained more fully in the following paragraphs.

Epithelial Tissue

When you think of epithelial tissue, think of a covering, lining, or gland. Epithelial tissue covers the body and most organs in the body. It lines the body's tubes, such as blood vessels and the esophagus, and the body's hollow organs, such as the stomach and heart. This type of tissue also lines body cavities, such as the thoracic cavity and the abdomino-pelvic cavity.

Glandular tissue also is classified as a type of epithelial tissue. It is composed of cells that make and secrete (give off) substances. If a gland secretes its product into a duct, as does a sweat or oil (sebaceous) gland, it is called an *exocrine gland.* If a gland secretes its product directly into surrounding tissue fluids or blood, it does not have ducts and is called an *endocrine gland.* The pancreas and thyroid are considered endocrine glands because they release their hormones directly into the bloodstream.

Epithelial tissues are avascular, which means they lack blood vessels. However, these tissues have a nerve supply and are very mitotic, meaning they divide constantly. In addition, the cells within epithelial tissues are packed together tightly. Epithelial tissues have many different functions, depending on their location in the body. For example, those covering the body protect against invading pathogens and toxins. Those that line the digestive tract secrete a variety of enzymes needed for digestion. They often possess microvilli—tiny, finger-like projections that allow the body to absorb nutrients. Epithelial tissues lining the respiratory tract have goblet cells and cilia. The goblet cells produce mucus, which traps small particles that enter the respiratory tract. The cilia constantly push the mucus and trapped particles away from the lungs (see Figure 21-2). Epithelial cells within the kidneys act as filters to help remove waste products from the blood.

Connective Tissue

Connective tissue is the most abundant tissue in the body. The cells of connective tissue are not packed together tightly. Instead, a matrix separates the cells. Think of the matrix simply as the matter between the cells of connective tissue. The matrix may contain fibers, water, proteins, inorganic salts, and other substances. The components of the matrix vary, depending on the type of connective tissue. Connective tissue generally has a rich blood supply, except for cartilage and some dense connective tissues that contain a very poor blood supply.

Many different cell types are located in connective tissue; the most common are fibroblasts, mast cells, and macrophages. Fibroblasts are responsible for secreting collagen and making fibers. They are essential for the normal development and repair of connective tissue. Mast cells

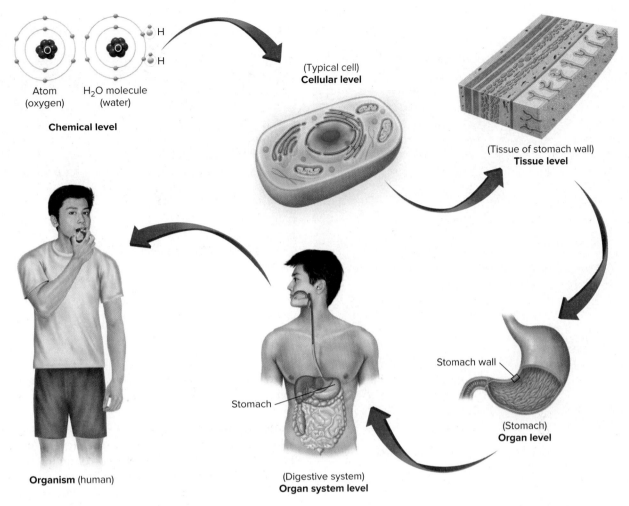

Chemical level

Atom (oxygen) H_2O molecule (water)

(Typical cell)
Cellular level

(Tissue of stomach wall)
Tissue level

Stomach wall

(Stomach)
Organ level

Stomach

(Digestive system)
Organ system level

Organism (human)

FIGURE 21-1 The human body is organized in levels, beginning with the chemical level and progressing to the cellular, tissue, organ, organ system, and organism (whole body) levels.

secrete substances such as heparin and histamine that promote inflammation when tissue is damaged. Macrophages are cells that destroy unwanted material, such as bacteria or toxins.

The following sections discuss the various types of connective tissue in more detail.

Blood This tissue is composed of red blood cells, white blood cells, platelets, and plasma. Plasma is the matrix of blood. Unlike other connective tissues, this matrix does not contain fibers. Blood transports substances throughout the body. Blood and its cell functions will be discussed in depth in the chapter *The Blood*.

Osseous (Bone) Tissue The matrix of osseous tissue contains mineral salts that make it a very hard tissue. Contrary to popular belief, bone is a living tissue—it is metabolically active.

Cartilage The matrix of cartilage is rigid, although it is not as hard as osseous tissue. Cartilage gives shape to structures such as the ears and nose. It also protects the ends of long

bones and forms the discs between the vertebrae of the neck and spine.

Dense Connective Tissue The matrix of dense connective tissue is packed with tough fibers that make it a soft but very strong tissue. Ligaments, tendons, and joint capsules have large amounts of this tissue type. Ligaments connect bones to bones, tendons connect muscles to bones, and joint capsules surround moveable joints in the body. Dense connective tissue also makes up a large part of the skin's dermis. When skin is damaged, this tissue "fills in" the damaged space and forms a scar.

Adipose (Fat) Tissue Within adipose tissue, unique cells—adipocytes—store fats. This tissue type stores energy for body cells, cushions body parts and organs, and insulates the body against excessive heat or cold (see Figure 21-3).

Muscle Tissue

Muscle is a specialized type of tissue that contracts and relaxes. The three types of muscle tissue are skeletal, visceral (smooth), and cardiac.

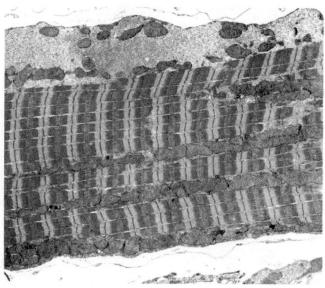
FIGURE 21-4 Skeletal muscle tissue.
©Science Photo Library-STEVE GSCHMEISSNER/Getty Images

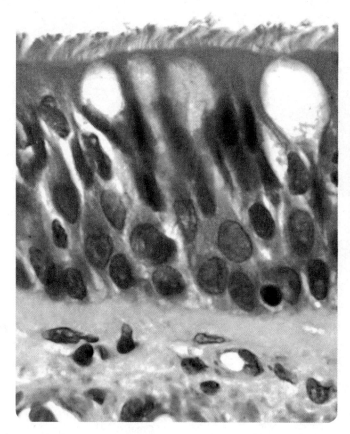
FIGURE 21-2 Epithelial tissue lining the respiratory tract.
©McGraw-Hill Education/Al Telser, Photographer

Skeletal Muscle Tissue As its name suggests, skeletal muscle tissue is attached to the skeleton. This type of tissue is voluntary because we can consciously control its movement. For example, we can consciously decide to contract the skeletal muscles attached to our arm bones and make them move. It also is referred to as striated because the cells of this muscle

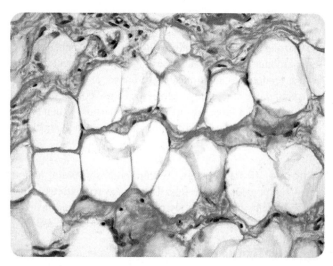
FIGURE 21-3 Adipose tissue.
©McGraw-Hill Education/Al Telser, Photographer

tissue type have striations, or stripes, in their cytoplasm (see Figure 21-4).

Visceral Muscle Tissue This smooth muscle tissue is located in the walls of hollow organs (except the heart), the walls of blood vessels, and the dermis of skin. It is involuntary—we cannot consciously control its movement. For example, you do not consciously decide when the visceral muscle of your stomach contracts. This tissue also is called *smooth muscle* because its cells do not have striations in their cytoplasm.

Cardiac Muscle Tissue This specialized muscle tissue is located in the wall of the heart. Like skeletal muscle tissue, cardiac muscle is striated. Like smooth muscle tissue, it is not under voluntary control; it is involuntary.

Nervous Tissue

Nervous tissue is located in the brain, spinal cord, and peripheral nerves. This tissue specializes in sending impulses, or electrical messages, to the neurons, muscles, and glands in the body (see Figure 21-5). Nervous tissue contains two types of cells: neurons and neuroglial cells. Neurons are the largest cells, and they transmit impulses. Although neuroglial cells are smaller, they are more abundant and act as support cells for the neurons. They do not transmit impulses.

▶ Body Organs and Systems   LO 21.4

Organs are structures formed by the organization of two or more different tissue types that work together to carry out specific functions. For example, the heart is made up of cardiac muscle tissue, connective tissue, and epithelial tissue. These

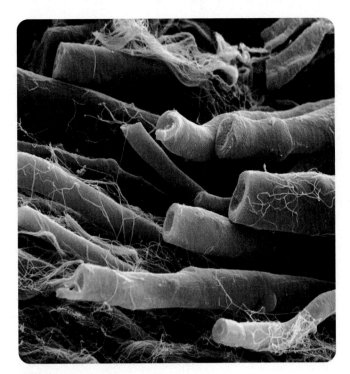

FIGURE 21-5 Nervous tissue.
©Science Photo Library-STEVE GSCHMEISSNER/Getty Images

tissues work together to carry out the heart's function—to effectively pump blood into blood vessels. Organ systems are formed when organs join together to carry out vital functions. For example, the heart and blood vessels unite to form the cardiovascular system. The organs of the cardiovascular system circulate blood throughout the body to ensure that all body cells receive enough nutrients. See Figure 21-6 for a summary of the human body's organ systems, their general functions, and the organs within each.

Understanding Medical Terminology

LO 21.5

Unlike the English language, in which word meanings often seem to have no rhyme or reason—like the overly used "whatever" and various difficult-to-translate modern slang—medical terminology often can be broken down into word parts that make the meaning concrete and easy to understand. All medical terms must have a **word root** (WR) that contains the base meaning for the term and a **suffix** at the end of the term that alters the word root's meaning. In the term *appendectomy,* for example, the word root *append* refers to the appendix and is combined with the suffix *-ectomy,* which means "surgical removal." So *appendectomy* means "surgical removal of the appendix." The word parts' meanings stay consistent, making it easier to learn new terms containing already understood word parts. Using your new knowledge, if you are told that the word root *hyster* means "uterus," you can easily see that *hysterectomy* means "surgical removal of the uterus."

In addition to word roots and suffixes, some terms also contain a **prefix,** which comes at the beginning of the term

and, like the suffix, alters the term's meaning. Let's take the terms *premenstrual* and *postmenstrual.* In defining terms, the general rule is to start with the suffix, then add the prefix (if present), and finally the word root(s); for example,

- The suffix *-al* means "pertaining to."
- The prefix *pre-* means "before."
- The prefix *post-* means "after."

The word root *menstru* refers to the menstrual period. Putting them together, *premenstrual* means "pertaining to *before* the menstrual period" and *postmenstrual* is "pertaining to *after* the menstrual period."

For terms in which the suffix begins with a consonant, a combining vowel—often an "o"—is used between the word root and the suffix to ease pronunciation. An example of this is the term *tracheotomy.* The word root *trache* ("windpipe") is joined to the suffix *-tomy* ("to cut into"). The letter "o" is inserted between the two to make pronunciation easier. When a combining vowel is added to a word root, it becomes a combining form (CF). In this case, the CF is *tracheo-.* Unlike prefixes and suffixes, combining vowels do not change the meaning of the term. The word parts *trache* and *tracheo* have exactly the same meaning. *Appendix I* contains commonly used word roots, suffixes, and prefixes. Table 21-1 summarizes information on understanding medical terminology.

Understanding how to build and dissect medical terms is a necessary part of the practice of a medical assistant. Throughout the anatomy and physiology chapters you will find medical terminology examples in a box like the one below. Review these features and then complete the *medical terminology practice section* found at the end of each chapter to improve your knowledge of medical terminology.

Medical terms are built and dissected using prefixes, word roots/combining form, and suffixes. For example, we can build the term *endocrine* by placing the parts of the term in the puzzle pieces where P = prefix, WR/CF = word root or combining form, and S = suffix.

endocrine

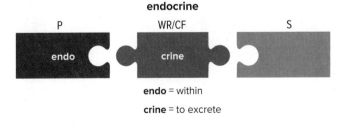

endo = within

crine = to excrete

Endocrine means to secrete within the body, such as an endocrine gland. Learn additional medical terms in the **Medical Terminology Practice** section at the end of this chapter.

Anatomical Terminology

LO 21.6

Anatomical terms describe the locations of body parts and various body regions. To correctly use these terms, it is assumed that the body is in the anatomical position.

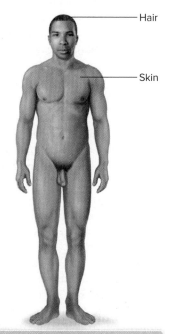

Integumentary System

Serves as a sense organ for the body, provides protection, regulates temperature, prevents water loss, and produces vitamin D precursors. Consists of skin, hair, nails, and sweat glands.

Hair
Skin

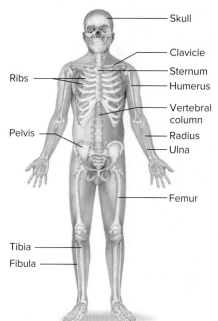

Skeletal System

Provides protection and support, allows body movements, produces blood cells, and stores minerals and fat. Consists of bones, associated cartilages, ligaments, and joints.

Skull
Clavicle
Sternum
Humerus
Ribs
Vertebral column
Pelvis
Radius
Ulna
Femur
Tibia
Fibula

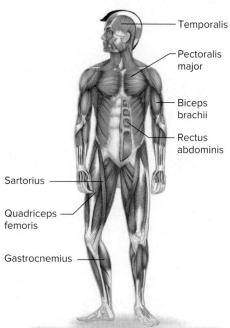

Muscular System

Produces body movements, maintains posture, and produces body heat. Consists of muscles attached to the skeleton by tendons.

Temporalis
Pectoralis major
Biceps brachii
Rectus abdominis
Sartorius
Quadriceps femoris
Gastrocnemius

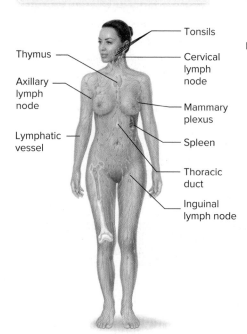

Lymphatic System

Removes foreign substances from the blood and lymph, combats disease, maintains tissue fluid balance, and absorbs fats from the digestive tract. Consists of the lymphatic vessels, lymph nodes, and other lymphatic organs.

Thymus
Axillary lymph node
Lymphatic vessel
Tonsils
Cervical lymph node
Mammary plexus
Spleen
Thoracic duct
Inguinal lymph node

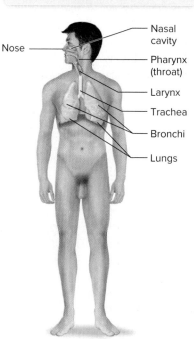

Respiratory System

Exchanges oxygen and carbon dioxide between the blood and air and regulates blood pH. Consists of the lungs and respiratory passages.

Nose
Nasal cavity
Pharynx (throat)
Larynx
Trachea
Bronchi
Lungs

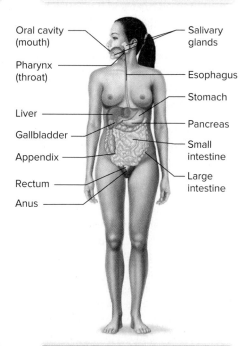

Digestive System

Performs the mechanical and chemical processes of digestion, absorption of nutrients, and elimination of wastes. Consists of the mouth, esophagus, stomach, intestines, and accessory organs.

Oral cavity (mouth)
Pharynx (throat)
Liver
Gallbladder
Appendix
Rectum
Anus
Salivary glands
Esophagus
Stomach
Pancreas
Small intestine
Large intestine

FIGURE 21-6   Organ systems of the body.

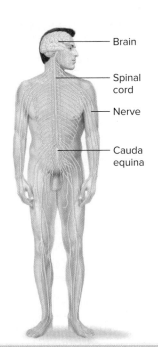

Nervous System

A major regulatory system that detects sensations and controls movements, physiologic processes, and intellectual functions. Consists of the brain, spinal cord, nerves, and sensory receptors.

Labels: Brain, Spinal cord, Nerve, Cauda equina

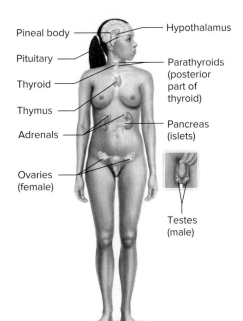

Endocrine System

A major regulatory system that influences metabolism, growth, reproduction, and many other functions. Consists of glands, such as the pituitary, that secrete hormones.

Labels: Pineal body, Pituitary, Thyroid, Thymus, Adrenals, Ovaries (female), Hypothalamus, Parathyroids (posterior part of thyroid), Pancreas (islets), Testes (male)

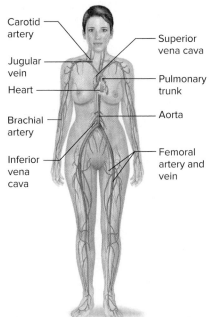

Cardiovascular System

Transports nutrients, waste products, gases, and hormones throughout the body; plays a role in the immune response and the regulation of body temperature. Consists of the heart, blood vessels, and blood.

Labels: Carotid artery, Jugular vein, Heart, Brachial artery, Inferior vena cava, Superior vena cava, Pulmonary trunk, Aorta, Femoral artery and vein

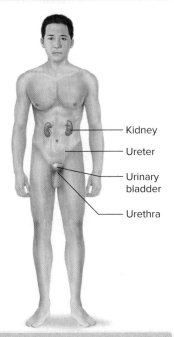

Urinary System

Removes waste products from the blood and regulates blood pH, ion balance, and water balance. Consists of the kidneys, urinary bladder, and ducts that carry urine.

Labels: Kidney, Ureter, Urinary bladder, Urethra

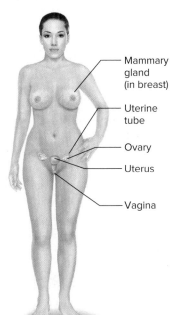

Female Reproductive System

Produces oocytes and is the site of fertilization and fetal development; produces milk for the newborn; produces hormones that influence sexual function and behaviors. Consists of the ovaries, vagina, uterus, mammary glands, and associated structures.

Labels: Mammary gland (in breast), Uterine tube, Ovary, Uterus, Vagina

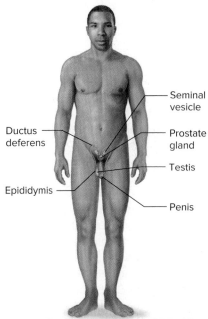

Male Reproductive System

Produces and transfers sperm cells to the female and produces hormones that influence sexual functions and behaviors. Consists of the testes, accessory structures, ducts, and penis.

Labels: Ductus deferens, Epididymis, Seminal vesicle, Prostate gland, Testis, Penis

FIGURE 21-6   Organ systems of the body. (*Continued*)

TABLE 21-1 Understanding Medical Terminology

Word Part	Description	Term Using Word Part	Term Meaning
Word root	Base meaning of the term	Colostomy	*Colo* = colon; *-stomy* = to cut (or create) a new opening colostomy: to cut a new opening for the colon
Suffix	Ending of term; alters meaning of the word root	Cardiology	*Cardi* = heart; *-logy* = knowledge of cardiology: knowledge (specialty) of the heart (with the combining vowel "o" between the two to ease pronunciation)
Prefix	Beginning of the term; alters the meaning of the word root	Tachycardia	*Tachy-* = rapid; *cardi* = heart; *-ia* = condition of tachycardia: condition of rapid heart (beat)
Combining vowel	Placed between word root and suffix to ease pronunciation	Cardiologist	*Cardi* = heart; *o* = combining vowel to ease pronunciation; *-logist* = specialist in knowledge of cardiology: specialist in the knowledge of the heart

TABLE 21-2 Directional Anatomical Terms

Term	Definition	Example
Superior (cranial)	Above or close to the head	The thoracic cavity is superior to the abdominal cavity.
Inferior (caudal)	Below or close to the feet	The neck is inferior to the head.
Anterior (ventral)	Toward the front of the body	The nose is anterior to the ears.
Posterior (dorsal)	Toward the back of the body	The brain is posterior to the eyes.
Medial	Close to the midline of the body	The nose is medial to the ears.
Lateral	Farther away from the midline of the body	The ears are lateral to the nose.
Proximal	Close to a point of attachment or to the trunk of the body	The knee is proximal to the toes.
Distal	Farther away from a point of attachment or from the trunk of the body	The fingers are distal to the elbow.
Superficial	Close to the surface of the body	Skin is superficial to muscles.
Deep	More internal	Bones are deep to skin.

For example, picture yourself in the **anatomical position**: Your body is standing upright and facing forward, and your arms are at your sides with the palms of your hands facing forward. Even if patients are lying down, for consistency and correct communication when you use anatomical terms, always refer to patients as if they were in the anatomical position. Anatomical position is pictured in Figure 21-9.

Directional Anatomical Terms

The directional anatomical terms that identify the position of body structures compared to other body structures are *superior (cranial)*, *inferior (caudal)*, *anterior (ventral)*, *posterior (dorsal)*, *medial, lateral, proximal, distal, superficial,* and *deep.* For example, the eyes are medial to the ears but lateral to the nose. See Table 21-2 and Figure 21-7 for an explanation and illustration of these important directional terms.

Anatomical Terms That Describe Body Sections

Sometimes, in order to study internal body parts, it helps to imagine the body as being divided into sections. Medical professionals often use the following terms to describe how the body is divided into sections:

- A *sagittal plane* divides the body into left and right portions.
- A *midsagittal plane* runs lengthwise down the midline of the body and divides it into equal left and right halves.

- A *transverse plane* divides the body into superior (upper) and inferior (lower) portions.
- A *frontal,* or *coronal,* plane divides the body into anterior (frontal) and posterior (rear) portions.

Figure 21-8 illustrates these planes.

Anatomical Terms That Describe Body Parts

Many other anatomical terms describe different regions or parts of the body. For example, the term *brachium* refers to the arm and the term *femoral* refers to the thigh. Figure 21-9 illustrates anatomical position and many of the common anatomical terms that describe body parts.

▶ Body Cavities and Abdominal Regions   LO 21.7

Body cavities house and protect the internal organs. The largest body cavities are the dorsal cavity and the ventral cavity. The dorsal cavity is divided into the cranial cavity (which houses the brain) and the spinal cavity (which contains the spinal cord). The ventral cavity is divided into the thoracic cavity and the abdominopelvic cavity. The muscle called the *diaphragm* separates the thoracic and abdominopelvic cavities. The thoracic cavity contains the following:

- Lungs
- Heart

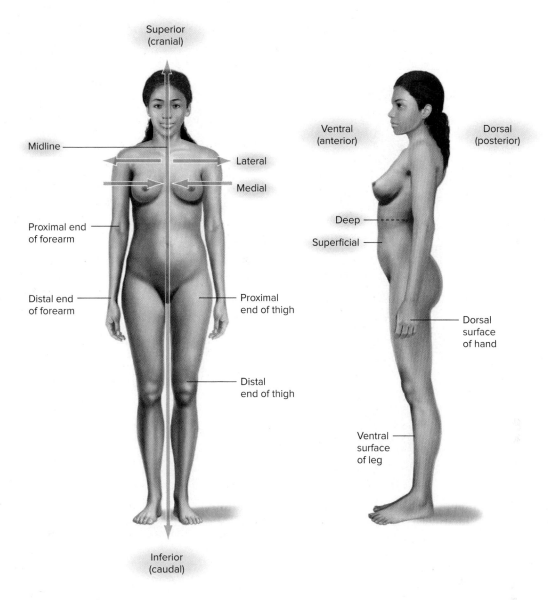

FIGURE 21-7 Directional terms provide mapping instructions for locating organs and body parts.

- Esophagus
- Trachea

The abdominopelvic cavity is divided into a superior abdominal cavity and an inferior pelvic cavity. It contains the following:

- Stomach
- Small and large intestines
- Gallbladder
- Liver
- Spleen
- Kidneys
- Pancreas

The bladder and internal reproductive organs are located in the pelvic cavity, which is depicted in Figure 21-10. The abdominal area is further divided into nine regions or four quadrants, which are illustrated in Figure 21-11.

Medical terms are built and dissected using prefixes, word roots/combining form, and suffixes. For example, we can build the term *epigastric* by placing the parts of the term in the puzzle pieces where P = prefix, WR/CF = word root or combining form, and S = suffix.

epigastric

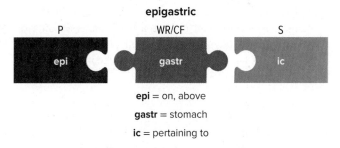

epi = on, above

gastr = stomach

ic = pertaining to

Learn additional medical terms in the **Medical Terminology Practice** section at the end of this chapter.

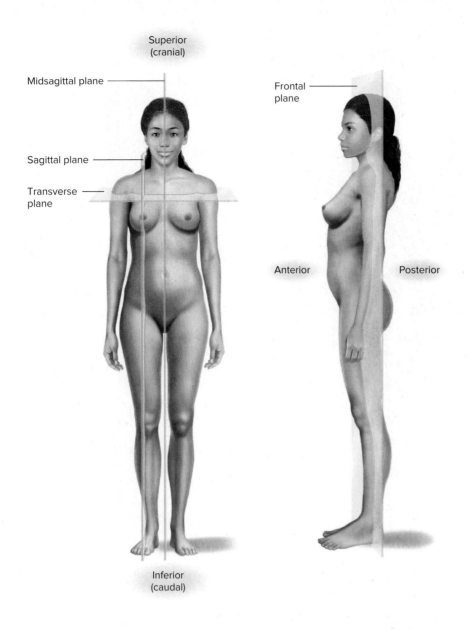

Superior
(cranial)

Midsagittal plane

Sagittal plane

Transverse
plane

Frontal
plane

Anterior   Posterior

Inferior
(caudal)

FIGURE 21-8   Spatial terms are based on imaginary cuts, or planes, through the body.

▶ Chemistry of Life   LO 21.8

Now that you have studied how the body is organized structurally, you need to learn about its chemical structure. **Chemistry** is the study of what matter is made of and how it changes. It is important to have a basic understanding of chemistry when studying anatomy and physiology because body structures and functions result from chemical processes that occur within body cells and fluids.

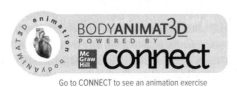

Go to CONNECT to see an animation exercise
about *Basic Chemistry (Organic Molecules).*

As you learned earlier in the chapter, the chemical level is the lowest level of organization. The building blocks of every living organism are the same chemical elements that make up all matter, liquids, solids, and gases. When two or more atoms are chemically combined, a molecule is formed. A compound is formed when two or more atoms of different elements are combined. For example, a molecule of oxygen (O_2) is not a compound because it is made up of only one element. In contrast, a water molecule is a compound because it is made up of atoms of two different elements—two hydrogen atoms and one oxygen atom. Water is critical to both chemical and physical processes in human physiology, and it accounts for approximately two-thirds of a person's body weight.

Metabolism is the overall chemical functioning of the body. It is a series of life-sustaining processes, including the

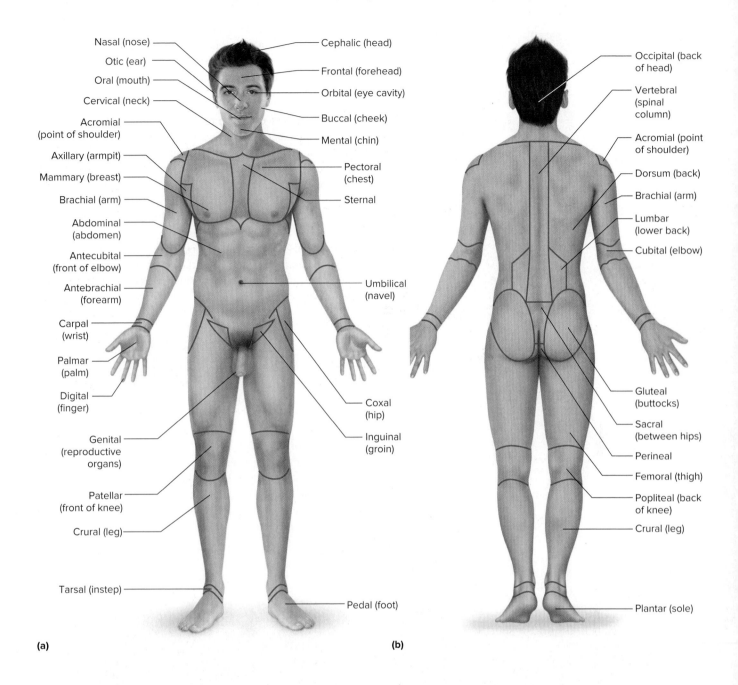

FIGURE 21-9 Numerous anatomical terms describe regions of the body: (a) anterior view and (b) posterior view.

breakdown of food and its transformation into energy. The two processes of metabolism are anabolism and catabolism. In anabolism, small molecules combine to form larger ones (for example, when amino acids combine to form proteins). In catabolism, larger molecules are broken down into smaller ones (for example, when stored glycogen is converted to glucose molecules for energy).

Electrolytes

When put into water, some substances release **ions,** which are either positively or negatively charged particles. These substances are called **electrolytes.** For example, when you put sodium chloride (NaCl) in water, it releases two electrolytes:

the sodium ion (Na) and the chloride ion (Cl). Electrolytes are critical because the movements of ions into and out of body structures regulate or trigger many physiologic states and activities in the body. For example, electrolytes are essential to fluid balance, muscle contraction, and nerve impulse conduction. Exercising makes you sweat, causing fluid and electrolyte loss. Drinking a sports drink after exercising helps you maintain fluid balance because sports drinks contain water and electrolytes such as sodium and potassium.

Acids and Bases Acids are substances that release hydrogen ions (H^+) in water. Many acids, such as lemon juice and vinegar, have a sour taste. Bases are substances that release

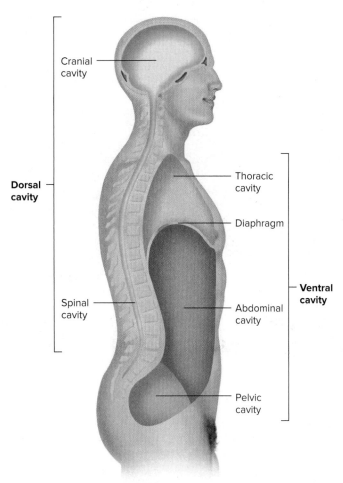

Cranial
cavity

Dorsal
cavity

Thoracic
cavity

Diaphragm

Ventral
cavity

Spinal
cavity

Abdominal
cavity

Pelvic
cavity

FIGURE 21-10   The two main body cavities are dorsal and ventral.

hydroxyl ions (OH⁻) in water. A basic substance also may be referred to as an alkali. Many basic substances are slippery and bitter to the taste. Laundry detergents, bleach, dish soaps, and many other household cleaning agents are examples of basic substances.

Testing Acids and Bases   In the clinical setting, litmus paper, pH indicator test strips, liquid pH indicator test kits, or a pH meter may be used to determine if a substance is acidic or basic. An acidic substance will turn blue litmus paper red, and a basic substance will turn red litmus paper blue. The pH scale runs from 0 to 14. If a solution has a pH of 7, the solution is neutral, which means it is neither acidic nor basic. If a solution has a pH less than 7, the solution is acidic. If a solution has a pH greater than 7, it is basic, or alkaline. The more acidic a solution is, the higher the concentration of hydrogen ions it contains. The pH values of some common substances are shown in Figure 21-12.

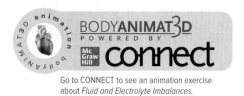

Go to CONNECT to see an animation exercise about *Fluid and Electrolyte Imbalances*.

Biochemistry

Biochemistry is the study of matter and chemical reactions in the body. Matter can be divided into two large categories: organic and inorganic matter. Organic matter contains carbon and hydrogen, and its molecules tend to be large. Organic matter is derived from or produced by living organisms. Most

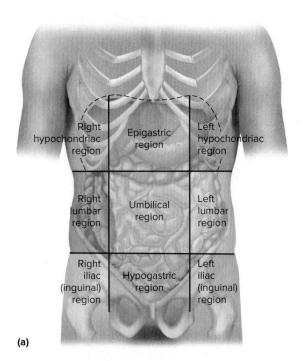

(a)

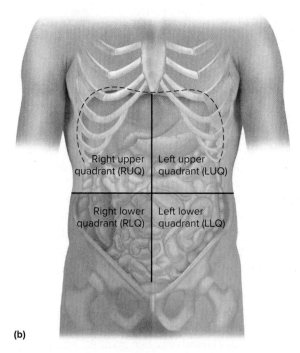

(b)

FIGURE 21-11   (a) The abdominal area divided into nine regions and (b) the abdominal area divided into four quadrants.

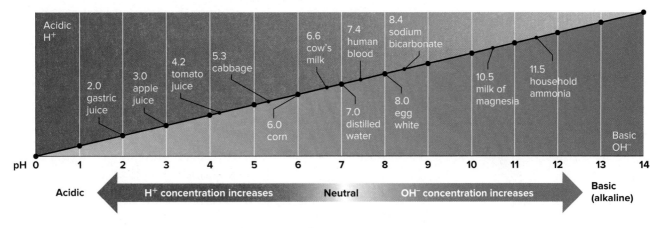

FIGURE 21-12 pH scale. As the concentration of hydrogen ions (H^+) increases, a solution becomes more acidic, and the pH decreases. As the concentration of hydroxyl ions (OH^-) increases, a solution becomes more basic and the pH increases.

inorganic matter does not contain carbon and carbon-hydrogen bonds; these molecules tend to be small. Inorganic matter is derived from nonliving sources. Examples of inorganic substances are water, oxygen, carbon dioxide, and salts such as sodium chloride. Water is the most abundant inorganic compound in the body. The four major classes of organic matter in the body are carbohydrates, lipids, proteins, and nucleic acids. These are outlined in the following sections.

Carbohydrates Body cells depend on carbohydrate molecules to make energy. The carbohydrate most commonly used by the body cells is glucose. A type of carbohydrate commonly found in potatoes, pastas, and breads is starch, which is broken down into glucose when needed.

Lipids Lipids are fats. Three types of lipids are found in the body: triglycerides, phospholipids, and steroids. Triglycerides store energy for cells and phospholipids primarily make cell membranes. Butter and oils are composed of triglycerides, and the body stores these molecules in adipose tissue (fat). Steroids are very large lipid molecules that make cell membranes and some hormones. Cholesterol is an example of an essential steroid for body cells.

Proteins Proteins have many functions in the body. Many proteins act as structural materials for the building of solid body parts. Other proteins act as hormones, enzymes, receptors, and antibodies.

Nucleic Acids DNA (deoxyribonucleic acid) and RNA (ribonucleic acid) are two examples of nucleic acids. DNA contains the genetic information of cells, and RNA makes proteins. Nucleic acids are made up of nucleotides, which are discussed in *section 21.12* of this chapter.

▶ Cell Characteristics

LO 21.9

Chemicals react to form the complex substances that make up cells, the basic unit of life. The human body is composed of trillions of cells. There are many kinds of cells, and each type

has a specific function. Most cells have three main parts: cell membrane, cytoplasm (liquid matrix containing each cell's organelles), and nucleus. Figure 21-13 shows the structure of a composite cell.

Cell Membrane

The cell membrane is the outer boundary of a cell. It is very thin and selectively permeable, which means that it allows some substances to pass through it while preventing other substances from passing through. Think of a fence and gate at an amusement park; people who have a ticket can enter through the gate, but those who do not have a ticket are kept behind the fence. The cell membrane is composed of two layers of phospholipids, different types of proteins, cholesterol, and a few carbohydrates.

Cytoplasm and Its Organelles

The cytoplasm is the "inside" of the cell. Mostly made up of water, proteins, ions, and nutrients, the cytoplasm houses organelles that perform many cell functions, and therefore body system functions. These organelles include cilia, the flagellum, ribosomes, the endoplasmic reticulum, mitochondria, the Golgi apparatus, lysosomes, and centrioles.

- Many cells contain hair-like projections on the outside of the cell membrane called *cilia*. Cilia assist with propelling matter throughout the body tracts, including the respiratory system. Cells with cilia often are found in the mucous membranes.

- A flagellum is a tail-like structure found on the human sperm cell and provides its "swimming" type of locomotion.

- Ribosomes, in conjunction with RNA molecules, are responsible for protein synthesis. Amino acids are connected together to form proteins through a specialized process involving different types of RNA molecules. The ribosome supports the protein chain as it is formed.

- The endoplasmic reticulum comes in two forms—smooth and rough. The rough endoplasmic reticulum is named for the presence of ribosomes on its surface, which give it a bumpy or rough appearance. Both types of endoplasmic

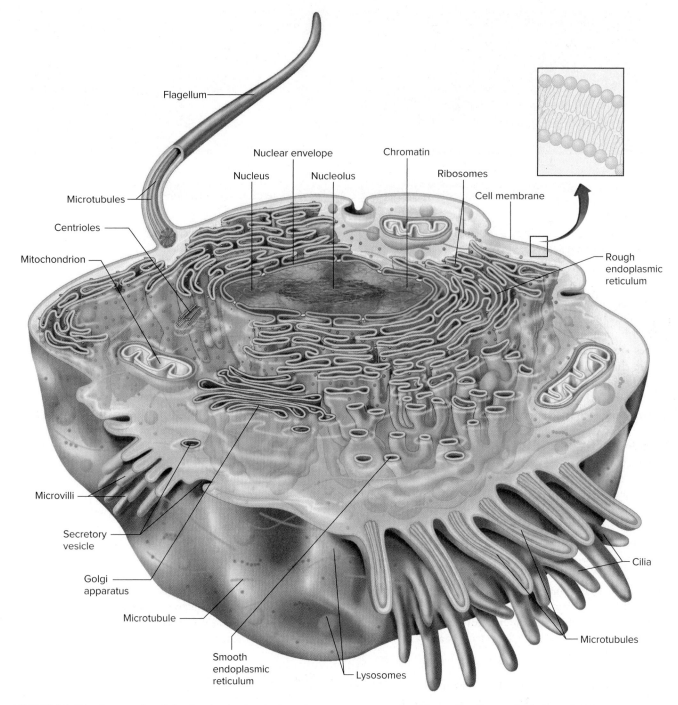

Flagellum

Nuclear envelope

Chromatin

Nucleus   Nucleolus   Ribosomes

Microtubules

Cell membrane

Centrioles

Rough
endoplasmic
reticulum

Mitochondrion

Microvilli

Cilia

Secretory
vesicle

Golgi
apparatus

Microtubule

Microtubules

Smooth
endoplasmic
reticulum

Lysosomes

FIGURE 21-13 A composite cell drawing showing the structures that are common to many cell types. Not all types of cells have all of these structures.

reticulum form networks, or passageways, for transporting substances throughout the cytoplasm.

- Mitochondria—the centers for cell respiration—provide energy for the cell. There may be only one mitochondrion in a cell or many, depending on how much energy each cell type requires.

- The cell's Golgi apparatus is known to process and sort proteins from the ribosome and to synthesize or produce carbohydrates. It is also thought to prepare and store secretions for discharge from the cell.

- The organelles known as lysosomes perform the cell's digestive function.

- The centrioles—two cylindrical organelles near the nucleus—are essential to cell division, as they equally distribute chromosomes to the resultant "daughter" cells.

Nucleus

The nucleus of a cell, a specialized organelle, is typically round and located near the center of a cell. It is enclosed by a nuclear membrane that contains nuclear pores, which allow larger substances to move into and out of the nucleus. It contains **chromosomes,** which are thread-like structures made up of DNA.

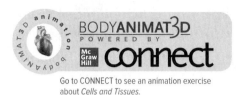

Go to CONNECT to see an animation exercise about *Cells and Tissues.*

▶ Movement Through Cell Membranes

LO 21.10

The selectively permeable cell membrane controls what moves into and out of a cell. Recall that selective permeability means there is some selection, or choice, in what substances cross the membrane. Some substances, such as oxygen and water, move across the cell membrane without the use of energy. These movements are called *passive mechanisms.* Sometimes the cell has to use energy to move a substance across its membrane in movements known as *active mechanisms.* Large molecules, such as glucose and proteins, move across the cell membrane by active transport.

Diffusion

Diffusion is the movement of a substance from an area of high concentration of that substance to an area of low concentration of the same substance; it can be described as the spreading out of a substance. Substances that easily diffuse across the cell membrane include gases, such as oxygen and carbon dioxide.

Osmosis

Osmosis is the diffusion, or movement, of water across a semipermeable membrane, such as a cell membrane. A semipermeable membrane lets water and other solvent liquids through but nothing else. Remember, water will always try to diffuse toward the higher concentration of solutes (solids in solution).

Filtration

In filtration, some type of pressure, such as gravity or blood pressure, forces substances across a membrane that acts as a filter. Filtration separates substances in solutions. For example, you could separate sand from water by pouring the sand/water mixture through a filter. In the body, capillaries in the kidneys act as filters to separate the components of blood.

Active Transport

In active transport, substances move across the cell membrane with the help of carrier molecules, from an area of low concentration of the substance to an area of high concentration of the substance. In other words, substances are gathered together, which is the opposite of diffusion. These molecules create channels in the cell membrane or otherwise change the membrane so that large substances can pass through. Think of these carrier, or transport, molecules as tiny doormen opening the door for large substances to enter an already crowded room. Some substances that move across the cell membrane through active transport are sugars; amino acids; and potassium, calcium, and hydrogen ions.

▶ Cell Division

LO 21.11

Cells can become damaged, diseased, or worn out, and replacements must be made. Also, new cells are needed for normal growth. Cells reproduce by cell division, a process that involves splitting the nucleus, through **mitosis** or **meiosis,** and splitting the cytoplasm, called **cytokinesis.**

A cell that carries out its normal daily functions and is not dividing is said to be in *interphase.* For example, if a liver cell is in interphase, it is making liver enzymes, detoxifying blood, and processing nutrients. During interphase, a cell prepares for cell division by duplicating its DNA and cytoplasmic organelles. For most body cells, each daughter cell will have an exact copy of the DNA and organelles in the original mother cell. Sometimes when the DNA is duplicated, errors called *mutations* occur. These mutations will be passed on to the descendants (daughter cells) of that cell and may or may not affect the cells in harmful ways. Mutations can be simple changes in the DNA sequence or complete deletions of a gene or part of a **gene.** A gene is a discrete section of DNA that contains a code for a specific protein or function. Think about this book as a gene; a simple mutation might be a misspelled word or the loss of a sentence, a chapter, or even the whole book.

Mitosis

Following interphase, a cell may enter mitosis—a part of cell division in which the nucleus divides. During this process, the cell membrane constricts to divide the cell's cytoplasm. This causes the organelles of the original cell to be distributed almost evenly into the two new cells. The stages of mitosis are listed here and pictured in Figure 21-14.

- *Prophase* occurs when the centrioles that have replicated just prior to the onset of mitosis move to opposite ends of the cell. As they separate, they create spindle fibers between them.
- During *metaphase,* the chromosomes line up in the middle of the cell between the centrioles on these spindle fibers.
- During *anaphase,* the centromeres divide, pulling the chromatids (now chromosomes) toward the centrioles at opposite sides of the cell.
- The final stage is called *telophase.* As the chromosomes reach the centrioles, each with its complete set, cytokinesis, or division of the cytoplasm, takes place and mitosis is complete.

Remember, during mitosis, the nucleus makes a complete copy of all 23 of its chromosome pairs (46 chromosomes

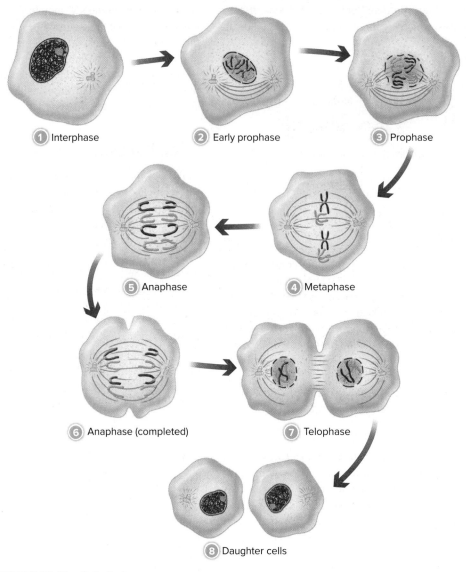

① Interphase   ② Early prophase   ③ Prophase

④ Metaphase   ⑤ Anaphase

⑥ Anaphase (completed)   ⑦ Telophase

⑧ Daughter cells

FIGURE 21-14   Cell mitosis.

altogether). As the cell divides, each new cell receives a complete set of chromosome pairs. The resulting cells are identical to each other.

Meiosis

Meiosis is reproductive cell division. It takes place only in the reproductive organs when the male and female sex cells are formed. During meiosis, the nucleus copies all 23 chromosome pairs, but two divisions take place. The four cells that are formed each contains only one of each chromosome pair, for a total of 23 chromosomes. This type of cell division must occur so that when the sex cells combine during fertilization, the resulting cell contains the usual number of chromosomes (46).

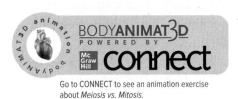

BODY**ANIMAT3D**
POWERED BY
Mc Graw Hill **connect**

Go to CONNECT to see an animation exercise
about *Meiosis vs. Mitosis.*

▶ Genetic Techniques   LO 21.12

DNA is the primary component of genes and is found in the nucleus of most cells within the body. As mentioned earlier in the chapter, a gene is a section of DNA that contains the code for a specific protein or function. Genetic techniques involve using or manipulating genes.

The chemical structure of every person's DNA is the same. The unique sequence of the *nucleotides* (groups of molecules that form the basic unit of DNA) determines an individual's characteristics. As an illustration, take the statement "my cat has blue eyes." Think of each letter as one nucleotide. If you change the letter "c" in the statement to an "r" you have an entirely different statement: "my rat has blue eyes." Many genetic differences—excessively large muscles in sheep, for instance—are caused by changes in just a few nucleotides. One DNA molecule contains hundreds or thousands of genes. Each gene occupies a particular location on the DNA molecule, making it possible to compare the same gene in a number of different samples. Two widely used genetic techniques in the clinical setting are the polymerase chain reaction (PCR) and DNA fingerprinting.

Polymerase Chain Reaction

The polymerase chain reaction (PCR) is a quick, easy method for making millions of copies of any fragment of DNA. This technique has been revolutionary in the study of genetics and has very quickly become a necessary tool for improving human health.

PCR can produce millions of gene copies from tiny amounts of DNA, even from just one cell. This method is especially useful for detecting disease-causing organisms that are impossible to culture, such as many kinds of bacteria, fungi, and viruses. For example, it can detect the AIDS virus sooner than other tests—during the first few weeks after infection. PCR is also more accurate than standard tests. The technique can detect bacterial DNA in children's middle ear fluid, which indicates an infection, even when culture methods fail to detect bacteria. Other diseases diagnosed through PCR include Lyme disease, stomach ulcers, viral meningitis, hepatitis, tuberculosis, and many sexually transmitted infections (STIs), including herpes and chlamydia.

PCR also is leading to new kinds of genetic testing because it easily can distinguish among the tiny variations in DNA that all people possess. This testing can diagnose people who have inherited disorders or who carry mutations that could be passed to their children. PCR also is used in tests that determine who may develop common disorders such as heart disease and various types of cancer. This knowledge helps individuals take steps to prevent those diseases.

DNA Fingerprinting

A DNA "fingerprint" comprises the unique sequences of nucleotides in a person's DNA and is the same for every cell, tissue, and organ of that person. Consequently, DNA fingerprinting is a reliable method for identifying and distinguishing among human beings to establish paternity and identify suspects in criminal cases (see Figure 21-15).

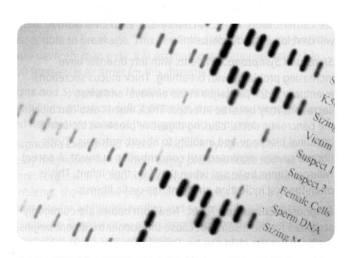

FIGURE 21-15 DNA fingerprinting can be used to establish paternity or identify a suspect in a criminal investigation.
©Martin Shields/Science Source

It also is used to diagnose genetic disorders such as cystic fibrosis, hemophilia, Huntington's disease, familial Alzheimer's, sickle cell anemia, thalassemia, and many others. Detecting genetic diseases early, or in utero, allows patients and medical staff to prepare for proper treatment. Researchers also use this information to identify DNA patterns associated with genetic diseases.

▶ Heredity and Common Genetic Disorders LO 21.13

Heredity is the transfer of genetic traits from parent to child. When a sperm cell and an ovum (egg) unite, a cell called a *zygote* forms. The zygote has 46 chromosomes, or 23 chromosomal pairs. One-half of each pair comes from the sperm and the other half, from the ovum. The first 22 pairs, which are the same size and shape, are called *homologous chromosomes,* also known as *autosomes.* The 23rd pair are called *sex chromosomes.* If the sex chromosomes are an X chromosome and a Y chromosome, the child is a male. If the sex chromosomes are both X chromosomes, the child is a female. Although the sex chromosomes determine a child's gender, they also determine other body traits. However, the autosomes determine most body traits such as eye color or freckles.

Each chromosome possesses many genes. Homologous chromosomes carry the same genes that code for a particular trait, but the genes may be of different forms, which are called *alleles.* Many times only one allele is actually expressed as a trait, even if another allele is present. The allele that is always expressed over the other is a dominant allele. The one that is not expressed is recessive. The only way a recessive allele can be expressed is if no dominant allele is present.

Detached earlobes are an example of a trait determined by a dominant allele. If a child inherits a dominant allele for this trait from one parent but inherits the recessive allele from the other parent, the child will have detached earlobes. If the child inherits recessive alleles from both parents, then he or she will have attached earlobes. See Figure 21-16.

Most traits in the body are determined by multiple alleles. For example, hair color, height, skin tone, eye color, and body build are each determined by many different genes. *Complex inheritance* is the term that describes inherited traits that are determined by multiple genes. It explains why different children within the same family can have different characteristics.

Sex-linked traits are carried on the sex chromosomes, X and Y. The Y chromosome is much smaller than the X chromosome and does not carry many genes. So if the X chromosome carries a recessive allele, it is likely to be expressed because there is usually no corresponding allele on the Y chromosome. For example, the presence of a recessive allele that is always found on the X chromosome determines red-green color blindness. This disorder (like most sex-linked disorders) primarily affects males because the corresponding Y chromosome does not have any allele to prevent the expression of the recessive allele. Genetic influences are known to contribute to many thousands of different health conditions.

CAAHEP

I.C.1	Describe structural organization of the human body
I.C.2	Identify body systems
I.C.4	List major organs in each body system
I.C.5	Identify the anatomical location of major organs in each body system
I.C.6	Compare structure and function of the human body across the life span
I.C.7	Describe normal function of each body system
I.C.8	Identify common pathology related to each body system including: (a) signs (b) symptoms (c) etiology
I.C.9	Analyze pathology for each body system including: (a) diagnostic measures (b) treatment modalities
V.C.9	Identify medical terms labeling the word parts
V.C.10	Define medical terms and abbreviations related to all body systems

ABHES

2. Anatomy and Physiology

a. List all body systems and their structures and functions

b. Describe the common diseases, symptoms, and etiologies as they apply to each system

c. Identify diagnostic and treatment modalities as they relate to each body system

3. Medical Terminology

a. Define and use the entire basic structure of medical terminology and be able to accurately identify the correct context (i.e. root, prefix, suffix, combinations, spelling, and definitions)

b. Build and dissect medical terminology from roots and suffixes to understand the word element combinations

c. Apply medical terminology for each specialty

d. Define and use medical abbreviations when appropriate and acceptable

▶ Introduction

Consider what you see when you stand undressed facing a full-length mirror. Pretty much everything you see in the reflection is part of the integumentary system. The integumentary system consists of skin and its accessory organs. Skin is the body's outer covering and its largest organ. Your skin accounts for approximately 15% of your entire body weight. The accessory organs of skin are hair follicles, nails, and skin glands.

▶ Functions of the Integumentary System   LO 22.1

People are often interested in the appearance of their skin—the color, the texture, the presence or absence of freckles, lines, wrinkles, puffiness, redness—but rarely consider its functions. The integumentary system serves many important purposes, including:

- *Protection.* As long as skin is intact, it is the body's first line of defense against bacteria and viruses. It also protects underlying structures from ultraviolet (UV) radiation and dehydration.

- *Body temperature regulation.* Skin plays a major role in regulating body temperature. When a person is hot, dermal blood vessels dilate, which is why a person's skin becomes pinkish. Because the dermal blood vessels are dilated, more blood than normal passes through the skin. This is beneficial because blood carries a lot of the body's heat.

When the blood gets close to the body's surface (to skin), the heat can escape. On the other hand, if a person is cold, the dermal blood vessels constrict, preventing the heat in blood from escaping.

- *Vitamin D production.* When exposed to sunlight, the skin produces a molecule that is turned into vitamin D. The body needs vitamin D for calcium absorption.

- *Sensation.* The skin is packed with sensory receptors that can detect touch, heat, cold, and pain.

- *Excretion.* Small amounts of waste products, such as water and salts, are lost through skin when a person perspires. This is why hydration is so important when exercising or during exposure to high temperatures, as the amount of perspiration increases and higher amounts of water and salts are lost.

▶ Skin Structure   LO 22.2

The skin is a complex organ that consists of three layers. The **epidermis** (top layer) and the dermis (middle layer) sit on a third layer called the subcutaneous layer or hypodermis (see Figure 22-1).

Epidermis

The epidermis is the most superficial layer of skin. It is made up of many layers of tightly packed cells and can be divided into two major sublayers: the stratum corneum and the stratum basale.

The **stratum corneum** is the most superficial layer of the epidermis. Most of the cells in this layer are dead and very

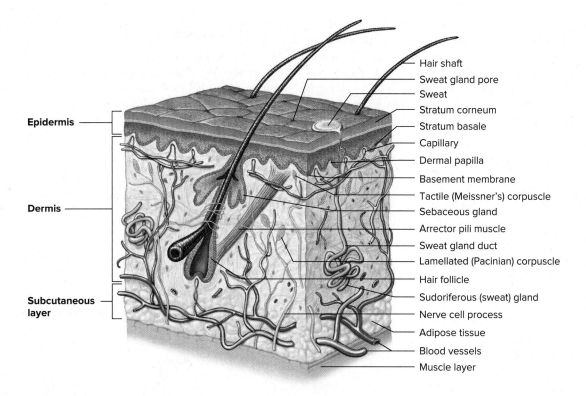

Hair shaft
Sweat gland pore
Sweat
Stratum corneum
Stratum basale
Capillary
Dermal papilla
Basement membrane
Tactile (Meissner's) corpuscle
Sebaceous gland
Arrector pili muscle
Sweat gland duct
Lamellated (Pacinian) corpuscle
Hair follicle
Sudoriferous (sweat) gland
Nerve cell process
Adipose tissue
Blood vessels
Muscle layer

Epidermis

Dermis

Subcutaneous layer

FIGURE 22-1 Section of skin.

flat. Because they have accumulated a tough protein called **keratin,** the cells in this layer stick together and form an impermeable layer for skin. Most bacteria, viruses, and water cannot penetrate the stratum corneum.

The **stratum basale,** also known as the *stratum germinativum,* is the deepest layer of the epidermis. The cells in this layer are constantly dividing (or germinating), which pushes older cells up toward the stratum corneum.

The most common cell type in the epidermis is the **keratinocyte.** This cell makes and accumulates keratin, which makes the epidermis waterproof and resistant to bacteria and viruses. Another cell type of the epidermis is the **melanocyte,** which makes the pigment **melanin.** Melanin is deposited throughout the layers of the epidermis. This pigment absorbs UV radiation from sunlight and prevents the radiation from harming structures in the skin's underlying layers. The amount of melanin inherited in combination with sun exposure is responsible for the freckles that "appear" after sun exposure.

Dermis

Lying below the epidermis is the dermis. The **dermis** is living tissue that binds the epidermal top layer to the underlying subcutaneous tissue layer. As living tissue, the dermal layer includes all major tissue types, as well as the following:

- Epithelial, connective, muscle, and nervous tissues.
- Sudoriferous (sweat) glands.
- Sebaceous (oil) glands.
- Hair follicles.
- The arrector pili muscles.
- Collagen fibers, elastin fibers, nerve fibers, and many blood vessels.

Subcutaneous Layer

The **subcutaneous** layer of skin, or **hypodermis,** is largely made up of adipose and loose connective tissue. Like the dermis, the subcutaneous layer also contains blood vessels and nerves. The adipose, or fat, tissue acts as a storage facility. It also cushions and insulates the underlying structures and organs. The amount of adipose tissue varies from body region to body region and from person to person.

▶ Skin Color   LO 22.3

The amount of melanin in the skin's epidermis is what most determines skin color. Melanin can range in color from yellowish to brownish. The more melanin a person has in the skin, the darker the skin color. All people have about the same number of melanocytes, regardless of skin color. What varies from person to person is how active the melanocytes are in producing melanin. For example, a person with dark skin has very active melanocytes. Sunlight, UV lamps, and X-rays stimulate melanin production. This is why your skin darkens when you go to a tanning bed or to the beach for the day. Patients undergoing radiation therapy often have tanned skin in the treatment area.

As you studied in the chapter *Organization of the Body,* your inherited characteristics come from your parents. So your skin color—meaning the activity of the melanocytes—is directly related to the genes you received from your parents. As the gene pool is varied between ethnic backgrounds, it is also varied within families, which explains the differences in skin color not only among races but also within families.

Another factor that determines skin color is the amount of **oxygenated** blood in the skin's dermis. Oxygen is carried by a pigment called *hemoglobin* in the red blood cells (RBCs). *Oxygenation* refers to the amount of oxygen dissolved in the hemoglobin. Well-oxygenated hemoglobin is bright red, whereas poorly oxygenated hemoglobin is darker red. A person with a rich supply of oxygenated blood will have skin that is a pinkish hue. When the supply of oxygen in the blood is low, the skin looks rather pale or bluish. A bluish color of skin is called *cyanosis*.

▶ Skin Lesions LO 22.4

The term *skin lesion* may be loosely defined as any variation in or on the skin (see Figure 22-2). Many of us have skin lesions; even a freckle is a lesion because it is a skin variation. Other lesions, such as ulcers and tumors, are more troublesome types of lesions. Skin lesions are classified into three major categories: primary, secondary, and vascular.

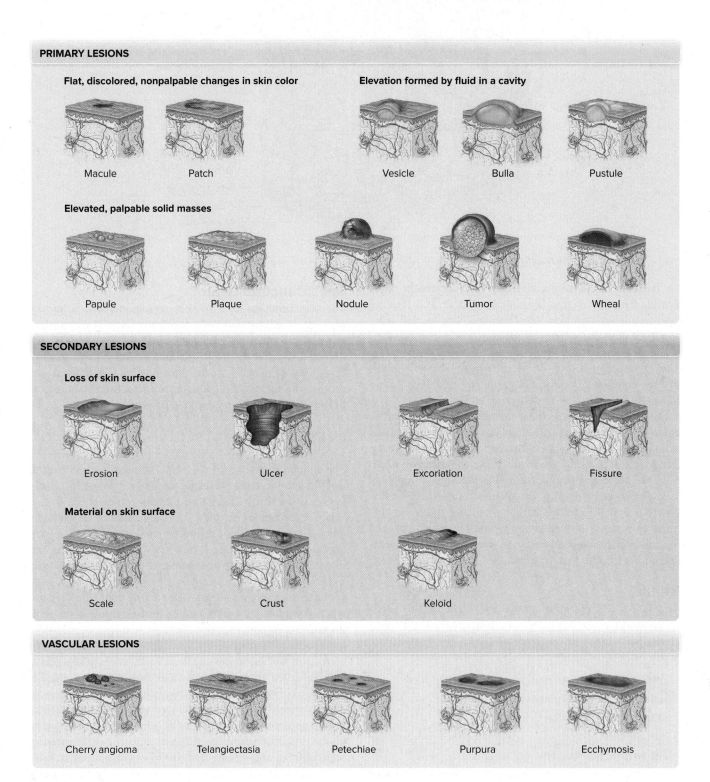

PRIMARY LESIONS

Flat, discolored, nonpalpable changes in skin color

Macule Patch

Elevation formed by fluid in a cavity

Vesicle Bulla Pustule

Elevated, palpable solid masses

Papule Plaque Nodule Tumor Wheal

SECONDARY LESIONS

Loss of skin surface

Erosion Ulcer Excoriation Fissure

Material on skin surface

Scale Crust Keloid

VASCULAR LESIONS

Cherry angioma Telangiectasia Petechiae Purpura Ecchymosis

FIGURE 22-2 Types of skin lesions.

- Primary lesions such as macules and vesicles originate from disease or body changes.
- Secondary lesions, which include ulcers and keloids, are caused by a reaction to external traumas such as scratching or rubbing, some are caused by healing processes, or they also may be caused by primary lesions.
- Vascular lesions are anomalies of the blood vessels and include telangiectasias, which are small, dilated blood vessels on the skin's surface; hemangiomas, which are benign blood vessel tumors; and ecchymoses, commonly called bruises.

Medical terms are built and dissected using prefixes, word roots/combining form, and suffixes. For example, we can build the term *hemangioma* by placing the parts of the term in the puzzle pieces where P = prefix, WR/CF = word root or combining form, and S = suffix.

hemangioma

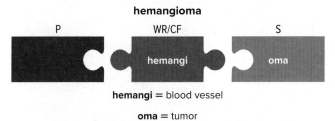

hemangi = blood vessel

oma = tumor

A hemangioma is a tumor of a blood vessel. Learn additional medical terms in the **Medical Terminology Practice** section at the end of this chapter.

Table 22-1 lists some of the common types of skin lesions.

▶ Accessory Organs

LO 22.5

The skin's accessory organs include hair follicles, **sebaceous** (oil) glands, nails, and **sudoriferous** (sweat) glands. Technically, breasts are considered an accessory organ of the integumentary system, but because they are more closely associated with the female reproductive system, they will be discussed in *The Reproductive Systems* chapter.

Hair Follicles

Hair **follicles** are tube-like structures in the skin's dermis; they are made up of epithelial tissue. Their function is to generate hairs (see Figure 22-3). Keratinocytes make up most of the hair follicle. As hair follicles produce new keratinocytes, old ones are pushed toward the skin's surface. The old keratinocytes stick together to produce a hair. The portion of the hair embedded in the skin is called the *root* and the portion of the hair extending from the surface of skin is called the *shaft*.

Melanocytes also are found in hair follicles. They produce and distribute pigments to create hair color. A person develops gray hair when these melanocytes produce less pigment than normal.

When a hair follicle goes into a resting cycle, the hair falls out. Most of the time, the hair follicle will begin a growing cycle again and produce a new hair. However, sometimes hair follicles completely die, and **alopecia** (baldness) develops.

Arrector pili muscles are attached to most hair follicles. When a person is cold or nervous, these muscles pull on hair follicles and cause hairs to stand erect. These muscles also pull on fibers in the skin's dermis, causing goose bumps (see Figure 22-3).

Sudoriferous Glands

Most sudoriferous glands are located in the skin's dermis. However, their ducts open onto the skin's epidermis. There are two types of sweat glands: eccrine and apocrine.

- **Eccrine glands** are the most numerous sweat glands. They produce a watery type of sweat and are activated primarily by heat. Once sweat is deposited onto skin, it evaporates and carries heat away from the body. Eccrine sweat glands are most concentrated on the forehead, neck, and back.
- **Apocrine glands** produce a thicker type of sweat that contains more proteins than the type of sweat produced by eccrine sweat glands. Apocrine glands are most concentrated in areas of skin with coarse hair, such as the armpit and groin areas. They become active during puberty and

TABLE 22-1	Common Skin Lesions and Descriptions
Lesion Name	**Description**
Bulla	A large blister or cluster of blisters
Cicatrix	A scar, usually inside a wound or tissue
Crust	Dried blood or pus on the skin
Ecchymosis	A black and blue mark, or bruise
Erosion	A shallow area of skin worn away by friction or pressure
Excoriation	A scratch; may be covered with dried blood
Fissure	A crack in the skin's surface
Keloid	An overgrowth of scar tissue
Macule	A flat skin discoloration, such as a freckle or a flat mole
Nodule	A large pimple or small node (larger than 6 cm)
Papule	An elevated mass similar to but smaller than a nodule
Petechiae	Pinpoint skin hemorrhages that result from bleeding disorders
Plaque	A small, flat, scaly area of skin
Purpura	Purple-red bruises, usually the result of clotting abnormalities
Pustule	An elevated (infected) lesion containing pus
Scale	Thin plaques of epithelial tissue on the skin's surface
Tumor	A swelling of abnormal tissue growth
Ulcer	A wound that results from tissue loss
Verrucae	Another term for warts
Vesicle	A blister
Wheal	Another term for hive

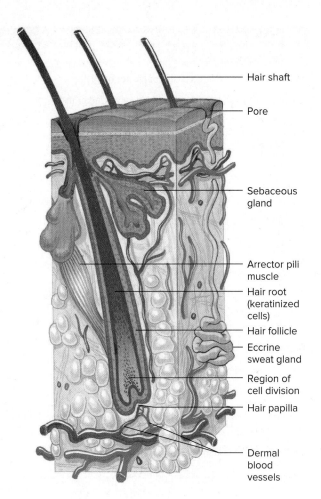

FIGURE 22-3 The hair follicle extends into the dermis.

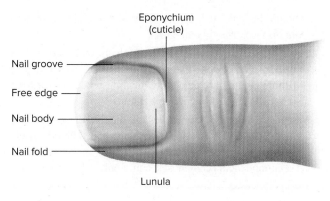

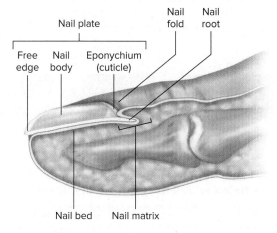

FIGURE 22-4 Anatomy of a nail.

are primarily activated by nervousness, pain, or stress, but they also can be activated by heat. Remember the last time you watched a scary movie that really frightened you? These glands were responsible for producing your cold sweat. Bacteria often break down the proteins in the sweat produced by apocrine glands. As the proteins are digested, the bacteria release a foul-smelling waste product that is responsible for the smell of body odor.

Sebaceous Glands

Sebaceous glands—more commonly called *oil glands*—produce an oily substance called **sebum.** Sebum is secreted onto hairs to keep them soft and pliable, and it is eventually deposited onto skin to keep it soft as well. Sebum also prevents bacteria from growing on skin (see Figure 22-1).

Nails

Nails protect the ends of the fingers and toes. They are formed by epithelial cells with hard keratin, which is more permanent than the softer keratin found in your skin. For this reason, the nails must be cut because they do not slough off by themselves as your skin cells do. The portion of a nail that you can see is the nail body and the portion embedded in skin is the nail root. The nail root contains active keratinocytes that constantly divide to produce nail growth. The white, half-moon-shaped area at the base of a nail is called a *lunula.* The lunula also

contains very active keratinocytes. Beneath each nail is a layer called the **nail bed,** which holds the nail down to underlying skin and provides nutrients to the nail from the blood supply under the nail bed (see Figure 22-4). Extending from the nail bed beyond the fingertip is the free edge of the nail. This is the part that you cut and file so that your nails look neat and trimmed.

▶ Skin Healing   LO 22.6

When skin is injured, it becomes inflamed. Redness, swelling, localized warmth, and pain are characteristics of inflammation. An inflamed area looks red because nearby blood vessels dilate. The inflamed area also swells because the dilated blood vessels "leak" and fluids seep into spaces between cells. Inflamed areas are often painful because the excess fluid activates pain receptors. However, inflammation promotes healing because more blood travels to the area, and this extra blood carries more nutrients needed for skin repair. It also carries defensive cells to clear up the cause of inflammation.

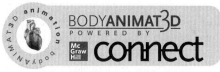

CAUTION: HANDLE WITH CARE

Preventing and Treating Scars

One of the skin's major functions is to protect your underlying tissues from injury and infection. Whether skinning your knees as a child or cutting yourself in the kitchen while preparing food, you have most likely injured your skin at some time in your life. Your skin responds to this injury by forming a scab and then a scar. Many scars simply retract and go away in time. The size and extent of the scar depend on the following:

- *Extent of the wound.* Deep or jagged wounds may produce a larger scar.
- *Wound location.* Wounds over mobile areas such as the knees and elbows often have larger scars because they are constantly under tension.

It is important that you seek medical attention for wounds that:

- Bleed profusely.
- Are larger than ½ inch deep or wide.
- Are located on the face.
- Are caused by a rusty tool or nail.
- Are jagged in appearance.
- Are caused by an animal bite.
- Show signs of infection.

These basic tips may help prevent the formation of lasting scars:

- Wash wounds with mild soap and water and clean out any debris left in the wound.
- Do not use harsh soaps, hydrogen peroxide, or alcohol to clean a wound, as these can damage tissues and delay healing.

- Cover the wound to keep out bacteria, dirt, and debris to reduce the possibility of infection.
- Keep the wound moist by applying an antibiotic ointment. This keeps the bandage from sticking to the wound and may reduce the likelihood of infection.
- Do not pick or pull at a scab. This reopens the wound and may cause infection or larger scar formation.
- Use medical honey. Honey has antibacterial properties and has been found to accelerate healing. Special medical products are available for hard-to-heal wounds.

If a scar forms, numerous treatments are available:

- *Sunscreen.* Protecting a newly healed wound from UV radiation by using sunscreen with an SPF of 30 or higher helps reduce scar thickening and hyperpigmentation.
- *Silicone gel sheeting.* Studies show that covering a wound with a silicone gel sheet reduces healing time and scar formation. These sheets may be used for surgical and nonsurgical wounds.
- *Dermabrasion.* This procedure literally "sands" the surface of the skin and scar and is most often used for raised scars.
- *Surgical scar repair.* A large or hyperpigmented scar can be reduced in size by removing it surgically. Scar reduction surgical procedures include the following:

  - Z-plasty—a specialized plastic surgical technique that alters the pull on a tightened scar by lengthening it.
  - Scar shaving—a technique for shaving off a raised scar.
  - Scar removal—making an elliptical incision around the scar and removing it, which results in a scar that is thinner than the original scar.

When structures and blood vessels of the dermis are injured, a blood clot initially forms. A scab, which is basically clotted blood and other dried tissue fluids, eventually replaces the blood clot. The scab is normally replaced by collagen fibers that bind the edges of the wound together. Collagen fibers are whitish and serve as the major component of scars.

Sometimes skin scars are replaced with new skin, but if the wound is extensive, a scar will persist. Scars can be merely a cosmetic nuisance or they can cause problems with underlying structures. For example, a large scar over a joint can cause loss of movement in that joint. See the *Caution: Handle with Care* feature for more information on preventing and treating scars.

PATHOPHYSIOLOGY

LO 22.7

Common Diseases and Disorders of the Skin

BURNS

Although many of the skin conditions discussed in this chapter can be extremely serious and even life-threatening (such as skin cancer), the skin also is prone to burns. In fact, burns are a leading cause of accidental death in the United States, where there are approximately 150 burn care centers devoted to this type of skin injury.

It is also important to note that an estimated 450,000 people seek medical treatment for burn injuries each year; 45,000 require hospitalization; and more than 3,500 patients die annually from burn injuries. Worldwide, more than a million people each year suffer from burn injuries that cause significant or permanent disability.

The extent of the affected body surface area and the severity (degree) of a burn are the most important factors in predicting the risk of death associated with burn injuries. The rule of nines

stress, diet, and medications can exacerbate or worsen the signs and symptoms of this disease.

Signs and Symptoms. The rashes of eczema are red, scaly, and itchy.

Diagnostic Exams and Tests. Physical examination of the skin is typically the only examination required to diagnose eczema.

Treatment. Treatments include topical steroids and other types of anti-inflammatory drugs. Antibiotics may be needed for any secondary infections that develop. Avoiding known factors that trigger eczema, such as stress, also can be helpful.

FOLLICULITIS, sometimes called "swimmer's rash," is an inflammation of hair follicles. See Figure 22-10.

Causes. This disorder usually results from shaving or excess rubbing of skin areas. It also may be caused by bacteria and fungi, which may develop from prolonged wearing of wet swimwear or using undertreated hot tubs.

Signs and Symptoms. Follicles become red and itchy and often look like pimples.

Diagnostic Exams and Tests. Often folliculitis is diagnosed based on skin examination, but a biopsy may be done to determine the cause of the inflammation.

Treatment. Treatments include regular cleansing of skin, topical antibiotics, and the use of electric razors instead of razor blades. Wearing wet swimwear for prolonged periods of time also should be avoided.

HERPES SIMPLEX types 1 and 2 are the most common types of herpes simplex.

Causes. Herpes simplex types 1 and 2 are both caused by a virus. Herpes simplex type 1 causes cold sores. It is very contagious and is spread through saliva. Herpes simplex type 2, known as *genital herpes,* is sexually transmitted.

Signs and Symptoms. Herpes simplex type 1 causes painful sores on the lips, mouth, and face. Herpes simplex type 2 normally causes painful sores on genital areas.

Diagnostic Exams and Tests. Examination of the affected area often results in a diagnosis, but lab tests for the herpes virus also may be performed.

Treatment. There is no cure for herpes simplex, and its skin lesions usually recur throughout life. However, antiviral drugs such as acyclovir (Zovirax®) prevent frequent outbreaks. Patients also should be instructed to get adequate rest and nutrition and to control stress as much as possible.

HERPES ZOSTER is a disorder commonly known as *shingles.* See Figure 22-11.

Causes. Herpes zoster is caused by the *Varicella* virus, which also causes chickenpox. After a person has chickenpox, the virus becomes dormant in the spine's dorsal nerve root but can become active again later in life to cause shingles.

Signs and Symptoms. Herpes zoster causes a painful, blistering rash usually on one side of the body following the *dermatome*—the skin area along the pathway of the affected nerve root. Shingles usually starts as a tingling or pain on the torso or neck, followed by a rash that eventually blisters.

Diagnostic Exams and Tests. Physical examination and a confirmed prior history of chickenpox is normally all that is required for diagnosis.

Treatment. Some antiviral medications, such as Zovirax®, shorten the duration of the disease, and pain medications assist with pain control. Recovery is usually complete, but recurrences of the disease do occur. Some patients suffer from the complication known

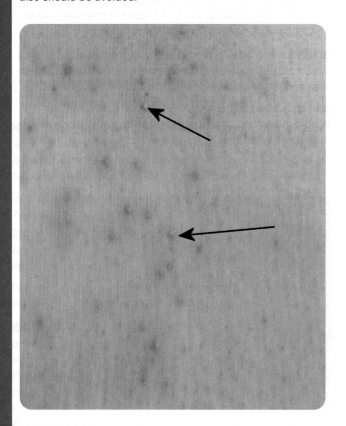

FIGURE 22-10 Folliculitis can be caused from shaving or rubbing of the skin and often looks like pimples.
©McGraw-Hill Education

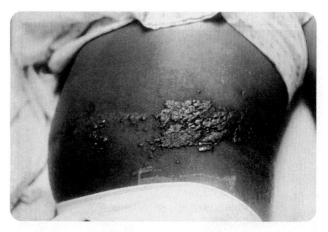

FIGURE 22-11 Herpes zoster, more commonly known as shingles, is a painful, blistering rash that follows the pathway of an affected nerve root.
Source: Centers for Disease Control and Prevention.

as *post-herpetic pain syndrome,* where nerve pain continues even though the rash is no longer present. It is uncertain whether the chickenpox vaccine prevents herpes zoster. The vaccine Zostavax® by Merck Pharmaceuticals is a preventive alternative for patients 60 years of age and older with a history of having had chickenpox. Patients considering Zostavax® should know that it is advertised as reducing the risk of developing shingles; it does not guarantee that shingles will not occur.

IMPETIGO causes the formation of oozing skin lesions that eventually crust over. It is highly contagious for those who come in contact with the lesions or the exudates (exuded substances) from them.

Causes. This disease is caused by staphylococcal and streptococcal bacteria.

Signs and Symptoms. The skin develops itchy, oozing lesions that eventually crust over with a distinctive, honey-colored crust from the drying exudates.

Diagnostic Exams and Tests. Physical examination is normally all that is required for a diagnosis, but skin biopsy or scraping may be performed to confirm the causative agent.

Treatment. This condition is treated with antibiotics. Washing the lesions two or three times a day with soap and water will help remove the exudates and decrease the spread to other skin areas.

PEDICULOSIS is more commonly known as *lice* and comes in three forms: head lice (*Pediculosis capitis*), body lice (*Pediculosis corporis*), and pubic lice (*Pediculosis pubis*).

Causes. All forms are caused by parasitic lice and are associated with overcrowded conditions causing person-to-person contact. Pubic lice also are spread by sexual contact.

Signs and Symptoms. Skin itches and can become irritated from scratching. Head lice also are identifiable by the dandruff-like nits that cannot be shaken off.

Diagnostic Exams and Tests. Physical exam, confirming the presence of lice, is all that is required.

Treatment. Prescription medications and shampoos are often necessary. For head lice, some patients find equal success with over-the-counter (OTC) treatments such as Nix®.

PSORIASIS is a common chronic, inflammatory skin condition.

Causes. This skin disorder is most likely an inherited autoimmune disorder.

Signs and Symptoms. Patients with psoriasis have recurring episodes of itching and redness with outbreaks of distinctive silvery, scaly skin lesions. Some people also have joint pain with this condition, known as psoriatic arthritis.

Diagnostic Exams and Tests. Typically, psoriasis is diagnosed based on the patient's symptoms and an examination of the skin.

Treatment. Mild cases are treated with anti-inflammatory drugs and therapeutic ointments such as creams with vitamins A and D, hydrocortisone creams, and retinoids. Some patients also experience relief with controlled UV ray treatments. Some patients with moderate to severe plaque psoriasis have more recently found treatment success with TNF (tumor necrosis factor)-blocking medications such as Enbrel®. Severe cases may require hospitalization.

RINGWORM is a fungal skin infection, commonly occurring in three forms: *Tinea corporis* (body), *Tinea capitis* (scalp), and *Tinea pedis* (feet), which is commonly known as athlete's foot. See Figure 22-12.

Causes. All forms of ringworm are caused by fungi called *dermatophytes.*

Signs and Symptoms. Flat, circular lesions that may be dry and scaly or moist and crusty are the hallmarks of ringworm. *Tinea capitis* is characterized by small papules that may cause small, patchy areas of baldness.

Diagnostic Exams and Tests. Normally a physical exam is the only requirement to make a diagnosis.

Treatment. Topical and oral antifungal agents are used to treat all forms of ringworm. The spread is contained by not sharing sheets, towels, and other personal care items.

ROSACEA is a skin disorder that commonly appears as facial redness, predominantly over the cheeks and nose.

Causes. Rosacea results from dilation of small facial blood vessels, but the cause of this dilation is unknown. It occurs most frequently in fair-skinned people.

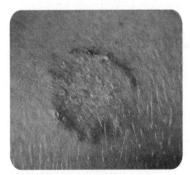
(a) *Tinea corporis* affects the body.

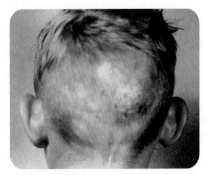
(b) *Tinea capitis* affects the scalp.

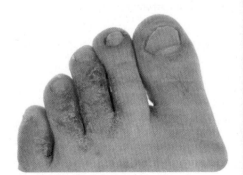
(c) *Tinea pedis* affects the feet.

FIGURE 22-12 Ringworm is a fungal infection that affects the body in three places.

Source: (a) CDC/Dr. Lucille K. Georg; (b) Source: Centers for Disease Control; (c) ©carroteater/Getty Images

Signs and Symptoms. Redness and acne-like symptoms on the face are the most common symptoms.

Diagnostic Exams and Tests. Diagnosis is made on physical examination.

Treatment. Although it is not curable, rosacea is usually managed well with topical cortisone or antibiotic creams. In severe cases, electrolysis may be useful in destroying large or dilated blood vessels.

SCABIES is a highly contagious skin condition.

Causes. Scabies is caused by an itch mite that burrows beneath skin and lays its eggs. Sometimes the burrows of the mites can be seen and look like red pencil marks.

Signs and Symptoms. Redness and severe itching, especially at night, are usually the only symptoms of scabies.

Diagnostic Exams and Tests. Often physical examination alone can confirm a diagnosis of scabies. Skin biopsy can be performed to confirm the presence of the mite.

Treatment. Most cases are easily treated with prescription medications such as Elimite™, which is left on the skin for 6 to 10 hours and followed by a bath. Antipyretic (anti-itching) or steroid creams may control the itching. Because scabies is contagious, it is wise to treat an entire family if one member is infected.

WARTS (verrucae) are harmless skin growths that can appear almost anywhere on the body surface but most commonly occur on the hands, feet, and face.

Causes. These growths are caused by a virus.

Signs and Symptoms. Warts vary greatly in appearance; they can be smooth, flat, rough, raised, dark, small, or large.

Diagnostic Exams and Tests. Verrucae are typically diagnosed by a physical examination of the skin.

Treatment. Warts are often removed with OTC medications but also can be treated through surgery, lasers, freezing, or burning.

SUMMARY OF LEARNING OUTCOMES

OUTCOME	KEY POINTS
22.1 Describe the functions of skin.	The functions of skin include protection, body temperature regulation, vitamin D production, sensation, and excretion.
22.2 Describe the layers of skin and the characteristics of each layer.	The topmost layer of the skin is the epidermis. The dermis is the complex middle layer. The innermost layer attaching the skin to muscle is the subcutaneous layer.
22.3 Explain the factors that affect skin color.	The amount of melanin affects and determines skin color. The amount of oxygen-carrying hemoglobin in the blood also affects skin color.
22.4 Summarize types of common skin lesions.	Skin lesions are split among three main types: primary lesions such as macules and vesicles; secondary lesions, which include ulcers and keloids; and vascular lesions, which involve blood vessels and include telangiectasias and ecchymoses.
22.5 Describe the accessory organs of skin along with their structures and functions.	The accessory organs of skin include hair follicles, arrector pili muscles, sebaceous glands, sudoriferous glands, and keratin-filled nails.
22.6 Explain the process of skin healing, including scar production.	Injured skin becomes inflamed from dilating blood vessels that leak and cause swelling. A blood clot is formed, which is replaced by a scab, which is then replaced by collagen fibers that produce scar tissue.
22.7 Describe the causes, signs and symptoms, diagnosis, and treatments of various diseases and disorders of the integumentary system.	There are many common diseases and disorders of the skin with varied signs, symptoms, diagnosis, and treatments. Some of these include acne, alopecia, cellulitis, dermatitis, eczema, folliculitis, herpes simplex, herpes zoster, impetigo, pediculosis, psoriasis, ringworm, rosacea, scabies, and warts.

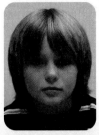

Recall Chris Matthews from the case study at the beginning of the chapter. Now that you have completed the chapter, answer the following questions regarding his case.

©McGraw-Hill Education

1. Considering the information you already have on Chris Matthews' feet and his behavior, what is the likely diagnosis?
2. What is the clinical name for this condition? During and after treatment, what are some tips you can give Chris Matthews to avoid a recurrence?

EXAM PREPARATION QUESTIONS

1. (LO 22.2) Which protein gives skin its protective quality?
   a. Melanin
   b. Vitamin D
   c. Keratin
   d. Hemoglobin
   e. Collagen

2. (LO 22.4) Which of the following lesions is a vascular lesion?
   a. Tumor
   b. Macule
   c. Ecchymosis
   d. Wheal
   e. Plaque

3. (LO 22.7) The patient has burned his left arm front and back from elbow to fingertips as well as his left chest and abdomen (approximately half of his trunk). Using the rule of nines, what percentage of his body is burned?
   a. 27%
   b. 18%
   c. 13.5%
   d. 9.5%
   e. 22.5%

4. (LO 22.5) The medical term for hair loss is
   a. Folliculitis
   b. Alopecia
   c. Pediculosis
   d. Impetigo
   e. Excoriation

5. (LO 22.4) Which medical condition is more commonly known as a *hive*?
   a. Cicatrix
   b. Vesicle
   c. Pustule
   d. Wheal
   e. Erosion

6. (LO 22.4) *Verrucae* is a medical term meaning
   a. Bruises
   b. Warts
   c. Nodules
   d. Wrinkles
   e. Moles

7. (LO 22.1) Which of the following is *not* a function of skin?
   a. Temperature regulation
   b. Protection
   c. Excretion
   d. Sensation
   e. Vitamin B production

8. (LO 22.7) Scabies is caused by
   a. Fungi
   b. Lice
   c. Mites
   d. Bed bugs
   e. Bacteria

9. (LO 22.2) The most superficial layer of the epidermis is the
   a. Stratum basale
   b. Stratum corneum
   c. Stratum germinativum
   d. Stratum dermis
   e. Stratum keratin

10. (LO 22.5) The part of the nail that holds it down to the underlying tissues and provides nutrients to the nail is the
   a. Lunula
   b. Nail bed
   c. Cuticle
   d. Free edge
   e. Nail root

Analyze the following medical terms, presented throughout the chapter. Using a medical dictionary (or Appendix I), place a / mark between each word part. Define each word part and then define the whole word.

EXAMPLE: **chemo/therapy** = chemo means "chemical" + therapy means "treatment"
CHEMOTHERAPY means "treatment with chemicals."

1. cellulitis
2. cyanosis
3. dermatitis
4. dermatome
5. epidermis

6. folliculitis
7. hemoglobin
8. hypodermis
9. keratinocyte
10. lunula

11. melanocyte
12. pediculosis
13. sebaceous
14. subcutaneous
15. sudoriferous

The Skeletal System

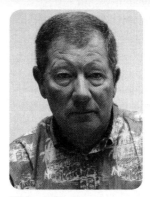
LEARNING OUTCOMES

After completing Chapter 23, you will be able to:

23.1 Describe the structure of bone tissue.

23.2 Explain the functions of bones.

23.3 Compare intramembranous and endochondral ossification.

23.4 Describe the skeletal structures and one location of each structure.

23.5 Locate the bones of the skull.

23.6 Locate the bones of the spinal column.

23.7 Locate the bones of the rib cage.

23.8 Locate the bones of the shoulders, arms, and hands.

23.9 Locate the bones of the hips, legs, and feet.

23.10 Describe the three major types of joints and give examples of each.

23.11 Describe the causes, signs and symptoms, diagnosis, and treatments of various diseases and disorders of the skeletal system.

KEY TERMS

appendicular	patella
articulations	pectoral girdle
axial	pelvic girdle
clavicle	radius
diaphysis	scapula
dislocation	sternum
epiphysis	suture
femur	temporal mandibular joint (TMJ)
fibula	tibia
metacarpal	ulna
metatarsal	
ossification	

CAAHEP

I.C.1	Describe structural organization of the human body
I.C.2	Identify body systems
I.C.4	List major organs in each body system
I.C.5	Identify the anatomical location of major organs in each body system
I.C.6	Compare structure and function of the human body across the life span
I.C.7	Describe the normal function of each body system
I.C.8	Identify common pathology related to each body system including: (a) signs (b) symptoms (c) etiology
I.C.9	Analyze pathology for each body system including: (a) diagnostic measures (b) treatment modalities
V.C.9	Identify medical terms labeling the word parts
V.C.10	Define medical terms and abbreviations related to all body systems

ABHES

2. **Anatomy and Physiology**
   a. List all body systems and their structures and functions
   b. Describe common diseases, symptoms, and etiologies as they apply to each system
   c. Identify diagnostic and treatment modalities as they relate to each body system

3. **Medical Terminology**
   a. Define and use the entire basic structure of medical terminology and be able to accurately identify the correct context (i.e., root, prefix, suffix, combinations, spelling, and definitions)
   b. Build and dissect medical terminology from roots and suffixes to understand the word element combinations
   c. Apply medical terminology for each specialty
   d. Define and use medical abbreviations when appropriate and acceptable

▶ Introduction

Imagine that you are walking along a bustling city sidewalk and someone behind you calls your name. As you pause and turn your head to see who it is, you catch a glimpse of your profile in the reflection of a coffee shop window. You stand taller than you think you are, with one leg in front of the other as if pivoting. You bring your right hand up to your forehead and quickly rub your brow, then let it drop to your side. Your friend then appears beside you, and the two of you hug. Although it may seem as if your body is simply made of only the surface features you can see reflected in this window, dressed for the day in nice clothing and hugging your friend, of course, there is much more to this picture. After all, your bones are behind this picture, scattered all throughout your body to provide it with the structure and support you need for daily functioning.

In this chapter, you will learn about the bones of the body, their structure, and how the joints of the body work. The skeletal system is composed of 206 bones as well as joints and related connective tissues. Now, picture this many bones hiding within that person—you!—reflected earlier in the coffee shop window.

The skeleton has two major divisions—the **axial** skeleton and the **appendicular** skeleton (see Figure 23-1). These divisions differ in the following ways:

- The axial skeleton contains 80 bones, including the bones of the skull, vertebral column, and rib cage. It supports the head, neck, and trunk, and it protects the brain, spinal cord, and organs in the thorax. The hyoid bone, which anchors the tongue, is also included in the axial skeleton.

- The body's other 126 bones belong to the appendicular skeleton, which includes the bones of the arms, legs, **pectoral girdle,** and **pelvic girdle.** The pectoral girdle attaches the arms to the axial skeleton, and the pelvic girdle attaches the legs to the axial skeleton.

▶ Bone Structure   LO 23.1

Bones contain various kinds of tissues, including osseous tissue, blood vessels, and nerves. Osseous tissue can be compact or spongy (see Figure 23-2). At the microscopic level, spongy, or cancellous, bone has more spaces within it than compact bone does. Spongy bone looks a lot like a natural sea sponge with the spaces filled with *red bone marrow*. Compact bone looks solid, like granite or marble. However, the following structures within these bones can be observed with a microscope:

- *Osteons,* also known as the *Haversian system,* are elongated cylinders that run up and down the bone's long axis. Each osteon has a central canal that contains blood vessels and nerves.

- *Bone matrix,* made of inorganic salts, collagen fibers, and proteins, is the substance between bone cells. Bone cells are called *osteocytes.* The primary salt of the matrix is calcium phosphate, which makes bone matrix very hard.

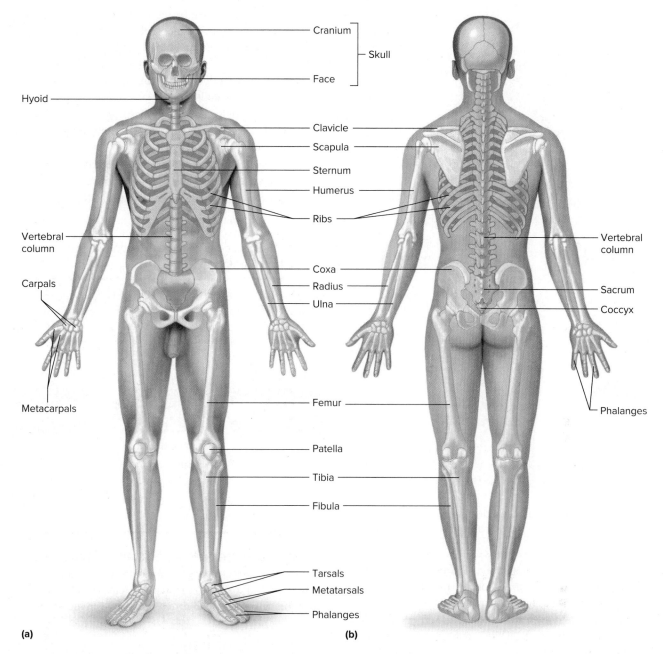

FIGURE 23-1 Major bones of the skeleton: (a) anterior view and (b) posterior view. The axial skeleton is shown in orange and the appendicular skeleton is shown in yellow.

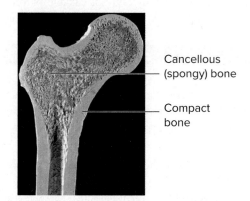

FIGURE 23-2 Cross section of bone showing compact and cancellous (spongy) bone tissue.
©ALFRED PASIEKA/SCIENCE PHOTO LIBRARY/Getty Images

- *Lamellae* are layers of bone surrounding the canals of osteons.
- *Lacunae* are holes in the matrix of bone that hold osteocytes.
- *Canaliculi* are tiny canals that connect lacunae to each other and allow osteocytes to spread nutrients to each other.

All bones are made up of both compact and cancellous bone. They are classified according to their shape (see Figure 23-3):

- *Long bones* are located primarily in the arms and legs. Examples include the **femur** (thighbone, see Figure 23-4) and the humerus (upper arm bone). Long bones have the following parts (see Figure 23-5):
  - **Diaphysis**—the shaft of a long bone. It is tubular and consists of a thick collar of compact bone that surrounds the central medullary cavity.

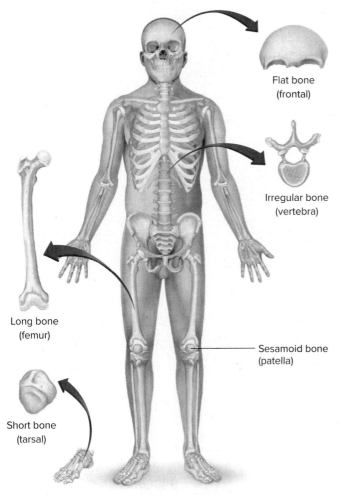

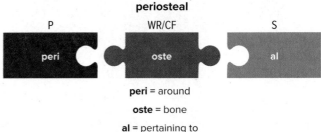

Flat bone
(frontal)

Irregular bone
(vertebra)

Sesamoid bone
(patella)

Long bone
(femur)

Short bone
(tarsal)

FIGURE 23-3 Classification of bone by shape: Five different classes of bone are recognized according to shape—long, short, flat, irregular, and sesamoid.

- **Epiphysis**—the expanded end of a long bone. It consists of a thin layer of compact bone surrounding cancellous bone. Long bones have an epiphysis at both ends.
- *Articular cartilage*—the cartilage that covers the epiphyses of long bones. It cushions bones and absorbs stress during bone movements.
- *Medullary cavity*—the canal that runs through the center of the diaphysis. In adults, it contains *yellow bone marrow* (mostly fat).

- *Periosteum*—a membrane that surrounds the diaphysis. It contains bone-forming cells, dense fibrous connective tissue, nerves, and blood vessels.
- *Endosteum*—a membrane that lines the medullary cavity and the holes of cancellous bone. It contains bone-forming cells.
- *Short bones* are located in the wrists and ankles. Examples include the carpals (wrist bones) and some of the tarsals (ankle bones).
- *Flat bones* are primarily located in the skull and rib cage. Examples include the ribs and frontal bone.
- *Irregular bones* include the vertebrae and the pelvic girdle bones.
- *Sesamoid bones* are small, rounded bones usually found next to joints or embedded in a tendon. An example is the patella, or kneecap.

Medical terms are built and dissected using prefixes, word roots/combining form, and suffixes. For example, we can build the term *periosteal* by placing the parts of the term in the puzzle pieces where P = prefix, WR/CF = word root or combining form, and S = suffix.

periosteal

| P | WR/CF | S |
| peri | oste | al |

peri = around

oste = bone

al = pertaining to

Learn additional medical terms in the **Medical Terminology Practice** section at the end of this chapter.

Gender Differences in Skeletal Structure

You may wonder how physicians, pathologists, and archeologists can tell if a skeleton is male or female. Table 23-1 outlines some of the skeletal differences between the sexes.

▶ Functions of Bones   LO 23.2

Bones have many functions. Without bones, the body would be more like a glob of jelly and not capable of very much. Bones give shape to body parts such as the head, legs, arms,

TABLE 23-1	Differences Between the Male and Female Skeletons
Part	**Differences**
Skull	Male skull is larger and heavier, with more conspicuous muscular attachments. Male forehead is shorter, facial area is less round, jaw is larger, and mastoid processes are more prominent than those of a female.
Pelvis	Male pelvic bones are heavier, thicker, and have more obvious muscular attachments. The obturator foramina and the acetabula are larger and closer together than those of a female.
Pelvic cavity	Male pelvic cavity is narrower in all diameters and is longer, less roomy, and more funnel-shaped. The distances between the ischial spines and between the ischial tuberosities are less than in a female.
Sacrum	Male sacrum is narrower, sacral promontory projects forward to a greater degree, and sacral curvature is bent less sharply posteriorly than in a female.
Coccyx	Male coccyx is less movable than that of a female.

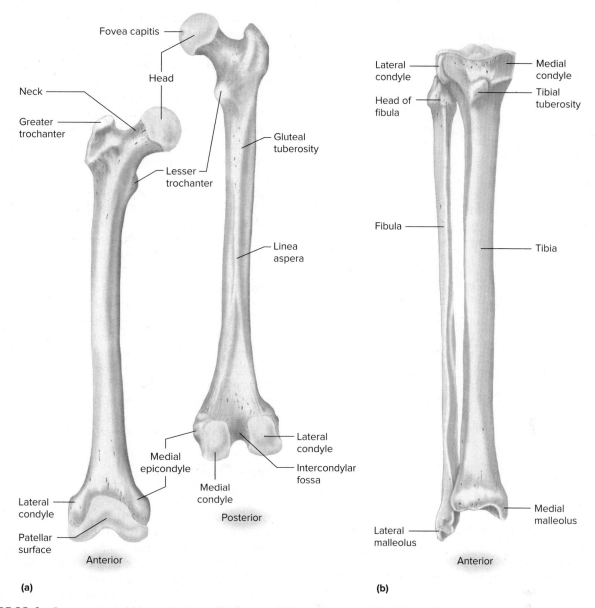

FIGURE 23-4 Bone structures: (a) bone structures of the femur and (b) bone structures of the tibia and fibula.

and trunk. They also support and protect soft structures in the body. For example, the skull protects the brain. Bones also function in body movement because skeletal muscles attach to them, allowing you to create willful, or voluntary, movements.

The red marrow within cancellous bone produces new blood cells in a process called *hematopoiesis.* Blood cells have a limited lifespan, so they need to be replaced. Red blood cells, for example, need replacing as often as every 90 to 120 days. Your red marrow is actively making more blood cells 24 hours a day. Bones also store calcium for the body. Every cell in the body needs calcium, so the body must have a large supply readily available.

▶ Bone Growth   LO 23.3

Bones grow through a process called **ossification.** Ossification is the process of creating bone from either fibrous membranes or cartilage. These two types of ossification are called intramembranous and endochondral ossification.

In *intramembranous* ossification, bones begin as tough, fibrous membranes. Eventually, bone-forming cells called *osteoblasts* secrete bone matrix into the membrane, changing the membrane to bone. Except for the lower jaw bone, the bones of the skull are formed by intramembranous ossification.

In *endochondral* ossification, bones start out as cartilage models. Eventually, the osteoblasts form a bone collar around the diaphysis of the cartilage model. Think of a sculptor who first builds a framework or model of soft material before applying sculpting clay over the framework. Eventually, when the clay hardens, either through drying or firing in a kiln, there is more hard material than there is soft framework. Then bone is formed in the diaphysis of the bone. This area is called the *primary ossification center.* Later, the epiphyses turn to bone (secondary ossification centers), and the medullary cavity and spaces in cancellous bone are formed. The cells that form holes in bone are called *osteoclasts.* As long as a bone

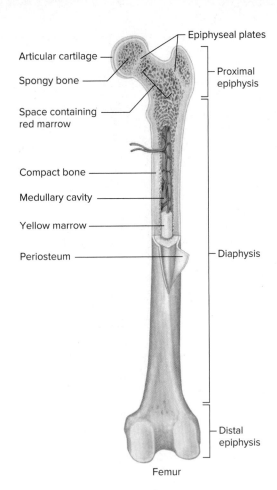

Articular cartilage
Spongy bone
Space containing
red marrow
Compact bone
Medullary cavity
Yellow marrow
Periosteum

Epiphyseal plates

Proximal
epiphysis

Diaphysis

Distal
epiphysis

Femur

FIGURE 23-5 Parts of a long bone.

contains some cartilage between an epiphysis and the diaphysis, it can continue to grow in length. This plate of cartilage is called an *epiphyseal disk* or *growth plate.* Once the cartilage is gone, bone growth stops. For most people, bone growth stops between the ages of 18 and 25.

Even after bone growth stops, osteoclasts and osteoblasts continually remodel bone tissue. Throughout life, osteoclasts break down bone when the body needs more calcium in the blood, and osteoblasts replace the bone when there is excess calcium in the blood.

Building Better Bones

Many factors influence bone health, including diet, exercise, and a person's overall lifestyle. You can help patients improve or maintain their bone health by teaching them about behaviors that will support it.

Bone-Healthy Diet Good nutrition is essential for proper bone growth during childhood and the teen years. It is equally important in adulthood in order to maintain healthy bones. Bone-building nutrients are found in dairy products, broccoli, kale, spinach, salmon, sardines, egg yolks, whole grains, and fruits—especially bananas and oranges. Calcium and vitamin D are particularly important for healthy bones. Without vitamin D, the bloodstream cannot absorb calcium from the digestive tract. Without calcium, bone tissue will slowly wear

away. Supplements can always be taken if a person's diet does not include adequate amounts of calcium and vitamin D.

Bone-Healthy Exercises Weight-bearing and strength-training exercises are best for bone health. When your muscles contract, they pull on your bones. This tension stimulates bones to thicken and strengthen. Lifting weights is an effective way to increase the tension on bones. Other activities such as jogging, walking briskly, or playing a sport regularly also will stimulate your bones to increase in density.

Bone-Healthy Lifestyle A person with a bone-healthy lifestyle avoids smoking and alcohol. Smoking rids the body of calcium, which is necessary for bone growth. Alcohol prevents calcium absorption in the digestive tract. Smokers are almost twice as likely to develop osteoporosis as nonsmokers.

Bone Tests

Bone density tests and bone scans are currently the most useful tools in determining bone health. Bone density tests are painless procedures used to determine the density of a person's bones. Because osteoporosis shows no symptoms in early stages, it is important to have these tests done when your doctor recommends them. Bone scans help diagnose the causes of bone pain, arthritis, bone infections, and bone cancers. These scans use radioactive tracers that are injected into the patient and concentrate in bone tissue.

▶ Bony Structures   LO 23.4

The skeletal bones act as your body's rigid foundation. By design, they are not perfectly smooth or perfectly rounded. Bones have projections and processes for muscle and ligament attachment. For bones to come together at joints, or **articulations,** there are depressions and hollows. In addition, blood vessels and nerves need openings within bones for entrances and exits. Each of these structures has a specific name and design. Table 23-2 lists some of these common terms to describe skeletal structures and directs you to the appropriate figures throughout this chapter.

▶ The Skull   LO 23.5

Skull bones are divided into two types: cranial and facial bones. Cranial bones form the top, sides, and back of the skull (see Figure 23-6). Facial bones form the face (see Figure 23-7). The skull bones of an infant are not completely formed. The "soft spots" felt on an infant's skull are actually *fontanels,* which are tough membranes that connect the incompletely developed bones. These structures allow the infant's skull to be somewhat moldable to assist with delivery through the birth canal. As the fontanels close, the sutures of the skull are formed.

The major cranial bones are the following:

- The *frontal bone* forms the anterior portion of the cranium. It is also called the forehead bone.
- *Parietal bones* form most of the top and sides of the skull.

TABLE 23-2 Terms Used to Describe Skeletal Structures

Term	Definition	Examples
Condyle	A rounded process that usually articulates with another bone	Medial and lateral condyles of the femur (see Figure 23-4a)
Crest	A narrow, ridge-like projection	Iliac crest of the ilium (see Figure 23-11)
Epicondyle	A projection situated above a condyle	Medial epicondyle of the femur (see Figure 23-4a)
Foramen	An opening through a bone that is usually a passageway for blood vessels, nerves, or ligaments	Mental foramen of the mandible (see Figure 23-7)
Fossa	A relatively deep pit or depression	Olecranon fossa of the humerus (see Figure 23-10c)
Head	An enlargement on the end of a bone	Head of the femur (see Figure 23-4a)
Process	A prominent projection on a bone	Mastoid process of the temporal bone (see Figure 23-6)
Suture	An interlocking line of union between bones	Lambdoidal suture between the occipital and parietal bones (see Figure 23-6)
Trochanter	A relatively large process	Greater trochanter of the femur (see Figure 23-4a)
Tubercle	A small, knob-like process	Greater tubercle of the humerus (see Figure 23-10b)
Tuberosity	A knob-like process usually larger than a tubercle	Tibial tuberosity of the tibia (see Figure 23-4b)

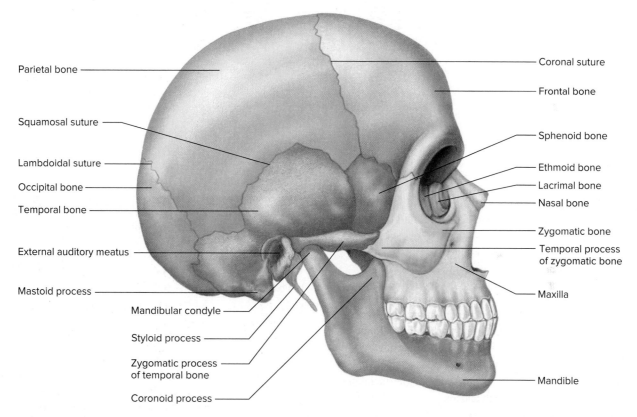

FIGURE 23-6 Lateral view of the skull.

- The *occipital bone* forms the back of the skull. The large hole at the base of the occipital bone is called the *foramen magnum*. It allows the spinal cord to connect to the brain. Two bumps called occipital *condyles* are on either side of the foramen magnum. They sit on top of the first vertebra. When you nod your head, your occipital condyles are rocking back and forth on the first vertebra of the spinal column.
- Two *temporal bones* form the lower sides of the skull.
  - A canal called the *external auditory meatus* (commonly called the ear canal) runs through each temporal bone.

- A large bump called the *mastoid process* is located on each temporal bone just behind each ear. Major neck muscles attach to your skull at the mastoid processes.
- A *sphenoid bone* forms part of the floor of the cranium. It is shaped like a butterfly. In the center is a deep depression called the *sella turcica*. The pituitary gland sits in this deep depression.
- *Ethmoid bones* are between the sphenoid bone and the nasal bones. They also form part of the floor of the cranium.

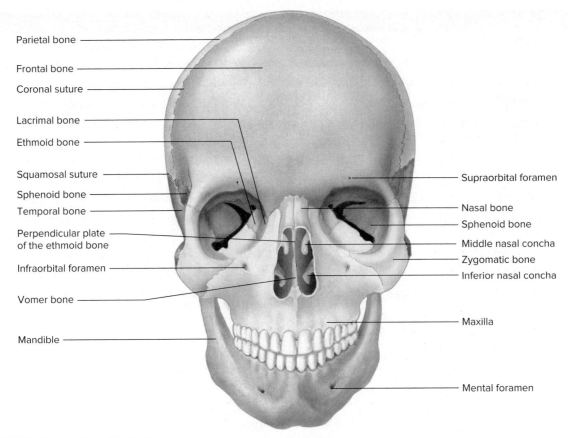

Parietal bone

Frontal bone

Coronal suture

Lacrimal bone

Ethmoid bone

Squamosal suture

Sphenoid bone

Temporal bone

Perpendicular plate of the ethmoid bone

Infraorbital foramen

Vomer bone

Mandible

Supraorbital foramen

Nasal bone

Sphenoid bone

Middle nasal concha

Zygomatic bone

Inferior nasal concha

Maxilla

Mental foramen

FIGURE 23-7 Anterior view of the skull.

- *Ear ossicles* are the body's smallest bones. They are the malleus, incus, and stapes and are in the middle ear cavities of the temporal bones.

The following are major facial bones:

- The *mandible* is the lower jaw bone and is the only movable bone in the skull. It attaches to the temporal bone in front of the external auditory meatus in an area known as the **temporal mandibular joint (TMJ)** (also known as the temporomandibular joint). The mandible anchors the lower teeth and forms the chin.
- The *maxillae* form the upper jaw bone of the facial skeleton to which the upper teeth anchor.
- The *zygomatic bones* are the cheekbones.
- Several thin *nasal bones* fuse together to form the bridge of the nose.
- *Palatine bones* form the hard palate, which is the roof of the mouth.
- The *vomer* is a thin bone that divides the nasal cavity.

▶ The Spinal Column   LO 23.6

The spinal column consists of 7 cervical vertebrae, 12 thoracic vertebrae, 5 lumbar vertebrae, a sacrum, and a coccyx (see Figure 23-8 and Table 23-3):

TABLE 23-3	The Spinal Column	
Vertebrae Name	**Number**	**Description**
Cervical	7	Smallest and lightest
Thoracic	12	Posterior attachments for ribs
Lumbar	5	Form the small of the back
Sacrum	5	Bones are fused.
Coccyx	3 to 5	Bones are fused.

- *Cervical vertebrae,* which are located in the neck, are the smallest and lightest vertebrae. The first cervical vertebra is called the *atlas* and the second is called the *axis.* When you rotate your head from side to side, your atlas is pivoting around your axis.
- *Thoracic vertebrae* are the posterior attachment for the 12 pairs of ribs. They have long, sharp spinous processes that you can feel when you run your finger down someone's spine.
- *Lumbar vertebrae* are very sturdy structures. They form the small of the back and bear the most weight of all the vertebrae.
- The *sacrum* is a triangular-shaped bone that consists of five fused vertebrae.
- The *coccyx* (commonly called the tailbone) is a small, triangular-shaped bone made up of three to five fused vertebrae; it is considered nonessential in humans.

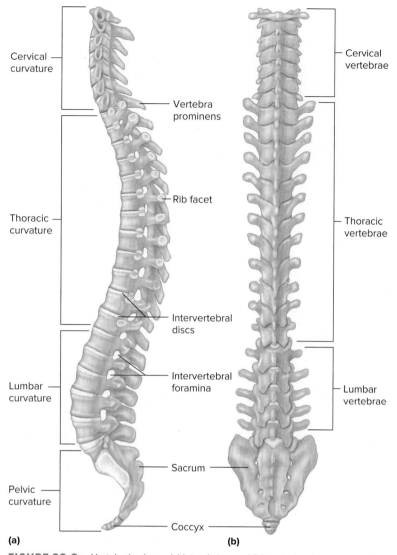

Cervical
curvature

Vertebra
prominens

Cervical
vertebrae

Thoracic
curvature

Rib facet

Thoracic
vertebrae

Intervertebral
discs

Lumbar
curvature

Intervertebral
foramina

Lumbar
vertebrae

Pelvic
curvature

Sacrum

Coccyx

(a)   **(b)**

FIGURE 23-8   Vertebral column: (a) lateral view and (b) posterior view.

▶ The Rib Cage

LO 23.7

The rib cage is made of 12 pairs of ribs and the **sternum** (see Figure 23-9). The sternum—often called the breastplate—forms the front middle portion of the rib cage. The cartilaginous tip of the sternum is known as the *xiphoid process*. The sternum joins with the clavicles and most ribs. All 12 pairs of ribs are attached posteriorly to thoracic vertebrae. The ribs themselves are classified in three groups based on their anterior attachment:

- True. The first seven pairs of ribs are *true ribs*. They attach directly to the sternum through pieces of cartilage called *costal cartilage*.

- False. Rib pairs 8, 9, and 10 are called *false ribs*. They do not attach directly to the sternum by individual cartilage but instead attach to the costal cartilage of rib pair number 7.

- Floating. Rib pairs 11 and 12 are called *floating ribs* because they do not attach anteriorly to the sternum or to any other structure.

Medical terms are built and dissected using prefixes, word roots/combining form, and suffixes. For example, we can build the term *intercostal* by placing the parts of the term in the puzzle pieces where P = prefix, WR/CF = word root or combining form, and S = suffix.

intercostal

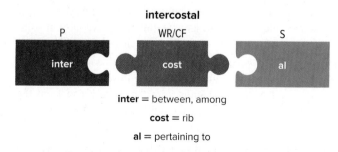

P — inter
WR/CF — cost
S — al

inter = between, among

cost = rib

al = pertaining to

Intercostal means pertaining to between the ribs. Learn additional medical terms in the **Medical Terminology Practice** section at the end of this chapter.

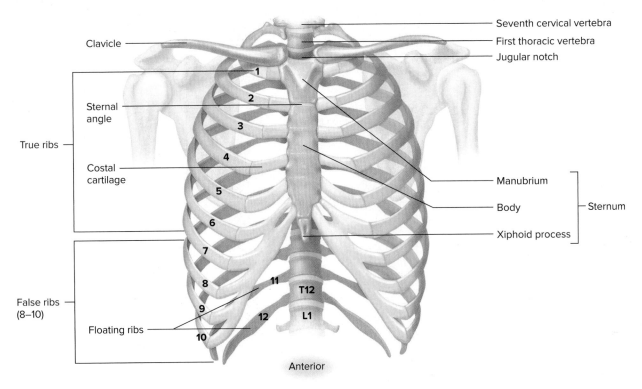

Clavicle

Seventh cervical vertebra

First thoracic vertebra

Jugular notch

Sternal angle

True ribs

Costal cartilage

Manubrium

Body

Sternum

Xiphoid process

False ribs (8–10)

Floating ribs

Anterior

FIGURE 23-9   Thoracic rib cage showing pectoral girdle attachment of upper extremities.

Bones of the Shoulders, Arms, and Hands

LO 23.8

The bones of the shoulders make up the pectoral girdle and include the clavicles and the scapulae (see Figure 23-10). They attach the arms to the axial skeleton.

- The **clavicles,** or collar bones, are slender in shape. Each joins with the sternum and a scapula.
- **Scapulae** (or shoulder blades) are thin, triangular-shaped flat bones located on the dorsal surface of the rib cage. Each scapula joins with the head of a humerus and a clavicle.

The upper limb, or arm, bones include the humerus, radius, and ulna:

- The *humerus* is located in the upper part of the arm. Its proximal end joins with the scapula and its distal end attaches at the radius and the ulna.
- The **radius** is the lateral bone of the forearm. It is on the same side of the arm as your thumb. Proximally, it joins with the humerus and the ulna, and distally with the carpal (wrist) bones.
- The **ulna** is the medial bone of the lower arm. The proximal end of the ulna joins with the humerus to form the elbow joint. Distally, it also joins with the radius and some of the carpal bones of the wrist.

The bones of the hand include carpals, metacarpals, and phalanges:

- *Carpals* are wrist bones. Each wrist contains eight marble-sized carpal bones.

- **Metacarpals** form the palms of the hands. Each hand has five metacarpals.
- *Phalanges* are the bones of the fingers. There are 14 phalanges in each hand—3 for each finger and 2 per thumb.
- The joints between the phalangeal bones are the proximal and distal *interphalangeal* (PIP and DIP) joints.
- The joints that join the phalanges to the metacarpals are called the *metacarpophalangeal* (*MCP*) joints. You probably know these joints as the knuckles.

Refer to Figure 23-10 for the bones of the shoulders, arms, and hands.

Bones of the Hips, Legs, and Feet

LO 23.9

The hip bones, also called *coxal* bones, attach the legs to the axial skeleton. They also protect pelvic organs. Each coxal bone has three parts: the ilium, the ischium, and the pubis.

- The *ilium* is the most superior part of a coxal bone. When you put your hands on your hips, you are touching the part of the ilium called the *iliac crest.*
- The *ischium* forms the lower part of a coxal bone and the pubis forms the front.
- The *pubis* bones of each coxal bone join together to form the *symphysis pubis.*

These three bones also are referred to as the *pelvic girdle* (see Figure 23-11).

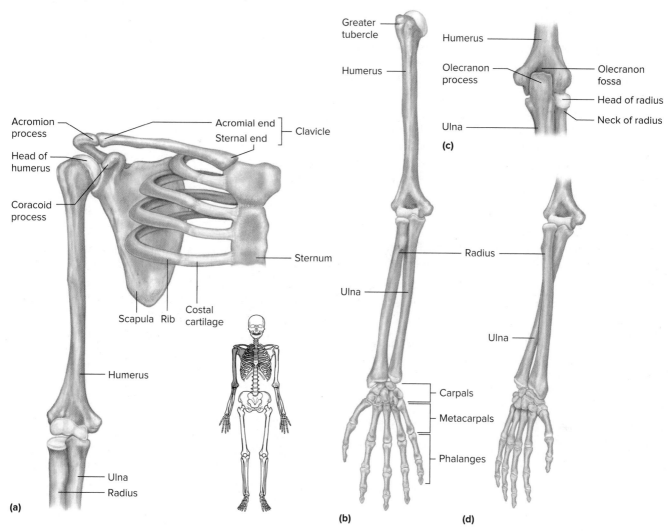

FIGURE 23-10 (a) The pectoral girdle with upper limb attached. (b) Frontal view of upper limb (palm anterior). (c) Posterior view of right elbow. (d) Frontal view of upper limb (palm posterior).

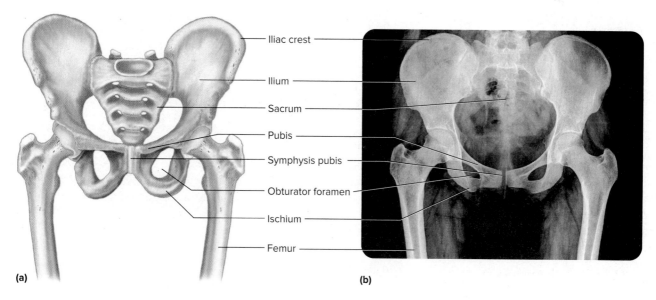

FIGURE 23-11 (a) Pelvic girdle. (b) Radiograph of the pelvic girdle.
(b) ©thailoei92/Shutterstock

The bones of the lower limb, or leg, include the femur, the patella, the tibia, and the fibula.

- The femur is the thigh bone and the largest bone in the body. Its proximal end joins with the hip bone at the *acetabulum* (or hip socket). Ligaments and muscles hold it in place.
- The distal end of the femur attaches to the tibia and the **patella** (kneecap). The patella is a sesamoid bone that literally resembles a sesame seed—a small, rounded bone in front of the knee joint.
- The **tibia** (or shinbone) is the medial bone of the lower leg. Its proximal end joins with the femur and fibula, and distally it joins to the ankle bones.
- The **fibula** is the lateral bone of the lower leg. It is much thinner than the tibia. It joins with the ankle bones at its distal end. Figure 23-12 illustrates the bones of the lower extremity.

The bones of the foot include the tarsals, the metatarsals, and the phalanges.

- The *tarsal* bones form the back of the foot. The *calcaneus,* or heel bone, is the largest tarsal bone. There are seven tarsal bones per foot.

- **Metatarsals** are bones that form the front of the foot. There are five metatarsals per foot.
- The bones of the toes are called *phalanges.* Each foot contains 14—2 for each big toe and 3 in all the other toes. The joints between these lower phalanges are interphalangeal joints, just like those of the fingers.
- The joints that join the toes to the foot are called *metatarsophalangeal* (*MTP*) joints.

▶ Joints   LO 23.10

Joints are the junctions between bones. Based on their structure, joints can be classified as fibrous, cartilaginous, or synovial.

- The bones of *fibrous joints* are connected together with short fibers. So the bones of this type of joint do not normally move against each other. Most fibrous joints are found between cranial bones and facial bones. Fibrous joints in the skull are called **sutures.**
- The bones of *cartilaginous joints* are connected together with a disc of cartilage. This type of joint is slightly movable. The joints between vertebrae are cartilaginous joints.
- The bones of *synovial joints* are covered with hyaline cartilage and are held together by a fibrous joint capsule (see Figure 23-13). The joint capsule is lined with a synovial membrane, which secretes a slippery fluid called *synovial fluid.* This fluid allows the bones to move easily against each other. Bones also are held together through tough, cord-like structures called *ligaments.* Synovial joints are freely movable. Examples of synovial joints are the elbows, knees, shoulders, and knuckles.

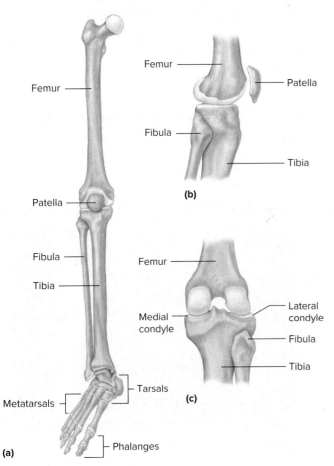

FIGURE 23-12   (a) Anterior view of the right lower limb. (b) Lateral view of the right knee. (c) Posterior view of the right knee.

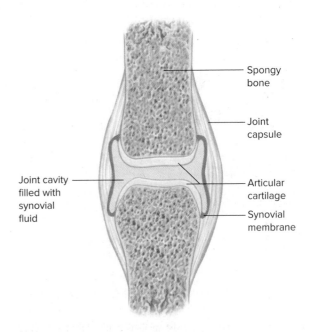

FIGURE 23-13   Structure of a synovial joint.

PATHOPHYSIOLOGY

Common Diseases and Disorders of the Skeletal System

Arthritis is a general term meaning "joint inflammation." Although there are more than 100 types of arthritis, we will discuss the two most common types: osteoarthritis and rheumatoid arthritis.

OSTEOARTHRITIS, also known as *degenerative joint disease (DJD),* is the most common type of joint disorder, affecting nearly everyone to some degree by the age of 70. DJD primarily affects the weight-bearing joints of the hips and knees, and the cartilage between the bones and the bones themselves begin to break down.

Causes. Research points to inflammatory processes or metabolic disorders as the etiology of DJD.

Signs and Symptoms. These include joint stiffness, aching, and pain, especially with weather changes. There is often fluid around the joint and grating noises with joint movement. The grating noise is usually caused by bone-on-bone contact.

Diagnostic Exams and Tests. X-rays of the affected joint are used to determine if osteoarthritis is present. Blood tests are used to rule out rheumatoid arthritis.

Treatment. Anti-inflammatory drugs, including aspirin and nonsteroidal anti-inflammatory drugs (NSAIDs) such as naproxen and Feldene®, may be used. Intra-articular steroid injections may be tried for severe cases. In some cases, a series of injections of hyaluronic acid–containing medications is used when other treatments do not work. These injections serve as joint fluid replacement. Some success has been found with transplanting harvested cartilage cells from the patient's healthy knee cartilage, which are then grown in the lab and reinjected into the patient's diseased joint. Surgical scraping of the joint also may be done to remove deteriorated bone fragments. As a last resort, joint replacement may be recommended.

Joint replacement prostheses can be metal, plastic, or a combination of both. The physician can surgically replace part of the joint (partial) or the entire joint (total). An example of a partial hip replacement is the Birmingham Hip Resurfacing prosthesis. In this procedure, the head of the femur is replaced by an all-metal prosthesis (see Figure 23-14). One of the advantages of partial joint replacement is that it conserves more bone than conventional total joint replacement. Conserving bone is important if additional surgery is needed in the future. The surgeon will have more natural bone to work with if a revision or new prosthesis is required.

RHEUMATOID ARTHRITIS (RA) is the second most common form of arthritis. RA is a chronic, systemic, inflammatory disease that first attacks the smaller joints, typically of the hands and feet, as well as the surrounding tissues of those joints. As the disease progresses, inflammation in larger joints occurs. There may be flares or attacks of pain and inflammation followed by periods of remission. RA is three times more common in women than in men.

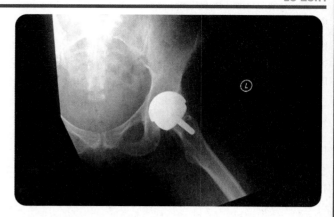

FIGURE 23-14 X-ray image of the Birmingham Hip Resurfacing prosthesis of the left hip.
©Total Care Programming, Inc.

Causes. RA is an autoimmune disease. The body's immune system attacks the synovium (lining) of the joints, triggering inflammation.

Signs and Symptoms. In this disease, immune system attacks cause edema (swelling), tenderness, and warmth in and around the joints. Tissue becomes granular and thick, eventually destroying the joint capsule and bone. Scar tissue forms, bones atrophy, and visible deformities become apparent due to the bone malalignment and immobility. Patients also have moderate to severe pain in the affected joints.

Diagnostic Exams and Tests. Magnetic resonance imaging (MRI) and X-rays in conjunction with blood tests are used to diagnose RA.

Treatment. Treatment includes anti-inflammatory drugs, exercise, heat or cold treatments, and cortisone injections. Researchers are working with genetic techniques to block the immune system reaction. Low-impact aerobic exercise may be helpful, and some patients find warm water exercises beneficial, too.

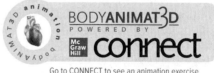

Go to CONNECT to see an animation exercise about *Osteoarthritis vs. Rheumatoid Arthritis*

BURSITIS is inflammation of a bursa, which is a fluid-filled sac that cushions tendons. It occurs most commonly in the elbow, knee, shoulder, and hip.

Causes. Overuse of and trauma to joints are the most common causes of this condition. Bacterial infections also can cause bursitis.

Signs and Symptoms. These include joint pain and swelling, as well as tenderness in the structures surrounding the joint.

Diagnostic Exams and Tests. Physical exam, patient history, X-rays, and MRI are used to diagnose bursitis. Lab tests on fluid withdrawn from the bursa also may be used to diagnose the cause.

Treatment. The most common treatments are bed rest, pain medications, steroid injections, aspiration of excess fluid from the bursa, and antibiotics.

EWING SARCOMA FAMILY OF TUMORS (ESFT) is a group of tumors that affect different tissue types. However, the tumors primarily affect bone.

Causes. Causes of ESFT are not clear, but it mostly affects Caucasians between the ages of 10 and 20. The tumors are usually located in the lower extremities but also may occur in the pelvis, chest wall, upper extremities, spine, and skull.

Signs and Symptoms. Fever, pain in the tumor location, fractures, and bruises in the tumor location are the primary symptoms.

Diagnostic Exams and Tests. ESFT is diagnosed with a combination of X-rays, MRI, computed axial tomography (CT) scans, blood tests, and biopsy.

Treatment. Treatment options include surgery, chemotherapy, radiation therapy, a bone marrow transplant, and stem cell transplant.

FRACTURES are cracks, breaks, or splintering of a bone. Fractures are categorized in several ways (Figure 23-15). Complete fractures go across the entire bone; incomplete fractures go through only part of the bone. Comminuted fractures are those in which the bone has broken into several fragments. In a greenstick fracture, the bone is bent, but only one side is fractured. Greenstick fractures occur most often in children

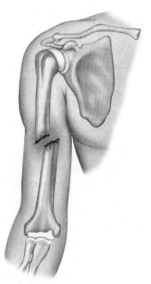
Complete fracture

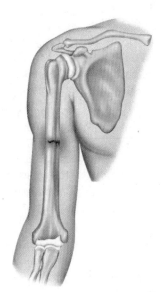
Incomplete fracture

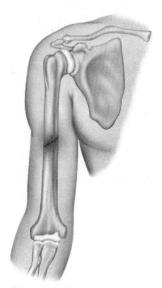
Closed fracture

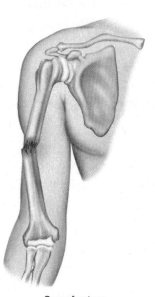
Open fracture

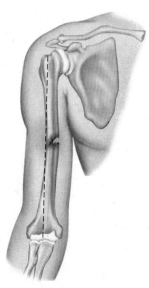
Greenstick fracture

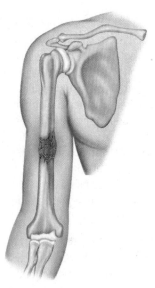
Comminuted fracture

FIGURE 23-15 Various types of fractures.

because their bones are still soft and pliable. A fracture is closed if it does not cause a break in the skin. In open fractures, the bone breaks through the skin. A **dislocation** is the displacement of a bone end from the joint.

Causes. Fractures and dislocations are most often caused by falls, automobile accidents, and sports injuries. Fractures also may occur in people with bone disorders such as tumors, osteoporosis, and Paget's disease.

Signs and Symptoms. After an accident or a fall, the patient may have intense pain, localized swelling, bruising, bleeding, a limb or joint that is deformed or out of place, numbness, and loss of use of the limb.

Diagnostic Exams and Tests. X-ray images and physical examination are used to diagnose fractures.

Treatment. Fractures and dislocations must be realigned (put back in place) and immobilized. This is usually accomplished by casting or splinting but may require surgical placement of plates, screws, or pins. For more information about emergency treatment of fractures, refer to the *Emergency Preparedness* chapter.

GOUT, also known as *gouty arthritis,* is a type of arthritis that usually occurs more frequently with age.

Causes. Gout is caused by deposits of uric acid crystals in the joints. People with gout cannot properly break down uric acid and remove it from their bloodstream.

Signs and Symptoms. Symptoms include sudden or chronic joint pain, commonly in the great toe; joint swelling and stiffness; and fever.

Diagnostic Exams and Tests. To diagnose gout, a specimen of joint fluid is aspirated from the affected joint and tested for urate crystals. Blood tests for high levels of uric acid and creatinine also may be performed.

Treatment. The most common treatments are pain medications and changes to the patient's diet. Patients should eliminate from their diet certain foods that cause the formation of uric acid (meats, fish, beer, and wine). There are medications available that increase uric acid elimination by the kidneys (uricosuric agents) or decrease uric acid production (xanthine oxidase inhibitors).

KYPHOSIS is an abnormal curvature of the spine, most often at the thoracic (chest) level. This condition is often referred to as humpback.

Causes. Adolescent kyphosis may result from growth retardation or improper development of the epiphyses as a result of rapid growth. Poor posture may exacerbate or worsen this condition. The adult form of kyphosis is frequently the result of aging and degenerative disc disease of the intervertebral discs and vertebral fracture from underlying osteoporosis.

Signs and Symptoms. In adolescent kyphosis, there may be no symptoms other than visible back curvature. There may be mild pain, tiredness, tenderness, or stiffness of the thoracic spine. In adult kyphosis, the upper back is rounded, and there may be pain, back weakness, and fatigue.

Diagnostic Exams and Tests. Kyphosis is diagnosed by physical examination, X-rays, MRI, and CT scans.

Treatment. Childhood kyphosis can be treated with exercise, a firm mattress, and a back brace if needed until growth is completed to keep the spine in alignment. Spinal fusion or grafting may be needed in rare cases of neurological damage or disabling pain. Harrington rods also may be used to keep the vertebrae aligned.

LORDOSIS is an exaggerated inward (convex) curvature of the lumbar spine. Sometimes this condition is called swayback.

Cause. Wearing high heels is a frequent cause. The positioning of the feet with the elevated heel height causes an inward positioning of the back as a counterbalancing measure.

Signs and Symptoms. The main sign is visual inward curvature of the lower back. There may be mild pain with this exaggerated curvature.

Diagnostic Exams and Tests. Spinal curvature disorders such as lordosis are diagnosed by physical exam, X-ray, CT, and MRI scans.

Treatment. Avoiding excessive heel height is the best prevention. Once the condition begins, exercise and appropriate footwear will at least keep the condition stable.

OSTEOGENESIS IMPERFECTA (OI) is more commonly called *brittle-bone disease.* People with this disease have decreased amounts of collagen in their bones, which leads to very fragile bones. There are eight types of this disease:

- Type I—the mildest form of OI, which occurs more often than any of the other types.
- Type II—the most severe form of OI, normally fatal within a few weeks of birth.
- Type III—also a severe type of OI; however, infants usually live longer than those with Type II.
- Type IV—a moderate form of OI that is usually diagnosed later in childhood.
- Type V—similar to Type IV except that large callouses form around bone fractures. This type accounts for only 5% of OI cases.
- Type VI—an extremely rare, moderate form of OI characterized by a defect in mineralization of the bone.
- Type VII—a moderate form caused by inheritance of a recessive gene mutation. Similar to Type IV. Moderately abnormal bone growth occurs in this type of OI.
- Type VIII—similar to OI Types II and III, and growth deficiency is severe; however, sclera are white in Type VIII.

Cause. The disorder is hereditary.

Signs and Symptoms. These include fractures (all types); blue sclera (types I, II, III, and IV); dental problems (types III and IV); hearing loss (type I); a triangular face (type III); abnormal spinal curves (types I, III, IV, V, and VI); very small stature (types II, III, IV, VII, and VIII); a small chest (types II and III); fractures at birth (types II and III); loose joints (type IV); muscle weakness (types I, III, and IV); and respiratory difficulties (types I, II, III, and VIII).

Diagnostic Exams and Tests. Genetic tests are used to determine if there are mutations in genes associated with OI.

Treatment. Because this disease has many symptoms, the list of treatments is extensive and includes fracture repair, surgery to strengthen bones by inserting metal rods into them, dental procedures, physical therapy, braces to prevent bone deformities, wheelchairs and other supportive aids, medications, and counseling. Other surgeries may be required to treat lung and heart problems that sometimes occur with this disease.

OSTEOPOROSIS is a condition in which bones become thin (more porous) over time. It is a very common disorder in the United States and affects women more than men and Caucasians more than any other race. This condition occurs because of hypocalcemia in which bone is broken down to release calcium and is not replaced in sufficient amounts; thus, bone density decreases.

Causes. These include hormone deficiencies (estrogen in women and testosterone in men), a sedentary lifestyle, a lack of calcium and vitamin D in the diet, bone cancers, corticosteroid excess (usually as a result of endocrine diseases), smoking, excess alcohol consumption, and steroid use.

Signs and Symptoms. There are usually no symptoms in the early stages of this disease. Patients in later stages of the disease may experience fractures (usually of the spine, wrists, or hips), back and neck pain, a loss of height over time, and an abnormal curving of the spine (kyphosis).

Diagnostic Exams and Tests. Patients at high risk, especially those with a family history of osteoporosis, should request bone densitometry studies to catch the disease before symptoms begin.

Treatment. The most common treatments include medications to prevent bone loss and relieve bone pain; hormone replacement therapy; lifestyle changes to prevent bone loss (including regular exercise and diets or supplements that include calcium, phosphorus, and vitamin D); moderation in use of alcohol; and stopping smoking.

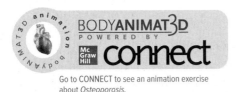

Go to CONNECT to see an animation exercise about *Osteoporosis.*

OSTEOSARCOMA is a type of bone cancer, usually affecting the leg bones, that originates from osteoblasts, the cells that make bony tissue. It occurs most often in children, teens, and young adults and more often in males than females.

Causes. The etiology of this type of cancer is unclear.

Signs and Symptoms. Primary symptoms include pain in affected bones (usually the legs), swelling around affected bones, and an increase in pain with movement of the affected bones.

Diagnostic Exams and Tests X-rays, MRI, CT scans, bone scans, and biopsy are all used to diagnose osteosarcoma.

Treatment. Treatments include surgery, chemotherapy, and radiation therapy. Amputation of the affected limb, followed by a prosthesis fitting, may be needed in some cases to prevent metastasis.

PAGET'S DISEASE causes bones to enlarge and become deformed and weak. It usually affects people over the age of 40.

Causes. This disease may be caused by a virus or various hereditary factors.

Signs and Symptoms. Bone pain, deformed bones, and fractures are common symptoms. Patients may experience headaches and hearing loss if the disease affects skull bones.

Diagnostic Exams and Tests. X-rays and bone scans are performed to visualize bone deformities common in people with Paget's disease.

Treatment. Treatments include surgery to remodel bones, hip replacements, medications to prevent bone weakening, and physical therapy.

SCOLIOSIS is an abnormal, S-shaped, lateral curvature of the thoracic or lumbar spine.

Causes. This disorder can develop prenatally when vertebrae do not fuse together. It also can result from diseases that cause weakness of the muscles that hold vertebrae together. Other causes of scoliosis are unknown, but they may be genetic.

Signs and Symptoms. A patient with scoliosis usually has a spine that looks bent to one side, with one shoulder or hip appearing to be higher than the other. Patients often experience back pain.

Diagnostic Exams and Tests. Scoliosis is diagnosed by physical exam and spinal X-rays.

Treatment. Treatment includes different types of back braces, surgery to correct spinal curves, and physical therapy to strengthen the muscles of the back and abdomen.

OUTCOME	KEY POINTS
23.1 **Describe the structure of bone tissue.**	Bones consist of the following substances: osteons (the Haversian system), bone matrix between osteocytes (bone cells), collagen fibers and proteins, lamellae, and canaliculi. Long bones include the femur and humerus; short bones include the carpals and tarsals; flat bones include the ribs and the frontal bone; irregular bones include the vertebrae and bones of the pelvic girdle. The diaphysis is the shaft of the long bone. The epiphysis is an end of a long bone. Articular cartilage covers the end of the long bones. The endosteum lines the medullary cavity. The periosteum is the membrane surrounding the diaphysis.
23.2 **Explain the functions of bones.**	Bone functions include giving shape to body parts, protecting soft structures of the body, and assisting in movement. The red bone marrow is responsible for hematopoiesis. Bones also store calcium.
23.3 **Compare intramembranous and endochondral ossification.**	Bones grow through two types of ossification: intramembranous ossification and endochondral ossification. The cartilage plate between the diaphysis and the epiphysis allows for growth of the long bone.
23.4 **Describe the skeletal structures and one location of each structure.**	Skeletal structures include the following: condyles, crests, epicondyles, foramina, fossae, heads, processes, sutures, trochanters, tubercles, and tuberosities.
23.5 **Locate the bones of the skull.**	The major bones of the skull are the frontal, parietal, temporal, and occipital bones. The fontanels are the membranous structures that connect the incompletely developed cranial bones. Within the skull are the mastoid processes, sphenoid, ethmoid, and ear ossicles. The facial bones include the mandible, maxillae, zygomatics, nasal and palatine bones, and vomer. Locations are shown in Figures 23-6 and 23-7.
23.6 **Locate the bones of the spinal column.**	The spinal column includes cervical, thoracic, and lumbar vertebrae; the sacrum; and the coccyx. Locations are shown in Figure 23-8.
23.7 **Locate the bones of the rib cage.**	There are 12 pairs of ribs, a sternum, and the xiphoid process. Locations are shown in Figure 23-9.
23.8 **Locate the bones of the shoulders, arms, and hands.**	Each upper extremity includes the clavicle, scapula, humerus, radius, ulna, carpals, metacarpals, and phalanges. Locations are shown in Figure 23-10.
23.9 **Locate the bones of the hips, legs, and feet.**	The bones of the hip, leg, and foot include the coxal bones, the femur, patella, tibia, fibula, metatarsals, tarsals, and phalanges. Locations are shown in Figures 23-11 and 23-12.
23.10 **Describe the three major types of joints and give examples of each.**	The three joint types are fibrous joints (for example, sutures of the skull), cartilaginous joints (for example, the joints between vertebrae), and synovial joints (for example, the elbow). A synovial joint consists of hyaline-covered bones held together by a fibrous joint capsule, which is lined by a synovial membrane that secretes synovial fluid. Ligaments hold the bones of these joints together.

OUTCOME	KEY POINTS
23.11 **Describe the causes, signs and symptoms, diagnosis, and treatments of various diseases and disorders of the skeletal system.**	There are many common diseases and disorders of the bones and the skeletal system with varied signs, symptoms, diagnosis, and treatments. Examples include arthritis, bursitis, ESFT, fractures, gout, kyphosis, lordosis, and scoliosis, as well as osteoporosis and osteosarcoma.

CASE STUDY CRITICAL THINKING

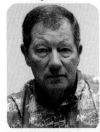

©McGraw-Hill Education

Recall John Miller from the case study at the beginning of the chapter. Now that you have completed the chapter, answer the following questions regarding his case.

1. Explain to John Miller what bursitis is and what causes it.

2. What treatment might the family nurse practitioner prescribe for John Miller's bursitis?

3. Why do you think John Miller's family nurse practitioner suspects bursitis and not a fracture?

4. John Miller's family nurse practitioner thinks that John may have bruised the sesamoid bone in front of his knee joint. What is the medical term for this bone?

5. The X-ray findings state that AP and lateral views of the knee and elbow showed no fractures. Describe the terms *AP* and *lateral*.

EXAM PREPARATION QUESTIONS

1. (LO 23.1) The tiny canals of cancellous bone that allow for the spread of nutrients are called
   a. Lamellae
   b. Lacunae
   c. Osteons
   d. Canaliculi
   e. Osteoblasts

2. (LO 23.3) Which substance is necessary for bone to absorb calcium?
   a. Vitamin C
   b. Phosporus
   c. Vitamin D
   d. Protein
   e. Carbohydrates

3. (LO 23.4) Articulation is another name for a
   a. Fossa
   b. Joint
   c. Foramen
   d. Suture
   e. Tubercle

4. (LO 23.5) Neck muscles attach to the skull via the
   _____ process.
   a. Mastoid
   b. Xiphoid
   c. Styloid
   d. Zygomatic
   e. Coracoid

5. (LO 23.9) The acetabulum is the
   a. Hip bone
   b. Knee joint
   c. Hip socket
   d. Shoulder bone
   e. Shoulder socket

6. (LO 23.11) A lateral curvature of the spine is known as
   a. Lordosis
   b. Kyphosis
   c. Osteoporosis
   d. Scoliosis
   e. Sarcoma

7. (LO 23.11) The medical term for brittle-bone disease is
   a. Ewing sarcoma family of tumors
   b. Osteogenesis imperfecta
   c. Rheumatoid arthritis
   d. Osteoporosis
   e. Paget's disease

8. (LO 23.1) Which of the following is the shaft of a long bone?
   a. Spine
   b. Epiphysis
   c. Crest
   d. Periosteum
   e. Diaphysis

9. (LO 23.1) The bones of the rib cage are
   a. Long bones
   b. Flat bones
   c. Irregular bones
   d. Short bones
   e. Sesamoid bones

10. (LO 23.4) Which of the following is an interlocking line of union between bones?
   a. Suture
   b. Condyle
   c. Process
   d. Articulation
   e. Fossa

MEDICAL TERMINOLOGY PRACTICE

Analyze the following medical terms, presented throughout the chapter. Using a medical dictionary (or Appendix I), place a / mark between each word part. Define each word part and then define the whole word.

EXAMPLE: **mast/oid** = mast means "breast" + oid means "resembling"
    MASTOID means "resembling a breast." (A mastoid process resembles a breast.)

1. arthritis
2. bursitis
3. scoliosis
4. costal
5. coxal
6. metacarpophalangeal

7. metatarsophalangeal
8. osteoblast
9. osteoclast
10. osteocyte
11. osteoporosis
12. osteosarcoma

13. hematopoiesis
14. interphalangeal
15. intramembranous
16. synovial
17. periosteum
18. temporal

The Muscular System

CASE STUDY

PATIENT INFORMATION

Patient Name	DOB	Allergies
Ken Washington	12/01/1958	Sulfa

Attending	MRN	Other Information
Paul F. Buckwalter, MD	00-AA-008	AFO brace ordered

Ken Washington has arrived for a follow-up visit from a recent hospitalization for a stroke. Until this hospitalization, he had no major health issues. However, he now has weakness in his left arm, and his speech is difficult to understand. He has left-leg weakness with foot drop, a condition characterized by an inability to raise the front part of the

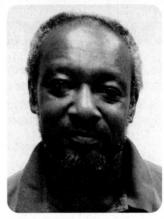
©McGraw-Hill Education

foot. The foot drop is causing him to trip when he walks more than a few steps. The physician has ordered a physical therapy evaluation and treatment as needed. The patient has been placed on an exercise regimen for his left-arm weakness. A special ankle foot orthosis (AFO) brace has been ordered to help Ken Washington with his foot drop.

Keep Ken Washington in mind as you study this chapter. There will be questions at the end of the chapter based on the case study. The information in the chapter will help you answer these questions.

LEARNING OUTCOMES

After completing Chapter 24, you will be able to:

24.1 Describe the functions of muscle.
24.2 Compare the three types of muscle tissue, including their locations and characteristics.
24.3 Explain how muscle tissue generates energy.
24.4 Describe the structure of a skeletal muscle.
24.5 Differentiate between the terms *origin* and *insertion*.
24.6 Identify the major skeletal muscles of the body, giving the action of each.
24.7 Summarize the changes that occur to the muscular system as a person ages.
24.8 Describe the causes, signs and symptoms, diagnosis, and treatments of various diseases and disorders of the muscular system.

KEY TERMS

acetylcholine
acetylcholinesterase
agonist
antagonist
aponeurosis
creatine phosphate
fascicle
insertion
lactic acid
multi-unit smooth muscle

myofibrils
origin
prime mover
sarcolemma
sarcoplasm
sarcoplasmic reticulum
sphincter
striations
synergist
visceral smooth muscle

I.C.1   Describe structural organization of the human body

I.C.2   Identify body systems

I.C.4   List major organs in each body system

I.C.5   Identify the anatomical location of major organs in each body system

I.C.6   Compare structure and function of the human body across the life span

I.C.7   Describe the normal function of each body system

I.C.8   Identify common pathology related to each body system including:
(a) signs
(b) symptoms
(c) etiology

I.C.9   Analyze pathology for each body system including:
(a) diagnostic measures
(b) treatment modalities

V.C.9   Identify medical terms labeling the word parts

V.C.10   Define medical terms and abbreviations related to all body systems

2. Anatomy and Physiology

a. List all body systems and their structures and functions

b. Describe common diseases, symptoms, and etiologies as they apply to each system

c. Identify diagnostic and treatment modalities as they relate to each body system

3. Medical Terminology

a. Define and use the entire basic structure of medical terminology and be able to accurately identify the correct context (i.e., root, prefix, suffix, combinations, spelling, and definitions)

b. Build and dissect medical terminology from roots and suffixes to understand the word element combinations

c. Apply medical terminology for each specialty

d. Define and use medical abbreviations when appropriate and acceptable

▶ Introduction

Your bones and joints do not produce movement all by themselves. Instead, your muscles—by alternating between contraction and relaxation—cause your bones and supported structures to move. The human body has more than 600 individual muscles. Although each muscle is a distinct structure, muscles act in groups to perform particular movements. In this chapter, you will explore the differences among three muscle tissue types, the structure of skeletal muscles, muscle actions, and the names of skeletal muscles.

▶ Functions of Muscle   LO 24.1

Muscle tissue is unique because it has the ability to contract. This contraction allows muscles to perform various functions. In addition to allowing the human body to move, muscles provide stability, control body openings and passages, and warm the body.

Movement

Skeletal muscles are attached to bones by tendons. Because skeletal muscles cross joints, when these muscles contract, the bones they attach to move. This allows for various body motions, such as walking or waving your hand. Facial muscles are attached to the skin of the face; when they contract, different facial expressions are produced, such as smiling or frowning. Smooth muscle is found in the walls of various organs, such as the stomach, intestines, and uterus. The contraction of smooth muscle in these organs produces the movement of their contents,

such as the movement of food material through the intestine or the birth of a child being pushed from the mother's uterus. Cardiac muscle of the heart produces the atrial and ventricular contractions that pump blood into the blood vessels.

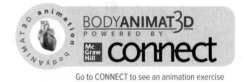

Go to CONNECT to see an animation exercise about *Muscle Contraction*.

Stability

You rarely think about it, but muscles are holding your bones tightly together so that your joints remain stable. There are also very small muscles holding your vertebrae together to stabilize your spinal column.

Heat Production

When muscles contract, heat is released, which helps the body maintain a normal temperature. This is why moving your body—say, jogging in place for a few seconds—can make you warmer if you are cold.

Control of Body Openings and Passages

In addition to providing important structural support for your bones and joints, muscles also form valve-like structures called **sphincters** around various body openings and passages. These sphincters control the movement of substances into and out of these passages. For example, a urethral sphincter prevents urination until you relax it to permit urination.

Muscle Cells and Tissue   LO 24.2

There are three types of muscle tissue: skeletal, smooth, and cardiac. Muscle tissue is made of muscle cells. Muscle cells, or *myocytes,* are called muscle fibers because of their long lengths. The cell membrane of a muscle fiber is called a **sarcolemma.** The cytoplasm of this cell type is called **sarcoplasm,** and the endoplasmic reticulum is called **sarcoplasmic reticulum.** Most of the sarcoplasm is filled with long structures called **myofibrils.** It is the arrangement of the actin and myosin

filaments in myofibrils that produces the **striations,** or stripes, observed in skeletal and cardiac muscle cells. Muscle fibers are controlled by motor neurons that release chemical substances called *neurotransmitters,* such as acetylcholine, dopamine, and epinephrine, onto the fibers. See Figure 24-1 for an illustration of the structure of a skeletal muscle. Study Table 24-1 to review the locations and features of the three types of muscle tissue.

Skeletal Muscle

Skeletal muscle fibers respond only to the neurotransmitter **acetylcholine,** which causes skeletal muscle to contract. Once contraction has occurred, skeletal muscles release an enzyme called **acetylcholinesterase,** which breaks down acetylcholine.

TABLE 24-1	Types of Muscle Tissue					
Muscle Group	**Major Location**	**Major Function**	**Striated (Yes/No)**	**Mode of Control**	**Characteristics of Contractions**	**Intercalated Discs**
Skeletal muscle	Attached to bones and the skin of the face	Produces body movements and facial expressions	Yes	Voluntary	Fast to contract and relax	No
Smooth muscle	Walls of hollow organs, blood vessels, and iris	Moves contents through organs; vasoconstriction	No	Involuntary	Slow to contract and relax	No
Cardiac muscle	Wall of the heart	Pumps blood through heart	Yes	Involuntary	Groups of muscle fibers contract as a unit	Yes

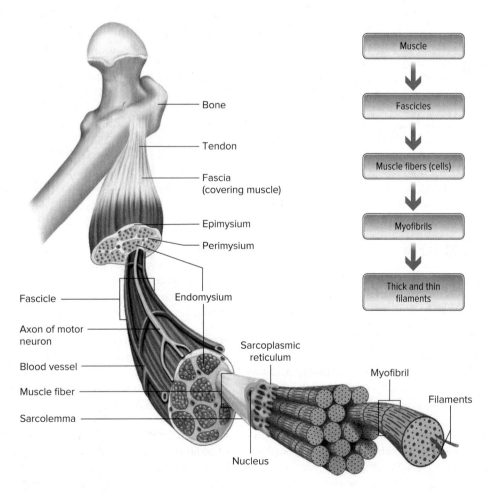

FIGURE 24-1   Structure of a skeletal muscle.

This allows the muscle to relax. Figure 24-2a shows a photomicrograph of skeletal muscle. These muscles are responsible for body movement, posture, and heat generation through shivering.

Smooth Muscle

There are two types of smooth muscle: multi-unit and visceral. **Multi-unit smooth muscle** is found in the iris of the eye and the walls of blood vessels. This muscle type contracts in response to neurotransmitters and hormones. **Visceral smooth muscle** contains sheets of muscle cells that closely contact each other. It is found in the walls of hollow organs such as the stomach, intestines, bladder, and uterus. Muscle fibers in visceral smooth muscle respond to neurotransmitters, but they also stimulate each other to contract, so the muscle fibers tend to contract and relax together. This type of muscle produces an action called peristalsis. *Peristalsis* is a rhythmic contraction that pushes substances through tubes of the body. For example, peristalsis in the lower two-thirds of the esophagus moves the *bolus* of food through the stomach; peristaltic muscle movements in the fallopian tubes propel the ovum (egg) through the tubes toward the uterus.

Two neurotransmitters are involved in smooth muscle contraction—acetylcholine and norepinephrine. Depending on the smooth muscle type, these neurotransmitters cause or inhibit contractions. Figure 24-2b is a photomicrograph of smooth muscle.

Cardiac Muscle

Groups of cardiac muscle are connected to each other through *intercalated discs*—discs with tunnels that physically connect the cardiac muscle cells. These discs allow the fibers in each group to contract and relax together—a design that allows the heart to work as a pump. First, the atria (holding chambers) contract and relax together; then the ventricles (pumping chambers) contract to send blood to the lungs and body, after which they relax and the cycle starts again. Cardiac muscle is also self-exciting, which means that it does not need nerve stimulation to contract. Nerves only speed up or slow down the contraction of the heart. Like smooth muscle, cardiac muscle responds to two neurotransmitters—acetylcholine and norepinephrine. Acetylcholine slows the heart rate and norepinephrine speeds it up. Figure 24-2c is a photomicrograph of cardiac muscle.

▶ Production of Energy for Muscle LO 24.3

Because a lot of adenosine triphosphate (ATP)—a type of chemical energy—is needed for sustained or repeated muscle contractions, a muscle cell must have multiple ways to store or make this substance. Muscle cells make this energy in three ways:

- **Creatine phosphate** production. Creatine phosphate production is a rapid way for a muscle to produce energy. When ATP is used during muscle contraction, it loses a phosphate and, therefore, energy. Imagine a desk toy that has five ball bearings suspended by strings. You create potential energy by lifting one of the ball bearings away from the others. When you release the ball bearing—breaking the bond between your fingers and the ball—the potential energy is released

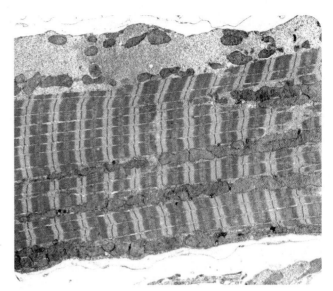

(a)

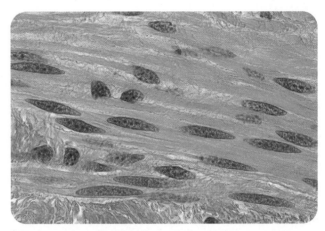

(b)

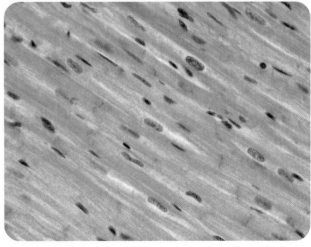

(c)

FIGURE 24-2 Photomicrographs of (a) skeletal, (b) smooth, and (c) cardiac muscle.

(a) ©Science Photo Library-STEVE GSCHMEISSNER/Getty Images; (b) ©McGraw-Hill Education/Dennis Street, photographer; (c) ©McGraw-Hill Education/Al Telser, Photographer

and the ball bearing hits the others, causing them to swing back and forth for several minutes. As with the ball bearing, energy stored in the phosphate bond is released when the bond is broken. Creatine phosphate "donates" a phosphate group, restoring energy potential.

- *Aerobic respiration*—an energy-forming biochemical process that requires oxygen—uses the body's store of glucose to make ATP. A cell breaks down glucose into pyruvic acid using oxygen (hence the term *aerobic*). The pyruvic acid is further converted into acetyl coenzyme A, which begins a series of reactions known as the *Krebs cycle,* or citric acid cycle. The oxygen needed for this method is stored in the muscle pigment called *myoglobin,* which also gives muscle its pinkish color.

- **Lactic acid** production occurs when a cell is low in oxygen and must convert pyruvic acid to lactic acid. This conversion produces a small amount of ATP for the cell, but because lactic acid is a waste product, it must then be released from the cell.

Oxygen Debt

Oxygen debt occurs when skeletal muscle is used strenuously for several minutes. When pyruvic acid is converted to lactic acid for energy production, the lactic acid builds up and causes muscle fatigue and soreness. The lactic acid is taken to the liver via the bloodstream to be converted back into glucose, which requires more energy. The amount of oxygen the liver cells need to make enough ATP for this conversion results in the oxygen debt. This process explains why your body still burns energy even after you are done exercising.

Muscle Fatigue

Muscle fatigue is a condition in which a muscle has lost its ability to contract. It usually develops because of an accumulation of lactic acid. It also can occur if the blood supply to a muscle is interrupted or if a motor neuron loses its ability to release acetylcholine onto muscle fibers. Cramps—painful, involuntary contractions of muscles—can accompany muscle fatigue. For this reason, if you have just finished an intense workout, it is important to replenish your electrolytes by drinking fluids and eating foods that are good sources of sodium, potassium, and calcium.

▶ Structure of Skeletal Muscles   LO 24.4

Skeletal muscles are the major organs that make up the muscular system. A skeletal muscle consists of connective tissue, skeletal muscle tissue, blood vessels, and nerves. When you see marbling in a steak, you are actually viewing connective tissue. The red portion of the steak is the muscle tissue.

The following connective tissue coverings are associated with skeletal muscles (see Figure 24-1):

- *Fascia.* Connective tissue located just below the skin that helps support and hold together muscles, bones, nerves, and blood vessels.

- *Tendon.* Tough, cord-like structure made of fibrous connective tissue that connects muscles to bones.

- **Aponeurosis.** Tough, sheet-like structure made of fibrous connective tissue. It typically attaches muscles to other muscles (See Figure 24-10).

- *Epimysium.* A thin covering that is just deep to the fascia of a muscle. It surrounds the entire muscle.

- *Perimysium.* A sheath of connective tissue surrounding a group of 10 to 100 muscle fibers. This grouping of muscle fibers is called a **fascicle.**

- *Endomysium.* The connective tissue that surrounds individual muscle cells.

▶ Attachments and Actions of Skeletal Muscles   LO 24.5

In order for skeletal muscle to produce movement, it must cross a joint and have at least two attachments to bone—one to the bone proximal to the joint and the second distal to the joint. Typically, one of the bones is more movable than the other when the muscle contracts. These attachments are known as the *origin* and *insertion.* An **origin** is an attachment site for the less movable bone during muscle contraction. An **insertion** is an attachment site for the more movable bone during muscle contraction. For example, the biceps brachii (the muscle on the anterior upper arm) attaches to two places on the scapula and to one site on the radius. When the biceps brachii contracts, the radius moves and the arm bends at the elbow. So the origin of the biceps brachii is where it attaches to the scapula. The insertion site of the biceps brachii is its attachment site on the radius (see Figure 24-3).

Most of the time, body movement is not produced by only one muscle but by a group of muscles. However, one muscle is responsible for most of the movement; this muscle is called the **prime mover** or **agonist.** Other muscles help the prime mover by stabilizing joints; these muscles are called **synergists.** An **antagonist** is a muscle that produces

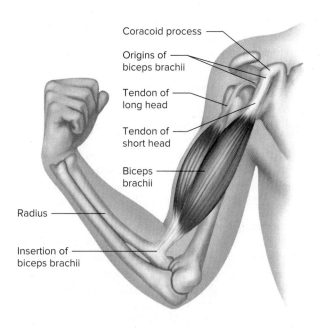

FIGURE 24-3 Origins and insertion of biceps brachii.

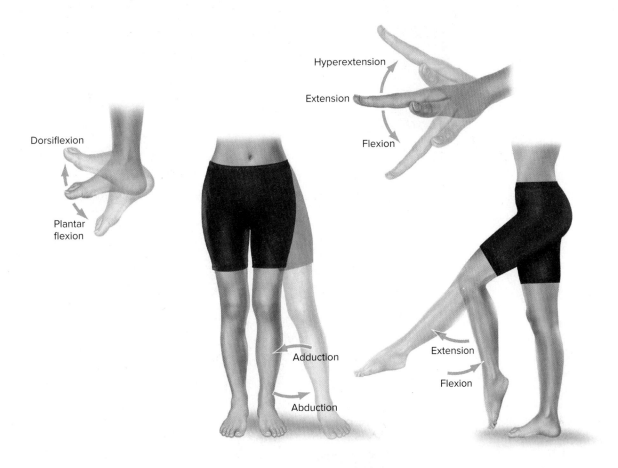

FIGURE 24-4 Adduction, abduction, dorsiflexion, plantar flexion, hyperextension, extension, and flexion.

a movement opposite to the prime mover. When the prime mover contracts, the antagonist must relax in order to produce a smooth body movement. For example, when you bend your arm at the elbow, the prime mover (agonist) is the biceps brachii. The synergist muscles are the brachialis and brachioradialis. The antagonist is the triceps brachii because its action is to extend the arm at the elbow. While the prime mover and synergists contract, the agonist relaxes; when the antagonist contracts, the prime mover and synergists relax.

The body movements produced by skeletal muscles include the following:

- *Flexion*—bending a body part or decreasing the angle of a joint.
- *Extension*—straightening a body part or increasing the angle of a joint.
- *Hyperextension*—extending a body part past the normal anatomical position.
- *Dorsiflexion*—pointing the toes up.
- *Plantar flexion*—pointing the toes down.
- *Abduction*—moving a body part away from the midline of the body.
- *Adduction*—moving a body part toward the midline of the body.
- *Rotation*—twisting a body part—for example, turning your head from side to side.

- *Circumduction*—moving a body part in a circle—for example, moving your arm in a circular motion.
- *Pronation*—turning the palm of the hand down or lying face down.
- *Supination*—turning the palm of the hand up or lying face up.
- *Inversion*—turning the sole of the foot medially.
- *Eversion*—turning the sole of the foot laterally.
- *Retraction*—moving a body part posteriorly.
- *Protraction*—moving a body part anteriorly.
- *Elevation*—lifting a body part—for example, elevating your shoulders as in a shrugging gesture.
- *Depression*—lowering a body part—for example, lowering your shoulders.

See Figures 24-4, 24-5, and 24-6 for illustrations of these types of movements. As a medical assistant, it is important to understand these movements so that you can assist with judging and measuring your patients' ability to perform range-of-motion (ROM) exercises when assessing injuries and illnesses.

▶ Major Skeletal Muscles   LO 24.6

The name of a skeletal muscle often describes it in some way. Usually, the name indicates the location, size, action, shape, or number of attachments of the muscle. For example, the

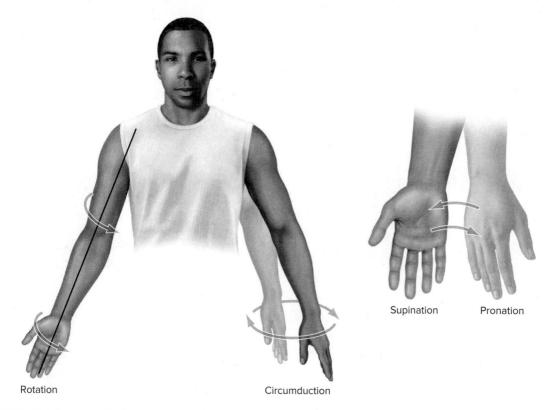

FIGURE 24-5 Rotation, circumduction, supination, and pronation.

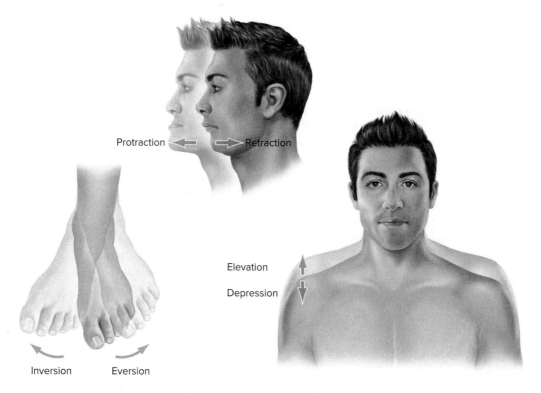

FIGURE 24-6 Eversion, inversion, protraction, retraction, elevation, and depression.

pectoralis major is named for its large size (major) and its location (pectoral, or chest, region). The sternocleidomastoid is named for its attachment sites—*sterno* (sternum), *cleido* (clavicle), and *mastoid* (the mastoid process of the temporal bone, located behind the ear). As you study muscles, you will find it easier to remember them if you think about what the name describes. Figures 24-7 and 24-8 show the anterior and posterior views of superficial skeletal muscles.

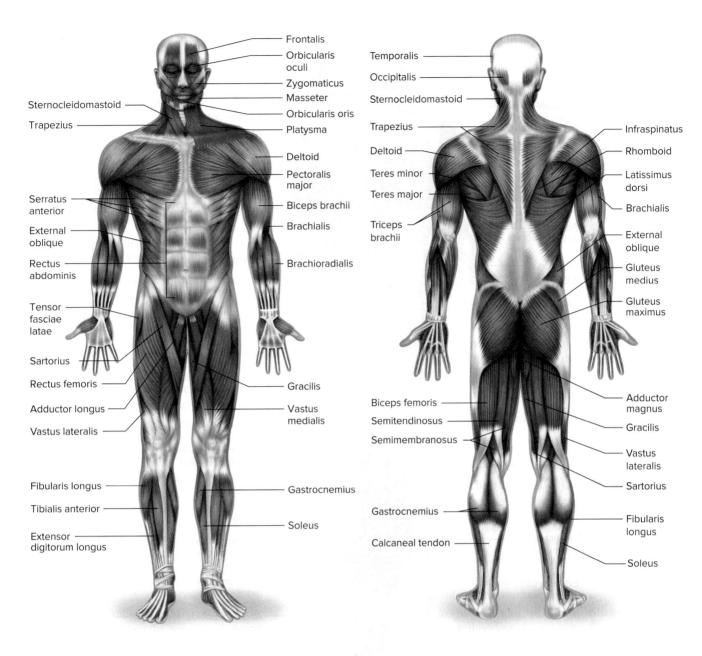

FIGURE 24-7 Anterior view of superficial skeletal muscles.

FIGURE 24-8 Posterior view of superficial skeletal muscles.

Muscles of the Head

The muscles of the head include those that move the head, provide facial expression, and move the jaw. Muscles that move the head include the following, and hints to assist you with remembering the locations for some of these muscles are provided in parentheses:

- Sternocleidomastoid. This muscle pulls the head to one side and pulls the head to the chest. (sterno = sternum, cleido = clavicle, mastoid = mastoid)

- Splenius capitis. This muscle rotates the head and allows it to bend to the side. (capit = head)

Muscles of facial expression include the following:

- Frontalis. This muscle raises the eyebrows. (frontal = pertaining to the front)

- Orbicularis oris. This muscle allows the lips to pucker. (oris = oro or mouth)

- Orbicularis oculi. This muscle allows the eyes to close. (oculi = eye)

- Zygomaticus. This muscle pulls the corners of the mouth up. (zygomat = cheekbone)

- Platysma. This muscle pulls the corners of the mouth down.

The muscles of the jaw allow for mastication (chewing) and include the following:

- Masseter and temporalis. These muscles close the jaw. (masseter, as in mastication or chewing; temporo = temple)

- Internal and external pterygoids. These muscles help position the jaw.

- Sternohyomastoid. This muscle opens the jaw. (hyo = hyoid bone)

OUTCOME	KEY POINTS
24.1 Describe the functions of muscle.	The functions of muscles include movement, stability, control of body openings and passages, and the production of heat. Valve-like muscular structures called sphincters control the passage of substances into and out of organs such as the stomach and bladder.
24.2 Compare the three types of muscle tissue, including their locations and characteristics.	The three types of muscle tissue are striated, voluntary skeletal muscle; smooth, involuntary visceral muscle; and specialized striated and involuntary cardiac muscle.
24.3 Explain how muscle tissue generates energy.	There are three ways muscles create energy. Creatine phosphate is a rapid method for muscles to create energy; aerobic respiration uses stored glucose to produce ATP in the Krebs cycle; and lactic acid production occurs when a cell is low in oxygen and converts pyruvic acid to lactic acid.
24.4 Describe the structure of a skeletal muscle.	Skeletal muscle is composed of connective tissue, skeletal muscle tissue, blood vessels, and nerves. The coverings of skeletal muscles include fascia, tendon, aponeurosis, epimysium, perimysium, and endomysium.
24.5 Differentiate between the terms origin and insertion.	The origin of a muscle is the attachment site of the muscle to the less movable bone during muscle contraction. The insertion of a muscle is the attachment site for the muscle to the more movable bone during muscle contraction.
24.6 Identify the major skeletal muscles of the body, giving the action of each.	The major muscles of the head are the sternocleidomastoid, splenius capitis, frontalis, orbicularis oris and oculi, zygomaticus, platysma, masseter, and temporalis. The upper extremity muscles include the pectoralis major, latissimus dorsi, deltoid, subscapularis, infraspinatus, biceps brachii, brachialis, brachioradialis, triceps brachii, supinator, pronator teres, flexor carpi radialis and ulnaris, plamaris longus, flexor digitorum profundus, extensor carpi radialis longus and brevis, extensor carpi ulnaris, and extensor digitorum. The major respiratory muscles are the diaphragm and the external and internal intercostals. The abdominal muscles include the external and internal obliques, transverse abdominis, and rectus abdominis. The pectoral girdle muscles include the trapezius and pectoralis minor. The muscles of the lower extremity include the iliopsoas major; gluteus maximus, medius, and minimus; adductor longus and magnus; biceps femoris; semitendinosus and semimembranosus; rectus femoris; vastus lateralis, medialis, and intermedius; sartorius; tibialis anterior; extensor digitorum longus; gastrocnemius; soleus; and flexor digitorum longus.
24.7 Summarize the changes that occur in the muscular system as a person ages.	The common diseases of aging include arthritis, fractures, osteoporosis, and muscular decline. Aging causes a decline in strength and speed of muscle contractions. Dexterity and gripping abilities lessen, and mobility often decreases related to skeletal and muscular decline.
24.8 Describe the causes, signs and symptoms, diagnosis, and treatments of various diseases and disorders of the muscular system.	There are many common diseases and disorders of the muscular system with varied signs, symptoms, methods of diagnosis, and treatments. Some of these are botulism, fibromyalgia, muscular dystrophy, myasthenia gravis, rhabdomyolysis, tendonitis, tetanus, torticollis, and trichinosis.

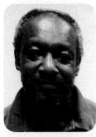

©McGraw-Hill Education

Recall Ken Washington from the case study at the beginning of the chapter. Now that you have completed the chapter, answer the following questions regarding his case.

1. Relate the benefits of exercise to the musculoskeletal system.

2. Identify the arm muscles Ken Washington will need to strengthen.

3. The physical therapist wants Ken Washington to strengthen the extensor digitorum longus muscle. Where is this muscle, and why does the therapist think this will help Ken's foot drop?

EXAM PREPARATION QUESTIONS

1. (LO 24.2) Groups of cardiac muscle are connected by
   a. Striations
   b. Multi-units
   c. Intercalated discs
   d. Fascia
   e. Myofibrils

2. (LO 24.2) Skeletal muscle responds to which of the following neurotransmitters?
   a. Epinephrine
   b. Acetylcholine
   c. Norepinephrine
   d. Dopamine
   e. Glucagon

3. (LO 24.5) Increasing the angle of a joint produces which of the following body movements?
   a. Extension
   b. Plantar flexion
   c. Flexion
   d. Hyperextension
   e. Elevation

4. (LO 24.6) Which muscle acts to abduct and extend the arm at the shoulder?
   a. Biceps brachii
   b. Gluteus maximus
   c. Triceps brachii
   d. Deltoid
   e. Brachioradialis

5. (LO 24.6) Which muscle separates the thoracic and abdominal cavities and assists in respiration?
   a. Internal/external obliques
   b. Internal/external intercostals
   c. Diaphragm
   d. Pectoralis major
   e. Serratus anterior

6. (LO 24.6) Which of the following muscles assists with mastication?
   a. Masseter
   b. Frontalis
   c. Platysma
   d. Zygomaticus
   e. Orbicularis oculi

7. (LO 24.8) The medical term for a condition known as wry neck is
   a. Tetanus
   b. Fibromyalgia
   c. Rhabdomyolysis
   d. Tendonitis
   e. Torticollis

8. (LO 24.8) Trichinosis is caused by a(n)
   a. Autoimmune disorder
   b. Parasitic worm
   c. Cervical deformity
   d. Soil bacterium
   e. Genetic mutation

9. (LO 24.5) The attachment site for the more movable bone during muscle contraction is the
   a. Origin
   b. Agonist
   c. Synergist
   d. Insertion
   e. Antagonist

10. (LO 24.5) Pointing the toes downward is known as
    a. Plantar flexion
    b. Abduction
    c. Inversion
    d. Dorsiflexion
    e. Pronation

Analyze the following medical terms, presented throughout the chapter. Using a medical dictionary (or Appendix I), place a / mark between each word part. Define each word part and then define the whole word.

EXAMPLE: **myo/globin** = myo means "muscle" + globin means "protein"
MYOGLOBIN means "muscle protein."

1. abduction
2. adduction
3. circumduction
4. dorsiflexion

5. eversion
6. fibromyalgia
7. hyperextension
8. inversion

9. tendonitis
10. myocytes
11. triceps
12. rhabdomyolysis

The Cardiovascular System

CASE STUDY

PATIENT INFORMATION		
Patient Name	**DOB**	**Allergies**
John Miller	12/05/1954	Bee stings
Attending	**MRN**	**Other Information**
Paul F. Buckwalter, MD	00-AA-005	Current Medications: Glyburide 2.5 mg daily, Captopril 25 mg bid, HCTZ 25 mg daily

John Miller was referred to the cardiologist's office for an evaluation. The patient has a history of hypertension and had a myocardial infarction (heart attack) 4 years ago. More recently, he was diagnosed with mild congestive heart failure (CHF). Three weeks ago, on the advice of his primary care physician, he started a light exercise program for

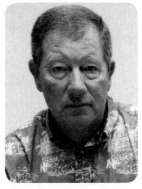

©McGraw-Hill Education

weight loss. Following exercise he has had a radiating chest pain (angina pectoris) that stopped after rest. The condition has worsened in the last week. The cardiologist ordered a stress echocardiogram (a test that visualizes the heart during increasing stress). The stress echocardiogram results suggested that the chest pain may be due to coronary artery disease (CAD). The patient was scheduled for a cardiac catheterization the next morning. It was noted in the patient's chart that he smokes two packs of cigarettes per day.

Keep John Miller in mind as you study this chapter. There will be questions at the end of the chapter based on the case study. The information in the chapter will help you answer these questions.

LEARNING OUTCOMES

After completing Chapter 25, you will be able to:

25.1 Describe the structures of the heart and the function of each.

25.2 Explain the cardiac cycle, including the cardiac conduction system.

25.3 Differentiate among the different types of blood vessels and their functions.

25.4 Compare the various types of circulation.

25.5 Explain blood pressure and tell how it is controlled.

25.6 Describe the causes, signs and symptoms, diagnosis, and treatments of various diseases and disorders of the cardiovascular system.

KEY TERMS

atrioventricular node (AV node)
bundle of His
cardiac output
chordae tendineae
coronary circulation
diastolic pressure
embolus
endocardium
epicardium
hepatic portal system

myocardium
pericardium
pulmonary circulation
Purkinje fibers
sinoatrial node (SA node)
stenosis
systemic circulation
systolic pressure
vasoconstriction
vasodilation
viscosity

I.C.1 — Describe structural organization of the human body

I.C.2 — Identify body systems

I.C.4 — List major organs in each body system

I.C.5 — Identify the anatomical location of major organs in each body system

I.C.6 — Compare structure and function of the human body across the life span

I.C.7 — Describe the normal function of each body system

I.C.8 — Identify common pathology related to each body system including:
(a) signs
(b) symptoms
(c) etiology

I.C.9 — Analyze pathology for each body system including:
(a) diagnostic measures
(b) treatment modalities

V.C.9 — Identify medical terms labeling the word parts

V.C.10 — Define medical terms and abbreviations related to all body systems

2. Anatomy and Physiology
a. List all body systems and their structures and functions
b. Describe common diseases, symptoms, and etiologies as they apply to each system
c. Identify diagnostic and treatment modalities as they relate to each body system

3. Medical Terminology
a. Define and use the entire basic structure of medical terminology and be able to accurately identify the correct context (i.e. root, prefix, suffix, combinations, spelling and definitions)
b. Build and dissect medical terminology from roots and suffixes to understand the word element combinations
c. Apply medical terminology for each specialty
d. Define and use medical abbreviations when appropriate and acceptable

Introduction

The cardiovascular system consists of the heart and blood vessels. It pumps blood to the lungs to pick up oxygen and to the digestive system to pick up nutrients. It then delivers the oxygen and nutrients to all of the body cells. At the same time, it picks up waste products from the body cells and transports them to the lungs, kidneys, and other organs for removal from the body.

The Heart
LO 25.1

The heart is a cone-shaped organ about the size of a loose fist. It is located within the mediastinum (central part of the chest) and extends from the level of the second rib to about the level of the sixth rib. Although many people think the heart is in the left side of the chest, it is located only slightly left of the midline of the body. The heart is bordered laterally by the lungs, posteriorly by the thoracic spine, and anteriorly by the sternum. Inferiorly, the heart rests on the diaphragm.

Cardiac Membranes

The heart is enclosed by a membrane called the **pericardium,** or pericardial sac (see Figure 25-1). The pericardium has two parts. The outer part, called the *fibrous pericardium,* consists of a tough, fibrous material that helps protect the heart and anchor it in the chest. The inner part of the pericardium,

which is called the *serous pericardium,* has two layers: the *parietal pericardium* and the *visceral pericardium.* The visceral pericardium is actually the outermost layer of the heart. It is also referred to as the epicardium or epicardial layer. The area between these two layers of the pericardium is known as the pericardial space. It contains pericardial fluid (about 10 to 20 mL), which reduces the friction between the membranes when the heart contracts and relaxes.

The Heart Wall

The wall of the heart (see Figure 25-2) is composed of the following three layers:

- **Epicardium.** This outermost layer is the visceral pericardium. It contains fat, which helps to cushion the heart.

- **Myocardium.** This middle layer is the thickest layer of the wall and is made primarily of cardiac muscle, which makes it the working layer of the heart.

- **Endocardium.** This innermost layer is thin and very smooth. This layer contains part of the cardiac electrical conduction system, which is discussed in *section 25.2* of this chapter.

Heart Chambers and Valves

The heart contains four hollow chambers, two on the left and two on the right (see Figure 25-3). The upper chambers of the heart are called *atria* (the singular form is *atrium*). They have

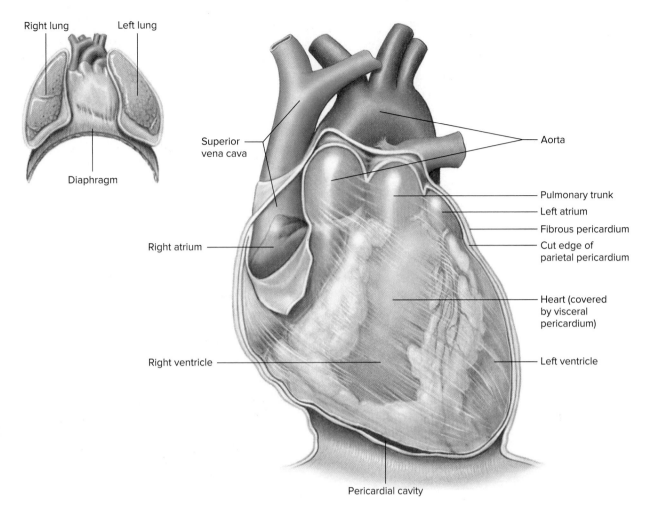

FIGURE 25-1   Location and membranes of the heart.

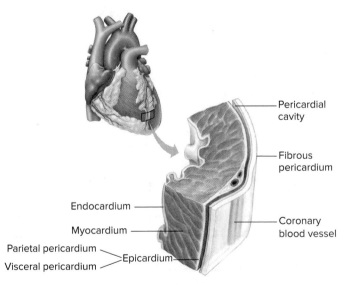

FIGURE 25-2   Layers of the wall of the heart.

thin walls and receive blood returning to the heart from the lungs and the body. The lower chambers of the heart called the *ventricles* pump blood into the arteries, which send the blood to the lungs and the body. The wall that separates the left and right sides of the heart is the septum. The septum between the atria is known as the interatrial septum. Likewise, the septum between the ventricles is called the interventricular septum.

For the heart to function properly, the blood must move through it in only one direction. The four valves within the heart that keep blood flowing in one direction are the tricuspid and the bicuspid (mitral) valves, which are located between the atria and ventricles, and the pulmonary semilunar and aortic semilunar valves, which are located between the ventricles and their arteries.

Tricuspid Valve   The *tricuspid valve* has three cusps and is located between the right atrium and the right ventricle (see Figure 25-4). It prevents blood from flowing back into the right atrium when the right ventricle contracts. This valve is also called the *right atrioventricular (AV) valve.* The cusps of this valve are attached to cord-like structures called **chordae tendineae** which are anchored to muscular mounds called *papillary muscles.* These muscles contract when the ventricles contract, closing the valve.

Bicuspid Valve   The *bicuspid valve* has two cusps and is located between the left atrium and the left ventricle. It prevents blood from flowing back into the left atrium when the left ventricle contracts. This valve is also known as the

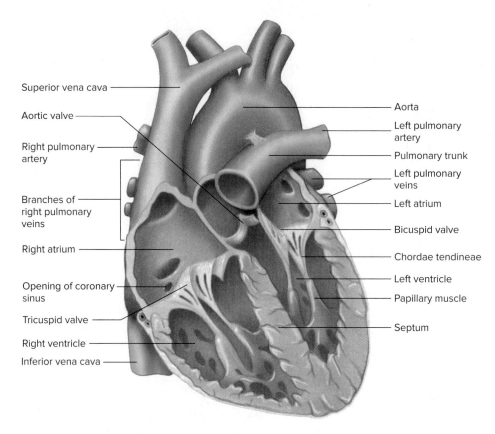

Superior vena cava

Aortic valve

Right pulmonary
artery

Branches of
right pulmonary
veins

Right atrium

Opening of coronary
sinus

Tricuspid valve

Right ventricle

Inferior vena cava

Aorta

Left pulmonary
artery

Pulmonary trunk

Left pulmonary
veins

Left atrium

Bicuspid valve

Chordae tendineae

Left ventricle

Papillary muscle

Septum

FIGURE 25-3 The chambers and valves of the heart are visible in this coronal section.

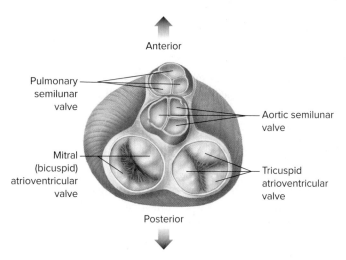

Anterior

Pulmonary
semilunar
valve

Aortic semilunar
valve

Mitral
(bicuspid)
atrioventricular
valve

Tricuspid
atrioventricular
valve

Posterior

FIGURE 25-4 Valves viewed from a cross section of the heart.

mitral valve and the *left AV valve*. Like the tricuspid valve, the bicuspid valve also has chordae tendineae attached to papillary muscles.

Pulmonary Semilunar Valve The *pulmonary semilunar valve* is located between the right ventricle and the trunk of the pulmonary arteries. It prevents blood from flowing back into the right ventricle. Because its cusps are shaped like a half moon, this valve is called a *semilunar valve*.

Aortic Semilunar Valve The *aortic semilunar valve* is between the left ventricle and the aorta. It prevents blood from flowing back into the left ventricle and is also known as a semilunar valve because of the shape of its cusps.

▶ Cardiac Cycle   LO 25.2

One heartbeat makes up one cardiac cycle. During the course of one cardiac cycle, all four heart chambers contract and then relax. The atria contract first, then the ventricles. Here are the actions that occur:

- Right atrium contracts → tricuspid valve opens → blood flows into the right ventricle.
- Left atrium contracts → bicuspid valve opens → blood flows into the left ventricle.
- Right ventricle contracts → tricuspid valve closes, pulmonary semilunar valve opens → blood is pushed into the trunk of the pulmonary artery.
- Left ventricle contracts → bicuspid valve closes, aortic semilunar valve opens → blood is pushed into the aorta.

The following factors influence the cardiac cycle:

- Exercise. Strenuous exercise increases the heart rate because skeletal muscles need more oxygen and nutrients.
- Parasympathetic nerves. The parasympathetic nerve to the heart is the vagus nerve. When stimulated, the vagus nerve causes slowing of the heart rate.

- Sympathetic nerves. The sympathetic nerves increase the heart rate during times of stress. Parasympathetic and sympathetic nerves are discussed in more detail in *The Nervous System* chapter.
- Cardiac control center. This center is located in the medulla oblongata, which is part of the brainstem. When blood pressure rises, this control center sends impulses to decrease the heart rate. When blood pressure falls, it sends impulses to increase the heart rate.
- Body temperature. An increase in body temperature usually increases the heart rate. This explains the high heart rate when a person runs a fever.
- Potassium ions. A low concentration of potassium ions in the blood may decrease the heart rate, but a high concentration causes a dysrhythmia (abnormal heart rate).
- Calcium ions. A low concentration of calcium ions in the blood depresses the contractile force, but a high concentration causes heart contractions called *tetanic contractions,* which are longer than normal heart contractions.

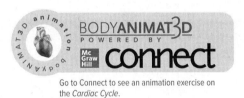

Go to Connect to see an animation exercise on the *Cardiac Cycle.*

Heart Sounds

During one cardiac cycle, you can hear two heart sounds. The sounds, commonly called *lubb* and *dubb,* are generated when valves in the heart snap shut. Lubb is the first heart sound and occurs when the ventricles contract and the tricuspid and bicuspid valves snap shut. Dubb is the second heart sound and occurs when the atria contract and the pulmonary and aortic semilunar valves snap shut.

Licensed practitioners listen to heart sounds to diagnose certain conditions. For example, if an AV valve (tricuspid or bicuspid) is damaged, it will not close completely. This allows blood to leak back into the atria when the ventricles contract and produces an abnormal heart sound called a *murmur.* Murmurs may indicate serious heart conditions, although many heart murmurs are harmless.

Cardiac Conduction System

The cardiac conduction system consists of a group of structures that send electrical impulses through the heart. When cardiac muscle receives an electrical impulse, it contracts (see Figure 25-5). The components of the cardiac conduction system are the sinoatrial node, atrioventricular node, bundle of His, left and right bundle branches, and the Purkinje fibers.

- **Sinoatrial node (SA node).** This node is located in the wall of the right atrium and generates an electrical impulse that flows to the atrioventricular node. The SA node also is known as the natural "pacemaker of the heart" because it generates the heart's rhythmic contractions.
- **Atrioventricular node (AV node).** This node is located between the atria, just above the ventricles. Once the wave of electrical energy reaches the AV node, there is a brief pause. During this pause the atria are completing their contraction pumping the remaining blood into the ventricles. Then the impulse continues to the bundle of His.
- **Bundle of His.** This structure, also known as the *atrioventricular,* or *AV, bundle,* is located between the ventricles

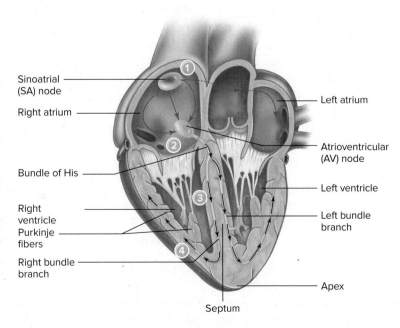

FIGURE 25-5 In the cardiac conduction system, impulses begin at the sinoatrial (SA) node and travel through the heart in the order shown here.

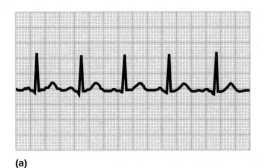

(a)

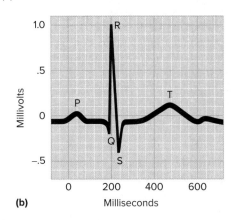

(b)

FIGURE 25-6 Electrocardiogram: (a) a normal ECG and (b) waves of a normal ECG pattern.

and splits into two branches, forming the left and right *bundle branches,* before sending the electrical impulse to the Purkinje fibers.

• **Purkinje fibers.** These fibers are located in the walls of the ventricles. As the electrical impulse flows through the Purkinje fibers, it delivers the electrical impulse to the ventricle muscle cells which causes the ventricles to contract.

Practitioners use a test called an electrocardiogram (ECG or EKG) to tell if the cardiac conduction system is working properly. In a normal ECG, the waves shown in Figure 25-6 are produced. The first wave (P wave) indicates that an electrical impulse was sent through the atria, causing them to contract (depolarization). The Q, R, and S waves occur in sequence and make up the QRS complex. This complex indicates that an electrical impulse was sent through the ventricles. This wave of electricity refers to an electrical event called depolarization. Depolarization is what causes the ventricles to contract. Finally, the T wave indicates electrical changes that occur in the ventricles as they relax (repolarization). You will learn more about the electrical conduction system of the heart and ECGs, including how to perform them, in the chapter *Electrocardiography and Pulmonary Function Testing.*

▶ Blood Vessels

LO 25.3

Blood circulation takes place in blood vessels that form a closed pathway to carry blood from the heart to cells and back again. These vessels include arteries, arterioles, veins, venules, and capillaries.

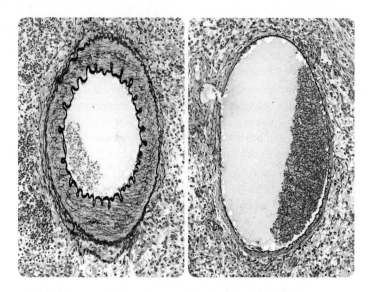

FIGURE 25-7 Arteries have much thicker walls than other blood vessels. (left) Cross section of an artery. (right) Cross section of a vein.
©MicroScape/Science Source

TABLE 25-1	Major Arteries of the Body
Artery	**Anatomical Location or Organ Supplied**
Lingual	Tongue
Facial	Face
Occipital	Back of scalp and neck
Maxillary	Teeth, jaw, and eyelids
Ophthalmic	Eye
Axillary	Armpit area
Brachial	Upper arm
Ulnar	Forearm and hand
Radial	Forearm and hand
Intercostals	Rib area
Lumbar	Posterior abdominal wall
External iliac	Anterior abdominal wall
Common iliac	Legs, gluteal area, and pelvic organs
Femoral	Thigh
Popliteal	Posterior knee
Tibial	Lower leg and foot

Arteries and Arterioles

Arteries carry blood away from the heart and are the strongest, thickest and most muscular of the blood vessels. They have a thick layer of smooth muscle that can withstand the high pressure the heart exerts on them (see Figure 25-7). This pressure is necessary to carry the blood throughout the body. Small branches of arteries are called *arterioles.*

The largest artery in the body is the aorta, which receives its blood directly from the left ventricle. The aorta branches into the coronary arteries and many other major arteries that supply blood to various parts of the body. Major arteries are summarized in Table 25-1 and illustrated in Figure 25-8.

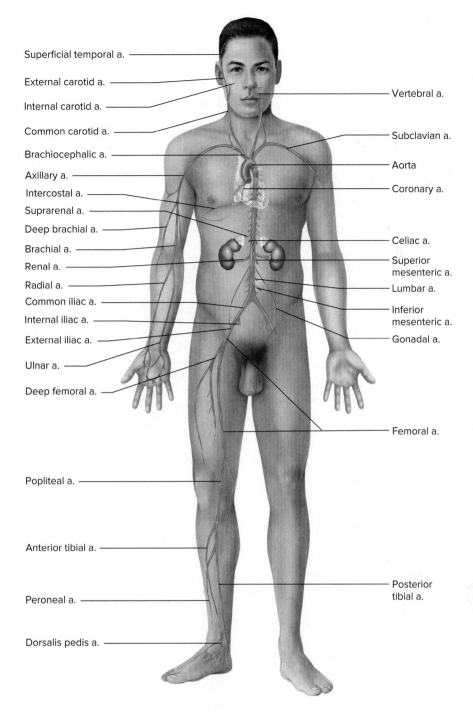

Superficial temporal a.

External carotid a.

Internal carotid a.

Common carotid a.

Brachiocephalic a.

Axillary a.

Intercostal a.

Suprarenal a.

Deep brachial a.

Brachial a.

Renal a.

Radial a.

Common iliac a.

Internal iliac a.

External iliac a.

Ulnar a.

Deep femoral a.

Popliteal a.

Anterior tibial a.

Peroneal a.

Dorsalis pedis a.

Vertebral a.

Subclavian a.

Aorta

Coronary a.

Celiac a.

Superior mesenteric a.

Lumbar a.

Inferior mesenteric a.

Gonadal a.

Femoral a.

Posterior tibial a.

FIGURE 25-8 Major arteries of the body (a. stands for *artery*).

Many arteries are paired, meaning there is a left and a right artery of the same name.

Most arteries carry oxygenated blood. The exceptions to this are the pulmonary arteries, which carry deoxygenated blood from the heart to the lungs.

Capillaries

Capillaries are the smallest type of blood vessel and they are the connecting vessel between the arterioles of the arterial system and venules of the venous system. They branch off of arterioles and have walls that are only about one cell layer thick. These thin walls make the exchange of oxygen, carbon dioxide, and nutrients possible between the blood and the body cells (see Figure 25-9). In fact, capillaries are the only type of blood vessels that allow substances to move into and out of the blood. Tissues that require a lot of oxygen, such as muscle and nervous tissues, have a lot of capillaries.

The substances that move through the capillary walls include oxygen, carbon dioxide, nutrients, water, and metabolic wastes. These substances move through the walls through one of three processes: diffusion, filtration, or osmosis. These processes are described in the *Organization of the Body* chapter.

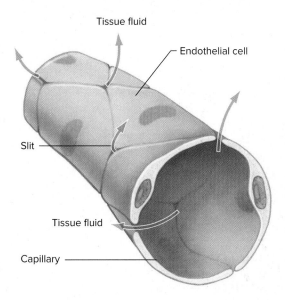

FIGURE 25-9 Structure of a capillary wall.

Veins and Venules

Veins are blood vessels that carry blood toward the heart. Unlike arteries, they are not under high pressure, so they do not need thick, muscular walls. Their walls are thinner than those of arteries. Because the blood in veins is not under pressure, veins have valves that prevent backflow and keep the blood moving toward the heart (see Figure 25-10).

Skeletal muscle contractions help move the blood through veins. When the muscles contract, they squeeze the veins and blood is pushed through them, much the way toothpaste is pushed out of a tube. The sympathetic nervous system also influences the flow of blood through veins. If blood pressure becomes abnormally low, the sympathetic nervous system causes vein walls to constrict, which forces blood through the veins. Small valves within veins keep blood from flowing back in the direction from which it came.

Venules are very small veins formed when capillaries merge together (see Figure 25-11). The venules then merge to form the veins.

Most veins carry deoxygenated blood. The exceptions to this are the pulmonary veins, which carry oxygenated blood

from the lungs to the left ventricle of the heart. Large veins often have the same names as the arteries they run next to, but there are exceptions. For example, the veins next to the carotid arteries are the jugular veins.

Large veins empty blood into the superior vena cava and the inferior vena cava (plural: *venae cavae*), which are the largest veins in the body. The superior vena cava generally collects blood from veins above the heart and the inferior vena cava collects blood from veins below the heart. The major veins are summarized in Table 25-2 and are illustrated in Figure 25-12.

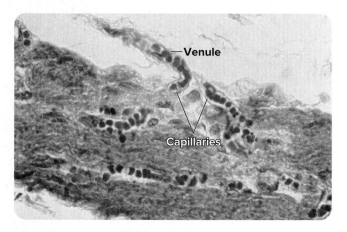

FIGURE 25-11 This light micrograph of a capillary network shows the capillaries merging to become venules.
©Biophoto Associates/Science Source

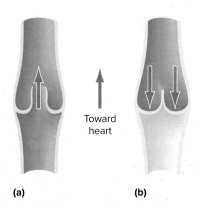

FIGURE 25-10 Venous valve: (a) valve opens when blood is flowing toward the heart and (b) valve closes to prevent blood from flowing away from the heart.

TABLE 25-2	Major Veins of the Body
Vein	**Anatomical Location or Organ Drained**
Jugular	Head and neck
Brachiocephalic	Head and neck
Axillary	Armpit area
Brachial	Upper arm
Ulnar	Lower arm and hand
Radial	Lower arm and hand
Intercostal	Rib area
Azygos	Thorax and abdomen
Iliac	Pelvic organs, legs, and gluteal areas
Femoral	Thighs
Popliteal	Knees
Saphenous	Legs
Hepatic	Liver to the inferior vena cava
Hepatic Portal System	
Gastric	Stomach to the liver
Splenic	Spleen, pancreas, and stomach to the liver
Mesenteric	Intestines to the liver
Hepatic portal	Gastric, splenic, and mesenteric veins to the liver

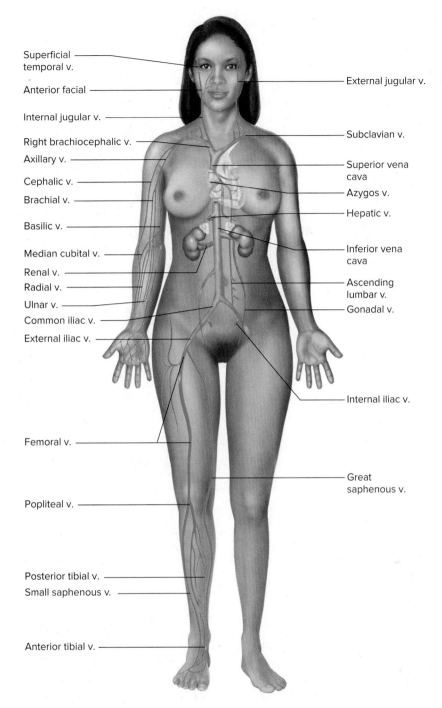

FIGURE 25-12   Major veins of the body (v. stands for *vein*).

The veins of the intestines carry blood from the digestive tract to the liver. The liver then processes nutrients in the blood and returns it to general circulation through the hepatic veins. The veins involved in this process are known as the **hepatic portal system.**

▶ Circulation

LO 25.4

Blood circulates through the body through three main circuits. The *pulmonary circuit* provides oxygen, the *systemic circuit* distributes the oxygen throughout the body, and the *coronary circuit* distributes the oxygen to the heart muscle.

Pulmonary Circulation

The pulmonary circuit, or **pulmonary circulation,** is the route blood takes from the heart to the lungs and back to the heart again (see Figure 25-13). The purpose of this circuit is to remove waste gases such as carbon dioxide and replenish the blood with oxygen. When blood returns to the heart from the body cells, it is low in oxygen (deoxygenated)

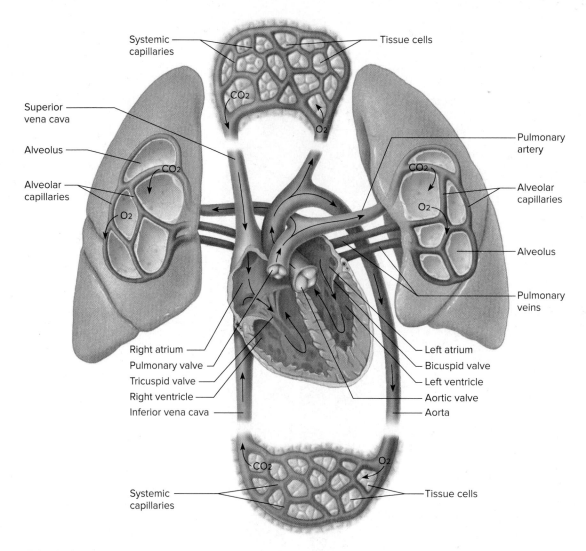

FIGURE 25-13 Pathway of blood through the heart and lungs and on to other body parts. The right side of the heart delivers blood to the lungs (pulmonary circulation), and the left side delivers blood to all other body parts (systemic circulation).

and rich in carbon dioxide. As described in *section 25.3* of this chapter, the deoxygenated blood enters the right atrium, which delivers it to the right ventricle. The right ventricle pumps the blood through the left and right pulmonary arteries to the lungs.

In the lungs, blood picks up oxygen and gets rid of carbon dioxide. Blood rich in oxygen and low in carbon dioxide then returns to the heart through the four pulmonary veins. The pulmonary veins empty the oxygenated blood into the left atrium.

Systemic Circulation

The systemic circuit, or **systemic circulation,** is the route blood takes from the heart through the body and back to the heart. The purpose of this circuit is to deliver oxygen and nutrients to the body cells. It also picks up carbon dioxide and waste products from the body cells (see Figure 25-13).

Blood that returns from the lungs and enters the left atrium is oxygen rich (oxygenated) and has a low level of carbon dioxide. It flows from the left atrium to the left ventricle,

which contracts to pump the oxygenated blood into the aorta, which branches off to various arteries to deliver the blood throughout the body.

The arteries branch into the smaller arterioles, and the arterioles branch into capillaries. In the capillaries, oxygen picked up from the lungs and nutrients picked up from the digestive system move from the blood into the body cells. Carbon dioxide and metabolic wastes move from the body cells into the blood. The blood then moves through the venules and veins and is collected into the vena cava, which delivers the blood back to the right atrium of the heart, and the whole process starts over again with pulmonary circulation.

Coronary Circulation

Coronary circulation is the part of systemic circulation that supplies oxygen and nutrients to the heart and removes carbon dioxide and other wastes. The coronary arteries branch directly off the aorta immediately after the blood leaves the left atrium (see Figure 25-14). Like all other arteries, the coronary arteries branch into smaller and smaller vessels, ending

Chest Pain

Chest pain, or angina, is a common reason for people to go to the emergency room or an urgent care center. Explain to patients that there are many causes of chest pain, both cardiac and noncardiac. Cardiac causes include myocardial infarction (MI, or heart attack), pericarditis, and coronary spasms. See the *Pathophysiology section* of this chapter for more detailed descriptions of these causes. Noncardiac causes include heartburn, panic attacks, lung conditions, broken ribs, inflammation of the gallbladder or pancreas, and even just sore muscles. However, tell patients that all chest pain should be taken seriously because some conditions, both cardiac and noncardiac, can be life-threatening if not treated.

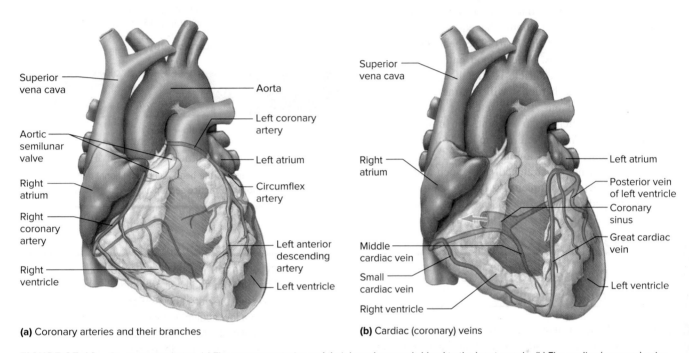

(a) Coronary arteries and their branches

(b) Cardiac (coronary) veins

FIGURE 25-14 Coronary circulation. (a) The coronary arteries and their branches supply blood to the heart muscle. (b) The cardiac (coronary) veins collect the deoxygenated blood and deposit it into the coronary sinus, which empties into the right atrium.

in capillaries, where oxygen and nutrients move into the heart cells and carbon dioxide and wastes move into the blood. The blood then travels through the venules and the cardiac veins, which merge to form a large vein called the *coronary sinus*. Unlike other veins, however, the coronary sinus does not empty into the vena cava. It empties directly into the right atrium.

Partial or complete blockage of one or more of the coronary arteries may cause chest pain, or angina, and may lead to myocardial infarction (MI, or heart attack) if not corrected. See the *Educating the Patient* feature and the *Pathophysiology section* of this chapter for more information about these disorders.

▶ Blood Pressure   LO 25.5

Blood pressure is the force that blood exerts on the inner walls of blood vessels. Blood pressure is highest in arteries and lowest in veins. In the clinical setting, *blood pressure* refers to the pressure in arteries.

Arterial blood pressure rises and falls as the ventricles of the heart contract and relax. It is highest when the ventricles contract. This highest point of pressure is called the **systolic pressure** or systole. When the ventricles relax, blood pressure in arteries is at its lowest. This pressure is called the **diastolic pressure** or diastole. Blood pressure is usually reported as the systolic pressure over the diastolic pressure. For example, in the blood pressure reading 120/80, 120 denotes the systolic pressure and 80 refers to the diastolic pressure.

You can feel the surge of blood through arteries when you take a pulse. The pulse is created as the artery expands when pressure increases and then subsequently relaxes as blood pressure decreases. Common places to feel a pulse are the carotid and radial arteries.

Many factors affect blood pressure, including cardiac output, blood volume, vasoconstriction, vasodilation, and blood viscosity. **Cardiac output** is the total amount of blood the heart pumps in 1 minute. As cardiac output increases, it causes an increase in blood pressure. When cardiac output decreases, blood pressure decreases accordingly.

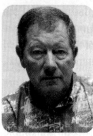
©McGraw-Hill Education

Recall John Miller from the case study at the beginning of this chapter. Now that you have completed this chapter, answer the following questions regarding his case.

1. What symptoms suggest that this patient is suffering from coronary artery disease and not some other disorder?

2. Why is it important to test the heart under stress rather than obtaining a resting echocardiogram?

3. Why is a cardiac catheterization needed in addition to the stress echocardiogram?

4. What lifestyle changes should John Miller make to prevent future heart attacks?

EXAM PREPARATION QUESTIONS

1. (LO 25.1) Which heart valve is between the left atrium and left ventricle?
   a. Tricuspid
   b. Bicuspid
   c. Pulmonary semilunar
   d. Aortic semilunar
   e. Right atrioventricular

2. (LO 25.2) Which part of the cardiac conduction system receives electrical impulses from the bundle branches?
   a. AV node
   b. SA node
   c. Bundle of His
   d. Purkinje fibers
   e. Chordae tendineae

3. (LO 25.3) In which blood vessels does the exchange of oxygen and waste gases occur?
   a. Arteries
   b. Arterioles
   c. Veins
   d. Venules
   e. Capillaries

4. (LO 25.4) Which chamber of the heart receives oxygenated blood from the lungs?
   a. Left atrium
   b. Right atrium
   c. Pulmonary trunk
   d. Left ventricle
   e. Right ventricle

5. (LO 25.6) Which of the following causes of chest pain is *not* cardiac in nature?
   a. Angina
   b. Pericarditis
   c. Heartburn
   d. Myocardial infarction
   e. Coronary spasms

6. (LO 25.5) The amount of pressure in the arteries when the ventricles contract is called
   a. Cardiac output
   b. Vasodilation
   c. Vasoconstriction
   d. Diastole
   e. Systole

7. (LO 25.1) The layer of the heart wall that is made mostly of cardiac muscle that allows the heart to contract and relax is the
   a. Pericardial space
   b. Myocardium
   c. Epicardium
   d. Visceral pericardium
   e. Endocardium

8. (LO 25.6) A condition in which a blood clot and inflammation develop in a vein is
   a. Mitral stenosis
   b. Varicose veins
   c. Thrombophlebitis
   d. Myocardial infarction
   e. Pericarditis

9. (LO 25.3) The largest veins in the body are the
   a. Hepatic portal veins
   b. Jugular veins
   c. Venae cavae
   d. Pulmonary veins
   e. Femoral veins

10. (LO 25.5) The total amount of blood pumped out of the heart in 1 minute is known as the
    a. Cardiac output
    b. Systolic pressure
    c. Systemic circulation
    d. Coronary sinus
    e. Diastolic pressure

Analyze the following medical terms, presented throughout the chapter. Using a medical dictionary (or Appendix I), place a / mark between each word part. Define each word part and then define the whole word.

EXAMPLE: **vaso / spasm** = vaso means "vessel" + spasm means "cramp or twitching"
VASOSPASM means "twitching or cramping of a vessel."

1. atherosclerosis
2. atrioventricular
3. baroreceptor
4. echocardiogram
5. electrocardiogram
6. intercostal
7. myocardium
8. pericarditis
9. stenosis
10. thrombophlebitis
11. vasoconstriction
12. ventricular

The Blood

CASE STUDY

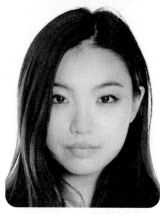

<table>
<tr><th>Patient Name</th><th>DOB</th><th colspan="2">Allergies</th></tr>
<tr><td>Cindy Chen</td><td>07/15/1993</td><td colspan="2">NKA</td></tr>
<tr><th>Attending</th><th>MRN</th><th colspan="2">Other Information</th></tr>
<tr><td>Alexis N. Whalen, MD</td><td>00-AA-001</td><td colspan="2">CD4 (T-cell) count: 480 cells/mm^3
CBC
   RBC: 3.9 million/mm^3
   Hgb: 12.1 g/dL
   Hct: 39%
   MCV: 98 fL
   Platelets: 90,000
   WBC: 4,100</td></tr>
</table>

PATIENT INFORMATION

Cindy Chen is complaining of inability to sleep and nervousness. She tested positive for HIV in 2014 and has been taking the antiviral drug Retrovir® as prescribed by her physician. She currently lives with her aunt and is going to school for phlebotomy. When looking at her chart, you notice that she has lost 20 pounds in the last 3 months. When she was in for a checkup a week ago, Dr. Whalen ordered a series of blood tests, including helper T-cell tests and CBC with platelet count. She is in the office today to discuss the results of the tests.

Keep Cindy Chen in mind as you study the chapter. There will be questions at the end of the chapter based on the case study. The information in the chapter will help you answer these questions.

LEARNING OUTCOMES

After completing Chapter 26, you will be able to:

26.1 Describe the components of blood, giving the function of each component listed.

26.2 Explain how bleeding is controlled.

26.3 Differentiate among blood types A, B, AB, and O related to their compatibility.

26.4 Explain the difference between Rh-positive blood and Rh-negative blood.

26.5 Describe the causes, signs and symptoms, diagnosis, and treatments of various diseases and disorders of the blood.

KEY TERMS

agglutination
agranulocyte
albumins
basophil
coagulation
eosinophil
erythrocyte
erythropoietin
fibrinogen
globulins
granulocyte

hematocrit (Hct)
hemoglobin (Hgb)
hemostasis
leukocyte
lymphocyte
monocyte
neutrophil
platelets
serum
thrombocytes
thrombus

CAAHEP

I.C.1 Describe structural organization of the human body

I.C.2 Identify body systems

I.C.4 List major organs in each body system

I.C.5 Identify the anatomical location of major organs in each body system

I.C.6 Compare structure and function of the human body across the life span

I.C.7 Describe the normal function of each body system

I.C.8 Identify common pathology related to each body system including:
    (a) signs
    (b) symptoms
    (c) etiology

I.C.9 Analyze pathology for each body system including:
    (a) diagnostic measures
    (b) treatment modalities

V.C.9 Identify medical terms labeling the word parts

V.C.10 Define medical terms and abbreviations related to all body systems

ABHES

2. Anatomy and Physiology
  a. List all body systems and their structures and functions
  b. Describe common diseases, symptoms, and etiologies as they apply to each system
  c. Identify diagnostic and treatment modalities as they relate to each body system

3. Medical Terminology
  a. Define and use the entire basic structure of medical terminology and be able to accurately identify the correct context (i.e. root, prefix, suffix, combinations, spelling, and definitions)
  b. Build and dissect medical terminology from roots and suffixes to understand the word element combinations
  c. Apply medical terminology for each specialty
  d. Define and use medical abbreviations when appropriate and acceptable

Introduction

Your blood is a type of connective tissue that is made up of multiple parts, including red and white blood cells, cell fragments called platelets, and plasma (the fluid part of the blood). The average-sized adult body contains approximately 4 to 6 liters of blood, or approximately 8% of the total body weight. Blood volume varies from person to person depending on the person's size, the amount of adipose tissue in the body, and the concentrations of certain ions in the blood. In general, partly because of their smaller size, females generally have less blood volume than males.

Blood performs many essential functions. It carries oxygen, nutrients, and hormones to cells throughout the body, and it carries carbon dioxide and other wastes away from the body cells. It also helps regulate body temperature, and some of its cells aid in immune function.

Components of Blood   LO 26.1

Red Blood Cells

Red blood cells (RBCs), also called **erythrocytes,** are biconcave-shaped cells, similar to a doughnut with a depression where the hole should be. RBCs are small enough to pass through capillaries (see Figure 26-1).

The percentage of red blood cells in a sample of blood is called the **hematocrit (Hct).** A healthy person normally has a hematocrit level of about 45%. Almost 99% of the "formed elements," or cells in blood, are red blood cells; white blood cells and platelets make up only about 1%. The rest of blood (approximately 55%) is plasma (see Figure 26-2).

Mature RBCs do not contain nuclei. They do, however, contain a pigment called **hemoglobin (Hgb).** The function of hemoglobin is to carry oxygen from the lungs to the body tissues and to carry carbon dioxide from the tissues to the lungs for release from the body. Hemoglobin that carries oxygen is called *oxyhemoglobin* and is bright red; hemoglobin that is not carrying oxygen is called *deoxyhemoglobin* and is a darker red. Often, because the deoxyhemoglobin is now carrying carbon dioxide, it is referred to as *carbaminohemoglobin.*

An RBC count consists of the number of red blood cells in 1 cubic millimeter (roughly 20 drops) of blood. A normal RBC count varies among laboratories, but a typical normal count is between 4.2 and 5.4 million RBC/cubic milliliter (mm^3) for adult males and between 3.6 and 5.0 million RBC/mm^3 for adult females. Because the function of an RBC is to transport oxygen throughout the body, a low count reflects a decreased ability to carry oxygen, causing a condition known as *anemia.* Likewise, if the RBC count is adequate but the amount of hemoglobin within the red blood cells is decreased, thus impairing the ability to carry adequate oxygen, anemia also may be diagnosed.

During fetal development, RBCs are made in the yolk sac, the liver, and the spleen. However, once a baby is born, most blood cells are produced in red bone marrow by cells called *hemocytoblasts.* The average lifespan of an RBC is only about 120 days, so red bone marrow is constantly making new cells. The hormone **erythropoietin,** produced by the kidneys, stimulates the red bone marrow and is responsible for regulating the production of RBCs. The kidneys release erythropoietin when oxygen concentrations in the blood get low.

Iron is necessary to make hemoglobin. In addition to iron, vitamin B_{12} and folic acid (vitamin B_9) are two dietary factors

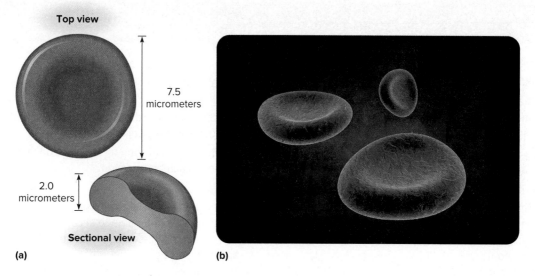

FIGURE 26-1 Red blood cells: (a) biconcave shape of red blood cells and (b) scanning electron micrograph of red blood cells.

(b) ©Cre8tive Studios/Alamy Stock Photo

that affect RBC production. These vitamins are necessary for DNA synthesis, so red bone marrow, like all actively dividing tissue, is affected when DNA cannot be produced. As stated earlier, too few RBCs or too little hemoglobin can result in one of the many types of anemia, which will be discussed in more detail in the *Pathophysiology: Common Diseases and Disorders of the Blood System* section of this chapter.

As RBCs age, macrophages in the liver and spleen destroy them. When an RBC is destroyed, a pigment called *biliverdin*

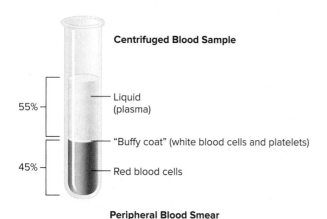

Centrifuged Blood Sample

55% — Liquid (plasma)

"Buffy coat" (white blood cells and platelets)

45% — Red blood cells

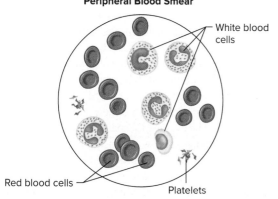

Peripheral Blood Smear

White blood cells

Red blood cells

Platelets

FIGURE 26-2 Centrifuged blood sample and peripheral blood smear slide seen through a microscope showing blood components.

is released from the cell. The liver usually converts biliverdin into an orange-colored pigment called *bilirubin*. Bilirubin is used to make bile, which is needed for the digestion of fats. However, when there is too much bilirubin, it builds up in the bloodstream. This causes the individual's skin and the sclera of the eyes to appear yellow-orange in color, a condition known as *jaundice* (or *icterus*).

Medical terms are built and dissected using prefixes, word roots/combining form, and suffixes. For example, we can build the term *hemocytoblasts* by placing the parts of the term in the puzzle pieces where P = prefix, WR/CF = word root or combining form, and S = suffix.

hemocytoblasts

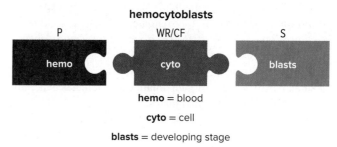

P   WR/CF   S

hemo   cyto   blasts

hemo = blood

cyto = cell

blasts = developing stage

Hemocytoblasts are blood cells in their developing stage. Learn additional medical terms in the **Medical Terminology Practice** section at the end of this chapter.

White Blood Cells

White blood cells (WBCs), commonly called **leukocytes**, are divided into two categories: granulocytes and agranulocytes. **Granulocytes** have granules (small particles) in their cytoplasm and include neutrophils, eosinophils, and basophils. **Agranulocytes** do not have granules in their cytoplasm and include monocytes and lymphocytes. The types of WBCs and their characteristics are described in Table 26-1.

A WBC count is the number of WBCs in 1 cubic millimeter of blood. This count is normally between 5,000 and 10,000 cells. A WBC count above normal is called *leukocytosis*. This condition often results from bacterial infections.

TABLE 26-1 Types of White Blood Cells

Cell Type	Description	Adult Normal Range % of Total WBC Count	Function
Granulocytes (Polymorphonuclear)			
©Ed Reschke	**Neutrophils** have distinct nuclei with 3 or 4 lobes. They show neutral staining: tan, lavender, or pink.	60–70%	Aid in immune system defense; release pyrogens (chemicals produced by leukocytes to cause fever); phagocytize (engulf) bacteria; use lysosomal enzymes to destroy bacteria; level increases during infection and inflammation
©Ed Reschke	**Eosinophils** have a bilobed nucleus and cytoplasmic granules that stain orange-red.	1–4%	Assist with inflammatory responses; secrete chemicals that destroy certain parasites; level increases with allergies and parasitic infection
©Ed Reschke	**Basophils** have a bilobed nucleus and cytoplasmic granules that stain deep blue.	0–1%	Assist with inflammatory response by releasing histamine; release heparin (anticoagulant) and produce a vasodilator; count increases with chronic inflammation and during healing from infection
Agranulocytes (Mononuclear)			
©Ed Reschke	**Monocytes** have large, kidney-shaped nuclei.	2–6%	Are the largest WBCs; become macrophages; phagocytize dying cells, microorganisms, and foreign substances; levels increase during chronic infections, such as tuberculosis (TB)
©Ed Reschke	**Lymphocytes** have round nuclei and a minimum amount of cytoplasm. Lymphocytes may be B cells, T cells, or natural killer (NK) cells.	20–30%	B-cell lymphocytes assist the immune system by producing antibodies; T-cell lymphocytes assist the immune system through interactions with other leukocytes; NK cells quickly respond to stressed cells; lymphocyte levels increase during viral infections; see the chapter *The Lymphatic and Immune Systems.*

A WBC count below normal is called *leukopenia* and is caused by some viral infections and various other conditions.

A differential WBC count lists the percentages of the different types of leukocytes in a sample of blood. This is a useful test because certain diseases and conditions change the usual balance among the different types of WBCs. For example, neutrophil numbers increase at the beginning of a bacterial or viral infection, but monocyte numbers do not increase until about 2 weeks after a bacterial infection. Eosinophil numbers increase during viral or worm infections as well as with allergic reactions. In AIDS, lymphocyte numbers fall, particularly lymphocytes known as T lymphocytes or T cells. You will gain more in-depth knowledge about T cells in the chapter *The Lymphatic and Immune Systems.*

Some WBCs stay in the bloodstream to fight infections, whereas others leave the bloodstream by squeezing through blood vessel walls to reach other tissues. This squeezing of a cell through a blood vessel wall, which is called *diapedesis,* is shown in Figure 26-3.

Blood Platelets

Platelets are fragments of cells that are found in the bloodstream (refer back to Figure 26-2). Platelets are also called **thrombocytes** (*thrombo* = clot; *cyte* = cell) and are important in the blood-clotting process. Platelets come from cells called *megakaryocytes* found in red bone marrow. A normal platelet count is between 150,000 and 450,000 platelets per microliter of blood.

Blood Plasma

Plasma is the liquid portion of blood. It is mostly water but also contains a mixture of proteins, nutrients, gases, electrolytes, and waste products. The three major types of proteins in plasma are:

- **Albumins**—the smallest plasma proteins; they pull water into the bloodstream to help maintain blood pressure.
- **Globulins**—transport lipids and some fat-soluble vitamins in plasma; some globulins become antibodies.
- **Fibrinogen**—an important protein for the blood-clotting process.

The term **serum** refers to the fluid that is left when all clotting factors are removed from plasma. You will learn more about serum in the *Collecting, Processing, and Testing Blood Specimens* chapter.

Nutrients in plasma are absorbed from the gastrointestinal tract and include amino acids, glucose, nucleotides, and lipids.

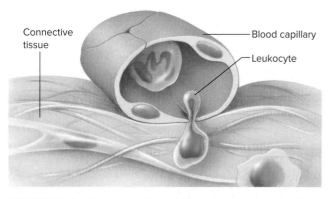

FIGURE 26-3 Diapedesis of white blood cells into surrounding tissue.

Labels: Connective tissue — Blood capillary — Leukocyte

Because lipids are not water soluble and because plasma is mostly water, lipids must combine with molecules called *lipoproteins* to be transported. The different types of lipoproteins are chylomicrons, very low-density lipoproteins (VLDL), low-density lipoproteins (LDL), and high-density lipoproteins (HDL). You will learn more about lipids and their effect on the body in the *Nutrition and Health* chapter.

The gases dissolved in plasma include oxygen, carbon dioxide, and nitrogen. Many electrolytes also are dissolved in plasma. They include sodium, potassium, calcium, magnesium, chloride, bicarbonate, phosphate, and sulfate. Molecules that contain nitrogen but are not proteins include amino acids, urea, and uric acid. Urea and uric acid are waste products produced by cells. Amino acids are the "building blocks" that combine to form proteins.

▶ Bleeding Control   LO 26.2

Hemostasis refers to the control of bleeding. The medical term *hemostasis* breaks down into *hemo,* meaning "blood," and *stasis,* meaning "stopping." Following an injury, four major events are involved in stopping the flow of blood at the injured site:

1. Blood vessel spasm.
2. Platelet plug formation.
3. Blood clotting.
4. Fibrinolysis, or dissolving of the clot and return of the vessel to normal function.

If the blood vessel is small and the injury is limited, a blood vessel spasm alone may stop the bleeding. At the time of injury, the involved blood vessel constricts (narrows in diameter), and this decreases the amount of blood flowing through the vessel, which stops or controls the bleeding. If bleeding continues in spite of the blood vessel spasms, platelets are called into action. The torn, inner lining of the blood vessels releases chemical signals, which stimulate platelets to gather at the injury site. These platelets clump together to form a platelet plug, which further decreases the flow of blood from the injured site. This process occurs within seconds after an injury and is known as primary hemostasis.

A blood clot eventually replaces the platelet plug. The formation of a blood clot is called blood **coagulation.** In this process, the plasma protein fibrinogen is converted to fibrin. Once fibrin forms, it sticks to the damaged area of the blood vessel, creating a mesh that entraps blood cells and platelets (Figure 26-4). The resulting mass—the blood clot—stops the bleeding entirely. The clot stimulates the growth of fibroblasts and smooth muscle cells within the vessel wall. This begins the repair process, which includes the final step in hemostasis, *fibrinolysis,* ultimately resulting in the dissolution of the clot. The vessel finally returns to normal. See Figure 26-5.

When a blood vessel is injured, it is normal for a blood clot to form. However, sometimes blood clots form on the side of a blood vessel with no known injury; this abnormal blood clot is called a **thrombus.** A thrombus is dangerous because a portion of it can break off and start moving through the bloodstream. The moving portion of the thrombus is called an *embolus.* An embolus is dangerous because, as discussed

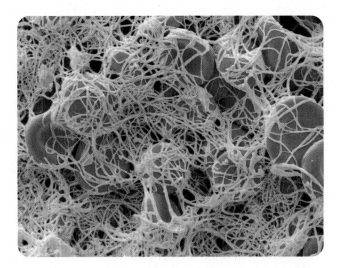

FIGURE 26-4 Scanning electron micrograph of a blood clot. Yellow fibrin threads are covering red blood cells.
©Science Photo Library/Alamy Stock Photo

in the chapter *The Cardiovascular System*, it can eventually block a small artery in the lungs, heart, or brain, causing pulmonary embolism, myocardial infarction, or CVA (stroke), respectively. All of these are serious and possibly fatal conditions if not treated, or if treatment cannot be initiated quickly enough to stop the condition from progressing.

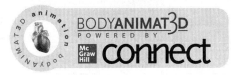

Go to CONNECT to see an animation exercise on *Strokes*.

▶ ABO Blood Types   LO 26.3

The most widely used system to determine blood typing and compatibility is the ABO blood group system. This system places blood into one of four groups, or types, based on the antigens present on the red blood cells.

- Type A—blood that has antigen A on the surface of its RBCs and antibody B in its plasma.

- Type B—blood that has antigen B on the surface of its RBCs and antibody A in its plasma.
- Type AB—blood that has both antigen A and antigen B on the surface of its RBCs but has neither antibody A nor antibody B in its plasma.
- Type O—blood that has neither antigen A nor antigen B on the surface of its RBCs but has both antibody A and antibody B in its plasma.

The reaction between these antigens and antibodies is very specific. Antibody A binds only to antigen A, and antibody B binds only to antigen B. If a person with type A blood is given type B blood, then the antibody B in the recipient's blood will bind with the RBCs of the donor blood because those cells have antigen B on their surfaces. As a result, **agglutination** occurs, and the donated RBCs are destroyed. This is why a person with type A blood should not be given type B blood (and vice versa). When this type of reaction occurs, it is called a transfusion reaction.

People with type AB blood are called *universal recipients* because most of them can receive all ABO blood types. They can receive these blood types because they lack antibody A and antibody B in their plasma, so there is no reaction with antigens A and B of the donor blood.

People with type O blood are called *universal donors* because their blood can be given to most people, regardless of the recipient's blood type. Type O blood will not agglutinate when given to other people because it does not have the antigens to bind to antibody A or antibody B. Table 26-2

TABLE 26-2	ABO Blood Type Overview		
Blood Type	**Antigen Present**	**Antibody Present**	**Blood Type That Can Be Received**
A	A	B	A and O
B	B	A	B and O
AB	A and B	None	All blood types
O	None	A and B	O only

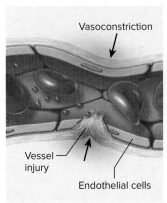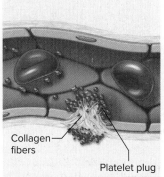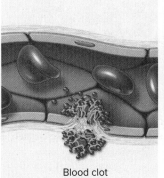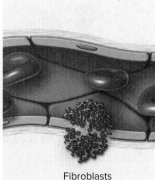

(a) Blood vessel spasm **(b)** Platelet plug formation **(c)** Blood clotting **(d)** Fibrinolysis

FIGURE 26-5 Events in hemostasis.

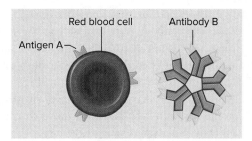

Type A blood

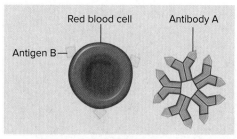

Type B blood

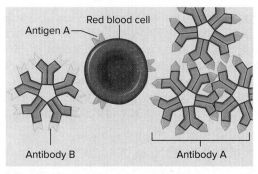

Type AB blood

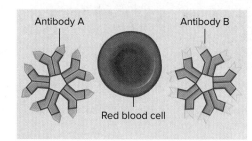

Type O blood

FIGURE 26-6 Blood Types A, B, AB, and O.

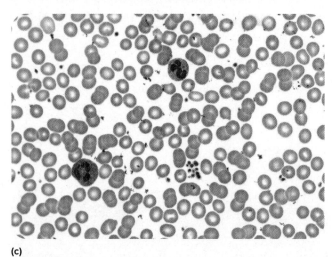

(a)

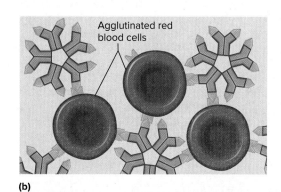

(b)

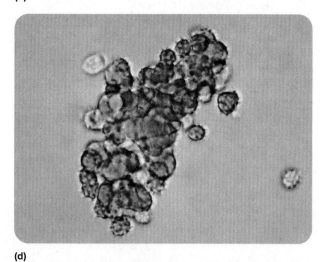

(c)

(d)

FIGURE 26-7 Agglutination: (a) red blood cells with antigen A are added to blood that contains antibody A; (b) antibody A reacts with antigen A, causing the agglutination of blood; (c) normal blood; and (d) agglutinated blood.

summarizes the ABO blood groups. Also see Figure 26-6 for a pictorial representation of each blood type.

When a patient needs a blood transfusion, the blood used in the transfusion must be compatible with the patient's blood type. If it is not, antigens on the patient's RBCs will bind to antibodies in the donor's plasma. This causes the RBCs to agglutinate, resulting in severe anemia. (see Figure 26-7).

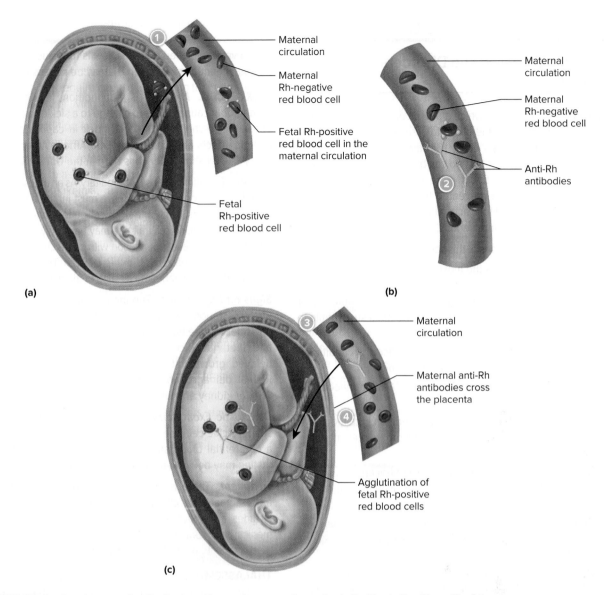

FIGURE 26-8 Development of antibodies in an Rh-negative woman in reaction to the blood of her Rh-positive fetus.

▶ The Rh Factor

LO 26.4

The *Rh antigen* is a protein first discovered on RBCs of the rhesus monkey, hence the name Rh. People who are Rh-positive have RBCs that contain the Rh antigen. People who are Rh-negative have RBCs that do not contain the Rh antigen. If a person who is Rh-negative is given Rh-positive blood, then the Rh-negative person's blood will make antibodies that bind to the Rh antigens. If the Rh-negative person is given Rh-positive blood a second time, the antibodies will bind to the donor cells and agglutination will occur.

Clinically, it is very important for a female to know her Rh type if she is pregnant or wishes to become pregnant. If an Rh-negative female mates with an Rh-positive male, there is a 50% chance her fetus will be Rh-positive. When the blood of an Rh-positive fetus mixes with the blood of a mother who is Rh-negative, the mother develops antibodies against the fetus's RBCs. Typically, the first Rh-positive fetus (infant) does not suffer any effects from these antibodies because it takes so long for the mother's body to generate them. However, if the mother conceives a second Rh-positive fetus, her antibodies will attack this fetus's blood right away. The second fetus then develops a condition called *erythroblastosis fetalis,* also known as hemolytic disease of the newborn. The baby is born severely anemic, often needing multiple blood transfusions at birth and often several times as a neonate (see Figure 26-8). Erythroblastosis fetalis is prevented by giving an Rh-negative woman the drug RhoGAM. RhoGAM prevents an Rh-negative mother from making antibodies against the Rh antigen.

OUTCOME	KEY POINTS
26.4 Explain the difference between Rh-positive blood and Rh-negative blood.	The Rh factor is an antigen that may be attached to any blood type. Its importance arises during transfusions (Rh-negative blood cannot receive Rh-positive blood) and during pregnancy if the mother is Rh-negative but the fetus received the Rh-positive antigen from the father. The first fetus will not be much affected; unless treated, however, any subsequent Rh-positive fetus will suffer effects of erythroblastosis fetalis because the mother's blood developed antibodies against the Rh-positive factor during the initial pregnancy.
26.5 Describe the causes, signs and symptoms, diagnosis, and treatments of various diseases and disorders of the blood.	The blood can be affected by many common diseases and disorders with varied signs, symptoms, diagnoses, and treatments. Some of these include anemia, leukemia, sickle cell anemia, polycythemia vera, and thalassemia.

CASE STUDY CRITICAL THINKING

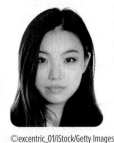

Recall Cindy Chen from the case study at the beginning of the chapter. Now that you have completed the chapter, answer the following questions regarding her case.

1. What information about Cindy Chen's blood can be gained by the CBC and platelet count?
2. A helper T cell is a type of white blood cell (WBC). Why would information about Cindy Chen's WBCs, particularly T cells, be of interest to her physician, considering her HIV status?

EXAM PREPARATION QUESTIONS

1. (LO 26.1) Which of the following is the hormone responsible for regulating the production of RBCs?
   a. Hemoglobin
   b. Erythropoietin
   c. Biliverdin
   d. Oxyhemoglobin
   e. Hematocrit

2. (LO 26.1) Which blood cell type does not normally contain a nucleus?
   a. RBCs
   b. Eosinophils
   c. Agranulocytes
   d. Basophils
   e. Neutrophils

3. (LO 26.2) Which term refers to control of bleeding?
   a. Hemoglobin
   b. Hematocrit
   c. Platelets
   d. Agglutination
   e. Hemostasis

4. (LO 26.2) The other term for blood coagulation is
   a. Plug
   b. Fibrin
   c. Clotting
   d. Granulation
   e. Agglutination

5. (LO 26.3) Which blood type is the universal donor?
   a. Blood type A
   b. Blood type B
   c. Blood type AB
   d. Blood type O
   e. Rh-negative

6. (LO 26.3) Which process could indicate a transfusion reaction because of a blood typing mismatch?
   a. Coagulation
   b. Clotting
   c. Hemorrhage
   d. Bleeding
   e. Agglutination

7. (LO 26.4) Which combination could be a problem for an unborn fetus?
  a. Rh-negative mom/Rh-positive dad/first pregnancy
  b. Rh-positive mom/Rh-negative dad/first pregnancy
  c. Rh-negative mom/Rh-positive dad/second pregnancy
  d. Rh-positive mom/Rh-negative dad/second pregnancy
  e. Rh-negative mom/Rh-negative dad/second pregnancy

8. (LO 26.4) RhoGAM is used to prevent
  a. Iron deficiency anemia
  b. Erythroblastosis fetalis
  c. Leukemia
  d. Transfusion reactions
  e. Hemophilia

9. (LO 26.5) Which of the following is *not* a cause of anemia?
  a. Vitamin B_{12} deficiency
  b. Blood loss
  c. RBC destruction
  d. Bone marrow destruction
  e. Low WBC count

10. (LO 26.5) Which blood disorder(s) is(are) hereditary?
  a. Sickle cell anemia
  b. Thalassemia
  c. Leukemia
  d. Sickle cell anemia and thalassemia
  e. Thalassemia and leukemia

MEDICAL TERMINOLOGY PRACTICE

Analyze the following medical terms, presented throughout the chapter. Using a medical dictionary (or Appendix I), place a / mark between each word part. Define each word part and then define the whole word.

EXAMPLE: **hemo / rrhage** = hemo means "blood" + rrhage means "excessive flow"
  HEMORRHAGE means "excessive flow of blood."

1. erythrocytes

2. leukocytes

3. granulocytes

4. agranulocytes

5. anemia

6. thrombocytes

7. hemostasis

8. erythroblastosis fetalis

9. leukemia

10. hemolytic

11. hematoma

12. venogram

CASE STUDY

PATIENT INFORMATION	Patient Name	DOB	Allergies
	Cindy Chen	07/15/1993	NKA
	Attending	**MRN**	**Other Information**
	Alexis N. Whalen, MD	00-AA-001	CBC is within normal limits; rapid influenza test is negative for A & B types. Oral temperature 100.8

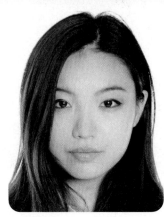

©excentric_01/iStock/Getty Images

Cindy Chen is a female patient in her twenties complaining of sore throat, congestion, coughing, fever, and malaise.

She tested positive for HIV in 2014 and is asymptomatic and on antiviral drugs. She currently lives with her aunt and is going to school to become a phlebotomist. When taking Cindy Chen's initial history, she tells you that she can feel large "tender, lumps" in her neck. Dr. Whalen has ordered a CBC and a rapid influenza A/B test.

Keep Cindy Chen in mind as you study the chapter. There will be questions at the end of the chapter based on the case study. The information in the chapter will help you answer these questions.

LEARNING OUTCOMES

After completing Chapter 27, you will be able to:

27.1 Describe the pathways and organs of the lymphatic system.

27.2 Compare the nonspecific and specific body defense mechanisms.

27.3 Explain how antibodies fight infection.

27.4 Describe the four different types of acquired immunities.

27.5 Describe the causes, signs and symptoms, diagnosis, and treatments of major immune disorders.

KEY TERMS

anaphylaxis
antibodies
antibody-mediated response
antigens
autoimmune disease
cell-mediated response
complements
cytokines
hapten
immunoglobulins
innate immunity
interstitial fluid
lymph
lymph nodes
lymphocytes
lymphokines
macrophages
major histocompatibility complex (MHC)
monokines
natural killer (NK) cells
phagocytosis
spleen
thymus
tonsils

▶ Introduction

Your immune system works as a personal coat of armor, responsible for protecting your body against bacteria, viruses, fungi, toxins, parasites, and cancer. This important system, present in every human being, works with the organs of the lymphatic system—the thymus, spleen, and lymph nodes—to clear the body of various disease-causing agents.

▶ The Lymphatic System   LO 27.1

The lymphatic system is a network of connecting vessels that collect the interstitial (or tissue) fluid found between cells. These lymphatic vessels then return this fluid, now called **lymph,** to the bloodstream. See Figure 27-1. The lymphatic system also picks up lipids and fat-soluble vitamins (A, D, E, and K) from the digestive tract and transports them to the bloodstream. The third function of the lymphatic system is to protect the body against disease-causing agents.

Interstitial (Tissue) Fluid and Lymph

Fluid constantly leaks out of blood capillaries into the spaces between cells. This fluid is high in nutrients, oxygen, and small proteins. Most of this fluid is picked up by body cells. However, some of the fluid persists between cells. Increased tissue hydrostatic pressure moves **interstitial (tissue) fluid** into the lymphatic vessels. This fluid is destined to become lymph.

Lymphatic Vessels and Lymph Circulation

The lymphatic vessels transport lymph and excess fluid away from the interstitial spaces toward the heart. Smaller lymphatic capillaries join to form larger lymphatic vessels.

Lymphatic Capillaries The lymphatic capillaries are similar in structure to blood capillaries except that lymphatic capillaries are larger in diameter and facilitate drainage of interstitial fluids—fluids between the cells—from the tissues. This is facilitated by the thin, very permeable lymphatic capillary walls, which are lined by a single layer of squamous epithelial cells called endothelium. The epithelial cells of the lymphatic capillary wall overlap, creating flap-like valves that allow fluid to enter the capillary but do not allow fluid to exit under normal conditions. However, under some conditions, lymph can leak out of the vessels, causing *edema,* or fluid buildup, in the interstitial spaces. Lymphatic capillaries converge to form lymphatic trunks, which in turn merge to form lymphatic ducts. This is similar to the structure of the venous system, but lymphatic vessels have thinner walls and more valves than do veins. The lymphatic pathway is illustrated in Figure 27-2.

Lymphatic Trunks and Ducts Lymphatic trunks are typically named after the region in which they are found. For example, the *jugular trunks* (left and right) drain the head and neck region. The *lumbar trunk* drains the lymph from the lower extremities, the *subclavian trunk* drains the upper limbs, and the *bronchomediastinal trunk* drains lymph from the thorax. The trunks eventually empty into the two lymphatic ducts. The *right lymphatic duct* receives lymph from the upper right side of the body. It empties its contents into the right internal jugular and right subclavian veins. These veins

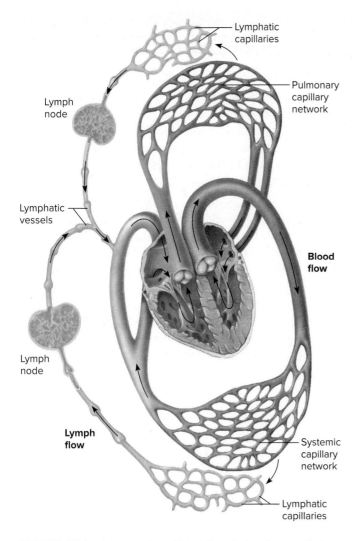

FIGURE 27-1 Schematic flow of lymph from the lymphatic capillaries to the bloodstream.

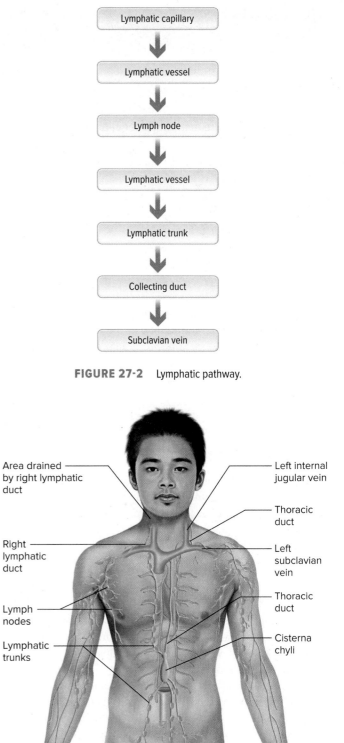

FIGURE 27-2 Lymphatic pathway.

(Figure 27-2 flowchart:)
Lymphatic capillary → Lymphatic vessel → Lymph node → Lymphatic vessel → Lymphatic trunk → Collecting duct → Subclavian vein

return the lymph to the right atrium by way of the superior vena cava. The other duct is the *thoracic duct,* which is the largest lymphatic vessel in the body. It drains lymph from all parts of the body that are not drained by the right lymphatic duct. The thoracic duct begins at the level of the second lumbar vertebra. The thoracic duct passes through the diaphragm beside the aorta and empties into the junction of the left internal jugular and left subclavian veins (see Figure 27-3).

Lymph is moved along by two pumps and flows in only one direction—toward the heart. The *skeletal muscle pump* utilizes skeletal muscle contractions to move the lymph toward the heart. The other pump is the *respiratory pump,* which utilizes pressure changes in the thorax to assist circulation. Along its way to the venous blood, lymph will pass through more than 600 *lymph nodes* throughout the body.

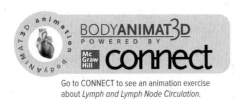

BODY**ANIMAT3D**
POWERED BY
Mc Graw Hill **connect**

Go to CONNECT to see an animation exercise about *Lymph and Lymph Node Circulation.*

FIGURE 27-3 Areas drained by the right lymphatic duct (shaded) and thoracic duct (not shaded).

Lymphoid Organs and Tissues

Lymphoid organs and tissues are widespread throughout the body and consist of lymph nodes, the thymus, and the spleen.

Lymph Nodes **Lymph nodes** are very small, glandular structures that usually cannot be felt, or palpated, very easily (Figure 27-4). They are located along the paths of larger lymphatic vessels and are spread throughout the body. A major exception is that no lymph nodes are found in the nervous system. There is a greater concentration of nodes in certain places in the body such as the cervical (neck), axillary (armpit), inguinal (groin), supratrochlear (medial side of the elbow), pelvic, thoracic, and aortic (thorax) nodes. The indented side of a lymph node is called the hilum. Nerves and blood vessels enter the node through the hilum. The lymphatic vessels that carry lymph to the node and are located opposite the hilum are called afferent (meaning "toward") lymphatic vessels. About four or five afferent vessels are associated with each node. The lymphatic vessels that carry lymph out of a node are called efferent (meaning "away from") vessels.

A lymph node usually has only one or two efferent vessels. Because more lymph enters the node than can exit at one time, lymph tends to concentrate in the node and pressure builds up that assists in the filtration process. Lymph nodes also are surrounded by a fibrous capsule of connective tissue. The lymph node is divided into an inner portion called the medulla and an outer portion called the cortex.

Two important cell types are found inside the nodes: macrophages and lymphocytes. Together these form the *lymph nodules,* the functional units of the lymph node. Lymph nodules are found in the cortex of the lymph node. **Macrophages** digest unwanted pathogens in the lymph and the **lymphocytes** are part of the immune response against the pathogen. Lymph nodes are also responsible for the generation of some lymphocytes.

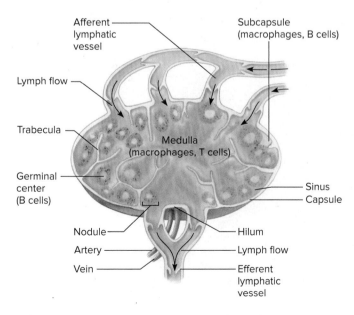

FIGURE 27-4   Section of a lymph node.

When someone has a viral or bacterial infection, he or she may have *lymphadenitis,* an inflammation of the lymph nodes. Any disease of the lymph nodes is called *lymphadenopathy.* The terms *lymphadenitis* and *lymphadenopathy* are often used interchangeably by healthcare professionals, but it is important to remember that the suffix *-itis* refers to inflammation and the suffix *-pathy* refers to disease. Other causes of lymphadenopathy are autoimmune disease and malignancy.

Thymus The **thymus** is a soft, bilobed organ located behind the sternum, just below the thyroid gland and above the heart in the mediastinum (a space between the right and left lungs) (see Figure 27-5). The thymus is large in the infant and reaches its maximum size of 1 to 2 ounces when the child is about 2 years of age. After adolescence, the thymus starts to atrophy (waste away) or *involute* (turn in on itself). In older adults, the thymus is tiny, almost nonexistent. Starvation or acute disease can sometimes accelerate this process. The outer portion of the thymus is called the cortex. This is where T lymphocytes (T cells) that have been produced in the bone marrow proliferate. They then move to a more central portion of the gland called the medulla, where they mature. The thymus also produces the hormone *thymosin,* which stimulates the production of mature lymphocytes.

Spleen The **spleen** is the largest lymphoid organ. It is located in the upper-left quadrant of the abdominal cavity, just below the diaphragm and behind the stomach. It is protected by the rib cage and normally is not palpable. The spleen is divided into lobules with two types of tissues: white pulp and red pulp. The white pulp is concentrated with lymphocytes similar to those seen in lymph nodes. Red pulp has an abundance of red blood cells, lymphocytes, and macrophages. The spleen filters blood in much the same way that lymph nodes filter lymph. The spleen also removes senescent (old), worn-out red blood cells from the bloodstream. If the spleen is injured or becomes enlarged due to disease, a condition known as *splenomegaly,* the spleen is often removed (a *splenectomy*) to prevent rupture of the spleen if trauma were to occur. When a splenectomy is performed, the patient's liver takes over most of its functions. Table 27-1 summarizes the characteristics of the major organs of the lymphatic system.

Lymph Nodules Lymph nodules are masses of lymphoid tissue not surrounded by a capsule. These are often referred to as *mucosa-associated lymphoid tissue (MALT)* because they are distributed in the connective tissue of mucosa. The **tonsils** are three sets of lymphoid tissue. These three sets include

- Pharyngeal tonsils, or adenoids, located at the junction of the mouth and oropharynx.
- Palatine tonsils, located at the junction of the nasal cavity and nasopharynx.
- Lingual tonsils, located at the base of the tongue.

The appendix, or *vermiform appendix,* is usually located in the lower-right quadrant at the junction of the large and small intestines. It was once thought that the appendix had no function. We now know it is part of the immune system.

TABLE 27-1 Major Organs of the Lymphatic System

Organ	Location	Functions
Thymus	In the mediastinum posterior to the upper portion of the body of the sternum	Houses lymphocytes; differentiates thymocytes into T lymphocytes
Spleen	In the upper-left portion of the abdominal cavity inferior to the diaphragm, posterior and lateral to the stomach	Blood reservoir; houses macrophages that remove foreign particles, damaged red blood cells, and cellular debris from the blood; contains lymphocytes
Lymph nodes	In groups or chains along the paths of the larger lymphatic vessels	Filter foreign particles and debris from lymph; produce and house lymphocytes that destroy foreign particles in lymph; house macrophages that engulf and destroy foreign particles and cellular debris carried in lymph

There are also lymph nodules in the small intestine. Peyer's patches are collections of lymph nodules, found mostly in the ileum of the small intestine. Peyer's patches act as immune sensors, identifying pathogens and other harmful agents taken into the small intestine and activating the immune system to neutralize these pathogens and agents. For more information regarding the small intestine, see the chapter *The Digestive System.*

▶ Defenses Against Disease LO 27.2

An infection is the presence of a pathogen—a disease-causing agent such as a bacterium, virus, toxin, fungus, or protozoan—in or on the body. The body has mechanisms called nonspecific defenses, or **innate immunity,** to protect itself from pathogens in general. The body also has mechanisms to protect itself against specific pathogens; these mechanisms, called immunities, are considered specific defenses.

Nonspecific Defenses

The nonspecific mechanisms that protect the body against pathogens include species resistance, mechanical and chemical barriers, and phagocytosis. Fever and inflammation

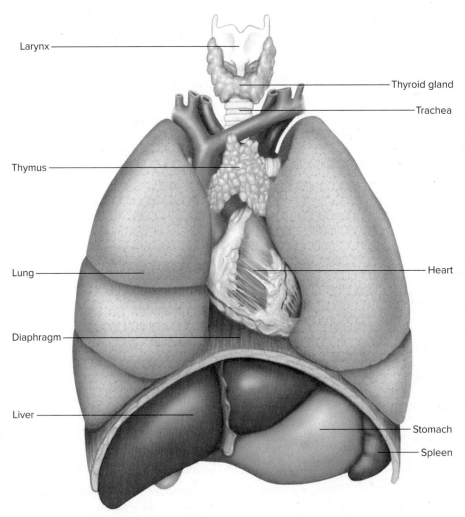

Larynx

Thyroid gland

Trachea

Thymus

Lung

Heart

Diaphragm

Liver

Stomach

Spleen

FIGURE 27-5 The bilobed thymus is located between the lungs and superior to the heart; the spleen is inferior to the diaphragm and posterior and lateral to the stomach.

TABLE 27-2 Nonspecific Defenses

Species resistance	A species is resistant to certain diseases to which other species are susceptible.
Mechanical barriers	Unbroken skin and mucous membranes prevent the entrance of some infectious agents; fluids wash away microorganisms before they can firmly attach to tissues.
Chemical barriers	Enzymes in various body fluids kill pathogens; pH extremes and high salt concentration also harm pathogens; interferons induce production of other proteins that block reproduction of viruses, stimulate phagocytosis, and enhance the activity of cells to resist infection and the growth of tumors; defensins damage bacterial cell walls and membranes; collectins attach to microbes; complement stimulates inflammation, attracts phagocytes, and enhances phagocytosis.
Phagocytosis	Neutrophils, monocytes, and macrophages engulf and destroy foreign particles and cells.
Fever	Elevated body temperature inhibits microbial growth and increases phagocytic activity.
Inflammation	Inflammation is a tissue response to injury that helps prevent the spread of infectious agents into nearby tissues.
Natural killer cells	Natural killer cells are a distinct type of lymphocyte that secretes perforins that lyse virus-infected cells and cancer cells.

are also effective in protecting the body from invading organisms. These defenses are described in this section and summarized in Table 27-2.

Species Resistance Species resistance means that a species typically gets only diseases unique to that species. For example, humans do not get diseases that affect plants. Humans also do not get most diseases that affect animals.

Mechanical Barriers The covering of the body (skin) and the linings of the tubes of the body (mucous membranes) provide mechanical barriers against pathogens. Intact skin is impermeable or resistant to most pathogens. Intact mucous membranes, although generally impermeable, do permit the entry of a few pathogens.

Chemical Barriers Chemicals and enzymes in body fluids provide chemical barriers that destroy pathogens. For example, acids in the stomach destroy most pathogens that are swallowed. Lysozymes in tears destroy pathogens on the surface of the eye. Salt in sweat kills bacteria and interferon in blood blocks viruses from infecting cells.

Phagocytosis Phagocytes are cells that surround and destroy pathogens and unwanted debris in the body. Neutrophils and monocytes are the most active phagocytes in blood. They also can leave the bloodstream to attack pathogens in other tissues.

When a monocyte leaves the bloodstream, it becomes a macrophage, which is simply a larger phagocytic cell. The process of destroying pathogens by this method is called **phagocytosis.**

Medical terms are built and dissected using prefixes, word roots/combining form, and suffixes. For example, we can build the term *phagocyte* by placing the parts of the term in the puzzle pieces where P = prefix, WR/CF = word root or combining form, and S = suffix.

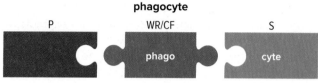

phagocyte

phago = eating, consuming, swallowing

cyte = cell

A *phagocyte* is a cell that consumes foreign matter. Learn additional medical terms in the **Medical Terminology Practice** section at the end of this chapter.

Fever An elevated body temperature is a fever. It causes the liver and spleen to take iron out of the bloodstream. Many pathogens need iron to survive in a body, so when their iron sources are gone, they die. Fever also activates phagocytic cells in the body to attack pathogens.

Inflammation When an area of the body becomes injured or infected with a pathogen, inflammation can result. In inflammation, blood vessels in the injured area dilate and become leaky. Because blood vessels dilate, more blood enters the area, bringing phagocytic white blood cells (WBC) to the area to attack the pathogen. The blood also brings proteins to replace injured tissues and clotting factors to stop any bleeding. The clotting factors also "wall off" the area so that pathogens cannot spread. Because blood vessels become leaky, more fluid accumulates in the injured area, which leads to edema. The excess fluid often irritates pain receptors. The four cardinal signs of inflammation are redness, heat, swelling, and pain.

Natural Killer Cells Natural killer **(NK) cells** are another type of lymphocyte. They primarily target cancer cells but also protect the body against many types of pathogens. Like cytotoxic T cells, NK cells kill harmful cells on contact. They secrete chemicals that produce holes in the membranes of harmful cells, which cause the cells to burst. Unlike B cells and T cells, NK cells do not have to recognize a specific antigen to start destroying pathogens. B cells and T cells are discussed later in the chapter.

Specific Defenses

Specific defenses are called immunities. They protect the body against specific pathogens. For example, a person who has chickenpox develops a specific defense that prevents him or her from getting chickenpox again. However, this specific defense does not protect the person from any other disease.

For example, a person who has measles will not get the measles again, but if she is exposed to the mumps virus and has not been vaccinated, she can get the mumps.

Antigens are simply defined as foreign substances in the body. Pathogens have many antigens on their surfaces. The immune system is programmed to recognize antigens in the body. Foreign substances in the body that are too small to start an immune response by themselves are called **haptens.** Haptens often attach to proteins in the blood, where they are then able to trigger an immune response. Penicillin is an example of a hapten.

Antibodies and complements are the major proteins involved in specific defenses. **Antibodies** are proteins the body produces in response to specific antigens and **complements** are proteins in serum that work with antibodies to eliminate or destroy antigens.

Lymphocytes and macrophages are the major WBCs involved in specific defenses. The cells of the lymphatic system produce proteins known as **cytokines,** which assist in immune response regulation. Cytokines are special messenger proteins that send signals to other parts of the immune system so that the immune response is coordinated. These messengers can act as on/off switches for certain immune cells or can attract immune cells to a specific area of need, such as a wound, that needs immune cells to heal. Lymphocytes and macrophages produce cytokines known as **monokines.** Monokines assist in regulation of the immune response by increasing B-cell production and stimulating red bone marrow to produce more WBCs.

B Cells and T Cells Two major types of lymphocytes are B cells and T cells. Although both B cells and T cells circulate in the blood, most of the lymphocytes in blood are T cells. B cells and T cells also are found in lymph nodes, the spleen, the thymus, the lining of digestive organs, and bone marrow.

Both T cells and B cells recognize antigens in the body; however, they respond to antigens in different ways. T cells bind to antigens on cells and attack them directly. This type of response is called a **cell-mediated response.** T cells also respond to antigens by secreting cytokines called **lymphokines,** which increase T-cell production and directly kill cells that have antigens.

B cells, on the other hand, do not attack antigens directly. They respond to antigens by becoming plasma cells. The plasma cells then make antibodies against the specific antigen. The antibodies attach to antigens in the humors (fluids) of the body; this response is called a humoral, or **antibody-mediated, response.** B cells become activated when a specific antigen binds to receptors on their surfaces. Each group of B cells recognizes only one type of antigen. Once activated, B cells divide to make plasma cells and memory B cells. Plasma cells make antibodies, which travel through the fluids of the body and bind to the antigens that activated the B cells. Memory B cells trigger a faster and stronger immune response the next time the person is exposed to the same antigen because they already know to respond to the antigen—just as you know what to expect the second time

you play a computer game and can thus play faster and better. (See Figures 27-6 and 27-7.)

As seen in Figure 27-6, before a T cell can respond to an antigen, it must be activated. T-cell activation begins when a macrophage ingests and digests a pathogen that has antigens on it. The macrophage then takes some of the antigens from the pathogen and puts them on its cell membrane next to a large protein complex called a **major histocompatibility complex (MHC).** Every human being has a unique MHC (similar to an internal fingerprint), and it is present on every cell in the body. A T cell that has a receptor for the antigen recognizes and binds to the antigen and the MHC on the surface of the macrophage. The T cell is now activated and begins to divide to form other types of T cells and T memory cells. It is important to note that T cells cannot be activated without macrophages and MHC proteins. MHC also is involved in recognizing foreign cells versus host cells. This is important in keeping the immune system from attacking the body's own cells by mistake.

Some activated T cells form cytotoxic T cells—known as CD8 cells due to the presence of the CD8 protein on their surface—that are important in protecting the body against viruses and cancer cells. Other activated T cells become helper T cells—known as CD4 cells due to the presence of the CD4 protein on their surface—that carry out many important roles in immunity. Helper T cells increase antibody formation, memory cell formation, B-cell formation, and phagocytosis. Some activated T cells become memory T cells that "remember" the pathogen that activated the original T cell. When a person is later exposed to the same pathogen, memory cells trigger an immune response that is more effective than the first immune response. The production of memory cells prevents a person from suffering from the same disease-causing organism twice. This is why if you have had chickenpox as a child you are unlikely to get the disease again.

▶ Antibodies   LO 27.3

Antibodies also are called **immunoglobulins.** The following is a list of different types of immunoglobulins (Ig):

- IgA is an antibody found in secretions of the body such as breast milk, sweat, tears, saliva, and mucus. It prevents pathogens from entering the body.
- IgD is an antibody found on the cell membranes of B cells. IgD has an important role in activating basophils, a type of white blood cell.
- IgE is an antibody found wherever IgA is located. It is involved in triggering allergic reactions.
- IgG is an antibody that primarily recognizes bacteria, viruses, and toxins. It also can activate complements.
- IgM is a large antibody that primarily binds to antigens on food, bacteria, or incompatible blood cells. It also activates complements.

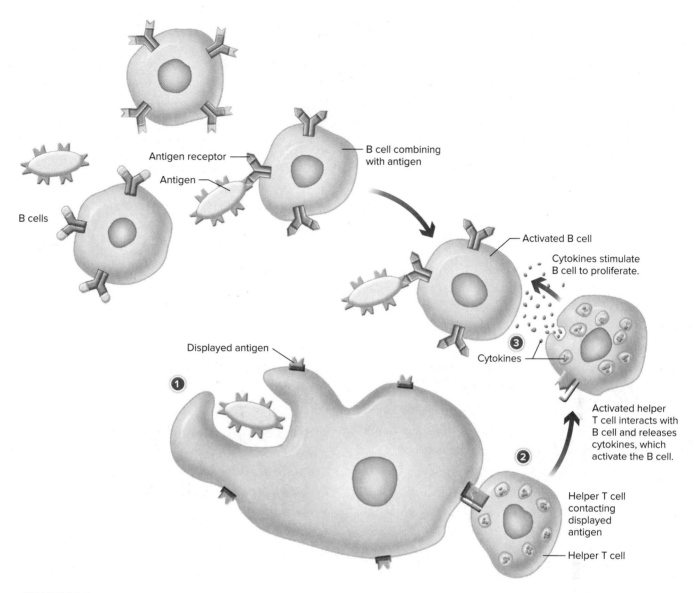

FIGURE 27-6 T-cell and B-cell activation. (1) A macrophage displays an antigen on its cell membrane. (2) A helper T cell binds to the antigen on the macrophage and becomes activated. (3) An activated helper T cell releases cytokines to help an activated B cell proliferate. Notice that the B cell also must bind to an antigen to become activated.

When antibodies bind to antigens, they take one of the following actions:

- They allow phagocytes to recognize and destroy antigens.
- They make antigens clump together, causing them to be destroyed by macrophages. This is how incompatible blood cells are destroyed.
- They cover the toxic portions of antigens to make them harmless.
- They activate complements, which are proteins in serum that attack pathogens by forming holes in them. Complement proteins also attract macrophages to pathogens and can stimulate inflammation.

▶ Immune Responses and Acquired Immunities

LO 27.4

A primary immune response occurs the first time a person is exposed to an antigen. This response is slow and takes several weeks to occur. In this response, memory cells are made. A secondary immune response occurs the next time a person is exposed to the same antigen. This response is quick and usually prevents a person from developing a disease from the antigen. Memory cells carry out the secondary immune response.

A person is born with very few immunities but normally develops or acquires them as long as his immune system is

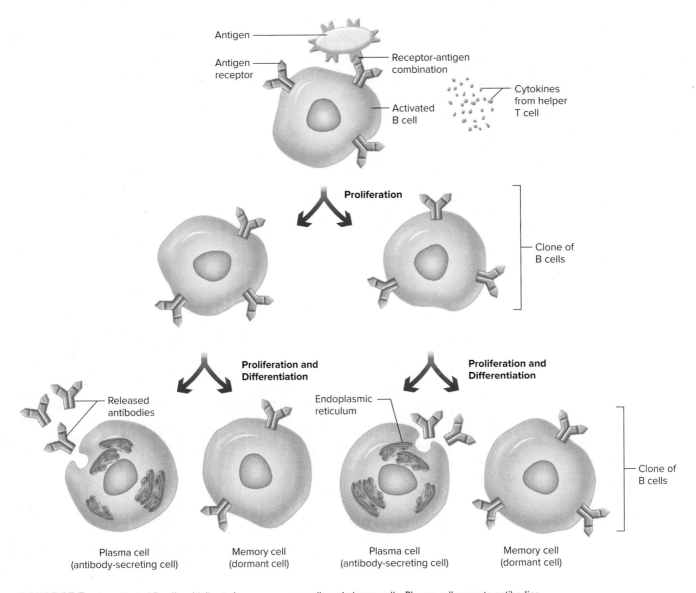

FIGURE 27-7 An activated B cell multiplies to become memory cells and plasma cells. Plasma cells secrete antibodies.

healthy. The four types of immunities a person can acquire are (1) naturally acquired active immunity, (2) artificially acquired active immunity, (3) naturally acquired passive immunity, and (4) artificially acquired passive immunity.

Naturally Acquired Active Immunity

A person develops this immunity by being naturally exposed to an antigen and subsequently making antibodies and memory cells against the antigen. Having an infectious disease caused by pathogens leads to the development of this type of immunity, which is usually long-lasting.

Artificially Acquired Active Immunity

A person develops this immunity by being injected with a pathogen and subsequently making antibodies and memory cells against the pathogen. Immunizations and vaccines cause this type of immunity, which is also usually long-lasting.

Naturally Acquired Passive Immunity

A person receives this immunity from his mother. When a mother breastfeeds, she passes antibodies to her baby through breast milk. A mother also passes antibodies to her baby across the placenta, which is a short-lived immunity.

Artificially Acquired Passive Immunity

A person receives this immunity when she is injected with antibodies made by another person or an animal. For example, if a person is exposed to hepatitis A at a restaurant, she can be given antibodies from a person who has previously had the disease. The treatment must be administered in the first 2 weeks after exposure. This type of immunity is short-lived.

Common Diseases and Disorders of the Immune System

As science and medicine develop a better understanding of the immune system and its relationship to causing disease, multiple diseases and disorders involving many body systems are now thought to have an autoimmune component.

An **autoimmune disease** is one in which the body begins to attack its own antigens. This happens when the immune system is no longer able to recognize itself and mounts an immune response against its own body cells. Examples of autoimmune diseases include scleroderma (integumentary system), rheumatoid arthritis (skeletal system), multiple sclerosis (nervous system), glomerulonephritis (urinary system), Crohn's disease (digestive system), and insulin-dependent (Type 1) diabetes mellitus (endocrine system). Although the reason is unknown, autoimmune disorders affect women almost 75% of the time, often during childbearing years.

A number of diseases and disorders can challenge the immune system. Among them, HIV infection, AIDS, cancer, and allergies are the most significant. HIV and AIDS are discussed in the *Microbiology and Disease* chapter. In this section, you will focus on specific immune system disorders. For other diseases with possible or probable autoimmune components, please refer to the appropriate body system in *Appendix III*.

CANCER is defined as the uncontrolled growth of abnormal cells. Healthy cells normally know when to stop reproducing, but cancer cells have lost this ability. Occasionally, normal cells create growths, but these are benign, which means they are not cancerous. Cancer cells, however, often form growths called malignant tumors, which may become fatal. In many cases, these cancerous cells or tumors damage normal cells of tissues and organs, causing organ systems to fail.

At least 200 different types of cancers are known. In the United States, the three most common cancer types in men are prostate, lung, and colorectal cancer. The three most common types in women are breast, lung, and colorectal cancer. Lung cancer kills more people in the United States than any other type of cancer.

Causes. The causes of cancer are mostly unknown, but certain risk factors have been identified, including a suppressed immune system, radiation, tobacco use, and some viruses. Many other factors are suspected. One of the best ways to prevent cancer is to avoid smoking and other known risk factors. A substance or agent known to cause the formation of cancer is called a carcinogen.

Signs and Symptoms. The symptoms of different types of cancer vary, but the following symptoms are usually observed in most types: fever, chills, unintended weight loss, fatigue, and a general sense of not feeling well.

Diagnostic Exams and Tests. Most cancers are diagnosed with a biopsy, which is a removal of tissues for examination. CT scans also are used to help diagnose most cancer types. Other diagnostic tests include blood counts, an analysis of blood chemistry, and X-rays.

Treatment. The treatment of cancer differs depending on the type and stage of cancer. The stage of cancer refers to how large a tumor is and how far cancer cells have spread throughout the body. Table 27-3 provides a summary of cancer staging.

If tumors are localized and have not spread, the cancer often can be treated successfully by surgically removing the tumor. Other treatment options are chemotherapy, radiation therapy, newer immune therapies, and transplants, such as bone marrow transplant, which may be successful for curing certain types of cancer. Even if a cancer cannot be cured, its progression can sometimes be slowed, allowing the patient to live additional years.

ALLERGIES cause an allergic reaction, which is an immune response to a substance, like pollen, that is not normally harmful to the body. An allergy also can be an excessive immune response. Substances that trigger allergic responses are called *allergens*. Allergic reactions involve IgE antibodies and mast cells. IgE antibodies increase and respond when exposed to an allergen (trigger). The IgE antibodies bind to these allergens and cause mast cells to release histamine and heparin. These chemicals trigger allergic reactions such as sneezing or wheezing, or worse.

To help prevent this reaction, a patient receiving allergy shots is injected with tiny amounts of the allergen. This causes the body to produce IgG antibodies that will prevent IgE antibodies from binding to the allergen. IgG antibodies do not trigger immune responses because they do not activate mast cells.

Most allergies do not cause life-threatening conditions, but some do. One life-threatening condition that can result is **anaphylaxis,** when blood vessels dilate so quickly that blood pressure drops too fast for organs to adjust. Without treatment, patients may go into anaphylactic shock and die.

Signs and Symptoms. The signs and symptoms of allergies vary depending on what part of the body is exposed to allergens. Inhaled allergens often cause a runny nose, sneezing,

TABLE 27-3	Cancer Staging
Stage	**Description**
Stage 0	Very early cancer. Cancer cells are localized in a few cell layers.
Stage I	Cancer cells have spread to deeper cell layers, or some may have spread to surrounding tissues.
Stage II	Cancer cells have spread to surrounding tissues but are considered contained in the primary cancer site.
Stage III	Cancer cells have spread beyond the primary cancer site to nearby areas.
Stage IV	Cancer cells have spread to other organs of the body.
Recurrent	Cancer cells have reappeared after treatment.

coughing, or wheezing. Ingested allergens may cause nausea, diarrhea, or vomiting. Skin allergens cause rashes. Allergens in the blood, such as penicillin, are often the most life-threatening for people who are allergic to them because the allergens can affect many organ systems.

Diagnostic Exams and Tests. A physical exam with a thorough history to determine allergic reaction triggers and allergy testing are used to diagnose allergies. Skin testing is the most common type of allergy testing.

Treatment. Many allergies are effectively treated with over-the-counter medications called antihistamines. Prescription-strength antihistamines are also available. Various types of nasal sprays and decongestants also can reduce allergy symptoms. When a person experiences anaphylaxis, an injection of epinephrine is usually an effective treatment. Epinephrine causes vasoconstriction, which increases blood pressure.

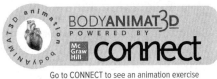

Go to CONNECT to see an animation exercise about *Immune Response: Hypersensitivity.*

CHRONIC FATIGUE SYNDROME (CFS) is a condition in which a person feels severe tiredness that cannot be relieved by rest and is not related to other illness.

Causes. The causes are primarily unknown, although some believe the cause may be viral. This condition also may be caused by an autoimmune response against the nervous system.

Signs and Symptoms. The most common symptom is severe fatigue. Other signs and symptoms include mild fever, sore throat, tender lymph nodes in the neck or armpit, general body aches, joint pain, sleep disturbances, and depression.

Diagnostic Exams and Tests. There is not a specific test used to diagnose CFS. A physical exam, complete history, and blood tests are used to rule out other diseases or disorders that could be the cause of the symptoms.

Treatment. There is no cure for CFS; however, medications to treat the symptoms associated with this condition, including antidepressants, often are prescribed. There is some evidence that cognitive therapy and light exercise can help alleviate the symptoms.

LYMPHEDEMA is the blockage of the lymphatic vessels that drain excess fluids from various areas of the body.

Causes. This condition may be caused by parasitic infections, trauma to the vessels, tumors, radiation therapy, cellulitis (a skin infection), and surgeries such as mastectomies and biopsies in which lymphoid tissues have been removed.

Signs and Symptoms. The common symptom is tissue swelling that lasts longer than a few days or increases over time.

Diagnostic Exams and Tests. Physical exam and medical history are used to diagnose lymphedema. If the cause is not apparent after examination and medical history, MRI, CT, Doppler ultrasound, or special radionuclide imaging may be performed to determine the cause.

Treatment. Treatment options include compression stockings for swelling in the legs or arms, elevation of the affected limb, and surgery to remove abnormal lymphoid tissue. Physical therapy and massage therapy are also helpful in the early stages of lymphedema to spread the fluid into surrounding tissues for reabsorption.

MONONUCLEOSIS is also known as mono. Because it frequently affects teenagers and is a highly contagious viral infection spread through the saliva of the infected person, it has earned the nickname "the kissing disease." Mono also is spread through coughing and sneezing.

Causes. Mononucleosis can be caused by either the Epstein-Barr virus or cytomegalovirus (CMV).

Signs and Symptoms. Unexplained fever, extreme fatigue, and sore throat are common. Other symptoms include weakness; headache; and swollen, tender lymph nodes (lymphadenopathy).

Diagnostic Exams and Tests. Mononucleosis is diagnosed by physical exam and blood tests to determine the presence of antibodies to the Epstein-Barr virus. A complete blood count also may be performed.

Treatment. Rest, proper nutrition, gargling with warm salt water, and taking acetaminophen for fever usually result in recovery from acute symptoms in a week or two, although complete recovery may take a month or longer.

SYSTEMIC LUPUS ERYTHEMATOSUS (SLE), commonly referred to as lupus, is an autoimmune disorder that affects a few or, sometimes, many organ systems of the body. In this condition, people produce antibodies that target their own cells and tissues. As with many autoimmune disorders, lupus affects women much more often than men.

Causes. This disorder may be caused by some drugs or by bacterial infections. Except for its autoimmune component, its actual cause is unknown.

Signs and Symptoms. The list of signs and symptoms is extensive and may include any or all of the following:

- Fatigue
- General body aches
- Fever
- Weight loss (anorexia)
- Hair loss
- Arthritis
- Numbness of the fingers and toes
- "Butterfly" rash on the face
- Sensitivity to sunlight (photosensitivity)
- Vision problems
- Nausea
- Dry eyes
- Headaches
- Seizures

- Abnormal blood clots
- Chest pains
- Inflammation of heart tissues (carditis)
- Anemia
- Shortness of breath
- Fluid accumulation around the lungs
- Renal failure
- Blood in the urine (hematuria)

Diagnostic Exams and Tests. Diagnosis of SLE is made by a combination of physical exam, urinalysis, and blood tests. Blood tests include a complete blood count, erythrocyte sedimentation rate to determine if inflammation is present, and a special test for the presence of antinuclear antibodies (ANA).

Medical terms are built and dissected using prefixes, word roots/combining form, and suffixes. For example, we can build the term *antinuclear* by placing the parts of the term in the puzzle pieces where P = prefix, WR/CF = word root or combining form, and S = suffix.

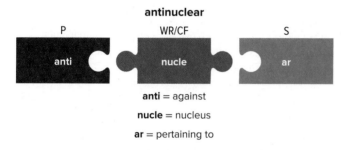

antinuclear

P	WR/CF	S
anti	nucle	ar

anti = against

nucle = nucleus

ar = pertaining to

Learn additional medical terms in the **Medical Terminology Practice** section at the end of this chapter.

Treatment. Treatment options include anti-inflammatory medications, including steroids, and protective clothing and creams to prevent damage from sunlight. Dialysis, immunosuppressive medications, and kidney transplants may be necessary for more serious cases.

CELIAC DISEASE is an immune reaction to eating gluten, making it a diagnosable autoimmune disorder. Gluten is a protein substance found in wheat, barley, and rye.

Causes. When a person with celiac disease eats more than 10 milligrams of gluten (about 1/8 of a teaspoon of flour), this triggers an autoimmune reaction that causes the individual's body to attack the small intestinal mucosa.

Signs and Symptoms. The intestinal damage from eating gluten can cause weight loss, bloating, stomach pain, and sometimes diarrhea. If left untreated, eventually the brain, nervous system, bones, liver, and other organs can be deprived of vital nutrients. In children, malabsorption in the small intestine can affect growth and development.

Diagnostic Exams and Tests. Diagnosis can be difficult but includes blood tests for specific antibodies and genetic testing. The licensed practitioner also may perform an endoscopy to examine the small intestine for damage caused by reaction to gluten and to obtain biopsies.

Treatment. A strict, lifelong gluten-free diet is the only treatment. This means not only eating gluten-free foods but also being aware of gluten cross-contamination. The FDA regulates product labeling for gluten-free foods. However, individuals with celiac disease should be aware that gluten can even be present in small quantities in more obscure additives, such as malt flavoring.

SUMMARY OF LEARNING OUTCOMES

OUTCOME	KEY POINTS
27.1 Describe the pathways and organs of the lymphatic system.	The lymphatic system is composed of pathways known as lymphatic vessels. In addition to the lymphatic vessels, the organs of the lymphatic system include lymph nodes, located throughout the body; the thymus, in the mediastinum; and the spleen, located in the upper-left quadrant of the abdominal cavity.
27.2 Compare the nonspecific and specific body defense mechanisms.	Nonspecific (innate) body defenses include species resistance, mechanical and chemical barriers, phagocytosis, fever, inflammation, and natural killer (NK) cells. Specific defenses are immunities, or defenses, against specific antigens created by B cells, and T cells.

OUTCOME	KEY POINTS
27.3 **Explain how antibodies fight infection.**	Antibodies work in the following ways: phagocytosis, antigen clumping, covering (inactivating) toxic portions of antigens, and activating complements. Antibodies also are known as immunoglobulins. IgA prevents pathogens from entering the body; IgD controls B-cell activity; IgE works with IgA in triggering allergic reactions; IgG recognizes bacteria, viruses, and toxins and activates complements; and IgM binds to antigens on food, bacteria, or incompatible blood cells. IgM also activates complements.
27.4 **Describe the four different types of acquired immunities.**	The four types of immune response are naturally acquired active immunity, such as when a person becomes ill and develops immunity; artificially acquired active immunity, as when an injection is given a vaccination against a pathogen, preventing illness; naturally acquired passive immunity, which occurs when an infant has its mother's immunity for a short while after birth and through breast milk; and artificially acquired passive immunity, which occurs after injection of antibodies such as antivenom.
27.5 **Describe the causes, signs and symptoms, diagnosis, and treatments of major immune disorders.**	There are many common diseases and disorders of the immune system with varied signs, symptoms, diagnosis, and treatments. Some of these include cancer, allergies, and other autoimmune diseases, in which the body attacks its own antigens.

CASE STUDY CRITICAL THINKING

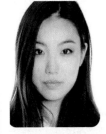

©excentric_01/iStock/Getty Images

Recall Cindy Chen from the case study at the beginning of the chapter. Now that you have completed the chapter, answer the following questions regarding her case.

1. Based on the negative rapid influenza test and the normal CBC, Dr. Whalen's diagnosis of Cindy Chen is that she has a common cold. What is Cindy Chen most likely feeling in her neck?

2. What is the medical term for this condition?

3. Based on your reading in this chapter, why does Cindy Chen have "tender lumps" in her neck?

4. Why do you think Cindy Chen has an elevated temperature?

5. What immune purpose does an elevated temperature serve for Cindy Chen? Is this a specific or nonspecific response?

EXAM PREPARATION QUESTIONS

1. (LO 27.1) The fluid found between cells is called
   a. Lymph
   b. Interstitial fluid
   c. Plasma
   d. CSF
   e. Cellular fluid

2. (LO 27.1) The thoracic duct collects lymph from which of the following areas of the body?
   a. Right side of the head and neck
   b. Right side of the chest
   c. Right leg
   d. Right arm
   e. Left side of the head and neck

3. (LO 27.2) Innate immunity is the other name for which type of body protection?
   a. Specific immunity
   b. Artificial immunity
   c. Humoral immunity
   d. Nonspecific immunity
   e. Temporal immunity

4. (LO 27.2) The types of white blood cells that are involved in specific defenses are lymphocytes and
   a. Macrophages
   b. Neutrophils
   c. Eosinophils
   d. Basophils
   e. Leukophils

5. (LO 27.3) Which of the following cells do not attack antigens directly?
   a. Lymphokines
   b. B cells
   c. T cells
   d. NK cells
   e. Alpha cells

6. (LO 27.3) Which antibody is involved in triggering *most* allergic reactions?
   a. IgA
   b. IgD
   c. IgE
   d. IgM
   e. IgG

7. (LO 27.4) A patient has been exposed to hepatitis A at a local restaurant and is treated with antibodies from a patient who previously had hepatitis A. What type of acquired immunity does this provide?
   a. Naturally acquired active immunity
   b. Artificially acquired active immunity
   c. Naturally acquired passive immunity
   d. Artificially acquired passive immunity
   e. Humorally acquired active immunity

8. (LO 27.5) Which of the following is a known carcinogen?
   a. Family history
   b. Weight gain
   c. Sedentary lifestyle
   d. Smoking
   e. Black vegetables

9. (LO 27.5) Which of the following is a life-threatening condition that can be caused by allergies?
   a. Anaphylaxis
   b. AIDS
   c. Lymphedema
   d. Mononucleosis
   e. HIV

10. (LO 27.5) An example of an autoimmune disease is
    a. Chickenpox
    b. Rheumatoid arthritis
    c. Influenza
    d. Atherosclerosis
    e. Strep throat

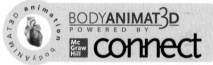

Go to CONNECT to see an animation exercise about *Inflammation*.

MEDICAL TERMINOLOGY PRACTICE

Analyze the following medical terms, presented throughout the chapter. Using a medical dictionary (or Appendix I), place a / mark between each word part. Define each word part and then define the whole word.

EXAMPLE: **patho / logy** = patho means "disease" + logy means "study of"
PATHOLOGY means "study of disease."

1. autoimmune
2. carcinogenic
3. cytotoxic
4. immunoglobulin

5. interstitial
6. leukocyte
7. lymphedema
8. lymphocyte

9. macrophage
10. mononucleosis
11. phagocytosis
12. thymectomy

The Respiratory System

CASE STUDY

PATIENT INFORMATION	Patient Name	DOB	Allergies
	Mohammad Nassar	05/17/2005	Animal dander
	Attending	**MRN**	**Other Information**
	Elizabeth H. Williams, MD	00-AA-007	History of asthma

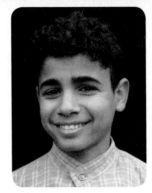
©David Sacks/Getty Images

Mohammad Nassar is a teenage male patient complaining of increased difficulty breathing over the last 2 days. From his chart, you see that Mohammad Nassar is on a maintenance dose of albuterol 4 mg extended-release tablets twice a day. Mohammad Nassar states that he spent the weekend with his girlfriend's family at their summer home with the family's two dogs and a cat. He is thinking that exposure to the pets may be connected to the worsening of his asthma. Dr. Williams has ordered a peak expiratory flow test and has referred Mohammad Nassar for allergy testing.

Keep Mohammad Nassar in mind as you study the chapter. There will be questions at the end of the chapter based on the case study. The information in the chapter will help you answer these questions.

LEARNING OUTCOMES

After completing Chapter 28, you will be able to:

28.1 Describe the structure and function of each organ in the respiratory system.

28.2 Describe the events involved in the inspiration and expiration of air.

28.3 Explain how oxygen and carbon dioxide are transported in the blood.

28.4 Compare various respiratory volumes and tell how they are used to diagnose respiratory problems.

28.5 Describe the causes, signs and symptoms, diagnosis, and treatments of various diseases and disorders of the respiratory system.

KEY TERMS

alveoli
bronchi
bronchioles
dyspnea
epiglottis
expiration
glottis
inspiration
laryngopharynx
larynx
morbidity
mortality
nares

nasal conchae
nasopharynx
oropharynx
paranasal sinuses
pharynx
pleura
respiratory capacity
respiratory volume
surfactant
thoracocentesis
thoracostomy
thorax
trachea

I.C.1	Describe structural organization of the human body
I.C.2	Identify body systems
I.C.4	List major organs in each body system
I.C.5	Identify the anatomical location of major organs in each body system
I.C.6	Compare structure and function of the human body across the life span
I.C.7	Describe the normal function of each body system
I.C.8	Identify common pathology related to each body system including: (a) signs (b) symptoms (c) etiology
I.C.9	Analyze pathology for each body system including: (a) diagnostic measures (b) treatment modalities
V.C.9	Identify medical terms labeling the word parts
V.C.10	Define medical terms and abbreviations related to all body systems

2. Anatomy and Physiology

a. List all body systems and their structures and functions

b. Describe common diseases, symptoms, and etiologies as they apply to each system

c. Identify diagnostic and treatment modalities as they relate to each body system

3. Medical Terminology

a. Define the entire basic structure of medical terminology and be able to accurately identify the correct context (i.e., root, prefix, suffix, combinations, spelling, and definitions)

b. Build and dissect medical terminology from roots and suffixes to understand the word element combinations

c. Apply medical terminology for each specialty

d. Define and use medical abbreviations when appropriate and acceptable

Introduction

The function of the respiratory system is to move air in and out of the lungs. This process may be called ventilation, respiration, or breathing. The respiration process works with the cardiovascular system to deliver oxygen (O_2) to body cells via the bloodstream. It also removes a waste product—carbon dioxide (CO_2)—from the blood. This exchange of oxygen and carbon dioxide in the lungs is called *external respiration.* This same exchange, when it occurs within the hemoglobin of the red blood cells (RBCs), is known as *internal respiration.*

Organs of the Respiratory System LO 28.1

The organs of the respiratory system are the nose, pharynx, larynx, trachea, bronchial tree (including the bronchi and bronchioles), and lungs (see Figure 28-1). The nose is made of bones and cartilage and the skin covering them. The openings of the nose are the nostrils, which in medicine are referred to as the **nares.** The hairs within the nares prevent large particles from entering the nose.

The Nasal Cavity and Paranasal Sinuses

The nasal cavity is simply the hollow space behind the nose. The nasal cavity is divided into left and right portions by the cartilaginous (made of cartilage) nasal septum. Most of the nasal cavity is lined with a mucous membrane that warms and moistens air as it passes through the cavity. Three structures called **nasal conchae** extend from the lateral walls of the nasal cavity and increase the surface area of the nasal cavity, which increases the effectiveness of the mucous membrane. The three conchae are simply named by their position, as superior, middle, and inferior nasal conchae.

The nasal cavity also is lined with cells that possess *cilia,* which are microscopic, hair-like projections from the mucous membrane. As mucus traps dust and other particles in the nasal cavity, the cilia push the mucus toward the pharynx, where it is swallowed. The enzymes of the stomach then destroy these foreign particles and pathogens, thus helping to protect the respiratory system from disease.

The **paranasal sinuses** are air-filled spaces within the skull bones that open into the nasal cavity. The paranasal sinuses reduce the weight of the skull and equalize pressure between the inside of the skull and the outside environment. The sinuses also give your voice its tone. When your paranasal sinuses are "stopped up" with mucus, they cause the tone of your voice to change. The bones of the skull that contain the sinuses include the frontal, sphenoid, ethmoid, and maxillae bones. See Figure 28-2. When sinus membranes become inflamed due to allergies or infection (sinusitis), they swell, which results in a sinus headache.

The Pharynx

The **pharynx** is an organ of both the respiratory system and the digestive system. It consists of three separate sections: The **nasopharynx** is located at the junction of the nasal cavity and

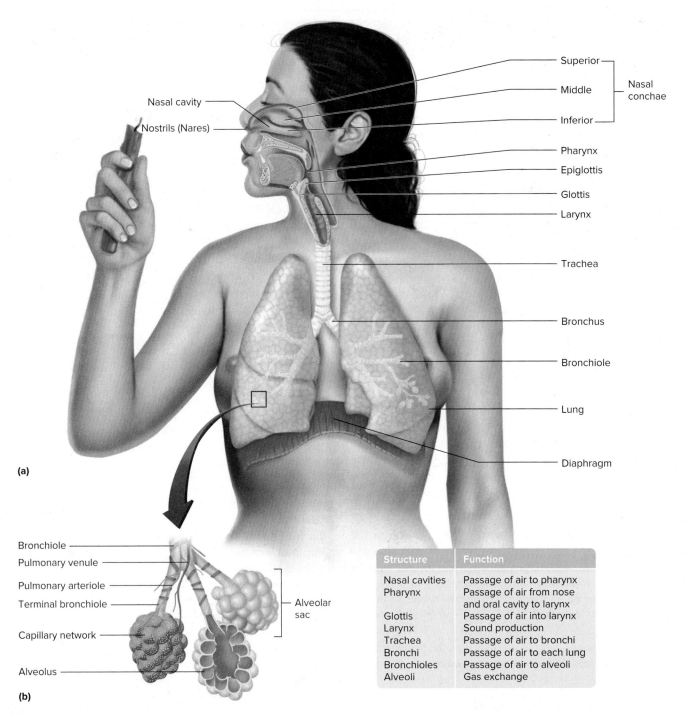

Superior ─┐
Middle ─┤ Nasal conchae
Inferior ─┘

Nasal cavity

Nostrils (Nares)

Pharynx
Epiglottis
Glottis
Larynx
Trachea
Bronchus
Bronchiole
Lung
Diaphragm

(a)

Bronchiole
Pulmonary venule
Pulmonary arteriole
Terminal bronchiole
Capillary network
Alveolus

Alveolar sac

(b)

Structure	Function
Nasal cavities	Passage of air to pharynx
Pharynx	Passage of air from nose and oral cavity to larynx
Glottis	Passage of air into larynx
Larynx	Sound production
Trachea	Passage of air to bronchi
Bronchi	Passage of air to each lung
Bronchioles	Passage of air to alveoli
Alveoli	Gas exchange

FIGURE 28-1 (a) Organs of the respiratory system and (b) a bronchiole with alveolar sac, covered by capillary network, in cross section, and whole (left to right).

the pharynx; the **oropharynx** is the area at the junction of the oral cavity (mouth) and pharynx; and, finally, the **laryngopharynx** is the area of the pharynx that contains the larynx, or "voice box." During inspiration, air flows from the nasal or oral cavity into the pharynx. From the pharynx, air flows into the larynx.

The Larynx and Vocal Cords

The **larynx** sits superior to and is continuous with the trachea, or windpipe. It moves air into and out of the trachea and produces the sounds of a person's voice. The larynx consists mostly of cartilage and muscle tissue. There are three cartilages in the larynx (see Figure 28-3). The uppermost

cartilage is the *epiglottic cartilage,* which forms the framework of the **epiglottis,** the flap-like structure that closes off the larynx during swallowing so that food and liquids do not enter the respiratory system. The second cartilage is a larger structure called the *thyroid cartilage,* which forms the anterior wall of the larynx. During the puberty of a male, testosterone causes the thyroid cartilage to enlarge to produce the "Adam's apple." The third cartilage of the larynx is called the *cricoid cartilage.* It forms most of the posterior wall of the larynx and a small part of the anterior wall.

The vocal cords stretch between the thyroid cartilage and the cricoid cartilage. The opening between the vocal cords is called

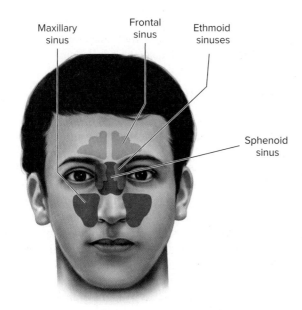

FIGURE 28-2   The human skull contains sets of two sinuses, or air spaces, in the sphenoid, ethmoid, maxillary, and frontal bones.

Source: Adapted from Paranasal Sinuses, 2009 Nucleus Medical Media, Inc.

in pitch. Males tend to have thicker vocal cords, which is why their voices are generally deeper than female voices.

The Trachea, Bronchi, and Bronchioles

The **trachea** (windpipe) is a tubular organ made of rings of cartilage and smooth muscle. It extends from the larynx to the bronchi. The trachea is lined with cells that possess cilia that constantly move mucus up to the pharynx and the esophagus, where it is swallowed. Mucus traps bacteria, viruses, and other harmful substances a person inhales. The digestive juices of the stomach then destroy the harmful substances.

Smoking destroys cilia, so the only way a smoker can get mucus out of his trachea is to cough. Smokers feel the urge to cough more frequently than nonsmokers in an effort to move mucus to the pharynx.

The distal end of the trachea branches and starts a series of tubes called the *bronchial tree*. The first branches off the trachea are called primary, or main stem, **bronchi.** The branches of the primary bronchi are called secondary bronchi. The secondary bronchi branch into tertiary bronchi. Tertiary bronchi then branch into **bronchioles.** At the ends of the bronchioles are air sacs called alveoli (see Figure 28-1b).

Alveoli are thin sacs made of only one layer of simple squamous epithelial cells and are surrounded by capillaries. They are considered the "working tissue" of the lung because it is in the alveoli that the exchange of oxygen and carbon dioxide takes place. Many physicians refer to the alveoli as the *pulmonary parenchyma* (*parenchyma* means "working tissue"). Through

the **glottis** (see Figure 28-3c). The upper vocal cords are referred to as *false vocal cords* because they do not produce sound. The lower vocal cords are called *true vocal cords* because muscles stretch and relax them to produce different types of sounds. When the true vocal cords are stretched, the voice becomes higher in pitch. When they are relaxed, the voice becomes lower

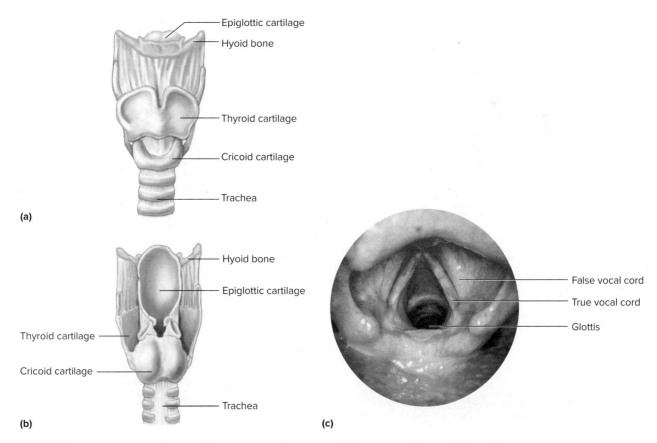

FIGURE 28-3   (a) Anterior view of larynx, (b) posterior view of larynx, and (c) photograph of the vocal cords and glottis.

(c) ©CNRI/Phototake

the process of diffusion, red blood cells in the capillaries release carbon dioxide into the alveoli. Conversely, the alveoli release oxygen into the blood through the thin walls of the capillaries. This exchange is known as *internal* or *cellular respiration.*

The Lungs

The lungs are two cone-shaped organs that contain connective tissue, the bronchial tree, nerves, lymphatic vessels, and many blood vessels. The right lung is larger than the left because the heart is also located in the left **thorax,** or chest area. The right lung is divided into three lobes, known as the right upper, middle, and lower lobes. The left lung is divided into the left upper and lower lobes. The double-walled membrane that surrounds the lungs is called the **pleura.** The outer membrane is known as the parietal pleura, and the innermost membrane is the visceral pleura. The pleura produces a slippery, serous fluid called *pleural fluid* that helps decrease friction as the membranes move against each other during breathing.

The lungs contain the bronchial tree and alveoli. Some alveolar cells secrete a fatty substance called **surfactant** that helps maintain the inflation of the alveoli so that they do not collapse in on themselves between inspirations. Premature infants often suffer from respiratory distress syndrome (RDS) (formerly known as hyaline membrane disease—see the *Pathophysiology section*) because their lungs do not yet create enough surfactant. This often causes them to have great difficulty maintaining adequate lung inflation.

▶ The Mechanisms of Breathing   LO 28.2

Breathing, or pulmonary ventilation, consists of two events: **inspiration** and **expiration.** During inspiration, or inhalation, air, which is 21% oxygen, enters through the naso- or oropharynx and travels through the sinuses into the larynx, trachea, and bronchial tree, eventually reaching the alveoli in the lungs. Air flows into the airways during inspiration because the thoracic cavity enlarges. When the thoracic cavity enlarges, pressure decreases in the cavity. The atmospheric pressure outside the body is greater than the pressure inside the cavity, and air passively flows from an area of high pressure to an area of low pressure. The following events enlarge the thoracic cavity and therefore lead to inspiration (see Figure 28-4a):

- The diaphragm contracts. As it does so, it flattens, which increases the amount of space in the thoracic cavity.
- The intercostal muscles raise the ribs, further enlarging the thoracic cavity.

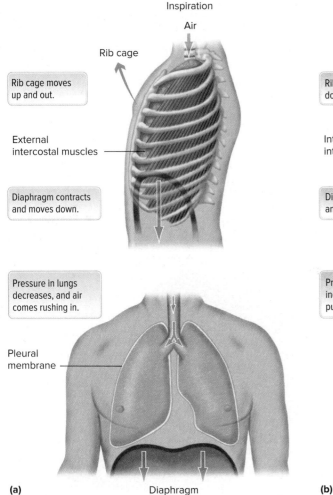
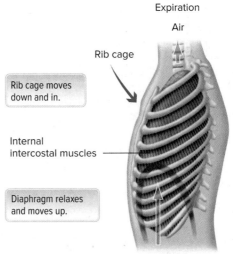
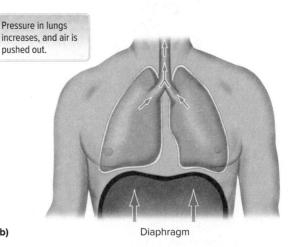

FIGURE 28-4 (a) Events of inspiration and (b) events of expiration.

During expiration, or exhalation, air rich with carbon dioxide flows out of the airways. Air flows out because the thoracic cavity becomes smaller, which increases the pressure inside the cavity. When the pressure inside the cavity becomes greater than the atmospheric pressure, air flows out. The following events lead to expiration (see Figure 28-4b):

- The diaphragm relaxes. As it does so, it domes up into the thoracic cavity, which decreases the space in the cavity.
- The intercostal muscles lower the ribs; this further decreases the size of the thoracic cavity.

Breathing is controlled by the respiratory center of the brain, which is located in the pons and medulla oblongata. The medulla oblongata controls both the rhythm and the depth of breathing. The pons controls the rate of breathing.

Other factors that affect breathing are the carbon dioxide levels in the blood and the pH of the blood. When carbon dioxide levels rise in the blood, the rate and depth of breathing increase. The rate and depth of breathing also increase when the blood pH drops. Fear and pain also increase the breathing rate. Breathing rapidly and deeply is called *hyperventilation,* which decreases the amount of carbon dioxide in the blood. However, it should be noted that in patients with chronic obstructive pulmonary disease (COPD), decreased oxygen levels stimulate respiratory rates. Therefore, giving a patient with COPD a high level of oxygen may actually decrease his or her breathing reflex.

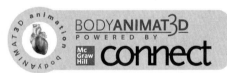

Go to CONNECT to see animation exercise about *Acid-Base Balance: Acidosis* and *Acid-Base Balance: Alkalosis.*

The inflation reflex also helps to regulate the depth of breathing. Stretch receptors in pleural membranes are activated when the lungs are stretched past a certain point. This triggers a decrease in the depth of breathing to prevent over-inflation of the lungs.

Normal, everyday situations also alter our breathing patterns. Consider these common occurrences:

- Coughing. A deep inspiration occurs and the glottis is closed. As the air forces the glottis open, a rush of air is forced up to clear the lower respiratory passages.
- Sneezing. The same process occurs as in coughing except that air is moved to the nasal passages by lowering the uvula. This causes a clearing of the upper respiratory passages.
- Laughing. A deep breath is expelled in short bursts, expressing happiness.
- Crying. The same respiratory process occurs as in laughing, but the expression is one of sadness.
- Hiccups. Also spelled hiccoughs, these are spasmodic contractions of the diaphragm against a closed glottis. Interestingly, the purpose for this is not known.
- Yawning. A deep inspiration that increases the amount of air brought to the alveoli aids in blood oxygenation.

- Speaking. Air is forced through the larynx, vibrating the vocal cords. Words are formed by the tongue, lips, and teeth, allowing for verbal communication.

Also, consider the common patient complaint of snoring. See the feature *Educating the Patient* for more information.

▶ The Transport of Oxygen and Carbon Dioxide in the Blood LO 28.3

Once oxygen gets into the bloodstream, most of it binds to the heme portion of hemoglobin in red blood cells. Hemoglobin bound to oxygen is called *oxyhemoglobin* and is bright red in color. Some oxygen stays dissolved in plasma and does not bind to hemoglobin, but this is generally a lesser amount than that which attaches to the RBCs. Carbon dioxide also binds to hemoglobin, but at the globin or protein portion of the hemoglobin, forming *carbamino-hemoglobin.* However, unlike oxygen, much of the carbon dioxide enters the plasma for transport through the body, after being converted into carbonic acid by the RBCs. Carbonic acid can be converted quickly into the buffer bicarbonate as needed by the blood to maintain its narrow, constant pH level of 7.35 to 7.45 (see *The Cardiovascular System* chapter).

Carbon monoxide is a colorless, odorless gas. Poisonous to humans, it is particularly dangerous because it binds to the same heme area of hemoglobin as does oxygen. In fact, it binds more tightly to this molecule than oxygen. When hemoglobin is exposed to carbon monoxide, the carbon monoxide "overrules" oxygen, leading to carbon monoxide poisoning.

Medical terms are built and dissected using prefixes, word roots/combining form, and suffixes. For example, we can build the term *carboxyhemoglobin* by placing the parts of the term in the puzzle pieces where P = prefix, WR/CF = word root or combining form, and S = suffix.

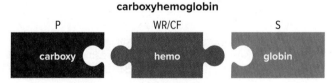

carboxyhemoglobin

carboxy = containing carbon and oxygen

hemo = blood

globin = protein

Carboxyhemoglobin is a blood protein that contains carbon and oxygen. Unlike carbaminohemoglobin, when carbon monoxide binds to hemoglobin it is called carboxyhemoglobin. Learn additional medical terms in the **Medical Terminology Practice** section at the end of this chapter.

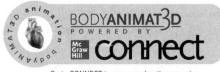

Go to CONNECT to see an animation exercise about *Oxygen Transport and Gas Exchange.*

EDUCATING THE PATIENT

Snoring

Snoring occurs when the muscles of the palate, tongue, and throat relax. Airflow then causes these soft tissues to vibrate. These vibrating tissues produce the harsh sounds characteristic of snoring.

Snoring causes daytime sleepiness and is sometimes associated with a condition known as obstructive sleep apnea (OSA). In OSA, the relaxed throat tissues cause airways to collapse, which prevents a person from breathing. Snoring affects approximately 50% of men and 25% of women older than age 40. The common causes of snoring include the following:

- Enlargement of the tonsils or adenoids
- Being overweight
- Alcohol consumption
- Nasal congestion
- A deviated (crooked) nasal septum

The severity of snoring varies among people. The Mayo Clinic's Sleep Disorders Center uses the following scale to specify the severity of snoring:

- Grade 1: Snoring can be heard from close proximity to the face of the snoring person.

- Grade 2: Snoring can be heard from anywhere in the bedroom.
- Grade 3: Snoring can be heard just outside the bedroom with the door open.
- Grade 4: Snoring can be heard outside the bedroom with the door closed.

You can educate patients about making lifestyle modifications and using aids to help reduce their snoring:

- Lose weight.
- Change the sleeping position from the back to the side.
- Avoid the use of alcohol and medications that cause sleepiness.
- Use nasal strips to widen the nasal passageways.
- Use dental devices to keep airways open.

In addition, patients may benefit from a continuous positive airway pressure (CPAP) machine if OSA is diagnosed as the underlying cause of the snoring. A CPAP machine consists of a mask attached to a pump that forces air into their passageways while they sleep. If these therapies are not effective, patients may need surgery such as a uvulotomy to trim excess tissues in the throat or laser surgery to remove a portion of the soft palate.

▶ Respiratory Volumes

The amount of air that moves into and out of the lungs when a person breathes is called **respiratory volume.** A person's respiratory volume varies depending on the depth and intensity of the breaths the person is taking. **Respiratory capacity,** or the amount of air the lungs can hold, is another common measure of respiratory health. It can be calculated by adding certain respiratory volumes together. In fact, several different measurements related to respiratory volume and capacity are commonly used to assess a person's lungs, which is part of pulmonary function testing (see Table 28-1). You will learn more about these respiratory volumes and the process of measuring them in the *Electrocardiography and Pulmonary Function Testing* chapter.

TABLE 28-1 Respiratory Air Volumes and Capacities		
Name	**Volume**	**Description**
Tidal volume (TV)	500 mL	Volume moved into or out of the lungs during a respiratory cycle
Inspiratory reserve volume (IRV)	3,000 mL	Volume that can be inhaled during forced breathing in addition to resting tidal volume
Expiratory reserve volume (ERV)	1,100 mL	Volume that can be exhaled during forced breathing in addition to resting tidal volume
Residual volume (RV)	1,200 mL	Volume that remains in the lungs at all times
Inspiratory capacity (IC)	3,500 mL	Maximum volume of air that can be inhaled following exhalation of resting tidal volume: IC = TV + IRV
Functional residual capacity (FRC)	2,300 mL	Volume of air that remains in the lungs following exhalation of resting tidal volume: FRC = ERV + RV
Vital capacity (VC)	4,600 mL	Maximum volume of air that can be exhaled after taking the deepest breath possible: VC = TV + IRV + ERV
Total lung capacity (TLC)	5,800 mL	Total volume of air that the lungs can hold: TLC = VC + RV
Forced vital capacity (FVC)	Varies depending on gender, age, and height	Amount of air exhaled with force after inhaling as deeply as possible
Peak expiratory flow (PEF)	Varies depending on gender, age, and height	Greatest rate of flow during forced exhalation

Common Diseases and Disorders of the Respiratory System

ALLERGIC RHINITIS is a hypersensitivity reaction to various airborne allergens.

Causes. There are many causes, which may be seasonal, such as hay fever, or continual, such as those caused by dust, molds, colognes, cigarette smoke, animal dander, or mites.

Signs and Symptoms. There are numerous signs and symptoms, which may include sneezing; itchy, watery eyes; red, swollen eyelids; congested nasal mucous membranes; and nasal discharge.

Diagnostic Exams and Tests. Allergic rhinitis is often diagnosed using skin tests for allergies, as well as blood tests that test for antibodies to specific allergens. In some cases, sinus involvement is ruled out by performing a nasal endoscopy or computerized tomography (CT) scan.

Treatment. Treatment commonly includes the use of over-the-counter (OTC) antihistamines and decongestants. Patients also should avoid known allergens. Air filters and air conditioners assist in keeping allergen counts down. Seeking the assistance of an allergist for desensitization injections may be an option for long-term management.

ASTHMA is a condition in which the tubes of the bronchial tree become obstructed as a result of inflammation.

Causes. The causes include allergens (pollen, pets, dust mites, etc.), cigarette smoke, pollutants, perfumes, cleaning agents, cold temperatures, and exercise (in susceptible individuals).

Signs and Symptoms. Symptoms include difficulty breathing, a tight feeling in the chest, wheezing, and coughing, all of which can cause a feeling of suffocation and increased anxiety.

Diagnostic Exams and Tests. Asthma is usually diagnosed using pulmonary function tests such as spirometry and peak flow tests. See the *Electrocardiography and Pulmonary Function Testing* chapter for more information about these tests. Imaging tests, allergy tests, and other tests for specific triggers, such as methacholine, also may be used.

Treatment. Treatment includes avoiding allergens, using steroidal and nonsteroidal inhalers such as Advair® and Flovent®, and taking oral medications such as Singulair® and other bronchodilators to reduce inflammation. See Figure 28-5. Patients who have asthma should avoid smoky environments; those who smoke should stop. Strongly scented items such as perfumes, hair products, and cleaning agents also should be avoided.

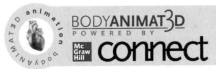

Go to CONNECT to see an animation exercise about *Asthma*.

ATELECTASIS is more commonly called collapsed lung. It may occur after abdominal or thoracic surgery or because of pleural effusion, which may consist of blood, fluid, air, or pus in the pleural cavity. The medical names for these conditions are hemothorax (blood in the pleural cavity), hydrothorax (fluid in the pleural cavity), pneumothorax (air in the pleural cavity), and pyothorax (pus in the pleural cavity).

Causes. Underlying cystic fibrosis may cause atelectasis. In some forms of COPD, patients may have a chronic form of atelectasis. Cancer patients and those with inflammatory conditions such as pleurisy (pleuritis) also may be subject to chronic atelectasis. Acute atelectasis may occur after any injury to the ribs or trauma to the thorax. Postsurgical patients are also susceptible.

Signs and Symptoms. These include **dyspnea** (difficulty breathing), cyanosis (a blue coloration of skin and mucous membranes), diaphoresis (excessive perspiration), anxiety, tachycardia, and intercostal muscle retraction. Depending on the cause of the atelectasis, there also may be chest pain.

Diagnostic Exams and Tests. Testing for atelectasis often focuses on determining the underlying cause so that it can be

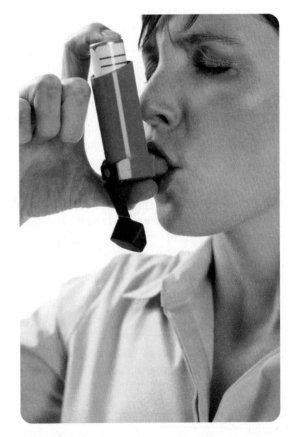

FIGURE 28-5 Individuals with asthma may use an inhaler with steroidal or nonsteroidal medication for treatment.
©Radius Images/Getty Images

treated. Common diagnostic tests include chest X-rays, oximetry (a measure of oxygen saturation in the blood), bronchoscopy, and CT scans.

Treatment. In acute cases, **thoracocentesis,** in which fluid and/or pus is removed using a needle through the chest wall, may be needed to drain the pleural cavity. For chronic atelectasis, treatment may include chest percussion, postural drainage, coughing, deep breathing exercises, and intermittent positive-pressure breathing (IPPB).

BRONCHITIS is inflammation of the bronchi and often follows a cold. Bronchitis that occurs frequently may indicate more serious underlying conditions, such as asthma or emphysema. Smokers are much more likely to develop bronchitis than are nonsmokers. Repeated episodes of bronchitis are one of the risk factors that increase a person's chance of developing lung cancer.

Causes. This condition can be caused by viruses and gastroesophageal reflux disease (GERD), a condition in which acids move from the stomach into the esophagus. Exposure to cigarette smoke, pollutants, and household cleaner fumes also can contribute to the development of bronchitis.

Signs and Symptoms. The signs and symptoms include chills, fever, coughing up yellow-gray or green mucus, tightness in the chest, wheezing, and dyspnea.

Diagnostic Exams and Tests. Because bronchitis can be caused by many different factors, diagnostic tests are generally aimed at determining whether an underlying illness or condition is causing the bronchial inflammation. Tests may include a chest X-ray to rule out pneumonia, pulmonary function tests to check for asthma or emphysema, and various sputum tests for allergies or conditions that can be treated using antibiotics.

Treatment. This condition can be treated with rest, fluids, nonprescription and prescription cough medicines, the use of a humidifier, and possibly antibiotics. Patients who also have asthma may need to use inhalers. They also should wear masks if they may be exposed to lung irritants.

CHRONIC OBSTRUCTIVE PULMONARY DISEASE (COPD) is a group of lung disorders that limit airflow to the lungs and usually cause enlargement of the alveoli in the lungs. Emphysema and chronic bronchitis are the most common types of COPD.

Causes. The primary causes are smoking and air pollution.

Signs and Symptoms. Common signs and symptoms include dyspnea, hypoxia (inadequate oxygenation of the cells), fatigue, and frequent coughing.

Diagnostic Exams and Tests. Pulmonary function tests, including spirometry, oximetry, and various lung volume and capacity tests, are performed to diagnose various forms of COPD. CT scans and chest X-rays also are commonly performed. An arterial blood gas analysis may be used to determine how well the patient's respiratory system is transporting both oxygen and carbon dioxide.

Treatment. Treatment should be focused first on lifestyle changes, especially smoking cessation. Other treatment options include respiratory therapy and the use of inhalers. In more serious cases, a lung transplant may be necessary.

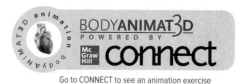

Go to CONNECT to see an animation exercise about *COPD*.

EMPHYSEMA is a chronic condition that damages the alveoli of the lungs. It is heavily associated with smoking, which causes stretching of the spaces between the alveoli and paralyzes the cilia of the respiratory system.

Causes. The most common causes are cigarette smoking and exposure to cigarette smoke; pollutants; and the dust from grains, cotton, wood, or coal.

Signs and Symptoms. Symptoms include shortness of breath that progresses over time, chronic cough, unintended weight loss, and fatigue. In advanced cases, patients develop the characteristic barrel chest caused by the muscular changes in the chest as the patient struggles to breathe.

Diagnostic Exams and Tests. The diagnostic tests for emphysema are similar to those for bronchitis. Pulmonary function tests and arterial blood gases become increasingly more abnormal as the disease progresses. CT scans and chest X-rays also may be ordered.

Treatment. Smoking cessation and prevention of exposure to cold environments and pollutants should be the first treatment measures. Vaccinations to prevent the flu and pneumonia as well as antibiotics to control the respiratory infections associated with emphysema also may be administered. In addition, patients can be treated with bronchodilators, supplemental oxygen, inhaled steroids, and respiratory therapy. The most serious cases may require either surgery to remove damaged lung tissue or a lung transplant, without which patients will develop respiratory and/or heart failure, resulting in death.

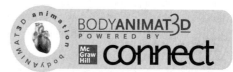

Go to CONNECT to see animation exercise about *Respiratory Tract Infections* and *Respiratory Failure.*

INFLUENZA is more commonly called the flu. Babies, the elderly, people with suppressed immune systems, and those with chronic respiratory illnesses such as COPD are at the highest risk of developing influenza. The flu normally lasts between 5 and 10 days.

Causes. This disease is caused by a number of different viruses that attack the respiratory system. It can be prevented, or at least the course shortened and symptoms lightened, by obtaining a yearly flu vaccination. Note that each year there are multiple strains of influenza. Therefore, the vaccine available each year is for the known strains for that year. Explain this to patients so that they understand they need a flu shot each year for that year's specific viral strains.

Signs and Symptoms. Common symptoms include a runny nose (rhinorrhea), sore throat (pharyngitis), sneezing, fever or chills, dry cough, muscle pain, fatigue, anorexia (loss of appetite), and diarrhea.

Diagnostic Exams and Tests. Because flu symptoms are so similar to those of the common cold, most people do not see a doctor immediately, and many are not tested at all. However, there are some tests, called *rapid influenza diagnostic tests (RIDTs),* that can quickly determine whether a patient has any of several different strains of influenza. These tests are now commonly used to detect influenza.

Treatment. OTC analgesics and antipyretics can alleviate the aches and pains as well as the fever associated with the flu. Other treatment options include bed rest, fluids, and antiviral medications.

LARYNGITIS is an acute inflammation of the larynx. Chronic laryngitis is associated with lung cancer.

Causes. The causes of this condition are varied. They include viruses; bacteria; polyp formation in the larynx; excessive talking, shouting, or singing; allergies; smoking; frequent heartburn; the frequent use of alcohol; damage to nerves that supply the larynx; and a stroke (cerebrovascular accident, or CVA) that paralyzes vocal cord muscles.

Signs and Symptoms. Signs and symptoms include a hoarse voice (dysphonia), a sore throat (pharyngitis), a dry cough and throat, and tickling sensations in the throat.

Diagnostic Exams and Tests. Laryngitis is usually diagnosed from symptoms and treated accordingly. However, if the symptoms do not improve, laryngoscopy, with or without a fiber-optic camera, may be used to determine its cause. If the laryngoscopy reveals a polyp or other suspicious-looking tissue, the physician may perform a biopsy and send the specimen for testing to rule out cancer.

Treatment. The most common treatment options are antibiotics, the management of heartburn, the avoidance of cigarettes and alcohol, and voice rest. The treatment of more serious cases includes the removal of laryngeal polyps and surgery to tighten the vocal cords.

LEGIONNAIRE'S DISEASE is an acute type of bacterial pneumonia. As with many respiratory diseases, smokers are much more susceptible to pneumonia than are nonsmokers.

Causes. This disease is caused by *Legionella* bacilli that usually grow in the standing water of air-conditioning systems.

Signs and Symptoms. The symptoms include fever, which may spike as high as 105.8°F; fatigue; anorexia; dyspnea; frequent coughing; chest pain; muscle aches; and headache. Complications may include hypotension, arrhythmia, respiratory and renal failure, and shock, which is often fatal.

Diagnostic Exams and Tests. The most common test for Legionnaire's disease is a urine test to determine whether *Legionella* antigens are present. Blood and sputum tests often are performed as well. A brain CT scan may be ordered for patients who have confusion or other neurological symptoms.

Treatment. Treatments include antibiotics, antipyretics, and respiratory therapy, including oxygen and ventilator support if needed. Supportive therapy, such as IV fluids, also is used.

LUNG CANCER kills more people in the United States than any other type of cancer. Although other causes of cancer exist, smoking is the most prevalent risk factor leading to **morbidity** (disease state) and **mortality** (death) due to lung cancer. Smoking and secondhand smoke account for approximately 85% of all lung cancer cases. See Figure 28-6.

Causes. The primary causes of lung cancer are smoking and exposure to radon, asbestos, and industrial carcinogens.

Signs and Symptoms. The respiratory symptoms include a cough that worsens over time, hemoptysis (coughing up blood), dyspnea, wheezing, shortness of breath, and recurrent bronchitis. Other symptoms are chest pain, dysphonia, unintended weight loss, and bone pain if the cancer has spread.

Classification. Lung cancer is classified as follows:

- *Small cell lung cancer.* This type occurs almost exclusively in smokers. It is the most aggressive type and spreads readily to other organs. Small cell lung cancer that spreads to other organs is termed *extensive.*
- *Squamous cell lung cancer.* This type of lung cancer arises from the epithelial cells that line the bronchi and bronchioles of the lungs. It occurs most commonly in men.
- *Adenocarcinoma.* This type arises from the mucus-producing cells of the lungs. It develops most commonly in women and nonsmokers.
- *Large cell carcinoma.* This type of lung cancer arises from the peripheral parts of the lungs.

Stages. Squamous cell lung cancer, adenocarcinoma, and large cell carcinoma are staged as follows:

- Stage 0: Cancer is found only in the lining of the bronchi and bronchioles of the lungs.
- Stage 1: Cancer has spread from the lining of the bronchi and bronchioles to lung tissues.
- Stage 2: Cancer has spread to the lymph nodes or the chest wall.
- Stage 3: Cancer has spread to the lymph nodes and to other organs within the chest.
- Stage 4: Cancer has spread to organs outside the chest.

Small cell lung cancer is staged as follows:

- Limited-stage small cell lung cancer: Cancer is found in one lung, the tissues between the lungs, and nearby lymph nodes only.
- Extensive-stage small cell lung cancer: Cancer has spread outside of the lung in which it began or to other parts of the body.

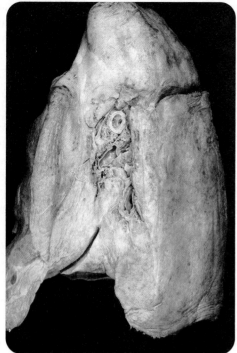

(a) Healthy lung, mediastinal surface

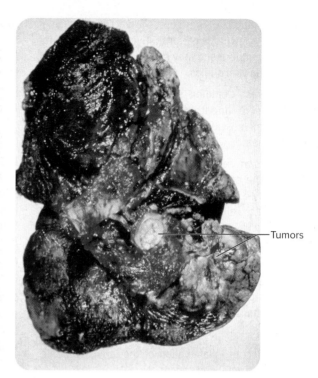

Tumors

(b) Smoker's lung with carcinoma

FIGURE 28-6 (a) A healthy lung is pink, unlike (b) a lung with cancer caused by smoking.

(a) ©McGraw-Hill Education/Dennis Strete, Photographer; (b) ©Biophoto Associates/Science Source

Diagnostic Exams and Tests. An X-ray and/or CT scan may be performed to detect abnormal masses in the lungs. Sputum from patients with a severe cough may be examined for cancer cells. A lung biopsy, performed either during bronchoscopy or as a needle biopsy, can confirm the presence of cancer.

Treatment. Treatment varies, depending on the type of cancer and the stage. Stopping smoking and avoiding exposure to secondhand smoke should be the first treatment considerations. Common treatment options include chemotherapy and radiation therapy. More serious cases may require the surgical removal of tumors (if they are confined), a lobectomy (the removal of a lung lobe or lobes), or a pneumonectomy (the removal of an entire lung).

PLEURISY AND PLEURAL EFFUSION are conditions that affect the pleura that surrounds the lungs. Pleurisy, also called *pleuritis,* is an inflammation that causes the two layers of the pleura to rub painfully against each other. Sometimes pleurisy is accompanied by a buildup of fluid between the layers; this buildup is known as *pleural effusion.*

Causes. Pleurisy has many causes, including viruses, pneumonia, autoimmune diseases such as lupus or rheumatoid arthritis, tuberculosis, a pulmonary embolism, inflammation of the pancreas, and trauma to the chest. Pleural effusion often occurs in pleurisy but also may be caused by either an overproduction of pleural fluid or an inadequate absorption of the fluid. These often result from an underlying disease, such as congestive heart failure, cirrhosis, tuberculosis, cancer, lupus, or rheumatoid arthritis.

Signs and Symptoms. Pleurisy symptoms include fever or chills; a dry cough; shortness of breath; and a sharp, stabbing chest pain during respiration. In pleural effusion, as the fluid builds in the pleural space, the lungs begin to compress, reducing the gaseous exchange of oxygen and carbon dioxide. Infections may result in a pus buildup, which is known as *empyema.*

Diagnostic Exams and Tests. The diagnostic tests for pleurisy and pleural effusion are similar. To rule out other causes of chest pain, blood tests, an electrocardiogram (ECG), or a computerized tomography (CT) scan may be ordered. In addition, a chest X-ray or ultrasound may be ordered to detect pleural effusion. Pleuroscopy (thoracoscopy) may be performed to help rule out cancer or tuberculosis. Thoracocentesis may be performed to obtain fluid or lung tissue for further testing.

Treatment. Analgesics may be prescribed to relieve chest pain associated with pleurisy. Anti-inflammatory drugs, antibiotics, and the removal of excess fluid around the lungs by thoracocentesis are the primary treatment options. **Thoracostomy,** which involves the insertion of a tube to continually drain the fluid, may be required to maintain drainage during the acute phase of pleural effusion. Oxygen may be administered to increase the oxygen concentration in the lung.

PNEUMOCONIOSIS is lung disease that results from years of exposure to different environmental or occupational types of dust. There are three basic types: *anthracosis, asbestosis,* and *silicosis.*

Causes. Anthracosis (black lung disease) results from exposure to coal dusts. Asbestosis results from lung exposure to asbestos. Silicosis arises from exposure to silica sand from sand blasting and ceramic manufacture.

Signs and Symptoms. These include tachypnea, nonproductive cough, progressive dyspnea on exertion, pulmonary hypertension, recurrent respiratory infections, and eventual right ventricular hypertrophy. In all cases, fibrous tissue takes over healthy lung tissue, which destroys the alveoli and takes over the air passageways.

Diagnostic Exams and Tests. Initial diagnosis is often based on the patient's symptoms and a work history. A chest X-ray, CT scan of the chest, arterial blood gas analysis, and pulmonary function tests may be ordered for symptomatic patients who have worked near sources of coal dust, asbestos, or silica. A biopsy may be ordered to confirm the disease.

Treatment. Treatment for all types includes avoiding respiratory infections, using bronchodilators, and using supplemental oxygen as needed. Respiratory therapy also can be useful in helping patients rid themselves of respiratory secretions.

PNEUMONIA, also known as *pneumonitis,* is an inflammation of the lungs caused by a bacterial, viral, or fungal infection. There are at least 50 different types of pneumonia, and they range from mild to serious. *Double pneumonia* refers to inflammation of both lungs.

Causes. Pneumonia can be caused by bacteria, viruses, fungi, and parasites. It also can be caused by foreign matter that enters the lungs (for example, stomach contents that enter the lungs after vomiting), known as aspiration pneumonia. Some types of pneumonia may be prevented by not smoking; other types of pneumonia may be prevented by pneumococcal vaccinations.

Signs and Symptoms. Common signs and symptoms include fever or chills; headache; chest or muscle pain; fatigue; dyspnea; and sputum consisting of rust-colored, green, or yellowish mucus.

Diagnostic Exams and Tests. The presence of pneumonia is usually confirmed using a chest X-ray. Further testing is necessary to determine the cause of pneumonia, including blood and sputum tests to identify the organism responsible for the infection. In some severe cases, a CT scan or culture of pleural fluid also may be performed.

Treatment. Rest, fluids, OTC pain medications, and antibiotics are the most common treatments. In severe cases, oxygen and ventilator support may be required.

PNEUMOTHORAX is a collection of air in the chest around the lungs, which may cause atelectasis.

Causes. Some causes of this disorder are unknown. Various respiratory diseases and trauma to the chest, such as a stabbing wound, also can contribute to the development of pneumothorax.

Signs and Symptoms. The primary symptoms include tightness in the chest or a sharp chest pain, shortness of breath, and a rapid heart rate.

Diagnostic Exams and Tests. Chest X-ray is the most commonly used diagnostic tool. A CT scan of the chest may be ordered in some cases if more detail is needed.

Treatment. The insertion of a chest tube (thoracostomy) to remove air from the chest and surgery to repair chest wounds are the primary treatments.

PULMONARY EDEMA is a condition in which fluids fill spaces within the lungs. This disorder makes it very difficult for the lungs to oxygenate the blood. It most commonly occurs when the heart cannot pump all the blood it receives from the lungs. Left heart failure occurs when blood then backs up in the lungs, causing fluids to seep into lung spaces.

Causes. The many causes of this condition include the following: congestive heart failure, myocardial infarction (heart attack), cardiomyopathy, heart valve disorders, lung infections, allergic reactions, smoke inhalation, drowning, various drugs such as narcotics and heroin, chest injuries, and high altitudes. This disorder may be prevented by avoiding high altitudes and smoking. Preventing heart disease also may reduce the chance of developing this disorder.

Signs and Symptoms. The symptoms of pulmonary edema are shortness of breath; difficulty breathing, especially when lying down (a condition known as *orthopnea*); a feeling of suffocating; wheezing; a productive cough that produces pink mucus; rapid weight gain; pallor; and profuse sweating, which is known as diaphoresis.

Diagnostic Exams and Tests. Initial diagnosis is generally made based on symptoms, a chest X-ray, and an electrocardiogram. Further testing is then performed to detect the reason for the condition, including any underlying diseases. These tests depend on symptoms and the result of a physical exam. They may include blood tests, echocardiogram, cardiac catheterization, or pulmonary artery catheterization.

Treatment. Treatment includes oxygen therapy, diuretics to eliminate excess fluids, and morphine to reduce anxiety and shortness of breath.

PULMONARY EMBOLISM is a blockage in an artery in the lungs. Usually, the artery is blocked by a blood clot that has traveled from a vein in the legs. If an artery in the lungs is completely blocked, death can occur quickly from resultant respiratory failure.

Causes. People at the highest risk of developing this condition are those who have had previous heart attacks, cancer, a fractured hip, or chronic lung diseases. Women who use birth control pills and individuals who have a pacemaker may be at risk for developing a pulmonary embolism. In addition, long periods of inactivity, increased levels of clotting factors in the blood (usually caused by certain cancers), injury to veins, or a stroke that causes paralysis of the arms or legs may cause this condition. A sedentary lifestyle as well as auto or airplane travel— or any activity that requires prolonged sitting or standing—are also major risk factors for developing a pulmonary embolism. A half-dose aspirin (formerly known as a baby aspirin) taken daily, as well as plenty of fluids and frequent movement of the arms and legs, may help prevent the development of a pulmonary embolism.

Signs and Symptoms. Symptoms include fainting, a sudden shortness of breath, hemoptysis (coughing up blood), wheezing, tachycardia (a rapid heartbeat), diaphoresis (profuse sweating), and chest pain that may spread to a shoulder, an arm, or the face.

Diagnostic Exams and Tests. Tests may include a chest X-ray and blood tests for D-dimer (a substance in the blood that dissolves clots), oxygen and carbon dioxide levels, and genetic testing for an inherited clotting disorder. In addition, a spiral (helical) CT scan, ultrasound, or a pulmonary angiogram may be performed. MRI is used instead of chest X-ray on pregnant women and patients with kidney conditions.

Treatment. Support stockings can be used to promote circulation. The patient should rest until the blood clot has dissolved and may be prescribed thrombolytic (clot-dissolving) medications, such as tissue plasminogen activator (tPA). Anticoagulants, typically warfarin, may be used to prevent new blood clots from forming in the deep veins of the body. Finally, a filter may be surgically implanted in the vena cava to prevent blood clots from reaching the lungs.

RESPIRATORY DISTRESS SYNDROME (RDS), which was formerly known as hyaline membrane disease, kills apparently healthy infants. At highest risk are newborns to infants 8 months of age, especially "preemies."

Causes. The underlying problem is known to be a lack of surfactant in the lungs. Surfactant helps prevent the alveoli from totally collapsing on expiration. Without it, the alveoli collapse, resulting in poor oxygenation due to difficulty with reinflation of the alveoli.

Signs and Symptoms. RDS is usually diagnosed soon after birth, when the infant's breathing becomes rapid and shallow. The infant's nares flare, and the accessory muscles are used to aid in respiration. The infant also will exhibit "grunting" noises in an attempt to breathe.

Diagnostic Exams and Tests. Blood tests, including a blood gas analysis, and a chest X-ray are used to diagnose RDS in infants who display signs and symptoms or who are known to be at high risk for the condition.

Treatment. Treatment must be immediate, preferably in a neonatal intensive care unit (NICU). Oxygen therapy, an endotracheal tube, ventilator support, and artificial surfactant all are used in an attempt to keep the alveoli inflated. Infants who survive RDS may be at higher risk for respiratory infections later, but this threat lessens as their lungs continue to mature.

SINUSITIS is an inflammation of the membranes lining the sinuses of the skull.

Causes. Bacteria, excess mucus production in the sinuses (often from the "common cold"), the blockage of sinus openings, and the destruction of cilia that move mucus out of sinuses can cause this disorder.

Signs and Symptoms. Fever, cough, headache, pharyngitis, facial pain, and nasal congestion are the common signs and symptoms.

Diagnostic Exams and Tests. Diagnosis is commonly made after a physical exam of the nose and face. In some cases, allergy testing, a nasal endoscopy, or nasal cultures may be performed, as well as a CT scan or MRI.

Treatment. Treatment options include the use of nasal decongestants, nasal steroid sprays, a humidifier, applications of heat to the face, and antibiotics. Surgery to clear the sinuses or unblock sinus openings may be required.

SUDDEN INFANT DEATH SYNDROME (SIDS) claims the lives of infants less than 1 year old. There were 3,700 sudden unexpected infant deaths in 2015 in the United States, 1,600 of which were due to SIDS. The baby with SIDS simply goes to sleep and never wakes up.

Risk Factors. The causes of SIDS are unknown, but certain risk factors have been identified:

- Male babies are more likely to die of SIDS.
- Babies are most susceptible between the ages of 2 and 4 months.
- Premature or low-birth-weight babies are more likely to have SIDS.
- A baby with a sibling who died of SIDS is more likely to also die of this disorder.
- Nonwhite infants are more likely to develop SIDS.
- Babies who live with smokers have a higher risk of SIDS.

Prevention. Placing the baby on his or her back is the best sleeping position to help prevent SIDS. At-risk infants also may be sent home with an apnea monitor that will sound an alarm if breathing ceases. There are numerous other steps that based upon research appear to reduce the risk of SIDS. These steps include breastfeeding, keeping immunizations up to date, using a pacifier for sleep, avoiding overheating the infant, using a firm bed with no soft toys or thick bedding, and no smoking around the infant. These steps should be discussed with all new parents. Support groups are available and are suggested for families who have experienced the tragedy of losing a child to SIDS.

TUBERCULOSIS (TB) kills more than 2 million people worldwide each year. Although it primarily affects the lungs, it can spread to other parts of the body.

Causes. This disease is caused by various strains of the bacterium *Mycobacterium tuberculosis*. Widespread tuberculosis may be complicated by the following factors:

- HIV infection. HIV infection makes a person more vulnerable to TB.
- Crowded living conditions. This factor allows TB to spread easily; TB, therefore, is found in some prisons and homeless shelters.
- Poverty. Poverty prevents some patients with TB from seeking or completing therapy.
- Drug-resistant bacterium. Drug-resistant strains of the bacterium that causes TB have increased.

- Long-term therapy. Current treatments require antibiotic therapy for many months, which some patients with TB do not complete.

Signs and Symptoms. The symptoms include a cough that lasts more than 3 weeks, unintended weight loss, fever or chills, fatigue, night sweats, pain when breathing or difficulty breathing, and pain in other affected areas.

Diagnostic Exams and Tests. The standard test for tuberculosis is a tuberculin skin test. Blood tests also have been developed to confirm tuberculosis, even in its latent form. Sputum tests, chest X-rays, or CT scans also may be performed if the skin test is positive for TB.

Treatment. The first step should be TB testing to detect carriers of this disease, who should then be treated. Therapy for TB normally lasts 6 months to a year, but drug-resistant cases of TB may require years of drug therapy. Isolating the patient during the contagious phase of the disease (usually 2 to 4 weeks after treatment begins) is required. Also, during the initial stages of treatment, the patient should be encouraged to receive adequate bed rest and maintain an adequate, nutritious diet.

UPPER RESPIRATORY (TRACT) INFECTION (URI) is the term often used for *coryza,* or the common cold.

Causes. URIs are caused by a family of viruses known as *rhinovirus.* The viruses are airborne and transmitted by contact with contaminated surfaces and on the hands. Children are frequent sources of transmission.

Signs and Symptoms. This is a generally self-limiting condition of approximately 1 week's duration, which follows an initial incubation period of 2 to 5 days. Symptoms include pharyngitis, nasal congestion, rhinitis, headache, fever, and general malaise. There may be a nonproductive cough, especially at night.

Diagnostic Exams and Tests. In most cases, a common cold is diagnosed by the physician based on the patient's signs and symptoms. Diagnostic tests such as blood tests and a chest X-ray are typically performed only if the physician suspects that another, underlying condition may be present, such as a bacterial infection.

Treatment. Care is usually symptomatic and includes antipyretics, analgesics, decongestants, and cough suppressants. Adequate rest and plenty of fluids to flush the system are also helpful. Antibiotics are ordinarily prescribed only for patients with an underlying illness or complication.

SUMMARY OF LEARNING OUTCOMES

OUTCOME	KEY POINTS
28.1 Describe the structure and function of each organ in the respiratory system.	The function of the respiratory system is to move air into and out of the lungs in a process known as ventilation, respiration, or breathing. The larynx contains the vocal cords, which stretch between the thyroid and cricoid cartilages. The lungs contain connective tissue, the bronchial tree, nerves, lymphatic vessels, and blood vessels. The bronchial tree consists of the primary, secondary, and tertiary branches of the bronchi; the bronchioles; and the alveoli.
28.2 Describe the events involved in the inspiration and expiration of air.	During inspiration, the diaphragm contracts and the intercostal muscles raise the ribs, increasing the space in the thoracic cavity. This decreases the pressure within the cavity so that the air outside the body passively flows into the thoracic cavity. During expiration, the diaphragm relaxes, pushing up into the thoracic cavity, and the intercostal muscles lower the ribs, forcing the air to flow out of the body. Breathing is controlled by the respiratory center of the brain, located in the pons and medulla oblongata.
28.3 Explain how oxygen and carbon dioxide are transported in the blood.	Most of the oxygen in the bloodstream binds to the hemoglobin within red blood cells, resulting in oxyhemoglobin, although a small amount does not bind to hemoglobin and remains dissolved in the plasma. Carbon dioxide binds to hemoglobin, resulting in carboxyhemoglobin. Most of the carbon dioxide that enters the blood reacts with water in plasma and cerebrospinal fluid to form carbonic acid. As carbonic acid ionizes, it releases hydrogen and bicarbonate ions, which attach to hemoglobin making its way back to the lungs to be exhaled.

OUTCOME	KEY POINTS
28.4 **Compare various respiratory volumes and tell how they are used to diagnose respiratory problems.**	Respiratory volumes are measured to check the health of the respiratory system. The volumes are tidal volume, inspiratory and expiratory reserve volumes, residual volume, inspiratory capacity, functional residual capacity, vital capacity, and total lung capacity. The normal capacities are found in the chapter.
28.5 **Describe the causes, signs and symptoms, diagnosis, and treatments of various diseases and disorders of the respiratory system.**	There are many common diseases and disorders of the respiratory system with varied signs, symptoms, diagnostic tests, and treatments. Some of these include allergic rhinitis, asthma, atelectasis, bronchitis, chronic obstructive pulmonary disease (COPD), emphysema, influenza, laryngitis, Legionnaire's disease, lung cancer, pleurisy and pleural effusion, pneumoconiosis, pneumonia, pneumothorax, pulmonary edema, pulmonary embolism, respiratory distress syndrome (RDS), sinusitis, sudden infant death syndrome (SIDS), tuberculosis (TB), and upper respiratory (tract) infection (URI).

CASE STUDY CRITICAL THINKING

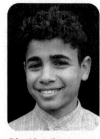

©David Sacks/Getty Images

Recall Mohammad Nassar from the case study at the beginning of the chapter. Now that you have completed the chapter, answer the following questions regarding his case.

1. Why is asthma considered a life-threatening condition?

2. Why did the doctor refer Mohammad Nassar for allergy testing?

3. In addition to the prescribed medication, what can Mohammad Nassar do to help reduce his symptoms?

EXAM PREPARATION QUESTIONS

1. (LO 28.1) Which of the following is/are known as the pulmonary parenchyma?
   a. Nares
   b. Bronchi
   c. Bronchioles
   d. Alveoli
   e. Larynx

2. (LO 28.2) What is responsible for raising and lowering the rib cage during respiration?
   a. Diaphragm
   b. Lungs
   c. Intercostal muscles
   d. Respiratory center
   e. Spinal cord

3. (LO 28.5) Lack of surfactant is responsible for which of the following in premature infants?
   a. Pleurisy
   b. RDS
   c. COPD
   d. Pneumonia
   e. Asthma

4. (LO 28.1) Which structure covers the larynx during swallowing?
   a. Epiglottis
   b. Glottis
   c. Conchae
   d. Hyoid
   e. Uvula

5. (LO 28.5) Which condition is commonly known as a collapsed lung?
   a. Bronchitis
   b. Pleuritis
   c. Coryza
   d. Pneumonia
   e. Atelectasis

6. (LO 28.3) Most of the carbon dioxide in the blood remains in the plasma in which of the following forms?
   a. Carboxyhemoglobin
   b. Carbon monoxide
   c. Bicarbonate
   d. Carbonic acid
   e. Oxyhemoglobin

7. (LO 28.4) Which term refers to the total amount of air the lungs can hold?
   a. Total lung capacity
   b. Vital capacity
   c. Tidal volume
   d. Expiratory reserve volume
   e. Inspiratory reserve volume

8. (LO 28.2) Which of the following everyday occurrences alters our breathing patterns?
   a. Blinking
   b. Swallowing
   c. Yawning
   d. Watching TV
   e. Studying

9. (LO 28.5) The most common types of COPD are emphysema and which other disorder?
   a. Pleuritis
   b. Chronic bronchitis
   c. Asthma
   d. Pleural effusion
   e. Legionnaire's disease

10. (LO 28.2) Which of the following occurs during expiration?
    a. Air flows into the lungs.
    b. The diaphragm contracts.
    c. The diaphragm flattens.
    d. The thoracic cavity enlarges.
    e. The intercostal muscles lower the ribs.

M E D I C A L   T E R M I N O L O G Y   P R A C T I C E

Analyze the following medical terms, presented throughout the chapter. Using a medical dictionary (or Appendix I), place a / mark between each word part. Define each word part and then define the whole word.

EXAMPLE: **pharyng/itis** = pharyng means "throat" + itis means "inflammation"
   PHARYNGITIS means "inflammation of the throat."

1. anthracosis
2. bronchitis
3. epiglottis
4. lobectomy

5. pneumothorax
6. pulmonary
7. pyothorax
8. rhinitis

9. thoracostomy
10. uvulotomy
11. costochondritis
12. dyspnea

The Nervous System

CASE STUDY

Patient Name	DOB	Allergies
Nancy Evans	01/29/1948	Amoxicillin

Attending	MRN	Other information
Elizabeth H. Williams, MD	00-AA-010	PET scan: Minor restrictions of blood flow in some areas MRI: WNL Lumbar puncture: WNL FH: Negative for Alzheimer's disease

PATIENT INFORMATION

In preparing for the patient interview, you check the chart and notice that at Nancy Evans' previous visit, the physician ordered an MRI, a PET scan, and a lumbar puncture. She is here for a follow-up visit to find out the results of these tests. During the patient interview, you ask the patient her name and date of birth. She states, "I am Nancy Evans, I am Welsh, and I was born in January but I don't remember

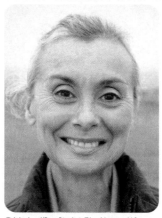

what year." You look at the chart and note that her name is Nancy Evans and she was born on January 29, 1948. Her husband is in the waiting room; after obtaining Nancy Evans' permission, you ask him to come to the interview area. He confirms Nancy Evans' complete name and date of birth and then states, "She seems to forget everything these days. I sure hope these tests last week will help you find out what is causing it."

Keep Nancy Evans in mind as you study the chapter. There will be questions at the end of the chapter based on the case study. The information in the chapter will help you answer these questions.

LEARNING OUTCOMES

After completing Chapter 29, you will be able to:

29.1 Describe the general functions of the nervous system.

29.2 Summarize the structure of a neuron.

29.3 Explain the function of nerve impulses and the role of synapses in their transmission.

29.4 Describe the structures and functions of the central nervous system.

29.5 Compare the structures and functions of the somatic and autonomic nervous systems in the peripheral nervous system.

29.6 Recognize common tests that are performed to determine neurologic disorders.

29.7 Describe the causes, signs and symptoms, diagnosis, and treatments of various diseases and disorders of the nervous system.

KEY TERMS

afferent nerves
autonomic nervous system
axon
cell body
central nervous system (CNS)
cerebrospinal fluid (CSF)
dendrite
dermatome
efferent nerves
ganglia
interneurons
meninges

myelin sheath
neuroglia
neurotransmitter
parasympathetic branch
paresthesia
peripheral nervous system (PNS)
plexus
Schwann cells
somatic nervous system
sympathetic branch
synaptic knob

▶ Introduction

The nervous system is highly complex. It controls all other organ systems and is important for maintaining balance within those systems. Disorders of the nervous system are often difficult to diagnose and treat because of this system's complexity.

▶ General Functions of the Nervous System

LO 29.1

The nervous system is divided into two major parts: the **central nervous system (CNS)** and the **peripheral nervous system (PNS).** The CNS consists of the brain and the spinal cord; the peripheral nervous system consists of peripheral nerves, which are located throughout the rest of the body.

The peripheral nervous system is further divided into two separate sections: the **somatic nervous system,** which governs your body's skeletal (or voluntary) muscles, and the **autonomic nervous system,** which is in charge of your body's automatic functions, such as breathing and digesting food.

Three different types of nerve cells carry out the functions of the nervous system:

- **Afferent nerves**—sensory nerves responsible for detecting information from the environment or from inside the body and taking it to the CNS for interpretation.

- **Efferent nerves**—motor nerves that take information or impulses from the CNS to the PNS to control the movement or action of a muscle or gland.

- **Interneurons**—neurons in the brain and spinal cord that lie between the sensory and motor nerves and act as go-betweens, or interpreters, between the afferent and efferent nerves

One example of how the nervous system works is noting a red light while driving. The afferent (sensory) neurons in your eyes note the color and send the information to the brain's cerebral cortex, where the interpretation takes place. The interneurons pick up the signal, interpret it, and send the information to the efferent (motor) neurons that you are supposed to stop your vehicle, which in turn send the instructions to your right foot to step on the brake pedal of your vehicle. This entire transaction, of course, takes place in milliseconds, allowing you to stop in time.

The nervous system also includes *neuroglial cells,* or **neuroglia.** These cells do not transmit impulses. Instead, they function as support cells for neurons. (See Figure 29-1.) Unlike neurons, neuroglial cells never lose their ability to divide. The three types of neuroglia are:

- *Astrocytes*—star-shaped cells that anchor blood vessels to the nerve cells.

- *Microglia*—small cells that detect, engulf, and destroy invaders.

- *Oligodendrocytes*—cells that assist in the production of the myelin sheath, which will be discussed in further detail later.

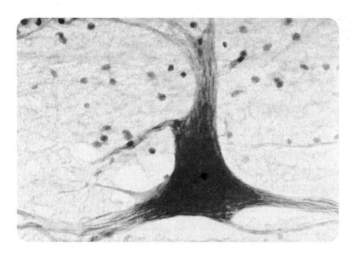

FIGURE 29-1   A typical neuron surrounded by neuroglial cells.
©Allen Bell/Corbis

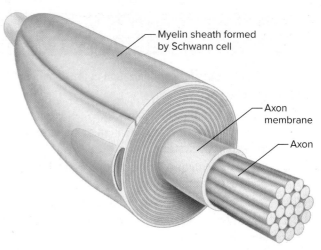

FIGURE 29-2   Schwann cells wrap around the axons of some neurons to create an insulating sheath that speeds up impulse transmission.

Neuron Structure   LO 29.2

Neurons are the functional cells of the nervous system. They transmit electrochemical messages called *nerve impulses* to other neurons and *effectors* (muscles or glands that react to nerve impulses). An important characteristic of neurons is that they lose their ability to divide. Therefore, when neurons are destroyed by disease, they cannot be replaced.

All neurons have a **cell body** and nerve fibers that extend from the cell body. The cell body is the portion of the neuron that contains the nucleus and the organelles typical of any cell. (Refer to the *Organization of the Body* chapter.) It is responsible for generating a large amount of protein and energy the neuron needs to carry out its functions.

Extending from the cell body are two types of nerve fibers: **axons** and **dendrites.** A neuron may have one or more dendrites but typically has only one axon. Dendrites are usually short and branch profusely near the cell body. Their function is to receive information for the neuron. Axons are typically long and branch profusely after they have extended far away from the cell body. Their function is to send information (nerve impulses) away from the cell body.

In the PNS, cells called **Schwann cells** wrap themselves around the axons of some of the neurons (see Figure 29-2). Schwann cells contain a large amount of myelin, a fatty substance that insulates the axons. This insulation, called a **myelin sheath,** allows nerve impulses to move more quickly through the axons.

Nerve Impulse and Synapse   LO 29.3

Neuron cell membranes have a *cell membrane potential*. This means the membrane is *polarized.* Just as a battery is polarized—one end is negative and the other end is positive—neuron cell membranes are polarized because the inside is negatively charged

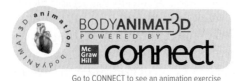

BODYANIMAT3D
animation
POWERED BY
Mc Graw Hill **connect**

Go to CONNECT to see an animation exercise about *Nerve Impulse.*

and the outside is positively charged. This is true in most other types of body cells as well. The outside of cell membranes is positively charged because more positive ions are on the outside. The inside of cell membranes is negatively charged because more negative ions are on the inside. This membrane potential is very important for the function of neurons (see Figure 29-3).

Potassium and sodium ions are both positively charged and play important roles in generating nerve impulses. When a neuron is at rest or without stimulation, the outside of its membrane is relatively positive and the inside is relatively negative because the number of sodium and potassium ions is greater outside the membrane. As long as the neuron is at rest, it remains in this polarized state.

When a neuron detects a stimulus, such as heat or pressure, some of the sodium ions on the outside of the membrane move inside. This changes the polarization of the cell membrane, making the outside less positive and the inside more positive. There is now less difference between the inside and outside of the membrane, so it is said to be *depolarized.* The depolarization creates a nerve impulse, or electric current. The nerve impulse moves along the length of the axon as small areas along the axon become depolarized and then almost immediately repolarize, as shown in Figure 29-4. Repolarization begins when potassium moves outside the membrane, followed by sodium. Then the potassium moves back inside the membrane and the cell is once again polarized (see Figure 29-3).

The speed of a nerve impulse depends on several factors. Myelinated axons conduct impulses faster than those that do not have a myelin sheath. The diameter of the axon also affects the speed of transmission. The larger the diameter, the faster the nerve impulse travels through the axon.

At the end of the axon branches, a nerve impulse reaches the **synaptic knob.** Synaptic knobs contain small sacs called *vesicles* that produce chemicals called **neurotransmitters.** Neurotransmitters are released by the synaptic knob to transport the nerve impulse from the end of the axon to the dendrites of other neurons (see Figure 29-5). This allows the impulse to be conducted along a chain of neurons to reach its destination.

There are about 50 different neurotransmitters. In addition to helping transmit nerve impulses, many neurotransmitters

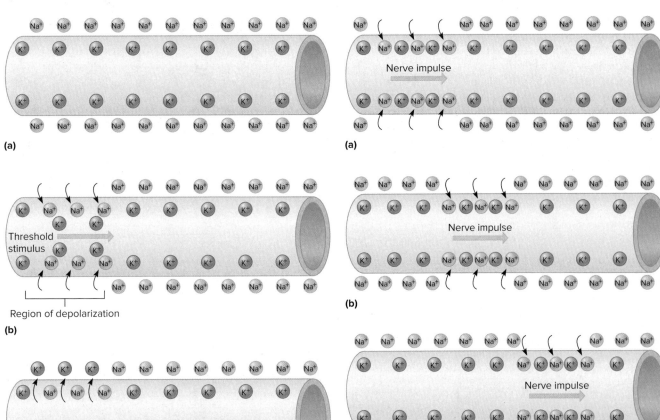

FIGURE 29-3   Nerve impulse: (a) At rest, or in its polarized state, more sodium (Na⁺) is on the outside of the membrane, which makes the outside positive and the inside relatively negative (less positive). (b) When Na⁺ moves into the cell, the membrane depolarizes and the inside becomes more positive. (c) The membrane repolarizes when potassium (K⁺) and later Na⁺ move to the outside of the cell membrane.

perform other functions. These include causing muscles to contract or relax, causing glands to secrete products, activating neurons to send nerve impulses, and inhibiting neurons from sending nerve impulses.

▶ Central Nervous System   LO 29.4

The CNS includes the spinal cord and brain (see Figure 29-6). The tissues of the CNS are so delicate that a *blood-brain barrier* and layers of membranes protect them. Tight capillaries form the blood-brain barrier, which prevents certain substances from entering the tissues of the CNS. For example, various waste products and drugs do not cross the blood-brain barrier well. Inflammation, however, can make this barrier more permeable.

Meninges are membranes that protect the brain and spinal cord. The three layers of meninges are the dura mater, arachnoid mater, and pia mater. *Dura mater* is the toughest and outermost layer of the meninges. The space above the dura mater is called the *epidural space;* below the dura mater is the *subdural space.*

FIGURE 29-4   The depolarization that causes a nerve impulse moves rapidly through the axon, with only a small portion of the axon depolarizing at a time. *Note:* For clarity, the repolarization process is not shown in this illustration.

The middle layer, named for its spider web–like appearance, is the *arachnoid mater. Pia mater* is the innermost and most delicate layer. It sits directly on top of the brain and spinal cord and holds blood vessels onto the surface of these structures. Between the arachnoid mater and pia mater is an area called the *subarachnoid space.* It contains **cerebrospinal fluid (CSF),** sometimes referred to simply as *spinal fluid,* which cushions the CNS.

Medical terms are built and dissected using prefixes, word roots/combining form, and suffixes. For example, we can build the term *epidural* by placing the parts of the term in the puzzle pieces where P = prefix, WR/CF = word root or combining form, and S = suffix.

epidural

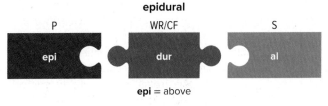

P	WR/CF	S
epi	dur	al

epi = above

dur = dura matter or the brain

al = pertaining

Epidural means pertaining to above the dura matter of the brain. Learn additional medical terms in the **Medical Terminology Practice** section at the end of this chapter.

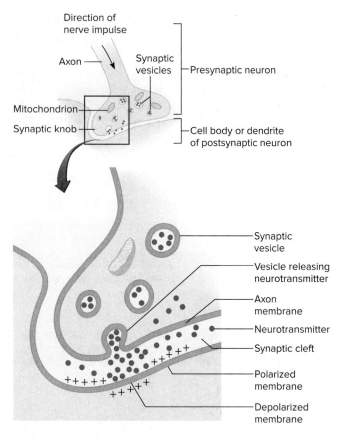

FIGURE 29-5   Synapse. When a nerve impulse reaches a synaptic knob, it releases a neurotransmitter that transports the impulse to the dendrites of the next neuron.

Spinal Cord

The spinal cord is a slender structure that is continuous with the brain. The spinal cord descends into the vertebral canal and ends around the level of the first or second lumbar vertebra. The spinal cord is divided into 31 spinal segments: 8 cervical segments, 12 thoracic segments, 5 lumbar segments, 5 sacral segments, and 1 coccygeal segment. The thickening of the spinal cord in the neck region is called the *cervical enlargement* and contains the motor neurons that control the arm muscles. Another thickening of the spinal cord occurs in the lumbar region. Called the *lumbar enlargement,* this thickening contains the motor neurons that control the leg muscles (see Figure 29-6).

Gray Matter and White Matter   When you view a cross section of the spinal cord, you observe two differently colored areas (see Figure 29-7). The inner tissue is termed *gray matter* because it is darker than the outer tissue, which is termed *white matter.* The white matter contains the myelinated axons of neurons. It is divided into columns that contain groups of axons called *nerve tracts.* The gray matter contains the neuron cell bodies and dendrites, as well as unmyelinated axons. A canal called the *central canal* contains CSF and runs through the center of the gray matter down the entire length of the spinal cord.

Ascending and Descending Tracts   One function of the spinal cord is to carry sensory information up to the brain. The tracts that carry sensory information up to the brain are

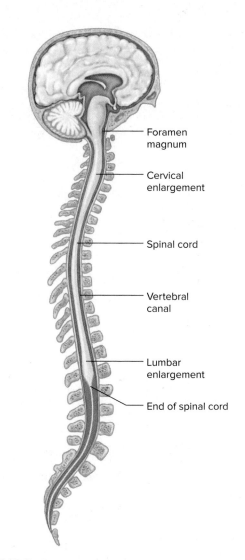

FIGURE 29-6   The central nervous system (CNS) consists of the brain and spinal cord. The spinal cord ends at the level of the third lumbar vertebra.

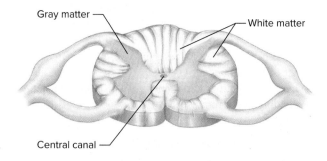

FIGURE 29-7   A cross section of the spinal cord shows the gray matter and the white matter that surrounds it. The central canal is located at the center of the spinal cord, in the gray matter.

called *ascending tracts.* Another function of the spinal cord is to carry motor information down from the brain to muscles and glands in tracts called *descending tracts.*

Reflexes   Another important function of the spinal cord is to provide reflexes. A *reflex* is a predictable, automatic response to a stimulus. For example, if you touch something hot, the predictable response is that you will pull your finger away from the hot surface in a withdrawal reflex. The information that flows through a typical reflex moves in the following order: from receptors to sensory neurons to interneurons to motor neurons to effectors. Figure 29-8 shows what happens in a typical reflex action. When a person steps on a tack, the receptors at the ends of the sensory neurons generate a nerve impulse that travels through the sensory neurons directly to the interneurons in the spinal cord. The interneurons interpret the impulse and determine which muscles must be activated to remove the foot from the tack. They immediately trigger the motor neurons to act, inhibiting some muscle movements and stimulating others and coordinating the muscle movements to move the foot away from the painful stimulus.

Brain

The brain is divided into four major parts: the cerebrum, the diencephalon, the brainstem, and the cerebellum (see Figure 29-9).

Cerebrum The cerebrum is the largest part of the brain. It is divided into two halves called *cerebral hemispheres.* A thick bundle of nerve fibers called the *corpus callosum* connects the two hemispheres. The grooves on the surface of the cerebrum are called *sulci.* The "bumps" of brain matter between the sulci are called *gyri,* or convolutions. A deep groove called the *longitudinal fissure* runs between the two longitudinal hemispheres.

Lobes Each cerebral hemisphere is divided into *lobes*—frontal, parietal, temporal, and occipital. The right and left frontal lobes contain motor areas that allow a person to consciously decide to produce a body movement such as walking or tapping a pencil. Somatosensory areas are located in the parietal lobes. These areas interpret sensations felt on or within the body. For example, if you feel a light touch on your right hand, the somatosensory area interprets the sensation and where it is occurring. The temporal lobes contain auditory areas that interpret sounds. Visual areas are located in the occipital lobes and interpret what a person sees.

Cortex The outermost layer of the cerebrum is called the *cerebral cortex.* It is composed of gray matter and therefore contains neuron cell bodies and dendrites. This layer contains nearly 75% of all neurons in the entire nervous system. Beneath the cerebral cortex is white matter. Besides interpreting sensory information and initiating body movements, the cortex also stores memories and creates emotions.

Ventricles The *ventricles* are the cavities in the brain that produce cerebrospinal fluid (CSF). The two lateral ventricles are the largest and are located in the cerebrum (see Figure 29-10). The third ventricle is located in the diencephalon and the fourth ventricle is located in the brainstem. All four ventricles are responsible for producing and circulating CSF to cushion and protect the brain and spinal cord. CSF also delivers nutrients to the brain and carries away wastes.

Diencephalon The *diencephalon* is located between the cerebral hemispheres and is superior to the brainstem. The diencephalon includes the thalamus and hypothalamus.

The *thalamus* serves as a relay station for sensory information that goes to the cerebral cortex for interpretation. If sensory

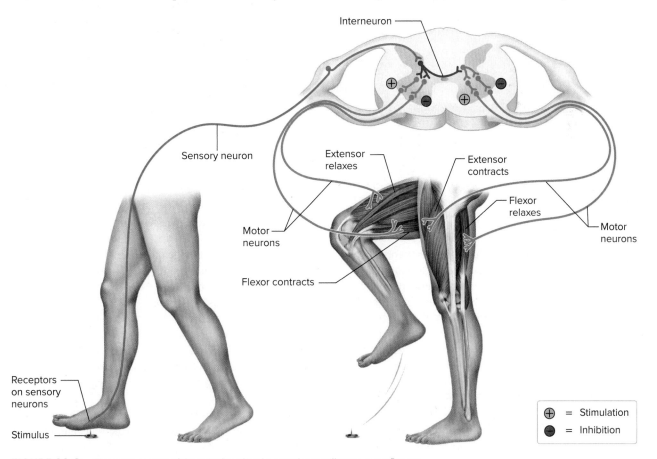

FIGURE 29-8 The cross section of the spinal cord and a spinal nerve illustrates a reflex arc.

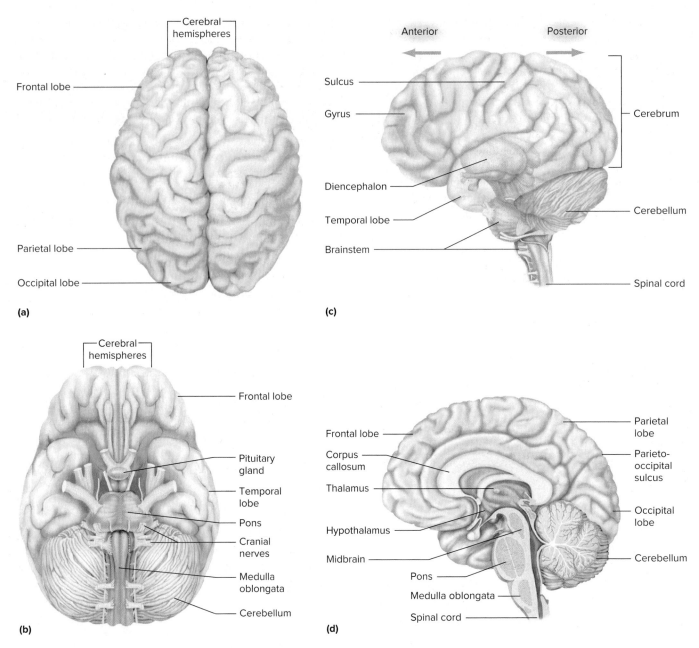

FIGURE 29-9 Four views of the brain: (a) superior, (b) inferior, (c) left lateral, and (d) sagittal section.

information does not pass through the thalamus before it reaches the cerebral cortex, it cannot be interpreted correctly. For example, say you are feeling pain in your left forearm. This information goes up the spinal cord and through the thalamus, and then to the cerebral cortex for interpretation. If the information did not go through the thalamus, the cerebral cortex might interpret that you are feeling cold instead of pain in your left forearm.

The *hypothalamus* maintains homeostasis by regulating hunger, thirst, and body temperature. It also provides a link between the nervous system and the endocrine system.

Brainstem The *brainstem* is a structure that connects the cerebrum to the spinal cord. The three parts of the brainstem are the midbrain, the pons, and the medulla oblongata. The *midbrain* lies just beneath the diencephalon. It controls both visual and auditory reflexes. Seeing something in your

peripheral vision and automatically turning your head to view it more clearly is an example of a visual reflex.

The *pons* is a rounded bulge on the underside of the brainstem between the midbrain and the medulla oblongata. It contains nerve tracts to connect the cerebrum to the cerebellum. The pons also regulates respiration.

The *medulla oblongata* is the most inferior portion of the brainstem and is directly connected to the spinal cord. It controls many vital activities such as heart rate, blood pressure, and respiration. It also controls reflexes associated with coughing, sneezing, and vomiting.

Cerebellum The cerebellum is inferior to the occipital lobes of the cerebrum and posterior to the pons and medulla oblongata. It coordinates the complex skeletal muscle contractions needed for body movements. For example, when you

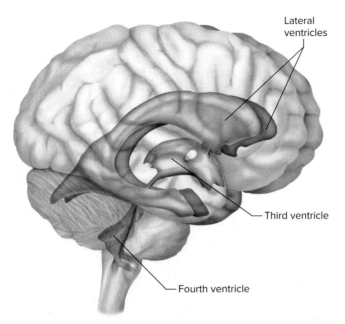

FIGURE 29-10 The CSF produced in the ventricles cushions and protects the brain and spinal cord.

walk, many muscles have to contract and relax at appropriate times. Your cerebellum coordinates these activities. The cerebellum also coordinates fine movements such as threading a needle, playing an instrument, and writing.

Maintaining the health of the central nervous system is vital. See the feature *Educating the Patient* for more information on preventing brain and spinal cord injuries.

▶ Peripheral Nervous System LO 29.5

The peripheral nervous system (PNS) consists of nerves that branch off the CNS. These *peripheral nerves* are classified into two types: cranial nerves and spinal nerves.

Cranial Nerves

Cranial nerves are peripheral nerves that originate from the brain. The 12 cranial nerves are identified using Roman numerals as well as descriptive names (see Figure 29-11):

I. *Olfactory nerves* carry smell information to the brain for interpretation.

II. *Optic nerves* carry visual information to the brain for interpretation.

III. *Oculomotor nerves* are found in the muscles that move the eyeball, eyelid, and iris.

IV. *Trochlear nerves* act in the muscles that move the eyeball.

V. *Trigeminal nerves* carry sensory information from the surface of the eye, the scalp, facial skin, the lining of the gums, and the palate to the brain for interpretation. They also are found in the muscles needed for chewing.

VI. *Abducens nerves* act in the muscles that move the eyeball.

VII. *Facial nerves* are found in the muscles of facial expression as well as in the salivary and tear glands. These nerves also carry sensory information from the tongue.

VIII. *Vestibulocochlear nerves* carry hearing and equilibrium information from the inner ear to the brain for interpretation.

EDUCATING THE PATIENT

Preventing Brain and Spinal Cord Injuries

In the United States alone, almost half a million people a year suffer brain and spinal cord injuries. The most common causes of these injuries are motor vehicle accidents, sports and recreational accidents—especially diving—and violence. People at the highest risk for spinal cord injuries are children and teens. However, most brain and spinal cord injuries can be prevented. Use the following tips to educate patients on preventing these types of injuries.

Prevention Tips

- Buy and use approved head gear or a helmet when riding a bike or motorcycle, or doing any sporting activity in which you might fall such as horse riding or skateboarding. Your risk of brain injury is 85% greater during a biking accident if you are not wearing a helmet. Make sure your helmet fits properly. Replace your helmet if you have hit your head while wearing it; the helmet may be compromised from the fall and thus unsafe.

- Know the depth of water into which you are diving. More than 90% of diving injuries occur in 5 feet of water or less.

- Explore diving areas before diving. For example, know where rocks are located before you dive.

- Do not drive or do any recreational activity while under the influence of alcohol or drugs. Both affect good judgment and control. Alcohol-related traffic crashes are the leading cause of disabling brain and spinal cord injuries.

- Always wear appropriate protective gear while playing any sport.

- Always wear your seat belt in the car.

- Make sure children use car seats appropriate for their age and weight.

- Be familiar with ways to get help quickly in emergencies.

- Follow traffic rules and signs while walking, biking, or driving.

- Follow safety rules posted on playgrounds, swimming pools, public beaches, and parks.

- Store firearms and ammunition in separate and locked places.

- Teach children the safety rules to follow if they find a gun.

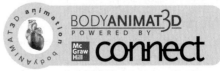

Go to CONNECT to see an animation exercise about *Spinal Cord Injury.*

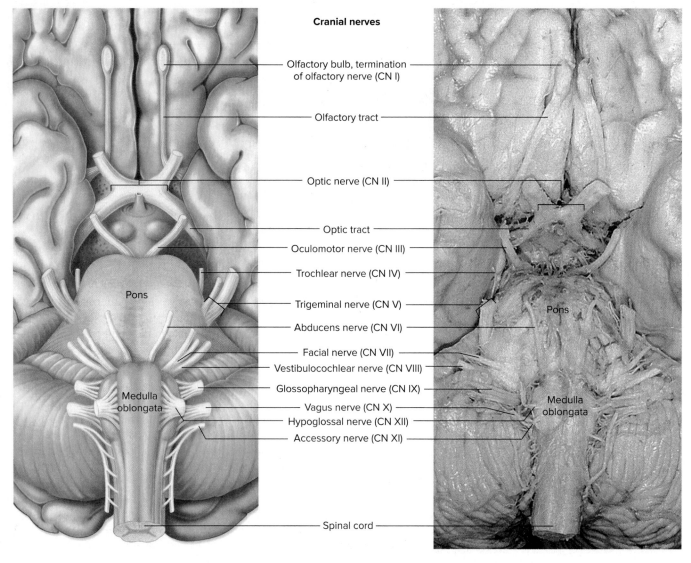

Cranial nerves

Olfactory bulb, termination of olfactory nerve (CN I)

Olfactory tract

Optic nerve (CN II)

Optic tract

Oculomotor nerve (CN III)

Trochlear nerve (CN IV)

Trigeminal nerve (CN V)

Abducens nerve (CN VI)

Facial nerve (CN VII)

Vestibulocochlear nerve (CN VIII)

Glossopharyngeal nerve (CN IX)

Vagus nerve (CN X)

Hypoglossal nerve (CN XII)

Accessory nerve (CN XI)

Spinal cord

Pons

Medulla oblongata

Pons

Medulla oblongata

FIGURE 29-11 A view of the inferior surface of the brain shows the 12 pairs of cranial nerves.

©McGraw-Hill Education/Rebecca Gray, Photographer

IX. *Glossopharyngeal nerves* carry sensory information from the throat and tongue to the brain for interpretation. They also act in the muscles of the throat.

X. *Vagus nerves* carry sensory information from the thoracic and abdominal organs to the brain for interpretation. These nerves also are found in the muscles in the throat, stomach, intestines, and heart.

XI. *Accessory nerves* are found in the muscles of the throat, neck, back, and larynx.

XII. *Hypoglossal nerves* are found in the muscles of the tongue.

Spinal Nerves

Spinal nerves are peripheral nerves that originate from the spinal cord (see Figure 29-12). There are 31 pairs of spinal nerves: 8 pairs of cervical nerves (numbered C1 through C8), 12 pairs of thoracic nerves (numbered T1 through T12), 5 pairs of lumbar nerves (numbered L1 through L5), 5 pairs of sacral nerves (numbered S1 through S5), and 1 pair of coccygeal nerves (Cx). Except for C1, each spinal nerve innervates a skin segment known as a **dermatome.** A map of the dermatomes with the spinal nerve responsible for the skin area is shown in Figure 29-13.

The spinal nerves are formed from two roots, or nerve fibers. The ventral, or anterior, root consists of efferent (motor) nerve fibers. The dorsal, or posterior, root consists of afferent (sensory) nerve fibers. Because these two roots combine to form the spinal nerves, these nerves can carry both sensory and motor information.

Except in the thoracic region, the main portions of spinal nerves fuse together to form complex networks called nerve **plexuses.** The major nerve plexuses are the cervical, brachial, and lumbosacral plexuses. Nerves coming off the cervical plexus supply the skin and the muscles of the neck. The phrenic nerve also originates from the cervical plexus. This nerve controls the diaphragm, which is a muscle needed for breathing.

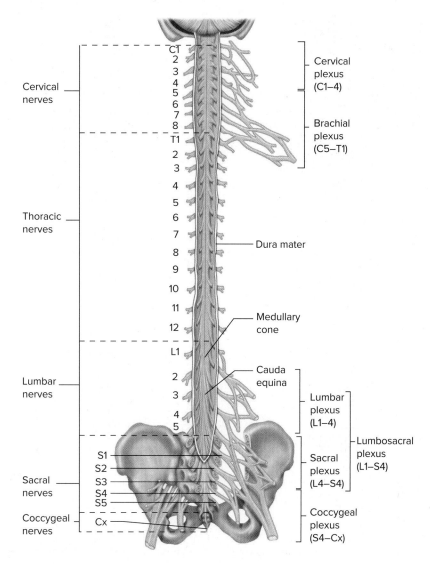

FIGURE 29-12 Spinal cord, spinal nerves, and plexuses.

The brachial plexus includes nerves that control muscles in the arms. The lumbosacral plexus supplies the lower abdominal wall, external genitalia, buttocks, thighs, legs, and feet. The largest nerve of the body, the sciatic nerve, originates from this plexus. This nerve controls the leg muscles. The coccygeal plexus is the source of the anococcygeal nerve, which controls the muscles in the anus and the back of the thighs.

Somatic and Autonomic Nervous Systems

The peripheral nervous system contains two subparts: the somatic nervous system (SNS) and the autonomic nervous system (ANS). The somatic nervous system consists of nerves that connect the central nervous system (CNS) to skin and skeletal muscle. Because it controls the skeletal muscles, which are under a person's direct (voluntary) control, this system is sometimes called the "voluntary" nervous system. The autonomic nervous system connects the central nervous system to body organs such as the heart, stomach, intestines, and bladder, as well as glands and blood vessels. Because these organs are not under a person's voluntary (direct) control, the autonomic nervous system is sometimes referred to as the "involuntary" nervous system.

In the autonomic nervous system, motor neurons from the brain and spinal cord communicate with other motor neurons located in ganglia. **Ganglia** are collections of neuron cell bodies outside the CNS. The motor neurons of ganglia then communicate with various organs and blood vessels.

The autonomic nervous system is further divided into the sympathetic and parasympathetic branches (see Figure 29-14). The **sympathetic branch** responds to stressful or emergency situations by increasing the heart rate. This is often called the "fight-or-flight" response because it increases blood flow throughout the body in preparation for immediate action. Most sympathetic neurons release the neurotransmitter norepinephrine into organs and glands. Norepinephrine increases heart and breathing rates; slows down the activity of the digestive glands, stomach muscles, and intestines; and dilates the pupils. It also constricts the blood vessels, increasing the blood pressure, which is a needed response during an emergency situation.

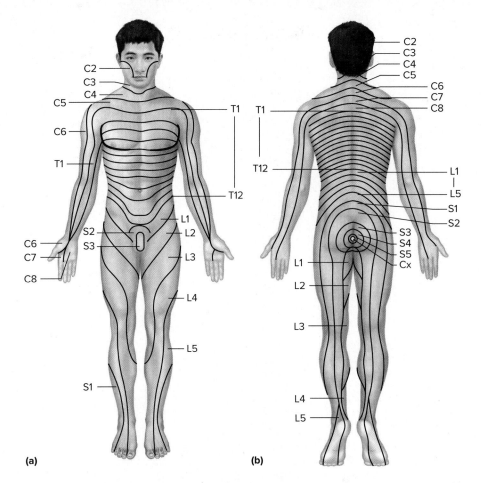

FIGURE 29-13 Dermatome maps. A dermatome is an area of skin supplied by a single spinal nerve. These diagrams only approximate the dermatomal distribution.

The **parasympathetic branch** of the autonomic nervous system does just the opposite. It keeps the heart rate relatively low, preparing the body for resting and digesting nutrients. Most of the body's organs are under parasympathetic control. All parasympathetic neurons release the neurotransmitter acetylcholine to organs and glands. Acetylcholine has the opposite effect from norepinephrine. It slows the heart and breathing rates; activates the digestive glands, stomach muscles, and intestines; and constricts the pupils. It has little effect on the blood vessels, however, because most blood vessels do not receive input from the parasympathetic nerves.

▶ Neurologic Testing   LO 29.6

Patients with nervous system disorders may have a wide variety of signs and symptoms, but the most common are headache, muscle weakness, and **paresthesia** (loss of feeling). A typical neurologic examination can determine the following:

- State of consciousness. This state can vary from normal to a state of coma. A patient in a coma cannot respond to stimuli and cannot be awakened. Other terms used to describe states of consciousness include *stupor* (difficulty being awakened), *delirium* (loss of function of the

cerebral cortex), *vegetative* (having no cortical function), and *asleep* (can be aroused with normal stimulation).

- Reflex activity. Reflex tests primarily determine the health of the peripheral nervous system.

- Speech patterns. Abnormal speech patterns include a loss of the ability to form words correctly or to form sentences that make sense.

- Motor patterns. Abnormal motor patterns include loss of balance; abnormal posture; and inappropriate, involuntary movements of the body. For example, *chorea* is a sudden, exaggerated jerking of a body part.

Diagnostic Procedures

Common diagnostic procedures to determine neurologic disorders include the following tests:

- Lumbar puncture (spinal tap). When a physician needs to examine cerebrospinal fluid (CSF), a lumbar puncture is performed. A needle is used to remove CSF from the subarachnoid space, usually below the third lumbar vertebra of the spinal column. Analysis of this fluid provides a great deal of information about the patient's health. For example, cancer cells in CSF often indicate a brain tumor or spinal cord tumor. White blood cells in

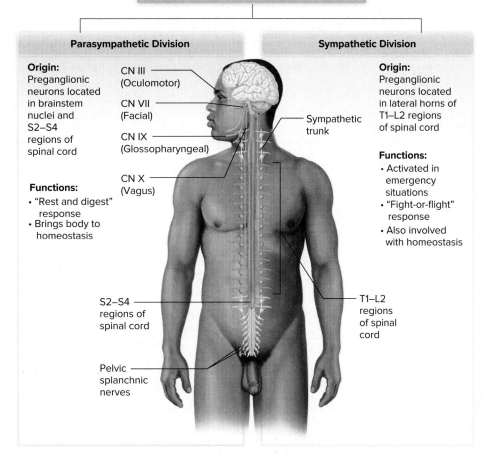

FIGURE 29-14 Comparison of the parasympathetic and sympathetic branches.

this fluid indicate infections such as meningitis. Red blood cells indicate abnormal bleeding.

- Magnetic resonance imaging (MRI). This procedure allows the brain and spinal cord to be visualized from many angles. It uses powerful magnets to generate images and is useful in detecting tumors, bleeding, and other abnormalities.
- Positron emission tomography (PET) scan. This procedure uses radioactive chemicals that collect in specific areas of the brain. These chemicals allow images of those areas to be generated. This test is useful in detecting brain tumors, checking blood flow to different areas of the brain, and helping to diagnose diseases such as Parkinson's and Alzheimer's.
- Cerebral angiography. This procedure uses contrast material that can be visualized in the blood vessels of the brain. It is useful in detecting aneurysms (abnormal, blood-filled bulges in blood vessels).
- Computerized tomography (CT) scan. This procedure produces images that provide more information than a standard X-ray. It is useful in detecting tumors, abnormal structures, and bleeding.
- Electroencephalogram (EEG). This test detects electrical activity in the brain. It is useful in diagnosing various states of consciousness.

- X-ray. This procedure is useful in detecting skull or vertebral fractures.

Cranial Nerve Tests

Disorders of the cranial nerves can be determined using the following tests:

- The olfactory nerves (I) are tested by asking a patient to smell various substances.
- Cranial nerves III, IV, and VI are tested by asking a patient to track the movement of the physician's finger. If a patient cannot move her eyeballs properly, there may be damage to one of these nerves. Recall that these nerves control the muscles that move the eyeballs.
- Cranial nerve V controls the muscles needed for chewing. To assess this nerve, a patient is asked to clench his teeth. The physician then feels the jaw muscles. If the muscles feel limp or weak, this nerve may be damaged.
- If a person can no longer make facial expressions, then cranial nerve VII may be damaged. This nerve controls the muscles needed to make facial expressions.
- If a patient cannot extend his tongue and move it from side to side, cranial nerve XII may be damaged. This nerve controls tongue movement.

Reflex Testing

Testing a patient's reflexes allows a physician to evaluate the components of a reflex as well as the overall health of the individual's nervous system. The absence of a reflex is called *areflexia. Hyporeflexia* is a decreased reflex, and *hyperreflexia* is a stronger-than-normal reflex. The following are common reflex tests:

- Biceps reflex. The absence of this reflex may indicate spinal cord damage in the cervical region.
- Knee reflex. The absence of this reflex may indicate damage to lumbar or femoral nerves.
- Abdominal reflexes. These reflexes are tested to evaluate damage to thoracic spinal nerves.

Common Diseases and Disorders of the Nervous System

ALZHEIMER'S DISEASE is a progressive, degenerative disease that occurs in the brain.

Causes. Fiber tangles within neurons, degenerating nerve fibers, and a decreased production of neurotransmitters cause the symptoms of this disorder. Alzheimer's is associated with advanced age, family history, certain genes, and possibly some environmental factors. Many causes have not yet been determined.

Signs and Symptoms. Common symptoms include memory loss, confusion, personality changes, language deterioration, impaired judgment, and restlessness.

Diagnostic Exams and Tests. Although Alzheimer's cannot actually be diagnosed until after the patient dies, tests are performed to determine risk factors and to rule out other causes of the symptoms. The physician performs a physical and mental examination, and may order a PET scan to assess blood flow in various parts of the brain. MRI may be used to rule out a brain tumor or stroke. A CT scan also may be ordered to determine any physical changes in the brain.

Treatment. There is no cure, but with medications such as Aricept®, Cognex®, Razadyne®, and Namenda®, as well as proper nutrition, physical exercise, social activity, and calm environments, the disease progress may be slowed and managed.

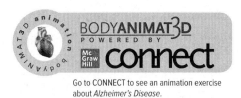

Go to CONNECT to see an animation exercise about *Alzheimer's Disease.*

AMYOTROPHIC LATERAL SCLEROSIS (ALS), commonly known as Lou Gehrig's disease, is a fatal disorder characterized by the degeneration of neurons in the spinal cord and brain.

Causes. Most causes are unknown, but researchers suspect that they involve hereditary and environmental factors.

Signs and Symptoms. Early symptoms include cramping of hand and feet muscles, persistent tripping and falling, chronic fatigue, and slurred speech. Signs and symptoms that appear in later stages include breathing difficulty and muscle paralysis.

Diagnostic Exams and Tests. There is no definitive test for ALS. Instead, it is diagnosed based on symptoms, after ruling out other causes. A neurological exam is usually performed, as well as electromyography and nerve conduction studies. Blood tests and MRI often are used to help rule out other reasons for the symptoms.

Treatment. There is no cure for this disorder; however, physical, speech, and respiratory therapies help to manage the symptoms. Some medications relieve muscle cramping, but currently only the drug riluzole is approved by the US Food and Drug Administration (FDA) specifically for ALS.

BELL'S PALSY is a disorder in which facial muscles are very weak or totally paralyzed.

Causes. This condition can result from damage to cranial nerve VII (the facial nerve), but many times the cause is unknown. It is more common in people with diabetes, the flu, or a cold.

Signs and Symptoms. The most common signs and symptoms are a loss of feeling in the face, the inability to produce facial expressions, headache, and excessive tearing or drooling.

Diagnostic Exams and Tests. A physical exam is performed, including a test for a characteristic eye movement when the eye is closed. However, there is no specific diagnostic test for Bell's palsy. The diagnosis is usually made after a CT scan, MRI, or skull X-ray rules out other conditions, such as stroke (CVA) or brain tumor.

Treatment. Treatments include the use of eyedrops, anti-inflammatory medications, and pain relievers. Symptoms usually diminish or go away within 5 to 10 days.

BRAIN TUMORS AND CANCERS are abnormal growths in the brain. A brain tumor with cancer cells is termed malignant. Malignant tumors that start in any tissue of the brain are called primary brain cancers. Those that start in other body parts and spread to the brain are classified as secondary brain cancers. The most common primary brain tumors are *gliomas* that arise from neuroglial cells.

Causes. Like most cancers, the causes are gene mutations. Factors associated with gene mutations include exposure to toxins, an impaired immune system, and hereditary factors.

Signs and Symptoms. The signs and symptoms depend on the size and location of the tumor. Common symptoms include headache, seizures, nausea, weakness in the arms or legs, fatigue, changes in speech patterns, and a loss of memory.

Diagnostic Exams and Tests. The two most widespread tests to diagnose brain tumors and cancers are the CT scan and the MRI. A CT scan is performed with contrast (a dye injected to improve the detail shown in the scan). Blood tests also are usually performed.

Treatment. Treatment options include surgery, radiation therapy, chemotherapy, and gene therapy. The success of the treatment depends on the type of tumor, the location and extent of the tumor, the tumor's response to treatment, and the patient's overall health.

EPILEPSY AND SEIZURES occur when parts of the brain receive a burst of electrical signals that disrupt normal brain functioning. Seizures may be either petit mal (partial) or grand mal (generalized). *Absence,* or *petit mal, seizures* may appear as loss of awareness of the present, whereas *grand mal seizures* result in the classic tonic-clonic seizure, in which the person becomes unconscious and muscles twitch sporadically. Epilepsy is the condition of having repeated seizures over a long period of time.

Causes. Causes vary but may include birth trauma, high fevers, alcohol and drug withdrawal, head trauma, infections, brain tumors, and certain medications. Many causes are unknown.

Signs and Symptoms. The most common sign of an absence seizure is a "vacant stare" that may last from 10 to 20 seconds. Other signs and symptoms include chewing movements of the jaws, finger rubbing or other small movements of the hands, and lip smacking, with no memory of the episode afterward. Signs and symptoms of grand mal seizure may include visual disturbances, nausea, generalized abnormal feelings, a loss of consciousness, and uncontrolled muscle contractions and tremors.

Diagnostic Exams and Tests. For both absence and grand mal seizures, an electroencephalogram (EEG) is commonly performed to determine any changes in the normal pattern of brain waves. A single-photon emission computerized tomography (SPECT) test may be performed to determine where in the brain the seizures begin. Blood tests and an MRI may be performed to help rule out other causes of the seizures. In some cases, a magnetic resonance spectroscopy (MRS) may be performed to show a part of the brain in greater detail.

Treatment. The primary treatment is medication to prevent seizures. Absence seizures in children may stop as the child becomes older, so medication use and dosage are monitored carefully.

GUILLAIN-BARRÉ SYNDROME is a disorder in which the body's immune system attacks part of the peripheral nervous system. It usually has a sudden and unexpected onset.

Causes. The destruction of myelin by the body's immune system produces the signs and symptoms. Viral infections, immunizations, and pregnancy sometimes trigger the disease.

Signs and Symptoms. Symptoms may include weakness or tingling sensations in the legs or arms that can progress to paralysis. Difficulty breathing and an abnormal heart rate are more dangerous signs and symptoms. The disease normally runs its course, and with proper medical treatment, it is not fatal.

Diagnostic Exams and Tests. A spinal tap may be performed to look for changes in spinal fluid that commonly occur in patients with this syndrome. Nerve conduction studies and electromyography also may be used to check for abnormalities in the nervous and muscular systems.

Treatment. Various supportive therapies, such as the use of respirators and heart machines, are necessary until the disease subsides. Physical therapy is used to keep muscles strong.

MENINGITIS is an inflammation of the meninges.

Causes. Causes include bacterial, viral, and fungal infections. Some types of meningitis can be prevented with vaccines.

Signs and Symptoms. Fever, headache, vomiting, stiffness in the neck, sensitivity to light, drowsiness, and joint pain usually accompany this disorder.

Diagnostic Exams and Tests. The definitive test for meningitis is a spinal tap. An increased WBC and low glucose levels are indications of meningitis. The practitioner also may order X-rays, a CT scan, or MRI of the head and/or chest, along with blood cultures to identify the microorganism causing the infection.

Treatment. The treatment varies depending on the type of meningitis. Intravenous antibiotics are used for bacterial meningitis, supportive therapy for viral meningitis, and antifungal drugs are given for fungal meningitis. Bacterial meningitis can be fatal.

MULTIPLE SCLEROSIS (MS) is a chronic disease of the central nervous system in which myelin is destroyed.

Causes. The causes are mostly unknown, but some known causes are viruses, genetic factors, and immune system abnormalities.

Signs and Symptoms. Depending on the type of MS, symptoms can range from mild to severe. In severe cases, a person loses the ability to walk or speak.

Diagnostic Exams and Tests. There are currently no direct tests for MS, although new tests are currently under development. Instead, tests are performed to rule out other causes of the symptoms. These tests may include blood tests, an MRI (with contrast), a spinal tap, and a complete neurological exam.

Treatment. There is no cure for MS, but supportive treatments may lessen the symptoms. Some medications, including interferon, Copaxone®, prednisone, and Solu-Medrol®, are available to treat and slow the progression of symptoms.

NEURALGIAS are a group of disorders commonly referred to as nerve pain. They most frequently occur in the nerves of the face.

Causes. There are many causes of neuralgia, including trauma, chemical irritation of the nerves, bacterial infections, and diabetes. Many times the causes are unknown.

Signs and Symptoms. Sudden and severe skin pain is the most common symptom. The pain occurs repeatedly in the same body area. Numbness of skin areas is also common.

Diagnostic Exams and Tests. A neurological exam, combined with the patient's description of the symptoms, is used to diagnose a neuralgia. In some cases, an MRI or a magnetic resonance angiogram may be used to rule out other conditions, such as a tumor or multiple sclerosis, that may be causing the pain.

OUTCOME	KEY POINTS
29.4 Describe the structures and functions of the central nervous system.	The brain consists of the cerebrum, diencephalon, brainstem, and cerebellum. The blood-brain barrier is a layer of tightly woven capillaries that protects the delicate brain tissues. The meninges are a triple-layered membrane protecting the brain and spinal cord. The spinal cord is continuous with the brain and consists of 31 spinal segments. The basic function of the spinal cord is to carry sensory information from the body to the brain and motor information from the brain to the muscles and glands of the body. Cerebrospinal fluid (CSF) is located within the subarachnoid space of the brain and within the central canal of the spinal cord. It cushions the brain and spinal cord.
29.5 Compare the structures and functions of the somatic and autonomic nervous systems in the peripheral nervous system.	The somatic nervous system connects the central nervous system to the skin and skeletal muscle (voluntary functions). The autonomic nervous system connects the CNS to the internal organs (involuntary functions). The autonomic nervous system is divided into the sympathetic branch, which prepares the body for "fight or flight" (stressful) situations, and the parasympathetic branch, which is the body's everyday "resting" system for normal situations.
29.6 Recognize common tests that are performed to determine neurologic disorders.	Tests commonly used to determine neurologic disorders include tests of the reflexes and cranial nerves, as well as diagnostic procedures such as lumbar puncture (spinal tap), MRI, PET, cerebral angiography, CT scan, EEG, and X-ray.
29.7 Describe the causes, signs and symptoms, diagnosis, and treatments of various diseases and disorders of the nervous system.	There are many common diseases and disorders of the nervous system with varied signs, symptoms, diagnosis, and treatments. Some of these include Alzheimer's disease, amyotrophic lateral sclerosis (ALS), Bell's palsy, brain tumors, cancer, epilepsy, seizures, Guillain-Barré syndrome, episodic and chronic tension headaches, migraines, cluster headaches, meningitis, multiple sclerosis (MS), neuralgias, Parkinson's disease, sciatica, and stroke (cerebrovascular accident or CVA).

CASE STUDY CRITICAL THINKING

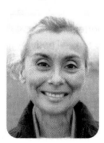

©John Lund/Sam Diephuis/
Blend Images LLC

Recall Nancy Evans from the case study at the beginning of the chapter. Now that you have completed the chapter, answer the following questions regarding her case.

1. Forgetfulness is a common sign of what types of neurologic disorders?

2. What are some of the possible causes of these disorders?

3. What information might the physician hope to gain from the ordered MRI, PET scan, and lumbar puncture?

4. What are the treatment options for these disorders?

1. (LO 29.6) Which of the following is *not* a common symptom of patients with neurologic disorders?
   a. Headache
   b. Paresthesia
   c. Fever
   d. Muscle weakness
   e. Numbness

2. (LO 29.6) Which of the following diagnostic procedures uses radioactive chemicals that collect in specific areas of the brain to generate images of those areas?
   a. MRI
   b. PET scan
   c. CT scan
   d. Cerebral angiography
   e. X-ray

3. (LO 29.4) The _____ are interconnecting cavities of the brain that produce and circulate CSF.
   a. Ventricles
   b. Lobes
   c. Convolutions
   d. Gyri
   e. Sulci

4. (LO 29.1) What kind of neurons connect the neurons that carry messages to the central nervous system with those that carry messages from the central nervous system to the muscles and glands?
   a. Efferent neurons
   b. Sensory neurons
   c. Afferent neurons
   d. Motor neurons
   e. Interneurons

5. (LO 29.2) Which type of neuroglial cells anchor blood vessels to the nerve cells?
   a. Microglia
   b. Oligodendrocytes
   c. Astrocytes
   d. Schwann cells
   e. Satellite cells

6. (LO 29.4) What is the name of the tough, outer layer of the meninges?
   a. Dura mater
   b. Epidural space
   c. Arachnoid mater
   d. Subdural space
   e. Pia mater

7. (LO 29.3) Which two ions are responsible for cell membrane depolarization and repolarization?
   a. Na^+ and Ca^{++}
   b. Na^+ and Cl^-
   c. Ca^{++} and Cl^-
   d. K^+ and Na^+
   e. K^+ and SO_4^-

8. (LO 29.5) Collections of neuron cell bodies outside the central nervous system that communicate with organs and blood vessels are called
   a. Ganglia
   b. Plexuses
   c. Dermatomes
   d. Ventral roots
   e. Dorsal roots

9. (LO 29.5) Which of the following cranial nerves are found in the muscles of the tongue?
   a. Olfactory nerves (I)
   b. Oculomotor nerves (III)
   c. Trigeminal nerves (V)
   d. Facial nerves (VII)
   e. Hypoglossal nerves (XII)

10. (LO 29.7) In which nervous system disorder are the facial muscles paralyzed?
    a. Amyotrophic lateral sclerosis
    b. Epilepsy
    c. Bell's palsy
    d. Guillain-Barré syndrome
    e. Meningitis

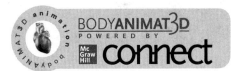

Go to CONNECT to see an animation exercise about *Strokes*

Analyze the following medical terms, presented throughout the chapter. Using a medical dictionary (or Appendix I), place a / mark between each word part. Define each word part and then define the whole word.

EXAMPLE: **crani/otomy** = crani means "skull" + otomy means "incision"
CRANIOTOMY means "incision into the skull."

1. angiography
2. areflexia
3. astrocyte
4. cerebral

5. electroencephalogram
6. hyperreflexia
7. hypothalamus
8. interneuron

9. neuralgia
10. neurotransmitter
11. meningitis
12. anesthesia

The Urinary System

CASE STUDY

	Patient Name	DOB	Allergies
	Peter Smith	03/28/1946	NKA
	Attending	**MRN**	**Other Information**
	Paul F. Buckwalter, MD	00-AA-003	Today's Vital Signs BP: 138/92 R: 18 P: 84 T: 101.2°

Peter Smith is a male patient with mild Type 2 diabetes. He states that he has needed to urinate more frequently during

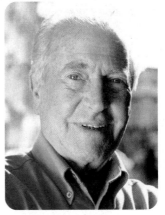

©Image Source/Getty Images

the last 2 weeks, and he feels a burning sensation when he urinates. He also has been very tired lately. Based on the vital signs you measured and Peter Smith's current complaints, the physician ordered a fasting blood glucose and a urinalysis.

Keep Peter Smith in mind as you study the chapter. There will be questions at the end of the chapter based on the case study. The information in the chapter will help you answer these questions.

LEARNING OUTCOMES

After completing Chapter 30, you will be able to:

30.1 Describe the structure, location, and functions of the kidneys.

30.2 Explain how nephrons filter blood and form urine.

30.3 Compare the locations, structures, and functions of the ureters, bladder, and urethra.

30.4 Describe the causes, signs and symptoms, diagnosis, and treatments of various diseases and disorders of the urinary system.

KEY TERMS

Bowman's capsule
detrusor muscle
distal convoluted tubule
glomerulus
hilum
lithotripsy
loop of Henle
metabolic wastes
micturition
nephrons
proximal convoluted tubule

renal columns
renal corpuscle
renal cortex
renal medulla
renal pelvis
renal pyramids
renal sinus
renal tubule
trigone
ureters
urethra

CAAHEP

I.C.1 Describe structural organization of the human body

I.C.2 Identify body systems

I.C.4 List major organs in each body system

I.C.5 Identify the anatomical location of major organs in each body system

I.C.6 Compare structure and function of the human body across the life span

I.C.7 Describe the normal function of each body system

I.C.8 Identify common pathology related to each body system including:
  (a) signs
  (b) symptoms
  (c) etiology

I.C.9 Analyze pathology for each body system including:
  (a) diagnostic measures
  (b) treatment modalities

V.C.9 Identify medical terms labeling the word parts

V.C.10 Define medical terms and abbreviations related to all body systems

ABHES

2. **Anatomy and Physiology**
  a. List all body systems and their structures and functions
  b. Describe common diseases, symptoms, and etiologies as they apply to each system
  c. Identify diagnostic and treatment modalities as they relate to each body system

3. **Medical Terminology**
  a. Define and use the entire basic structure of medical terminology and be able to accurately identify the correct context (i.e., root, prefix, suffix, combinations, spelling, and definitions)
  b. Build and dissect medical terminology from roots and suffixes to understand the word element combinations
  c. Apply medical terminology for each specialty
  d. Define and use medical abbreviations when appropriate and acceptable

▶ Introduction

The organs of the urinary system are the kidneys, ureters, urinary bladder, and urethra (see Figure 30-1). This system removes waste products from the bloodstream. These waste products are excreted from the body in the form of urine. **Nephrons** are microscopic structures within the kidneys that filter blood, remove waste products, and form urine.

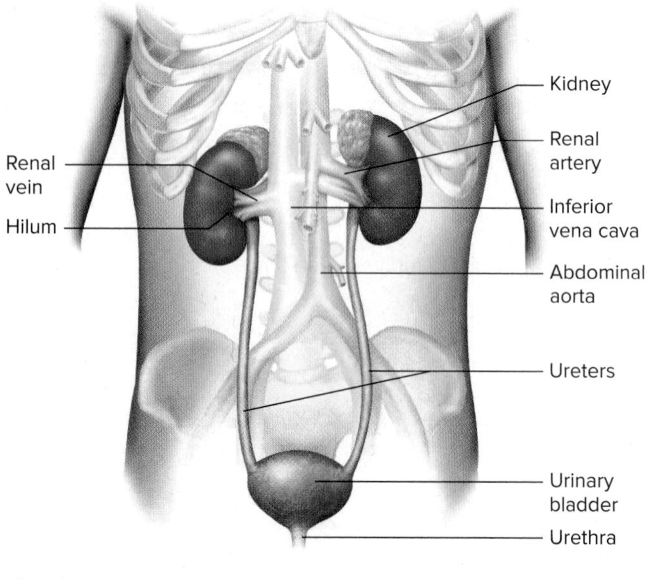

▶ The Kidneys   LO 30.1

The kidneys remove metabolic waste products from the blood. **Metabolic wastes** are the waste products produced during normal body operations such as converting food into a form that is usable by the body cells for energy. In the kidneys, metabolic wastes are combined with water and ions to form urine, which is excreted from the body. The kidneys also secrete the hormone *erythropoietin,* which stimulates the red bone marrow to produce red blood cells, and the hormone *renin,* which helps to regulate blood pressure. All three of these functions are important in maintaining the body's internal environment at homeostasis, which is a balanced, stable state within the body.

The kidneys are reddish-brown, bean-shaped organs that measure about 3.54 to 5 inches (9 to 12 centimeters) in adults. Tough, fibrous capsules cover them. (See Figure 30-2.) The kidneys are *retroperitoneal* in position, which means they lie behind the peritoneal cavity. They lie on either side of the vertebral column at about the level of the lumbar vertebrae; the left kidney is slightly higher than the right, which is displaced by the liver.

FIGURE 30-1 Organs of the urinary system.

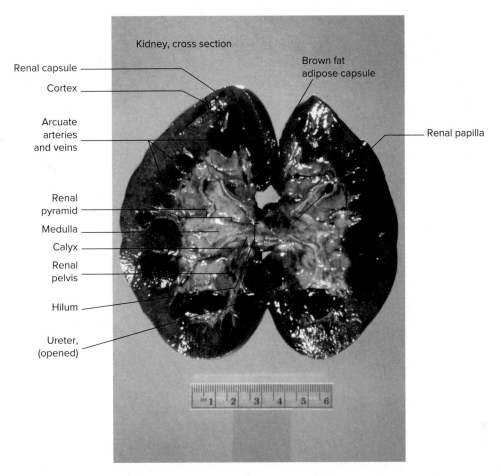

Kidney, cross section

Renal capsule
Cortex
Arcuate arteries and veins
Renal pyramid
Medulla
Calyx
Renal pelvis
Hilum
Ureter, (opened)

Brown fat adipose capsule
Renal papilla

FIGURE 30-2 Cross-section of a human kidney.
©Southern Illinois University/Science Source

The surface area of the concave depression of the kidney is called the **renal sinus**. The renal artery, renal vein, and ureter enter the kidney here in the area known as the **hilum**. The ureter is the tube that drains urine from the kidney, carrying it to the bladder. Inside the kidney, the same area is called the **renal pelvis**, formed by the expansion of the ureter inside the kidney. The renal pelvis further divides into small tubes known as *calyces* (*calyx* is the singular).

The outermost layer of the kidney is the **renal cortex** and the middle portion is the **renal medulla** (see Figure 30-3). The renal medulla is divided into triangular-shaped areas called **renal pyramids**. The renal cortex covers the pyramids and dips down between them. The portions of the cortex located between pyramids are called **renal columns**.

Blood enters the kidney through the renal artery and goes through the filtration process explained in the next section. It then exits the kidney via the renal vein.

Nephrons

Nephrons remove waste products from the blood. Each kidney contains about 1 million nephrons, which are located in the renal medulla. Nephrons are made up of a **renal corpuscle** and a **renal tubule** (see Figure 30-3). A renal corpuscle is composed of a mass of capillaries called a **glomerulus**; the capsule that surrounds the glomerulus is called the **Bowman's capsule**, or *glomerular capsule*. Blood filtration occurs in the renal corpuscle.

Renal tubules extend from the Bowman's capsule of a nephron. The three parts of a renal tubule are the **proximal convoluted tubule**, the **loop of Henle** (*nephron loop*), and the **distal convoluted tubule** (see Figure 30-4). The proximal convoluted tubule is directly attached to the Bowman's capsule and eventually straightens out to become the loop of Henle. The loop of Henle curves back toward the renal corpuscle and starts to twist again, becoming the distal convoluted tubule. Distal convoluted tubules from several nephrons merge to form collecting ducts. These ducts collect urine and deliver it to the renal pelvis, which in turn empties the urine into the ureters.

Afferent arterioles take blood to the tightly packed capillaries of the glomeruli. This narrowing causes the filtration of the blood. The blood is forced through the capillary walls, similar to what occurs when water drips through a coffee filter in a drip coffee-maker. Efferent arterioles deliver blood to *peritubular capillaries,* which are wrapped around the renal tubules of the nephron. Blood leaves the peritubular capillaries through the venules and veins of the kidneys. By the time the blood leaves the peritubular capillaries, it has been cleansed of waste products. Blood flows through a nephron in the following pathway:

afferent arteriole → glomerulus → efferent arteriole → peritubular capillaries → venules and veins of the kidney

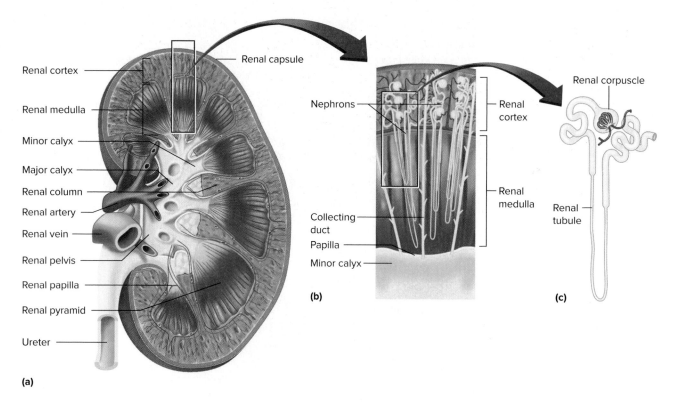

FIGURE 30-3 (a) Longitudinal section of a kidney, (b) the location of nephrons, and (c) a single nephron.

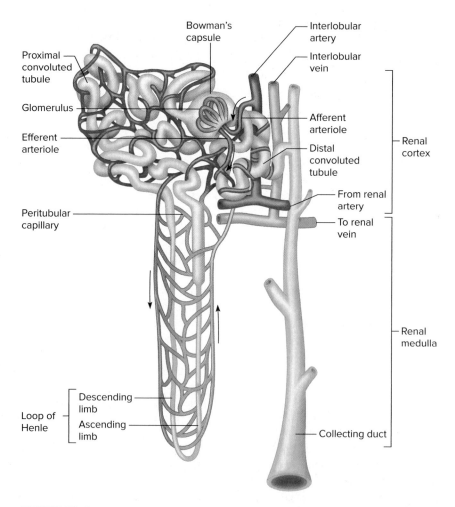

FIGURE 30-4 Structure of a nephron and its associated blood vessels.

▶ Urine Formation

LO 30.2

The three processes of urine formation are glomerular filtration, tubular reabsorption, and tubular secretion.

Glomerular Filtration

Glomerular filtration takes place in the renal corpuscles of nephrons. In this process, the fluid part of blood is forced from the glomerulus (the capillaries) into Bowman's capsule (see Figure 30-5). The fluid in Bowman's capsule is called the *glomerular filtrate.*

Glomerular filtration depends on filtration pressure, which is the pressure that forces substances (filtrate) out of the glomerulus into Bowman's capsule. Filtration pressure is largely determined by blood pressure. If a person's blood pressure is too low, glomerular filtrate will not form. If the blood pressure increases, filtration pressure also increases, causing the rate of filtration and the amount of glomerular filtrate to increase as well.

The sympathetic branch of the autonomic nervous system largely controls the rate of filtration. If blood pressure or blood volume drops, the sympathetic nervous system causes the afferent arterioles in the kidneys to constrict. When this constriction occurs, glomerular filtration pressure decreases and less glomerular filtrate is formed. When less glomerular filtrate is formed, less urine is ultimately formed. This allows the body to retain fluids that are needed to raise blood pressure and blood volume.

Tubular Reabsorption

Tubular reabsorption is the second process in urine formation. In this process, the glomerular filtrate flows into the proximal convoluted tubule (see Figure 30-6a). The body needs to keep many of the substances (nutrients, water, and ions) that are found in glomerular filtrate. In tubular reabsorption, all the substances to be kept pass through the wall of the renal tubule into the blood of the peritubular capillaries.

Water reabsorption varies depending on the level of two hormones: antidiuretic hormone (ADH) and aldosterone. Both of these hormones increase water reabsorption, which decreases urine production. This fluid retention and the resultant increase in blood pressure is one of the reasons diuretics, which rid the body of excess fluid, are successful in treating some forms of hypertension.

Tubular Secretion

Tubular secretion is the third process of urine formation. In tubular secretion, substances move from the blood in the peritubular capillaries into the renal tubules (see Figure 30-6b). Substances that are secreted include drugs, hydrogen ions, and waste products, all of which will be excreted in the urine.

Urine Composition

The final solution that reaches the collecting ducts of the kidneys is urine. Urine is mostly made of water but also normally contains urea, uric acid, trace amounts of amino acids, and various ions. *Urea* and *uric acid* are waste products formed by the breakdown of proteins and nucleic acids. The secretion of these waste materials helps maintain the body's acid-base balance.

▶ The Ureters, Urinary Bladder, and Urethra

LO 30.3

The remaining organs in the urinary system transport and store urine after it is formed in the kidneys.

The Ureters

The **ureters** are muscular tubes about 10 to 12 inches long that carry urine from the kidneys to the urinary bladder. They

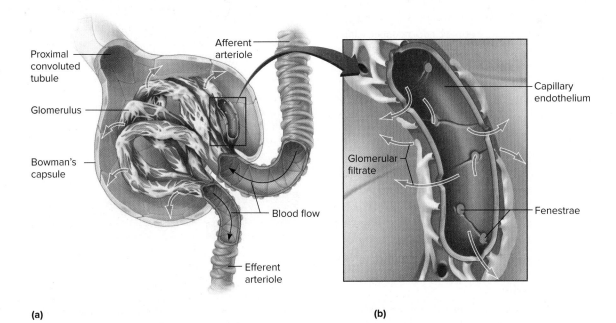

(a)

(b)

FIGURE 30-5 Glomerular filtration. (a) Substances move out of glomerular capillaries and into Bowman's capsule. (b) Glomerular capillaries have large holes called *fenestrae* that allow substances to move out of them and into Bowman's capsule.

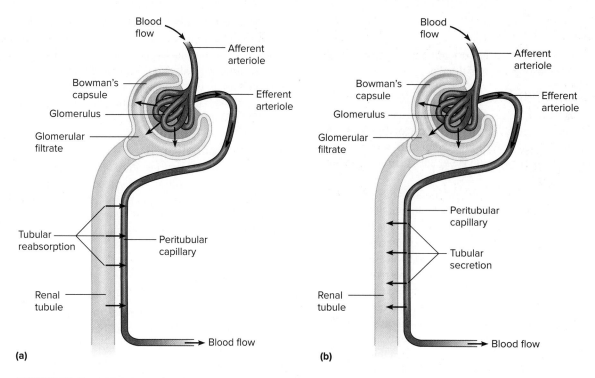

FIGURE 30-6 (a) Tubular reabsorption. Substances move from the glomerular filtrate into the blood of peritubular capillaries. (b) Tubular secretion. Substances move out of the blood of the peritubular capillaries into the renal tubule.

propel urine toward the bladder through rhythmic muscular contractions of the ureters called *peristalsis.*

The Urinary Bladder

The urinary bladder is a distensible (expandable) organ located in the pelvic cavity. Its function is to store urine (up to 600 mL on average) until it is eliminated from the body. The internal floor of the bladder contains three openings—one for the urethra and two for the ureters. These three openings form a triangle called the **trigone** of the bladder. The wall of the bladder contains smooth muscle, called the **detrusor muscle**. This muscle contracts to push urine from the bladder into the urethra (see Figure 30-7).

Micturition is the process of urination. The stretching of the bladder triggers this process—usually when the bladder contains approximately 150 mL of urine. The major events of micturition are the following:

1. The urinary bladder distends as it fills with urine.
2. The distension stimulates stretch receptors in the bladder wall, which sends a nerve impulse to the spinal cord.
3. Parasympathetic nerves stimulate the detrusor muscle, which begins rhythmic contractions that trigger the sense of the need to urinate.
4. The brainstem and cerebral cortex send impulses to voluntarily contract the external urethral sphincter and to inhibit the micturition impulse.
5. Upon the decision to urinate, the external urethral sphincter is relaxed and impulses from the pons and hypothalamus start the micturition reflex.

6. Contraction of the detrusor muscle occurs and urine is expelled through the urethra.

The Urethra

The **urethra** is a tube that moves urine from the bladder to the outside world. In females, the urethra is only about 1 to 1.5 inches long, which is much shorter than in males (about 8 inches long). This anatomical difference, combined with the fact that the anus, vagina, and urethra are in close proximity in females, makes females much more susceptible to urinary tract infections (UTIs).

Medical terms are built and dissected using prefixes, word roots/combining form, and suffixes. For example, we can build the term *urospasm* by placing the parts of the term in the puzzle pieces where P = prefix, WR/CF = word root or combining form, and S = suffix.

urospasm

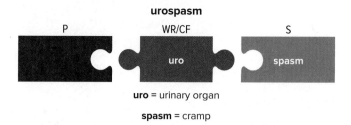

uro = urinary organ

spasm = cramp

Urospasm is a cramp of of an urinary organ such as the bladder. Learn additional medical terms in the **Medical Terminology Practice** section at the end of this chapter.

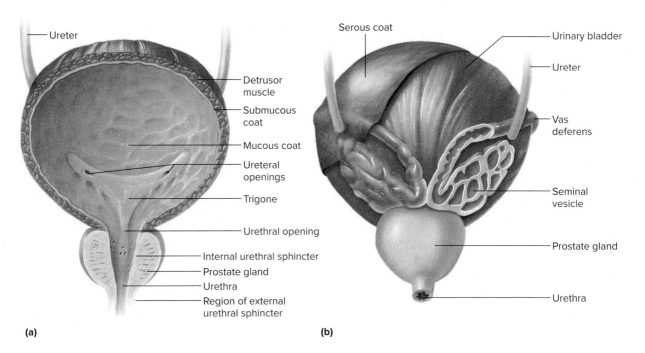

FIGURE 30-7 Male urinary bladder: (a) anterior view and (b) posterior view.

PATHOPHYSIOLOGY

LO 30.4

Common Diseases and Disorders of the Urinary System

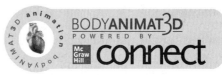

Go to CONNECT to see an animation exercise about *Renal Function.*

ACUTE KIDNEY (RENAL) FAILURE is a sudden loss of kidney function.

Causes. There are many causes and risk factors of kidney failure, including burns, dehydration, low blood pressure, hemorrhaging, allergic reactions, obstruction of the renal artery, various poisons, alcohol abuse, trauma to the kidneys and skeletal muscles, blood disorders, blood transfusion reactions, kidney stones, urinary tract infections, enlarged prostate, childbirth, immune system disorders, and food poisoning involving the bacterium *E. coli.*

Signs and Symptoms. The signs and symptoms include decreased or no urine production, excessive urination, swelling of the extremities, bloating, mental confusion, coma, seizures, hand tremors, nosebleeds, easy bruising, pain in the back or abdomen, hypertension, abnormal heart or lung sounds, abnormal urinalysis, and an increase in potassium levels.

Diagnostic Exams and Tests. Tests include a urinalysis, blood tests, and a 24-hour urine collection to check both the amount of urine the patient's body is producing and the components of the urine. Both the blood and the urine are checked for creatinine and urea levels. In some cases, a CT scan, ultrasound, or biopsy of the kidneys may be needed as well.

Treatment. The first treatment measure is modifying the diet to decrease the amount of protein consumed. Controlling fluid intake and potassium levels is recommended. Antibiotics and dialysis also may be needed. If the underlying cause can be treated, acute renal failure may be reversed and kidney function returned to normal.

CHRONIC KIDNEY (RENAL) FAILURE is a condition in which the kidneys slowly lose their ability to function. The patient may be asymptomatic until the kidneys have lost about 90% of their function.

Causes. This disorder results from diabetes, hypertension, glomerulonephritis, polycystic kidney disease, kidney stones, obstruction of the ureters, or acute kidney failure.

Signs and Symptoms. The list of signs and symptoms is extensive and includes headache, mental confusion, coma, seizures, fatigue, frequent hiccups, itching, easy bruising, abnormal bleeding, anemia, excessive thirst, fluid retention, nausea, hypertension, abnormal heart or lung sounds, weight loss, white spots on the skin or increased pigmentation, high potassium levels, an increased or decreased urine output, urinary tract infections, and abnormal urinalysis results.

Diagnostic Exams and Tests. The diagnostic tests for chronic kidney failure are similar to those for acute kidney failure. Blood and urine tests, including a 24-hour urine collection, are usually performed. In some cases, ultrasound or a CT scan is performed. A kidney biopsy may be performed as well.

Treatment. This disorder can be treated with antibiotics; blood transfusions; medications to control anemia; restriction of fluids, electrolytes, and protein; control of high blood pressure; and

Preventing Urinary Cystitis in Women

Urinary cystitis and other UTIs can cause pain (dysuria), urgency, and frequency of urination. Because the female anatomy makes women more prone to these problems, educate your female patients to take these steps:

1. *Urinate when the urge occurs.* When you "hold it," urine stays in the bladder and the upper urethra, allowing bacteria to grow and cause infection.

2. *Drink lots of clear fluids.* This is known as "pushing fluids." The more clear liquids you drink, the more urine is created and the system is flushed on a regular basis. Cranberry juice is highly recommended as a preventive fluid, as well as part of the treatment if infection does occur.

3. *Wipe front to back.* Teach your female patients they should wipe "front to back" after a bowel movement.

Doing so prevents contamination of both the vagina and urethra by gastrointestinal (GI) bacteria such as *E. coli.* Maintaining excellent hygiene in the perineal area is an important component of UTI and cystitis prevention.

4. *Urinate after sexual intercourse.* Explain to your sexually active patients that urinating immediately after sexual intercourse also will help prevent episodes of cystitis. The urine will flush out contamination that could enter the bladder, causing an infection.

If cystitis or UTI does strike despite preventive methods, reassure your patient that antibiotics and lots of fluids should take care of the problem. If the patient suffers from more than three infections during a year, a urologic workup may be advisable to look for underlying anatomical anomalies.

---

dialysis. The most serious cases may require surgery to repair a ureteral obstruction or a kidney (renal) transplant.

CYSTITIS is a urinary bladder infection. Women are much more likely to develop this disorder than men because of the short length of their urethras. The urethral opening in women is also close to the anal opening, allowing bacteria from this area to be more easily introduced into the urinary tract. For more information on preventing urinary cystitis in women, see the *Educating the Patient* feature.

Causes. This infection is caused by various types of bacteria (especially those found in the rectum), as well as by the placement of a catheter in the bladder. Good hygiene, urinating promptly when the urge occurs, and, for females, wiping from front to back can help to prevent this infection.

Signs and Symptoms. Common symptoms include fatigue; chills; fever; and a painful, frequent need to urinate, often with only small amounts of urine produced. Urine is often cloudy, and blood may be present in the urine.

Diagnostic Exams and Tests. A urinalysis is ordered to look for blood or bacteria in the urine. If bacteria are found, a urine culture is performed to identify the bacteria. In some cases, if a patient has had multiple infections, a cystoscopy is performed to examine the urethra and bladder. Cystoscopy allows the practitioner to look for disease and also take a biopsy if indicated.

Treatment. This infection is treated with antibiotics and, when needed, pain medication. The patient also should be urged to drink lots of clear liquids.

GLOMERULONEPHRITIS is an inflammation of the glomeruli of the kidney. Chronic glomerulonephritis is one of the causes of chronic renal failure.

Causes. This disorder is caused by renal diseases, immune disorders, and bacterial infections.

Signs and Symptoms. The signs and symptoms are hiccups, drowsiness, coma, seizures, nausea, anemia, high blood pressure, increased skin pigmentation, abnormal heart sounds, abnormal urinalysis results, blood in the urine, and a decreased or increased urine output.

Diagnostic Exams and Tests. The first indication of glomerulonephritis usually shows up in a urinalysis. Red or white blood cells in the urine require further diagnosis. Blood tests are then ordered to check the level of urea (blood urea nitrogen or BUN) and creatinine in the blood. In some cases, an X-ray or CT scan may be performed to rule out damage to the kidney. See Figure 30-8. However, the final diagnosis is usually made after biopsy of the kidney.

Treatment. Treatment begins with a low-sodium, low-protein diet. Medications to control high blood pressure, corticosteroids to reduce inflammation, and dialysis are other treatment options.

INCONTINENCE is a temporary or long-lasting condition in which a person (other than a child) cannot control urination. Women are more likely to develop incontinence than men are.

Causes. This condition can be caused by various medications, excessive coughing (for example, in smokers), UTIs, nervous system disorders, and bladder cancer. In men, prostate problems can lead to the development of this disorder. Weakness of the urinary sphincters from surgery, trauma, or pregnancy also can cause incontinence. It may be prevented by avoiding urinary bladder irritants such as coffee, cigarettes, diuretics, and various medications.

Signs and Symptoms. The primary symptom is the involuntary leakage of urine.

Diagnostic Exams and Tests. Diagnosis concentrates on determining the type of or cause for the incontinence. The physician conducts a history and physical exam, followed by a urinalysis. The patient may be asked to keep a "bladder diary"

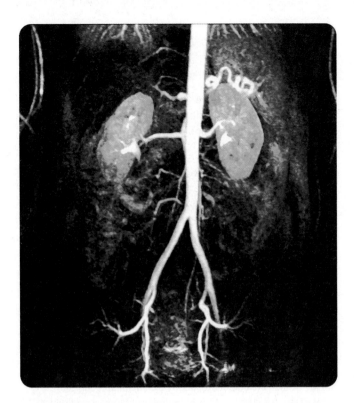

FIGURE 30-8 An X-ray may be used to check for kidney damage.
©Miriam Maslo/SPL/Getty Images

to help pinpoint the symptoms and causes. In some cases, a post-void residual measurement is performed to determine how much urine is left in the bladder after the patient urinates.

Treatment. Treatment depends on the reason for the incontinence and may include various medications, incontinence pads, removal of the prostate, Kegel exercises to increase the control of urinary sphincters, and surgery to repair damaged bladders or urethral sphincters.

POLYCYSTIC KIDNEY DISEASE is a disorder in which the kidneys enlarge because they are filled with cysts. The disease develops relatively slowly, with symptoms worsening over time.

Causes. The causes are hereditary (via an inherited dominant gene from a parent).

Signs and Symptoms. Fatigue, hypertension, anemia, pain in the back or abdomen, joint pain, heart murmurs, the formation of kidney stones, kidney failure, blood in the urine, and liver disease are the symptoms of this disorder.

Diagnostic Exams and Tests. Tests are performed to find out how many cysts are present, as well as how much healthy kidney tissue is present. These tests usually include an ultrasound, CT scan, or, in some cases, an MRI.

Treatment. Treatment includes medications to control anemia and high blood pressure, blood transfusions, draining of the cysts, dialysis, and surgery to remove one or both kidneys.

PYELONEPHRITIS is a complicated UTI. It begins as a bladder infection and spreads to one or both kidneys. This condition can develop suddenly, or it may be chronic.

Causes. This disorder is caused by bacteria, a bladder infection, kidney stones, or an obstruction of the urinary system ducts.

Signs and Symptoms. Signs and symptoms include fatigue, mental confusion, fever, nausea, pain in the back or abdomen, enlarged kidneys, painful urination, and cloudy or bloody urine.

Diagnostic Exams and Tests. Both urine and blood cultures may be performed to identify causative microorganisms. In addition, ultrasound or a CT scan may be ordered. A voiding cystourethrogram also is ordered in some cases. In this test, an X-ray is taken while the patient has a full bladder and again while the patient is urinating.

Treatment. Treatment includes intravenous fluids, pain medication, and antibiotics.

RENAL CALCULI are commonly called *kidney stones.* They can become lodged in the ducts within the kidneys or ureters, causing more severe disorders such as pyelonephritis and chronic kidney failure.

Causes. This condition is caused by gouty arthritis, defects of the ureters, overly concentrated urine, and UTIs.

Signs and Symptoms. The signs and symptoms include fever, nausea, severe back or abdominal pain, a frequent urge to urinate, blood in the urine, and abnormal urinalysis results.

Diagnostic Exams and Tests. Tests include blood tests for calcium and uric acid levels, as well as one or more 24-hour urine collections. X-rays, ultrasound, an intravenous pyelogram, or specialized CT scans may be performed. The practitioner also may send stones the patient has passed to a laboratory for analysis.

Treatment. Treatment includes pain medication, intravenous fluids, medications to decrease stone formation, surgery to remove kidney stones, and **lithotripsy** (a procedure that uses shock waves to break up stones).

OUTCOME	KEY POINTS
30.1 **Describe the structure, location, and functions of the kidneys.**	The retroperitoneal kidneys are composed of the outer renal cortex and inner renal medulla. Their function is to remove metabolic wastes from the body.
30.2 **Explain how nephrons filter blood and form urine.**	A nephron is a single kidney cell. It is composed of a renal corpuscle, which consists of the glomerulus and the Bowman's capsule, and the renal tubule, which has three parts: the proximal convoluted tubule, the loop of Henle, and the distal convoluted tubule. The nephrons filter blood and form urine through three consecutive processes: glomerular filtration, tubular reabsorption, and tubular secretion.
30.3 **Compare the locations, structures, and functions of the ureters, bladder, and urethra.**	The ureters are long tubes extending from each renal pelvis that bring urine to the bladder for storage. The urethra is the muscular tube extending from the bladder that transports urine to be expelled from the body.
30.4 **Describe the causes, signs and symptoms, diagnosis, and treatments of various diseases and disorders of the urinary system.**	There are many common diseases and disorders of the urinary system with varied signs, symptoms, diagnosis, and treatments. Some of these include acute kidney (renal) failure, chronic kidney (renal) failure, cystitis, glomerulonephritis, incontinence, polycystic kidney disease, pyelonephritis, and renal calculi.

CASE STUDY CRITICAL THINKING

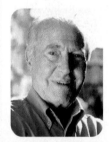

©Image Source/Getty Images

Recall Peter Smith from the case study at the beginning of the chapter. Now that you have completed the chapter, answer the following questions regarding his case.

1. What is the likely diagnosis for Peter Smith?
2. Why did the physician order both a urinalysis and a blood glucose test?
3. Why might Peter Smith's vital signs show that his temperature is slightly elevated?
4. Based on the laboratory test results, the physician prescribed an antibiotic for Peter Smith. What can you advise Peter Smith to do in addition to taking the antibiotic as prescribed?

EXAM PREPARATION QUESTIONS

1. (LO 30.4) _____ is a complicated UTI that begins as a bladder infection and spreads to one or both kidneys.
   a. Cystitis
   b. Glomerulonephritis
   c. Pyelonephritis
   d. Polycystic kidney disease
   e. Chronic renal failure

2. (LO 30.2) In which of the following processes do substances move into the renal tubules?
   a. Glomerular filtration
   b. Tubular secretion
   c. Tubular reabsorption
   d. Micturition
   e. Urination

3. (LO 30.2) Distal convoluted tubules from several nephrons merge together to form the
   a. Bowman's capsule
   b. Glomerulus
   c. Loop of Henle
   d. Collecting ducts
   e. Renal pyramids

4. (LO 30.2) Water reabsorption amounts vary depending on which two hormones?
   a. ADH and aldosterone
   b. ADH and erythropoietin
   c. Aldosterone and renin
   d. Angiotensin and ADH
   e. Erythropoietin and renin

5. (LO 30.1) _____ is the hormone from the kidneys that stimulates the bone marrow to produce RBCs.
   a. Renin
   b. ADH
   c. Aldosterone
   d. Hematopoietin
   e. Erythropoietin

6. (LO 30.1) The outermost layer of the kidney is the renal
   a. Cortex
   b. Pelvis
   c. Medulla
   d. Tubule
   e. Sinus

7. (LO 30.1) The _____ is the structure that surrounds the glomerulus.
   a. Loop of Henle
   b. Proximal convoluted tubule
   c. Distal convoluted tubule
   d. Bowman's capsule
   e. Renal pyramid

8. (LO 30.2) The rate of glomerular filtration is controlled mainly by the
   a. Blood pressure
   b. Sympathetic branch of the autonomic nervous system
   c. Somatic nervous system
   d. Parasympathetic branch of the autonomic nervous system
   e. Central nervous system

9. (LO 30.2) Which of the following is *not* a normal component of urine?
   a. Water
   b. Ions
   c. Glucose
   d. Uric acid
   e. Urea

10. (LO 30.3) The _____ is a triangular area formed by the urethral and ureteral openings into the bladder.
    a. Detrusor muscle
    b. Renal pyramid
    c. Trigone
    d. Hilum
    e. Calyx

M E D I C A L   T E R M I N O L O G Y   P R A C T I C E

Analyze the following medical terms, presented throughout the chapter. Using a medical dictionary (or Appendix I), place a / mark between each word part. Define each word part and then define the whole word.

EXAMPLE: **nephro/logy** = nephro means "kidney" + logy means "study of"
NEPHROLOGY means "study of the kidney."

1. antidiuretic
2. cystitis
3. dysuria
4. erythropoietin
5. glomerulonephritis
6. lithotripsy
7. nephritis
8. peristalsis
9. peritubular
10. pyelonephritis
11. retroperitoneal
12. uric

The Reproductive Systems

CASE STUDY

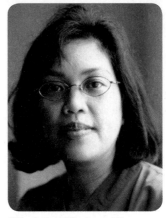

©ERproductions Ltd/Blend Images LLC

Raja Lautu has come to the office complaining of vaginal itching and a greenish vaginal discharge with a "fishy" smell. She is sexually active and recently changed partners, but she says her partner has no symptoms. Dr. Williams obtains a vaginal fluid specimen and sends it to the lab for testing.

Keep Raja in mind as you study the chapter. There will be questions at the end of the chapter based on the case study. The information in the chapter will help you answer these questions.

LEARNING OUTCOMES

After completing Chapter 31, you will be able to:

31.1 Summarize the organs of the male reproductive system, including the locations, structures, and functions of each.

31.2 Describe the causes, signs and symptoms, diagnosis, and treatment of various disorders of the male reproductive system.

31.3 Summarize the organs of the female reproductive system, including the locations, structures, and functions of each.

31.4 Describe the causes, signs and symptoms, diagnosis, and treatment of various disorders of the female reproductive system.

31.5 Explain the process of pregnancy, including fertilization, the prenatal period, and fetal circulation.

31.6 Describe the birth process, including the postnatal period.

31.7 Compare several birth control methods and their effectiveness.

31.8 Explain the causes of and treatments for infertility.

31.9 Describe the causes, signs and symptoms, diagnosis, and treatments of the most common sexually transmitted infections.

KEY TERMS

amnion
APGAR
Bartholin's glands
blastocyst
bulbourethral glands
Cowper's glands
ductus arteriosus
ductus venosus
embryo
fetus
foramen ovale

infundibulum
menarche
menopause
oogenesis
ovulation
placenta
primary germ layers
seminiferous tubules
spermatogenesis
testes
zygote

▶ Introduction

The male and female reproductive systems function together to produce offspring. The female reproductive system nurtures a developing offspring. If a female breast-feeds, her breasts, considered accessory organs of both her reproductive and integumentary systems, are used to nurture the newborn baby. The male and female reproductive systems also produce a number of important hormones before and during the reproductive years.

▶ The Male Reproductive System   LO 31.1

The male reproductive system is responsible for developing sperm. Accessory organs also produce substances that provide an environment for the sperm that allows them to reach the female ova (eggs).

Testes

Testes are considered the primary organs of the male reproductive system because they produce the male sex cells (sperm) (see Figure 31-1). They also produce the male hormone *testosterone*. Most males have two testes that are held just below the pelvic cavity in the *scrotum*. During the fetal stage, the testes develop in the abdominopelvic cavity of the fetus. Shortly before or soon after birth, the testes descend into the scrotal sac. A fibrous capsule encloses each testis and invades the testis to divide it into lobules. Each lobule is filled with **seminiferous tubules,** which are filled with *spermatogenic cells*. These cells give rise to sperm cells. Between the seminiferous tubules are the *interstitial cells,* which are the cells within the testes that produce testosterone.

Sperm Cell Formation Spermatogenic cells of the seminiferous tubules begin the process of making sperm cells, but the sperm cells do not mature until they travel to the *epididymis*. **Spermatogenesis** is the process of sperm cell formation. At the beginning of spermatogenesis, the cells are called *spermatogonia*. Spermatogonia contain 46 chromosomes. These cells undergo mitosis, as discussed and shown in the *Organization of the Body* chapter, and the resulting cells are called *primary spermatocytes*. Primary spermatocytes also contain 46 chromosomes. At about the time of puberty, primary spermatocytes undergo a process called *meiosis* (see Figures 31-2 and 31-3a). In meiosis, each primary spermatocyte divides to make two secondary

Medical terms are built and dissected using prefixes, word roots/combining form, and suffixes. For example, we can build the term *spermatogenesis* by placing the parts of the term in the puzzle pieces where P = prefix, WR/CF = word root or combining form, and S = suffix.

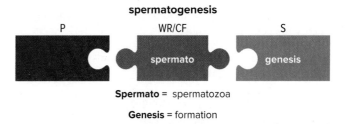

spermatogenesis

P   WR/CF   S

spermato   genesis

Spermato = spermatozoa

Genesis = formation

Spermatogenesis is the formation of spermatozoa. Learn additional medical terms in the **Medical Terminology Practice** section at the end of this chapter.

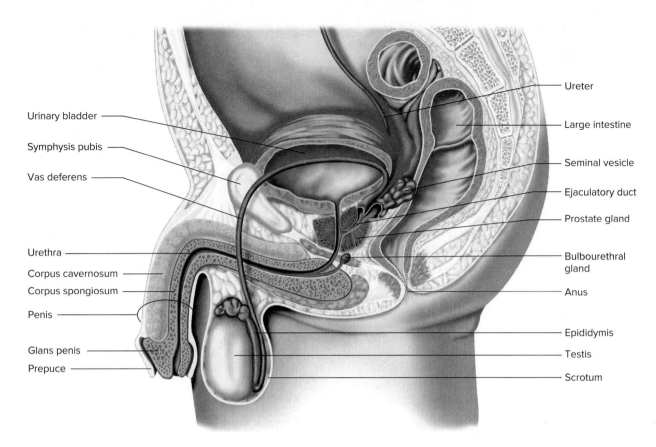

FIGURE 31-1 Sagittal view of male reproductive organs. The male reproductive system produces sperm and delivers them in a form that keeps them viable long enough to fertilize an ovum.

spermatocytes. Each secondary spermatocyte divides to make two *spermatids.* Therefore, from one primary spermatocyte, four spermatids are formed. In the last part of spermatogenesis, called *spermiogenesis,* the spermatids develop flagella to become mature sperm cells. Each sperm cell contains only 23 chromosomes.

Structure of Sperm Cells A mature sperm (see Figure 31-3b) has the following three parts: the head, the midpiece, and the tail.

The Head The head is oval and holds a nucleus with 23 chromosomes. The head is covered with an enzyme-filled sac called an *acrosome,* which helps the sperm penetrate an ovum at the time of fertilization.

The Midpiece This portion of the sperm is between the head and tail. It is filled with mitochondria that generate the energy the cell needs to move.

The Tail The tail is a flagellum that propels the sperm forward in the female reproductive tract.

Internal Accessory Organs of the Male Reproductive System

The internal accessory organs of the male reproductive system are the epididymis; vas deferens; seminal vesicles; prostate gland; and bulbourethral, or Cowper's, glands.

Epididymis An epididymis sits on top of each testis. It is a highly coiled tube that receives spermatids from seminiferous tubules as the spermatids are formed. Inside the epididymis, spermatids mature to become sperm cells.

Vas Deferens A tube called a *vas deferens* is connected to each epididymis. These tubes carry sperm cells from the epididymis to the urethra in the male pelvic cavity. When a male has a vasectomy, these tubes are cut and tied to prevent sperm from reaching the ovum.

Seminal Vesicles Seminal vesicles are sac-like organs that secrete an alkaline *seminal fluid* that is rich in sugars and *prostaglandins.* Sperm cells use the sugars to make energy and the prostaglandins stimulate muscular contractions in the female reproductive system. These muscular contractions, known as *peristalsis,* help to propel sperm forward in the female reproductive tract. Seminal vesicles release their product into the vas deferens just before ejaculation. Seminal fluid makes up approximately 60% of semen volume.

Prostate Gland The muscular prostate gland surrounds the proximal portion of the urethra. It produces a milky, alkaline fluid and secretes this fluid into the urethra just before ejaculation. The alkaline nature of this fluid helps to protect the sperm when they enter the acidic environment of the female vagina.

First Meiotic Division (Meiosis I)

Second Meiotic Division (Meiosis II)
(continued from the bottom of previous column)

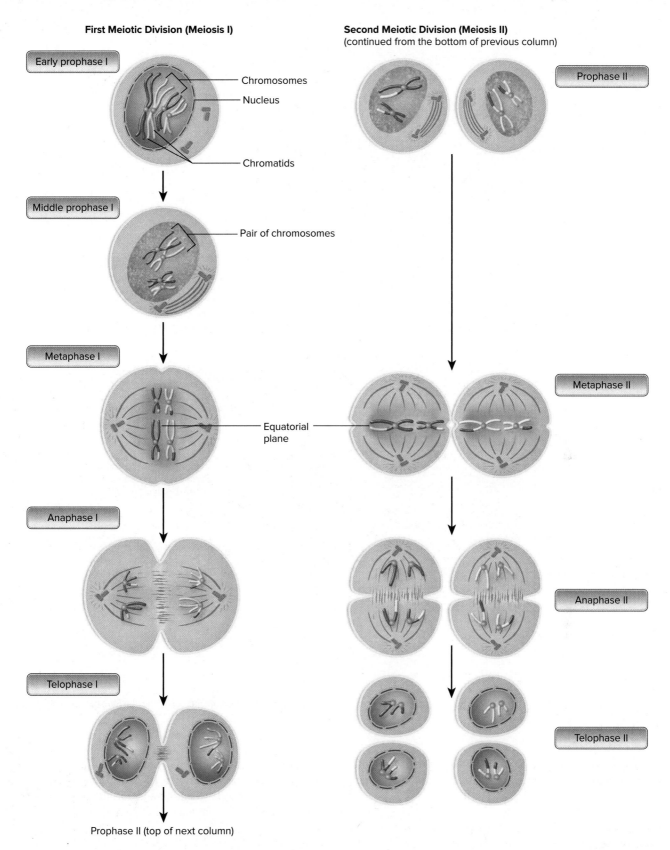

Early prophase I

Chromosomes

Nucleus

Chromatids

Middle prophase I

Pair of chromosomes

Metaphase I

Equatorial plane

Anaphase I

Telophase I

Prophase II (top of next column)

Prophase II

Metaphase II

Anaphase II

Telophase II

FIGURE 31-2 The process of meiosis, including prophase, metaphase, anaphase, and telophase.

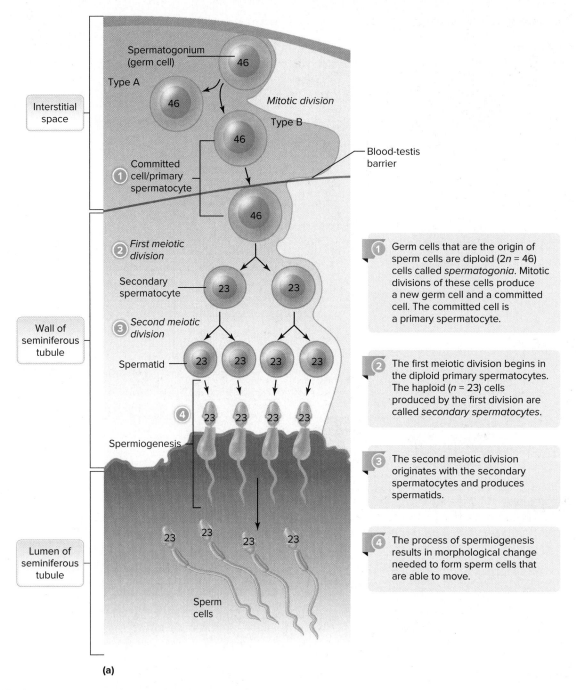

FIGURE 31-3 Spermatogenesis: (a) The process of spermatogenesis takes place in the wall of the seminiferous tubule. (b) Structural changes occur as a sperm cell forms from a spermatid.

The callout labels within the figure read:

Spermatogonium (germ cell)

Type A

Interstitial space

Mitotic division

Type B

Blood-testis barrier

① Committed cell/primary spermatocyte

② First meiotic division

Secondary spermatocyte

③ Second meiotic division

Wall of seminiferous tubule

Spermatid

④ Spermiogenesis

Lumen of seminiferous tubule

Sperm cells

(a)

① Germ cells that are the origin of sperm cells are diploid (2n = 46) cells called *spermatogonia*. Mitotic divisions of these cells produce a new germ cell and a committed cell. The committed cell is a primary spermatocyte.

② The first meiotic division begins in the diploid primary spermatocytes. The haploid (n = 23) cells produced by the first division are called *secondary spermatocytes*.

③ The second meiotic division originates with the secondary spermatocytes and produces spermatids.

④ The process of spermiogenesis results in morphological change needed to form sperm cells that are able to move.

Prostatic fluid makes up approximately 40% of semen volume. During ejaculation, the muscular contractions of the prostate help expel semen.

Bulbourethral Glands Bulbourethral glands, or **Cowper's glands,** are inferior to the prostate gland. They produce a mucus-like fluid that is secreted into the urethra before ejaculation. This fluid lubricates the end of the penis in preparation for sexual intercourse.

Semen Semen is a mixture of sperm cells and fluids from the seminal vesicles, prostate gland, and bulbourethral glands.

This alkaline mixture contains nutrients and prostaglandins. Total semen volume is between 1.5 and 5.0 mL per ejaculate, with a sperm count between 40 and 250 million/mL. A normal sperm count is more than 80 million.

External Organs of the Male Reproductive System

The two male external reproductive organs are the scrotum and the penis (see Figure 31-1).

Scrotum The scrotum is a pouch of skin that holds the testes. It is lined with a serous membrane that secretes fluid

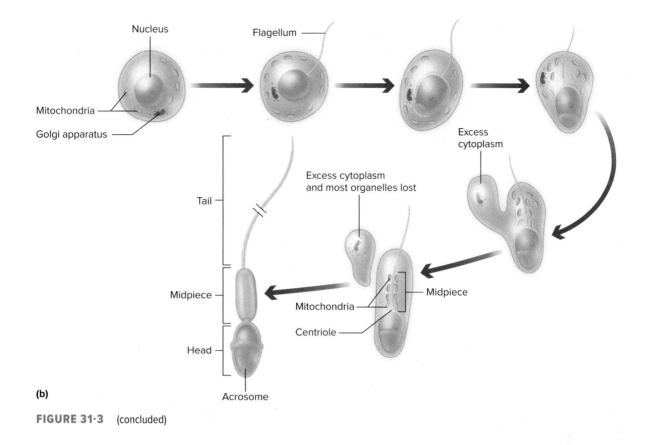

(b)

FIGURE 31-3 (concluded)

to ensure that the testes move freely within it. The scrotum holds the testes away from the body, keeping their temperature about 1 degree lower than the rest of the body, which is necessary for sperm viability.

Penis The penis is a cylindrical organ that moves urine and semen out of the body. The shaft, or body, of the penis contains specialized *erectile tissue* that surrounds the urethra, which runs the length of the penis. The end of the penis is enlarged into a cone-shaped structure called the *glans penis.* If a male has not been circumcised, a piece of skin, called the *prepuce,* covers the glans penis. The reproductive function of the penis is to deliver sperm to the female reproductive tract. The penis is also part of the urinary system because it contains the urethra, which drains urine from the bladder.

Erection, Orgasm, and Ejaculation

During sexual arousal, the parasympathetic nervous system causes erectile tissue of the penis to become engorged with blood, which produces erection of the penis. During orgasm, sperm cells are propelled out of the testes toward the urethra. The secretions of the prostate, seminal vesicles, and bulbourethral glands also are released into the urethra. The movement of the sperm and secretions into the urethra is called *emission.* The process of *ejaculation* occurs when semen is forced out of the urethra. After ejaculation, sympathetic nerve fibers cause the erectile tissue

to release blood, and the penis gradually returns to a flaccid, or nonerect, state.

Male Reproductive Hormones

The hypothalamus, the anterior pituitary gland, and the testes secrete hormones that regulate male reproductive functions. At the onset of puberty and throughout life, the hypothalamus releases a hormone called *gonadotropin-releasing hormone (GnRH).* GnRH stimulates the anterior pituitary gland to release *follicle-stimulating hormone (FSH)* and *luteinizing hormone (LH).* FSH causes spermatogenesis to begin and LH stimulates interstitial cells to produce *testosterone.*

Testosterone is responsible for the development of male secondary sex characteristics that are typically unique to males. Examples of these characteristics include chest hair, thick facial hair, a thickening and strengthening of muscles and bones, and the thickening of vocal cords that produce a deeper voice. Testosterone also stimulates the maturation of male reproductive organs.

Testosterone levels are regulated by negative feedback in the following cycle: Blood testosterone levels increase to above normal levels, which causes the hypothalamus to stop releasing GnRH. In response, the anterior pituitary stops secreting LH and FSH, in turn causing the testosterone level to fall. When the testosterone level falls below normal, GnRH is again secreted by the hypothalamus, triggering the release of LH and FSH by the anterior pituitary, and the cycle begins again.

Common Diseases and Disorders of the Male Reproductive System

BENIGN PROSTATIC HYPERTROPHY, ALSO CALLED BENIGN PROSTATIC HYPERPLASIA, OR BPH, is the nonmalignant enlargement of the prostate gland. This condition is common in older men.

Causes. BPH is related to the hormonal changes that occur as part of the aging process.

Signs and Symptoms. Men with BPH often complain of frequent urination, especially at night, as well as painful urination and difficulty starting or stopping the urinary stream, including "dribbling" at the end of urination.

Diagnostic Exams and Tests. Diagnosis often is confirmed by digital rectal exam (DRE), in which the licensed practitioner inserts a gloved finger into the rectum and palpates the prostate. Blood tests (PSA) and a biopsy may be done to rule out cancer. In some cases, more advanced tests, such as a transrectal ultrasound, cystoscopy, or CT urogram, may be ordered as well.

Treatment. Once cancer is ruled out, medications such as Avodart® or Flomax® may manage the problem, or a *transurethral resection of the prostate (TURP)* may be performed to remove the enlarged tissue.

EPIDIDYMITIS is inflammation of an epididymis. Most cases start out as an infection of the urinary tract that spreads to an epididymis.

Causes. The causes include the use of certain medications, placement of a catheter in the urethra, and bacteria—especially those that cause gonorrhea and chlamydia.

Signs and Symptoms. Signs and symptoms include fever, pain in the testes, a lump in the testes, swelling of the scrotum, painful ejaculation, blood in the semen, pain during urination, discharge from the urethra, and enlarged lymph nodes in the pelvic area.

Diagnostic Exams and Tests. A physical exam is performed to check for enlargement of lymph nodes or the testes. Tests also may be performed to rule out sexually transmitted infections such as chlamydia or gonorrhea. An ultrasound is sometimes ordered to check blood flow to the testes, in order to rule out testicular torsion.

Treatment. Treatment includes pain medication, antibiotics for both the patient and his sexual partner, elevation of the scrotum, and ice packs applied to the scrotum.

IMPOTENCE, OR ERECTILE DYSFUNCTION (ED), is a disorder in which a male cannot achieve or maintain an erect penis to complete sexual intercourse. It is estimated that half of all men between the ages of 40 and 70 years have some degree of impotence. Most causes are physical and not psychological.

Causes. Psychological causes include anxiety, stress, and depression. Common physical causes include diabetes; high blood pressure; anemia; coronary artery disease (CAD); peripheral vascular disease (PVD); low testosterone production; various medications; smoking; excessive alcohol consumption; and drugs such as cocaine, marijuana, and heroin.

Signs and Symptoms. Signs and symptoms include an inability to achieve an erection and an inability to maintain an erection long enough to complete sexual intercourse.

Diagnostic Exams and Tests. Diagnosis is usually based on a history and physical exam. If the practitioner suspects that the impotence is due to an underlying medical cause, additional tests may be ordered, including blood and urine tests for diabetes and heart disease.

Treatment. The first treatment step should be lifestyle changes to quit smoking and stop using alcohol and/or drugs. Counseling to reduce anxiety and depression also may be helpful. Other treatment options include oral medications such as Viagra® or Cialis®, penile injections of medications, and penile implants if oral medications do not work.

PROSTATE CANCER is one of the most common cancers in men older than age 40, and the risk of developing prostate cancer increases with age. Awareness about this malignancy is growing, and access to screenings such as digital rectal exam (DRE) is becoming widely available. Therefore, many cases in the United States are being diagnosed even before symptoms occur.

Causes. The causes are mostly unknown, although decreased testosterone production may contribute to the development of this disease, explaining why risk increases with age.

Diagnostic Exams and Tests. The first indication of prostate cancer may come from a DRE or a prostate-specific antigen (PSA) blood test. If either of these is abnormal, diagnostic tests include a transrectal ultrasound or a prostate biopsy.

Signs and Symptoms. Common symptoms include anemia, weight loss, incontinence, difficulty starting or stopping urination, painful urination, pain in the lower back or abdomen, pain during bowel movements, high levels of prostate-specific antigen (PSA) in the blood, blood in the urine, and bone pain in advanced cases when cancer cells have spread (metastasized) to the bone.

Treatment. Treatments include hormone therapy, chemotherapy, radiation therapy to shrink or destroy the tumor, and surgery to remove the prostate, known as prostatectomy.

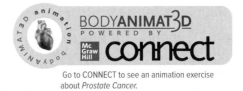

Go to CONNECT to see an animation exercise about *Prostate Cancer.*

PROSTATITIS is an inflammation of the prostate gland. If it develops suddenly, it is called *acute prostatitis.* The slow development of this condition is termed *chronic prostatitis.*

Causes. This condition can be caused by excessive alcohol consumption, bacterial infection, a catheterization, trauma to the urethra or urinary bladder, and scarring of the urethra or prostate because of frequent infections. Urinating frequently can help to prevent this infection.

Signs and Symptoms. Signs and symptoms include fever; pain in the scrotum, pelvic area, or abdomen; difficult, frequent, and/or painful urination; blood in the urine; painful ejaculation; blood in the semen; discharge from the urethra; a low sperm count; and white blood cells in urine or semen.

Diagnostic Exams and Tests. Initial diagnosis is based on a history and physical exam and tests to rule out other causes. Blood and urine tests are performed to determine whether infection is present. If prostatitis is diagnosed, additional tests are performed to determine the type of prostatitis: bacterial, nonbacterial/chronic, or inflammatory.

Treatment. This condition is treated with antibiotics if the cause is bacterial. Surgery also may be required to repair any damage to the urethra.

TESTICULAR CANCER is a malignant growth in one or both testicles. Unlike prostate cancer, which tends to occur in older males, testicular cancer occurs in males ages 15 to 30 and is a much more aggressive malignancy.

Causes. Predisposing factors include cryptorchidism (undescended testicles during infancy). Family history also may be a factor.

Signs and Symptoms. A hard, painless lump in one testicle is a common early symptom. Patients may complain of groin or abdominal pain as the disease progresses.

Diagnostic Exams and Tests. Ultrasound is performed to examine lumps in the testes. Blood tests are usually done to check for elevated levels of tumor markers.

Treatment. Orchiectomy, or removal of the involved testis, is usually performed, followed by radiation therapy and chemotherapy. Caught in the early stages, testicular cancer has up to a 95% success rate. It is therefore very important for males to perform testicular self-exams on a monthly basis. You will learn how to instruct patients in this important exam technique in the *Assisting in Reproductive and Urinary Specialties* chapter.

▶ The Female Reproductive System LO 31.3

Ovaries and Ovum Formation

The ovaries are considered the primary female sex organs because they produce the female sex cells, called *ova* (see Figures 31-4 and 31-5). They also produce *estrogen* and *progesterone,* the female hormones. Most females have two ovaries. They are oval in shape and are located in the pelvic cavity. Each ovary is divided into an inner area called the *medulla* and an outer area called the *cortex.* The medulla contains nerves, lymphatic vessels, and many blood vessels. The cortex contains small masses of cells called *ovarian follicles.* Epithelial tissue and dense connective tissue cover each ovary.

Before a female child is born, *primordial follicles* develop in her ovarian cortex. Each primordial follicle contains a large cell called a *primary oocyte* (immature ovum) and smaller cells called *follicular cells.* Unlike males, who make sperm cells throughout their entire life, a female is born with the maximum number of primary oocytes she will ever produce.

Oogenesis is the process of ovum formation. At the onset of puberty, some primary oocytes are stimulated to continue meiosis (see Figure 31-2). When a primary oocyte divides, it produces one *polar body* (a nonfunctional cell) and a *secondary oocyte.* A secondary oocyte is released from an ovary each month during a process called **ovulation.** When the secondary oocyte is fertilized, it divides to form a mature, fertilized ovum. Therefore, the process of meiosis begins before a female is born and is completed only if a secondary oocyte is fertilized. The mature ovum contains 23 chromosomes; when it combines with a sperm cell, the resulting cell contains 46 chromosomes.

Medical terms are built and dissected using prefixes, word roots/combining form, and suffixes. For example, we can build the term *oophorectomy* by placing the parts of the term in the puzzle pieces where P = prefix, WR/CF = word root or combining form, and S = suffix.

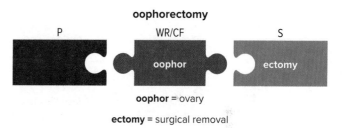

oophorectomy

oophor = ovary

ectomy = surgical removal

Learn additional medical terms in the **Medical Terminology Practice** section at the end of this chapter.

Internal Accessory Organs of the Female Reproductive System

The female reproductive internal accessory organs are the fallopian tubes, uterus, and vagina.

Fallopian Tubes A fallopian tube, or *oviduct,* opens near each ovary, and the other end connects to the uterus. The fringed, expanded end of a fallopian tube near an ovary is called an **infundibulum.** The infundibulum ends in *fimbriae,* or finger-like projections. The infundibulum and its fimbriae "catch" an ovum as it leaves an ovary. Fallopian tubes are muscular tubes that are lined with mucous membrane and cilia. This construction allows the tube to propel the ovum toward the uterus using peristalsis and the sweeping motions of cilia.

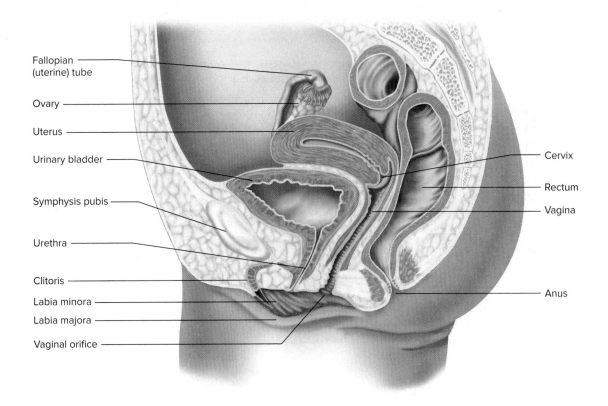

FIGURE 31-4 Sagittal view of female reproductive organs. The female reproductive system produces ova for fertilization and provides the place and means for a fertilized ovum to develop.

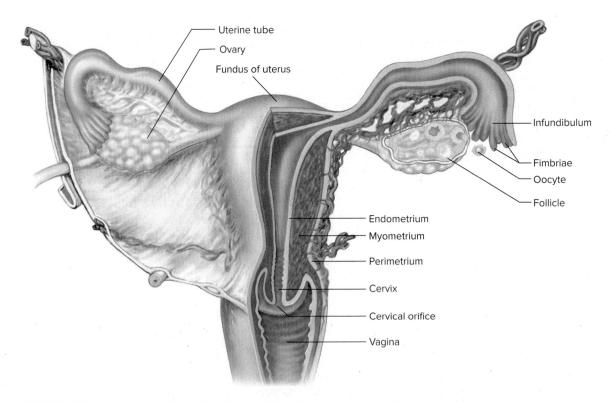

FIGURE 31-5 Anterior view of internal female reproductive organs, showing ovulation of an oocyte.

Uterus The uterus is a hollow, muscular organ that receives a developing embryo and sustains its development. The upper, domed portion of the uterus is called the *fundus;* the main portion is called the *body;* and the narrow, lower portion that extends into the vagina is called the *cervix.* The opening of the cervix is called the *cervical orifice.*

The wall of the uterus has three layers: the endometrium, myometrium, and perimetrium. The *endometrium* is the innermost lining of the uterus. It is vascular with a rich blood supply and contains numerous tubular glands that secrete mucus. The *myometrium* is the middle, thick, muscular layer. The *perimetrium* is a thin layer that covers the myometrium. It secretes serous fluid that coats and protects the uterus.

Vagina The vagina is a tubular, muscular organ that extends from the uterus to the outside of the body. The muscular folds of the vagina, called *rugae,* allow it to expand to receive an erect penis during sexual intercourse and to provide a passageway for delivery of offspring as well as for uterine secretions. The opening of the vagina is posterior to the urinary opening and anterior to the anal opening. The wall of the vagina has three layers: an innermost, mucosal layer that secretes mucus; a middle, muscular layer; and an outermost, fibrous layer. The opening of the vagina to the outside is known as the *vaginal os,* the *vaginal orifice,* or the *vaginal introitus.*

External Accessory Organs of the Female Reproductive System

Mammary glands are accessory organs of both the female reproductive system and the integumentary system (see Figure 31-6).

Their reproductive function is the secretion of milk for newborn offspring.

Mammary glands are located beneath the skin in the breast area. A nipple is near the center of each breast. The pigmented area that surrounds the nipple is called the *areola.* Each gland is made of 15 to 20 lobes and contains *alveolar glands* that make milk under the influence of the hormone *prolactin.* The hormone *oxytocin (OT)* induces *lactiferous ducts* to deliver milk through openings in the nipples. If a woman wants to breast-feed, she must produce adequate amounts of prolactin and oxytocin.

External Genitalia of the Female Reproductive System

The female external genitalia, collectively known as the *vulva,* include the following structures: mons pubis, labia majora, labia minora, clitoris, urethral meatus, vaginal orifice, Bartholin's glands, and perineum.

Labia Majora The labia majora are rounded folds of adipose tissue and skin that protect the other external female reproductive organs. At their anterior ends, the labia majora form the *mons pubis,* which is a fatty area that overlies the symphysis pubis. The labia majora and mons pubis are typically covered in pubic hair in postpubescent females.

Labia Minora The labia minora are folds of skin between the labia majora. They are pinkish in color because of their high degree of vascularity. They merge together anteriorly to form a hood over the clitoris.

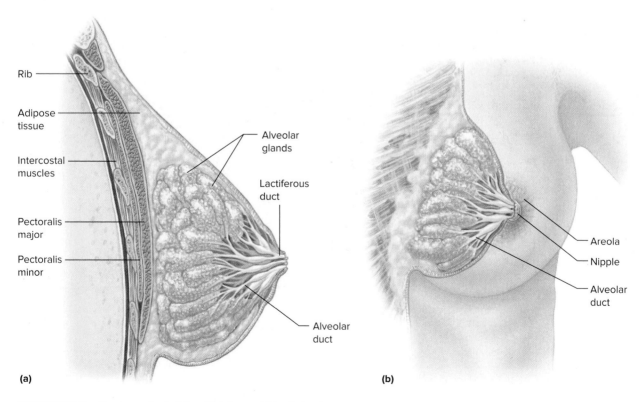

FIGURE 31-6 Mammary glands: (a) sagittal view and (b) anterior view.

The space enclosed by the labia minora is called the *vestibule.* The **Bartholin's glands,** sometimes referred to as the *vestibular glands,* secrete mucus into this area during sexual arousal. This mucus eases insertion of the penis into the vagina.

Clitoris The clitoris is anterior to the urethral meatus. It contains the female erectile tissue and is rich in sensory nerves.

Perineum The perineum is the area between the vagina and the anus. This is the area that is sometimes "clipped" during the birth process, in a procedure known as an *episiotomy.*

Erection, Lubrication, and Orgasm
During sexual arousal, nervous stimulation causes the clitoris to become erect and the Bartholin's glands to become active. At the same time, the vagina elongates. If the clitoris is sufficiently stimulated, an orgasm occurs. During orgasm, the walls of the uterus and fallopian tubes contract to help propel sperm toward the upper ends of the fallopian tubes.

Female Reproductive Hormones
Beginning at puberty, the hypothalamus secretes increasing amounts of GnRH. This causes the anterior pituitary gland to release FSH and LH, which stimulate the ovary to produce estrogen and progesterone, as well as to mature the ovarian follicles. Estrogen and progesterone are responsible for the female secondary sex characteristics: breast development; increased vascularization of the skin; and increased fat deposits in the breasts, thighs, and hips.

Female Reproductive Cycle
The female reproductive cycle is also called the *menstrual cycle.* See Figure 31-7. It consists of regular changes in the uterine lining that lead to a monthly "period," or shedding of the uterine lining, along with bleeding. The first menstrual period is known as **menarche. Menopause** is the termination of the menstrual cycle because of normal aging of the ovaries. The following steps are the major hormonal changes that occur during one reproductive cycle:

1. The anterior pituitary gland releases FSH, which stimulates an ovarian follicle to mature.
2. The maturing follicle secretes estrogen. Estrogen causes the uterine lining to thicken.
3. The anterior pituitary gland releases a sudden surge of LH, which triggers ovulation.
4. Following ovulation, follicular cells of the follicle become a *corpus luteum.*
5. The corpus luteum secretes progesterone, which causes the uterine lining to become more vascular and glandular.
6. If the released oocyte is not fertilized, the corpus luteum degenerates, causing estrogen and progesterone levels to fall.
7. The decline in estrogen and progesterone levels causes the uterine lining to break down, and menses (elimination of the uterine lining, with bleeding) starts.
8. When the anterior pituitary releases FSH, the reproductive cycle begins again.

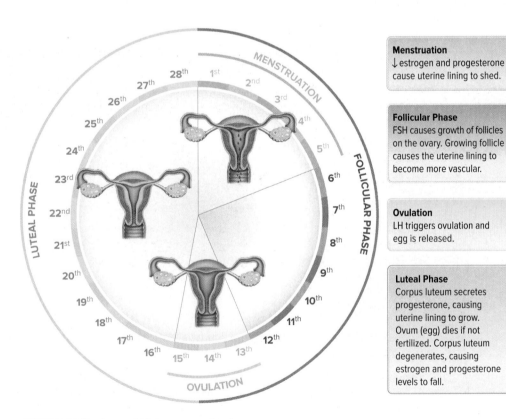

Menstruation
↓estrogen and progesterone cause uterine lining to shed.

Follicular Phase
FSH causes growth of follicles on the ovary. Growing follicle causes the uterine lining to become more vascular.

Ovulation
LH triggers ovulation and egg is released.

Luteal Phase
Corpus luteum secretes progesterone, causing uterine lining to grow. Ovum (egg) dies if not fertilized. Corpus luteum degenerates, causing estrogen and progesterone levels to fall.

FIGURE 31-7 A typical 28-day menstrual cycle.

Common Diseases and Disorders of the Female Reproductive System

BREAST CANCER, according to the American Cancer Society, is the second leading cause of cancer deaths in women after lung cancer. Depending on tumor size and how far cancer cells have spread, breast cancer is classified in stages from 0 to 4, with stage 4 cancer being the most serious. Early diagnosis through regular mammograms and breast self-exams greatly increases the success of treatment. Teaching female patients about breast self-exam and its importance in the early detection of breast cancer is an important aspect of being a medical assistant. You will learn how to teach women this technique in the *Assisting in Reproductive and Urinary Specialties* chapter.

Causes. The causes are largely unknown, although breast cancer may be related to hormonal changes or the presence of certain genes.

Signs and Symptoms. Signs and symptoms include a lump in the breast that is usually painless and firm, a lump in the armpit, discharge from the nipples, dimpled skin on the breast or nipple, and breast pain. Swelling of the breast into the adjacent arm and bone pain may be present in advanced cases. Inflammatory breast cancer may present only as a painless rash of the affected breast with none of the other typical symptoms.

Diagnostic Exams and Tests. If a routine mammogram or breast self-exam indicates an abnormality, a diagnostic mammogram (which is more detailed than the routine screening mammogram) and ultrasound may be performed. An MRI may be ordered and a biopsy is performed if a suspicious lump is found.

Treatment. Nonsurgical treatment methods include hormone therapy, radiation therapy, and chemotherapy. Surgical options include surgery to remove affected lymph nodes, lumpectomy (surgery to remove a lump), and mastectomy (surgery to remove a breast).

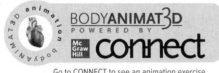

Go to CONNECT to see an animation exercise about *Breast Cancer.*

CERVICAL CANCER generally develops slowly, although adenocarcinoma of the cervix, which tends to be a more rapidly spreading cancer, is the exception to this rule. With early detection by a yearly Pap smear (a test looking for abnormal cervical cells), treatment is often successful. Note that the new recommendation for Pap smear screenings is now every other year if a woman's previous screenings have been negative for 5 years and if the woman is in a monogamous relationship and not on birth control pills.

Causes. A weak immune system may be a factor in the development of this cancer. Risk factors also include sexual intercourse early in life, multiple sexual partners, and infection with the human papillomavirus (HPV).

Signs and Symptoms. Primary symptoms include frequent vaginal discharge, sporadic vaginal bleeding, vaginal bleeding after sexual intercourse, and abnormal cells in the cervix. Patients who are in later stages of this disease may experience pain in the pelvic area or legs, or bone fractures.

Diagnostic Exams and Tests. If a Pap smear indicates abnormal cells, a colposcopy is usually performed to examine the cervix and a biopsy is performed if suspicious areas are found.

Treatment. Radiation therapy, chemotherapy, the removal or destruction of diseased tissue with cryosurgery or laser surgery, and the removal of the uterus (hysterectomy) are the treatments for this disease.

CERVICITIS is an inflammation of the cervix, which is usually caused by an infection.

Causes. Causes include bacterial or viral infections and allergic reactions to spermicidal creams and latex condoms.

Signs and Symptoms. Frequent vaginal discharge, pain during intercourse, and vaginal bleeding after intercourse are common signs and symptoms.

Diagnostic Exams and Tests. A pelvic exam is usually performed and may include an analysis of vaginal or cervical fluid. A urinalysis also may be ordered to check for bacterial infection.

Treatment. This condition is treated with antibiotics and by changing the contraception method.

DYSMENORRHEA is the condition of experiencing severe menstrual cramps that limit normal daily activities.

Causes. Causes include anxiety, endometriosis, pelvic inflammatory disease (PID), fibroid tumors in the uterus, ovarian cysts, abnormally high levels of prostaglandins, and multiple sexual partners.

Signs and Symptoms. Common symptoms are abdominal pain, including sharp or dull pain in the pelvic area just prior to and during the menstrual period.

Diagnostic Exams and Tests. A history and physical exam are performed, including a pelvic exam. If the cramping is severe, an ultrasound, MRI, or laparoscopy may be ordered to check for underlying causes.

Treatment. Nonsurgical treatments include pain medication, anti-inflammatory drugs, medications that inhibit prostaglandin formation, oral contraceptives, and antibiotics in the case of PID. Surgical treatments include hysterectomy and surgery to remove cysts or fibroids.

ENDOMETRIOSIS is a condition in which tissues that make up the lining of the uterus grow outside the uterus.

Causes. The cause of this disorder is unknown; it may be inherited.

Signs and Symptoms. Signs and symptoms include infertility, heavy bleeding from the uterus, pain in the abdomen or pelvis, painful periods, spotting between periods, and pain during sexual intercourse.

Diagnostic Exams and Tests. A pelvic exam and ultrasound are usually performed, but laparoscopy is needed for a definite diagnosis of endometriosis.

Treatment. Oral contraceptives, pain medications, and various hormone therapies may be prescribed. Surgical treatments include laser surgery to remove endometrial tissue outside the uterus and hysterectomy.

FIBROCYSTIC BREAST DISEASE is the presence of abnormal cystic tissues in the breasts. The cysts vary in size related to the menstrual cycle. It is a common disorder and occurs in more than 60% of women in the United States between age 30 and 50. It is rare in women who have gone through menopause because it is related to hormonal changes occurring during the menstrual cycle. It is important to note that fibrocystic breast disease is not considered to put a woman at higher risk of breast cancer.

Causes. This disorder is caused by hormonal changes associated with the menstrual cycle and ingestion of various dietary substances, including caffeine, nicotine, and sugar. Birth control pills also may aggravate this condition.

Signs and Symptoms. Common symptoms include breasts that feel "lumpy," breast tenderness or pain, itchy nipples, and dense tissues as seen in a mammogram.

Diagnostic Exams and Tests. A clinical breast exam is performed. If the practitioner finds changes or lumps, a diagnostic mammogram and/or ultrasound are ordered. A fine-needle aspiration may be performed on any lumps discovered.

Treatment. Treatments include changing one's diet and taking supplements such as vitamin E, B complex vitamins, and magnesium. Wearing support bras may help with pain control. Fine-needle aspiration also may be tried to collapse large cysts that are causing pain.

UTERINE FIBROIDS are benign (noncancerous) tumors that grow in the uterine wall. They are known to affect one out of four women in their thirties and forties and appear to be more common in women of African descent.

Causes. The causes are mostly unknown, although it has been found that the tumors enlarge as estrogen levels increase. Heredity appears to play a role.

Signs and Symptoms. The signs and symptoms are pressure in the abdomen, severe menstrual cramps, abdominal gas, heavy menstrual bleeding, and intermenstrual bleeding. Back and leg pain also may occur.

Diagnostic Exams and Tests. Uterine fibroids are often detected during routine pelvic exams and are confirmed by ultrasound or MRI. Blood tests, such as a CBC, may be ordered if the patient has heavy bleeding. In some cases, imaging tests such as *hysterosonography* (sonography after saline has been used to expand the uterus) or *hysterosalpingography* (X-ray taken after dye is injected to show the uterus and fallopian tubes more clearly) may be ordered as well.

Treatment. Treatment includes pain medications, hormone treatments to shrink tumors, surgery to remove tumors, hysterectomy, and surgery to decrease the blood supply to the uterus.

OVARIAN CANCER is considered more deadly than other types of cancer because its signs and symptoms are usually mild or indistinct until the disease has spread to other organs, making early detection difficult. Current statistics suggest that about 1 woman in 67 will develop ovarian cancer. Women with a family history of ovarian cancer may be counseled to consider prophylactic *oophorosalpingectomy* (removal of the ovaries and fallopian tubes) prior to actually developing ovarian cancer.

Causes. The causes are unknown, although the presence of certain genes has been indicated as a risk factor. Some oral contraceptives may lower the risk of developing this disease.

Signs and Symptoms. Abdominal and pelvic discomfort, unusual menstrual cycles, indigestion, bloating, nausea, and excessive hair growth are signs and symptoms.

Diagnostic Exams and Tests. Diagnosis is made using ultrasound, a CA-125 blood test, and an ovarian biopsy.

Treatment. Treatment options include radiation therapy, chemotherapy, and surgery to remove the ovaries and reproductive organs.

PREMENSTRUAL SYNDROME (PMS) is a collection of symptoms that occur just before a menstrual period.

Causes. The causes are mostly unknown, although hormone fluctuations during the menstrual cycle are implicated.

Signs and Symptoms. The signs and symptoms include anxiety, depression, irritability, acne, fatigue, food cravings, bloating, aches in the head or back, abdominal pain, breast tenderness, muscle spasms, diarrhea, weight gain, and loss of sex drive.

Diagnostic Exams and Tests. There are no specific tests available to diagnose PMS. The patient often is asked to keep a record or diary for a few months to establish the relationship of the symptoms to her menstrual cycle. If a definite pattern is seen, the diagnosis of PMS is made.

Treatment. PMS is commonly treated with pain medications, diuretics, medications to treat depression or anxiety, and oral contraceptives. Many women also have found changes in diet to be helpful, including limiting caffeine, sugar, and sodium. The addition of B complex vitamins also may be helpful.

UTERINE (ENDOMETRIAL) CANCER is most common in postmenopausal women. In the United States, it accounts for approximately 6% of cancer deaths in women.

Causes. The causes are mostly unknown, although it may be related to increased levels of estrogen.

Signs and Symptoms. Signs and symptoms include abdominal pain; abnormal bleeding from the uterus; pelvic pain; and a thin, white vaginal discharge in postmenopausal women.

Diagnostic Exams and Tests. A pelvic exam is performed; if abnormalities are noted, a transvaginal ultrasound and/or hysteroscopy is ordered. An endometrial biopsy is obtained of suspicious tissue and sent to the lab for analysis.

Treatment. Treatment includes radiation therapy; chemotherapy; and surgery to remove the uterus, fallopian tubes, and ovaries.

VULVOVAGINITIS (inflammation of the vulva and vagina) and **VAGINITIS** (inflammation of the vagina) are usually associated with an abnormal vaginal discharge. Some vaginal discharge is normal for all women, and it varies throughout the menstrual cycle. Normal vaginal discharge is clear, whitish, or yellowish in color.

Causes. This condition can be caused by yeast infections, tampon use, poor hygiene, bacteria, antibiotics, and sexually transmitted infections (STIs). Vaginitis may be prevented through good hygiene and safe sex practices.

Signs and Symptoms. Common symptoms include fever, vulvar and vaginal itching and swelling, an abnormal increase or decrease in the amount of vaginal discharge, an abnormal color of vaginal discharge (brown, green, or pinkish), a change in the consistency of vaginal discharge (frothy or cheese-like), and vaginal discharge that has an abnormal odor.

Diagnostic Exams and Tests. A history and physical exam are performed, including a pelvic exam, and the patient is asked about previous STIs. A sample of the discharge often is sent to a lab to determine the specific type of vaginitis—bacterial, fungal (yeast), or parasite (trichomoniasis)—so that treatment can be targeted correctly.

Treatment. The patient may be given medications for fungal or bacterial infections, or the patient and her sexual partner may be treated for STIs.

▶ Pregnancy

LO 31.5

Pregnancy is defined as the condition of having a developing offspring in the uterus. Pregnancy results when a sperm cell unites with an ovum in a process called fertilization (see Figure 31-8).

Fertilization

Prior to fertilization, an ovum is released from an ovary and travels through a fallopian tube. During sexual intercourse, the male deposits semen into the vagina. Sperm cells must travel up through the uterus to the fallopian tubes to fertilize the ovum.

Prostaglandins in semen stimulate the flagella of sperm cells to undulate, causing the swimming action of sperm.

Prostaglandins also stimulate muscles in the uterus and fallopian tubes to contract. These contractions (peristalsis) help the sperm reach the ovum. Normally about 10 to 14 days after ovulation, high estrogen levels stimulate the uterus and cervix to secrete a thin, watery fluid that also promotes the movement of sperm toward the ovum.

Although many sperm cells may reach an ovum, only one sperm cell unites with the ovum, penetrating the follicular cells and a layer called the *zona pellucida,* which surrounds the cell membrane of the ovum. The acrosome of this sperm releases enzymes to help the sperm penetrate the membrane of the ovum. Once a sperm unites with an ovum, the ovum releases enzymes to prevent other sperm from invading it. The enzymes cause the zona pellucida to become hard and therefore impenetrable to other sperm.

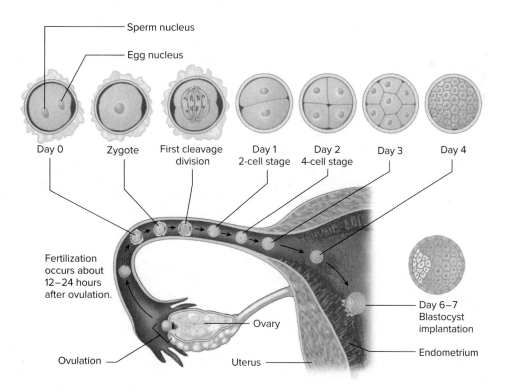

FIGURE 31-8   Stages of early embryo development.

The nucleus of the ovum (with 23 chromosomes) and the nucleus of the sperm (with 23 chromosomes) fuse together to make one nucleus that contains 46 chromosomes. The cell that is formed by this union is called a **zygote.**

The Prenatal Period

The prenatal period is the time before the offspring is born. It is divided into an *embryonic period* (weeks 2 through 8 of pregnancy) and a *fetal period* (week 9 to the delivery of the offspring). It is further divided into three periods known as trimesters, which consist of 3 calendar months each. See *Points on Practice: The Pregnant Patient.*

About 1 day after the zygote forms, it begins to undergo mitosis at a relatively rapid rate. This rapid cell division is called *cleavage,* and the resulting ball of cells is called a *morula.* The morula travels down the fallopian tube to the uterus. Fluid then invades the morula and the organism is called a **blastocyst.** The blastocyst implants in the endometrial wall of the uterus. The process of moving from zygote formation to implantation of the blastocyst takes about 1 week. Once the blastocyst implants, a group of cells in the blastocyst, called the *inner cell mass,* gives rise to an **embryo.** Other cells in the blastocyst, along with cells of the uterus, eventually form the **placenta.**

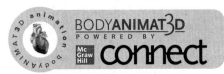

Go to CONNECT to see an animation exercise about *Meiosis vs. Mitosis.*

The Embryonic Period The embryonic period extends from the second week of pregnancy to the end of the eighth week of development. During this stage, the placenta, *amnion, umbilical cord,* and *yolk sac* form, along with most of the internal organs and external structures of the embryo

(see Figure 31-9). The cells of the inner cell mass organize into layers called **primary germ layers.** All organs are formed from the primary germ layers, which include the ectoderm, mesoderm, and endoderm.

- The *ectoderm* develops into nervous tissue and some epithelial tissue.
- The *mesoderm,* the middle layer, develops into connective tissues and some epithelial tissue.
- The *endoderm* develops into epithelial tissues only.

The placenta allows nutrients and oxygen from maternal blood to pass to embryonic blood. It also allows waste products from the fetal blood to pass into maternal blood. The **amnion** is a protective, fluid-filled sac that surrounds the embryo. The *umbilical cord* contains three blood vessels—one umbilical vein that carries oxygenated blood from the placenta to the embryo and two umbilical arteries that carry deoxygenated blood from the embryo back to the placenta.

The yolk sac makes new blood cells for the fetus, as well as cells that eventually become the sex cells of the baby. By the end of the embryonic stage, the baby closely resembles a human because all external structures (arms, hands, legs, feet, etc.) have formed.

The Fetal Period The fetal period begins at the end of the eighth week of development and ends at birth. During this period, the growth of the offspring, which is now called a **fetus,** is rapid. By the twelfth week, bones have begun to harden and the external reproductive organs are distinguishable as male or female.

The growth rate of the fetus slows down in the fifth month, but skeletal muscles become active. In the sixth month, the fetus starts to gain substantial weight. In the seventh month, the eyelids open. In the last 3 months of pregnancy, fetal brain cells divide rapidly and organs continue to grow. The testes of the male descend into the scrotum. The last organ systems to

POINTS ON PRACTICE
The Pregnant Patient

The pregnant patient goes through three distinct stages known as *trimesters.* Each trimester has specific events associated with it.

First Trimester
The first trimester is from week 1 to week 12. During weeks 1 to 8, the product of conception is an embryo; after week 8, it is a fetus. Week 12 marks the end of the first trimester, or one-third of the pregnancy. It is usually during the first trimester that women confirm they are pregnant. "Morning sickness" commonly occurs during this stage.

Second Trimester
Fine, soft hair (lanugo) appears on the shoulders, back, and head of the fetus during the fourth month. By the 20th week,

fetal movement may be felt, and the pregnant woman begins to show fullness in the abdomen. Identifiable periods of fetal sleep and wakefulness occur as the second trimester ends at the completion of the sixth month.

Third Trimester
The last trimester encompasses the most noticeable period of growth, both in the fetus and in the mother. By the end of 30 weeks, the fetus most likely has assumed a head-down position and has a 50% chance of survival if it is born at this time. The fetus is said to have come full term after it is approximately 9 months (40 weeks) old.

More information about caring for a pregnant patient is found in the *Assisting in Reproductive and Urinary Specialties* chapter.

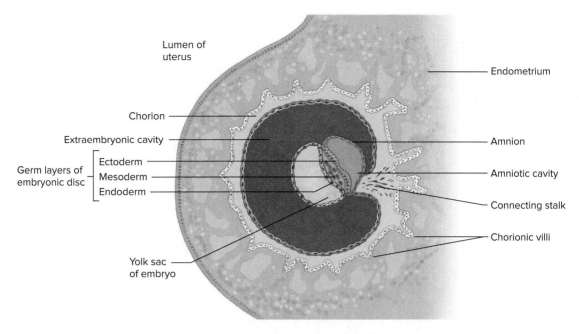

Lumen of uterus

Endometrium

Chorion

Extraembryonic cavity

Amnion

Germ layers of embryonic disc
- Ectoderm
- Mesoderm
- Endoderm

Amniotic cavity

Connecting stalk

Chorionic villi

Yolk sac of embryo

FIGURE 31-9   Primary germ layers and membranes associated with an embryo.

completely develop are the digestive and respiratory systems. By the end of the ninth month, the fetus is usually positioned upside down in the uterus in preparation for delivery.

Fetal Circulation

Throughout prenatal development, the placenta and umbilical blood vessels carry out the exchange of nutrients, oxygen, and waste products between maternal and fetal blood. Therefore, the fetus does not need to send blood to the lungs to pick up oxygen, nor does it need to send blood to the liver to process nutrients.

Fetal circulation has some important differences from normal circulation, which are illustrated in Figure 31-10. In the adult heart, blood flows from the right atrium into the right ventricle so that it can be pumped to the lungs. In the fetal heart, a hole called the **foramen ovale** is located between the right and left atria. This hole allows most of the fetal blood to flow from the right atrium into the left atrium. However, some fetal blood does flow from the right atrium into the right ventricle, and the right ventricle then delivers the blood to the pulmonary trunk.

In the fetus, there is also a connection between the pulmonary trunk and the aorta called the **ductus arteriosus.** This connection allows blood to flow from the pulmonary trunk into the aorta. In the adult, this connection closes and blood flows from the pulmonary trunk to the lungs. The fetus also contains a blood vessel called the **ductus venosus** that allows most of the blood to bypass the liver. After a baby is born, the foramen ovale, ductus arteriosus, and ductus venosus normally close.

Hemoglobin within the fetus has a much higher affinity for oxygen than does the normal hemoglobin that is found after birth and during growth. Therefore, the fetus's blood is adapted to carry more oxygen.

Hormonal Changes During Pregnancy

Many hormonal changes take place when a woman is pregnant. Following implantation of the embryo, the embryo cells begin to secrete *human chorionic gonadotropin (HCG).* HCG maintains the corpus luteum in the ovary so it will continue to secrete estrogen and progesterone. The placenta also secretes large amounts of progesterone and estrogen.

Progesterone and estrogen stimulate the uterine lining to thicken and inhibit the anterior pituitary gland from secreting FSH and LH, which prevents ovulation during pregnancy. Estrogen and progesterone also stimulate the development of the mammary glands, inhibit uterine contractions, and stimulate the enlargement of female reproductive organs.

A hormone called *relaxin,* which comes from the corpus luteum, inhibits uterine contractions and relaxes the ligaments of the pelvis in preparation for childbirth. The placenta also secretes *lactogen,* a hormone that stimulates the enlargement of mammary glands. *Aldosterone,* which is secreted by the adrenal gland, increases sodium and water retention. The secretion of *parathyroid hormone (PTH)* increases, helping to maintain high calcium levels in the blood.

▶ The Birth Process   LO 31.6

The birth process ends pregnancy. This process begins when progesterone levels fall. When this happens, uterine contractions are no longer inhibited and the uterus secretes prostaglandins that stimulate uterine contractions, which cause the posterior pituitary gland to release oxytocin. Oxytocin stimulates stronger uterine contractions until the birth process ends. The birth process itself occurs in three stages after the fetus settles into position in the mother's pelvis (see Figure 31-11a).

1. *Dilation* (see Figure 31-11b). The cervix thins and softens, known as *effacement,* dilating to approximately 10 cm. Regular contractions occur at this stage, and the amniotic sac ruptures. If rupture does not occur, the sac may be surgically punctured. This stage normally lasts 8 to 24 hours.

2. *Expulsion* (see Figure 31-11c). Also known as *parturition,* this is the actual childbirth stage. Forceful contractions

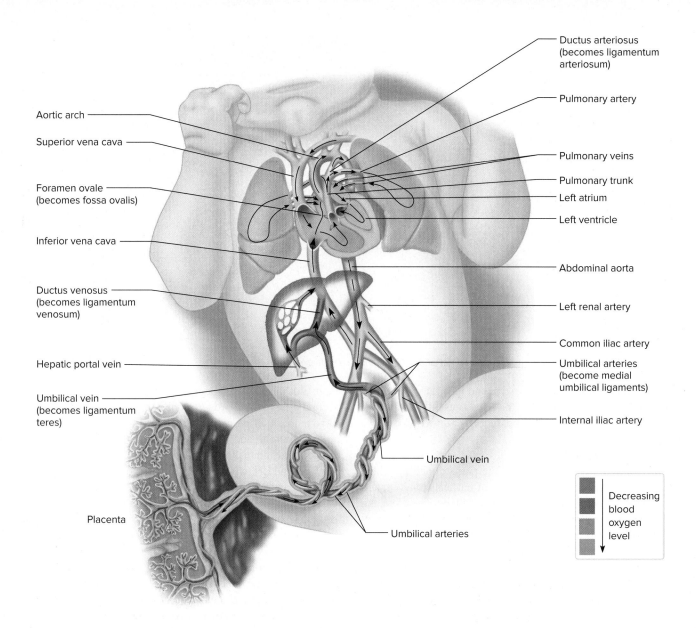

Aortic arch

Superior vena cava

Foramen ovale
(becomes fossa ovalis)

Inferior vena cava

Ductus venosus
(becomes ligamentum
venosum)

Hepatic portal vein

Umbilical vein
(becomes ligamentum
teres)

Placenta

Ductus arteriosus
(becomes ligamentum
arteriosum)

Pulmonary artery

Pulmonary veins

Pulmonary trunk

Left atrium

Left ventricle

Abdominal aorta

Left renal artery

Common iliac artery

Umbilical arteries
(become medial
umbilical ligaments)

Internal iliac artery

Umbilical vein

Umbilical arteries

Decreasing
blood
oxygen
level

FIGURE 31-10 Fetal circulation.

and abdominal compressions force the fetus from the uterus into the vagina. This stage may take 30 minutes or only a few minutes.

3. *Placental stage* (see Figure 31-11d). This stage also is referred to as the *afterbirth.* Approximately 10 to 15 minutes after the birth, the placenta separates from the uterine wall and is expelled. Uterine contractions continue during this stage and the blood vessels constrict to prevent hemorrhage. Normal blood loss is less than 350 mL (12 oz).

If the fetus is not in the usual head-down position, the child is said to be *breech,* in which the buttocks or feet present first. If the fetus cannot be turned manually, forceps may be used to assist in the birth. Alternately, a *cesarean section* (C-section) may be performed to deliver the infant through the abdominal wall.

At 1 minute and 5 minutes after the baby is born, an **APGAR** test is performed to determine how well the baby is

breathing and how well the heart is working. The test has five categories: respiratory effort, heart rate, skin color, reflexes, and muscle tone. In each category, the baby is given a score of 0, 1, or 2, with 2 being the best score. Table 31-1 shows how the scores are applied. The individual scores are added together to provide the APGAR score. A score of 7 to 9 is considered normal. Babies rarely score a 10 because their extremities are normally blue immediately after birth. An APGAR score below 7 indicates that the baby may need medical support, such as supplemental oxygen or physical stimulation.

The Postnatal Period

The *postnatal period* is the 6-week period following birth. The first 4 weeks of the postnatal period are called the *neonatal period* and the offspring is called a *neonate.* The neonatal period is marked by adjustment to life outside the uterus. The lungs of the neonate must expand, which is why the baby's first breath is forceful. The newborn's liver is immature, so

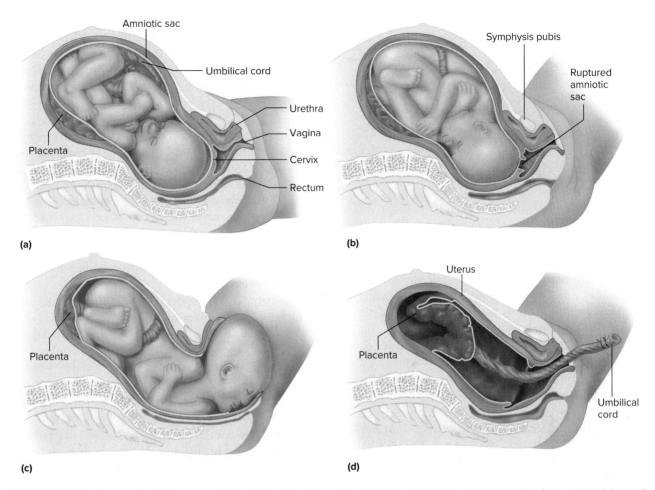

FIGURE 31-11 Stages of the birth process: (a) the fetal position before birth, (b) dilation of the cervix, (c) delivery of the fetus, and (d) delivery of the placenta.

TABLE 31-1	APGAR Scores		
	0	**1**	**2**
Respiratory Effort	Baby is not breathing.	Baby is breathing, but breaths are slow or irregular.	Baby is breathing well enough to cry successfully.
Heart Rate	Baby's heart is not beating.	Heart rate is less than 100 beats per minute.	Heart rate is 100 beats per minute or greater.
Skin Color	The skin is cyanotic (pale blue).	The skin is pink except in the extremities, which are cyanotic.	The skin is entirely pink.
Reflexes	Baby does not respond to stimulation such as a light pinch.	Baby grimaces in response to stimulation.	Baby grimaces and sneezes, coughs, or cries in response to stimulation.
Muscle Tone	Muscles are flabby or loose.	Muscles have some muscle tone.	The baby actively moves.

the baby must obtain most of its glucose from fat stores in the skin. The newborn urinates a lot because the kidneys are too immature to concentrate urine well. In addition, body temperature tends to be unstable. The newborn's umbilical vessels constrict and the foramen ovale, ductus arteriosus, and ductus venosus close.

Milk Production and Secretion

After childbirth, prolactin causes the mother's mammary glands to produce milk. The hormone oxytocin stimulates the ejection of milk from mammary gland ducts. As long as milk is removed from the mammary glands, milk production continues. Once a female stops breastfeeding, the hypothalamus inhibits the release of prolactin and oxytocin, and milk production stops.

▶ Contraception   LO 31.7

Birth control methods, also referred to as *contraception,* reduce the risk of pregnancy (see Figure 31-12). Although many birth control methods are available, some are more reliable than others. The following are the most commonly used birth control methods:

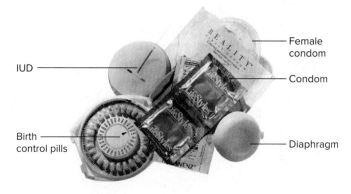

IUD

Female condom

Condom

Birth control pills

Diaphragm

FIGURE 31-12 Couples use various forms of contraception. To provide adequate patient teaching, you should be knowledgeable of these methods.
©Peter Ardito/Getty Images

- Coitus interruptus (withdrawal). The male physically withdraws the penis from the vagina before ejaculation. This method is not reliable because small amounts of semen may enter the vagina before ejaculation.
- Rhythm method (periodic abstinence). This method requires abstinence from sexual intercourse around the time a female is ovulating. However, predicting ovulation can be difficult; therefore, this type of contraception can be unreliable.
- Mechanical barriers. Mechanical barriers prevent sperm from entering the female reproductive tract. They include condoms, diaphragms, and cervical caps. Spermicides are often used in conjunction with barrier methods, particularly condoms and diaphragms.
- Chemical barriers. Chemical barriers destroy sperm in the female reproductive tract. They primarily include spermicides.
- Oral contraceptives. Birth control pills are oral contraceptives. They normally include low doses of estrogen or progesterone that prevent the LH surge necessary for ovulation. These pills therefore prevent ovulation. Newer oral contraceptives have been developed in which the woman

takes the pill daily for 3 months and then is off for 1 week, so that a period occurs only four times a year.
- Injectable contraceptives. Depo-Provera® is one brand of injectable contraceptive. It prevents ovulation and alters the lining of the uterus so that implantation of a blastocyst is not likely.
- Insertable contraceptives. NuvaRing® is one of the newest forms of contraception. The woman inserts the ring vaginally and leaves it in for 3 weeks. She removes the ring at the beginning of the fourth week to allow for menstruation on the same schedule she would experience using most oral contraceptives. However, this method has been associated with increased chances for blood clots, stroke, and heart attack, especially in women who smoke.
- Contraceptive implants. Contraceptive implants are small rods of progesterone that are implanted beneath the skin to prevent ovulation.
- Transdermal contraceptives. Commonly called "the patch," transdermal contraceptives are applied to the skin once a week and removed on the seventh day for a 3-week cycle. No patch is applied during the fourth week to allow for the menstrual period.
- Intrauterine devices. An intrauterine device (IUD) is a small, solid device that a licensed practitioner places in the uterus. It prevents the implantation of a blastocyst.
- Surgical methods. *Tubal ligation* is a surgical method used in females to prevent pregnancy. In this process, each fallopian tube is cut and tied to prevent sperm from reaching the oocyte. *Vasectomy* is a surgical method used in males in which each vas deferens is cut to prevent sperm from being ejaculated. Figure 31-13 illustrates these birth control methods.

▶ Infertility   LO 31.8

Infertility is the inability to conceive a child. A couple that has never been pregnant and has tried for 12 months to achieve pregnancy is said to have *primary infertility*. If a couple has

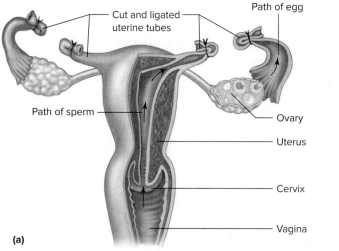

Cut and ligated uterine tubes

Path of egg

Path of sperm

Ovary

Uterus

Cervix

Vagina

(a)

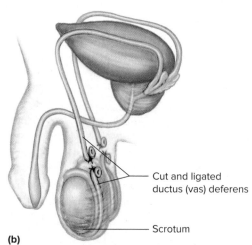

Cut and ligated ductus (vas) deferens

Scrotum

(b)

FIGURE 31-13 (a) Tubal ligation involves cutting and ligating each fallopian tube. (b) Vasectomy involves cutting and ligating the vas deferens.

had at least one pregnancy but has not been able to get pregnant again after 1 year, they are said to have *secondary infertility.*

In the United States, about 15% of infertility causes are unknown, about 35% are the result of problems in the male, and about 50% are because of problems in the female. Common causes of infertility as a result of male factors include the following:

- Impotence.
- Retrograde ejaculation.
- Low or absent sperm count.
- Use of various medications or drugs.
- Decreased testosterone production.
- Scarring of the male reproductive tract from sexually transmitted infections (STIs).
- Previous mumps infection that infected the testes.
- Inflammation of the epididymis or testes.

Infertility because of female factors includes these common causes:

- Scarring of fallopian tubes from STIs.
- Pelvic inflammatory disease (PID).
- Inadequate diet.
- Lack of ovulation.
- Lack of menstrual cycles.
- Endometriosis.
- Abnormal shape of the uterus or cervix.
- Hormone imbalances.
- Cysts in ovaries.
- Being older than age 40.

Women are most likely to get pregnant in their early twenties. By the time a woman reaches age 40, her chance of conceiving a child is less than 10% each month. In general, infertility in men is not age related.

Infertility Tests

A number of tests are used to diagnose infertility. They include the following:

- Semen analysis. This test determines the semen thickness and the number and motility of sperm cells in a sample.

- Monitoring morning body temperature. If a woman's body temperature does not rise slightly once a month, which is best determined by taking her temperature first thing in the morning, she may not be ovulating.
- Blood hormone measurements. In females, various hormone levels can be monitored to predict ovulation and the general health of the ovaries. In males, testosterone levels are measured.
- Endometrial biopsy. This test determines the health of the uterine lining.
- Urinary analysis for luteinizing hormone. The absence of this hormone in urine may indicate a lack of ovulation.
- Hysterosalpingogram. This type of X-ray uses contrast media to visualize the shape of the uterus and the fallopian tubes. If a woman has excess scar tissue in her fallopian tubes, the contrast cannot run through them.
- Laparoscopy. Laparoscopy is a procedure used to visualize pelvic organs.

Treatment of Infertility

Many treatments are available for infertility, but often there is no cure for this condition. Treatment depends on the reason for the infertility. Common treatments include:

- Changing habits or lifestyle. Both males and females may benefit from exercising regularly, stopping or reducing the use of harmful substances, and paying more attention to the timing of intercourse.
- Surgery. In females, a procedure may be performed to repair abnormal or scarred fallopian tubes or to remove obstructions such as polyps.
- Fertility drugs and hormone therapy. In females, medications are available to increase ovulation; in males, medication may improve sperm count.
- Assisted reproductive technology (ART). This refers to any treatment in which the ovum or the sperm (or both) are manipulated. The most common ART treatment is in vitro fertilization of the female's ovum with the male's sperm, but variations may be used in some cases. For example, a surrogate, or gestational carrier, may be used if a female cannot carry the fetus.

PATHOPHYSIOLOGY

LO 31.9

Sexually Transmitted Infections Occurring in Both Sexes

AIDS (ACQUIRED IMMUNODEFICIENCY SYNDROME) is covered in detail in the *Microbiology and Disease* chapter.

Causes. The human immunodeficiency virus (HIV) causes AIDS.

Signs and Symptoms. These are numerous and include decreased T-cell count; flu-like symptoms; and a host of opportunistic infections, including *Pneumocystis carinii* pneumonia (PCP), Kaposi's sarcoma (KS), and cytomegalovirus (CMV).

Diagnostic Exams and Tests. Diagnosis of AIDS begins with a positive diagnosis for HIV, which can be made by a healthcare professional or by using the FDA-approved home test. If the patient is HIV-positive, blood tests and cultures for T-cell count and opportunistic infections are ordered. Advanced testing checks for various complications, such as tuberculosis, urinary tract infections, hepatitis, or liver or kidney damage.

Treatment. Antiviral medications have been successful in decreasing the viral load and maintaining T-cell counts in some patients, but there are many side effects to these drugs and they require a strict medicine regime. Other treatments include

OUTCOME	KEY POINTS
31.4 Describe the causes, signs and symptoms, diagnosis, and treatment of various disorders of the female reproductive system.	The diseases of the female reproductive system range from simple inflammation to cancers, with varied signs, symptoms, diagnosis, and treatments. Some of these include breast cancer, cervical cancer, cervicitis, dysmenorrhea, endometriosis, fibrocystic breast disease, ovarian cancer, premenstrual syndrome (PMS), uterine (endometrial) cancer, vaginitis, and vulvovaginitis.
31.5 Explain the process of pregnancy, including fertilization, the prenatal period, and fetal circulation.	Fertilization occurs with the union of a sperm cell and an ovum, usually within the fallopian tubes, but it may occur anywhere in the female reproductive tract. The fertilized ovum becomes a blastocyst and implants in the endometrial wall of the uterus. The embryonic period occurs from week 2 through week 8 of the pregnancy; the fetal period is from week 9 through delivery.
31.6 Describe the birth process, including the postnatal period.	The birth process ends pregnancy and occurs in three stages: dilation (effacement), in which the cervix thins and softens and dilates up to 10 cm; expulsion (parturition), in which the baby is expelled from the vagina; and placental stage (afterbirth), in which the placenta is expelled through the vagina. The postnatal period is the 6-week period following birth, when the baby's organs continue to mature and the baby adjusts to life outside the uterus.
31.7 Compare several birth control methods and their effectiveness.	Some of the contraceptive methods include coitus interruptus; the rhythm method; mechanical barriers; chemical barriers; oral contraceptives; injectable, implantable, and insertable contraceptives; transdermal contraceptives; and surgical methods.
31.8 Explain the causes of and treatments for infertility.	The causes of infertility are varied, with about 15% of infertility from unknown causes. There are a number of infertility tests and treatments; the treatment plan depends on the reason for the infertility.
31.9 Describe the causes, signs and symptoms, diagnosis, and treatments of the most common sexually transmitted infections.	There are many sexually transmitted infections occurring in both sexes, all passed between sexual partners (both heterosexual and same-sex partners), with varied signs, symptoms, diagnosis, and treatments. Some of these include AIDS (acquired immunodeficiency syndrome), chlamydia, human papillomavirus (HPV), gonorrhea, pubic lice, syphilis, and trichomoniasis.

CASE STUDY CRITICAL THINKING

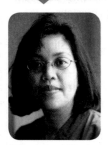

©ERproductions Ltd/Blend Images LLC

Recall Raja Lautu from the case study at the beginning of the chapter. Now that you have completed the chapter, answer the following questions regarding her case.

1. From Raja Lautu's symptoms, which STI might you suspect she is experiencing?

2. What causes this STI, and how is it treated?

3. Why is it important for her sexual partner to be treated?

1. (LO 31.1) Testosterone is produced in the _____ of the testes.
   a. Seminiferous tubules
   b. Epididymis
   c. Vas deferens
   d. Interstitial cells
   e. Bulbourethral gland

2. (LO 31.3) The innermost layer of the uterus is the
   a. Endometrium
   b. Myometrium
   c. Perimetrium
   d. Infundibulum
   e. Cervical orifice

3. (LO 31.4) In _____, the normal uterine lining is found outside of the uterus.
   a. PID
   b. Endometriosis
   c. PMS
   d. Dysmenorrhea
   e. Trichomoniasis

4. (LO 31.6) A newborn is described as a neonate until it reaches the age of
   a. 4 weeks
   b. 2 months
   c. 6 weeks
   d. 6 months
   e. 1 year

5. (LO 31.7) "The patch" is a _____ method of contraception.
   a. Barrier
   b. Mechanical
   c. Transdermal
   d. Chemical
   e. Surgical

6. (LO 31.2) An enlargement of the prostate gland due to normal hormonal changes as a man ages is known as
   a. Epididymitis
   b. Erectile dysfunction
   c. Prostatitis
   d. Testicular cancer
   e. BPH

7. (LO 31.5) The union of the nucleus of an ovum and the nucleus of a sperm to create one nucleus containing 46 chromosomes results in a(n)
   a. Blastocyst
   b. Embryo
   c. Zygote
   d. Inner cell mass
   e. Morula

8. (LO 31.8) Which of the following is *not* a test performed to diagnose infertility?
   a. Semen analysis
   b. Endometrial biopsy
   c. Hysterosalpingogram
   d. Amniocentesis
   e. Blood hormone measurement

9. (LO 31.9) The most commonly reported STI in the United States is
   a. Gonorrhea
   b. Chlamydia
   c. Syphilis
   d. AIDS
   e. Trichomoniasis

10. (LO 31.5) The structure in a fetus that allows most of the blood to bypass the liver is the
    a. Ductus venosus
    b. Foramen ovale
    c. Ductus arteriosus
    d. Fossa ovalis
    e. Ligamentum arteriosum

Analyze the following medical terms, presented throughout the chapter. Using a medical dictionary (or Appendix I), place a / mark between each word part. Define each word part and then define the whole word.

EXAMPLE: **spermato/cyte** = spermato means "sperm" + cyte means "cell"
SPERMATOCYTE means "sperm cell."

1. blastocyst
2. ectoderm
3. endometrium
4. episiotomy
5. hysterectomy
6. lactiferous
7. neonate
8. oogenesis
9. oviduct
10. vasectomy
11. vaginosis
12. oophorectomy

The Digestive System

PATIENT INFORMATION			
Patient Name	**DOB**	**Allergies**	
Sylvia Gonzales	09/01/1968	Penicillin	
Attending	**MRN**	**Other Information**	
Alexis N. Whalen, MD	00-AA-004	NIDDM blood sugars erratic	

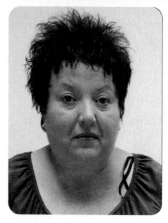

©McGraw-Hill Education

Yesterday afternoon, Sylvia Gonzales, went to a gastroenterologist's office complaining of severe pain in her upper right abdomen. She was nauseated and stated that for several months—and especially following meals—she had been having periodic abdominal pain. After several tests, she was diagnosed as having gallstones and was scheduled for the surgical removal of her gallbladder.

Keep Sylvia Gonzales in mind as you study this chapter. There will be questions at the end of the chapter based on the case study. The information in the chapter will help you answer these questions.

LEARNING OUTCOMES

After completing Chapter 32, you will be able to:

32.1 Describe the organs of the alimentary canal and their functions.

32.2 Explain the functions of the digestive system's accessory organs.

32.3 Identify the nutrients absorbed by the digestive system and where they are absorbed.

32.4 Describe the causes, signs and symptoms, diagnosis, and treatments of various common diseases and disorders of the digestive system.

KEY TERMS

alimentary canal	feces
bile	glycogen
bolus	lipid
cardiac sphincter	mechanical digestion
chemical digestion	nutrient
cholesterol	palate
chyme	peritoneum
diverticula	triglycerides
esophageal hiatus	uvula

CAAHEP

I.C.1 Describe structural organization of the human body

I.C.2 Identify body systems

I.C.4 List major organs in each body system

I.C.5 Identify the anatomical location of major organs in each body system

I.C.6 Compare structure and function of the human body across the life span

I.C.7 Describe normal function of each body system

I.C.8 Identify common pathology related to each body system including:
(a) signs
(b) symptoms
(c) etiology

I.C.9 Analyze pathology for each body system including:
(a) diagnostic measures
(b) treatment modalities

V.C.9 Identify medical terms labeling the word parts

V.C.10 Define medical terms and abbreviations related to all body systems

ABHES

2. **Anatomy and Physiology**
   a. List all body systems and their structures and functions
   b. Describe common diseases, symptoms and etiologies as they apply to each body system
   c. Identify diagnostic and treatment modalities as they relate to each body system

3. **Medical Terminology**
   a. Define and use entire basic structure of medical terminology and be able to accurately identify the correct context (i.e., root, prefix, suffix, combinations, spelling, and definitions)
   b. Build and dissect medical terminology from roots and suffixes to understand the word element combinations
   c. Apply medical terminology for each specialty
   d. Define and use medical abbreviations when appropriate and acceptable

▶ Introduction

Digestion is the mechanical and chemical breakdown of foods into forms that your body cells can absorb. The digestive system's organs carry out the digestive process and can be divided into two categories: organs of the alimentary (digestive) canal and accessory organs. Organs of the **alimentary canal** form a tube or pathway that extends from the mouth to the anus. These organs include the mouth, pharynx, esophagus, stomach, small intestine, large intestine, and anal canal. The accessory organs include the teeth, tongue, salivary glands, liver, gallbladder, and pancreas (Figure 32-1). You may find it helpful to review the *Organization of the Body* chapter to revisit the abdominal regions and quadrants while studying the organs described in this chapter.

▶ Characteristics of the Alimentary Canal

LO 32.1

The wall of the alimentary canal consists of four layers:

- *Mucosa.* The mucosa is the innermost layer of the canal wall. It is made mostly of epithelial tissue that secretes enzymes and mucus into the lumen, or passageway, of the canal. This layer also is active in absorbing nutrients.
- *Submucosa.* The submucosa is the layer just outside the mucosa. It contains loose connective tissue, blood vessels, glands, and nerves. The blood vessels in this layer carry absorbed nutrients throughout the body.

- *Muscular layer.* This layer lies between the submucosa and the canal's outermost layer. It is made of layers of smooth muscle tissue and contracts to move materials through the canal.
- *Serosa.* The serosa is the double-walled, outermost layer of the canal and is also known as the **peritoneum.** The innermost wall of the serosa is known as the *visceral peritoneum.* It secretes serous fluid to keep the outside of the canal moist, preventing it from sticking to other organs or to its outer layer, the *parietal peritoneum,* also called the abdominal lining.

Smooth muscle in the canal's wall can contract to produce two basic types of movements: churning and peristalsis. *Churning* mixes substances in the canal. *Peristalsis* propels substances through the tract (Figure 32-2).

The Mouth

The mouth, also known as the *buccal cavity,* takes in food and reduces its size through chewing—a process known as **mechanical digestion.** The mouth also starts the process of **chemical digestion** of food because saliva (spit) contains the enzyme amylase, which breaks down carbohydrates.

The cheeks consist of skin, adipose tissue, skeletal muscles, and an inner lining of moist, stratified squamous epithelium. The cheeks hold food in the mouth. The lips contain sensory nerve fibers that can judge the temperature of food before it enters the mouth. The tongue is made mostly of skeletal muscles and is covered by a mucous membrane. The body of the tongue is held to the floor of the oral cavity by a flap

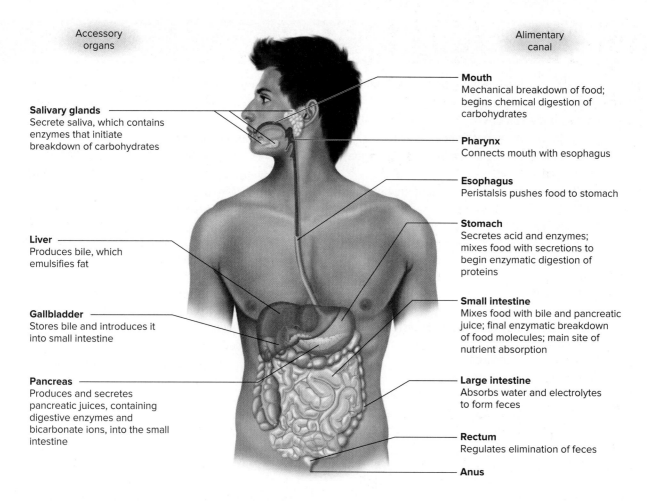

Accessory organs

Salivary glands
Secrete saliva, which contains enzymes that initiate breakdown of carbohydrates

Liver
Produces bile, which emulsifies fat

Gallbladder
Stores bile and introduces it into small intestine

Pancreas
Produces and secretes pancreatic juices, containing digestive enzymes and bicarbonate ions, into the small intestine

Alimentary canal

Mouth
Mechanical breakdown of food; begins chemical digestion of carbohydrates

Pharynx
Connects mouth with esophagus

Esophagus
Peristalsis pushes food to stomach

Stomach
Secretes acid and enzymes; mixes food with secretions to begin enzymatic digestion of proteins

Small intestine
Mixes food with bile and pancreatic juice; final enzymatic breakdown of food molecules; main site of nutrient absorption

Large intestine
Absorbs water and electrolytes to form feces

Rectum
Regulates elimination of feces

Anus

FIGURE 32-1   Major organs of the digestive system.

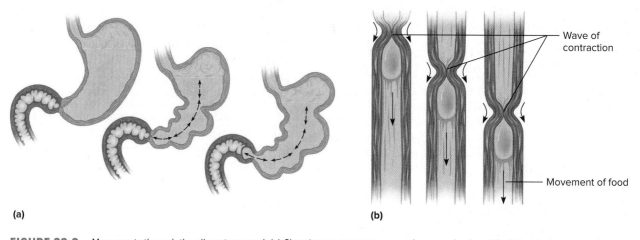

(a)

(b)

Wave of contraction

Movement of food

FIGURE 32-2   Movements through the alimentary canal: (a) Churning movements move substances back and forth to mix them.
(b) Peristalsis moves contents along the canal.

of mucous membrane called the *lingual frenulum.* The tongue mixes food in the mouth and holds it between the teeth. It also contains taste buds. The back of the tongue contains two lumps of lymphoid tissue called *lingual tonsils,* which destroy bacteria and viruses on the back of the tongue.

The **palate** is the roof of the mouth. It separates the oral cavity from the nasal cavity. The front of the palate, known as the

hard palate, is rigid because it has bony plates in it. The back of the palate, or soft palate, lacks bony material, so it is not rigid. The back of the soft palate hangs down into the throat. This portion of the soft palate is called the **uvula.** It prevents food and liquids from entering the nose during swallowing (Figure 32-3).

At the back of the mouth, where the oral cavity joins the pharynx in the area known as the *oropharynx,* are two masses

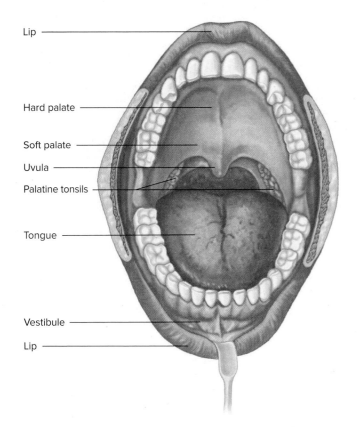

FIGURE 32-3 Structures of the mouth.

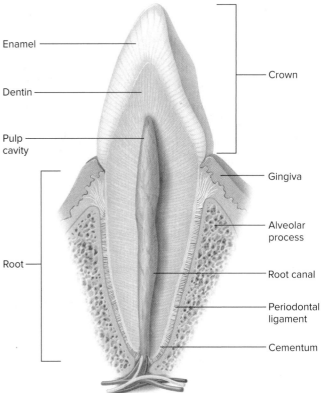

FIGURE 32-4 Structure of a cuspid tooth.

of lymphoid tissue called *palatine tonsils.* Just above the palatine tonsils, in the area known as the *nasopharynx* (the nasal cavity joins the pharynx here), are two more masses of lymphoid tissue called the *pharyngeal tonsils,* or *adenoids.* These masses of lymphoid tissue protect the area from bacteria and viruses.

Humans have 32 teeth—16 on the upper jaw and 16 on the lower jaw—which through mastication (chewing) work to decrease the size of food particles. Different types of teeth are adapted to handle food in different ways. The most medial teeth, called *incisors,* act as chisels to bite off food pieces. Teeth called *cuspids,* also known as the canines, are the sharpest teeth and designed to tear tough food (Figure 32-4). The back teeth, called *bicuspids* and *molars,* are flat and designed to grind food (Figure 32-5).

Salivary glands secrete saliva—a mixture of water, enzymes, and mucus—and are made of two types of cells: serous cells and mucous cells. Serous cells secrete a fluid made mostly of water, and they secrete amylase. Mucous cells secrete mucus. The mass created by food mixed with the saliva and mucous mixture is called a **bolus.**

All major salivary glands are paired (Figure 32-6):

- *Parotid glands* are the largest of the salivary glands, located beneath the skin just in front of the ears.
- *Submandibular glands* are located in the floor of the mouth just inside the surface of the mandibles (jaws).
- *Sublingual glands* are the smallest of the salivary glands, located in the floor of the mouth beneath the tongue.

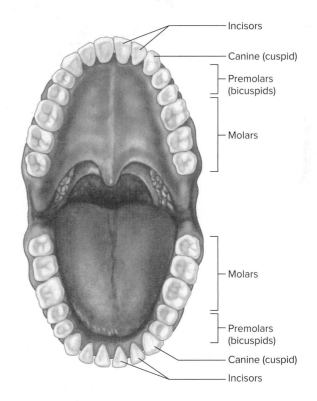

FIGURE 32-5 Types of teeth.

The Pharynx

The pharynx, commonly called the throat, is a long, muscular structure that extends from the area behind the nose to the esophagus. It connects the nasal cavity with the oral cavity for breathing through the nose. It also pushes food into the esophagus (Figure 32-7).

The divisions of the pharynx are as follows:

- *Nasopharynx:* the portion behind the nasal cavity.
- *Oropharynx:* the portion behind the oral cavity.
- *Laryngopharynx:* the portion behind the larynx. The laryngopharynx continues as the esophagus.

Swallowing is largely a reflex. In other words, it is an automatic response that does not require much thought. The following events occur during swallowing:

1. The soft palate rises, causing the uvula to cover the opening between the nasal cavity and the oral cavity.
2. The epiglottis covers the opening of the larynx so that food does not enter it (see Figure 32-7).
3. The tongue presses against the roof of the mouth, forcing food into the oropharynx.
4. The muscles in the pharynx contract, forcing food toward the esophagus.
5. The esophagus opens.
6. The muscles of the pharynx push food into the cardiac sphincter.

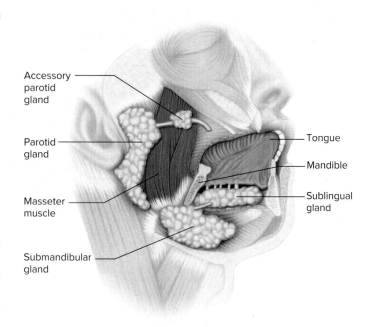

FIGURE 32-6   Major salivary glands.

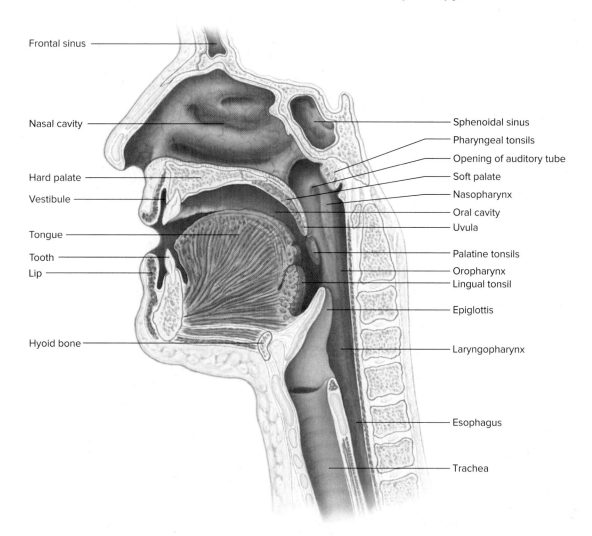

FIGURE 32-7   Sagittal section of the mouth, nasal cavity, and pharynx.

The Esophagus

The esophagus is a muscular tube that connects the pharynx to the stomach (Figures 32-7 and 32-8). It descends through the thoracic cavity, through the diaphragm, and into the abdominal cavity, where it joins the stomach. The hole in the diaphragm that the esophagus goes through is called the **esophageal hiatus.** This hiatus is a place where hernias commonly occur. A hernia develops when an organ pushes through a wall that contains it. A hiatal hernia occurs when the stomach gets pushed up into the thoracic cavity through the esophageal hiatus.

The **cardiac sphincter,** also known as the *lower esophageal sphincter,* controls the movement of food into the stomach. As stated in earlier chapters, sphincters are circular bands of muscle located at the openings of many tubes in the body. They open and close to allow or prevent the movement of substances out of a tube.

The Stomach

The stomach lies below the diaphragm in the left upper quadrant of the abdominal cavity. The folds of the inner lining of the stomach are called *rugae.* The stomach receives the food bolus from the esophagus, mixes food with gastric juice (secretions of the stomach lining), starts protein digestion, and moves food into the small intestine. The mixture of food and gastric juices is called **chyme.** Once chyme is well mixed, stomach contractions push it into the small intestine a little at a time. It takes 4 to 8 hours for the stomach to empty following a meal. The stomach does not absorb many substances, but it can absorb alcohol, water, and some fat-soluble drugs.

The beginning portion of the stomach that is attached to the esophagus is called the *cardiac region.* The portion of the stomach that balloons over the cardiac region is the *fundus.* The main part of the stomach is called the *body,* and the narrow portion connected to the small intestine is the *pylorus.* The *pyloric sphincter* controls the movement of substances from the pylorus of the stomach into the small intestine (Figure 32-8).

The lining of the stomach contains gastric glands, which are made of the following cell types:

- *Mucous cells:* secrete mucus to protect the lining of the stomach.
- *Chief cells:* secrete pepsinogen, which becomes *pepsin* in the presence of acid; pepsin digests proteins.
- *Parietal cells:* secrete hydrochloric acid, which is necessary to convert pepsinogen to pepsin; they also secrete *intrinsic factor,* which is necessary for vitamin B_{12} absorption.

When a person smells, tastes, or sees appetizing food, the parasympathetic nervous system stimulates the gastric glands to secrete their products. A hormone called *gastrin,* made by the stomach, also stimulates the gastric glands to become active. The opposing hormone, called *cholecystokinin (CCK),* is made by the small intestine and inhibits the gastric glands.

If a patient is unable to swallow for any reason, a gastrostomy tube, or G tube, may be inserted into the patient's stomach so that he can be fed liquid meals, such as Ensure®, through this tube.

The Small Intestine

The small intestine is a coiled, tubular organ that extends from the stomach to the large intestine (Figure 32-9). It fills most of the abdominal cavity. The small intestine carries out most of the actual digestion in the body and is responsible for absorbing most of the nutrients into the bloodstream.

The beginning of the small intestine is called the *duodenum.* It is C-shaped and relatively short. The middle portion of the small intestine is called the *jejunum.* It is coiled and forms the majority of the small intestine. If a patient's stomach is diseased or removed, a jejunostomy, or J, tube may be inserted into the jejunum to allow her to receive nutrition.

The last portion of the small intestine is called the *ileum,* and it is directly attached to the large intestine. The jejunum and ileum

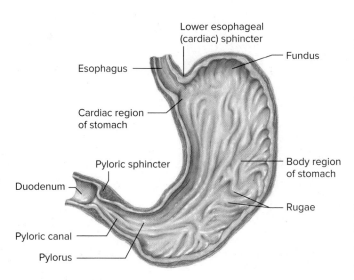

FIGURE 32-8 Regions of the stomach.

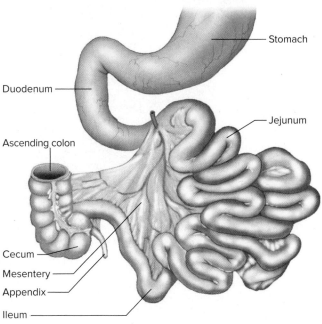

FIGURE 32-9 Parts of the small intestine.

are held in the abdominal cavity by a fan-like tissue called the *mesentery,* which attaches to the posterior wall of the abdomen.

The lining of the small intestine contains cells that have *microvilli.* Microvilli greatly increase the surface area of the small intestine so that it can absorb nutrients more efficiently. The lining of the small intestine also contains glands that secrete various substances, including mucus and water. Water aids in digestion, but infections or exposure to some toxins causes the secretion of too much water, and this leads to diarrhea—which in turn aids the body in eliminating the toxins. It also means, however, that needed nutrients are not absorbed in the small intestine as usual. The mucus secreted by the small intestine helps protect its lining. The parasympathetic nervous system and the stretching of the wall of the small intestine as it fills are the primary factors that trigger the small intestine to secrete its products. The following are the major enzymes the small intestine secretes:

- *Peptidases.* These enzymes digest proteins.
- *Sucrase, maltase, and lactase.* These enzymes digest sugars. A person who cannot produce lactase will not be able to digest lactose, which is the sugar in dairy products. This causes a condition called *lactose intolerance.*
- *Intestinal lipase.* This enzyme digests fats.

The small intestine absorbs almost all nutrients (water, glucose, amino acids, fatty acids, glycerol, and electrolytes) as the wall of the small intestine contracts to mix chyme and to propel it toward the large intestine. The *ileocecal sphincter* controls the movement of chyme from the ileum to the *cecum,* which is the beginning of the large intestine.

The Large Intestine

The large intestine begins at the ileum of the small intestine and ends where it opens to the outside of the body as the anus (Figure 32-10). The beginning of the large intestine is called the cecum. Projecting off the cecum is the *vermiform appendix,* which is made mostly of lymphoid tissue. It was once thought to have no function, but it is now thought to have a role in immunity. The cecum eventually gives rise to the ascending colon, which is the portion of the large intestine

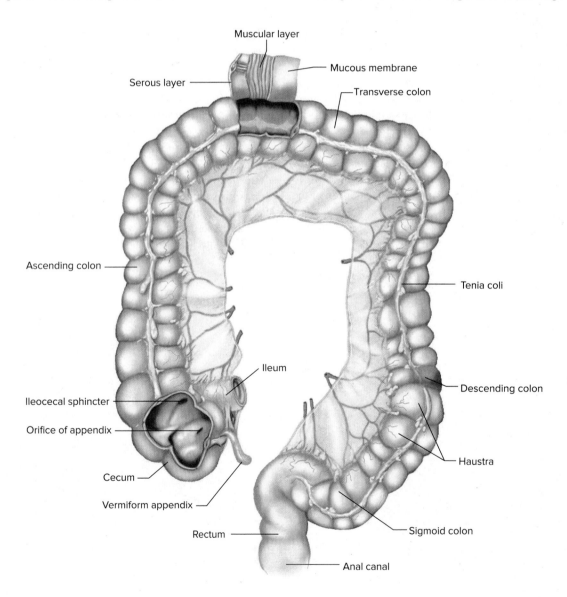

FIGURE 32-10   Parts of the large intestine.

that runs up the right side of the abdominal cavity. If you remember that the appendix is in the right lower quadrant (RLQ), it will be easy to remember that the ascending colon also goes up the right side of the abdomen. The ascending colon becomes the transverse colon as it crosses the abdominal cavity; from there, it becomes the descending colon as it descends the left side of the abdominal cavity. In the pelvic cavity, the descending colon then forms the S-shaped tube called the *sigmoid colon.*

The Rectum and Anal Canal

Eventually, the sigmoid colon straightens out to become the *rectum.* The last few centimeters of the rectum are known as the *anal canal,* and the opening of the anal canal to the outside of the body is called the *anus* (Figure 32-10).

The lining of the large intestine secretes mucus to aid in the movement of substances. As chyme leaves the small intestine and enters the large intestine, the proximal portion of the large intestine absorbs water and a few electrolytes from it. The leftover chyme is then called **feces,** which are made of undigested solid materials, a little water, ions, mucus, cells of the intestinal lining, and bacteria.

The contractions of the large intestine propel feces forward, but these contractions normally occur periodically and as mass movements. Mass movements trigger the *defecation reflex,* which allows the anal sphincters to relax and feces to move through the anus in the process of elimination. The squeezing actions of the abdominal wall muscles also aid in emptying the large intestine.

▶ Characteristics of the Digestive Accessory Organs   LO 32.2

Although they do not form part of the alimentary canal, the digestive system's accessory organs play important roles in digestion. They deliver enzymes and other substances to the alimentary canal to assist with the digestive process.

The Liver

The liver is a large organ that fills most of the upper-right abdominal quadrant. It is reddish-brown in color and enclosed by a tough capsule that divides the liver into a large right lobe and a small left lobe (Figure 32-11). Each lobe is separated into smaller divisions called *hepatic lobules.* Branches of the *hepatic portal vein* carry blood from the digestive organs to the hepatic lobules. These hepatic lobules contain macrophages that destroy bacteria and viruses in the blood. Most people associate the liver with cleansing and detoxifying the blood, but it also has other functions important to the digestive system. Each lobule contains many cells called *hepatocytes* (*hepato* = liver and *cytes* = cells). Hepatocytes process the nutrients in blood and make **bile,** which is used in the digestion of fats. Bile leaves the liver through the hepatic duct. The *hepatic duct* merges with the *cystic duct* (the duct from the gallbladder) to form the *common bile duct.* This duct delivers bile to the duodenum. Another important function of the liver is to store vitamins and iron.

The Gallbladder

The gallbladder is a small, sac-like structure located beneath the liver (Figures 32-11 and 32-12). Its only function is to store bile, which leaves the gallbladder through the cystic duct. The hormone cholecystokinin causes the gallbladder to release bile. The salts in bile break large fat globules into smaller ones so that the digestive enzymes can more quickly digest them. Bile salts also increase the absorption of fatty acids, cholesterol, and fat-soluble vitamins into the bloodstream.

The Pancreas

The pancreas is located behind the stomach. Pancreatic *acinar cells* produce pancreatic juices, which ultimately flow through the pancreatic duct to the duodenum (Figure 32-12). Pancreatic juices contain the following enzymes:

- *Pancreatic amylase,* which digests carbohydrates.
- *Pancreatic lipase,* which digests lipids.

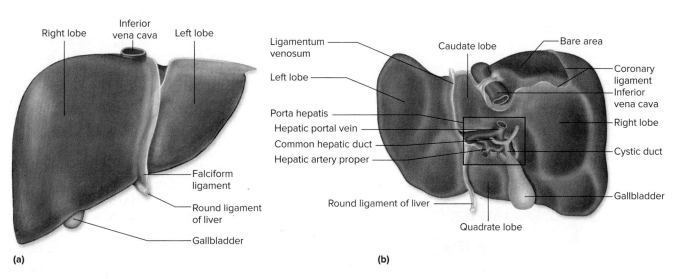

(a)

(b)

FIGURE 32-11   The liver is located in the right upper quadrant of the abdomen. (a) Anterior and (b) posteroinferior views show the two lobes of the liver, gallbladder, inferior vena cava, hepatic portal vein, and hepatic artery.

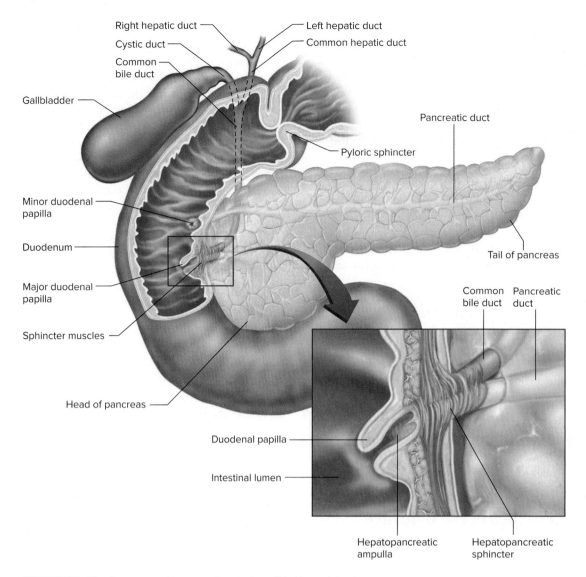

Labels in figure:
- Right hepatic duct
- Cystic duct
- Common bile duct
- Gallbladder
- Minor duodenal papilla
- Duodenum
- Major duodenal papilla
- Sphincter muscles
- Head of pancreas
- Left hepatic duct
- Common hepatic duct
- Pyloric sphincter
- Pancreatic duct
- Tail of pancreas
- Common bile duct
- Pancreatic duct
- Duodenal papilla
- Intestinal lumen
- Hepatopancreatic ampulla
- Hepatopancreatic sphincter

FIGURE 32-12   Pancreas and its connections to the gallbladder and duodenum.

- *Nucleases,* which digest nucleic acids.
- *Trypsin, chymotrypsin,* and *carboxypeptidase,* which digest proteins.

The pancreas also secretes bicarbonate ions into the duodenum that neutralize the acidic chyme arriving from the stomach. The parasympathetic nervous system stimulates the pancreas to release its enzymes. The hormones secretin and cholecystokinin also stimulate the pancreas to release digestive enzymes. Secretin and cholecystokinin come from the small intestine.

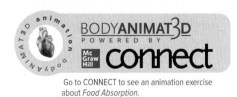

Go to CONNECT to see an animation exercise about *Food Absorption.*

▶ The Absorption of Nutrients   LO 32.3

Necessary food substances are known as **nutrients.** They include carbohydrates, proteins, lipids, vitamins, minerals, and water.

Three types of carbohydrates that humans ingest are starches (polysaccharides), simple sugars (monosaccharides and disaccharides), and cellulose. Starches come from foods such as pasta, potatoes, rice, and breads.

Monosaccharides and disaccharides are obtained from sweet foods and fruits. Most body cells use the monosaccharide glucose to make adenosine triphosphate (ATP). ATP provides a type of chemical energy needed by the body. When a person has an excess of glucose, it can be stored in the liver and skeletal muscle cells as **glycogen.**

Cellulose is a type of carbohydrate that humans cannot digest; it is found in many vegetables. It is necessary for digestion because it provides fiber or bulk for the large intestine, which helps the large intestine to empty more regularly. According to Harvard Medical International, a connection has been made between higher-fiber diets and a decrease in colon diseases, including cancer. This may be because fiber increases water absorption and bulk, causing more rapid emptying of the colon and decreasing the production of benign growths, such as adenomas or polyps, which increase the risk of cancer. Fiber also may neutralize toxins produced by gastrointestinal (GI) tract bacteria.

Lipids (fats) are obtained through various foods. The most abundant dietary lipids are **triglycerides.** They are found in meats, eggs, milk, and butter. **Cholesterol** is another common dietary lipid and is found in eggs, whole milk, butter, and cheeses. Lipids are used by the body primarily to make energy when glucose levels are low. Excess triglycerides are stored in adipose tissue. Cholesterol is essential to cell growth and function; cells use it to make cell membranes and some hormones. People should have the essential fatty acid linoleic acid in their diet because the body cannot make it. This fatty acid is found in corn and sunflower oils. People also need a certain amount of fat to absorb fat-soluble vitamins.

The fat-soluble vitamins are vitamins A, D, E, and K; the water-soluble vitamins are all the B vitamins and vitamin C. The many functions of vitamins are summarized in Table 32-1.

Minerals—primarily found in bones and teeth—make up about 4% of total body weight. Cells use minerals to make enzymes, cell membranes, and various proteins such as hemoglobin. The most important minerals to the human body are calcium, phosphorus, sulfur, sodium, chlorine, and magnesium. The body needs trace elements, including iron, manganese, copper, iodine, and zinc, in very small amounts.

Foods rich in protein include meats, eggs, milk, cheese, fish, chicken, turkey, nuts, seeds, and beans. Protein requirements vary from individual to individual, but all people must take in proteins that contain certain amino acids (called *essential amino acids*) because the body cannot make them. The body uses proteins for growth and tissue repair.

Keep in mind that an individual's ability to absorb nutrients changes over the course of his or her lifetime. See the feature *Caution: Handle with Care* for more information.

Medical terms are built and dissected using prefixes, word roots/combining form, and suffixes. For example, we can build the term *hyperlipidemia* by placing the parts of the term in the puzzle pieces where P = prefix, WR/CF = word root or combining form, and S = suffix.

hyperlipidemia

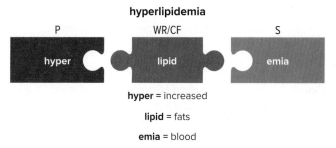

hyper = increased

lipid = fats

emia = blood

Hyperlipidemia is an increased amount of blood fats. Learn additional medical terms in the **Medical Terminology Practice** section at the end of this chapter.

TABLE 32-1	Common Vitamins and Their Importance in the Body
Vitamin	**Function**
Vitamin A	Needed for the production of visual receptors, mucus, the normal growth of bones and teeth, and the repair of epithelial tissues
Vitamin B_1 (thiamine)	Needed for carbohydrate metabolism
Vitamin B_2 (riboflavin)	Needed for carbohydrate and fat metabolism and for the growth of cells
Vitamin B_6	Needed for protein, antibody, and nucleic acid synthesis
Vitamin B_{12} (cyanocobalamin)	Needed for myelin production and carbohydrate and nucleic acid metabolism
Biotin	Needed for protein, fat, and nucleic acid metabolism
Folic acid	Needed for the production of amino acids, DNA, and red blood cells
Pantothenic acid	Needed for carbohydrate and fat metabolism
Niacin	Needed for carbohydrate, protein, fat, and nucleic acid metabolism
Vitamin C (ascorbic acid)	Needed for the production of collagen, amino acids, and hormones and for iron absorption
Vitamin D	Needed for calcium absorption
Vitamin E	Antioxidant that prevents the breakdown of certain tissues
Vitamin K	Needed for blood clotting

PATHOPHYSIOLOGY

LO 32.4

Common Diseases and Disorders of the Digestive System

APPENDICITIS is an inflammation of the appendix. If not treated promptly, it can be life-threatening.

Causes. This disorder may be caused by an appendix blocked by feces or tumor, infection, or other *idiopathic* (unknown) cause.

Signs and Symptoms. The signs and symptoms include lack of appetite, pain in the right lower quadrant (RLQ) that may radiate throughout the abdomen and even down the right leg, nausea, slight fever, and an increased white blood cell (WBC) count.

Diagnostic Exams and Tests. Often, the presenting symptoms are enough for diagnosis, but CBC (with an elevated WBC) and abdominal ultrasound or exploratory laparascopy can confirm the diagnosis. If exploratory laparoscopy is used, it will become a laparoscopic appendectomy when the inflamed appendix is removed.

Treatment. The primary treatments are antibiotics to prevent infection and an *appendectomy* to remove the appendix.

CIRRHOSIS is a chronic liver disease in which normal liver tissue is replaced with nonfunctional scar tissue.

Causes. This disease is often an autoimmune disease. It also may be caused by some medications and alcohol consumption. Hepatitis B and C infections also can contribute to the development of cirrhosis.

Signs and Symptoms. This disease has many symptoms, including anemia, fatigue, mental confusion, fever, vomiting, blood in the vomit, an enlarged liver, jaundice, unintended weight loss, swelling of the legs or abdomen, abdominal pain, decreased urine output, and pale feces.

Diagnostic Exams and Tests. Abdominal ultrasound and liver biopsy can confirm the diagnosis of cirrhosis.

Treatment. Alcohol consumption should be discontinued. A patient with cirrhosis may be given various medications, including antibiotics and diuretics. A liver transplant may be needed for the most seriously ill patients.

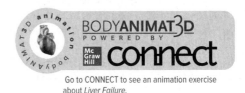

Go to CONNECT to see an animation exercise about *Liver Failure.*

CHOLELITHIASIS, or gallstones, are hard deposits that usually consist of either cholesterol or bilirubin. They are more common in women than in men.

Causes. Gallstones can be caused by a variety of factors, including diabetes, cirrhosis, and other medical conditions; rapid weight loss; failure of the gallbladder to empty completely, which may occur during pregnancy; and organ transplant.

Signs and Symptoms. Some people who have gallstones do not have symptoms. If symptoms do occur, they may include pain in the right upper quadrant (RUQ) of the abdomen, fever, jaundice, nausea and vomiting, and clay-colored feces.

Diagnostic Exams and Tests. An ultrasound of the gallbladder and CT scan or MRI may be done to confirm the diagnosis.

Treatment. Surgery to remove the stones is the most common treatment for people who have symptoms associated with gallstones. The most commonly used procedure is *laparoscopic cholecystectomy.* Another procedure, *lithotripsy,* is also a treatment option. It uses electrohydraulic shock waves to dissolve or break up the stones without the need for surgery. Medications also are used in some cases, but they take a long time to work.

COLITIS is inflammation of the large intestine. This condition can be chronic or short-lived, depending on the cause.

Causes. Colitis can be caused by a viral or bacterial infection or the use of antibiotics. Ulcers in the large intestine, Crohn's disease, various other diseases, and stress also may contribute to the development of this disorder.

Signs and Symptoms. The primary symptoms are abdominal pain, bloating, and diarrhea.

Diagnostic Exams and Tests. Upper and lower GI series may be performed in addition to colonoscopy (often with biopsy) to confirm a diagnosis of colitis.

Treatment. The first goal of therapy is to treat the underlying causes. Changing antibiotics, treating existing ulcers, and drinking plenty of fluids are treatment options. In advanced cases, surgery to remove the affected area of the colon, known as a *colectomy,* may be recommended. If too much of the colon is affected, a *colostomy* may be performed. In this procedure, the majority of the colon is removed and the opening to the outside of the body is moved to the abdomen, where an appliance known as an ostomy, usually with a collecting device commonly called a bag, collects fecal material.

COLORECTAL CANCER usually comes from the lining of the rectum or colon. This type of cancer is curable if treated early.

Causes. The causes are mostly unknown, although research is putting some blame on high-fat/low-fiber diets. Polyps in the colon or rectum can become cancerous, leading to this disease. Colorectal cancer may be prevented through regular screenings for polyps, which is done with a procedure known as a colonoscopy.

Signs and Symptoms. Anemia, unintended weight loss, abdominal pain, blood in the feces, narrow feces, or changes in bowel habits are all common symptoms.

Diagnostic Exams and Tests. In addition to lab tests, colonoscopy is most often performed to confirm a diagnosis of colon cancer.

Treatment. Chemotherapy is the first line of treatment. Surgery to remove a cancerous tumor or the affected portions of the colon or rectum (colectomy or colostomy) may be needed in more advanced cases.

CONSTIPATION is the condition of difficult defecation, which is the elimination of feces.

Causes. The primary causes are lack of physical activity, lack of fiber and adequate water in the diet, the use of certain medications, and thyroid and colon disorders.

Signs and Symptoms. Common signs and symptoms include infrequent bowel movements (for example, no bowel movement for 3 days), bloating, abdominal pain and pain during bowel movements, hard feces, and blood on the surface of feces.

Diagnostic Exams and Tests. Diagnosis is usually made based on the patient's signs and symptoms. A bowel motility test may be done if usual treatments are not helpful.

Treatment. Treatment includes an increase in dietary fiber; adequate fluid intake; regular exercise; and the use of stool softeners, laxatives, and enemas (for extreme cases only).

CROHN'S DISEASE is a common disorder called *inflammatory bowel disease.* It typically affects the end of the small intestine.

Causes. This is an autoimmune disorder.

Signs and Symptoms. The signs and symptoms of Crohn's disease include fever, tender gums, joint pain, GI ulcers, abdominal pain and gas, constipation or diarrhea, abnormal abdominal sounds, weight loss, intestinal bleeding, and blood in the feces.

Diagnostic Exams and Tests. Upper and lower GI series may be performed in addition to lab tests and colonoscopy. Many times Crohn's disease is diagnosed when no other diagnosis is apparent after testing.

Treatment. The first treatment is to change the patient's diet. Other treatments include medications to reduce inflammation, including steroids, as well as antibiotics and bowel "rest" in which IV (intravenous) feedings are given so that the patient's digestive system is not used. For the most serious cases, surgery to remove the affected part of the intestine may be needed. This procedure is known as an *enterectomy.*

DIARRHEA is the condition of watery and frequent feces. Many cases of diarrhea do not require treatment because they usually stop within a day or two.

Causes. The causes of diarrhea include bacterial, viral, or parasitic infections of the digestive system. It also may be caused by the ingestion of toxins; food allergies, including lactose intolerance; ulcers; Crohn's disease; laxative use; antibiotics; chemotherapy; and radiation therapy. Diarrhea related to infections may be prevented by washing hands thoroughly and cooking food properly.

Signs and Symptoms. The symptoms include abdominal cramps, watery feces, and the frequent passage of feces.

Diagnostic Exams and Tests. Labs, stool exams for ova and parasites, as well as barium enema and colonoscopy may be performed.

Treatment. Patients should drink fluids to prevent dehydration. The underlying causes, if known, should be treated. Medications and dietary changes are the primary treatment options. In severe cases, antidiarrheal medications such as Lomotil® may be prescribed.

DIVERTICULITIS is inflammation of diverticula in the intestine. **Diverticula** are abnormal dilations or pouches in the intestinal wall. When the diverticula are not inflamed, the condition is known as **DIVERTICULOSIS**.

Causes. The causes are mostly unknown. Lack of fiber in the diet and a bacterial infection of the diverticula can cause this disorder. Patients may find that certain foods, such as peanuts and seeds, aggravate this disorder.

Signs and Symptoms. Signs and symptoms include fever, nausea, abdominal pain, constipation or diarrhea, blood in the feces, and a high WBC.

Diagnostic Exams and Tests. In addition to labs, barium enema and colonoscopy often will be performed.

Treatment. Treatments include following a high-fiber diet, taking antibiotics, and keeping a food diary to track foods that cause flare-ups. A *colectomy* (surgery to remove the affected portion of the intestine) may be necessary in severe cases.

GASTRITIS is an inflammation of the stomach lining. It is often referred to as an "upset stomach."

Causes. Gastritis can be caused by bacteria or viruses, some medications, alcohol use, spicy foods, excessive eating, poisons, and stress. Cooking food properly to kill harmful bacteria and viruses can help to prevent this condition.

Signs and Symptoms. Symptoms include nausea, lack of appetite, heartburn, vomiting, and abdominal cramps.

Diagnostic Exams and Tests. Upper endoscopy may be done to confirm diagnosis and rule out other conditions such as ulcer or cancer.

Treatment. Lifestyle changes should be implemented to avoid foods or medications that irritate the stomach lining. Treatment with various medications to reduce the production of stomach acids, such as Pepcid® and Nexium®, can provide relief from the symptoms of this disorder.

GASTROESOPHAGEAL REFLUX DISEASE (GERD) is more commonly known as heartburn. It occurs when stomach acids are pushed into the esophagus.

Causes. Alcohol, some foods, a defective cardiac sphincter, pregnancy, obesity, a hiatal hernia, and repeated vomiting can contribute to the development of this disease.

Signs and Symptoms. Common symptoms include frequent burping, difficulty swallowing, a sore throat, a burning sensation in the chest following meals, nausea when lying down, and blood in the vomit.

Diagnostic Exams and Tests. Upper GI series and ultrasound may be done to confirm the diagnosis of GERD.

Treatment. Treatment includes losing weight, making dietary changes; reducing alcohol consumption; taking medications such as Pepcid® and Nexium®; and elevating the head, neck, and chest when lying down.

HEMORRHOIDS are varicose veins of the rectum or anus.

Causes. Hemorrhoids are caused by constipation, excessive straining during bowel movements, liver disease, pregnancy, and obesity.

Signs and Symptoms. Signs and symptoms include itching in the anal area, painful bowel movements, bright red blood on feces, and veins that protrude from the anus.

Diagnostic Exams and Tests. Physical exam usually confirms the diagnosis. For internal hemorrhoids, confirmatory proctosigmoidoscopy may be performed

Treatment. Constipation can be avoided or lessened by eating a high-fiber diet. Other treatments include stool softeners, medications to reduce hemorrhoid inflammation, and the surgical removal of hemorrhoids (*hemorrhoidectomy*).

HEPATITIS is inflammation of the liver. There are many different types of hepatitis.

Causes. Causes include bacteria, viruses, parasites, immune disorders, alcohol and drug use, and an overdose of acetaminophen. Preventive measures include getting hepatitis B (HBV) vaccinations, practicing safer sex, avoiding undercooked food (especially seafood), and using prescription or over-the-counter drugs (especially those containing acetaminophen) at their recommended dosages or as prescribed by a physician.

Signs and Symptoms. Symptoms include mild fever, bloating, lack of appetite, nausea, vomiting, abdominal pain, weakness, jaundice, itching in various body parts, an enlarged liver, dark urine, and breast development in males.

Diagnostic Exams and Tests. Lab studies, abdominal ultrasound, and liver biopsy all may be done to confirm the diagnosis of hepatitis and ascertain the type (A, B, C, nonA/nonB).

Treatment. Patients should avoid using alcohol and drugs as the inflamed liver cannot detoxify them. Various medications may be prescribed.

A **HIATAL HERNIA** occurs when a portion of the stomach protrudes into the chest cavity through an opening in the diaphragm.

Causes. The causes are mostly unknown, although obesity and smoking are considered risk factors. Eating small meals can be an effective preventive measure.

Signs and Symptoms. Signs and symptoms include excessive burping, difficulty swallowing, chest pain, and heartburn.

Diagnostic Exams and Tests. Upper endoscopy may be performed to confirm the hiatal hernia diagnosis.

Treatment. Treatments are weight reduction, medications to reduce stomach acid production, and surgical repair of the hernia.

INGUINAL HERNIAS occur when a portion of the large intestine protrudes into the inguinal canal (groin), which is located where the thigh and the body trunk meet. In males, the hernia also can protrude into the scrotum.

Causes. The causes are mostly unknown, although these hernias may be caused by weak muscles in the abdominal walls.

Signs and Symptoms. A lump in the groin or scrotum and pain in the groin that gets worse when bending or straining are the common symptoms.

Diagnostic Exams and Tests. Diagnosis is typically made during a physical examination.

Treatment. Pain medications may be prescribed. Surgery to repair the hernia is needed, in which the large intestine is pushed back into the abdominal cavity.

ORAL CANCER usually involves the lips or tongue but can occur anywhere in the mouth. This type of cancer tends to spread rapidly to other organs.

Causes. The causes are mostly unknown, although the use of tobacco products and alcohol are known risk factors. Poor oral hygiene and ulcers in the mouth also can cause oral cancer.

Signs and Symptoms. Signs and symptoms include difficulty tasting; problems swallowing; and ulcers on the tongue, lip, or other mouth structures. Leukoplakia, or hardened white patches in the mucous membrane of the mouth, are considered precancerous lesions.

Diagnostic Exams and Tests. Suspicious areas should be examined and biopsied to confirm any diagnosis of leukoplakia or oral neoplasm.

Treatment. Radiation therapy, chemotherapy, and surgical removal of the malignant area are the treatment options.

PANCREATIC CANCER is the fourth leading cause of cancer deaths in the United States.

Causes. The causes are mostly unknown, although smoking and alcohol consumption are considered risk factors.

Signs and Symptoms. Common signs and symptoms include depression, fatigue, lack of appetite, nausea or vomiting, abdominal pain, constipation or diarrhea, jaundice, and unintended weight loss.

Diagnostic Exams and Tests. Abdominal ultrasound and CT scans as well as biopsies may be done to confirm the diagnosis.

Treatment. Treatment includes radiation therapy, chemotherapy, and surgical removal of the tumor.

STOMACH CANCER most commonly occurs in the uppermost, or cardiac, portion of the stomach. It appears to occur more frequently in Japan, Chile, and Iceland than in the United States.

Causes. The causes are mostly unknown, although stomach ulcers may contribute to the development of stomach cancer.

Signs and Symptoms. Signs and symptoms include frequent bloating, lack of appetite, feeling full after eating small amounts, nausea, vomiting (with or without blood), abdominal cramps, excessive gas, and blood in the feces.

Diagnostic Exams and Tests. Upper and lower GI series may be performed in addition to stomach ultrasound and biopsy.

Treatment. Treatment includes radiation therapy, chemotherapy, and surgical removal of the tumor.

STOMACH ULCERS occur when the lining of the stomach breaks down.

Causes. Bacteria (particularly *Helicobacter pylori*), smoking, alcohol, excessive aspirin use, and hypersecretion of stomach acid all can cause stomach ulcers. They may be prevented by stopping smoking and avoiding aspirin, certain foods, and alcohol.

Signs and Symptoms. Symptoms include nausea, abdominal pain, vomiting (with or without blood), and weight loss.

Diagnostic Exams and Tests. Diagnosis can be confirmed by upper endoscopy and testing for the *H. pylori* bacteria.

Treatment. Treatment options include antibiotics, medications to reduce stomach acid production, *partial gastrectomy* (surgery to remove the affected portion of the stomach), and *vagotomy* (cutting the vagus nerve) to reduce the production of stomach acid.

SUMMARY OF LEARNING OUTCOMES

OUTCOME	KEY POINTS
32.1 Describe the organs of the alimentary canal and their functions.	The pathway of food through the alimentary canal starts with the mouth and continues through the pharynx, esophagus, stomach, small intestine, large intestine, and anal canal. The mouth takes in food and the teeth assist in reducing its size through chewing. The tongue mixes food and holds it between the teeth. The salivary glands produce saliva to moisten and break down food. The pharynx is a long, muscular tube connecting the oral and nasal cavities. It pushes food into the esophagus. The esophagus is a muscular tube that pushes food toward the stomach through muscular contractions. The stomach receives the food, mixes it with gastric juices to start protein digestion, and moves it into the small intestine. The small intestine carries out most of the nutrient absorption. The large intestine's primary job is to rid the body of solid waste by defecation.

OUTCOME	KEY POINTS
32.2 Explain the functions of the digestive system's accessory organs.	The accessory organs to the digestive system include the liver, gallbladder, and pancreas. As a digestive organ, the liver stores vitamins and iron and produces macrophages to fight infection. It also secretes bile for fat digestion. The gallbladder stores the bile produced by the liver. The pancreas produces pancreatic juices that assist in carbohydrate, lipid, and protein digestion.
32.3 Identify the nutrients absorbed by the digestive system and where they are absorbed.	Nutrients absorbed by the body include carbohydrates, proteins, lipids, vitamins, minerals, and water. Most of the absorption takes place in the small intestine.
32.4 Describe the causes, signs and symptoms, diagnosis, and treatments of various common diseases and disorders of the digestive system.	There are many common diseases and disorders of the digestive system with varied signs, symptoms, diagnosis, and treatments. Some of these include appendicitis, cirrhosis, cholelithiasis, colitis, colorectal cancer, constipation, Crohn's disease, diarrhea, diverticulitis, diverticulosis, gastritis, gastroesophageal reflux disease or GERD (commonly known as heartburn), hemorrhoids, hepatitis, hiatal hernia, inguinal hernia, oral cancer, pancreatic cancer, stomach cancer, and stomach ulcers.

CASE STUDY CRITICAL THINKING

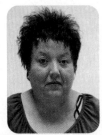

© McGraw-Hill Education

Recall Sylvia Gonzales from the case study at the beginning of this chapter. Now that you have completed the chapter, answer the following questions regarding her case.

1. What is the function of the gallbladder?

2. If Sylvia Gonzales does not want to have surgery, what other treatment options are available?

3. Will Sylvia Gonzales need to change her diet once her gallbladder is removed?

EXAM PREPARATION QUESTIONS

1. (LO 32.1) Which layer of the digestive tract is the most active in absorbing nutrients?
   a. Mucosa
   b. Submucosa
   c. Muscular
   d. Serosa
   e. Visceral

2. (LO 32.2) Which of the following is an accessory organ of the digestive process?
   a. Stomach
   b. Small intestine
   c. Liver
   d. Esophagus
   e. Pharynx

3. (LO 32.1) Although it hangs from the soft palate, the _____ is not one of the tonsils.
   a. Lingual
   b. Uvula
   c. Palatine
   d. Pharyngeal
   e. Adenoid

4. (LO 32.1) When an organ pushes through the wall that contains it, a(n) _____ develops.
   a. Sphincter
   b. Aneurysm
   c. Ulcer
   d. Hernia
   e. Bolus

5. (LO 32.4) Also known as inflammatory bowel disease, _____ often affects the end of the small intestine.
   a. Diverticulitis
   b. Crohn's disease
   c. GERD
   d. Colitis
   e. Cholelithiasis

6. (LO 32.2) Which of the following is made by the liver?
   a. Amylase
   b. Trypsin
   c. Secretin
   d. Bilirubin
   e. Bile

7. (LO 32.3) Which of the following is *not* a type of carbohydrate?
   a. Monosaccharides
   b. Polysaccharides
   c. Cellulose
   d. Disaccharides
   e. Triglycerides

8. (LO 32.3) Why do people need to include fiber in their diet?
   a. To help the large intestine empty more regularly
   b. To make energy when glucose levels are low
   c. To make cell membranes and hormones
   d. To help the body absorb fat-soluble vitamins
   e. To help synthesize antibodies and nucleic acids

9. (LO 32.4) Which of the following terms is used to describe difficult defecation?
   a. Cirrhosis
   b. Constipation
   c. Cholelithiasis
   d. Diarrhea
   e. Crohn's disease

10. (LO 32.4) Which disorder is commonly referred to as an "upset stomach"?
    a. GERD
    b. Diverticulitis
    c. Gastritis
    d. Hiatal hernia
    e. Crohn's disease

M E D I C A L   T E R M I N O L O G Y   P R A C T I C E

Analyze the following medical terms, presented throughout the chapter. Using a medical dictionary (or Appendix I), place a / mark between each word part. Define each word part and then define the whole word.

EXAMPLE: **gastr/oid** = gastr means "stomach" + oid means "resembling"
   GASTROID means "resembling the stomach."

1. bicuspid
2. carboxypeptidase
3. diverticulosis
4. hepatocyte

5. idiopathic
6. laryngopharynx
7. nuclease
8. polysaccharide

9. pyloric
10. sublingual
11. hematemesis
12. gastroenteritis

The Endocrine System

CASE STUDY

PATIENT INFORMATION	Patient Name	DOB	Allergies
	Ken Washington	12/01/1958	Sulfa
	Attending	**MRN**	**Other Information**
	Paul F. Buckwalter, MD	00-AA-008	Recent CVA w/ residual foot drop

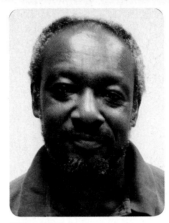
©McGraw-Hill Education

Ken Washington comes to the office today complaining of feeling "odd." His symptoms include weight loss for no apparent reason, "jitteriness" with a feeling like his heart is racing, and overall irritability. You notice that the patient's eyes appear more prominent than normal. Ken Washington is particularly concerned about his new symptoms, as he was only recently discharged from the hospital after suffering a CVA. He has a residual foot drop, for which he wears a brace and is receiving physical therapy.

Keep Ken Washington in mind as you study this chapter. There will be questions at the end of the chapter based on the case study. The information in the chapter will help you answer these questions.

LEARNING OUTCOMES

After completing Chapter 33, you will be able to:

33.1 Describe the general functions of hormones and the endocrine system.

33.2 Identify the hormones released by the pituitary gland, thyroid gland, parathyroid glands, adrenal glands, pancreas, and other hormone-producing organs and give the functions of each.

33.3 Explain the effect of stressors on the body.

33.4 Describe the causes, signs and symptoms, diagnosis, and treatments of various endocrine disorders.

KEY TERMS

endocrine gland
exocrine gland
feedback loop
gonads
G-protein
hormone
islets of Langerhans
nonsteroidal hormone

parathyroid glands
pineal body
prostaglandins
steroidal hormone
stressor
thymus
thyroid gland

I.C.1   Describe structural organization of the human body

I.C.2   Identify body systems

I.C.4   List major organs in each body system

I.C.5   Identify the anatomical location of major organs in each body system

I.C.6   Compare structure and function of the human body across the life span

I.C.7   Describe the normal function of each body system

I.C.8   Identify common pathology related to each body system including:
(a) signs
(b) symptoms
(c) etiology

I.C.9   Analyze pathology for each body system including:
(a) diagnostic measures
(b) treatment modalities

V.C.9   Identify medical terms labeling the word parts

V.C.10   Define medical terms and abbreviations related to all body systems

2. **Anatomy and Physiology**

   a. List all body systems and their structures and functions

   b. Describe common diseases, symptoms and etiologies as they apply to each system

   c. Identify diagnostic and treatment modalities as they relate to each body system

3. **Medical Terminology**

   a. Define and use the entire basic structure of medical terminology and be able to accurately identify the correct context (i.e., root, prefix, suffix, combinations, spelling, and definitions)

   b. Build and dissect medical terminology from roots and suffixes to understand the word element combinations

   c. Apply medical terminology for each specialty

   d. Define and use medical abbreviations when appropriate and acceptable

▸ Introduction

The endocrine (*endo-,* meaning "within," and *-crine,* meaning "to secrete") system includes the organs of the body that secrete hormones directly into body fluids such as blood. Hormones help to regulate the chemical reactions within cells. They therefore control the functions of the organs, tissues, and other cells. In this chapter, you will learn about the processes and organs of the endocrine system. Figure 33-1 shows the organs of the endocrine system, as well as the heart and kidney, both of which secrete a hormone, although hormone secretion is not the primary function of either of them. As shown, the gastrointestinal (GI) tract also secretes hormones, but again hormone secretion is not its primary function.

▸ Hormones
LO 33.1

Endocrine glands are ductless glands. This means they release their hormones directly into the tissues they act upon or into the bloodstream, which carries the hormone to the target cells. As you study each gland discussed in this chapter, refer to Figure 33-1 for its location.

   Hormones are chemicals secreted by a cell that affect the functions of other cells. Once released, most hormones enter the bloodstream, which transports them to their target cells. A hormone's target cells are those that contain the receptors for the hormone. A hormone cannot affect a cell unless the cell has receptors for it, in much the same way that a locked door needs the key specifically cut to open its lock. Table 33-1

outlines the endocrine glands, the hormone(s) secreted by each, and the action resulting from each hormone.

Types of Hormones

Many hormones in the body are derived from steroids. Steroids are soluble in lipids (fats) and therefore can cross cell membranes easily. Once a **steroidal hormone** is inside a cell, it binds to its receptor, which is commonly in the cell's nucleus. The hormone-receptor complex turns a gene on or off. When new genes are turned on or off, the cell begins to carry out new functions, and this is ultimately how steroidal hormones affect their target cells. Examples of steroidal hormones are estrogen, progesterone, testosterone, and cortisol.

   Nonsteroidal hormones are made of amino acids or proteins. Proteins cannot easily cross the cell membrane. Therefore, these hormones bind to receptors on the cell's surface. The hormone-receptor complex in the membrane usually activates a G-protein. The **G-protein** causes enzymes inside the cell to be turned on. Different chemical reactions then begin inside the cell, and the cell takes on new functions.

   Prostaglandins (tissue hormones) are local hormones. They are derived from lipid molecules and typically do not need to travel in the bloodstream to find their target cells. This is because the prostaglandin hormone is created in the same area of tissue that is home to that specific hormone's target cells. Prostaglandins, just like all other hormones, affect cell function and are produced by many body organs, including the kidneys, stomach, uterus, heart, and brain.

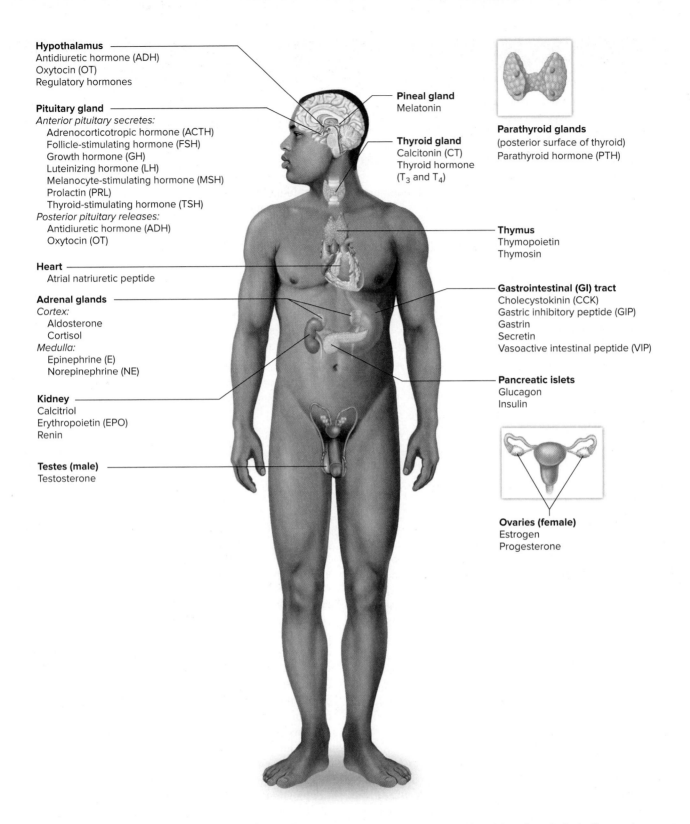

Hypothalamus
Antidiuretic hormone (ADH)
Oxytocin (OT)
Regulatory hormones

Pituitary gland
Anterior pituitary secretes:
  Adrenocorticotropic hormone (ACTH)
  Follicle-stimulating hormone (FSH)
  Growth hormone (GH)
  Luteinizing hormone (LH)
  Melanocyte-stimulating hormone (MSH)
  Prolactin (PRL)
  Thyroid-stimulating hormone (TSH)
Posterior pituitary releases:
  Antidiuretic hormone (ADH)
  Oxytocin (OT)

Heart
  Atrial natriuretic peptide

Adrenal glands
Cortex:
  Aldosterone
  Cortisol
Medulla:
  Epinephrine (E)
  Norepinephrine (NE)

Kidney
Calcitriol
Erythropoietin (EPO)
Renin

Testes (male)
Testosterone

Pineal gland
Melatonin

Thyroid gland
Calcitonin (CT)
Thyroid hormone
(T_3 and T_4)

Parathyroid glands
(posterior surface of thyroid)
Parathyroid hormone (PTH)

Thymus
Thymopoietin
Thymosin

Gastrointestinal (GI) tract
Cholecystokinin (CCK)
Gastric inhibitory peptide (GIP)
Gastrin
Secretin
Vasoactive intestinal peptide (VIP)

Pancreatic islets
Glucagon
Insulin

Ovaries (female)
Estrogen
Progesterone

FIGURE 33-1   Endocrine system—endocrine glands and other organs that secrete hormones are found throughout the body. They produce various types of hormones.

Negative and Positive Feedback Loops

Hormone levels are controlled by a mechanism known as a **feedback loop,** which can be negative or positive (see Figure 33-2). In a negative feedback loop, a stimulus such as eating raises blood sugar levels. This increase is detected by the pancreas, which secretes the hormone insulin in response.

As cells of the liver take up glucose to store it as glycogen and the body cells take up glucose for energy, the blood glucose levels decline and the insulin release stops as blood glucose levels normalize.

In a positive feedback loop, a stimulus also begins the process, as when a nursing infant suckles at the mother's

TABLE 33-1 Endocrine Glands: Their Hormones and Actions

Gland	Hormone	Action Produced
Hypothalamus (produces)	Antidiuretic hormone (ADH)	Stored and released by posterior pituitary
	Oxytocin (OT)	Stored and released by posterior pituitary
Anterior pituitary	Growth hormone (GH)	Promotes growth and tissue maintenance
	Melanocyte-stimulating hormone (MSH)	Stimulates pigment regulation in epidermis
	Adrenocorticotropic hormone (ACTH)	Stimulates adrenal cortex to produce its hormones
	Thyroid-stimulating hormone (TSH)	Stimulates the thyroid to produce its hormones
	Follicle-stimulating hormone (FSH)	(F) Stimulates ovaries to produce ova and estrogen (M) Stimulates spermatogenesis
	Luteinizing hormone (LH)	(F) Stimulates ovaries for ovulation and estrogen production (M) Stimulates testes to produce testosterone
	Prolactin (PRL)	(F) Stimulates breasts to produce milk (M) Works with and complements LH
Posterior pituitary (releases)	Antidiuretic hormone (ADH)	Stimulates kidneys to retain water
	Oxytocin (OT)	Stimulates uterine contractions for labor and delivery and breast milk ejection
Pineal body	Melatonin	Regulates biological clock; linked to onset of puberty
Thyroid	T_3 and T_4	Protein synthesis and increased energy production for all cells
	Calcitonin	Increases bone calcium and decreases blood calcium
Parathyroid	Parathyroid hormone (PTH)	Agonist to calcitonin; decreases bone calcium and increases blood calcium
Thymus	Thymosin and thymopoietin	Both hormones stimulate the production of T lymphocytes
Adrenal cortex	Aldosterone	Stimulates body to retain sodium and water
	Cortisol	Decreases protein synthesis; decreases inflammation
Adrenal medulla	Epinephrine and norepinephrine	Prepare the body for stress; increase heart rate, respiration, and blood pressure
Pancreas (islets of Langerhans)	Alpha cells—glucagon	Increases blood sugar; decreases protein synthesis
	Beta cells—insulin	Decreases blood sugar; increases protein synthesis
Gonads: Ovaries (Female)	Estrogen and progesterone	Secondary sex characteristics; female reproductive hormones
Testes (Male)	Testosterone	Secondary sex characteristics; male reproductive hormone

breast. The suckling sends an impulse to the hypothalamus, which in turn signals the posterior pituitary to release oxytocin. The oxytocin stimulates milk production and ejection from the mammary glands. Milk continues to be released as long as the infant continues to nurse.

▶ Hormone Production LO 33.2

Hormones are produced in various organs and glands throughout the body. For example, the brain has several sites of hormone production, including the hypothalamus, pituitary gland, and pineal body. The pancreas, kidneys, stomach, and reproductive organs also produce important hormones. In this section, we will discuss the individual endocrine organs and the hormones they produce and/or store.

The Hypothalamus

The hypothalamus is located in the diencephalon of the brain (see the chapter *The Nervous System*) and produces the

hormones *oxytocin* and *antidiuretic hormone* (*ADH*). These hormones are transported to the posterior pituitary, where they are stored and released as directed by the hypothalamus.

The Pituitary Gland

The pituitary gland, also known as the *hypophysis*, is located at the base of the brain and controlled by the hypothalamus. This gland is well protected by a bony structure called the sella turcica. The pituitary is divided into two lobes: the anterior lobe and the posterior lobe (see Figures 33-1 and 33-3).

Anterior Lobe of the Pituitary Gland
The anterior lobe of the pituitary gland, also known as the *adenohypophysis*, secretes the following hormones:

- *Growth hormone (GH).* As its name suggests, this hormone stimulates an increase in the size of the body's muscles and bones. It is important in childhood for growth. It also stimulates tissue repair. Growth hormone is also known as *somatotropin.*

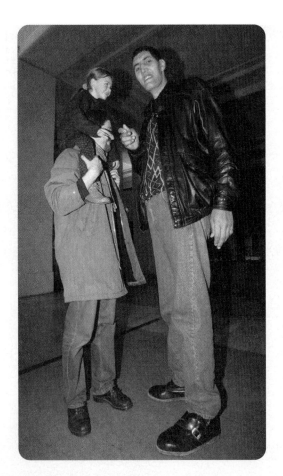

FIGURE 33-8   Gigantism results from hypersecretion of growth hormone.
©Eric Robert/Sygma/Getty Images

GRAVES' DISEASE is a disorder in which a person develops antibodies that attack the thyroid gland (see Figure 33-10). This attack causes the thyroid to produce too many thyroid hormones. Graves' disease is the most common type of hyperthyroidism in the United States.

Causes. This disease is caused by an overproduction of thyroid hormones. It also is considered an autoimmune disorder.

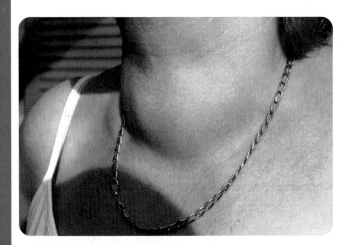

FIGURE 33-9   An iodine deficiency causes simple (endemic) goiter and results in high levels of TSH.
©Chris Pancewicz/Alamy Stock Photo

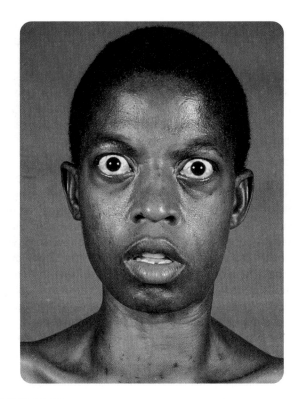

FIGURE 33-10   Signs of Graves' disease, a form of hyperthyroidism, include protruding eyes and goiter.
©Dr M.A. Ansary/Science Source

Signs and Symptoms. The most common signs and symptoms include exophthalmos (protrusion of the eyes) and goiter (thyroid enlargement). Other symptoms include insomnia, unexplained weight loss, anxiety, muscle weakness, increased appetite, excessive sweating, vision problems, and an increased heart rate.

Diagnostic Exams and Tests. Testing may include thyroid studies and radioactive iodine uptake testing.

Treatment. Treatment includes medications to reduce heart rate, sweating, and nervousness; radiation to destroy the thyroid gland; surgery to remove the thyroid gland (thyroidectomy); and supplemental thyroid hormones if the gland is destroyed or removed.

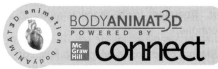

Go to CONNECT to see an animation exercise about *Hyperthyroidism.*

CRETINISM is an extreme form of hypothyroidism that is present prior to or soon after birth (see Figure 33-11).

Causes. The cause is hypothyroidism at birth (a congenital anomaly) related to the absence or malformation of the thyroid gland, abnormal formation of thyroid hormones, or pituitary failure that results in a lack of thyroid stimulation.

Signs and Symptoms. Stunted growth, abnormal bone formation, mental retardation, low body temperature, and overall sluggishness are the primary signs and symptoms.

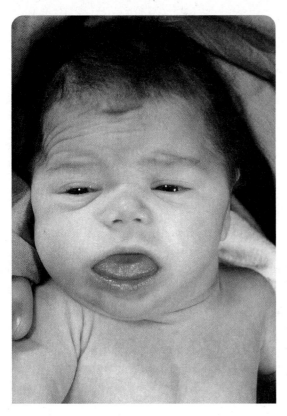

FIGURE 33-11 Cretinism is the result of an underactive thyroid gland during infancy and childhood.
©Alamy Stock Photo

Diagnostic Exams and Tests. Physical examination reveals typical features of cretinism. Thyroid studies will confirm diagnosis.

Treatment. The treatment is thyroid hormone replacement.

MYXEDEMA is a disorder in which the thyroid gland does not produce adequate amounts of thyroid hormone. It is a severe type of hypothyroidism that is most common in females over age 50.

Causes. Causes include the removal of the thyroid, radiation treatments to the neck area, and obesity. This disorder may be congenital.

Signs and Symptoms. Signs and symptoms include weakness, fatigue, weight gain, depression, general body aches, dry skin and hair, hair loss, puffy hands or feet, a decreased ability to taste food, abnormal menstrual periods, pale or yellow skin, a slow heart rate, low blood pressure, anemia, an enlarged heart, high cholesterol levels, and coma.

Diagnostic Exams and Tests. Physical exam and history will be the starting point. Thyroid testing will confirm the diagnosis.

Treatment. Treatment consists of giving supplemental thyroid hormones intravenously or orally and closely monitoring the levels of thyroid hormones.

SUMMARY OF LEARNING OUTCOMES

OUTCOME	KEY POINTS
33.1 Describe the general functions of hormones and the endocrine system.	Endocrine glands are ductless glands, releasing hormones directly into the bloodstream and tissues. The organs of the endocrine system produce hormones that regulate the chemical reactions within cells, controlling the functions of organs, tissues, and other cells. Hormone levels are controlled by positive and negative feedback loops.
33.2 Identify the hormones released by the pituitary gland, thyroid gland, parathyroid glands, adrenal glands, pancreas, and other hormone-producing organs and give the functions of each.	The pituitary gland releases the following hormones: GH, MSH, ACTH, TSH, FSH, LH, PRL, ADH, and OT. The thyroid gland releases calcitonin, T_3, and T_4, which are important in growth and protein synthesis. The parathyroid gland releases PTH, which balances the action of calcitonin. The adrenal medulla secretes epinephrine and norepinephrine, which work with the sympathetic nervous system. The adrenal cortex produces many hormones, but the two major ones are aldosterone and cortisol. The two types of hormone-releasing cells in the pancreas are alpha cells, which release glucagon, and beta cells, which release insulin. The pineal body releases melatonin; the thymus releases thymosin and thymopoietin; ovaries (females) release estrogen and progesterone; and the testes (males) release testosterone. The kidneys produce erythropoietin and the heart produces atrial natriuretic peptide. Each hormone's specific function may be found in Table 33-1.

OUTCOME	KEY POINTS
33.3 Explain the effect of stressors on the body.	Stressors are stimuli that produce a stress response, a physiologic response to the stimulus that changes the body's functioning in some way.
33.4 Describe the causes, signs and symptoms, diagnosis, and treatments of various endocrine disorders.	The diseases and disorders of the endocrine system are as varied as the organs and hormone dysfunctions that cause them. An overview of these conditions is found in Table 33-2.

CASE STUDY CRITICAL THINKING

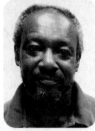

©McGraw-Hill Education

Recall Ken Washington from the case study at the beginning of the chapter. Now that you have completed this chapter, answer the following questions regarding his case:

1. What gland is likely to be causing Ken Washington's problems?

2. Based on what you have learned in this chapter, what diagnosis do you think Dr. Buckwalter will have for Ken Washington?

3. What treatment options are available?

4. What other condition is often caused by treating this condition, and how is it managed?

EXAM PREPARATION QUESTIONS

1. (LO 33.1) Which of following hormone types is also known as a tissue hormone?
   a. Steroidal hormones
   b. Nonsteroidal hormones
   c. G-proteins
   d. Prostaglandins
   e. Thyroid hormones

2. (LO 33.2) Which endocrine organ also has a digestive function?
   a. Adrenal medulla
   b. Adrenal cortex
   c. Pancreas
   d. Pineal body
   e. Thymus

3. (LO 33.2) Which hormone assists the kidneys in retaining fluid?
   a. ACTH
   b. ADH
   c. PTH
   d. FSH
   e. MSH

4. (LO 33.2) The numeral in "T_3" and "T_4" stands for the number of _____ atoms needed for the hormones to work properly.
   a. Chloride
   b. Potassium
   c. Calcium
   d. Iodine
   e. Sodium

5. (LO 33.4) From which endocrine disease did President John F. Kennedy suffer?
   a. Cushing's syndrome
   b. Addison's disease
   c. Acromegaly
   d. Hypothyroidism
   e. Graves' disease

6. (LO 33.3) Which hormone is released when a person is under prolonged stress?
   a. Glucagon
   b. Aldosterone
   c. Melatonin
   d. Oxytocin
   e. Cortisol

7. (LO 33.2) Which of the following hormones is not produced by the anterior pituitary?
   a. Growth hormone
   b. Follicle-stimulating hormone
   c. Oxytocin
   d. Luteinizing hormone
   e. Prolactin

8. (LO 33.1) Nonsteroidal hormones require which of the following to turn on enzymes inside target cells?
   a. Amino acids
   b. Prostaglandins
   c. Calcitonin
   d. G-protein
   e. Prolactin

9. (LO 33.4) A condition in which the body produces too much cortisol is
   a. Cushing's syndrome
   b. Graves' disease
   c. Myxedema
   d. Gigantism
   e. Diabetes insipidus

10. (LO 33.4) When too much growth hormone is produced in adults, the result is
    a. Dwarfism
    b. Gigantism
    c. Cretinism
    d. Myxedema
    e. Acromegaly

M E D I C A L   T E R M I N O L O G Y   P R A C T I C E

Analyze the following medical terms, presented throughout the chapter. Using a medical dictionary (or Appendix I), place a / mark between each word part. Define each word part and then define the whole word.

EXAMPLE: **aden/ oma** = aden means "gland" + oma means "tumor"
ADENOMA means "tumor of a gland."

1. acromegaly
2. adrenocorticotropic
3. antidiuretic
4. exocrine
5. hypothalamus

6. melanocyte
7. natriuretic
8. nonsteroidal
9. parathyroid
10. thymopoietin

11. hyperparathyroidism
12. endocrine

Special Senses

CASE STUDY

PATIENT INFORMATION	Patient Name	DOB	Allergies
	Valarie Ramirez	08/04/1986	Penicillin
	Attending	**MRN**	**Other Information**
	Paul F. Buckwalter, MD	00-AA-006	Current medications: Cyclafem 7/7/7 Lipitor® 10 mg daily

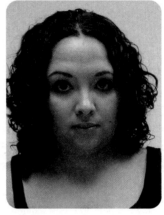

Valarie Ramirez is brought to the office by her boyfriend because she has something in her eye. While riding her motorcycle yesterday, something flew up under her helmet visor. She has been using Visine® eyedrops, but when she woke up this morning, her eye felt worse. She says she thinks a tiny bug flew into her eye, but she cannot get it out. She has tried flushing the eye with water, but it did not help. You notice her right eye is red and swollen. You prepare Valarie Ramirez for the physician to examine her eye.

Keep Valarie Ramirez in mind as you study this chapter. There will be questions at the end of the chapter based on the case study. The information in the chapter will help you answer these questions.

LEARNING OUTCOMES

After completing Chapter 34, you will be able to:

34.1 Describe the anatomy of the nose and the function of each part.

34.2 Describe the anatomy of the tongue and the function of each part.

34.3 Describe the anatomy of the eye and the function of each part, including the accessory structures and their functions.

34.4 Explain the visual pathway through the eye and to the brain for interpretation.

34.5 Describe the causes, signs and symptoms, diagnosis, and treatments of various disorders of the eyes.

34.6 Describe the anatomy of the ear and the function of each part, and explain the role of the ear in maintaining equilibrium.

34.7 Explain how sounds travel through the ear and are interpreted in the brain.

34.8 Describe the causes, signs and symptoms, diagnosis, and treatments of various disorders of the ears.

KEY TERMS

auricle	organ of Corti
cerumen	ossicles
choroid	oval window
cochlea	papillae
conjunctiva	refraction
cornea	retina
eustachian tube	semicircular canals
external auditory canal	sensory adaptation
gustatory cortex	tympanic membrane
labyrinth	vestibule
lacrimal apparatus	

CAAHEP

I.C.1   Describe structural organization of the human body

I.C.2   Identify body systems

I.C.4   List major organs in each body system

I.C.5   Identify the anatomical location of major organs in each body system

I.C.6   Compare structure and function of the human body across the life span

I.C.7   Describe the normal function of each body system

I.C.8   Identify common pathology related to each body system, including:
(a) signs
(b) symptoms
(c) etiology

I.C.9   Analyze pathology for each body system, including:
(a) diagnostic measures
(b) treatment modalities

V.C.9   Identify medical terms labeling the word parts

V.C.10   Define medical terms and abbreviations related to all body systems

ABHES

2. **Anatomy and Physiology**
   a. List all body systems and their structures and functions
   b. Describe common diseases, symptoms, and etiologies as they apply to each system
   c. Identify diagnostic and treatment modalities as they relate to each body system

3. **Medical Terminology**
   a. Define and use the entire basic structure of medical terminology, and be able to accurately identify the correct context (i.e., root, prefix, suffix, combinations, spelling, and definitions)
   b. Build and dissect medical terminology from roots and suffixes to understand the word element combinations
   c. Apply medical terminology for each specialty
   d. Define and use medical abbreviations when appropriate and acceptable

▶ Introduction

The special senses are smell, taste, vision, hearing, and equilibrium. They are called special senses because their sensory receptors are located within relatively large sensory organs in the head—the nose, tongue, eyes, and ears. Although the skin also is considered a sense organ (in fact, it is the largest sense organ), touch is not considered a special sense but rather a generalized one (refer to the chapter *The Integumentary System*). This chapter introduces the structure and function of the special sense organs.

As a medical assistant, you will likely be asked to assist with or perform examinations and treatments for common disorders of the eyes and ears, so you will need to understand how these important sense organs function.

▶ The Nose and the Sense of Smell   LO 34.1

Smell receptors, also called *olfactory receptors,* are located in the olfactory organ, found in the upper part of the nasal cavity. See Figure 34-1. Smell receptors are chemoreceptors, which means that they respond to changes in chemical concentrations. Chemicals that activate smell receptors must be dissolved in the mucus of the nose. To process odors, smell receptors must be activated, then they send their information to the olfactory nerves. Refer to the chapter *The Nervous System* for more information about these nerves and the various parts of the brain. The olfactory nerves send the information along olfactory bulbs and tracts to different areas of the cerebrum in the brain. The cerebrum interprets the information as a particular type of smell.

Consider the following information related to our sense of smell.

- When individuals have either a "dry nose" or excessive mucus related to an upper respiratory tract infection or allergies, they may have trouble smelling. This is due to the inability of the chemicals (odors) that cause our sense of smell to be dissolved in the mucus of the nose.

- Humans have a relatively poor sense of smell compared to certain animals for two reasons. The chemicals (odors) that activate smell must diffuse all the way up the nasal cavity.

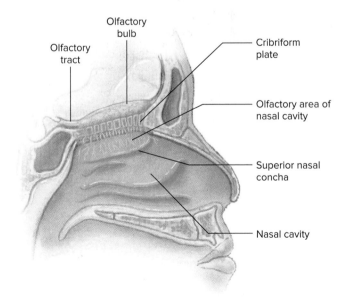

FIGURE 34-1   The olfactory area (organ) is located in the superior part of the nasal cavity.

Also, the human nose has fewer smell receptors than most animal noses.

- Our sense of smell undergoes **sensory adaptation,** which means that the same chemical can stimulate smell receptors for only a limited amount of time. In a relatively short period of time, the smell receptors fatigue and no longer respond to the same chemical (odor), so it can no longer be smelled. Sensory adaptation explains why you smell a strong odor, such as perfume, when you first encounter it, but after a few minutes, you cannot smell it or may be less aware of it.

Medical terms are built and dissected using prefixes, word roots/combining form, and suffixes. For example, we can build the term *rhinorrhea* by placing the parts of the term in the puzzle pieces where P = prefix, WR/CF = word root or combining form, and S = suffix.

rhinorrhea

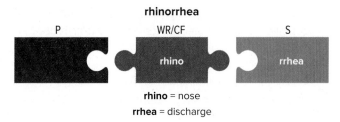

rhino = nose
rrhea = discharge

Rhinorrhea is discharge from the nose. Learn additional medical terms in the **Medical Terminology Practice** section at the end of this chapter.

▶ The Tongue and the Sense of Taste LO 34.2

Taste, or gustatory, receptors are located on taste buds. Taste buds are microscopic structures found mostly on the **papillae** (bumps) of the tongue. They cannot be seen with the naked eye. Some taste buds also are scattered on the roof of the mouth and in the walls of the throat. Recent research has indicated that a few taste receptors also are found in the lungs.

Each taste bud is made of taste cells and supporting cells (see Figure 34-2). The taste cells function as taste receptors, and the supporting cells simply fill in the spaces between the taste cells. Like the olfactory cells of smell, taste cells are types of chemoreceptors. They are activated by chemicals found in food and drink that must be dissolved in saliva as part of the digestive process.

There are five types of taste sensations. Each sensation is recognized by a different type of taste cell:

- Sweet: taste cells with receptors that respond to "sweet" chemicals
- Sour: taste cells with receptors that respond to "sour" chemicals
- Salty: taste cells with receptors that respond to "salty" chemicals
- Bitter: taste cells with receptors that respond to "bitter" chemicals
- Umami: taste cells with receptors that respond to a savory, meaty sensation

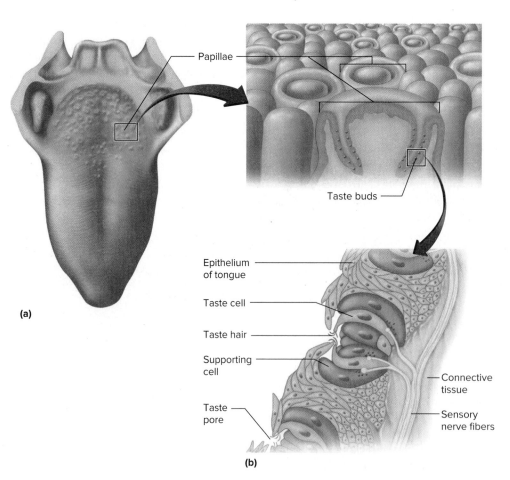

FIGURE 34-2 (a) Taste buds are located on and near the papillae on the tongue. (b) Each taste bud has several taste cells corresponding to the various taste sensations.

For many years, it was thought that each type of taste cell was concentrated in a different area on the tongue. However, research has shown that all five types of taste cells are typically located within each taste bud. The sensory nerve at each taste bud is responsible for transmitting all of the taste sensations to the cranial nerves in the brain. There, the information is processed by the **gustatory cortex,** an area of the brain that is responsible for interpreting taste sensations. The gustatory cortex integrates information from the taste cells with other information to provide a more complete interpretation. For example, eating spicy foods may activate pain receptors on the tongue that are interpreted by the gustatory cortex as "spicy."

▶ The Eye and the Sense of Sight   LO 34.3

The sense of sight comes from the eyes and is supported by visual accessory organs.

Vision

Your visual system consists of the eyes; the optic nerve, which connects the eyes to the vision center of the brain; and several accessory structures. If these parts of the system are healthy and normal, you are able to see normally.

Structure of the Eye

The eye is a complex organ that processes light to produce images. It is made up of three main layers, two chambers, and a number of specialized parts, as shown in Figure 34-3.

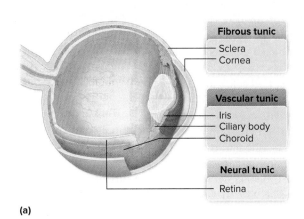

(a)

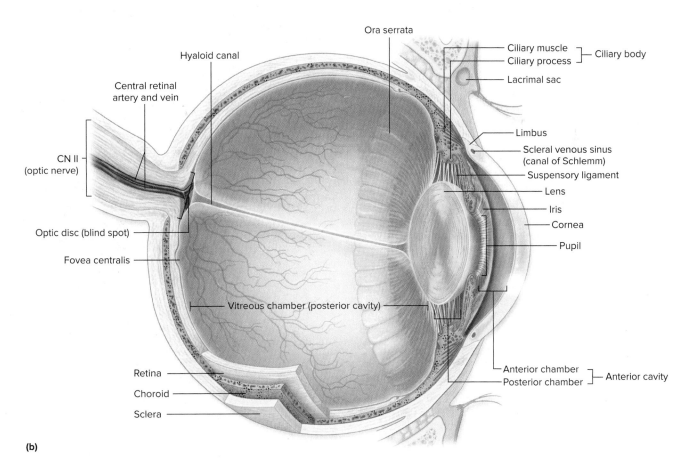

(b)

FIGURE 34-3   Anatomy of the internal eye: sagittal views depict (a) the three layers of the eye and (b) internal eye structures.

The Outer Layer The white of the eye—the *sclera*—is the tough, outermost layer of the eye. This layer, through which light cannot pass, covers all except the front of the eye. Here, the sclera gives way to the cornea in an area known as the corneal-scleral junction, or *limbus*. The **cornea** is a transparent area on the front of the eye that acts as a window to let light into the eye. Although there are no blood vessels in the sclera, numerous sense receptors detect even the smallest particles on the eyeball's surface.

The Middle Layer The **choroid** is the middle layer of the eye, which contains most of the eye's blood vessels. In the anterior part of the choroid are the iris and the ciliary body. The iris is the colored part of the eye. It is made of muscular tissue. As this tissue contracts and relaxes, the opening at its center (the pupil) grows larger or smaller. The size of the pupil regulates the amount of light that enters the eye. In bright light, the pupil becomes constricted (smaller). In dim light, it becomes dilated (larger).

The ciliary body is a wedge-shaped thickening in the eyeball's middle layer. Muscles in the ciliary body control the shape of the lens—making the lens more or less curved for viewing either near or distant objects. The lens is a clear, circular disk located just posterior to the iris. Because the lens can change shape, it helps the eye focus images of near or faraway objects. This process is called *accommodation*. Clouding and hardening of the lens, which often occur with aging, lead to a condition known as *cataracts*. This condition will be discussed in more detail later in the *Assisting with Eye and Ear Care* chapter.

The Inner Layer The eye's inner layer consists of the **retina.** Nerve cells at the posterior of the retina sense light. The area where the optic nerve enters the retina is known as the optic disc. This area contains no sensory nerves and is called the *blind spot.* There are two types of nerve cells, each named for its shape. *Rods* are highly sensitive to light. They function in dim light but do not provide a sharp image or detect color, only black, white, and shades of gray. They give you your limited "night vision" as well as peripheral vision. *Cones* function best in bright light. They are sensitive to color and provide sharper images. They are responsible for the ability to differentiate tones and hues of color. Deficiencies in the number or types of cones are responsible for the various types of color blindness, which is generally an inherited condition.

The Cavities of the Eye Each eyeball is divided into two cavities: anterior and posterior.

The Anterior Cavity The anterior cavity consists of an anterior and a posterior chamber. The chambers are segregated by the iris. Both chambers are filled with a watery fluid called *aqueous humor.* Aqueous humor provides nutrients to and bathes the structures in the anterior chamber of the eyeball. When there is an accumulation of aqueous humor, a person develops a visual condition known as *glaucoma.* This disorder will be discussed in more detail in the *Assisting with Eye and Ear Care* chapter.

The Posterior Cavity The posterior cavity also known as the vitreous chamber of the eyeball is behind the lens and is filled with a thick, jelly-like fluid called *vitreous humor.* Vitreous humor keeps the retina flat and helps to maintain the eye's shape.

Visual Accessory Organs

Visual accessory organs assist and protect the eyeball. They include the orbits, eyebrows, eyelids and eyelashes, conjunctiva, lacrimal apparatus, and extrinsic eye muscles.

Eye Orbits and Eyebrows The eye sockets, or *orbits,* form a protective shell around the eyes. Eyebrows protect the eyes by reducing the chance that sweat and direct sunlight will enter them.

Eyelids and Eyelashes Each eyelid is composed of skin, muscle, and dense connective tissue. The muscle in the eyelid is called the *orbicularis oculi* and is responsible for blinking and squinting. Blinking the eyelids prevents the mucous membrane surface of the eyeball from drying. A moist eyeball surface is much less likely to grow bacteria than a dry one is. Blinking also protects the eyes, keeping foreign material from entering them. The eyelashes catch foreign substances, including perspiration and dust.

Conjunctiva The **conjunctiva** is the mucous membrane that lines the inner surfaces of the eyelids and covers the anterior surface of each eyeball. Mucous membranes produce mucus, which keeps the surface of the eyeballs moist.

The Lacrimal Apparatus The **lacrimal apparatus** consists of lacrimal glands and nasolacrimal ducts (see Figure 34-4). *Lacrimal glands,* located on the lateral edge of each eyeball, produce tears. Tears are mostly water, but they also contain a *lysozyme,* an enzyme that can destroy bacteria and viruses. Tears

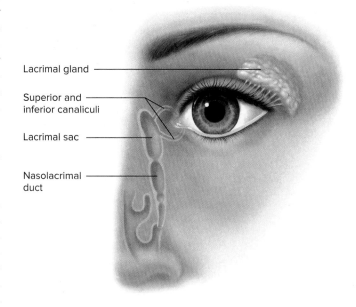

Lacrimal gland

Superior and inferior canaliculi

Lacrimal sac

Nasolacrimal duct

FIGURE 34-4 Lacrimal apparatus.

also have an outer, oily layer that prevents them from evaporating. *Nasolacrimal ducts,* located on the medial aspect of each eyeball, drain tears into the nose. When a person cries, the tears entering the nose produce the "runny nose" associated with crying.

Extrinsic Eye Muscles Extrinsic eye muscles are skeletal muscles that move the eyeball. Each eyeball has six extrinsic eye muscles attached to it that move the eyeball superiorly, inferiorly, laterally, or medially. (See Figure 34-5.)

▶ Visual Pathways

LO 34.4

The eye works much as a camera does. Light reflected from an object, or produced by one, enters the eye from the outside and passes through the cornea, pupil, lens, and fluids in the eye. The cornea, lens, and fluids help focus the light onto the retina by bending it in a process known as **refraction**. Light patterns carry an image of an object projecting it upside-down and on the retina in an eye (see Figure 34-6). The retina converts the light into nerve impulses. These impulses are transmitted along the optic nerve to the brain. This nerve, which consists of about a million fibers, serves as a flexible cable connecting the eyeball to the brain.

Parts of the optic nerve fuse together, then cross at a structure called the *optic chiasm*—an x-shaped structure located at the base of the brain. The visual area in the occipital lobes of the cerebrum is responsible for interpreting vision. Because visual information crosses in the optic chiasm, about half of the visual information detected in each eye is interpreted on

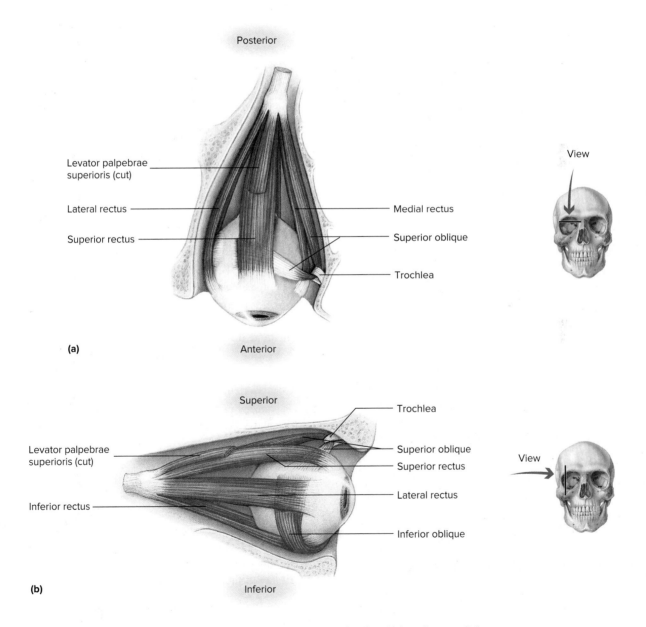

FIGURE 34-5 The six extrinsic eye muscles move the eyeball superiorly, inferiorly, laterally, or medially.

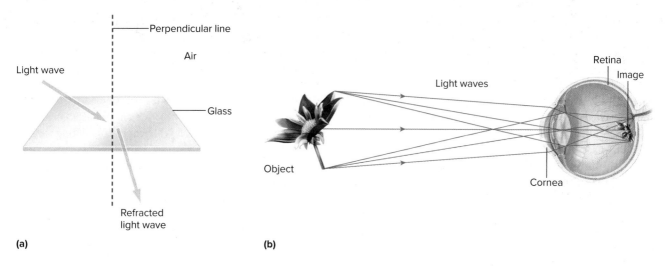

FIGURE 34-6 Visual pathways. (a) Refraction is the process of bending light. (b) The image forms upside-down on the retina.

(a)

(b)

the opposite side of the brain. So half of what a person sees in the right eye is interpreted in the left side of the brain and vice versa, where it is brought together as one image. The brain interprets these impulses, turns the image right-side up, and "develops" a picture of the object from which the light originally came. See Table 34-1 for a summary of the parts of the eye and their functions.

TABLE 34-1	The Functions of the Parts of the Eye
Structure	**Function**
Aqueous humor	Nourishes and bathes structures in the anterior eye cavity
Vitreous humor	Holds the retina in place; maintains the shape of the eyeball
Sclera	Protects the eye
Cornea	Allows light to enter the eye; bends light as it enters the eye (refraction)
Choroid	Supplies nutrients and provides a blood supply to the eye
Ciliary body	Holds the lens; controls the shape of the lens for focusing
Iris	Controls the amount of light entering the eye
Lens	Focuses light onto the retina (accommodation)
Retina	Contains visual receptors
Rods	Allow vision in dim light; detect black, white, and gray images; detect broad outlines of images
Cones	Allow vision in bright light; detect colors; detect details
Optic nerve	Carries visual information (stimuli) from rods and cones toward the brain

The Aging Eye

With age, a number of changes occur in the structure and function of the eye, including the following:

- The amount of fat tissue diminishes; this loss may cause the eyelids to droop.
- The quality and quantity of tears decrease.
- The conjunctiva becomes thinner and may be drier because of a decrease in tear production.
- The cornea begins to appear yellow and a ring of fat deposits may appear around it.
- The sclera may develop brown spots.
- Changes in the iris cause the pupil to become smaller, limiting the amount of light entering the eye.
- The lens becomes denser and more rigid; this trend reduces the amount of light that reaches the retina and makes focusing more difficult.
- Yellowing of the lens causes problems in distinguishing colors.
- Changes in the retina may make vision fuzzy.
- The ability of the eye to adapt to changes in light intensities may be reduced; glare can become painful as this ability diminishes.
- Night vision may be impaired.
- Peripheral vision is reduced, limiting the area a person can see and reducing depth perception.
- The vitreous humor breaks down, producing tiny clumps of gel or cellular material that cause floaters—dark spots or lines—that appear in a person's field of vision.
- Rubbing of the vitreous humor on the retina produces flashes of light, or "sparks."

Because of changes that impair vision—such as reductions in the field of vision, in depth perception, and in visual clarity—elderly people may fall more often than younger people.

Common Diseases and Disorders of the Eyes

As with all the body's organs, the sense organs are susceptible to various diseases and disorders. Many eye injuries, however, are preventable. See the *Educating the Patient* feature for general tips about eye safety and protection. The following common diseases and disorders are specific to the eyes. Additional information about diseases and disorders of the eyes is found in the chapter *Assisting with Eye and Ear Care*.

ASTIGMATISM occurs when the lens has an abnormal shape or the cornea is unevenly curved. This abnormality causes blurred images in near or distant vision. Astigmatism may cause vertical or horizontal lines to appear out of focus.

Causes. This condition is considered to be congenital.

Signs and Symptoms. There are no symptoms with this condition other than blurred vision.

Diagnostic Exams and Tests. Astigmatism is diagnosed by an eye care professional during an eye exam.

Treatment. Treatment includes corrective lenses or surgery, such as photorefractive keratectomy (PRK) or, more commonly now, laser-assisted in situ keratomileusis (LASIK) to reshape the cornea (see Figure 34-7). This procedure—done on an outpatient basis under local anesthesia—involves reshaping the cornea with a special laser. After LASIK surgery, 70% of patients have normal vision. A very small percentage of patients have postsurgical complications that cause their vision to worsen.

DRY EYE SYNDROME is one of the most common eye problems physicians treat. This syndrome results from a decreased production of the oil within tears, which occurs normally with age.

Causes. Dry eye can be caused by cigarette smoke; air conditioning; eye strain created by long hours at a computer monitor; some medications; contact lenses; hormonal changes associated with menopause; and hot, dry, or windy climates.

Signs and Symptoms. The common eye symptoms include burning, irritation, redness, itching, and excessive tearing.

Diagnostic Exams and Tests. The initial diagnosis is made based on patient symptoms. For further analysis, a Schirmer test may be performed to determine the amount of tear production. Other tests measure the quality of the tears produced, including the amount of oil present.

EDUCATING THE PATIENT
Eye Safety and Protection

Almost 90% of all eye injuries could be prevented by eye safety practices or proper protective eyewear. You can educate patients about preventing eye injuries in the home, at work, and during recreational activities.

Eye Safety in the Home
Patients should follow these suggestions to protect their eyes in the home:

- Pad or cushion the sharp corners and edges of furniture and home fixtures.
- Make sure adequate lighting and handrails are available on stairs.
- Keep personal use items (such as cosmetics and toiletries), kitchen utensils, and desk supplies out of the reach of children.
- Keep toys with sharp edges out of the reach of children. Also, make sure toys intended for older children are kept away from younger children.
- Remove dangerous debris from the lawn before mowing it.
- Wear safely goggles when operating any type of power equipment.
- Keep dangerous solvents, paints, cleaners, fertilizers, and other chemicals out of the reach of children.
- Never mix cleaning agents.

Eye Safety at Work
Approximately 15% of eye injuries in the workplace lead to temporary or permanent vision loss. Eye injuries at work can be diminished if patients take the following precautions:

- Choose safety eyewear according to the type of work being performed and the type of eye protection needed.
- Wear safety eyewear whenever there is a chance of flying objects from machines.
- Wear safety eyewear whenever there is possible exposure—by splash or splatter—to harmful chemicals, body fluids, or radiation.

Eye Safety During Sports and Recreational Activities
Eye injuries that commonly occur while playing a sport include scratched corneas, inflamed irises and retinas, bleeding in the anterior chamber of the eye, traumatic cataracts, and fractures of the eye socket. Wearing sports eye guards or goggles can prevent most sports eye injuries. These guards are recommended for baseball, basketball, soccer, football, rugby, and hockey. Protective goggles are recommended for mountain biking, motocross, and snow skiing. Virtually any type of contact sport requires appropriate eye protection.

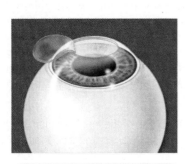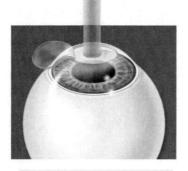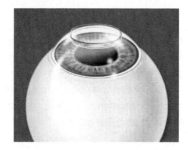

1 Cornea is sliced with a sharp knife. Flap of cornea is reflected, and deeper corneal layers are exposed.

2 A laser removes microscopic portions of the deeper corneal layers, thereby changing the shape of the cornea.

3 Corneal flap is put back in place, and the edges of the flap start to fuse within 72 hours.

FIGURE 34-7 LASIK laser vision correction procedure.

Treatment. Artificial tears may provide relief to many patients, and drugs such as Restasis® have helped patients with this condition make more of their own tears. People with this condition should drink 8 to 10 glasses of water a day and make a conscious effort to blink more frequently and avoid rubbing their eyes. In addition, punctal plugs can be inserted to trap tears on the eyes, which prevents the tears from entering the nasolacrimal duct and being drained.

ECTROPION is the eversion (turning inside-out) of the lower eyelid.

Causes. Aging and skin relaxation or scar tissue may cause this condition.

Signs and Symptoms. Common signs and symptoms include redness, irritation, and drying of the conjunctiva. Poor tear drainage through the nasolacrimal system also may be present.

Diagnostic Exams and Tests. The eye care professional diagnoses ectropion during a routine eye exam and/or physical exam.

Treatment. Surgery to repair the defect may be needed if the condition is bothersome to the patient.

ENTROPION is characterized by an inversion (turning outside-in) of the lower eyelid.

Causes. Aging and scar tissue may cause this condition.

Signs and Symptoms. Signs include irritation of the sclera as the lashes brush against it, which may lead to corneal ulceration or scarring.

Diagnostic Exams and Tests. The eye care professional diagnoses ectropion during a routine eye exam and/or physical exam.

Treatment. Surgery is the only treatment option to permanently correct this problem. Short-term remedies to ease the symptoms include sutures or skin tape to reposition the eyelid, or soft contact lenses.

NYSTAGMUS is rapid, involuntary eye movements.

Causes. Alcohol and some drug use may cause nystagmus. Inner ear disturbances also may result in involuntary eye movements. Brain lesions and injury (including those that may occur during birth) and cerebrovascular accidents (CVA), or strokes, also may cause nystagmus.

Signs and Symptoms. These include rapid, irregular eye movements that may be horizontal, vertical, or rotary, depending on the underlying cause of the nystagmus.

Diagnostic Exams and Tests. A physical exam and vision test are performed. A neurological exam or ear exam also may be performed, depending on the suspected cause. Eye movements may be recorded to determine the specific type of nystagmus. In some cases, a CT scan or MRI of the brain is performed as well.

Treatment. Treatment focuses on the underlying cause of the disorder.

RETINAL DETACHMENT occurs when the layers of the retina separate. It is considered a medical emergency and, if not treated right away, leads to permanent vision loss. Retinal detachment is rare; however, it is more common as people age.

Causes. This disorder is sometimes caused by fluids that seep between layers of the retina; this occurs most commonly in nearsighted people. In diabetics, vitreous body or scar tissue pulls the retina loose. Another cause is eye trauma that causes fluid to collect underneath the layers of the retina.

Signs and Symptoms. Signs and symptoms include light flashes, wavy vision, a sudden loss of vision (particularly of peripheral vision), and a larger amount of floaters.

Diagnostic Exams and Tests. A retinal examination is performed to scan the retina and the back of the eye for holes, tears, or other abnormalities. If blood has accumulated in the eye, an ultrasound may be done to help visualize the retina.

Treatment. When detected early, a hole in the retina can be "sealed" so that the retina does not completely detach. Sealing the hole is usually accomplished through the use of lasers or a procedure called cryopexy—surgical fixation with cold.

If the retina has already detached, some vision often can be restored with the following procedures:

- Pneumatic retinopexy, which involves injecting a gas bubble into the posterior segment of the eye; the pressure from the

gas bubble flattens the retina, and the retina is later fixed in place with a laser.

- Scleral buckle, which involves using a silicone band to hold the retina in place.

- Replacing the vitreous body with silicone oil to reattach the retina.

▶ The Ear and the Senses of Hearing and Equilibrium   LO 34.6

The ear is the organ of hearing. In addition to providing the sense of hearing, the ear aids the body in maintaining balance, or equilibrium. To assist with ear exams and procedures, you need to understand ear anatomy and the hearing process.

Structure of the Ear
The ear is divided into three parts: the external ear, middle ear, and inner ear (see Figure 34-8).

External Ear The external ear is composed of the **auricle,** or pinna, and the **external auditory canal.** The auricle is the flap of skin and cartilage that extends from the side of the head. It collects sound waves. The external auditory canal is more commonly

called the ear canal and is lined with skin that contains hairs and glands that produce **cerumen,** a wax-like substance commonly known as earwax. Cerumen lubricates the ear and protects it by trapping dirt, dust, and microbes. This canal carries sound waves to the **tympanic membrane,** or eardrum. The tympanic membrane is a fibrous partition located at the inner end of the external auditory canal. It separates the external ear from the middle ear.

Middle Ear The middle ear includes the tympanic membrane, the ossicles, and the oval window. The tympanic membrane is thin and vibrates when sound waves hit it. On the other side of the tympanic membrane are three tiny bones called ear **ossicles**—the *malleus* (hammer), *incus* (anvil), and *stapes* (stirrup). When the tympanic membrane vibrates, it causes the ossicles to vibrate and hit a membrane called the **oval window.** The oval window ends the middle ear and marks the beginning of the inner ear.

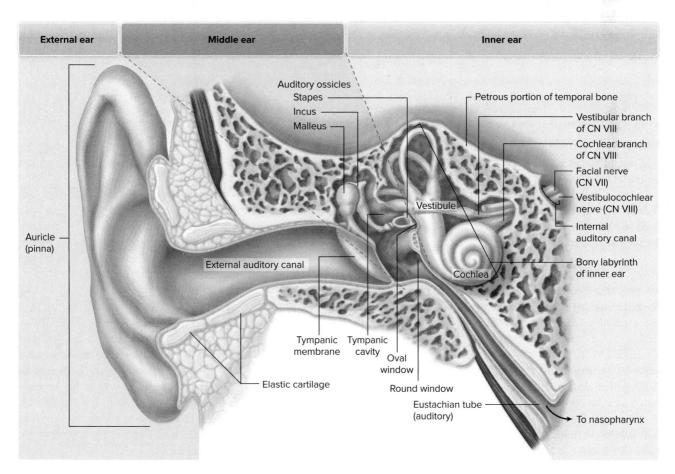

FIGURE 34-8   Anatomical regions of the right ear—the ear is divided into external, middle, and inner regions.

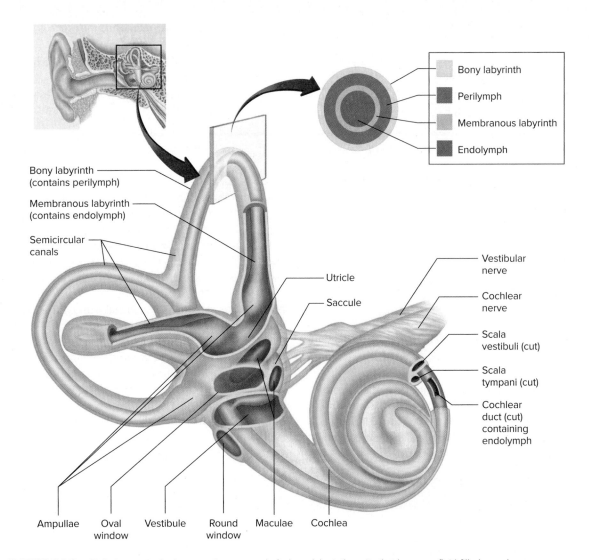

Bony labyrinth

Perilymph

Membranous labyrinth

Endolymph

Bony labyrinth
(contains perilymph)

Membranous labyrinth
(contains endolymph)

Semicircular
canals

Utricle

Saccule

Vestibular
nerve

Cochlear
nerve

Scala
vestibuli (cut)

Scala
tympani (cut)

Cochlear
duct (cut)
containing
endolymph

Ampullae   Oval   Vestibule   Round   Maculae   Cochlea
            window   window

FIGURE 34-9   Right inner ear: the inner ear is composed of a bony labyrinth cavity that houses a fluid-filled, membranous labyrinth. Within the bony labyrinth are the vestibular organs for equilibrium and balance and the cochlea for hearing.

The middle ear is connected to the throat by a tube called the **eustachian** (auditory) **tube.** This tube helps maintain equal pressure on both sides of the eardrum, which is important for normal hearing. Because the middle ear is connected to the throat by this tube, any throat infection can easily spread to the ear and vice versa.

Inner Ear The inner ear is a complex system of communicating chambers and tubes known as the **labyrinth.** It is divided into three portions: **semicircular canals,** a **vestibule,** and a **cochlea** (see Figure 34-9). Each ear has three semicircular canals that detect the body's balance. The cochlea is shaped like a snail's shell and contains hearing receptors, including the **organ of Corti,** which is known as the organ of hearing. The vestibule is the area between the semicircular canals and the cochlea. Like the semicircular canals, it functions in equilibrium. When the head moves, the *perilymph* and *endolymph* fluids in the semicircular canals and vestibule move. This activates both equilibrium and hearing receptors. The equilibrium receptors send the information along vestibular nerves to the cerebrum for interpretation. The cerebrum

can then advise the body if it needs to make any adjustments to prevent a fall.

When sound waves of different volumes and frequencies activate the hearing receptors in the cochlea, they send their information to auditory nerves. Auditory nerves (vestibulocochlear nerves) deliver the information to the auditory cortex in the cerebrum's temporal lobe. The auditory cortex interprets the information as sounds.

▶ The Hearing Process   LO 34.7

A sound consists of waves of different frequencies that move through the air. The external ear initiates sound conduction when it collects these waves and channels them to the tympanic membrane. Here, the waves make the tympanic membrane vibrate. The vibrations, in turn, are amplified by the middle ear's ossicles. The amplified waves enter the inner ear and the cochlea. These waves cause tiny hairs that line the cochlea to bend. Movements of the hairs trigger nerve impulses. The auditory nerve transmits these impulses to the brain, where they are perceived as sound.

Sound waves also are conducted through the bones of the skull directly to the inner ear—a process called *bone conduction*. This alternative pathway for sound bypasses the external and middle ears. When you hear your own voice, the sound has reached your inner ear mainly through bone conduction. By comparing a person's ability to sense sounds by bone conduction and through the entire ear, doctors often can identify what part of the ear is causing a hearing problem. For example, if bone conduction is normal, a hearing problem likely involves the middle or external ear rather than the inner ear.

The Aging Ear

As a person grows older, a number of changes occur in the ear. The external ear appears larger because of continued cartilage growth and loss of skin elasticity. The earlobe gets longer and may have a wrinkled appearance. The glands that produce cerumen become less efficient, producing earwax that is much drier and prone to impaction. The ear canal also becomes narrower.

In the middle ear, changes in the eardrum cause it to shrink and appear dull and gray. The joints between the bones of the middle ear degenerate, so they do not move as freely. In the inner ear, the semicircular canals become less sensitive to changes in position, and this reduced sensitivity affects balance.

Problems with equilibrium make the elderly prone to falls. Some ear disorders, such as hearing loss and Ménière's disease, are also more common in older individuals. Additional information about diseases and disorders of the ear are found in the chapter *Assisting with Eye and Ear Care*.

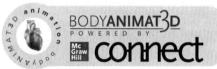

Go to CONNECT to see an animation exercise about *Hearing Loss: Sensorineural*.

How to Recognize Hearing Problems in Infants

Hearing problems in infants are not easy to recognize. The following general guidelines can be used to teach parents how to identify normal hearing in infants. Any deviations from these guidelines may indicate a hearing loss.

Infants Up to 4 Months Old

- They should be startled by loud noises (barking dog, hand clap, and so on).
- When sleeping in a quiet room, they should wake up at the sound of voices.
- Around the fourth month of age, they should turn their head or move their eyes to follow a sound.
- They should recognize the mother's or primary caregiver's voice better than other voices.

Infants 4 to 8 Months of Age

- They should regularly turn their head or move their eyes to follow sounds.
- Their facial expressions should change at the sound of familiar voices or loud noises.
- They should begin to enjoy certain sounds such as rattles or ringing bells.
- They should begin to babble at people who talk to them.

Babies 8 to 12 Months of Age

- They should turn quickly to the sound of their name.
- They should begin to vary the pitch of the sounds they produce in their babbling.
- They should begin to respond to music.
- They should respond to the instruction "no."

PATHOPHYSIOLOGY

LO 34.8

Common Diseases and Disorders of the Ears

The following common diseases and disorders are specific to the ears.

ACOUSTIC NEUROMA is a benign tumor of the cranial nerve involved in hearing and balance.

Causes. Acoustic neuroma is caused by a malfunction in a gene responsible for controlling the growth of Schwann cells—a type of neuroglial cell. (See the chapter *The Nervous System* for more information.) This gene is found on chromosome 22.

Signs and Symptoms. Gradual hearing loss in one ear is the most common symptom. Patients also may experience balance problems and tinnitus—ringing in the ears.

Diagnostic Exams and Tests. After performing a physical ear exam, the practitioner may order audiometry (a hearing test of each ear independently) to assess hearing loss, as well as an MRI to determine whether a tumor is present.

Treatment. Because acoustic neuromas often grow slowly, the physician may monitor the tumor if the patient is not experiencing severe symptoms. Large tumors or those causing severe symptoms may be treated with radiation therapy or surgical removal.

CERUMEN IMPACTION is a condition that consists of the buildup of earwax within the external auditory canal.

Causes. Cerumen impaction may be caused by improper cleaning of cerumen from the ear canal—using cotton-tipped applicators—or by overactive ceruminous glands producing more than the normal amount of cerumen. More information about caring for the ears is found in the chapter *Assisting with Eye and Ear Care*.

Signs and Symptoms. The most common sign is some degree of hearing loss because of the blockage of sound waves. Some patients also may complain of ear pain, ringing in the ear, or a feeling that the ear is stopped up.

risk factors are associated with increased incidence of HAI in both outpatient and inpatient facilities:

- Use of catheters and other indwelling (fixed within the body for a period of time) devices.
- Surgical procedures.
- Healthcare environment contamination.
- Communicable disease transmission (for example, influenza) between patients and healthcare workers.
- Improper antibiotic use.
- Immunocompromised patients.

Common Healthcare-Associated Infections in Outpatient Settings

As you learned in the *Infection Control Fundamentals* chapter, touching is the most common means of transmission of infectious agents. As a medical assistant, your duties will include activities that require you to touch patients. If standard precautions are not followed during procedures that require touching, such as obtaining vital signs, changing a dressing, and removing sutures, you and the patient are at risk for infection. HAI also are associated with the devices used during medical procedures and testing; surgical site infections; and improper use of needles, syringes, and blood collection devices. You should use the utmost care when performing any patient procedure or test, no matter how small the risk.

Methicillin-Resistant *Staphylococcus aureus*

Methicillin-resistant *Staphylococcus aureus* (MRSA) is an infection caused by a specific type of staph bacteria. These bacteria have become resistant to most of the antibiotics used to treat the infection. For this reason, MRSA infections are difficult to treat and can have devastating consequences. Skin infections, the most common type of infection caused by MRSA, can begin as small bumps or pimples and quickly develop into a large abscess (Figure 35-1). Additionally, MRSA infections can occur in the bloodstream, lungs, heart, bones, or joints. Anyone who has an **invasive procedure** (any procedure that requires entry into a body cavity or cutting into skin or mucous membranes) is at risk for MRSA infection.

The key to stopping the transmission of MRSA in the healthcare setting is proper hand hygiene and contact precautions (discussed in the *Infection Control Fundamentals* chapter). When assisting a patient with a known or suspected MRSA infection, put on gloves and a gown prior to entering the exam room. Once you are finished assisting with the patient care, remove your gloves and gown (in that order) before leaving the room. Perform proper hand hygiene immediately after removing your PPE.

***Clostridium difficile* Infection** *Clostridium difficile,* also known as C. diff, is a type of bacterium that causes diarrhea. It is of great concern in the elderly but can affect anyone taking antibiotics for prolonged periods of time and receiving medical care. It is transmitted by the fecal/oral route (touching a surface or patient contaminated with feces and then touching the mouth or mucous membranes). Symptoms of C. diff include watery diarrhea, fever, loss of appetite, nausea, and abdominal pain. Healthcare workers can transmit C. diff to patients by touching if proper hand hygiene is not followed. Because C. diff is found in feces, any surface or device contaminated with feces is a potential source of infection. This includes toilets, sinks, and rectal thermometers. For this reason, proper environmental cleaning in the healthcare facility is essential. Bathrooms and surfaces that may be contaminated

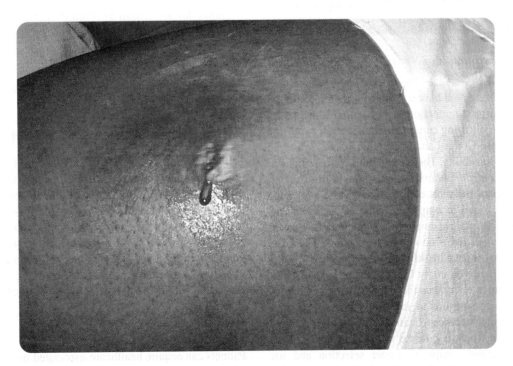

FIGURE 35-1 A wound infected with MRSA is difficult to treat and can lead to tissue loss and sepsis.
Source: Centers for Disease Control and Prevention (CDC)

with C. diff must be thoroughly decontaminated. You should wear gloves when assisting with a patient with known or suspected C. diff infection or when cleaning and disinfecting the exam room and equipment. Alcohol does not kill C. diff; therefore, the CDC recommends handwashing with soap and water after caring for a patient with C. diff. If C. diff is diagnosed or suspected, alcohol hand disinfectants are not recommended. Surfaces and equipment that are likely to be contaminated should be cleaned and disinfected. A solution of 1:10 bleach or an EPA-approved disinfectant with sporicidal (able to kill spores) properties is recommended. (See the *Examination and Treatment Areas* chapter for more information about mixing a 1:10 bleach solution.)

Central Line-Associated Bloodstream Infections

Central line-associated bloodstream infections (CLABSI) are caused by the entry of infectious microorganisms into the bloodstream by way of a **central line.** A central line is a catheter placed in a large vein, usually in the neck, chest, or groin, used to give fluids or medications. A central line differs from a normal intravenous (IV) catheter in several ways. IVs are usually placed for short amounts of time and are located in surface veins, whereas central lines are generally left in place for longer periods of time (weeks or months) and are placed in deep veins that are close to the heart. Though central lines are most often used in intensive care settings, they also are seen in patients receiving outpatient treatments such as chemotherapy.

Healthcare practitioners must follow strict infection control practices when inserting, checking, or changing a bandage of a central line:

- Following hand hygiene procedures.
- Performing appropriate skin antisepsis at the site of insertion.
- Allowing the skin prep agent to dry thoroughly before inserting the catheter.
- Wearing gloves, gown, cap, and mask when inserting the catheter.
- Using a large drape to cover the site during the procedure.
- Washing hands before and after checking the central line.

The CDC recommends removing the central line as soon as it is no longer needed.

As a medical assistant, you should instruct patients with central lines to contact the office immediately if:

- The dressing covering the central line comes off or becomes wet or dirty.
- The site around the central line becomes red, hot, or sore.
- They have a fever or chills.

Additionally, you should instruct patients to:

- Not touch the catheter insertion site.
- Avoid touching the tubing as much as possible.
- Not let visiting family and friends touch the tubing or site.
- Ask visiting family and friends to wash their hands when they arrive and before they leave.

- Tell the healthcare practitioner if they have concerns about the central line or the infection control practices of the healthcare personnel caring for them.

Catheter-Associated Urinary Tract Infections Anyone who uses urinary catheters on a long-term basis is at risk for **catheter-associated urinary tract infections (CAUTI).** Bacteria can enter the urinary tract by way of the catheter. The longer a catheter is in place, the more chance a patient has of contracting a CAUTI. For this reason, the CDC recommends that catheters be used for the least possible amount of time and only when necessary and no alternative is available. Catheters must be placed only by trained individuals using aseptic techniques. As a medical assistant, you can help patients with indwelling catheters to avoid CAUTI by teaching them to take the following precautions:

- Wash hands thoroughly with soap and water before and after touching the catheter.
- Ensure that the urine collection bag is always below the level of the bladder.
- Do not pull on the tubing.
- Do not kink or twist the tubing.

▶ Infection Control Methods   LO 35.2

As you learned in section 35.1, there are numerous healthcare-associated infections that patients can be exposed to. The best way to keep patients from being infected is to consistently apply infection control methods. As a medical assistant, you must have a thorough knowledge of the two types of asepsis:

- **Medical asepsis,** or clean technique, is based on maintaining cleanliness to prevent the spread of microorganisms and to ensure that there are as few microorganisms in the medical environment as possible. The goal of medical asepsis is to reduce/control microorganisms after they leave the body.
- **Surgical asepsis,** or sterile technique, depends on a completely sterile environment that eliminates all microorganisms. The goal of surgical asepsis is to keep organisms from entering the body. (More information about surgical asepsis can be found later in this chapter and in the *Assisting with Minor Surgery* chapter.)

Medical asepsis and surgical asepsis are required by law. Each individual who works in a medical setting must recognize the importance of asepsis and strictly adhere to aseptic procedures in daily routines.

Medical Asepsis

Because the medical office can be a host to many pathogens, strict, controlled asepsis is crucial. All employees in the medical office must observe and practice the principles of asepsis to ensure a safe environment for patients and staff.

You can promote asepsis through vigilant cleanliness. Every day before patients arrive, you must inspect the office for any surfaces or objects that may be dirty or contaminated. Keeping the office clean reduces the number of microorganisms on surfaces.

Transmission from Healthcare Workers

There may be times when a healthcare worker has a serious infection that could be transmitted to a patient. OSHA has special recommendations for workers who perform procedures that could result in a patient's exposure to disease. Although the risk of a healthcare worker's transmitting an infection to a patient is small if OSHA standards are followed, these additional precautions are advised for high-risk procedures. High-risk procedures include the following:

- Those that are thought to have caused the transmission of infection from a medical worker to a patient in the past.
- Those that may carry a high risk of infection, such as oral, obstetric, and gynecologic procedures.
- Those that involve needles, especially if a needle is in a body cavity or a body space that is difficult to see and the healthcare worker's fingers are nearby (if the worker's skin is cut, the patient could be exposed to the worker's blood).

Workers who perform high-risk procedures should know their HIV and HBV status. HBV vaccination is strongly recommended. Also, workers who have skin conditions characterized by sores that secrete fluid should forgo direct patient care and the handling of equipment used for exposure-prone procedures until their condition has healed.

HIV or HBV infection should not necessarily keep an individual from practicing as a healthcare worker, but some special measures may need to be taken. A member of the medical staff who is infected with HIV or HBV should not perform procedures that might result in exposure for the patient without the advice of an expert review panel. This panel could include the healthcare worker's own physician, someone with expert knowledge about the transmission of infectious disease, a medical professional with expert knowledge about the procedures in question, public health officials, and a member of the infection control committee of the institution, if applicable.

The panel advises the worker on whether procedures may be performed. The advice includes requiring the worker to inform potential patients of the infection before the procedure. Each medical facility has policies in place outlining if and how patients will be notified of a healthcare professional's HIV or HBV status. The notification may be in writing from the panel, or the healthcare worker may speak directly to the patient. It is the healthcare worker's ethical duty to protect a patient from known exposure to bloodborne pathogens. However, the panel also must protect the healthcare worker's confidentiality if possible.

Although great controversy has surrounded the subject of required testing of all healthcare workers for HIV or HBV, no recommendations are in place for such testing. The risk of infection transmission from worker to patient is not considered great enough to justify the extensive resources that mandatory testing would require.

Office Procedures

Other physical aspects of the medical office that contribute to asepsis include:

- A reception room that has designated waiting areas for well and sick people. If there is not enough space, sick patients should be led immediately to an examination room. You may need to explain this policy to well people who have been waiting so that no one thinks other patients are getting preferential treatment.
- An office that is cleaned daily.
- An office that is well lit and ventilated, has no drafts, and has a temperature of approximately 72°F.
- Furniture that is kept in good repair and is replaced when necessary.
- A strict "no eating or drinking" policy in the lab, clinical, and other patient areas.
- Trash that is emptied as necessary, at least once daily.
- An insect-free environment.
- A sign stating that any safety or health hazard should be reported to the receptionist.
- A sign asking that patients use tissues for coughs or sneezes, put all waste in the trash can, and tell the receptionist if they are nauseated or have to use the restroom. (Ideally, the reception area should be equipped with a restroom for emergencies.) See Figure 35-2.

Asepsis During Medical Assistant Procedures

Many of the procedures you perform require aseptic techniques to prevent cross-contamination from one place to another. For instance, when opening a sterile container, you should rest its lid face-up instead of facedown. Placing it facedown contaminates the inside of the lid by picking up materials on the surface of the counter such as dust, dirt, blood, or body fluids, making it unsuitable to be put back on the sterile container. When administering tablets or capsules, you should pour them into the bottle cap or a cup rather than into your hand to prevent the transfer of microorganisms from your hand onto the medication. To prevent cross-contamination, you also must follow guidelines about the types of protective gear to wear during a procedure. (Personal protective equipment is discussed later in this section.)

Other Aseptic Precautions

You need to make certain precautions part of your daily routine. For example, take these safeguards:

- Avoid leaning against sinks, supplies, or equipment.
- Avoid touching your face or mouth.
- Use tissues when you cough or sneeze, and always wash your hands afterward.
- Whenever possible, avoid working directly with patients when you have a cold.
- Wear gloves and a mask if you have a cold and must work with patients.
- Stay home if you have a fever, and remain there until you have maintained a normal temperature for 24 hours.

Personal Protective Equipment

Employers are required by law to supply **personal protective equipment (PPE)** at no charge to their employees. PPE is any type of protective gear worn to guard against physical

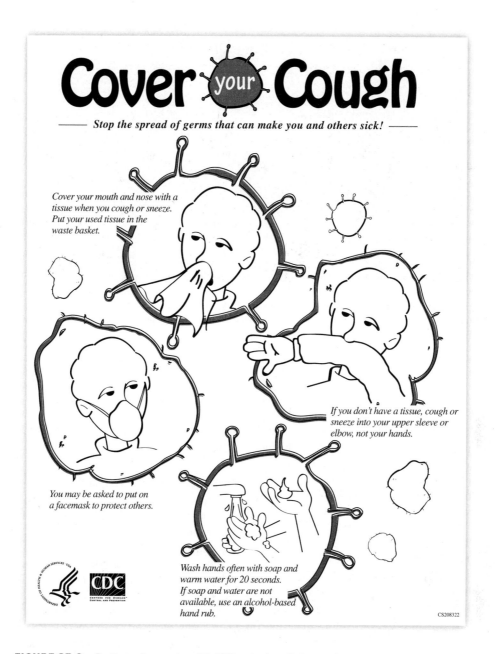

FIGURE 35-2 Posting notices such as this CDC poster in patient reception areas reminds patients to use tissues and cover their coughs to reduce the spread of infectious agents.
Source: Centers for Disease Control and Prevention

hazards. Healthcare workers require many kinds of personal protective equipment to do their jobs, including gloves, masks and protective eyewear or face shields, and protective clothing (Figure 35-3). During each procedure, keep in mind that the greater your chances of exposure to blood or other body fluids, the more pieces of PPE you will need to wear.

Gloves You must wear gloves for all procedures that involve exposure to blood, other body fluids, or broken skin. Several kinds of gloves for different situations are:

- Disposable gloves—worn once and discarded. They cannot be used if they are torn, punctured, or otherwise damaged. Both examination and sterile gloves are disposable.

- Examination gloves—worn during procedures that do not require a sterile environment.
- Sterile gloves—used for sterile procedures such as minor surgery or urinary catheterization.
- Utility gloves—used when cleaning up. They are stronger than disposable gloves and may be decontaminated and reused if they show no signs of deterioration (including discoloration) after use.

Masks and Protective Eyewear or Face Shields
You must wear appropriate masks and protective eyewear or face shields for procedures in which your eyes, nose, and mouth may be exposed. These procedures are ones that have

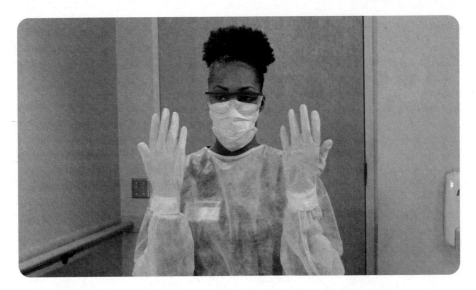

FIGURE 35-3 Healthcare workers may need to use various types of personal protective equipment, including gloves, masks and protective eyewear or face shields, gowns, and other protective clothing.
©McGraw-Hill Education

a potential for spraying or splashing blood, such as surgery or dental procedures.

Protective Clothing If you are likely to have blood or body fluids sprayed or splashed on your clothing during a procedure, you must wear a protective laboratory coat, gown, or apron. You also may wear a hair covering and/or shoe coverings for such procedures. You should always have a change of work clothing available in the event that blood or body fluids penetrate your regular clothes around or through the protective clothing.

Use of Multiple Types of PPE There may be situations that require you to wear more than one type of PPE. You may have to wear gloves, a gown, and a mask/face shield. The order in which you put these on and take them off is important. because the gloves must go over the sleeves of the gown, the gown must go on first. The proper placement order for multiple PPE is gown, mask/face shield, and gloves. To reduce the possibility of cross-contamination, remove contaminated PPE in the opposite order; that is, gloves, mask/face shield, and gown. Procedure 35-1, at the end of this chapter, demonstrates the correct method for removing contaminated gloves and Procedure 35-2, also at the end of this chapter, demonstrates the proper method for removing a contaminated gown.

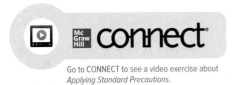

Go to CONNECT to see a video exercise about *Applying Standard Precautions.*

▶ Safe Injection Practices and Sharps Safety

LO 35.3

According to the World Health Organization (WHO), a safe injection does not cause injury to the patient, expose the provider to an avoidable risk, or create dangerous environmental/community waste. As a medical assistant, you may perform tasks, such as giving an injection, that require you to use needles or other sharp devices. During the course of these tasks, you must protect the patient, your coworkers, and yourself by always adhering to safe injection and sharps safety practices, correctly using engineered sharps safety devices, and properly disposing of all sharps.

Safe Injection Practices

Recently, several large outbreaks of hepatitis B and hepatitis C were linked to outpatient settings in the United States. In response to these outbreaks, the CDC began the One and Only campaign to reemphasize and reinforce safe injection practices. The hallmark of the campaign is "One Needle, One Syringe, Only One Time," reminding healthcare providers of the core of injection safety (Figure 35-4).

Recommendations for safe injection practices are part of the CDC's *Guideline for Isolation Precautions: Preventing Transmission of Infectious Agents in Healthcare Settings 2007* and include the following:

- Use aseptic technique to avoid contamination of sterile injection equipment.
- Clean the top of medication vials with 70% isopropyl alcohol before withdrawing medications.
- Do not administer medications from a syringe to multiple patients.
- Use single-dose vials for parenteral medications whenever possible.
- Do not administer medications from single-dose vials or ampules to multiple patients or combine leftover contents for later use.
- If multidose vials must be used, both the needle or cannula and syringe used to access the multidose vial must be sterile.
- Do not keep multidose vials in the immediate patient treatment area and store in accordance with the manufacturer's

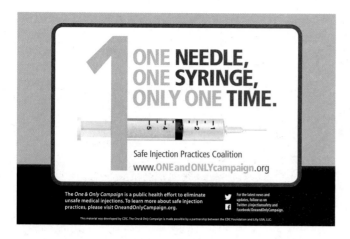

FIGURE 35-4 Posting notices such as this CDC One and Only poster reminds healthcare providers to follow safe injection practices.
Source: The Safe Injection Practices Coalition (SIPC)

recommendations; discard if sterility is compromised or questionable.

Protecting Against Needlestick Injuries

OSHA estimates that there are approximately 800,000 needlestick injuries each year and 2% of these are most likely contaminated with human immunodeficiency virus (HIV). Needlestick injuries are completely preventable if you follow OSHA and CDC guidelines. In order to protect yourself from exposure to bloodborne pathogens when handling contaminated sharps, there are certain work practice controls that you should always follow:

- Do not recap needles unless there is no alternative. If no alternative exists, use a one-handed "scoop" technique.
- Do not bend or break needles.
- Use engineered safety devices whenever possible.
- Engage safety devices on needles and scalpels immediately after use.
- Dispose of sharps promptly using approved sharps containers.
- Have sharps containers easily accessible and as close as is feasible for patient safety.
- Use only OSHA-approved sharps containers.
- Do not overfill sharps containers.
- Close sharps containers before removing for disposal so that the contents do not spill.
- Never try to open a sharps container.

If you treat any needle or sharp device as if it were contaminated with a bloodborne pathogen, you have a greater chance of staying safe in the medical office.

Safety-Engineered Devices As you learned in the *Infection Control Fundamentals* chapter, work practice and engineering controls are the key to any needlestick safety program. There are a variety of safety-engineered devices (devices specifically engineered to reduce the incidence of needlesticks) available, including self-sheathing, retractable, and self-blunting needles; re-sheathing scalpels; needleless devices; and needles with hinged safety features. According to OSHA, healthcare employers are required to evaluate new safety-engineered devices on a yearly basis and implement the use of devices that reasonably reduce the risk of needlestick injuries. Employers also must solicit input from employees using the devices. As a medical assistant, you may be asked to evaluate and provide input about safety-engineered devices. It is important that you familiarize yourself with the various types and categories of safety-engineered devices.

Self-Sheathing Needles Self-sheathing needles have a sheath over the barrel of the syringe. After injecting the patient, the user slides the sheath forward over the needle and locks it into place. The sheath completely covers the needle and, once locked, cannot be slid back over the barrel (Figure 35-5a). The disadvantage of this type of safety device is that it requires two hands to activate.

Retractable Needles and Capillary Puncture Devices Syringes with **retractable needles** such as the BD Integra™ have a needle that retracts inside the barrel of the syringe after it is activated. Once the medication is injected, the plunger is pushed again and the needle withdraws inside the syringe (Figure 35-5b). Capillary puncture devices are single-use devices. The lancet retracts into the device after use, keeping it away from the user (Figure 35-5c).

Self-Blunting Needles Self-blunting, or **blunt tip, blood-drawing needles** have a blunt tip that slides forward through the needle past the sharp point. This puts the sharp point of the needle below the blunt tip, removing the danger of a needlestick injury. Once the tube is filled with blood, the device can be activated while still in the patient's vein and then removed (Figure 35-5d). Blunt tip devices are available for blood collection systems and winged steel needles.

Re-sheathing Scalpels Re-sheathing scalpels are single-use, disposable devices. After use, the healthcare practitioner slides a sheath over the blade, locking it in place. This is done using one hand, keeping the hands clearly away from the blade. Once the sheath is activated, the blade is safely out of the way and the blade is discarded in a sharps container (Figure 35-5e).

Needles with Add-On Safety Devices Injection, phlebotomy, and winged steel needles are available with **add-on safety features.** The device is either a hinged or sliding sheath attached to the needle. Activating the device is done with one hand by either moving the hinged sheath into place or sliding the sheath up and over the needle tip. This keeps the user's hands behind the needle (Figure 35-5f).

▶ Respiratory Hygiene/Cough Etiquette Practices   LO 35.4

As you learned in the *Infection Control Fundamentals* chapter, many infectious diseases can be transmitted through respiratory droplets. Influenza, measles, whooping cough, and

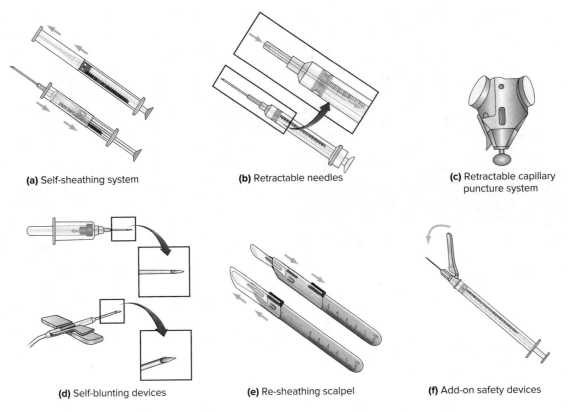

(a) Self-sheathing system

(b) Retractable needles

(c) Retractable capillary puncture system

(d) Self-blunting devices

(e) Re-sheathing scalpel

(f) Add-on safety devices

FIGURE 35-5 These are some of the safety-engineered devices available for use in healthcare settings.

meningitis are all transmitted through respiratory droplets. A sneeze or a cough can send virus-filled droplets into the air and onto surfaces several feet away, putting anyone in the area at risk for exposure. Anyone who coughs or sneezes into her hand and then touches surfaces such as doorknobs, light switches, pens, papers, and exam tables is spreading viruses throughout the environment. As a medical assistant, you will need to take measures to protect patients, coworkers, and yourself from exposure to infectious agents transmitted by droplets. **Respiratory hygiene/cough etiquette** practices are simple and effective, commonsense approaches to defending yourself and others against infectious agents spread by respiratory droplets.

Using Reminders, Alerts, and Education to Stop the Spread of Respiratory Infection

Patients, their family members, and office staff all need to be reminded what they should do in case they are ill with a fever, cough, and sneezing. As mentioned earlier, posters should be displayed at the front door of the medical office reminding patients and their families to let the staff know if they suspect they have a respiratory illness. They also may be posted in exam rooms, bathrooms, and reception areas. The CDC has a variety of posters in several languages that may be obtained either free of charge or for a nominal fee. These posters should remind everyone to:

- Cough and sneeze into a disposable tissue and immediately discard the tissue in an appropriate waste receptacle.
- Perform hand hygiene after coughing or sneezing to prevent the spread of germs.

Healthcare facilities should have tissues and alcohol-based hand rubs readily accessible in the reception area and in exam rooms and laboratory areas. No-touch waste receptacles should be placed so that patients can easily access them. Additionally, give patients educational materials to take home, reminding them of ways to reduce the spread of respiratory infection to family and friends.

Masks, Isolation, and Decontamination

During local or regional outbreaks of respiratory illness, special precautions may be necessary. Ask patients who are coughing to wear a mask. Have masks readily available for patients, including in sizes that fit children. If possible, isolate patients who are coughing in a separate reception area. If this is not possible, ask patients who are coughing to sit at least 3 feet away from other patients. If a patient is coughing and has a high fever, ask him to put on a mask and move him to an exam room as quickly as possible.

When assisting with a patient who is coughing, put on a mask before entering the room. If a patient is coughing uncontrollably and there is considerable spray, you should wear gloves, a gown, and goggles. Perform hand hygiene before and after touching the patient or items or surfaces likely contaminated with respiratory droplets. Once the patient has left the room, you should wash your hands, put on gloves, and thoroughly clean and disinfect the exam room using an EPA-approved disinfectant or a 1:10 bleach solution. Include any surface the patient may have touched, including the doorknob, chair, desk, and exam table. If you are unsure if a patient touched a surface or an item, treat it as contaminated and clean and disinfect it. Medical equipment used to examine the patient should be disinfected according to office policy and procedure.

▶ Infection Control Practices with Medical Equipment LO 35.5

There is a vast array of medical equipment used in patient care. Much of it is single use, meaning it is designed to be used for one patient during one test or procedure and then discarded in an approved container. Some equipment is reusable and must be appropriately disinfected or sterilized. This equipment is categorized based on the level of disinfection or sterilization necessary for reuse. Equipment is categorized as one of the following:

- Noncritical (such as blood pressure cuffs and reflex hammers)—these items only come in contact with intact skin and require low-level disinfection.
- Semi-critical (such as endoscopes)—these items come in contact with mucous membranes and nonintact skin and require high-level disinfection at a minimum.
- Critical (such as surgical instruments)—these items enter sterile tissue, body cavities, and veins and arteries and must be sterilized prior to use.

CDC key recommendations for cleaning, disinfecting, and/or sterilizing medical equipment in ambulatory care settings include the following:

- Reusable medical equipment should be cleaned and reprocessed prior to use with each patient.
- Cleaning and reprocessing reusable equipment must be done according to the manufacturer's recommendations. If no recommendations exist, the device may not be considered appropriate for use on multiple patients.
- Equipment reprocessing should be done only by trained professionals.
- Copies of the manufacturer's reprocessing recommendations should be kept on file and posted in the reprocessing area.
- Equipment reprocessing should be routinely monitored.
- Personnel responsible for reprocessing equipment should wear appropriate PPE.
- Equipment must be cleaned to remove organic material (blood and tissue) prior to disinfection.
- Single-use equipment should never be used on more than one patient. It is not designed for reprocessing and reuse.

▶ Surgical Site Infections (SSIs) LO 35.6

An infection that occurs after a surgical procedure at the site of surgery is considered a **surgical site infection (SSI)**. Approximately 3% of patients will develop an infection at the surgical site. The most common microorganism associated with SSIs is the bacterium *Staphylococcus aureus;* however, other bacteria also can cause infections at surgical sites. Most SSIs are endogenous—caused by microorganisms found on the skin or in the body of the patient—but they also can be exogenous—brought into the surgical site by medical

instruments or equipment. Classifications of SSIs are dependent on the location and extent of the surgical wound. The three classifications are:

- Superficial incisional—involves only the skin and subcutaneous tissue.
- Deep incisional—involves deep tissues such as fascia and muscle.
- Organ/space—excludes skin, fascia, and muscle; includes organs or body cavities.

In the medical office, you will most often see superficial incisional SSIs. Symptoms of superficial infections include:

- Purulent drainage from the surgical wound.
- Positive wound culture from the site.
- Redness, swelling, and heat at the wound site.

Adherence to CDC guidelines, careful sterile technique during office procedures and comprehensive patient education are the keys to preventing SSIs in the medical office. For more information about sterile technique, see the *Assisting with Minor Surgery* chapter.

Educating the Patient Prior to Surgery

Because most SSIs are endogenous, it is important that the patient be involved in reducing the occurrence of infection. You can help patients avoid an infection after surgery by giving them clear instructions about what to do before and after the surgical procedure:

Before the Procedure

- Report any previous postsurgical infections to the healthcare practitioner.
- Stop smoking as soon as possible before the surgery.
- Tell your doctor if you have diabetes.
- Eat well and get plenty of rest.
- Shower with an antibacterial soap before the procedure.
- Do not shave near the surgical site before your surgery.
- Stay warm while on the way to the hospital by starting the car and getting it warm before leaving for your surgery, wearing warm clothes, and covering with a blanket if needed.

The Day of Surgery

- Take any prescribed medications as instructed by your healthcare practitioner.
- Do not be afraid to speak up if you see healthcare workers fail to wash their hands.
- If a healthcare worker tells you she is going to shave the site with a razor, question her and ask to speak to the surgeon before allowing her to shave you. (The CDC recommends the use of clippers for hair removal, not razors.)

After the Surgery

- Do not allow family or friends to touch the wound.
- Care for the wound as directed by your healthcare practitioner.

- Wash your hands before and after caring for your wound.
- Call the office if you see any signs of infection.

You should give the patient all instructions in writing and verbally before the surgical procedure. Provide enough time for the patient to ask questions of you and the healthcare practitioner. Well-informed patients will be better prepared to care for themselves after surgery. Knowing how to care for their surgical wounds helps reduce the incidence of SSIs.

▶ Sterilization   LO 35.7

Sterilization is required for all instruments and supplies that will penetrate a patient's skin or come in contact with any other normally sterile areas of the body. Sterilization also is required for all instruments that will be used in a sterile field, even if they will not be used on a patient. An item is considered either sterile or unsterile. If you doubt the status of an item, consider it unsterile.

Before sterilizing an item, you must first sanitize it and, sometimes, disinfect it. Instruments and equipment that need to be sterilized include the following:

- Curettes (spoon-shaped instruments for removing material from a cavity wall or other surface).
- Instruments used during surgical procedures.
- Suture removal instruments.
- Vaginal specula (instruments used to enlarge the opening of the vagina and allow examination of the vagina and cervix).

Sterilize instruments and equipment by one of the following methods:

- Autoclaving
- Chemical (cold) processes

The Autoclave

The primary method for sterilizing instruments and equipment is the use of pressurized steam in an **autoclave** (Figure 35-6). This device forces the temperature of steam above the boiling point of water (212°F, or 100°C). Sterilization by autoclave is a widely accepted method of sterilization for two reasons:

1. Steam autoclaves can operate at a lower temperature than is required for dry heat sterilization. The moist heat from steam more quickly permeates the clean, porous wrappings in which all instruments are placed prior to loading them into the unit.
2. The moisture causes coagulation of proteins within microorganisms at a much lower temperature than is possible with dry heat. When cells containing coagulated protein cool, their cell walls burst; this kills the microorganisms.

General Autoclave Procedures In general, the sterilization process using an autoclave involves the following steps:

1. Prepare sanitized and disinfected instruments and equipment for loading into the autoclave by wrapping them in muslin, special porous paper, plastic bags, or envelopes and labeling each pack. (Include sterilization indicators.)

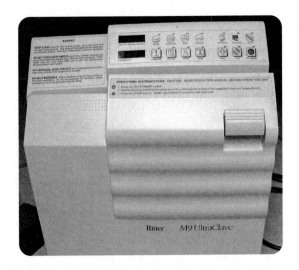

FIGURE 35-6 Steam autoclaving is the most common method of sterilizing instruments and equipment. Understanding the gauges and timer is essential to proper operation of an autoclave.
©Total Care Programming, Inc.

2. Check the water level in the autoclave; add distilled water if necessary.
3. Preheat the autoclave according to the manufacturer's guidelines. (Some models require putting instruments in before preheating.)
4. Perform any required quality control procedures (in addition to sterilization indicators in instrument packs).
5. Load the instruments and equipment into the autoclave. Allow adequate space around the items to ensure that steam reaches all areas.
6. Choose the correct setting based on the load type (unwrapped items, pouches, packs, liquids, and so on). If the autoclave is not automatic, set the autoclave for the correct time after the correct temperature and pressure have been reached.
7. Run the autoclave through the sterilization cycle, including drying time.
8. Remove the instruments and equipment from the autoclave.
9. Store the instruments and equipment properly for the next use. Rotate stored items so that packages with the oldest date are used first. Do not use packages past their expiration date.
10. Clean the autoclave and the surrounding work area.

During the autoclave process, assume the instruments and equipment are contaminated and follow standard precautions:

- Wear gloves to avoid contamination by blood, body fluids, or tissues.
- Take measures to protect against needlesticks or cuts—for example, use forceps to handle sharps.
- Wash your hands thoroughly after all cleaning procedures.

Wrapping and Labeling All Items Wrap items in porous fabric, paper, or plastic before placing them in the autoclave. This material helps surround the items with the correct levels of moisture and heat. Instruments and equipment to be used immediately after autoclaving can be placed on trays with material above and below the items. Items that must be stored in a sterile state for later use are wrapped and sealed before autoclaving. Refer to Procedure 35-3, at the end of this chapter, for wrapping and labeling instructions.

A number of products are available for wrapping items for sterilization. Muslin (140 count) may be used. However, because it is woven, it is more susceptible to contamination. All packs wrapped in muslin must be double wrapped. Other products include permeable paper, disposable nonwoven fabric, and clear plastic envelopes with one side made of permeable material. Figure 35-7 shows several common wrapping products and sterilization indicators.

Instruments that will be used together should be wrapped together to form a sterile pack. Wrap the pack loosely so that the steam can reach the instruments inside. After using a pack, consider all items (even those not used) unsterile and return them for sanitization, disinfection, and sterilization.

Clearly label each pack with a nontoxic, indelible, and nonbleeding marker to identify the item or items inside the wrapping and the person who completed the procedure. The label also must include the date to prevent use after expiring.

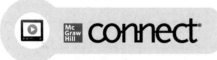

Go to CONNECT to see a video exercise about *Wrapping and Labeling Instruments for Sterilization in the Autoclave.*

Preheating the Autoclave Check for solutions that may have boiled over and for deposits that may have formed on any of the inner surfaces. Make sure the water reservoir is filled to the proper level with distilled water. Also check the discharge lines and valves to make sure there are no obstructions. If lines or valves are blocked, air may remain trapped inside the chamber, rendering the load unsterile.

Following this inspection, preheat the unit according to the manufacturer's guidelines. Loading cold instruments into an overheated chamber can cause excess condensation, so be sure to understand and follow the preheating instructions.

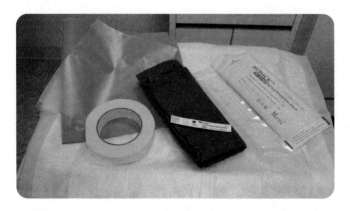

FIGURE 35-7 Common wrapping products and sterilization indicators.
©McGraw-Hill Education

Understanding Autoclave Settings Modern autoclaves are designed to operate as automatically as possible; however, manual autoclaves still are used. Because you are responsible for the sterility of the items processed by the autoclave, you must be able to identify the various gauges and interpret their readings correctly.

Manual autoclaves have three gauges and a timer. The jacket pressure gauge shows the outer chamber's steam pressure. The chamber pressure gauge shows the inner chamber's steam pressure. The temperature gauge shows the temperature inside the inner, or sterilization, chamber. The timer allows you to control the number of minutes the load is exposed to the high-temperature, pressurized steam.

Exact temperature and pressure requirements vary with the model and type of autoclave, and with the instruments and packaging in the load. In general, the temperature must reach 250°F to 270°F (121°C to 132°C), and the chamber pressure gauge must show 15 to 30 pounds of pressure. Follow the manufacturer's instructions precisely for each autoclave load. Procedure 35-4, at the end of this chapter, describes the general steps to follow for running a load through the preheated autoclave.

Sterilization Indicators and Quality Control It is important to monitor all sterilization procedures. This is accomplished through the use of various types of indicators and quality control measures.

Sterilization indicators include special packages, tags, inserts, tapes, tubes, and strips that confirm the items in the autoclave have been exposed to the correct volume of steam at the correct temperature for the correct length of time. Several types of indicators are available (Figure 35-8).

For example, you place tags or inserts within the load, whereas you affix tapes to the outside of wrapped instrument packs. Indicators have designated areas or words that change color when the correct temperature, pressure, and proper length of time have been reached. Although it is generally acceptable to rely on indicators as a guarantee of sterility, in reality, they are only indicators that the load has been exposed to conditions that usually result in sterile surfaces. They do not guarantee that the autoclave contents are actually sterile.

Biological indicators—containing bacterial spores—are used as a quality control method to confirm that sterilization has occurred. Bacterial spores come in various forms, including strips, disks, and ampules. They are used because they are more resistant to common sterilization processes than nonspore-forming organisms. The general procedure for using biological indicators is as follows:

- Place a biological indicator in a load to be sterilized.
- Place another biological indicator outside the autoclave as a positive control.
- Run the load as usual.
- Interpret the biological indicator and positive control as directed by the manufacturer or send to an outside lab for processing.
- Incubate as recommended by the manufacturer.

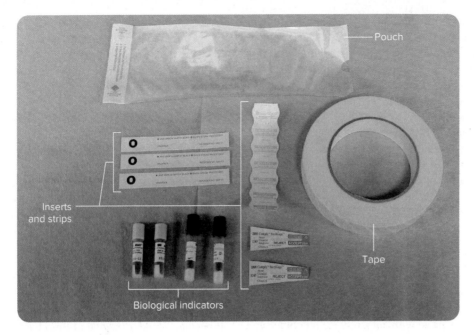

FIGURE 35-8 Sterilization indicators are manufactured in various types, sizes, and shapes.
©McGraw-Hill Education

In general, place indicators in a sufficient number of places in the load so that you can be reasonably confident of the sterility of all items in the chamber. The following locations are suitable for indicator positioning:

- Within instrument packs.
- On the outside of wrapped instrument packs.
- Inside containers, especially those that cannot be positioned to allow steam to surround the item.
- Near the air exhaust valve.
- In any other areas into which steam might not be able to flow freely.

For information on interpreting the results of a biological indicator, see the *Caution: Handle with Care* feature.

Preventing Incomplete Sterilization Although the autoclave is generally considered the simplest and most effective method for sterilizing instruments and equipment, certain pitfalls can cause incomplete sterilization. The four leading factors that cause incomplete sterilization are incorrect timing, insufficient temperature, overcrowding of packs, and inadequate steam levels. Once again, the manufacturer's guidelines provided with the autoclave unit are the best source of accurate information on how to operate it correctly.

Timing Guidelines After loading the autoclave, make sure the heating cycle lasts long enough to allow the steam to permeate all wrappings to reach the instruments and equipment inside. Timing for items to be sterilized should not be started until the unit has reached the proper temperature and

CAUTION: HANDLE WITH CARE

Interpreting the Results of a Biological Indicator

In some cases, you may be asked to interpret the results of a biological indicator. If the indicator exposed to the sterilization cycle is positive for bacterial growth, then sterilization has not occurred. The load should be held, the chemical indicators checked, and the biological indicator test repeated. If the second test is positive, have the sterilizer serviced. Once the sterilizer has been serviced, retest with three consecutive tests in an empty chamber. If all three tests are negative, the sterilizer can be returned to service. If the indicator exposed to the cycle shows no bacterial growth, check the growth of the positive control. The positive control should show bacterial growth

because it has not been exposed to the sterilization cycle. If there is no growth on the positive control, you should repeat the quality control procedure with biological indicators from another manufactured lot number. Record the results of each biological indicator monitoring procedure in the sterilization log. Biological indicators should be used at the following times:

- If a new type of packaging material is used.
- If you have a new autoclave.
- After autoclave maintenance or repair.
- On a weekly basis as a general quality control measure.

pressure. Automatic autoclaves have preset timing for each load type. You should keep up with the amount of time an automatic autoclave takes to complete a cycle, noting any differences between loads. Large differences in the amount of time it takes to complete a load cycle should alert you to a problem with the autoclave. Although following timing guidelines helps ensure sterilization, you also should use sterilization indicators.

If you have any doubt about the sterility of an instrument or a piece of equipment, do not use it. Instead, put it aside for another cycle of sanitization, disinfection, and sterilization. The risks to patients and to you are too great to take chances.

Temperature Guidelines The length of the sterilization cycle is only one factor that has an impact on the final quality of autoclave operations. If the autoclave is manual, the unit must operate at the correct temperature. Unit thermometers and sterilization indicators help confirm that correct temperatures have been reached.

Temperatures that are too high can cause problems as easily as those that are too low. If the temperature is too high inside the autoclave compartment, the steam does not have the correct level of moisture. The heat and moisture will not penetrate wrapped instrument packs, resulting in an unsterilized load.

If the temperature is too low, the steam contains too much moisture. Packs will be oversaturated and the drying cycle will be insufficient. Wet packs can easily pick up contaminants from surfaces they touch after you unload them from the autoclave. Common causes of low temperature are failing to preheat the autoclave chamber, loading cold instruments into an overheated chamber, opening the unit door too wide during drying, and overfilling the water reservoir. Always make sure you are familiar with the manufacturer's recommendations before running a load through an autoclave.

Overcrowding Packs or instruments placed in too close proximity in the autoclave chamber may not be sterilized because of the inability of the steam to penetrate or reach all surfaces.

Steam Level Guidelines Steam under pressure is necessary for sterilization. If the correct level of steam is not present during the autoclave cycle, items will not be sterile at the end of the cycle. It is vital that the unit force all air out of the chamber at the beginning of the sterilization cycle. It is also essential that you place items in the chamber in positions that will not cause the formation of air pockets.

To help ensure proper operation of the unit, check all release valves and discharge lines to make sure they are free from obstruction. Clogged valves and lines may prevent elimination of all air from the chamber.

To prevent the formation of air pockets, load items in the autoclave so that the steam can circulate freely around all sides of the items. Place containers on their sides to avoid trapping air. Besides allowing the free flow of steam, careful positioning helps ensure that all items dry thoroughly before you remove them from the autoclave.

Storing Sterilized Supplies Sterilized packs and instruments must be stored in a clean, dry location where they will not be disturbed or shuffled around. This keeps the wrapping material from being torn or otherwise compromised.

The method you use to wrap an item for sterilization determines the item's sterile shelf life. As a general rule, double-layer fabric- or paper-wrapped packages are considered sterile for 30 days. The manufacturers of other wrapping products provide their own guidelines for sterile shelf life.

Return items for sanitization, disinfection, and sterilization after the sterile shelf life period has elapsed. Do not reuse any wrapping or labeling products. Instead, open the packs or wrappings and process each item as if it had never been cleaned.

Cleaning the Autoclave and Work Area Clean the autoclave after each use to prevent accumulation of deposits that might affect the unit's operation. You may use a nontoxic all-purpose cleaner, although specific cleaning products are available for autoclave use.

You are responsible for ensuring that routine cleaning is done correctly and thoroughly. When you clean the unit, also check for signs of cracking or wear in gaskets, drain valves, and tubing. Check the level of distilled water in the reservoir. Service representatives who specialize in the maintenance of your unit should periodically clean and check all seals and gauges.

The work area around the autoclave unit should be divided into two clearly marked areas: one for nonsterile, not-yet-autoclaved items and one for sterile equipment as it is removed from the unit. Do not use supplies from one area in the other. Be sure to move any sterile packs or equipment to the correct storage areas when cleaning the counters and other work surfaces. If anything is spilled on a sterile pack or instrument, return the item for sanitization, disinfection, and sterilization.

Chemical Sterilization

Chemical, or cold, sterilization involves the use of liquids to eliminate microorganisms. It is used on instruments and equipment that are sensitive to heat and steam. For example, in a gastroenterologist's office, you may need to disinfect or sterilize an endoscope. Although each facility may perform this process differently, the process involves five steps after performing a leak test on the endoscope:

1. Clean: Mechanically clean internal and external surfaces, including brushing internal channels and flushing each internal channel with water and a detergent or enzymatic cleaners.

2. Disinfect: Immerse the endoscope in a high-level disinfectant or chemical sterilant and ensure contact of the germicide into all accessible channels, such as the suction/biopsy channel and air/water channel. Expose for the time recommended for specific products.

3. Rinse: Rinse the endoscope and all channels with sterile water, filtered water, or tap water (high-quality potable water that meets federal clean water standards at the point of use).

4. Dry: Rinse the insertion tube and inner channels with alcohol and dry with forced air after disinfection and before storage. Drying the endoscope is essential to greatly reduce the chance of recontamination of the endoscope by microorganisms that may be present in the rinse water.

5. Store: Store the endoscope in a way that prevents recontamination and promotes drying, such as hanging it vertically.

▶ Reporting Guidelines for Infectious Diseases   LO 35.8

The CDC requires the reporting of certain diseases to the state or county department of health. This information, which is forwarded to the CDC, helps research epidemiologists control the spread of infection. Table 35-1 lists diseases that must be reported to the National Notifiable Disease Surveillance System of the CDC through your state or county health department. When you report a communicable disease, you must fill out a report form either electronically or on a paper form. Your state health department may have a different form for each reportable disease. You must obtain the correct form (electronic or paper) and a disease identification number from the health department every time you report a communicable disease. To fill out such a form, you need access to the following information:

- Disease identification (usually a code number as well as the name of the disease)
- Patient identification (including name, address, date of birth, sex, ethnic origin, and occupational or educational status) if required
- Infection history (date of onset, vaccination history, laboratory results)
- Reporting-institution information (name of person completing report, title, contact information)

Each state and each medical facility has specific guidelines for filling out such a form. Procedure 35-5, at the end of this chapter, describes, in general, how to notify state and county agencies about reportable diseases. This procedure uses a paper form; however, electronic reporting may be available in the facility where you are employed.

Reporting guidelines also must be followed if a worker comes in contact with a substance that may transmit infection. These guidelines, which are explained in OSHA's Bloodborne Pathogens Standard, include reporting exposure incidents to employers immediately.

TABLE 35-1 The National Notifiable Disease Surveillance System	
Disease/Condition/Organism	**Disease/Condition/Organism**
Anthrax	Legionellosis
Arboviral diseases, neuroinvasive and non-neuroinvasive	Leptospirosis
California serogroup virus diseases	Listeriosis
Chikungunya virus disease	Lyme disease
Eastern equine encephalitis virus disease	Malaria
Powassan virus disease	Measles
St. Louis encephalitis virus disease	Meningococcal disease
West Nile virus disease	Mumps
Western equine encephalitis virus disease	Novel influenza A virus infections
Babesiosis	Pertussis
Botulism	Pesticide-related illness and injury, acute
Botulism, foodborne	Plague
Botulism, infant	Poliomyelitis, paralytic
Botulism, wound	Poliovirus infection, nonparalytic
Botulism, other	Psittacosis
Brucellosis	Q fever
Campylobacteriosis	Q fever, acute
Cancer	Q fever, chronic
Candida auris, clinical	Rabies, animal
Carbapenemase Producing Carbapenem-Resistant Enterobacteriaceae (CP-CRE)	Rabies, human
	Rubella
CP-CRE, Enterobacter spp.	Rubella, congenital syndrome
CP-CRE, Escherichia coli (E. coli)	*Salmonella* Paratyphi infection (*Salmonella* enterica serotypes Paratyphi A, B [tartrate negative], and C [*S.* Paratyphi])
CP-CRE, Klebsiella spp.	*Salmonella* Typhi infection (*Salmonella enterica* serotype Typhi)

(continued)

TABLE 35-1   The National Notifiable Disease Surveillance System

Disease/Condition/Organism	Disease/Condition/Organism
Carbon monoxide poisoning	Salmonellosis
Chancroid	Severe acute respiratory syndrome-associated coronavirus disease
Chlamydia trachomatis infection	Shiga toxin-producing *Escherichia coli*
Cholera	Shigellosis
Coccidioidomycosis	Silicosis
Congenital syphilis	Smallpox
Syphilitic stillbirth	Spotted fever rickettsiosis
Cryptosporidiosis	Streptococcal toxic shock syndrome
Cyclosporiasis	Syphilis
Dengue virus infections	Syphilis, primary
Dengue	Syphilis, secondary
Dengue-like illness	Syphilis, early non-primary non-secondary
Severe dengue	Syphilis, unknown duration or late
Diphtheria	Tetanus
Ehrlichiosis and anaplasmosis	Toxic shock syndrome (other than streptococcal)
Anaplasma phagocytophilum infection	Trichinellosis
Ehrlichia chaffeensis infection	Tuberculosis
Ehrlichia ewingii infection	Tularemia
Undetermined human ehrlichiosis/anaplasmosis	Typhoid fever
Foodborne Disease Outbreak	Vancomycin-intermediate *Staphylococcus aureus* and Vancomycin-resistant *Staphylococcus aureus*
Giardiasis	Varicella
Gonorrhea	Varicella deaths
Haemophilus influenzae, invasive disease	Vibriosis
Hanse's disease	Viral hemorrhagic fever
Hantavirus infection, non-Hantavirus pulmonary syndrome	Crimean-Congo hemorrhagic fever virus
Hantavirus pulmonary syndrome	Ebola virus
Hemolytic uremic syndrome, post-diarrheal	Lassa virus
Hepatitis A, acute	Lujo virus
Hepatitis B, acute	Marburg virus
Hepatitis B, chronic	New World arenavirus – Guanarito virus
Hepatitis B, perinatal virus infection	New World arenavirus – Junin virus
Hepatitis C, acute	New World arenavirus – Machupo virus
Hepatitis C, chronic	New World arenavirus – Sabia virus
Hepatitis C, perinatal infection	Waterborne Disease Outbreak
HIV infection (AIDS has been reclassified as HIV Stage III)	Yellow Fever
Influenza-associated pediatric mortality	Zika virus disease and Zika virus infection
Invasive pneumococcal disease	Zika virus disease, congenital
Latent TB Infection (TB Infection)	Zika virus disease, non-congenital
Lead, elevated blood levels	Zika virus infection, congenital
Lead, elevated blood levels, children (<16 Years)	Zika virus infection, non-congenital
Lead, elevated blood levels, adult (≥16 Years)	

Source: Adapted from Centers for Disease Control and Prevention Nationally Notifiable Infectious Conditions US 2019.

PROCEDURE 35-1 Removing Contaminated Gloves

Procedure Goal: To remove gloves contaminated with blood, body fluids, or other potentially hazardous substances while avoiding cross-contamination of your hands or other surfaces

OSHA Guidelines: This procedure does not involve exposure to blood, body fluids, or tissue if performed correctly.

Materials: Contaminated gloves, lined trash container or bio-hazardous waste container

Method:

1. Using your dominant hand, grasp the palm of the glove of your nondominant hand.
2. Gently pull the glove downward off the nondominant hand, turning it inside out and holding it in your dominant hand.

3. Encase the removed glove completely in the dominant hand. **RATIONALE:** *To contain any contaminants in the glove so that they are not accidentally transferred to your hands; encasing the glove also limits the possibility of splattering contaminants by flipping the glove.*
4. Place the thumb or two fingers of the ungloved hand under the cuff of the remaining glove, being careful not to touch the outside of the glove with your bare hand. **RATIONALE:** *The inside of the glove is most likely not contaminated.*
5. Pull the glove over your hand, turning it inside out over the other glove, leaving no outside surface exposed.
6. Throw the gloves away in the appropriate waste container.
7. Wash your hands.

PROCEDURE 35-2 Removing a Contaminated Gown

Procedure Goal: To remove a gown contaminated on the front and sleeves with blood, body fluids, or other potentially hazardous substances while avoiding cross-contamination of your hands, body, or other surfaces

OSHA Guidelines: This procedure does not involve exposure to blood, body fluids, or tissue if performed correctly.

Materials: Contaminated gown, lined trash container or bio-hazardous waste container

Method:

1. Unfasten ties from the neck, then from behind your back.

2. Peel the gown down and away from neck and shoulders, touching inside of gown only. **RATIONALE:** *You should always move from clean to dirty to avoid cross-contamination.*
3. Continue pulling the gown down from the neck and shoulders and away from your body.
4. Turn gown inside out, making sure you do not touch the outer surface of the gown. **RATIONALE:** *To avoid contaminating your hands.*
5. Slowly fold or roll into a bundle and discard.
6. Wash your hands if they become visibly contaminated; otherwise use an alcohol-based hand sanitizer.

PROCEDURE 35-3 Wrapping and Labeling Instruments for Sterilization in the Autoclave

Procedure Goal: To enclose instruments and equipment to be sterilized in appropriate wrapping materials to ensure sterilization and to protect supplies from contamination after sterilization

OSHA Guidelines:

Materials: Dry, sanitized, and disinfected instruments and equipment; wrapping material (paper, muslin, gauze, bags, envelopes); sterilization indicators; autoclave tape; labels (if wrapping does not include space for labeling); and a waterproof pen

Method:

For Wrapping Instruments or Equipment in Pieces of Paper or Fabric

1. Wash your hands and don gloves before beginning to wrap the items to be sterilized.
2. Place a square of paper or muslin on the table with one point toward you. With muslin, use a double thickness. The paper or fabric must be large enough to allow all four points to cover the instruments or equipment you will be wrapping. It also must be large enough to provide an overlap, which will be used as a handling flap.
3. Place each item to be included in the pack in the center area of the paper or fabric "diamond." Items that will be used together should be wrapped together. Make sure, however, that surfaces of the items do not touch each other inside the pack so that steam can penetrate

every surface of all instruments in the pack. Inspect each item to ensure it is operating correctly. Place hinged instruments in the pack in the open position. Wrap a small piece of paper, muslin, or gauze around delicate edges or points to protect against damage to other instruments or to the pack wrapping.

4. Place a sterilization indicator inside the pack with the instruments. Position the indicator correctly, following the manufacturer's guidelines (Figure a).
   RATIONALE: *A sterilization indicator always must be placed inside the pack to ensure the contents have been sterilized properly.*

5. Fold the bottom point of the diamond up and over the instruments in to the center (Figure b). Fold back a small portion of the point (Figure c).
   RATIONALE: *This "handle" will be used later, when the sterile pack is opened.*

6. Fold the right point of the diamond in to the center. Again, fold back a small portion of the point to be used as a handle (Figure d).

7. Fold the left point of the diamond in to the center, folding back a small portion to form a handle. The pack should now resemble an open envelope (Figure e).

8. Grasp the covered instruments (the bottom of the envelope) and fold this portion up, toward the top point (Figure f). Fold the top point down over the pack, making sure the pack is snug but not too tight.

9. Secure the pack with autoclave tape (Figure g). A "quick-opening tab" can be created by folding a small portion of the tape back onto itself. The pack must be snug enough to prevent instruments from slipping out of the wrapping or damaging each other inside the pack but loose enough to allow adequate steam circulation through the pack.

10. Label the pack with your initials and the date. Then list the contents of the pack. If the pack contains syringes, be sure to identify the syringe size(s). Use a labeling pen that is nontoxic, indelible, and nonbleeding to label the pack.
    RATIONALE: *Dating helps you keep up with the date the pack expires. Items should be easily identified without opening the pack. Using a pen that is nontoxic, indelible, and nonbleeding keeps the contents from being contaminated by the ink.*

11. Place the pack aside for loading into the autoclave.

12. Remove gloves, dispose of them in the appropriate waste container, and wash your hands.

For Wrapping Instruments and Equipment in Bags or Envelopes

1. Wash your hands and put on gloves before beginning to wrap the items to be sterilized.

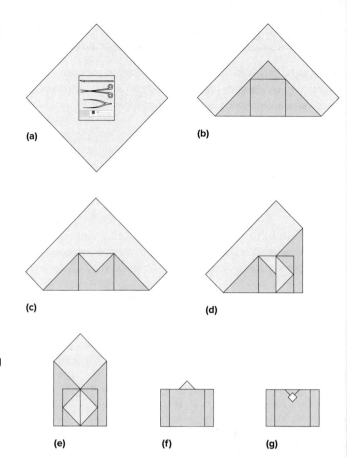

FIGURE Procedure 35-3 Steps 4 through 9   Follow the sequence in this figure when you wrap instruments in a paper or fabric pack for sterilization in an autoclave.

2. Insert the items into the bag or envelope as indicated by the manufacturer's directions. Hinged instruments should be opened before insertion into the package.
   RATIONALE: *This allows steam to penetrate inside the hinge.*

3. Close and seal the pack. Make sure the sterilization indicator is not damaged or already exposed.
   RATIONALE: *If the sterilization indicator is damaged or already exposed, you have no way of knowing if the sterilization cycle was completed.*

4. Label the pack with your initials and the date. Then list the contents of the pack. The pens or pencils used to label the pack must be nontoxic, indelible, and nonbleeding; otherwise, the contents of the pack and date of sterilization will be obliterated and could be contaminated by the ink.
   RATIONALE: *Dating helps you keep up with the date the pack expires. Items should be easily identified without opening the pack.*

5. Place the pack aside for loading into the autoclave.

6. Remove gloves, dispose of them in the appropriate waste container, and wash your hands.

PROCEDURE 35-4 Running a Load Through the Autoclave

Procedure Goal: To run a load of instruments and equipment through an autoclave, ensuring sterilization of items by properly loading, drying, and unloading them

OSHA Guidelines:

Materials: Dry, sanitized, and disinfected instruments and equipment, both individual pieces and wrapped packs; oven mitts; sterile transfer forceps; and storage containers for individual items

Method:

1. Wash your hands and don gloves before beginning to load items into the autoclave.
2. Rest packs on their edges and place jars and containers on their sides.
3. Place lids for jars and containers with their sterile sides down.
4. If the load includes plastic items, make sure no other item leans against them.
   RATIONALE: *Pressure that results from the high temperatures can cause plastic items to bend or warp.*
5. If your load is mixed—containing both wrapped packs and individual instruments—place the tray containing the instruments below the tray containing the wrapped packs.
   RATIONALE: *This arrangement prevents any condensation that forms on the instruments from dripping onto the wrapped packs and saturating the wrapping.*
6. Close the door and start the unit. For automatic autoclaves, choose the cycle based on the type of load you are running. Consult the manufacturer's recommendations before choosing the load type.
7. For manual autoclaves, start the timer when the indicators show the recommended temperature and pressure.
8. Right after the end of the steam cycle and just before the start of the drying cycle, open the door to the autoclave slightly (between ¼ and ½ inch).
   RATIONALE: *Opening the door more than ½ inch causes cold air to enter the autoclave, possibly creating excessive condensation in the chamber. This condensation would cause incomplete drying. Consult the manufacturer's recommendations regarding opening the door. Some automatic autoclaves do not require opening the door during the drying cycle.*
9. Dry according to the manufacturer's recommendations. Packs and large items may require up to 45 minutes for complete drying.
10. Unload the autoclave after the drying cycle is finished. Do not unload any packs or instruments with wet wrappings, or the objects inside will be considered unsterile and must be processed again.
    RATIONALE: *Wet wrappings can transfer bacteria from your hands to the interior of the pack.*
11. Unload each package carefully once they have cooled completely. Use sterile transfer forceps to unload unwrapped individual objects.
12. Inspect each package or item, looking for moisture on the wrapping, underexposed sterilization indicators, and tears or breaks in the wrapping. Consider the pack unsterile if any of these conditions are present.
13. Place sterile packs aside for transfer to storage.
14. Place individual items that are not required to be sterile in clean containers.
15. Place items that must remain sterile in sterile containers; close container covers tightly.
16. As you unload items, avoid placing them in an overly cool location; the cool temperature could cause condensation on the instruments or packs.
17. Remove gloves, dispose of them in the appropriate waste container, and wash your hands.

PROCEDURE 35-5 Notifying State and County Agencies About Reportable Diseases

WORK // DOC

Procedure Goal: To report cases of infection with reportable disease to the proper state or county health department

OSHA Guidelines: This procedure does not involve exposure to blood, body fluids, or tissues.

Materials: Communicable disease report form, pen, envelope, and stamp

Method:

1. Check to be sure you have the correct form (electronic or paper). Some states have specific forms for each reportable infectious disease or type of disease. CDC forms also may be used for reporting specific diseases.
2. Gather all necessary information, including:
   - Disease identification including code number
   - Patient identification information including name, address, date of birth, sex, ethnic origin, occupational and educational status
   - Infection history
   - Reporting-institution information including name of person completing the form, title, and contact information

MICHIGAN DEPARTMENT OF PUBLIC HEALTH
Division of Disease Surveillance

ENTERIC ILLNESS CASE INVESTIGATION
(Please check appropriate illness)

_____Shigellosis   _____Giardiasis
_____Non-typhoid Salmonellosis   _____Amebiasis
_____Campylobacter enteritis

CASE INFORMATION

Name: _____ Age or Birthdate: _____ Sex: _____ Race: _____

Address: _____ Phone: _____
       (Street)   (City)   (County)   (Zip)

Occupation: _____ *High Risk: Y N
              (What)   (Where)
    (If infant or student list school, nursery or day care center)

Attending   Address or   Was the patient
Physician: _____ Phone:_____ hospitalized: Y N

Hospital: _____ Dates:_____
                                       (Admission)   (Discharge)

Onset: _____ Date recovered: _____ Symptom Summary: _____
_____
_____

Suspected Causative Agent: _____
(include species or serotype if known)

HOUSEHOLD CONTACTS INFORMATION

Name	Age	Family Relationship	Occupation	*High Risk Y N	Provide date of onset for all household members with concurrent similar illness
1)					
2)					
3)					
4)					
5)					
6)					
7)					
8)					
9)					
10)					

*"High Risk" = occupation as food handler, direct patient care worker, day care center worker or person attending day care or who is institutionalized. Stool specimens should be obtained on "high risk" cases and "high risk" household contacts as appropriate for the illness. Results may be recorded in Laboratory Information Section of this form (see over).

Name of the person who completed this form:_____County:_____

Information obtained from: _____ Date:_____

Telephone Interview: _____ Home Visit: _____ Outbreak Investigation: _____

C-30 Rev. 10/83   AUTH: Act 368, P.A. 1978

FIGURE Procedure 35-5 Step 1   Some states have specific forms for use with particular communicable diseases or diseases of a certain type. (Continued)

NON-HOUSEHOLD CONTACTS WITH A CONCURRENT SIMILAR ILLNESS

Name	Approximate date of onset of symptoms	Address and/or Phone	Relationship to case (Nature of contact)
1)			
2)			
3)			
4)			
5)			

ADDITIONAL EXPOSURES OR COMMENTS

Home Sewage System: Municipal   Septic Tank   Other_____

Home drinking Water Type: Municipal   Private Well   Other_____

As appropriate for the illness, ask about meals eaten away from home, stores where groceries bought, brand of poultry, meat, dairy products consumed, overnight travel, recent foreign travel, group functions, exposure to raw milk, untreated water, animals, etc. within one incubation period before onset.

   (shigellosis to 7 days, salmonellosis - up to 3 days, Campylobacter enteritis - up to 10 days)

Be specific, provide place name(s) and date(s).

FOLLOW-UP FECAL CULTURE RESULTS FOR "HIGH RISK" CASE AND/OR CONTACTS.

Name or Initials	Date(s) Obtained and Findings
1)	
2)	
3)	
4)	
5)	

FIGURE Procedure 35-5 Step 1   Some states have specific forms for use with particular communicable diseases or diseases of a certain type.

3. Fill in all blank areas unless they are shaded (generally for local health department use).

4. Follow office procedures for submitting the report to a supervisor or physician before sending it out or submitting electronically.

5. If the form is paper, sign and date the form. Address the envelope, put a stamp on it, and place it in the mail. If the form is an electronic form, follow the online instructions for submitting the form.

SUMMARY OF LEARNING OUTCOMES

OUTCOME	KEY POINTS
35.1 Identify various healthcare-associated infections (HAI) specific to the ambulatory care setting.	The most common HAI specific to the ambulatory care setting is MRSA. Other types of HAI that occur in outpatient settings include *Clostridium difficile* (C. diff), central line–associated bloodstream infections (CLABSI), catheter-associated urinary tract infections (CAUTI), and surgical site infections (SSIs).

OUTCOME	KEY POINTS
35.2 Describe methods of infection control, including those for preventing healthcare-associated infections.	The two basic methods of infection control are medical asepsis (clean technique) and surgical asepsis (sterile technique). OSHA recommends that healthcare workers who work with high-risk patients know their HIV and HBV status, participate in an HBV vaccination program, and avoid direct patient contact if they have a skin condition characterized by sores that secrete fluid. Any healthcare worker who is HIV- or HBV-positive should not perform procedures that might expose a patient without first consulting an expert review panel.
35.3 Describe various methods of injection safety, including safety-engineered devices and work practice controls.	Injection safety procedures include always following strict aseptic procedures and standard precautions when administering injections. In addition, use safety-engineered devices whenever feasible.
35.4 Summarize proper respiratory hygiene/cough etiquette practices utilized in the medical office.	Post reminders for patients and staff to always cover their coughs and sneezes with a tissue and properly dispose of the tissue in an appropriate waste container. When assisting with patients who have symptoms of a respiratory infection, ask patients to wear masks and use isolation precautions to stop the spread of infections.
35.5 Describe infection control procedures related to medical equipment.	Multi-use medical equipment should be properly cleaned, disinfected, and sterilized according to the manufacturer's recommendations before use with every patient. Single-use medical equipment should be properly disposed of and never reused with a different patient.
35.6 Describe surgical site infections (SSIs) and ways to prevent them.	A surgical site infection (SSI) is an infection that occurs after a surgical procedure at the site of the surgery. The signs of an SSI include purulent drainage, heat and redness at the site, and fever. Giving patients clear instructions about what to do before and after surgery and always following surgical aseptic procedures reduces the incidence of SSI.
35.7 Discuss the procedures used in a medical office to sterilize surgical instruments and equipment.	Instruments and equipment that must be sterilized before use should be sanitized to remove blood and gross tissue and then sterilized either in an autoclave or by chemical means.
35.8 Describe Centers for Disease Control and Prevention (CDC) requirements for reporting cases of infectious disease.	The CDC requires the reporting of certain diseases to the state or county department of health, which then reports the information to the National Notifiable Disease Surveillance System of the CDC.

CASE STUDY CRITICAL THINKING

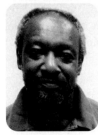

©McGraw-Hill Education

Recall Ken Washington from the case study at the beginning of the chapter. Now that you have completed the chapter, answer the following questions regarding his case.

1. Is it significant that Ken Washington had a urinary catheter in place for 6 days while he was in the hospital?

2. Dr. Buckwalter plans to send Ken Washington home with a urinary catheter in place. What information can you give him to help him prevent infection?

3. You note on the chart that Dr. Buckwalter wants to see Ken Washington again in 2 days. You ask him to schedule an appointment for that time. Ken Washington's wife states that they are going out of town for a week and will not be able to return until after that time. What should you tell Ken Washington about delaying the appointment more than a week?

1. (LO 35.2) When opening a sterile container, you should place the lid
   a. On the sterile field
   b. Facedown on the counter
   c. On a separate sterile field
   d. In your opposite hand
   e. Face-up on the counter

2. (LO 35.1) Which of the following best describes a CAUTI?
   a. An infection at the site of surgery
   b. An infection caused by microorganisms entering the bladder by way of a catheter
   c. A blood infection caused by a central line
   d. A procedure to stop bleeding
   e. A skin infection caused by antibiotic-resistant bacteria

3. (LO 35.4) All of the following are considered good respiratory hygiene *except*
   a. Isolating patients with respiratory infections in a separate reception area
   b. Placing a mask and goggles on anyone with symptoms of a respiratory infection
   c. Performing hand hygiene after coughing or sneezing
   d. Asking patients who are coughing to sit at least 3 feet away from other patients
   e. Immediately discarding used tissues into appropriate waste containers

4. (LO 35.6) A superficial incisional surgical site infection is one that involves
   a. Only the skin and subcutaneous tissue
   b. Organs and body cavities
   c. Muscles and fascia
   d. Bones and joints
   e. Intestinal tissue

5. (LO 35.8) All of the following are reportable diseases *except*
   a. Hantavirus
   b. Giardiasis
   c. Chickenpox
   d. Adenovirus
   e. Malaria

6. (LO 35.6) Which of the following is the term for surgical site infections caused by microorganisms found on the skin?
   a. Remote
   b. Exogenous
   c. Purulent
   d. Endogenous
   e. Extrinsic

7. (LO 35.1) A procedure that requires entry into a body cavity or cutting into skin or mucous membranes is known as
   a. Infectious
   b. Systemic
   c. Invasive
   d. Internal
   e. Vital

8. (LO 35.3) Self-blunting, or blunt tip, blood-drawing needles have
   a. A device that slides through the lumen of the needle past the sharp point
   b. A sheath that slides over the needle and locks
   c. A needle that retracts into the syringe
   d. A needle that automatically breaks off after removing from the patient
   e. A needle with a hinged safety cover

9. (LO 35.7) The sterile shelf life of a paper-wrapped surgical pack is
   a. 1 month
   b. 1 year
   c. 6 months
   d. 2 months
   e. 14 days

10. (LO 35.2) Another name for medical asepsis is
    a. Sterile technique
    b. Aseptic principles
    c. Safe technique
    d. Clean technique
    e. Surgical cleaning

SOFT SKILLS SUCCESS

Recall Ken F. Washington from the case study at the beginning of the chapter. While you are giving Ken F. Washington care instructions for urinary catheterization, his wife states that she is not happy that Ken F. Washington has to have another urinary catheter. She tells you that she thinks that the "man in the hospital" did not insert his urinary catheter properly and that is what has caused Ken F. Washington's problem. She asks you if you think it is possible that Ken F. Washington was "damaged" at the hospital when he had his urinary catheter inserted. What should you tell Ken F. Washington's wife?

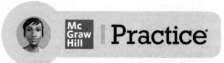

Go to PRACTICE MEDICAL OFFICE and complete the module Admin Check Out: Privacy and Liability.

Patient Interview and History

CASE STUDY

PATIENT INFORMATION			
	Patient Name	**DOB**	**Allergies**
	Peter Smith	03/28/1946	NKA
	Attending	**MRN**	**Other Information**
	Paul F. Buckwalter, MD	00-AA-003	Sleep study scheduled with Metro Sleep Specialists

Peter Smith, a male patient over 70 with mild Type 2 diabetes, calls to schedule an appointment. He states that he is feeling very anxious and fatigued and is having difficulty eating and sleeping. He arrives at the clinic with his wife.

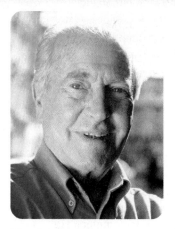

©Image Source/Getty Images

During the patient interview, he states that he wakes up in the middle of the night almost nightly. He also has many nights when he cannot even fall asleep. In addition, he has lost about 8 pounds in the last month. His symptoms started when his son died 6 months ago.

Keep Peter Smith in mind as you study this chapter. There will be questions at the end of the chapter based on the case study. The information in the chapter will help you answer these questions.

LEARNING OUTCOMES

After completing Chapter 36, you will be able to:

36.1 Identify the skills necessary to conduct a patient interview.

36.2 Recognize the signs of anxiety; depression; and physical, mental, or substance abuse.

36.3 Use the six Cs for writing an accurate patient history.

36.4 Carry out a patient history using critical thinking skills.

KEY TERMS

addiction
clarification
mirroring
objective data
reflection

restatement
subjective data
substance abuse
verbalizing

I.P.3	Perform patient screening using established protocols
I.A.1	Incorporate critical thinking skills when performing patient assessment.
V.C.2	Identify types of nonverbal communication
V.C.4	Identify techniques for overcoming communication barriers
V.C.15	Differentiate between adaptive and non-adaptive coping mechanisms
V.C.16	Differentiate between subjective and objective information
V.P.1	Use feedback techniques to obtain patient information including: (a) reflection (b) restatement (c) clarification
V.P.2	Respond to nonverbal communication
V.P.3	Use medical terminology correctly and pronounced accurately to communicate information to providers and patients
V.A.1	Demonstrate: (a) empathy (b) active listening (c) nonverbal communication
X.P.2	Apply HIPAA rules in regard to: (a) privacy (b) release of information
X.P.3	Document patient care accurately in the medical record
X.P.4	Apply the Patient's Bill of Rights as it relates to: (a) choice of treatment (b) consent for treatment (c) refusal of treatment
X.A.1	Demonstrate sensitivity to patient rights

3. Medical Terminology
   d. Define and use medical abbreviations when appropriate and acceptable

4. Medical Law and Ethics
   a. Follow documentation guidelines
   b. Institute federal and state guidelines when:
      (1) Releasing medical records or information
   f. Comply with federal, state, and local health laws and regulations as they relate to healthcare settings
   g. Display compliance with the Code of Ethics of the profession

5. Human Relations
   a. Respond appropriately to patients with abnormal behavior patterns
   c. Assist the patient in navigating issues and concerns that may arise (i.e. insurance policy information, medical bills, and physician/provider orders)

8. Clinical Procedures
   b. Obtain vital signs, obtain patient history, and formulate chief complaint

10. Career Development
   b. Demonstrate professional behavior

▶ Introduction

As a medical assistant, it is your job to prepare the patient and the patient's chart before the physician enters the exam room to examine the patient. You are the first contact with the patient in the exam room. How you conduct yourself during those first few moments can make a major difference in the patient's attitude and perception of the medical office. The patient must cooperate fully to provide the information the physician needs for an accurate diagnosis and successful treatment. Conducting the patient interview and recording the necessary medical history are essential to the practitioner's exam process.

▶ The Patient Interview and History LO 36.1

The first step in the exam process is the patient interview. A well-conducted initial interview in the exam room helps establish a beneficial relationship between you and the new patient while providing a detailed exchange of pertinent information. Subsequent interviews with established patients may take less time; however, all patient interviews require good communication skills.

When you interview a patient, you will ask the patient (or if the patient is a child, an attending family member) for specific information about the reason for his or her visit. If the visit is for a medical problem, you will ask about his or her symptoms and determine the patient's chief complaint. The chief complaint is a subjective statement made by the patient describing the patient's most significant symptoms or signs of illness. Medicare and most insurers require this information. When a patient makes an office visit for a routine checkup, you will ask the patient about general health and lifestyle and about any changes in health status since the last visit.

A patient's medical and health history is the basis for all treatment rendered by the practitioner. The history also provides information for research, reportable diseases, and insurance claims. The information contained on the chart becomes a legal record of the treatment rendered to the patient. It must be complete and accurate to be a good defense in case of legal action. Document all information regarding the patient precisely and accurately.

Patient Rights, Responsibilities, and Privacy

It is important to remember that all the data you obtain are subject to legal and ethical considerations. Most states have adopted a version of the American Hospital Association's (AHA) Patient's Bill of Rights, written in 1973 and revised in 1992. Although AHA has replaced this bill of rights with "The Patient Care Partnership: Understanding Expectations, Rights, and Responsibilities," each state encourages healthcare workers to be aware of and provide for the patient's rights. Familiarize yourself with the information about patient rights contained in the following list. All patients have the right to:

- Receive considerate and respectful care.
- Receive complete and current information concerning his or her diagnosis, treatment, and prognosis.
- Know the identity of physicians, nurses, and others involved with his or her care as well as know when those involved are students, residents, or trainees.
- Know the immediate and long-term costs of treatment choices.
- Receive information necessary to give informed consent prior to the start of any procedure or treatment.
- Have an advance directive concerning treatment or be able to choose a representative to make decisions.
- Refuse treatment to the extent permitted by law.
- Receive every consideration of his or her privacy.
- Be assured of confidentiality.
- Obtain reasonable responses to requests for services.
- Obtain information about his or her healthcare and be allowed to review his or her medical record and to have any information explained or interpreted.
- Know whether treatment is experimental and be able to consent or decline to participate in proposed research studies or human experimentation.
- Expect reasonable continuity of care.
- Ask about and be informed of the existence of business relationships between the hospital and others that may influence the patient's treatment and care.
- Know which hospital policies and practices relate to patient care, treatment, and responsibilities.

- Be informed of available resources for resolving disputes, grievances, and conflicts, such as ethics committees or patient representatives.
- Examine his or her bill and have it explained, and be informed of available payment methods.

Medical assistants also should know that patients have certain responsibilities when they seek medical care. Patients are responsible for:

- Providing information about past illnesses, hospitalizations, medications, and other matters related to their health status. If an incorrect diagnosis is made because a patient fails to give the physician the proper information, the physician may not be liable.
- Participating in decision making by asking for additional information about their health status or treatment when they do not fully understand information and instructions.
- Providing healthcare agencies with a copy of their written advance directive if they have one.
- Informing physicians and other caregivers if they anticipate problems in following a prescribed treatment.
- Following the physician's orders for treatment. If a patient willfully or negligently fails to follow the physician's instructions, that patient has little legal recourse.
- Providing healthcare agencies with necessary information for insurance claims and working with the healthcare facility to make arrangements to pay fees when necessary.

Additionally, in April 2003, enforcement of the Health Insurance Portability and Accountability Act (HIPAA) began. If this act is not followed, individual healthcare workers can be subject to fines up to $250,000 and 10 years in jail. The privacy standards of this act ensure the following:

- Healthcare facilities must provide patients with a written notice of their practices regarding the use and disclosure of all individually identifiable health information.
- Healthcare facilities may not use or disclose protected health information for any purpose that is not in the privacy notice.
- Patient consent is required when protected information is used or disclosed for purposes of treatment, payment, or health operations.
- Written authorization is required for other types of disclosures.
- Hospitals must make the privacy notice available either prior to or at the time of the delivery of care.
- A privacy notice must be posted in a clear and prominent location within the hospital facility.

Communicating with Professionalism

Remember, the first impression you make with patients in the exam room can be everlasting, as it can affect the way patients view the entire office's practice, including the physicians'. As a medical assistant, communicating with professionalism is key. In addition to your awareness of patient rights, responsibilities, and privacy, your overall professionalism and poise can be a direct result of your verbal communication skills. If you use improper language skills, such as poor grammar or slang, or appear to have sloppy body language, you may give the patient the perception that you are not educated or intelligent. Your communication skills will have a direct impact on your career. Take care and pride in what you know and how you communicate. Think before you speak or react and you will learn to avoid communication pitfalls.

Interviewing Skills

To conduct a successful patient interview and obtain history and health information, you will need to apply a variety of skills, including the following:

- Using effective listening.
- Being aware of nonverbal clues and body language.
- Using a broad knowledge base.
- Summarizing to form a general picture.

Using Effective Listening Listening attentively is one of the most important skills you will need for a successful interview. When you listen to what the patient is saying, you not only listen for details but also try to get an overall view of the patient's situation. As you become more experienced in conducting patient interviews, these skills will improve. One way to be a good listener is to hear, think about, and respond to what the patient has said. This technique is called *active listening*. Passive listeners simply sit back and hear. When you are an active listener, you look at the patient, pay attention, and provide feedback. For example, you may use the technique of **restatement**. Simply repeat what the patient says, in your own words, back to the patient. This helps to ensure that you have understood the meaning of the patient's words.

Being Aware of Nonverbal Clues and Body Language
Verbal communication is the asking and answering of questions. To conduct a successful interview, you also must be aware of nonverbal communication. The patient's tone of voice, facial expression, and body language are examples of nonverbal communication. These signs often communicate more than words could ever say. For example, a patient who has difficulty making eye contact may be embarrassed by some symptoms and may need your extra patience and encouragement to report symptoms fully. A child or adolescent may deny or exaggerate pain. Pay attention to the patient's facial expression and how much the patient guards the area in question.

Using a Broad Knowledge Base To conduct a successful interview, you must have a broad knowledge base so that you can ask questions that will elicit the most meaningful information about the patient. You must take every opportunity to expand your knowledge base by learning more about medical terminology, anatomy and physiology, symptoms, and diseases.

Summarizing to Form a General Picture You will gather a variety of subjective and objective data as you conduct a patient interview. You must consider the relative importance of each piece of information so that you can summarize the data to formulate a general picture of the patient. It is always a good idea to repeat back a summary of information to the patient. This will ensure that all important data are recorded. Patients will sometimes forget to add something, and repeating the summary may jog their memory.

Interviewing Successfully

One of the main goals of the patient interview is to give the patient an opportunity to fully explain, in her own words, the reason for the current office visit. These eight steps will help you conduct a successful interview.

1. Do your research before the patient interview.
2. Plan the interview.
3. Approach the patient and request the interview.
4. Make the patient feel at ease.
5. Conduct the interview in private without interruptions.
6. Deal with sensitive topics with respect.
7. Do not diagnose or give a diagnostic opinion.
8. Formulate the general picture.

Doing Research Before the Patient Interview
Before the interview, review the patient's medical record for history, medications, and chronic problems (for example, diabetes or high blood pressure). Note whether the patient has family problems that might have an impact on health issues. Make sure that all currently ordered diagnostic testing, laboratory work, and consultation results are in the chart. If you discover that you are missing a result, you have some time to retrieve it from the facility while the patient is in the office.

Planning the Interview Develop an interview plan by having a general idea of the questions you will ask. For example, if a patient is being treated for high blood pressure, you might ask about headaches or tinnitus (ringing in the ears), which are common signs of high blood pressure. Planning the interview helps you maintain your focus and ensures that you will obtain all the necessary information.

It is important to be organized before the interview takes place. Follow the office policies when gathering patient information. For example, you may record the patient's height, weight, and vital signs before you begin the interview. Make sure that you follow office policy on the types of information you will need to ask the patient during the interview. For example, some physicians prefer that you record the patient's medication list before the exam, whereas others prefer to record the medication list themselves. Planning for the types of information that you need to collect will save time for the visit itself.

Approaching the Patient and Requesting the Interview Ask the patient for permission before conducting the interview. You may need to explain that questions about the reason for the visit and the patient's current health situation are necessary to plan the most effective care. It is more courteous to seek permission to ask questions than to say that you "need to take a history." Asking permission helps the patient feel more comfortable and emphasizes the importance of the interview process. It also makes the patient feel more like a participant in the medical care being provided.

Making the Patient Feel at Ease Using certain words or phrases known as icebreakers can help set the stage for the interview. Icebreakers put the patient at ease and create a relaxed atmosphere. Examples of icebreakers include acknowledging the patient's reason for the visit, introducing yourself, and commenting about the weather. Icebreakers that also convey a sincere and sensitive interest in the patient are asking the patient how she prefers to be addressed and clarifying the pronunciation of a difficult name.

Another way to convey an image of a professional who is sensitive to the patient's needs is to sit with the patient and appear relaxed. By appearing relaxed, you help the patient relax and encourage a more open and comfortable interview. Eye contact is important when interviewing a patient. Sometimes patients will feel intimidated if they are forced to look up at you. If the patient sits in a chair, then it is best that you sit; if the patient sits on the examining table, then it is appropriate to stand while recording the visit. Remember, if you are entering data into an electronic record, there is a patient in the room with you. If you pay more attention to inputting information into the computer than looking at and speaking with your patient, she may feel as if she is just another patient and not an individual being cared for by you.

Conducting the Interview in Private Without Interruptions After setting the stage for the interview, ensure privacy by showing the patient to a private room or area or by closing the door if the patient is already in a private room. You can then begin to ask relevant questions. Some approaches are more effective than others, as shown in Table 36-1. Listening carefully to the patient's responses may lead you to ask questions other than those in your interview plan.

Developing a rapport with the patient is essential. Keep the atmosphere relaxed, do not rush, maintain eye contact, and use

TABLE 36-1 Methods of Collecting Patient Data	
Effective Methods	**Characteristics**
Asking open-ended questions	Requires more than a yes or no answer; allows the patient to more fully explain the situation, resulting in more relevant data. Instead of asking, "Do you have a cough?" ask, "Can you tell me about your symptoms?"
Asking hypothetical questions	Allows you to determine the patient's knowledge of the situation and whether it is accurate. For example, ask a patient who has been prescribed nitroglycerin for chest pain, "What would you do if you had chest pain?"
Mirroring patient's responses and verbalizing the implied	Allows non-threatening ways for the patient to discuss the situation further and to provide underlying meaning. **Mirroring** means restating what the patient says almost exactly as the patient says it. **Verbalizing** means stating what you believe the patient is suggesting by his response. If the patient says, "I have been hurting for 3 days and it is just getting worse and worse. It hasn't quit all day," you might say, "So the pain started about 3 days ago and has been getting worse each day, and today it has not let up at all."
Focusing on patient	Shows the patient that you are really listening to what he is saying. You maintain eye contact (as culturally appropriate), assume a relaxed and open body posture, and use the proper responses.
Encouraging patient to take the lead	Motivates the patient to discuss or describe the situation in his own way. Ask a question such as "Where would you like to begin?"
Encouraging patient to provide additional information	Conveys sincere interest in the patient by continuing to explore topics in more detail when appropriate. You might ask the patient if he has experienced a symptom before or if he associates it with a change in routine. This provides for **clarification**, or increased understanding of the problem.
Encouraging patient to evaluate his situation	Provides an idea of the patient's point of view about the situation; allows you to determine the patient's knowledge of the situation and possible fears. Ask the patient, "What do you think is going on here?" This will allow you and the patient to use **reflection**. Reflection is when a thought, an idea, or an opinion is formed as a result of deeper thought, in this case stimulated by a question.
Ineffective Methods	**Characteristics**
Asking closed-ended questions	Provides little information because closed-ended questions offer the patient little freedom to explain his answers. Closed-ended questions require only yes or no answers.
Asking leading questions	Leading questions suggest a desired response instead of the patient's true response. The patient tends to agree with such statements instead of elaborating on them. An example of a leading question is "You seem to be making progress, don't you agree?" This type of question limits the patient's response.
Challenging patient	The patient may feel you are disagreeing with what he is saying if you ask an emotional or challenging question or use a certain tone of voice. The patient may become defensive, which might block further communication. An example of challenging the patient is "You are not having that much pain from this small wound, are you?"
Probing	Continuing to question a patient after he appears to have finished giving information can make him feel that you are invading his privacy. The patient may become defensive and withhold information.
Agreeing or disagreeing with patient	When you agree or disagree with a patient, it implies that the patient is either "right" or "wrong." This action can block further communication.

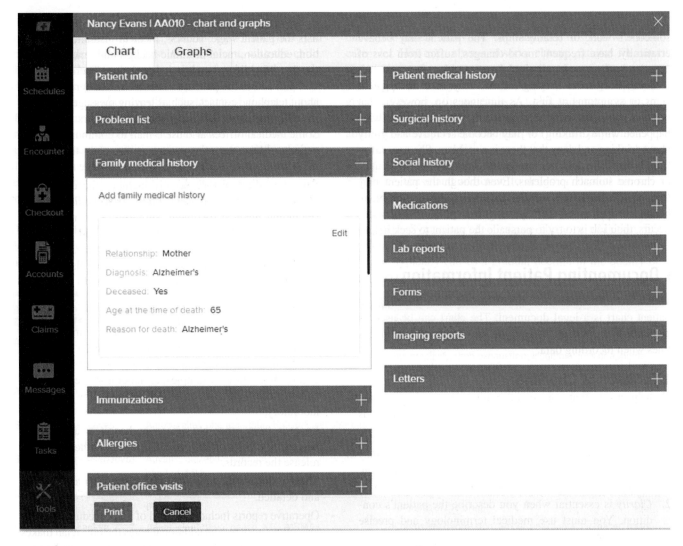

FIGURE 36-1 Medical history forms in an electronic health record, such as this one from ⱷEHRclinic, allow you to select, enter, or delete items based upon your patient interview.

©McGraw-Hill Education

Diagnostic Labs
976 Heirloom Ave*Madison*XY*56764*(555)478-6783*www.diagnosticlabsxy.com

LAB REPORT

Date: 4/6/2020

Patient Name: John Miller

MRN: 869-392942

Ordering Provider: Paul Buckwalter, M.D.

Test	Results	Reference Range
Cholesterol	240 mg/dL	120-200 mg/dL
Triglycerides	252	40-200 mg/dL
HDL Cholesterol	52 mg/dL	>40 mg/dL
LDL Cholesterol	146 mg/dL	70-130 mg/dL
VLDL	42	

FIGURE 36-2 Laboratory reports. (a) EHR laboratory reports include normal ranges appropriate for the laboratory's testing procedures.

©McGraw-Hill Education

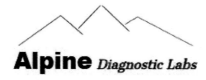

Alpine *Diagnostic Labs*

39452 Apollo Blvd Hanson XY 10365 (555) 267-8453 alpinediagnosticlabsxy.com

LAB REPORT

Date: 7/13/2020

Patient Name: Shenya Jones

MRN: 64-17984

Ordering Provider: Alexis Whalen, MD

BASIC METABOLIC PROFILE - Details

Component	Your Value	Standard Range
Sodium	**138** mmol/L	135 - 145 mmol/L
Potassium	**3.9** mmol/L	3.5 - 5.0 mmol/L
Chloride	**103** mmol/L	98 - 111 mmol/L
Carbon Dioxide	**24** mmol/L	21 - 35 mmol/L
Anion Gap	**11**	3 - 13
Blood Urea Nitrogen	**19** mg/dL	10 - 25 mg/dL
Creatinine IDMS Standardized.	**0.57** mg/dL	<1.16 mg/dL
Glucose	**103** mg/dL	50 - 140 mg/dL
Calcium Method change. Please note new reference interval.	**9.0** mg/dL	8.6 - 10.4 mg/dL
GFR nonafrican american	**114** ml/min/1.73m2	>60 ml/min/1.73m2
GFR african american	**>120** ml/min/1.73m2	>60 ml/min/1.73m2

GFR results reported as >60 can be regarded as normal, i.e., above minimum reference level for renal function. (NOTE)

GFR formula was clinically validated in metabolically stable patients, age 18 to 70. GFR calculated using the CKD-EPI equation. The GFR calculation may not be reliable in metabolically unstable patients.

FIGURE 36-2 Laboratory reports. (b) Laboratory results paper reports also include normal ranges. All laboratory reports provide valuable information about patients' health.

©McGraw-Hill Education

information. These steps are referred to as the SOAP method of documentation (Figure 36-3). Understanding the parts of SOAP will help you document information in a logical manner.

1. *Subjective data.* You obtain **subjective data** from conversation with the patient or an attending family member. Subjective data include thoughts, feelings, and perceptions, including the chief complaint. Such data are based on the patient's interpretation and opinion. They are not measurable by an outside observer; however, you should remember that they are real to the patient. An example of subjective information is the patient's statement about his or her chief complaint: "I have an itchy, red rash on my left hand that I noticed 3 days ago." The patient states that the rash is itchy; because itchiness cannot be observed

or measured by the physician, it is considered subjective. The chief complaint should always be recorded in the patient's own words.

2. *Objective data.* **Objective data** are readily apparent and measurable, such as vital signs, test results, and the physician's exam. An example of objective data is the examination of the rash by the physician.

3. *Assessment.* Assessment is the physician's diagnosis or impression of the patient's problem.

4. *Plan of action.* Options for treatment, the type of treatment chosen, medications, tests, consultations, patient education, and follow-up are included in a plan of action. The plan of action may include an order for injection or other treatment that you as the medical assistant will need to perform.

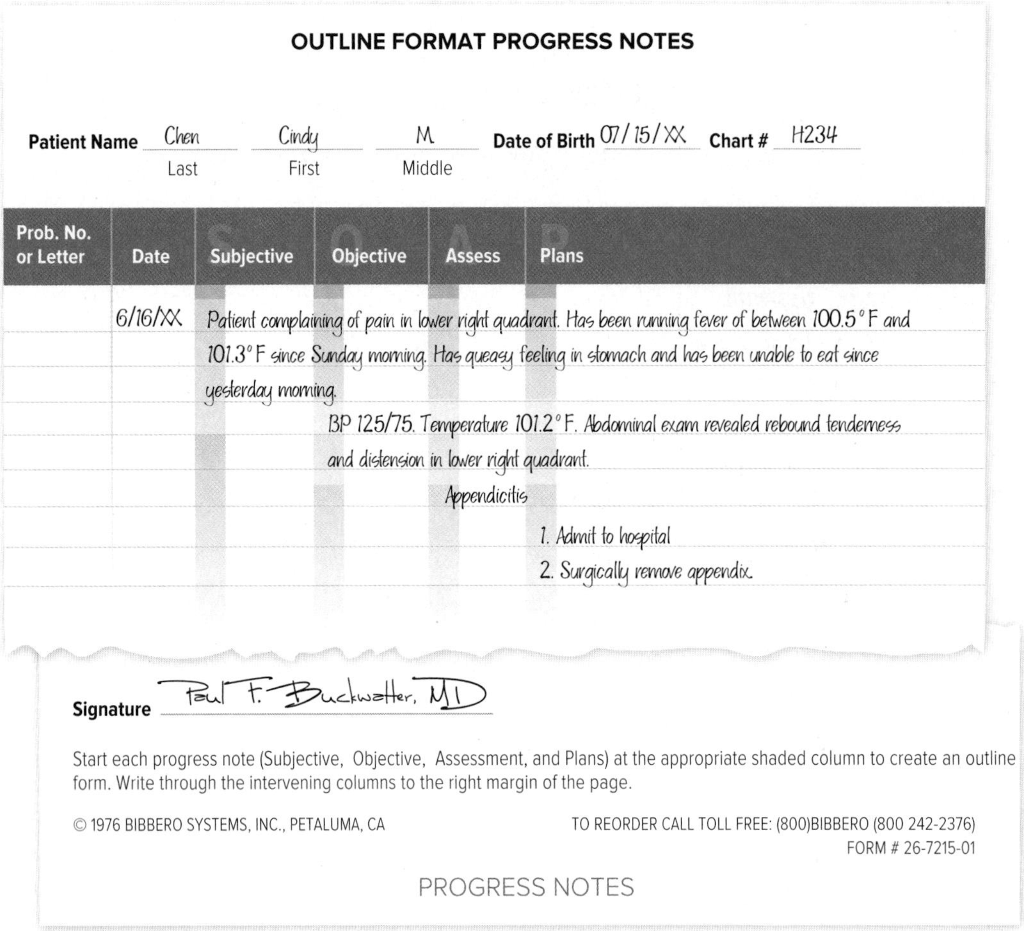

OUTLINE FORMAT PROGRESS NOTES

Patient Name __Chen__ __Cindy__ __M__ Date of Birth 07/15/XX Chart # __H234__
                Last   First   Middle

Prob. No. or Letter	Date	Subjective	Objective	Assess	Plans
	6/16/XX	Patient complaining of pain in lower right quadrant. Has been running fever of between 100.5°F and 101.3°F since Sunday morning. Has queasy feeling in stomach and has been unable to eat since yesterday morning.			
			BP 125/75. Temperature 101.2°F. Abdominal exam revealed rebound tenderness and distension in lower right quadrant.		
				Appendicitis	
					1. Admit to hospital
					2. Surgically remove appendix.

Signature _Paul F. Buckwalter, MD_

Start each progress note (Subjective, Objective, Assessment, and Plans) at the appropriate shaded column to create an outline form. Write through the intervening columns to the right margin of the page.

© 1976 BIBBERO SYSTEMS, INC., PETALUMA, CA

TO REORDER CALL TOLL FREE: (800)BIBBERO (800 242-2376)
FORM # 26-7215-01

PROGRESS NOTES

FIGURE 36-3 When you use the SOAP approach to documenting patient information, start each progress note at the appropriate shaded column to create an outline form. Write through the intervening columns to the right margin of the page.

Reprinted with permission from Bibbero Systems, Inc., An InHealth Company, Petaluma, CA (800) 242-2376, www.bibbero.com.

The following are three common methods for maintaining notes on a patient chart:

1. Conventional or source-oriented medical records (SOMR). Information is arranged according to who supplied the data, or the source. This could be the patient, the doctor, a specialist, or someone else. The medical form may have a space for patient remarks followed by a section for the doctor's comment.

2. Problem-oriented medical records (POMR). This method is used more extensively by large clinics or practices that may have more than one physician who may see the same patient. POMR includes a problem list that is dated, and numbers are assigned to each patient condition or problem. At the patient's initial visit, conditions or problems are identified by a number throughout the record until the problem is resolved. The POMR has four components:

   • *Database.* This includes the patient's medical history, diagnostic and laboratory results, and physical exam reports. This is the foundation of the problem-oriented medical record.

   • *Problem list.* Each patient condition or problem is listed individually, assigned a number, and dated.

   • *Diagnostic and treatment plan.* Laboratory and other diagnostic tests are completed, and the physician's treatment plan for the condition is documented.

   • *Progress notes.* The physician enters notes on every condition or problem recorded on the problem list. Progress notes are entered chronologically and include the chief complaint, problems, conditions, treatments, and responses to treatment.

3. Computerized medical records. This method uses a combination of SOMR and POMR but provides accessibility by the physician or other healthcare workers at any time from a computer terminal. This accessibility enhances the patient's continuity of care between departments and specialty physicians in other practices because everyone is looking at the same record.

Common Chart Terminology and Abbreviations

Most of the information that you collect verbally from a patient will be documented in the patient's medical record. Table 36-3 lists some of the most common abbreviations used in the medical chart. Abbreviations used must be accepted by the facility where you are employed as well as The Joint Commission (TJC).

The Joint Commission and the Institute for Safe Medication Practice (ISMP) are two healthcare organizations whose mission includes promotion of patient safety. These organizations have identified frequently misinterpreted abbreviations, acronyms, and symbols that have contributed to harmful medical errors. TJC, in has published an *Official "Do Not Use" List,* a standardized list of abbreviations, acronyms, and symbols that are not to be used. See Table 36-4. The ISMP publishes the more comprehensive *ISMP's List of Error-Prone Abbreviations, Symbols, and Dose Designations,* which is updated periodically. This list includes all of the abbreviations on TJC's "Do Not Use" list, denoting them with a double asterisk (**). It is found at https://www.ismp.org/recommendations/error-prone-abbreviations-list/tools/abbreviations/. Although you may see some of these on pre-printed order sheets, *do not use* the error-prone abbreviations when charting.

TABLE 36-3		Common Medical Abbreviations	
Abortion	Ab	Growth and development	G&D
Abnormal	Abnl	Headache	HA
Antibiotics	Abx	History of	H/O
Against medical advice	AMA	History and physical	H&P
As much as possible	AMAP	Hypertension	HTN
Awake and oriented	A&O	Left	L
Both	B	Right	R
Biopsy	BX	Low back pain	LBP
Chief Complaint	CC	Low birth weight	LBW
Childhood diseases	CHD	Last menstrual period	LMP
Complaints of	C/O	No known allergies	NKA
Cause of death	COD	Packs per day	PPD
Chest X-ray	CXR	Rule out	R/O
Date of birth	DOB	Range of motion	ROM
Date of conception	DOC	Shortness of breath	SOB
Diagnosis	Dx	Sudden unexplained/unexpected death	SUD
Digital rectal exam	DRE	Seizure	Sz
Estimated delivery date	EDD	Tonsillectomy and adenoidectomy	T & A
Follow-up	F/U	Within normal limits	WNL
Fracture	FX	Years Old	Y/O

▶ Recording the Patient's Medical History

LO 36.4

A patient's medical history includes pertinent information about the patient and the patient's family. Age, previous illnesses, surgical history, allergies, medication history, and family medical history are key items.

When recording a patient history, you must do more than just fill out the form (Figure 36-4). You must review the pieces of information, organize them, determine their importance, and document the facts. When you write your first histories, you may find it to be a lengthy process. When you become more experienced, however, you will be able to write histories more quickly. Whenever you write information on the chart, you must consider its completeness and accuracy. First determine the chief complaint or the main reason for the patient visit. For example, the patient may have a rash or pain. Then ask more questions. A good interview technique is the "PQRST" interview technique. It will help you remember the types of questions that are appropriate for the condition. Each letter stands for a word that will remind you to ask more specific questions about the chief complaint or problem the patient is having:

P: Provoke or Palliative
Q: Quality or Quantity
R: Region or Radiation
S: Severity Scale
T: Timing

See Table 36-5 for questions and charting examples using the PQRST interview technique.

You will need to chart other information prior to the physician visit. Figure 36-5b shows a form used by the medical assistant and the licensed practitioner when seeing a patient. When keying information in an electronic record, it is just as important to correctly type the information into the record. Pay special attention to spelling when entering data into the chart or electronic record. If you do not know how to spell a word, look it up. Use only TJC-approved and office-recognized abbreviations (see Tables 36-3 and 36-4). Many facilities have a document identifying these abbreviations. Electronic health records often use drop-down menus with common medical information provided. Take care to click the correct box when using drop-down menus. Remember, the chart is a legal document, so special attention to detail is required when charting.

The Progress Note

Many offices use a variation of the progress note for established patients who are seen for routine visits or follow-ups for such conditions as hypertension, arthritis, or flu (see Figures 36-3 and 36-5). The medical history form is primarily used for new patients the physician is seeing for the first time. The following are some important guidelines to consider when using a progress note:

- It must be arranged in reverse chronological order.
- Every entry must be initialed and signed by the person making the entry. Typically, the first initial, last name,

TABLE 36-4 TJC "Do Not Use" Abbreviations, Acronyms, and Symbols

Abbreviation	Potential Problem	Preferred Term
U (for unit)	Mistaken as zero, four, or cc	Write "unit."
IU (for international unit)	Mistaken as IV (intravenous) or 10 (ten)	Write "international unit."
Q.D., QD, qd, q.d., Q.O.D., QOD, q.o.d, qod (Latin abbreviation for once daily and every other day)	Mistaken for each other. The period after the Q can be mistaken for an "I" and the "O" can be mistaken for "I."	Write "daily" and "every other day."
Trailing zero (X.0 mg), lack of leading zero (.X mg) except when trailing zero is used to indicate a level of precision when reporting a lab value	Decimal point is missed.	Never write a zero by itself after a decimal point (X mg), and always use a zero before a decimal point (0.X mg) when writing medication documentation.
MS MSO_4 $MgSO_4$	Confused for one another; can mean morphine sulfate or magnesium sulfate	Write "morphine sulfate" or "magnesium sulfate."
Other Abbreviations, Acronyms, and Symbols to Avoid		
µg (for microgram)	Mistaken for mg (milligrams), resulting in one-thousand-fold dosing overdose	Write "mcg."
c.c. (for cubic centimeter)	Mistaken for U (units) when poorly written	Write "mL" for milliliters.
> (greater than) < (less than)	Misinterpreted as the number "7" or the letter "L"; confused for one another	Write "greater than" and "less than."
Abbreviations for drug names	Misinterpreted due to similar abbreviations for multiple drugs	Write drug names in full.
Apothecary units	Unfamiliar to many practitioners; confused with metric units	Use metric units.
@	Mistaken for the number "2" (two)	Write "at."
H.S. (for half-strength or Latin abbreviation for bedtime)	Mistaken for either half-strength or hour of sleep (at bedtime). qH.S. mistaken for every hour. All can result in a dosing error.	Write out "half-strength" or "at bedtime."
T.I.W. (for three times a week)	Mistaken for three times a day or twice weekly, resulting in an overdose	Write "3 times weekly" or "three times weekly."
S.C. or S.Q. (for subcutaneous)	Mistaken as SL for sublingual, or "5 every"	Write "Sub-Q," "subQ," or "subcutaneously."
D/C (for discharge)	Interpreted as discontinue whatever medications follow (typically discharge meds)	Write "discharge."
A.S., A.D., A.U. (Latin abbreviation for left, right, or both ears)O.S., O.D., O.U. (Latin abbreviation for left, right, or both eyes)	Mistaken for each other (such as AS for OS, AD for OD, AU for OU, etc.)	Write "left ear," "right ear," or "both ears"; "left eye," "right eye," or "both eyes."

and credentials are used—for example, K. Haddix, RMA (AMT).

- Entries most commonly made on progress notes include documentation for prescription refills, follow-up visits, telephone conversations with patients, appointment cancellations or no-shows, and referrals and consultation efforts made by the office for the patient.

- The patient name must be recorded on every progress note along with any other identifying information such as birth date or chart number.

- All entries must be dated. All entries typically include the time and must always include the date.

Procedure 36-2, at the end of this chapter, will guide you in how to use a progress note.

Polypharmacy

Many patients will take a variety of medications to treat several conditions, such as hypertension, elevated cholesterol, and diabetes. Some patients take several medications for the same condition, with each one treating a different aspect of the condition. The chapters *Principles of Pharmacology* and *Medication Administration* provide detailed information regarding various medications. During the patient interview, it is important to document medications the patient is currently taking. The patient often will see several physicians or specialists, and it is important for your office to be up to date on the treatments a patient is receiving. This reduces the likelihood of polypharmacy or unnecessarily repeating medical tests.

HEALTH HISTORY
(Confidential)

Name _____ Today's Date _____

Age _____ Birthdate _____ Date of last physical examination _____

What is your reason for visit? _____

SYMPTOMS Check (✓) symptoms you currently have or have had in the past year.

GENERAL
- ☐ Chills
- ☐ Depression
- ☐ Dizziness
- ☐ Fainting
- ☐ Fever
- ☐ Forgetfulness
- ☐ Headache
- ☐ Loss of sleep
- ☐ Loss of weight
- ☐ Nervousness
- ☐ Numbness
- ☐ Sweats

MUSCLE/JOINT/BONE
Pain, weakness, numbness in:
- ☐ Arms ☐ Hips
- ☐ Back ☐ Legs
- ☐ Feet ☐ Neck
- ☐ Hands ☐ Shoulders

GENITO-URINARY
- ☐ Blood in urine
- ☐ Frequent urination
- ☐ Lack of bladder control
- ☐ Painful urination

GASTROINTESTINAL
- ☐ Appetite poor
- ☐ Bloating
- ☐ Bowel changes
- ☐ Constipation
- ☐ Diarrhea
- ☐ Excessive hunger
- ☐ Excessive thirst
- ☐ Gas
- ☐ Hemorrhoids
- ☐ Indigestion
- ☐ Nausea
- ☐ Rectal bleeding
- ☐ Stomach pain
- ☐ Vomiting
- ☐ Vomiting blood

CARDIOVASCULAR
- ☐ Chest pain
- ☐ High blood pressure
- ☐ Irregular heart beat
- ☐ Low blood pressure
- ☐ Poor circulation
- ☐ Rapid heart beat
- ☐ Swelling of ankles
- ☐ Varicose veins

EYE, EAR, NOSE, THROAT
- ☐ Bleeding gums
- ☐ Blurred vision
- ☐ Crossed eyes
- ☐ Difficulty swallowing
- ☐ Double vision
- ☐ Earache
- ☐ Ear discharge
- ☐ Hay fever
- ☐ Hoarseness
- ☐ Loss of hearing
- ☐ Nosebleeds
- ☐ Persistent cough
- ☐ Ringing in ears
- ☐ Sinus problems
- ☐ Vision – Flashes
- ☐ Vision – Halos

SKIN
- ☐ Bruise easily
- ☐ Hives
- ☐ Itching
- ☐ Change in moles
- ☐ Rash
- ☐ Scars
- ☐ Sore that won't heal

MEN only
- ☐ Breast lump
- ☐ Erection difficulties
- ☐ Lump in testicles
- ☐ Penis discharge
- ☐ Sore on penis
- ☐ Other

WOMEN only
- ☐ Abnormal Pap smear
- ☐ Bleeding between periods
- ☐ Breast lump
- ☐ Extreme menstrual pain
- ☐ Hot flashes
- ☐ Nipple discharge
- ☐ Painful intercourse
- ☐ Vaginal discharge
- ☐ Other

Date of last menstrual period _____

Date of last Pap smear _____

Have you had a mammogram? _____

Are you pregnant? _____

Number of children _____

CONDITIONS Check (✓) conditions you have or have had in the past.

- ☐ AIDS
- ☐ Alcoholism
- ☐ Anemia
- ☐ Anorexia
- ☐ Appendicitis
- ☐ Arthritis
- ☐ Asthma
- ☐ Bleeding Disorders
- ☐ Breast Lump
- ☐ Bronchitis
- ☐ Bulimia
- ☐ Cancer
- ☐ Cataracts

- ☐ Chemical Dependency
- ☐ Chickenpox
- ☐ Diabetes
- ☐ Emphysema
- ☐ Epilepsy
- ☐ Glaucoma
- ☐ Goiter
- ☐ Gonorrhea
- ☐ Gout
- ☐ Heart Disease
- ☐ Hepatitis
- ☐ Hernia
- ☐ Herpes

- ☐ High Cholesterol
- ☐ HIV Positive
- ☐ Kidney Disease
- ☐ Liver Disease
- ☐ Measles
- ☐ Migraine Headaches
- ☐ Miscarriage
- ☐ Mononucleosis
- ☐ Multiple Sclerosis
- ☐ Mumps
- ☐ Pacemaker
- ☐ Pneumonia
- ☐ Polio

- ☐ Prostate Problem
- ☐ Psychiatric Care
- ☐ Rheumatic Fever
- ☐ Scarlet Fever
- ☐ Stroke
- ☐ Suicide Attempt
- ☐ Thyroid Problems
- ☐ Tonsillitis
- ☐ Tuberculosis
- ☐ Typhoid Fever
- ☐ Ulcers
- ☐ Vaginal Infections
- ☐ Venereal Disease

MEDICATIONS List medications you are currently taking

_____
_____
_____

Pharmacy Name _____ Phone _____

ALLERGIES To medications or substances

_____
_____
_____

FAMILY HISTORY Fill in health information about your family.
(All information is strictly confidential)

Relation	Age	State of Health	Age at Death	Cause of Death	Check (✓) if your blood relatives had any of the following:
					Disease / Relationship to You
Father					Arthritis, Gout
Mother					Asthma, Hay Fever
Brothers					Cancer
					Chemical Dependency
					Diabetes
Sisters					Heart Disease, Strokes
					High Blood Pressure
					Kidney Disease
					Tuberculosis
					Other

HOSPITALIZATIONS

Year	Hospital	Reason for Hospitalization and Outcome

Have you ever had a blood transfusion? ☐ Yes ☐ No
If yes, please give approximate dates.

SERIOUS ILLNESS/INJURIES

	DATE	OUTCOME

PREGNANCY HISTORY

Year of Birth	Sex of Birth	Complications if any

HEALTH HABITS Check (✓) which substances you use and describe how much you use.

- Caffeine _____
- Tobacco _____
- Drugs _____
- Other _____

OCCUPATIONAL CONCERNS Check (✓) if your work exposes you to the following.

- ☐ Stress
- ☐ Hazardous Substances
- ☐ Heavy Lifting
- ☐ Other

Your occupation: _____

I certify that the above information is correct to the best of my knowledge. I will not hold my doctor or any members of his/her staff responsible for any errors or omissions that I may have made in the completion of this form.

_____ _____
Signature   Date

_____ _____
Reviewed By   Date

FIGURE 36-4 The health history form must be complete and accurate. The patient should start the form, and the medical assistant should check and complete it.

TABLE 36-5	Example Questions When Using the PQRST Interview Technique		
PQRST Interview Technique	**Chief Complaint:** *Itching/ Rash Under Arms*	**Chief Complaint:** *Pain in the Left Shoulder*	**Chief Complaint:** *Persistent Cough*
P: Provoke or Palliative	• What causes the itching to occur? • Does anything make the itching go away?	• When did you first notice the pain? • Is there anything you do that reduces the pain?	• When is the cough worse? Morning? Night? • Is there anything that relieves the cough? Aggravates it?
Q: Quality or Quantity	• How severe is the rash/itching? • How often does the itching occur?	• Can you describe the pain: dull, aching, burning, or sharp? • When does the pain occur?	• Is the cough productive or nonproductive? • Are you coughing anything up? If so, does it have any color? • Do you have pain when you cough?
R: Region or Radiation	• Where is the itching/rash?	• Where do you feel the pain? • Does the pain move from one location to another?	• Is the pain on one side of the chest or both? • Does the pain radiate?
S: Severity Scale	• Is the rash/itching interfering with your daily life?	• Is the area red or tender to the touch? • Is there any swelling? • Rate the pain on a scale of 1 to 10, with 10 being the worst. (See Figure 36-6.)	• Rate the pain on a scale of 1 to 10, with 10 being the worst. • Does the cough disturb your sleep?
T: Timing	• When did you first notice the rash/itching?	• How long have you had the pain? • Is the pain intermittent or continuous? • How long does the pain last?	• Does the cough come in bouts or fits or is it continuous? • How long have you had the cough?

Some offices may use a medication flowsheet for the physicians to record patient medication histories. In some cases, the medical assistant gathers the information for the current medication flowsheet (see Figure 36-7). A helpful hint for organizing this task is to develop a form or card for the patient to use (if the office does not already have a form) and gather the initial medication history. Then instruct the patient to use the list and to have it updated by the other physicians whom he or she sees. A drug reference guide or the Internet will assist you with the spelling of medications.

The Health History Form

The medical office usually has a standard medical history form that is used for all patients. The specific arrangement and wording of items on this form, however, may vary from office to office. The following sections contain brief descriptions of each of the parts of this form. Procedure 36-3, at the end of this chapter, will assist in your practice of obtaining medical histories.

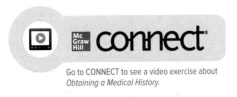

Go to CONNECT to see a video exercise about *Obtaining a Medical History.*

Personal Data This information is obtained from the administrative sheet and includes the patient's name, birth date, and other basic data.

Chief Complaint Abbreviated as CC, the chief complaint is the reason the patient came to visit the practitioner. It should be short and specific and should cover subjective and/ or objective data stated by the patient.

History of Present Illness This history includes detailed information about the chief complaint, including when the problem started and what the patient has done to treat the problem (including any medications taken). For example, a chief complaint might be "sore throat" and the history of the present illness would include when the sore throat started (such as 3 days ago), how severe the pain is on a scale of 1 to 10 (such as pain scale rating of 6 out of 10), and what treatments have been used (such as throat lozenges and four to six aspirin daily).

Past Medical History The past medical history includes any and all health problems both present and past, including major illnesses and surgery. The past medical history also includes important information about medications and allergies. It should list any medications taken by the patient, including their dosages and the reasons for taking them. Over-the-counter and herbal medications should be listed as well. Known or suspected allergies to medications or other substances should be listed and clearly visible. Some facilities use a red sticker or other means on charts to identify allergies immediately. Most electronic health record programs automatically run drug allergy and drug-drug interaction checks. If you are entering medication data into an

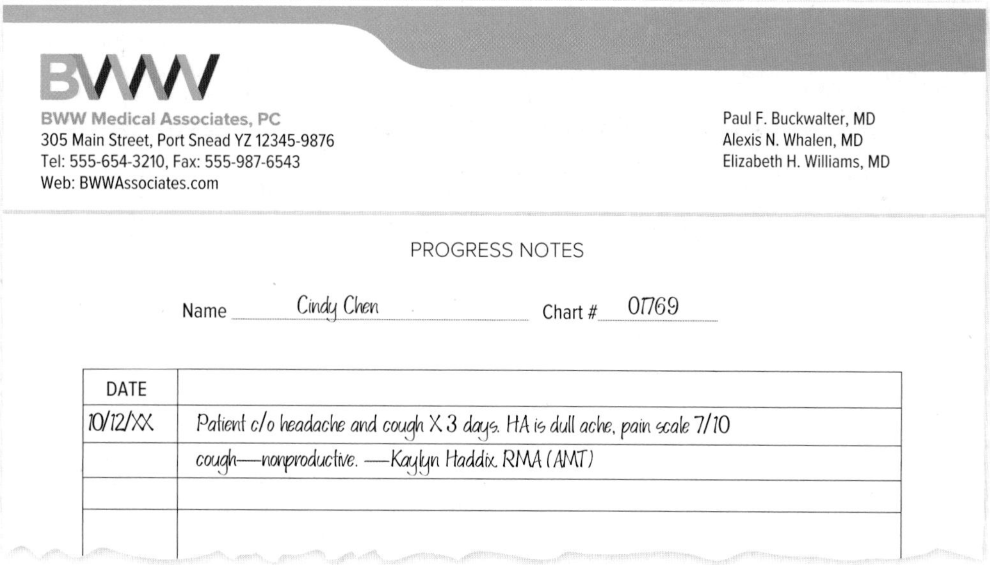

BWW

BWW Medical Associates, PC
305 Main Street, Port Snead YZ 12345-9876
Tel: 555-654-3210, Fax: 555-987-6543
Web: BWWAssociates.com

Paul F. Buckwalter, MD
Alexis N. Whalen, MD
Elizabeth H. Williams, MD

PROGRESS NOTES

Name _____ Cindy Chen _____   Chart # _____ 07769 _____

DATE	
10/12/XX	Patient c/o headache and cough X 3 days. HA is dull ache, pain scale 7/10
	cough—nonproductive. —Kaylyn Haddix RMA (AMT)

(a)

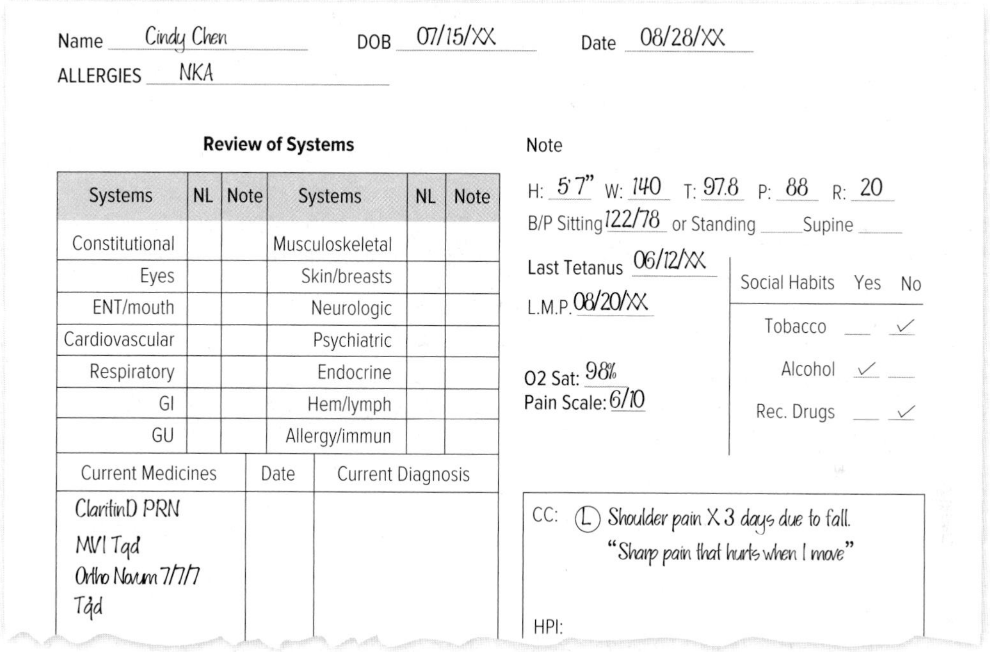

Name _____ Cindy Chen _____   DOB _____ 07/15/XX _____   Date _____ 08/28/XX _____
ALLERGIES _____ NKA _____

Review of Systems

Systems	NL	Note	Systems	NL	Note
Constitutional			Musculoskeletal		
Eyes			Skin/breasts		
ENT/mouth			Neurologic		
Cardiovascular			Psychiatric		
Respiratory			Endocrine		
GI			Hem/lymph		
GU			Allergy/immun		

Current Medicines	Date	Current Diagnosis
ClaritinD PRN		
MVI Tqd		
Ortho Novum 7/7/7 Tqd		

Note

H: 5'7" W: 140 T: 97.8 P: 88 R: 20
B/P Sitting 122/78 or Standing _____ Supine _____

Last Tetanus 06/12/XX
L.M.P. 08/20/XX

O2 Sat: 98%
Pain Scale: 6/10

Social Habits	Yes	No
Tobacco		✓
Alcohol	✓	
Rec. Drugs		✓

CC: Ⓛ Shoulder pain X 3 days due to fall.
"Sharp pain that hurts when I move"

HPI:

(b)

FIGURE 36-5   These forms are completed by the medical assistant prior to the physician visit. All information must be complete and accurate. (a) Progress note. (b) Medical visit form.

EHR program that does not have this feature, make sure you flag patient drug allergies according to office policy.

Family History This section includes information about the health of the patient's family members. Many times, the family history can help lead a practitioner to the cause of a current medical problem. Obtain specific information about family members' current ages and medical conditions or, if deceased, their age at death and the cause. Ask open-ended questions about the siblings, parents, and grandparents. Because the death of a parent or sibling or the limited knowledge of an adopted child can be difficult to discuss, use great care and sensitivity when asking these questions.

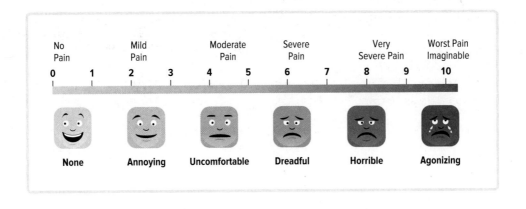

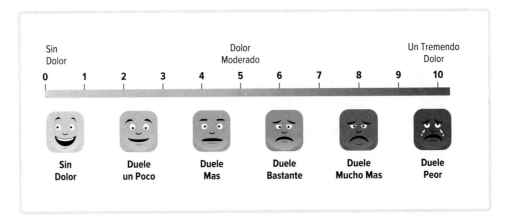

FIGURE 36-6 Assessing a patient's pain, considered the fifth vital sign, is part of the interview and history-taking process. A chart similar to this is used to make the process easier for the patient and the medical assistant.

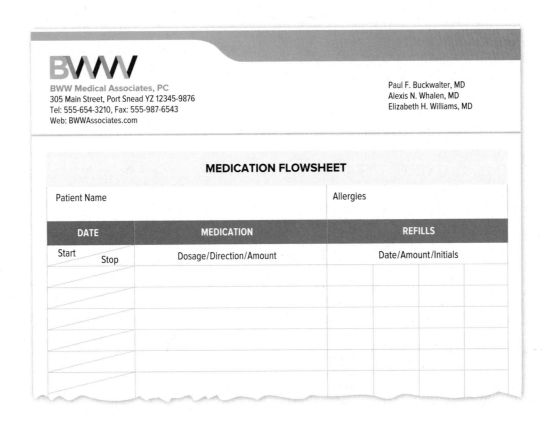

FIGURE 36-7 Medication flowsheet.

Social and Occupational History Information such as marital status, sexual behaviors and orientation, occupations, hobbies, and the use of chemical substances helps determine a patient's risk for disease. Patients should be asked about their use of alcohol, tobacco, recreational drugs, or other chemical substances. Be aware that patients may feel uncomfortable or may refuse to provide certain information. Depending on the circumstances, you may ask the question later in the interview. For example, an adolescent child may not want to answer questions about his sexual behaviors in front of his parents. Occupational information regarding the patient's level of stress, exposure to hazardous substances, and heavy lifting also may be included here.

Review of Systems Some of this information may be started by the patient but is completed by the practitioner. This systematic review of each of the body systems includes questions and an exam by the practitioner. The information is obtained in an orderly fashion but may vary depending on the physician or practitioner.

PROCEDURE 36-1 Using Critical Thinking Skills During an Interview

WORK // DOC

Procedure Goal: To be able to use verbal and nonverbal clues and critical thinking skills to optimize the process of obtaining data for the patient's chart

OSHA Guidelines: This procedure does not involve exposure to blood, body fluids, or tissues.

Materials: Progress note, patient chart or electronic health record, pen (if using a paper record)

Method:

Example 1: Getting at an Underlying Meaning

1. You are interviewing a female patient with Type 2 diabetes who has recently started insulin injections. She is in the office for a follow-up visit.

2. Use open-ended questions such as "How are you managing your diabetes?"
   RATIONALE: *Open-ended questioning allows the patient to explain the situation in her own words and often provides more information than closed-ended questioning.*

3. The patient states that she "just can't get used to the whole idea of injections."

4. To encourage her to verbalize her concerns more clearly, you can mirror her response or restate her comments in your own words. For example, you might say, "You seem to be having some difficulty giving yourself injections."
   RATIONALE: *This response should encourage her to verbalize the specific area in which she is having problems such as loading the syringe, injecting herself, finding the time for the injections, and so on.*

5. Verbalize the implied, which means that you state what you think the patient is suggesting by her response.
   RATIONALE: *Restating her response ensures you have understood.*

6. After you determine the specific problem, you will be able to address it in the interview or note it in the patient's chart for the doctor's attention.

Example 2: Dealing with a Potentially Violent Patient

1. You are interviewing a 60-year-old male patient who is new to the office. He appears agitated. You ask his reason for seeing the doctor today.

2. The patient explains that he does not want to talk to "some assistant" about his problem. He just wants to see the doctor.

3. You say that you respect his wish not to discuss his symptoms but explain that you need to ask

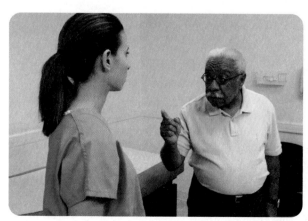

FIGURE Procedure 36-1 Example 2 Step 4   Do not try to handle by yourself a patient who may become violent. Ask for help from other staff members.
©McGraw-Hill Education

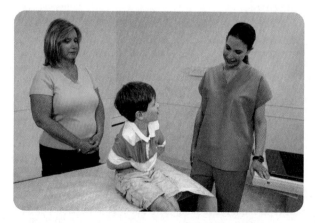

FIGURE Procedure 36-1 Example 3 Step 2   Gather any symptom information you can from the child. Then ask the parent or caregiver similar questions.
©McGraw-Hill Education

him a few questions so that the doctor can be prepared to provide the proper medical care. Ask questions that help the patient reflect on his or her situation.
RATIONALE: *The patient has the right to refuse to answer a question, even if it is a reasonable one.*

4. The patient begins to yell at you, saying he wants to see the doctor and does not "want to answer stupid questions."

5. The fact that the patient appears agitated and begins to raise his voice in anger should be a warning to you that he may become violent. It would be best not to handle this patient by yourself.

6. If you are alone with the patient, leave the room and request assistance from another staff member.

Example 3: Gathering Symptom Information About a Child

1. A parent brings a 5-year-old boy to the office because the child is complaining about stomach pain.

2. To gather the pertinent symptom information, ask the child various types of questions.
   RATIONALE: *Talking to the child first allows him to feel that his view of the problem is important.*
   a. Can he tell you about the pain?
   RATIONALE: *Open-ended questioning allows him to tell you about his problem in his own words.*
   b. Can he tell you exactly where it hurts?
   c. Is there anything else that hurts?

3. To clarify the child's answers, ask the parent to answer similar questions.

4. You should then ask the parent additional questions. Begin with an open-ended question, as above. Follow up with specific questions such as these:
   a. How long has he had the pain?
   b. Is the pain related to any specific event (such as going to school)?

5. Ask the child to confirm the parent's answers. He may be able to provide additional information at this time.

PROCEDURE 36-2 Using a Progress Note

WORK // DOC

Procedure Goal: To accurately record a chief complaint on a progress note

OSHA Guidelines: This procedure does not involve exposure to blood, body fluids, or tissues.

Materials: Progress note, patient chart or electronic health record, pen (if using a paper record)

Method:

1. Wash your hands.

2. Review the patient's chart notes from the patient's previous office visit. Verify that all results for any previously ordered laboratory work or diagnostics are in the chart.
   RATIONALE: *Ensures that all reports have been reviewed by the physician.*

3. Greet the patient and escort her to a private exam room.

4. Introduce yourself and ask the patient her name.

5. Using open-ended questions, find out why the patient is seeking medical care today.
   RATIONALE: *Asking open-ended questions such as "What is the reason for your visit today?" and "How long have you been feeling this way?" will encourage the patient to provide more details.*

6. Accurately document the chief complaint on the progress note. Document vital signs. Initial or sign the chart entry according to office policy.

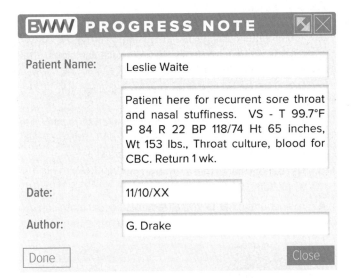

BWW PROGRESS NOTE

Patient Name:	Leslie Waite
	Patient here for recurrent sore throat and nasal stuffiness. VS - T 99.7°F P 84 R 22 BP 118/74 Ht 65 inches, Wt 153 lbs., Throat culture, blood for CBC. Return 1 wk.
Date:	11/10/XX
Author:	G. Drake

Done   Close

7. File the progress note in chronological order within the patient's chart if the record is a paper record (refer to Progress Note).
   RATIONALE: *This ensures that the most current patient information is reviewed by the physician and the medical staff.*

8. Thank the patient and offer to answer any questions she may have. Explain that the physician will come in soon to examine her.

9. Wash your hands.

PROCEDURE 36-3 Obtaining a Medical History

Procedure Goal: To obtain a complete medical history with accuracy and professionalism

OSHA Guidelines: This procedure does not involve exposure to blood, body fluids, or tissues.

Materials: Medical history form, physical examination form, patient chart, pen or electronic medical record

Method:

1. Wash your hands.
2. Assemble the necessary materials. Review the medical history form and plan your interview.
   RATIONALE: *This saves time and improves the effectiveness of the visit; plus, it will assist in determining the appropriate questions to ask.*
3. Invite the patient to a private exam room, and correctly identify the patient by introducing yourself and asking his or her name and date of birth.
4. Explain the medical history form while maintaining eye contact. Make the patient feel at ease.
5. Using language that the patient can understand, ask appropriate, open-ended questions related to the medical history form. Listen actively to the patient's response using reflection, restatement, and clarification.
6. Accurately document the patient's responses.
7. Thank the patient for his or her participation in the interview. Offer to answer any questions.
8. Sign or initial the medical history form and file it in the patient's chart.
9. Inform the physician that you are finished with the medical history according to the physician's office policy.
10. Wash your hands.

SUMMARY OF LEARNING OUTCOMES

OUTCOME	KEY POINTS
36.1 Identify the skills necessary to conduct a patient interview.	The skills necessary to conduct an interview include effective listening, awareness of nonverbal cues, use of a broad knowledge base, and the ability to summarize a general picture.
36.2 Recognize the signs of anxiety; depression; and physical, mental, or substance abuse.	Anxiety can range from a heightened ability to observe to a difficulty in being able to focus. Depression can be demonstrated through severe fatigue, sadness, difficulty sleeping, and loss of appetite. Abuse can be physical (such as an injury) or psychological (such as neglect).
36.3 Use the six Cs for writing an accurate patient history.	The six Cs for writing an accurate patient history are client's words, clarity, completeness, conciseness, chronological order, and confidentiality.
36.4 Carry out a patient history using critical thinking skills.	When obtaining a patient history, you can use open-ended questions, active listening, clarification, restatement, reflection, and the PQRST interview technique; review the information obtained; determine the importance; and then document the facts accurately.

CASE STUDY CRITICAL THINKING

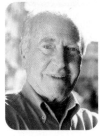

©Image Source/Getty Images

Recall Peter Smith from the case study at the beginning of the chapter. Now that you have completed the chapter, answer the following questions regarding his case.

1. What diagnosis will the licensed practitioner most likely give this patient?

2. What specific symptoms make you suspect this condition?
3. Peter Smith complains of not being able to fall asleep. Is this information objective or subjective data?
4. Why do you think a sleep study was ordered?

1. (LO 36.3) Which of the following represents objective data?
   a. Headache
   b. Pain
   c. Itching
   d. Rash
   e. Nausea

2. (LO 36.1) Which of the following is an open-ended question?
   a. How long have you had the rash under your arm?
   b. So, have you had a headache for 3 days on the left side of your head?
   c. Can you tell me more about your symptoms?
   d. How long does your pain last?
   e. Does your left arm hurt?

3. (LO 36.1) Which of the following is the most effective question to use during a patient interview?
   a. Do you agree that you are getting better when you use the medicine?
   b. Have you had a headache every day this week?
   c. Do you agree you should not have taken so much medication?
   d. What do you think is going on here?
   e. You haven't been taking your medicine, have you?

4. (LO 36.2) Which type of patient is the *least* likely victim of abuse?
   a. A 2-year-old child
   b. A 48-year-old male
   c. A 78-year-old male
   d. A 35-year-old female
   e. An 85-year-old female

5. (LO 36.3) Which of the following is an accepted abbreviation?
   a. HA
   b. OU
   c. HS
   d. ASA
   e. AU

6. (LO 36.4) In the PQRST interview technique, the "P" stands for
   a. Prescription
   b. Problem
   c. Provoke
   d. Plan
   e. Prevent

7. (LO 36.2) The intentional use of a medication or other substance in a way that is not medically approved is known as
   a. Medication error
   b. Substance abuse
   c. Polypharmacy
   d. Addiction
   e. Palliation

8. (LO 36.3) Which of the following is considered subjective data?
   a. Rash
   b. Fever
   c. Increased pulse rate
   d. Headache
   e. Hypertension

9. (LO 36.1) "You seem to be having trouble taking your medication, don't you agree?" is an example of
   a. Asking a leading question
   b. Asking an open-ended question
   c. Asking a hypothetical question
   d. Focusing on the patient
   e. Mirroring the patient's response

10. (LO 36.4) Asking a patient if his pain moves from one location to another is an example of which part of the PQRST interview technique?
    a. P
    b. Q
    c. R
    d. S
    e. T

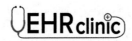

Go to CONNECT to complete the EHRclinic exercises: 36.01 Record a Patient's Interview and History in an EHR and 36.02 Record a Patient's Review of Systems (ROS) in an EHR.

SOFT SKILLS SUCCESS

Mrs. Smithers, an 83-year-old established patient, is in today for follow-up after falling and breaking her arm 2 weeks ago. Her daughter is with her and insists on going back to the exam room. During the patient interview, you notice that each time you ask Mrs. Smithers a question, her daughter answers before Mrs. Smithers is able to. How should you handle this situation?

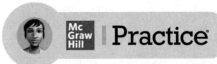

Go to PRACTICE MEDICAL OFFICE and complete the module Clinical: Interactions.

Vital Signs and Measurements

CASE STUDY

	Patient Name	DOB	Allergies
PATIENT INFORMATION	Mohammad Nassar	05/17/2005	Animal dander
	Attending	**MRN**	**Other Information**
	Elizabeth H. Williams, MD	00-AA-007	Current medication: albuterol 4 mg bid

Mohammad Nassar comes to the office because he has had several episodes of what he describes as "my heart is beating too fast." Mohammad has a known history of asthma that is being managed using albuterol. You measure his vital signs and record the following: BP 104/62, P 88 beats per minute, T 99.1°F orally, and R 18 breaths per minute. He is 5'10" tall and weighs 140 lb. When you ask about the episodes he has experienced, he says they often occur in the evening while he is studying for a big exam. He says he drinks coffee in order to stay awake and is worried about keeping his grades up so that his parents will continue to allow him to play sports.

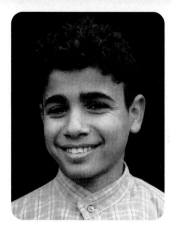
©David Sacks/Getty Images

Keep Mohammad Nassar in mind as you study this chapter. There will be questions at the end of the chapter based on the case study. The information in the chapter will help you answer these questions.

LEARNING OUTCOMES

After completing Chapter 37, you will be able to:

37.1 Describe the vital signs.

37.2 Identify various methods of taking a patient's temperature.

37.3 Describe the process of obtaining pulse and respirations.

37.4 Carry out blood pressure measurements.

37.5 Illustrate various body measurements.

KEY TERMS

afebrile	hypoxemia
apnea	orthostatic hypotension
auscultated blood pressure	palpatory method
body mass index (BMI)	positive tilt test
bradycardia	postural hypotension
calibrate	rales
dyspnea	rhonchi
febrile	sleep apnea
hyperpnea	sphygmomanometer
hyperpyrexia	stethoscope
hypertension	tachycardia
hyperventilation	tachypnea
hypotension	thermometer

CAAHEP

I.P.1 Measure and record:
    (a) blood pressure
    (b) temperature
    (c) pulse
    (d) respiration
    (e) height
    (f) weight
    (i) pulse oximetry

II.C.6 Analyze healthcare results as reported in:
    (a) graphs
    (b) tables

V.P.11 Report relevant information concisely and accurately

X.P.3 Document patient care accurately in the medical record

ABHES

2. **Anatomy and Physiology**
    c. Identify diagnostic and treatment modalities as they relate to each body system

4. **Medical Law and Ethics**
    f. Comply with federal, state, and local health laws and regulations as they relate to healthcare settings

8. **Clinical Procedures**
    b. Obtain vital signs, obtain patient history, and formulate chief complaint
    e. Perform specialty procedures including but not limited to minor surgery, cardiac, respiratory, OB-GYN, neurological, and gastroenterology
    j. Make adaptations for patients with special needs (psychological or physical limitations)

Introduction

Vital signs are important assessments you can make when preparing the patient to be examined by the practitioner. Temperature, pulse, respirations, and blood pressure give information about how a patient will adjust to changes within the body and in the environment. Changes in the vital signs can indicate an abnormality.

Measurements such as height and weight are used to monitor health. These measurements also are used to evaluate health problems such as obesity. Other measurements are completed to evaluate a patient's condition. For example, you may need to measure the size of a wound or bruise or the diameter of an arm or a leg. Head circumference, length, and weight indicate physical growth and development in infants and children. In all cases, you must be accurate when performing and recording vital signs and body measurements. The practitioner uses your results when evaluating the patient and making a diagnosis.

Vital Signs
LO 37.1

As a medical assistant, you usually will take the vital signs before the doctor examines the patient. Vital signs include temperature, pulse, respirations, and blood pressure. Pain assessment, which was discussed in the *Patient Interview and History* chapter, is considered by some practitioners to be the "fifth vital sign." Pain level is typically evaluated during the patient interview and recorded along with the vital signs. These measurements provide the doctor with information about the patient's overall condition.

In some offices, pre-exam procedures such as vital signs are performed in a general area outside the patient exam room. In other offices and in most pediatric offices, these measurements are taken in the exam room. In either case, you

typically take the measurements before the patient disrobes. Follow the standard procedure used in your office and provide for the privacy of your results.

Vital signs are usually measured at every office visit. There is a standard range of values for each measurement. Temperature ranges, discussed in *section 37.2* of this chapter, vary based upon the method used to take them. Table 37-1 shows the other vital sign ranges for ages 1 and older. Each patient has an individual baseline value that is normal for that patient. The difference between a patient's current values and normal values can help the licensed practitioner in making a diagnosis.

You must follow closely the guidelines from the Department of Labor's Occupational Safety and Health Administration (OSHA) for taking measurements of vital signs (Table 37-2). These guidelines are intended to prevent transmission of disease to or from the patient. They help protect the patient and you, and they keep the workplace safe.

TABLE 37-1   Vital Sign Ranges by Age

Age	Blood Pressure	Pulse (beats/min)	Respirations (breaths/min)
> 12 years	Systolic: 110–130 Diastolic: 65–80	60–100	12–20
6–12 years	Systolic: 100–120 Diastolic: 60–75	60–110	16–22
3–6 years	Systolic: 95–110 Diastolic: 60–75	70–120	20–24
1–3 years	Systolic: 90–105 Diastolic: 55–70	80–150	22–30

Source: Adapted from PALS Algorithms 2017

TABLE 37-2	OSHA Guidelines for Taking Measurements of Vital Signs
Situation	**OSHA Guidelines**
Before and after all patient contact	• Examination area cleaned according to OSHA standards • Aseptic handwashing
Temperature by oral or rectal route Contact with patient with lesions Contact with patient suspected of having infectious disease	• Gloves always worn for rectal route • Gloves worn for oral route if contact precautions exist • Biohazard bags used for disposal of used thermometer sheaths, otoscope tips, alcohol swabs, dressings, and bandages
In presence of patient suspected of having an airborne infectious disease (particularly sneezing)	• Mask worn • Patient weighed, measured, and examined in room away from staff and other patients • Protective clothing (laboratory coat, gown, or apron) worn • Biohazard bags used as above

▶ Temperature
LO 37.2

When you take a patient's temperature, you will determine whether the patient is **febrile** (has a body temperature above the patient's normal range) or **afebrile** (has a body temperature within the patient's normal range). A fever is usually a sign of inflammation or infection. An exceptionally high fever is known as **hyperpyrexia.** Body temperature is the balance between heat produced by metabolic processes and heat lost from the body; it varies based on numerous factors. These factors include the time of day (usually higher at night due to exercise and food intake), age, gender, physical exercise, emotion, ovulation, pregnancy, drugs, food, environmental changes, and metabolism (a slow metabolism, as seen in hypothyroidism, would cause a lower temperature).

Temperature is typically measured with an electronic **thermometer.** A disposable thermometer also may be used.

You can take a temperature in one of five locations: mouth (oral), ear (tympanic), rectum (rectal), armpit or axilla (axillary), and temporal artery (temporal). The body location where the temperature is taken affects the result. Temperature can be measured in degrees Fahrenheit (°F) or degrees Celsius (°C). Normal adult oral temperature is considered to be about 98.6°F (37.0°C). A temperature over 100°F (38°C) is generally considered a fever. Table 37-3 gives temperature methods and expected values. See the *Points on Practice* box to review formulas and example conversions between Fahrenheit and Celsius.

Electronic Digital Thermometers

Electronic digital thermometers are used most commonly in medical offices. These thermometers provide a digital readout of the patient's temperature (Figure 37-1). They are accurate, fast, easy to read, and comfortable for the patient. Separate

TABLE 37-3	Temperature Methods and Expected Values

Oral

• Range adults: 97°F (36.1°C) to 99°F (37.2°C)
• Range children: 97°F (36.1°C) to 100°F (37.8°C)
• Method can be used on adults and children over 4.
• More accurate

Rectal

• Range: 97.8°F (36.6°C) to 100.4°F (38°C)
• Preferred method for infants and children under 4
• More accurate

Axillary

• Range: 97.8°F (36.5°C) to 99°F.5 (37.5°C)
• Preferred method for infants and children under 4

Tympanic

• Range: 96.4°F (35.8°C) to 100.4°F (38°C)
• Not used on children under 2 because of narrow ear canal
• Less accurate, used for screening

Temporal

• Range: 97.8 (36.6°C) to 100.4°F (38°C)
• Measures arterial blood temperature

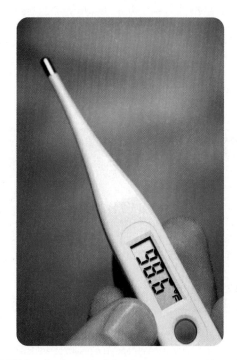

FIGURE 37-1 An electronic digital thermometer provides a digital readout of the patient's temperature.

©Purestock/Getty Images

probes and tips are available for oral and rectal use. Most units beep or have another audible indicator to let you know when the temperature has registered and is displayed.

Another type of electronic thermometer is the tympanic thermometer, which is designed for use in the ear. See Figure 37-2. This thermometer measures infrared energy emitted from the tympanic membrane (eardrum). This energy is converted into a temperature reading. The tip is covered with a disposable sheath to prevent cross-contamination.

A third type of electronic thermometer is a temporal scanner (Figure 37-3). This thermometer measures the infrared heat of the temporal artery and the ambient temperature (the temperature around the area) at the site where the temperature is taken. These two readings are processed to calculate the body temperature, which is then displayed on the screen.

Disposable Thermometers

Disposable, single-use thermometers are usually made of thin strips of plastic with specially treated dot or strip indicators (Figure 37-4). The indicators change color according to the temperature. This type of thermometer is used for oral and axillary or skin temperature measurements, particularly in children. Although not as accurate, disposable thermometers are useful for patients in their homes and for screening.

Taking Temperatures

Using the proper instrument and technique provides the most accurate temperature readings and prevents the spread of infection. All temperature measurements should be recorded to the nearest one-tenth of a degree. The procedure for taking temperatures is described in Procedure 37-1 at the end of this chapter.

Measuring Oral Temperatures To take an oral temperature, make sure the patient is able to hold the thermometer

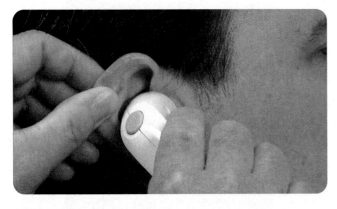

FIGURE 37-2 The tympanic thermometer measures infared energy emitted from the tympanic membrane. The result, converted to body temperature, is displayed within seconds of insertion of the shielded tip into the ear.
©McGraw-Hill Education

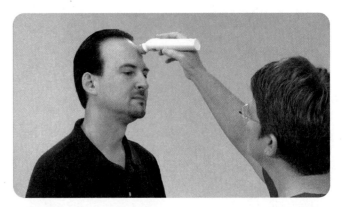

FIGURE 37-3 This temporal scanner is passed across the forehead to measure the temperature of the blood in the temporal artery.
©McGraw-Hill Education

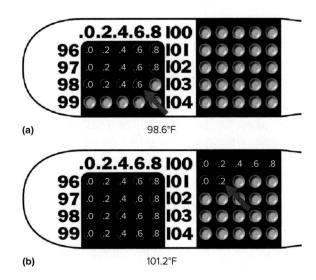

(a) 98.6°F

(b) 101.2°F

FIGURE 37-4 A disposable thermometer like this one is a convenient method for taking temperature. Thermometer reading after taking (a) a normal temperature and (b) an elevated temperature.

in the mouth. The patient also must be able to breathe through the nose. Place the thermometer under the tongue in either pocket just off-center in the lower jaw (Figure 37-5). The patient should hold the thermometer with lips closed. Wait at least 15 minutes after a patient has been eating, drinking, or smoking before taking an oral temperature; otherwise, you may obtain an inaccurate result.

Measuring Tympanic Temperatures Tympanic thermometers are easy to use, but you must follow manufacturers' instructions precisely. First, remove the thermometer from its recharging cradle and then wait for the indicator light to show that the unit is ready. Attach a disposable sheath and place the thermometer in the opening of the ear so that the fit is snug. To make sure you have a tight fit and the thermometer is pointing at the eardrum, pull the ear up and back for adults; pull the ear

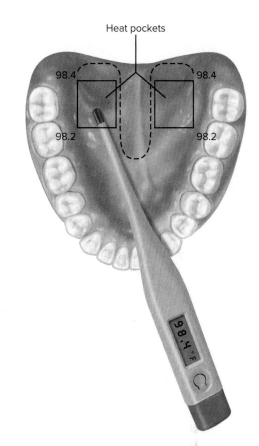

Heat pockets

98.4 98.4
98.2 98.2

FIGURE 37-5 When taking an oral temperature, place the thermometer under the tongue to the side of the mouth, as shown here.

down and back for children. The thermometer must be aiming directly at the eardrum. Press the button and the result will be displayed within seconds. Be certain to press the correct button to read the temperature. Another button on the thermometer releases the sheath. Do not release the sheath into the patient's ear. See the *Caution: Handle with Care* box for problems that can occur with tympanic thermometers.

CAUTION: HANDLE WITH CARE

Tympanic Thermometers: Where Problems Can Occur

Most tympanic thermometer units have an indicator to let you know when the thermometer is ready for use. Some units require taking the temperature within a certain period after removing the thermometer from its charging base. Read the manufacturer's instructions for specific information.

If the outer opening of the ear is not sealed completely when the probe is placed at the ear canal or the thermometer is not aimed at the eardrum, the results may be inaccurate. You will need to tug gently on the ear to position the thermometer properly and aim it at the eardrum.

If the thermometer has been charging for several hours before use, the initial reading may be inaccurately high. Some experts believe you should take two measurements on the first patient after charging the unit and record only the second reading.

Even with good technique, problems sometimes can occur. For example, excessive or impacted cerumen (earwax) or otitis media (ear infection) may prevent an accurate reading. If you obtain a reading that does not appear to match the patient's general condition, repeat the temperature measurement or use a different method to be sure. The tympanic method should not be used right after swimming or bathing or when ear pain is present.

Measuring Rectal Temperatures Rectal temperatures are usually 1°F higher than oral temperatures and are considered the most accurate measurement of body temperature. Temperatures are measured rectally in infants and in adults in whom an oral temperature cannot be taken. Gloves are always worn, and the patient is placed on his or her side. The left side is the preferred position because the rectum is angled in this direction. This position promotes comfort and prevents accidental puncture of the rectal wall. The tip of the thermometer should be inserted slowly and gently until it is covered or until you feel resistance, at approximately 1 inch for adults and ½ inch for infants and small children. For safety, always hold the thermometer in place while taking the temperature.

Measuring Axillary Temperatures To take an axillary temperature, first have the patient sit or lie down. Place the tip of the thermometer in the middle of the axilla (armpit), with the shaft facing forward. The patient's upper arm should be pressed against his side and his lower arm should be crossed over the stomach to hold the thermometer in place. Make sure the tip of the thermometer touches skin on all sides of the probe. The axillary temperature is 0.5 to 1°F lower than the oral temperature and 1 to 2°F lower than the rectal temperature. Therefore, if the patient's axillary temperature is 99°F or higher, verify the patient's temperature using another method because the patient may have a fever. Be sure to note the location of the temperature measurement on the patient's chart.

Measuring Temporal Temperatures The temporal scanner is a quick, noninvasive procedure for taking temperatures. You gently stroke the thermometer across the forehead, crossing over the temporal artery (on the side of the forehead at the temple) then touching the neck. An infrared scanner measures the difference in the temperature of the forehead and that of the temporal artery and then electronically calculates the patient's body temperature. As with all electronic devices, check the manufacturer's instructions before using.

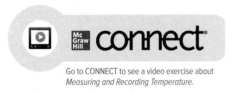

Go to CONNECT to see a video exercise about *Measuring and Recording Temperature.*

▶ Pulse and Respiration

LO 37.3

Pulse and respiration are related because the circulatory and respiratory systems work together. Pulse is measured as the number of times the heart beats in 1 minute. Respiration is the number of times a patient breathes in 1 minute. One breath, or respiration, equals one inhalation and one exhalation. Usually, if either the pulse or respiration rate is high or low, the other is also. In general, the younger the patient, the higher the normal pulse and respiration rate. Additionally, adult female rates tend to be faster than those for males. You should be familiar with these rates and how to perform the procedure. See Table 37-1 and Procedure 37-2 at the end of this chapter.

Pulse

A pulse rate gives information about the patient's cardiovascular system. It is an indirect measurement of the patient's cardiac output or the amount of blood the heart is able to pump in one minute. The average adult pulse rate is 60 to 100 BPM (beats per minute). If the pulse is weak or irregular or if the patient has **tachycardia** (abnormally fast pulse) or **bradycardia** (abnormally slow pulse), the patient may have a medical problem.

Measure the pulse of adults at the radial artery, where it can be felt in the groove on the thumb side of the inner wrist. Press lightly on this pulse point with your fingers and not your thumb (a pulse is located in your thumb, and you may feel it instead of the patient's pulse). Count the number of beats you feel in a set period of time (up to 1 minute). Also note the rhythm and volume. The rhythm can be regular or irregular. The volume can be weak, strong, or bounding. A bounding pulse feels like it is leaping out and then quickly disappearing with each pulse beat and sometimes can be seen at the pulse site. You may be asked to document the pulse volume on a numerical scale from 0 to 4+. Following are the characteristics of this scale.

- 0 = no palpable pulse
- 1+ = weak
- 2+ = faint pulse
- 3+ = normal pulse
- 4+ = bounding pulse

Count the pulse for 30 seconds and, if the beat is regular, multiply the results by 2 to obtain the beats per minute. If the pulse is irregular, weak, or bounding, you must count for a full minute and document the irregularities. In some cases, you may be able to count the pulse for as little as 15 seconds and multiply by 4 to obtain the beats per minute. However, this only should be done when you are comfortable with the procedure and you are certain the pulse is normal (3+) and regular.

Pulse sites other than the radial pulse may be used for various reasons. For example, in young children, the radial artery may be hard to feel. You may instead take the pulse at the brachial artery, which is in the medial aspect of the antecubital fossa (the bend of the elbow) or on the medial (inner) side of the upper arm. If you cannot feel the brachial pulse, then take the pulse over the apex (the left lower corner) of the heart, where the strongest heart sounds can be heard. Count the apical pulse (the heartbeat at the apex of the heart) while you listen with a **stethoscope,** an instrument that amplifies body sounds. The apex is located in the fifth intercostal space between the ribs on the left side of the chest, directly below the center of the clavicle. Consult Figure 37-6 for placement of the stethoscope. You also may use other locations to take a pulse. Figure 37-7 shows the location of common pulse points.

Pulse Oximetry Pulse oximetry is a noninvasive test that measures the pulse electronically and the saturation of oxygen in a patient's arterial blood. The pulse oximeter includes

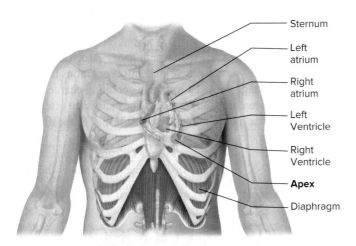

- Sternum
- Left atrium
- Right atrium
- Left Ventricle
- Right Ventricle
- **Apex**
- Diaphragm

FIGURE 37-6 A stethoscope is used over the apex of the heart to listen for the heart sounds and measure the heart rate in patients in whom pulse is not otherwise detectable.

a sensor and a monitoring device. The sensor is placed on a patient's finger, earlobe, toe, or bridge of the nose. Figure 37-8 shows pulse oximetry as part of an electronic blood pressure machine. A separate pulse oximeter machine also may be used (Figure 37-9).

When using these devices, be certain to attach the clip firmly to the finger, lobe, or nose. There must be a good blood supply at the site where the sensor is placed to detect the oxygen level. For the fingers or toes, you may need to check the capillary refill to determine if the blood supply is adequate. The finger clip also works best when no nail polish is present

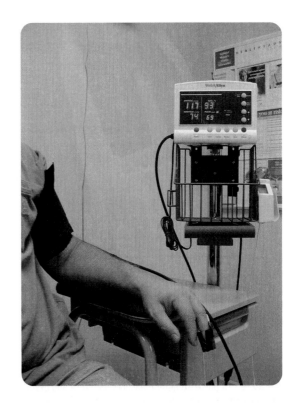

FIGURE 37-8 Pulse, blood pressure, and oxygen saturation all can be measured with this electronic blood pressure device.
©Total Care Programming, Inc.

on the patient's finger. When using a nose bridge pulse oximeter, make sure there is good skin contact. The nose bridge pulse oximeter should only be used with patients who have

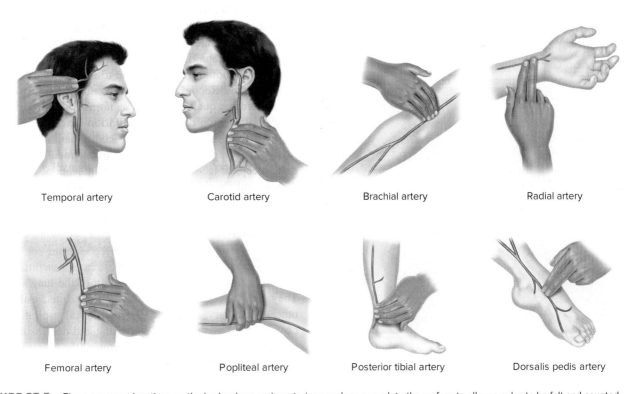

Temporal artery   Carotid artery   Brachial artery   Radial artery

Femoral artery   Popliteal artery   Posterior tibial artery   Dorsalis pedis artery

FIGURE 37-7 There are many locations on the body where major arteries are close enough to the surface to allow a pulse to be felt and counted.

4. Measure and record the blood pressure and pulse rate at 1 and 3 minutes. Note: Sometimes the sitting step is eliminated.

5. Have the person stand.

6. Measure and record the blood pressure and pulse rate at 1 and 3 minutes.

7. Document the results in the chart including any associated symptoms. See Figure 37-15.

▶ Body Measurements

LO 37.5

Certain measurements are obtained before the patient is seen by the practitioner. These include height and weight for adults and older children and weight, length, and head circumference for infants. Usually, these measurements are taken before or after the vital signs, depending on the office policy. In some cases, you may choose to take the patient's vital signs first. For example, if a patient could become upset about her weight, you should take her vital signs first so that the patient's vital signs will not be affected by the weight results. Anxiety can cause a patient's pulse, respirations, and blood pressure to increase. Follow the policy at your facility.

Measurements taken at each visit provide baseline values for a patient's current condition. Any extreme or abnormal changes may indicate a disease or disorder and should be noted for the practitioner. For children and adolescents, these measurements should be taken at each office visit, which allows the licensed practitioner to follow growth and development.

Measurements are also important in determining the extent of an injury or illness and help define certain treatment regimens. For example, dosages of some medications are based on patient weight; a wound or bruise may be measured to determine how well it is healing. If a patient has a swollen arm, for example, both arms may be measured and compared. Body measurements may be necessary for correct interpretation of certain diagnostic tests, such as electrocardiography.

In some cases when measurements are performed, they will need to be converted to a different system of measurement.

POSITION	TIME	BP	ASSOCIATED SYMPTOMS
Lying Down	5 Mins.	BP ___/___ HR ___	
Sitting	1 Mins.	BP ___/___ HR ___	
Sitting	3 Mins.	BP ___/___ HR ___	
Standing	1 Mins.	BP ___/___ HR ___	

FIGURE 37-15   Recording orthostatic vital signs.

For example, the scale you are using may only measure a patient's weight in pounds (household system) and it will need to be converted to kilograms (metric system). With other body measurements, depending upon the equipment, you may need to convert inches to centimeters or vice versa. Some equipment will make the conversion electronically; you also can check conversion tables that are readily available online. There are various conversions that may be necessary. To complete these conversions, you should review the *Points on Practice* feature Body Measurement Conversions.

Measuring the Weight and Height of Adults

Measure the weight of adults and older children at each office visit. Weight should be listed in the patient's chart to the nearest quarter of a pound. The height of an adult should be

POINTS ON PRACTICE
Body Measurement Conversions

When performing body measurements, certain basic math conversions may be required. Review the following formulas and examples in preparation for practice.

To convert kg to lb, use this formula:

lb = kg × 2.205

Example: Convert 52.4 kg to lb:

lb = 52.4 × 2.205

lb = 115.542, rounded to the nearest tenth equals 115.5

To convert lb to kg, use this formula:

kg = lb × 0.454

Example: Convert 134 lb to kg:

kg = 134 × 0.454

kg = 60.836, rounded to the nearest tenth equals 60.8

To convert inches to feet and inches:

Divide the number of inches by 12 and carry the remainder. The answer is the number of feet, and the remainder indicates the number of inches. For example, $\frac{66}{12} = 5$ with a remainder of 6, so a person who is 66 inches tall is 5 feet, 6 inches tall.

measured at the patient's initial visit and whenever a complete physical exam is performed or at least yearly. Height for older children is typically measured at each visit. Height should be measured to the nearest quarter of an inch. Measure the patient's height after weighing the patient. Most office scales have a height bar located in the center of the scale. This bar is calibrated in inches and quarter inches but may be in centimeters. The steps for measuring the height of adults and children are described in Procedure 37-5.

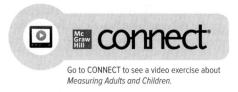

Go to CONNECT to see a video exercise about *Measuring Adults and Children.*

Body Mass Index

A reliable indicator of healthy weight is **body mass index (BMI),** which is calculated based on height and weight. If you are asked to calculate a patient's BMI, use the CDC's BMI chart (Figure 37-16). Handheld BMI calculators and smartphone apps are also available. See the chapter *Nutrition and Health* for more information on healthy weight management.

Other Body Measurements

In some facilities, you may be asked to obtain other body measurements. For example, if a patient has edema (swelling) of an arm or a leg, you might be asked to measure the diameter. You should measure both arms or legs to determine the difference in size. If a patient has a wound, bruise, or other injury,

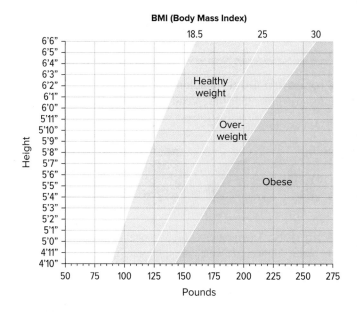

FIGURE 37-16 Use a BMI chart to calculate a patient's body mass index.

you may need to measure its length and width to evaluate the healing process. Additionally, sometimes an infant will need her head and chest circumference measured or an adult may require a measurement around his abdomen, which is known as *abdominal girth.* Infant vital signs and measurements are described in more detail in the *Assisting in Pediatrics* chapter.

All vital signs and measurements should be documented accurately and immediately (Figure 37-17).

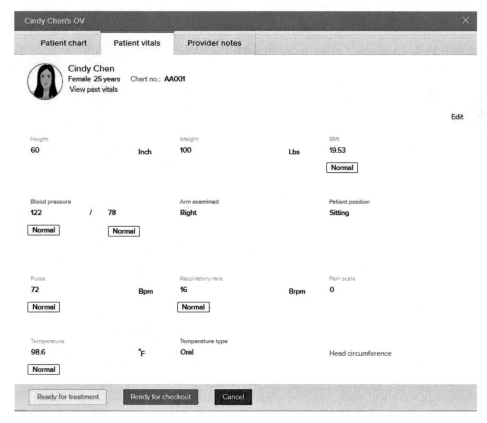

FIGURE 37-17 ꙨEHRclinic allows the user to document the vital signs and measurements on one screen.

©McGraw-Hill Education

PROCEDURE **37-1** Measuring and Recording Temperature

Procedure Goal: To accurately measure patient temperature while preventing the spread of infection

OSHA Guidelines:

Materials: Thermometer, probe cover if required by thermometer, lubricant for rectal temperature, gloves, trash receptacle, and the patient's vital signs flow sheet or medical record

Method:

1. Gather the equipment and make sure the thermometer is in working order.

2. Identify the patient and introduce yourself.

3. Wash your hands and explain the procedure to the patient.

4. Prepare the patient.

   a. *Oral.* If the patient has had anything to eat or drink, or has been smoking, wait at least 15 minutes before measuring the temperature orally.
   RATIONALE: *Inaccurate reading could result.*

   b. *Rectal.* Have the patient remove the appropriate clothing; assist as needed. Have the patient lie on his or her left side and drape for comfort.
   RATIONALE: *Proper positioning is necessary for the patient's safety and comfort.*

   c. *Axillary.* Assist the patient to expose the axilla. Provide for privacy and comfort. Pat dry the axilla.
   RATIONALE: *Perspiration or heavy deodorant prevents the thermometer from coming in direct contact with the skin.*

   d. *Temporal or tympanic.* If a hat is worn, ask the patient to remove it. Brush aside any hair that is blocking the ear canal or temporal artery.

5. Prepare the equipment.

   a. Prepare an electronic thermometer by inserting the probe into the probe cover if necessary.
   RATIONALE: *Probe covers are needed to prevent contamination of the probe.*

   b. Prepare a disposable thermometer by removing the wrapper to expose the handle end. Avoid touching the part of the thermometer that goes in the mouth or on the skin.
   RATIONALE: *Touching the thermometer could interfere with an accurate reading.*

   c. Prepare a temporal scanner by removing the protective cap and making sure the lens is clean.
   RATIONALE: *This will ensure an accurate reading.*

6. Measure the temperature.

   a. *Oral.* Place the thermometer under the tongue in the back of the mouth on one side. Have the patient

hold it in place with his or her lips and tongue. Wait for the electronic thermometer to beep or indicate completion. For a disposable thermometer, wait the required time, usually 60 seconds.

   b. *Rectal.* Put on gloves. Lubricate the thermometer tip. Raise the buttock with one hand to expose the anus and insert the thermometer into the anal canal using your other hand, approximately 1 inch for adults and ½ inch for infants and children. Hold the thermometer securely in place until the indicator beeps or blinks.
   RATIONALE: *Injury could occur if the thermometer is inserted too far or if the patient moves during the procedure.*

   c. *Axillary.* Place the thermometer into the axilla, making sure the tip is in direct contact with the top of the axilla and is touching skin on all sides. Hold the arm firmly against the body until the indicator light blinks or beeps or the proper amount of time has passed.
   RATIONALE: *Ensures accuracy.*

   d. *Tympanic.* Hold the outer edge of the ear (pinna) with your free hand. Gently pull the pinna up for adults and down for children (see figure). Insert the probe into the ear canal directed toward the eardrum and sealing the ear canal. Press the scan button.
   RATIONALE: *Ensures accuracy.*

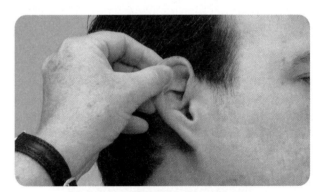

(a)

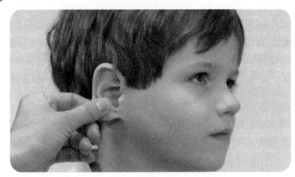

(b)

FIGURE Procedure 37-1 Step 6d   When placing a tympanic thermometer, seal the ear canal by holding the pinna (outer ear) upward and outward for an adult (a) and downward and backward for a child (b).
©McGraw-Hill Education

e. *Temporal.* Position the probe flat on the center of the exposed forehead. Press and hold the SCAN button and then slide the thermometer straight across the forehead until it beeps and the red light blinks.

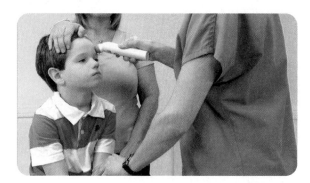

FIGURE Procedure 37-1 Step 6e   A temporal scanner is a safe, fast, and noninvasive method for taking temperature.
©McGraw-Hill Education

7. Remove and read the measurement in the display or on the thermometer. Discard the disposable thermometer.

Eject and discard the probe cover for an electronic thermometer. Replace the cap and/or place the thermometer into the charging base.
RATIONALE: *Contaminated items should be removed and the thermometer should be protected and charged until the next use.*

8. Record the results. Chart by including the date and location where the temperature was taken.
- Oral: 98.6
- Rectal: 99.6 R
- Axillary: 97.6 Ax
- Temporal: 97.6 Temp or TA
- Tympanic: 97.6 Tymp

RATIONALE: *The temperature varies depending upon the location; this location should be charted to ensure an accurate diagnosis.*

9. Help the patient to replace clothing as necessary. Clear the area and provide for safety and comfort for the patient.

10. Wash your hands.

11. Report any results that are outside the normal values found in Table 37-3.

PROCEDURE 37-2 Measuring and Recording Pulse and Respirations

WORK // DOC

Procedure Goal: To accurately measure a patient's pulse and respirations while keeping the patient unaware the respirations are being counted

OSHA Guidelines:

Materials: Watch with a second hand and the patient's vital signs flow sheet or medical record

Method:
1. Gather the equipment and wash your hands.
2. Introduce yourself and identify the patient.
3. Explain the procedure, saying, "I am going to take your vital signs. We'll start with your pulse first." Do not tell him you are counting the respirations.
   RATIONALE: *If the patient is aware you are counting respirations, he may unconsciously change his breathing rate.*
4. Ask the patient to sit or lie in a comfortable position. Have the patient rest his arm on a table. The palm should be facing downward.
5. Position yourself so you can observe and/or feel the chest wall movements. You may want to lay the

patient's arm over the chest to feel the respiratory chest movements.

6. Place two or three fingers on the radial pulse site. Find the radial bone on the thumb side of the wrist; then slide your fingers into the groove on the inside of the wrist to locate the pulse.

7. Count the pulse for 30 seconds if regular. Note the rhythm and volume. If irregular, count for a full minute. Remember or note the number.
   RATIONALE: *An irregular pulse is counted for a full minute to ensure accuracy and to note abnormalities.*

8. Without letting go of the wrist, observe and feel the respirations, counting for 1 full minute. Observe for rhythm, volume, and effort.

9. Once you are certain of both numbers, release the wrist and record them. If the pulse was measured for less than 1 minute, obtain the number of beats per minute. Multiply the number of beats counted in 30 seconds by 2.

10. Document results with the date and time (example: 6/18/18 P 88 regular and strong R 16 regular).

11. Report any findings that are a significant change from a previous result or outside the normal values, as shown in Table 37-1.

PROCEDURE 37-3 Obtaining a Pulse Oximetry Reading

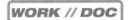

Procedure Goal: To obtain a pulse oximetry reading

OSHA Guidelines:

Materials: Pulse oximeter, patient chart/progress note

Method:

1. Assemble all the necessary equipment and supplies.
2. Wash your hands and correctly identify the patient.
3. Select the appropriate site to apply the sensor by assessing the capillary refill in the patient's toe or finger. This is done by applying pressure to the nail bed until it turns white, then releasing the pressure and watching for the return of blood flow. The pink color should return in less than 2 seconds.
   RATIONALE: *If the patient has poor circulation in his fingers or toes, use the bridge of his nose or an earlobe.*

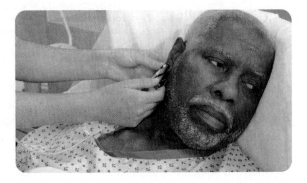

FIGURE Procedure 37-3 Step 3 The earlobe and bridge of the nose are alternative sites for placement of the sensor during pulse oximetry.

©McGraw-Hill Education

4. Prepare the selected site, removing nail polish or earrings if necessary. Wipe the selected site with alcohol and allow it to air-dry.
   RATIONALE: *Nail polish can alter the test results.*
5. Attach the sensor to the site (if a finger is used, place the finger in the clip).
6. Instruct the patient to breathe normally.
7. Attach the sensor cable to the oximeter and turn on the oximeter and listen to the tone if required.
8. Set the alarm limits for high and low oxygen saturations and high and low pulse rates, as directed by the physician's order, and turn on the oximeter, as needed.
9. Read the saturation level. If the result is less than 90%, have the patient take a few deep breaths and then recheck. Document the highest result. Report to the physician readings that are less than 95%.
10. Manually check the patient's pulse and compare it to the pulse oximeter. Document all the readings and the application site in the patient's chart/progress note.
11. Wash your hands.
12. Rotate the patient's finger sites every 4 hours if using a pulse oximeter long-term.

PROCEDURE 37-4 Taking the Blood Pressure of Adults and Older Children

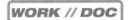

Procedure Goal: To accurately measure blood pressure in adults and older children

OSHA Guidelines:

Materials: Sphygmomanometer, stethoscope, alcohol gauze squares, and the patient's vital signs flow sheet or medical record

Method:

1. Gather the equipment and make sure the sphygmomanometer is in working order and correctly calibrated.
   RATIONALE: *Calibration helps ensure an accurate result.*

2. Identify the patient and introduce yourself.

3. Wash your hands and explain the procedure to the patient.

4. Have the patient sit in a quiet area. If she is wearing long-sleeved clothing, have her loosely roll up one sleeve. If she cannot, have her change into a gown.

5. Have the patient rest her bared arm on a flat surface so that the midpoint of the upper arm is at the same level as the heart.
   RATIONALE: *Doing so helps ensure an accurate reading.*

6. Select a cuff that is the appropriate size for the patient. The bladder inside the cuff should encircle 80% of the arm in adults and 100% of the arm in children younger than the age of 13. If you are not sure about the size, use a larger cuff.
   RATIONALE: *Using the proper cuff size helps ensure an accurate reading.*

7. Locate the brachial artery in the antecubital space.

8. Position the cuff so that the midline of the bladder is above the arterial pulsation. Then wrap and secure the cuff snugly around the patient's bare upper arm. The lower edge of the cuff should be 1 inch above the antecubital space, where the head of the stethoscope is to be placed.
   RATIONALE: *If the blood pressure cuff touches the stethoscope, it could interfere with your ability to hear.*

9. Place the manometer so that the center of the aneroid dial is at eye level and easily visible and so that the tubing from the cuff is unobstructed.

10. Close the valve of the pressure bulb until it is finger-tight.

11. Inflate the cuff rapidly to 70 mmHg with one hand and increase this pressure in 10 mmHg increments while palpating the radial pulse with your other hand. Note the level of pressure at which the pulse disappears and subsequently reappears during deflation. This procedure is the palpatory method.

12. Open the valve to release the pressure, deflate the cuff completely, and wait at least 30 seconds or remove and replace the cuff.
    RATIONALE: *If you do not deflate the cuff completely and wait, blood may pool in the artery and give a falsely high reading.*

13. Place the earpieces of the stethoscope in your ear canals and adjust them to fit snugly and comfortably. When placed in the ears, they should point toward the nose. Switch the stethoscope head to the diaphragm

position. Confirm the setting by listening as you tap the stethoscope head gently.

14. Place the head of the stethoscope over the brachial artery pulsation, just above and medial to the antecubital space but below the lower edge of the cuff. Hold the stethoscope firmly in place using your index and middle fingers, making sure the head is in contact with the skin around its entire circumference.
    RATIONALE: *Do not hold the stethoscope with your thumb because the pulse of your thumb can interfere with the reading.*

15. Inflate the bladder rapidly and steadily to a pressure 30 mmHg above the level previously determined by the palpatory method. Then partially open (unscrew) the valve and deflate the bladder at approximately 2 mm per second while you listen for the Korotkoff sounds.

16. As the pressure in the bladder falls, note the level of pressure on the manometer at the first appearance of repetitive sounds. This reading is the systolic pressure.

17. Continue to deflate the cuff gradually, noting the point at which the sound changes from strong to muffled.

18. Continue to deflate the cuff and note when the sound disappears. This reading is the diastolic pressure.

19. Continue to deflate the cuff for an additional 10 mmHg, listening carefully for a return of the repetitive sounds.
    RATIONALE: *Continue listening to ensure that the lack of sound is not the result of an auscultatory gap.*

20. Deflate the cuff completely and remove it from the patient's arm.

21. Record the systolic and diastolic numbers, separated by a slash, in the patient's chart. Chart the date and time of the measurement, the arm on which the measurement was made, the subject's position, and the cuff size when a nonstandard size is used. The value recorded is an exact measurement of the auscultated blood pressure.

22. Fold the cuff and replace it in the holder.

23. Inform the patient that you have completed the procedure.

24. Disinfect the earpieces and diaphragm of the stethoscope with gauze squares moistened with alcohol.

25. Properly dispose of the used gauze squares and wash your hands.

26. Report any blood pressure reading that is abnormal. See Table 37-1.

PROCEDURE 37-5 Measuring Adults and Children   [WORK // DOC]

Procedure Goal: To accurately measure weight and height of adults and children

OSHA Guidelines:

Materials: For an adult or older child, adult scale with height bar, disposable towel; for toddler, adult scale with height bar or height chart, disposable towel; and the patient's flow sheet or medical record

Method:

Adult or Older Child: Weight

1. Identify the patient and introduce yourself.

2. Wash your hands and explain the procedure to the patient.

3. Check to see whether the scale is in balance by moving all the weights to the left side. The indicator should be level with the middle mark. If not, check the manufacturer's directions and adjust it to ensure a zero balance. If you are using a scale equipped to measure either kilograms or pounds, check to see that it is set on the desired units and that the upper and lower weights show the same units.
   RATIONALE: *Proper functioning of the scale helps ensure an accurate result.*

4. Ask the patient to remove her shoes, if that is the standard office policy.
   RATIONALE: *Follow the policy and use the same procedure for all visits for consistency of results.*

5. Place a disposable towel on the scale or have the patient leave her socks on.
   RATIONALE: *Prevents cross-contamination of the scale from various patients' feet.*

6. Ask the patient to step on the center of the scale, facing forward. Assist as necessary.

7. Place the lower weight at the highest number that does not cause the balance indicator to drop to the bottom.
   RATIONALE: *To ensure accuracy.*

8. Move the upper weight slowly to the right until the balance bar is centered at the middle mark, adjusting as necessary.
   RATIONALE: *To ensure accuracy.*

9. Add the two weights together to get the patient's weight.

10. Record the patient's weight in the chart to the nearest quarter of a pound or tenth of a kilogram.

11. Return the weights to their starting positions on the left side.

Adult or Older Child: Height

12. With the patient off the scale, raise the height bar well above the patient's head and swing out the extension. (This also can be done before the patient steps on the scale for his weight measurement.)
    RATIONALE: *Doing so prevents hitting the patient with the extension bar.*

13. Ask the patient to step on the center of the scale and to stand up straight and look forward.
    RATIONALE: *Standing straight is necessary for accuracy.*

14. Gently lower the height bar until the extension rests on the patient's head.

15. Have the patient step off the scale while you hold the height bar before reading the measurement.
    RATIONALE: *To better visualize the height measurement.*

16. If the patient is fewer than 50 inches tall, read the height on the bottom part of the ruler; if the patient is more than 50 inches tall, read the height on the top, movable part of the ruler at the point at which it meets the bottom part of the ruler. Note that the numbers increase on the

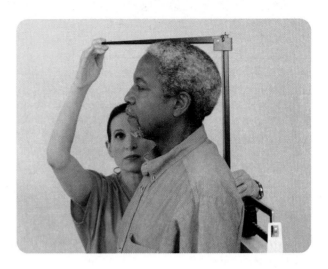

FIGURE Procedure 37-5 Step 14   The medical assistant adjusts the height bar to meet the top of the patient's head.
©McGraw-Hill Education

bottom part of the bar and decrease on the top, movable part of the bar. Read the height in the right direction.

17. Record the patient's height.

18. Have the patient put shoes back on, if necessary.

19. Properly dispose of the used towel and wash your hands.

Toddler: Weight

1. Identify the patient and obtain permission from the parent to weigh the toddler.

2. Wash your hands and explain the procedure to the parent.

3. Check to see whether the scale is in balance and place a disposable towel on the scale or have the patient wear shoes or socks, depending on the facility's policy.

4. Ask the parent to hold the patient and to step on the scale. Follow the procedure for obtaining the weight of an adult.

5. Have the parent put the child down or hand the child to another staff member.

6. Obtain the parent's weight.
   RATIONALE: *This is done to find the difference between the two weights.*

7. Subtract the parent's weight from the combined weight to determine the child's weight.

8. Record the patient's weight in the chart to the nearest quarter of a pound or tenth of a kilogram.

Toddler: Height

9. Measure the child's height in the same manner as you measure adult height, or have the child stand with her back against the height chart. Measure height at the crown of the head.

10. Record the height in the patient's chart.

11. Properly dispose of the towel (if used) and wash your hands.
    RATIONALE: *Doing so prevents infection.*

OUTCOME	KEY POINTS
37.1 Describe the vital signs.	Vital signs include temperature, pulse, respirations, and blood pressure; some practitioners also consider pain assessment to be one of the vital signs.
37.2 Identify various methods of taking a patient's temperature.	Using either an electronic digital or disposable thermometer, a patient's temperature may be measured by the oral, tympanic, rectal, axillary, or temporal method.
37.3 Describe the process of obtaining pulse and respirations.	Pressing lightly at the radial artery using your fingers, count the number of beats you feel in 1 minute to get the pulse. While still keeping fingers on the patient's pulse site, observe and feel the patient's respirations, and count the respirations for 1 full minute. See Procedure 37-2.
37.4 Carry out blood pressure measurements.	To obtain a blood pressure, have the patient sit in a quiet area, rest their bared arm on a flat surface at heart level, locate the brachial artery, snugly secure the cuff above the brachial artery, use the palpatory method to determine the approximate systolic pressure, and use a stethoscope to auscultate the systolic and diastolic blood pressure. Orthostatic, or postural, vital signs consist of taking the blood pressure and pulse in different positions, from lying to sitting to standing, then waiting 2 to 5 minutes between repositioning to allow the body's systems to adjust to the change.
37.5 Illustrate various body measurements.	For adults and older children, the measurements obtained are the height and weight; for infants, they are the weight, length, and head circumference. See Procedure 37-5. BMI, extremities, and wounds also are measured according to facility policy and patient condition.

CASE STUDY CRITICAL THINKING

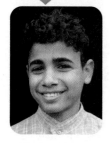

©David Sacks/Getty Images

Recall Mohammad Nassar from the case study at the beginning of the chapter. Now that you have completed the chapter, answer the following questions regarding his case.

1. Why is an accurate measurement and recording of Mohammad Nassar's vital signs critical in this case?

2. After examining Mohammad Nassar and ordering and reviewing the results of an ECG test, Dr. Williams indicates that Mohammad Nassar's heart appears to be normal. What factors might be contributing to Mohammad Nassar's episodes of tachycardia?

3. The physician is going to give Mohammad Nassar an injection and needs to know his weight in kilograms. You measured his weight as 140 pounds. Convert this weight to kilograms.

1. (LO 37.4) If a patient's blood pressure is 138/82, it is considered
   a. Normal
   b. Hypotension
   c. Prehypertension
   d. Stage 1 hypertension
   e. Stage 2 hypertension

2. (LO 37.1) When taking a patient's oral temperature, you should wear gloves if
   a. The patient is in for a routine physical exam
   b. There are contact precautions for the patient
   c. The patient is less than 5 years old
   d. You suspect the patient has a fever
   e. The patient cannot hold the thermometer in her mouth

3. (LO 37.2) Using the formula to convert degrees Fahrenheit to degrees Celsius, determine which of the following is equal to 99.8°F (round to the nearest tenth).
   a. 37.7°C
   b. 37.7°F
   c. 37.6°C
   d. 35.8°C
   e. 36.7°C

4. (LO 37.2) How would you abbreviate a rectal temperature of 99.7° Fahrenheit?
   a. T 97.9 R
   b. P 99.7 R
   c. T 99.7 Ax
   d. T 99.7 R
   e. T 99.7

5. (LO 37.3) The average ratio of the pulse rate to the respiration rate is
   a. 1:4
   b. 1:2
   c. 3:1
   d. 4:1
   e. 5:2

6. (LO 37.3) Abnormally rapid, deep, or labored breathing is known as
   a. Hyperpyrexia
   b. Hyperpnea
   c. Tachypnea
   d. Hypertension
   e. Bradypnea

7. (LO 37.3) Which of the following are crackling noises heard when the patient breathes?
   a. Rhonchi
   b. Apnea
   c. Cheyne-Stokes
   d. Asthma
   e. Rales

8. (LO 37.4) Low blood pressure is known as
   a. Papilledema
   b. Hypertension
   c. Tachycardia
   d. Hypotension
   e. Bradycardia

9. (LO 37.5) When measuring a patient's weight in pounds, it is important to round to the nearest
   a. $\frac{1}{4}$ pound
   b. Pound
   c. $\frac{1}{2}$ pound
   d. Ounce
   e. $\frac{1}{8}$ pound

10. (LO 37.4) Taking a patient's blood pressure in different positions is used to assess for
    a. Heart failure
    b. Hypertension
    c. Postural hypotension
    d. Vasoconstriction
    e. Kidney disease

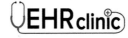

Go to CONNECT to complete the EHRclinic exercises 37.01 Record a Patient's Vital Signs and Measurements - A and 37.02 Record a Patient's Vital Signs and Measurements - B.

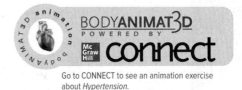

Go to CONNECT to see an animation exercise about *Hypertension*.

The electronic pulse oximeter is in use and, although you would rather not do it, you take the patient's pulse manually. While counting the pulse, you notice it seems irregular and every so often seems to feel stronger. You look at the patient, who appears pale and has a slight grimace on his face. What should you do?

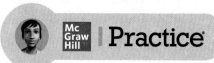

Go to PRACTICE MEDICAL OFFICE and complete the module Clinical: Office Operations.

Assisting with a General Physical Examination

CASE STUDY

PATIENT INFORMATION

Patient Name	DOB	Allergies
Valarie Ramirez	08/04/1986	Penicillin

Attending	MRN	Other Information
Paul F. Buckwalter, MD	00-AA-006	Previous eye injury Denies pain or blurred vision

Valarie Ramirez is at the office for a general physical exam. She has not had a physical exam for 3 years, so her exam today will include blood tests and a gynecological exam, as well as a screening electrocardiogram (ECG). Her vital

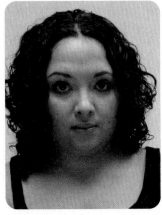
©McGraw-Hill Education

signs are BP 122/80, T 98.6, P 84, R 20, height 62 inches, and weight 140 pounds. While you are interviewing her, she states that she feels good in general and has no major complaints. She came in for a physical because she hasn't had one in a while.

Keep Valarie Ramirez in mind as you study this chapter. There will be questions at the end of the chapter based on the case study. The information in the chapter will help you answer these questions.

LEARNING OUTCOMES

After completing Chapter 38, you will be able to:

38.1 Identify the purpose of a general physical exam.

38.2 Describe the role of the medical assistant in a general physical exam.

38.3 Explain safety precautions used during a general physical exam.

38.4 Carry out the steps necessary to prepare the patient for an exam.

38.5 Carry out positioning and draping a patient in each of the nine common exam positions.

38.6 Apply techniques to assist patients from different cultures and patients with physical disabilities.

38.7 Identify the six examination methods used in a general physical exam.

38.8 List the components of a general physical exam.

38.9 Describe follow-up steps after a general physical exam.

KEY TERMS

auscultation
body mechanics
clinical diagnosis
cultural competence
culture
differential diagnosis
digital examination
fenestrated drape
hyperventilation
inspection
kyphosis
manipulation
mensuration
nasal mucosa
palpation
percussion
prognosis
quadrant
scoliosis
sign
stereotyping
symmetry
symptom

I.P.8	Instruct and prepare a patient for a procedure or a treatment
I.P.9	Assist provider with a patient exam
III.P.2	Select appropriate barrier/personal protective equipment (PPE)
V.P.3	Use medical terminology correctly and pronounced accurately to communicate information to providers and patients
V.P.5	Coach patients appropriately considering: (a) cultural diversity (c) communication barriers
X.P.3	Document patient care accurately in the medical record
XII.P.3	Use proper body mechanics

2. Anatomy and Physiology

  c. Identify diagnostic and treatment modalities as they relate to each body system.

5. Human Relations

  c. Assist the patient in navigating issues and concerns that may arise (i.e. insurance policy information, medical bills, and physician/provider orders)

7. Administrative Procedures

  g. Display professionalism through written and verbal communications

8. Clinical Procedures

  a. Practice standard precautions and perform disinfection/sterilization techniques

  b. Obtain vital signs, obtain patient history, and formulate chief complaint

  c. Assist provider with general/physical examination

  h. Teach self-examination, disease management and health promotion

  j. Make adaptations for patients with special needs (psychological or physical limitations)

▶ Introduction

Whether a patient comes for a regular checkup or to have a problem diagnosed and treated, the physical exam is the first step in the process for the physician or other licensed practitioner. As the medical assistant, your role during the physical exam is to make the patient comfortable and assist the physician as necessary. A skilled medical assistant who is sensitive to patient needs and proficient in performing these skills can create an atmosphere that results in a positive outcome for the patient and the healthcare facility where he/she is employed.

▶ The Purpose of a General Physical Exam

LO 38.1

General physical exams may be performed by physicians, nurse practitioners, physician assistants, or other licensed practitioners. These providers perform general physical exams for two purposes. The first is to examine a healthy patient to confirm an overall state of health and to provide baseline values for vital signs and measurements. The second is to examine a patient to diagnose a medical problem.

To confirm a patient's health status, physicians usually perform exams on a routine basis, such as once a year. Some exams are done to fulfill a requirement before an individual starts school, begins a new job, or starts an exercise program.

When a physician performs an examination to diagnose medical problems, she usually focuses on a particular organ system. The organ system is indicated to the physician by the patient's condition and chief complaint. Because organ systems are so interdependent, however, physicians generally perform an overall physical exam even when a specific medical problem exists.

During a general physical exam, physicians check all the major organs and body systems. They can determine much about a patient's general condition of health from the exam. If appropriate, they also try to make an initial, or **clinical, diagnosis**—a diagnosis based on the signs and symptoms of a disease, as well as the results of any ordered laboratory tests. A **sign** is objective information that can be detected by a person other than the affected person. Some examples of signs are blood in the stool and a rash. A **symptom** is subjective information supplied by the patient. Anxiety, back pain, abdominal pain, and fatigue are examples of symptoms. Only the patient can perceive these sensations, which are typically part of the chief complaint.

After forming an initial diagnosis of a patient's problem, physicians may order laboratory or other diagnostic tests. These tests are done to confirm a clinical diagnosis or to rule out other possible disorders and are necessary when a patient has symptoms that may indicate more than one condition. Determining the correct diagnosis when two or more diagnoses are possible is called making a **differential diagnosis.**

Laboratory and diagnostic tests also may aid physicians in developing a **prognosis,** or a forecast of the probable course and outcome of the disorder and the prospects of recovery. In addition, such tests help physicians formulate a treatment plan or appropriate drug therapy. Physicians may ask to have these tests repeated as part of the follow-up evaluation of a patient's progress.

▶ The Role of the Medical Assistant LO 38.2

Your job as a medical assistant is to assist both the licensed practitioner and the patient during the general physical exam. Your role starts before the actual exam. For example, you may be responsible for helping patients navigate insurance forms and other paperwork if necessary before they enter the exam room. After conducting the patient to an exam room, you will interview the patient, document an accurate history, determine vital signs, and measure weight and height.

Generally, your responsibilities during the exam include ensuring that all instruments and supplies are readily available to the licensed practitioner. You also ensure that patients are physically and emotionally comfortable during the exam by helping them into position and keeping them aware of what is going to happen. It is important to observe the patient for signs that indicate distress or the need for assistance. Providing comfort and safety to the patient and competent assistance to the physician are key during a general physical exam.

After the exam, you may be responsible for teaching patients how to perform self-examinations, such as a breast exam. You also may need to help patients understand physician orders for additional testing. In some cases, you may help the patient set up appointments for these tests.

▶ Safety Precautions LO 38.3

As you prepare for and assist with a general physical exam, you will practice safety measures. Some of these are outlined by the Department of Labor's Occupational Safety and Health Administration (OSHA) and the Department of Health and Human Services' Centers for Disease Control and Prevention (CDC). Recall that OSHA standards and guidelines are designed to protect employees and make the workplace safe. The CDC establishes the guidelines intended to protect both patients and healthcare professionals in the medical office and the hospital setting. Taken together, these safety measures help protect you, the physician, and the patient from disease transmission.

Safety measures that you must take before, during, and after a general physical exam include the following:

- Perform a thorough aseptic handwashing before and after contact with each patient and before and after each procedure. Waterless, alcohol-based hand cleanser may be used between patients if no gross contamination or visible soilage is on your hands. Refer to the chapter *Infection Control Fundamentals* for a review of these procedures.

- Wear gloves whenever there is a possibility that you may come in contact with blood, body fluids, nonintact skin, or moist surfaces, both during the patient exam and when handling specimens.

- Instruct symptomatic patients to maintain respiratory hygiene/cough etiquette by covering their mouth and nose with a tissue when coughing; using tissues and disposing

of them in a no-touch receptacle; observing hand hygiene; and wearing a surgical mask or maintaining a distance of greater than 3 feet if possible. See the chapter *Infection Control Practices* for more information about respiratory hygiene/cough etiquette.

- Wear a mask in the presence of a patient suspected of having an infectious disease that is transmitted by airborne droplets, such as tuberculosis (TB) or meningitis.

- Patients with highly contagious infectious diseases, such as diphtheria or chickenpox, must be examined under isolation precautions, such as in a private room. Wear personal protective equipment (PPE) during contact. Table 38-1 provides a summary of necessary PPE based on specific diseases. Refer to the chapter *Infection Control Practices* for additional information.

- Discard in biohazardous waste containers all disposable equipment and supplies that come in contact with a patient's blood or body fluids.

- Clean and disinfect the exam room following each patient's exam.

- Sanitize, disinfect, and sterilize equipment, as appropriate, after each patient's exam.

▶ Preparing the Patient for an Exam LO 38.4

As a medical assistant, you will need to prepare the patient both emotionally and physically.

Emotional Preparation

To prepare patients, begin by explaining exactly what will occur during the exam. Use simple, direct language that patients can understand. Describe what patients can expect to feel and how their cooperation can contribute to the procedure's success. As discussed in the *Assisting in Pediatrics* chapter, emotional preparedness is particularly important when dealing with children, who deserve to have the same sort of information and reassurance as adults. Mature adults may require special attention to communication during emotional preparation, as discussed in the *Assisting in Geriatrics* chapter.

If you are a male medical assistant, a female licensed practitioner may ask you to remain in the room when she examines a male patient. Likewise, if you are a female medical assistant, a male licensed practitioner may ask you to remain in the room when he examines a female patient. These measures are for the protection of both the patient and the physician. Such policies depend on the standard procedures in each medical practice or facility.

Physical Preparation

To ensure that the patient is physically prepared before the physician enters the exam room, give the patient an opportunity to empty his bladder and/or bowels in order to be more comfortable during the exam. Collect a urine specimen at this time, if needed.

Ensure that the room temperature is comfortable, and when the patient is ready, ask him to disrobe and put on an exam gown or cover himself with a drape. The extent of disrobing depends

TABLE 38-1 PPE for Infection and Precaution Type

Infection	Precaution Type	Appropriate PPE
Abscess	Contact	Gloves and gown
AIDS	Standard	Use appropriate PPE when exposed to blood or body fluids
Anthrax	Airborne/contact	Respirator (or mask and goggles) and gloves
Chickenpox (varicella)	Airborne/contact	Respirator (or mask and goggles) and gloves
Diphtheria • Cutaneous • Pharyngeal	Contact droplet	Gloves and gown Mask and goggles when working within 3 feet of patient
Gastroenteritis	Standard/contact	Use appropriate PPE when exposed to blood or body fluids; avoid contact with fecal material by donning gloves and gown
Hepatitis • A • B • C • E	 Contact Standard Standard Standard	 Gloves and gown Use appropriate PPE when exposed to blood or body fluids Use appropriate PPE when exposed to blood or body fluids Use appropriate PPE when exposed to blood or body fluids
Herpes zoster (shingles)	Contact	Gloves and gown; *note:* individuals who have not had chickenpox should avoid contact with patients with shingles
Influenza	Droplet	Mask and goggles when working within 3 feet of patient
Measles	Airborne	Mask and goggles or respirator
Meningitis	Standard/droplet	Use appropriate PPE when exposed to blood or body fluids; use mask and goggles when working within 3 feet of patient
Mumps	Droplet	Mask and goggles when working within 3 feet of patient
Pertussis	Droplet	Mask and goggles when working within 3 feet of patient
Poliomyelitis	Standard	Use appropriate PPE when exposed to blood or body fluids
Rotavirus	Contact	Gloves and gown
Rubella	Droplet	Mask and goggles when working within 3 feet of patient
Scabies	Contact	Gloves and gown
Staphylococcal disease	Contact	Gloves and gown
Streptococcal disease	Contact/droplet	Gloves, gown, mask, and goggles
Tuberculosis	Airborne	Mask and goggles or respirator

on the type of exam and the physician's preference. If the physician requests a gown for the patient, show the patient how to put on the gown. Include specific instructions on whether the gown should open in the back or front and whether it should be left open or tied. Leave the exam room while the patient disrobes to give him privacy, unless he needs and requests assistance.

Be aware of the patient's modesty and comfort at all times. Imagine what it feels like to visit a physician and, as you disrobe and put on the gown, you notice that it is too small and it's beginning to tear. In order to ensure patient comfort, make sure a variety of sizes are available for patient use. Use your critical thinking skills when selecting a patient gown. Your patient will remember this gesture and appreciate your consideration.

▶ Positioning and Draping   LO 38.5

During the exam, the patient may need to assume a variety of positions, which facilitate the physician's exam of certain areas of the body. The physician will indicate which positions are needed for specific exams. You may need to help the patient assume these positions. Depending upon the patient's mobility (ability to move), you may need to help transfer, lift, and move the patient. To protect yourself from injury when helping to position a patient, always follow the basic rules of good **body mechanics.** Body mechanics is the application of physical principles to help prevent stress and injury to healthcare practitioners who are lifting, moving, and positioning patients:

- Lifting with your strongest muscles, including your legs and arms, rather than your back.
- Keeping your feet apart.
- Bending from the hip and knees.

The steps for practicing good body mechanics while lifting and moving heavy objects are described in Procedure 38-1 at the end of this chapter.

Some positions are embarrassing or physically uncomfortable for patients. If you perceive embarrassment, explain the need for the position and help the patient assume the position when

exam. He may palpate the area first to locate the correct anatomical landmarks for placing the stethoscope. He may use percussion to check the heart's size. The patient should not speak while the physician auscultates the heart sounds with the stethoscope. The physician notes the heart's rate, rhythm, intensity, and pitch.

Breasts

During a general physical exam, every woman should have a complete breast exam to check for signs of cancer. The physician begins the exam with the patient in a sitting position. The physician asks the patient to hold her arms at her sides while he inspects the breasts for symmetry, contour, masses, and retracted areas. He then asks the patient to raise her arms above her head while he palpates the lymph nodes under her arms.

Next, the physician asks the patient to lie down and place her hand under her head on the first side to be examined. (The physician may ask you to place a small pillow or folded towel under the patient's shoulder blade on the same side.) This procedure allows the breast tissue to flatten evenly against the chest wall, permitting easier palpation. The physician then palpates the breast in a circular, systematic manner to check for lumps; examines the areola and nipple; and then repeats the procedure on the other side.

The breasts of men are also checked. When examining male patients, the physician palpates the patient's breasts and lymph nodes in the same manner that he does with his female patients. He also checks the breasts for lesions or swelling.

Abdomen

The physician examines the patient's abdomen while the patient is in a supine position with arms down at the sides. The abdominal muscles should be completely relaxed for this part of the exam. The physician may ask you to place a small pillow under the patient's head or knees (or both) to help keep the abdomen relaxed. If the patient is wearing a gown, it is raised to just under the breasts. If the patient is draped, the drape must be lowered to just above the genitalia to allow a complete view of the area. A separate drape should be placed to cover a female patient's breasts.

The order of exam methods for the abdomen should be followed correctly. The physician begins with inspection and auscultation, followed by percussion and palpation. Following this order allows the physician to listen to bowel sounds before palpating the abdominal organs. Palpation of the abdominal area can change bowel sounds in such a way that the physician could misdiagnose a patient's condition.

The physician begins with an inspection of the abdominal skin's color and surface and follows with an inspection of the abdomen's shape and symmetry. He then uses auscultation to check bowel and vascular sounds and uses percussion to note the size and position of the organs. Finally, he uses palpation to check muscle tone and to determine the presence of any tenderness or masses.

The physician describes observations based on a system of landmarks that map out the abdominal region. The abdomen is typically divided into four equal sections, or **quadrants.** Some physicians divide the abdomen into nine sections,

similar to a tic-tac-toe board. For example, if a patient has had her appendix removed, the physician might note that the patient has an abdominal scar on the right lower quadrant.

Female Genitalia

Female patients may feel self-conscious or anxious in the lithotomy position—most commonly used during examination of the genitalia. The medical assistant may help the patient relax during this procedure to assist the patient in maintaining the position. The procedure for a gynecologic exam is described in detail in the *Assisting in Reproductive and Urinary Specialties* chapter.

Male Genitalia

During the genitalia exam, men may be just as embarrassed or uncomfortable as women. If the physician performing the assessment is female, a male medical assistant, if available, should be in the room to protect both the patient and the physician from potential lawsuits.

The procedure begins with the patient in the supine position. The physician puts on gloves and visually inspects the patient's penis for signs of infection or structural abnormalities, palpating any lesions. The physician then examines the scrotum in the same manner, palpating the testicles for lumps. The patient is asked to stand while the physician checks for any bulges in the groin that may indicate a hernia. At the same time, the physician palpates the local lymph nodes to check for any abnormality.

Rectum

The physician usually examines the rectum after examining the genitalia. You may need to assist an adult patient into a dorsal recumbent or Sims' position. Female patients may already be in the lithotomy position for this exam. The physician normally examines a child when the child is in the prone position and inspects only the external areas of the rectum.

In adults, the physician may perform a **digital examination** to palpate the rectum for lesions or irregularities. Physicians recommend that patients older than age 40 have a yearly digital examination for early detection of colorectal cancer. For this exam, the physician puts on a clean pair of gloves. You may assist by applying lubricant to the physician's gloved index finger before the exam begins.

After performing the procedure, the physician may request that any stool found on the glove be tested for the presence of occult blood using a guaiac-based fecal occult blood test. The presence of occult blood in the stool is a possible indication of colorectal cancer or gastrointestinal bleeding. This test—often called by its brand name, Hemoccult® or Seracult® test—involves placing a sample of stool on a cardboard slide. You assist by presenting the slide to the physician. To produce an accurate test, three consecutive bowel movements are tested; this sample is usually the first. After the exam, you may be responsible for instructing the patient on how to collect the additional two samples. The procedure is outlined on the package of the occult blood-testing kit and in the *Collecting, Processing, and Testing Urine and Stool Specimens* chapter.

15. Still kee|
body me
back int

16. Unlock t

PROCE

Procedure
the various po

OSHA Guideli

Materials:
stepstool, exa

Method:

1. Identify

2. Wash yc

3. Explain

4. Provide
one, ani
after dis
and ass
RATION
patient
efficient

5. Explain
position

6. Ask the
the exa
the exa

7. Assist tl

a. *Sittir*
canr

b. *Supi*
patie
brea
head

c. *Dors*
som
patie

d. *Litho*
geni
Assi
neai
larg

e. *Fow*
ang
tabl
whic

f. *Pror*
It is

After the rectal exam, offer the patient the opportunity to clean the anal area before you adjust the drape. Dispose of gloves and soiled materials in a biohazardous waste container.

Musculoskeletal System

If the physician did not examine the patient's back during the chest exam, he does so during the musculoskeletal assessment. The physician checks for good posture from the back and side. He may ask the patient to walk so he can assess her gait. The physician always asks a child to bend at the waist so that he can check for the presence of **scoliosis,** a lateral curvature of the spine.

During the musculoskeletal assessment, the physician determines range of motion, the strength of various muscle groups, and body measurements. The physician also examines the arms, hands, legs, and feet for any lesions, deformities, or circulatory problems.

The physician checks a patient's range of motion to detect joint deformities and to learn whether the patient has any limitations in movement caused by an injury or other conditions, such as arthritis. Checking a patient's range of motion also allows the physician to follow a patient's progress during recovery from an injury or surgery.

Neurologic System

The physician's neurologic assessment includes an evaluation of the patient's reflexes, mental and emotional status (including intelligence, speech, and behavior), and sensory and motor functions. The physician often performs the neurologic assessment at the same time as the musculoskeletal assessment because both systems are involved in movement and coordination.

The physician may incorporate certain aspects of the neurologic assessment into other parts of the exam. For example, testing how a patient's pupils react to light is part of an eye exam, but because this test also examines the patient's light reflex, the test includes a neurologic assessment as

well. To check reflexes, the physician uses a reflex hammer to tap tendons in different areas of the patient's body.

Most exams of children also include an intellectual assessment, in which the physician asks the child general questions appropriate to the child's age. Physicians also may test the mental status and memory of older adults to detect disorders such as senility and Alzheimer's disease in patients who show signs of confusion or complain of memory loss.

▶ After the Exam   LO 38.9

After the physician completes the exam, you should assist in making the patient comfortable. Help her into a sitting position; then allow her to perform any necessary self-hygiene. Additionally, tests and procedures may be ordered. Depending upon what is ordered, you will complete them either before the patient dresses or after she is dressed. In addition, you may be responsible for patient education as well as follow-up care based on the physician's recommendations.

Additional Tests and Procedures

Post-exam procedures may include taking body fat measurements, obtaining blood samples, or preparing the patient for a diagnostic or therapeutic procedure, such as an X-ray, ECG, or physical therapy session. Other procedures medical assistants may perform before the patient dresses include administering cold or heat therapy, applying a bandage, collecting specimens, and administering certain medications.

If the physician has not ordered any additional procedures—or if wearing clothing does not interfere with the procedures ordered—the patient may dress. Help the patient get off the examining table and allow her to dress in privacy. Make sure she knows you are available to assist if she needs help dressing. Tests and procedures that can be done after the patient has dressed include urinalysis, pulmonary function tests, administration of oral medications, and eye or ear irrigation or medication administration. Finally, perform any patient

---

EDUCATING THE PATIENT

Assessing and Responding to Patient Educational Needs

The general physical exam provides you with the opportunity to assess the patient's educational needs. Based on the findings of the patient's interview, history, and exam, you may identify areas in which the patient will benefit from additional education.

Risk Factors

Pay special attention to educating patients about risk factors for disease. For example, women are often instructed about the risk factors for breast cancer and men are instructed about the risk factors for prostate cancer.

Self-Help and Diagnostic Techniques

The physician also may request that you teach patients how to administer certain medications or how to perform self-help

or diagnostic techniques. These procedures may involve collecting samples for occult blood testing or urine testing, applying cold or hot packs, or instilling eye drops. It is important to teach the patient the correct way to perform a diagnostic test. If a specimen is incorrectly obtained, the test results will be inaccurate.

Regardless of the type of instruction, be sure to address patients at a language level they can understand without talking down to them. To ensure that they understand fully, ask patients to repeat each instruction and to perform each demonstration. Give patients written instructions they can refer to at home.

Follow-Up

After the exam, you
of the physician's re
these actions:

- Scheduling the pa
- Making outside a
  such as mammog
  for therapeutic pr
- Helping the patie
  nursing care after

PROCEDU

Procedure Goal
ics when lifting or m
objects

OSHA Guidelines: Th
to blood, body fluids,

Materials: Wheelc
books or other heavy

Method:

Lifting a Heavy O

1. Stand with you
   inches apart. F
   and your shoul
   RATIONALE: M
   for using prope
2. Position your b
   lifted from the
3. Keeping your b
   from your hips
4. Lift the object,
   large muscles
   not to bend yo
   RATIONALE: Th
   than the muscl
   helps prevent r
5. Turn to face th
   back. Keep yo
6. Again using th
   weight, place t
   your arms to re
   table before pl

Moving a Heavy

7. Check to be su
   bed are firmly

---

21. Tell the patient you will lift on the count of 3 and ask the patient to support as much of her own weight as possible (if she is able).
22. At the count of 3, you should lift the patient together.
23. The stronger of the two of you should pivot the patient to bring the back of the patient's knees against the table.

PROCEDURE 38-5 Assisting with a General Physical Exam [WORK // DOC]

Procedure Goal: To effectively assist the physician with a general physical exam

OSHA Guidelines:

Materials: Supplies and equipment will vary depending on the type and purpose of the exam and the physician's practice preferences. Supplies may include the following: patient chart/progress note, gown, drape, adjustable examining table, gloves, laryngeal mirror, lubricant, nasal speculum, otoscope and ophthalmoscope, pillow, reflex hammer, tuning fork, sphygmomanometer, stethoscope, tape measure, tongue depressors, and a penlight

Method:

1. Wash your hands and adhere to standard precautions throughout the procedure.
   RATIONALE: *Safe, aseptic technique greatly reduces the transmission of an infectious disease.*
2. Gather and assemble the equipment and supplies.
3. Arrange the instruments and equipment in a logical sequence for the physician's use.

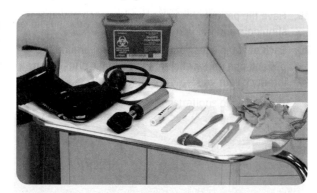

FIGURE Procedure 38-5 Step 3   Assemble and arrange equipment for a general physical exam.
©McGraw-Hill Education

4. Greet and properly identify the patient using at least two patient identifiers.
   RATIONALE: *To prevent treatment errors.*
5. Review the patient's medical history with the patient if office policy requires it.

---

24. Working together, gently lower the patient into a sitting position on the table. If the patient cannot sit unassisted, help her move into a supine position.
25. Move the wheelchair out of the way.
26. Assist the patient with disrobing as necessary, providing a gown and drape.

6. Obtain vital statistics according to the physician's preference.
7. Obtain the patient's weight and height (with shoes removed).
8. Obtain a urine specimen before the patient undresses for the exam.
9. Explain the procedure and exam to the patient.
   RATIONALE: *This builds the patient's confidence with the office and prepares the patient physically and emotionally.*
10. Obtain blood specimens or other laboratory tests according to the chart or verbal order.
11. Provide the patient with an appropriate gown and drape, and explain where the opening for the gown is placed.
12. Obtain the ECG if ordered by the physician.
13. Assist the patient to a sitting position at the end of the table with the drape placed across her legs.
14. Inform the physician the patient is ready and remain in the room to assist the physician.
15. You may be asked to shut off the light in the exam room to allow the patient's pupils to dilate sufficiently for a retinal exam.
16. Hand the instruments to the physician as requested.

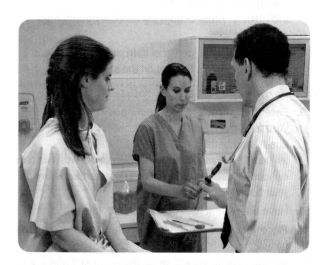

FIGURE Procedure 38-5 Step 16   Hand the instruments to the physician as needed.
©McGraw-Hill Education

17. Assist the patient to a supine position and drape her for an exam of the front of the body.

18. If a gynecologic exam is needed, assist and drape the patient in the lithotomy position.

19. If a rectal exam is needed, assist and drape the patient in the Sims' position.

20. Assist the patient to a prone position for a posterior body exam.

21. When the exam is complete, assist the patient to a sitting position and ask the patient to sit for a brief period of time.
RATIONALE: *Some patients experience dizziness when they first sit up.*

22. Ask the patient if she needs assistance in dressing.

23. After the patient has left, dispose of contaminated materials in an appropriate container.

24. Remove the table paper and pillow covering and dispose of them in the proper container.

25. Disinfect and clean the counters and the examining table.

26. Sanitize and sterilize the instruments, if needed.

27. Prepare the room for the next patient by replacing the table paper, pillowcase, equipment, and supplies.

28. Document the procedure (refer to Progress Note).

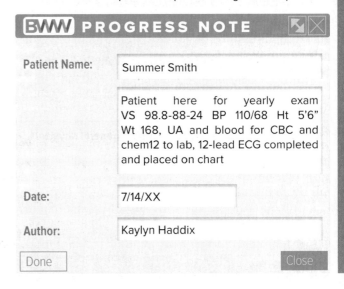

BWW PROGRESS NOTE

Patient Name: Summer Smith

Patient here for yearly exam VS 98.8-88-24 BP 110/68 Ht 5'6" Wt 168, UA and blood for CBC and chem12 to lab, 12-lead ECG completed and placed on chart

Date: 7/14/XX

Author: Kaylyn Haddix

Done   Close

SUMMARY OF LEARNING OUTCOMES

OUTCOME	KEY POINTS
38.1 Identify the purpose of a general physical exam.	A general physical exam is done either to confirm an overall state of health or to examine a patient to diagnose a medical problem.
38.2 Describe the role of the medical assistant in a general physical exam.	The medical assistant assists the patient and the physician during an exam. Making the patient physically and emotionally comfortable as well as providing materials and assistance to the physician are essential to a successful exam.
38.3 Explain safety precautions used during a general physical exam.	During an exam, the medical assistant should perform hand hygiene, wear gloves and other personal protective equipment, ensure respiratory hygiene/cough etiquette, use isolation precautions, dispose of biohazardous waste, and clean and disinfect the exam room as necessary to provide for safety.
38.4 Carry out the steps necessary to prepare the patient for an exam.	The medical assistant should prepare the patient for an exam emotionally, by using simple direct language, and physically, by providing for the patient's comfort and privacy when positioning him or her according to the type of exam or procedure and by modifying techniques to meet the needs of special patients.
38.5 Carry out positioning and draping a patient in each of the nine common exam positions.	The nine common exam positions include sitting, supine, dorsal recumbent, lithotomy, Fowler's, prone, Sims', knee-chest/knee-elbow, and proctologic.
38.6 Apply techniques to assist patients from different cultures and patients with physical disabilities.	When assisting with the physical exam, avoid judging and stereotyping patients from different cultures and obtain a translator for proper communication if necessary. Assist patients who have physical disabilities with transfers and other tasks they cannot accomplish themselves.

OUTCOME	KEY POINTS
38.7 Identify the six examination methods used in a general physical exam.	The six examination methods used in a general physical exam include inspection, auscultation, palpation, percussion, mensuration, and manipulation.
38.8 List the components of a general physical exam.	A general physical exam typically includes an evaluation of the general appearance, head, neck, eyes, ears, nose and sinuses, mouth and throat, chest and lungs, heart, breasts, abdomen, genitalia, rectum, musculoskeletal system, and neurologic system.
38.9 Describe follow-up steps after a general physical exam.	In order to assist the patient with follow-up after the exam, you may schedule future visits, schedule visits outside of the office, help plan for home care, and, if within your scope of practice, provide education related to the patient's condition.

CASE STUDY CRITICAL THINKING

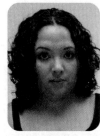

©McGraw-Hill Education

Recall Valarie Ramirez from the case study at the beginning of the chapter. Now that you have completed the chapter, answer the following questions regarding her case.

1. What things will you do during Valarie Ramirez's exam to make her more comfortable?

2. In which positions will she most likely be put during her examination, and why would these positions be used?

3. Because Valarie Ramirez is overweight, what position may be used for the gynecological exam if the lithotomy position is too uncomfortable or difficult for her?

4. If you were unable to communicate with Valarie Ramirez successfully, what measures should you take to improve communication and meet her privacy needs?

EXAM PREPARATION QUESTIONS

1. (LO 38.7) When the physician uses a stethoscope to listen to body sounds, he is performing
   a. Auscultation
   b. Percussion
   c. Inspection
   d. Palpation
   e. Mensuration

2. (LO 38.3) Which safety measure should the medical assistant perform with every patient?
   a. Wear gloves
   b. Use isolation precautions
   c. Perform hand hygiene
   d. Transfer the patient to the exam table
   e. Place all waste in a biohazardous container

3. (LO 38.5) Which of the following positions would be used to examine the female genitalia?
   a. Prone
   b. Sims'
   c. Fowler's

   d. Proctologic
   e. Lithotomy

4. (LO 38.1) The patient is complaining of pain in her left foot. This would be considered a
   a. Sign
   b. Symptom
   c. Prognosis
   d. Clinical diagnosis
   e. Differential diagnosis

5. (LO 38.2) You are asked to do all of the following during a general physical exam. Which one is outside your scope of practice?
   a. Prepare the instruments and supplies
   b. Give the patient a pillow while the physician conducts the exam
   c. Determine the vital signs, height, and weight
   d. Provide the patient with emotional support
   e. Check the patient's abdomen when he complains of pain

6. (LO 38.4) What would be your best response to a nervous, young female patient who is going to have a general physical exam by a male physician when she asks, "Will this hurt?"
   a. An exam is not painful; you don't need to worry.
   b. No, you just have to lie still; I will be here with you the whole time.
   c. Yes, you can expect a lot of pain, but I will be here with you the whole time.
   d. You won't have any discomfort; Dr. Buckwalter is very gentle.
   e. The exam may be uncomfortable at times, but I will be here to help keep you comfortable.

7. (LO 38.6) When assisting with a patient from another culture during an exam, which of the following would *least* likely be necessary?
   a. Extra drapes
   b. Translator
   c. Wheelchair
   d. Direct demonstrations
   e. Thorough explanations

8. (LO 38.8) What is the purpose of a digital examination?
   a. To check for blood in the urine
   b. To determine if a female patient has breast cancer
   c. To check for rectal lesions or irregularities
   d. To locate a landmark on the abdomen
   e. To listen to the patient's breathing

9. (LO 38.9) Which of the following would *not* be one of your duties after the physician has completed a general physical exam?
   a. Schedule a future visit to check the blood pressure
   b. Administer a medication
   c. Provide patient education
   d. Document a chief complaint
   e. Help the family plan for in-home care

10. (LO 38.3) A patient is suspected of having TB. What PPE should you wear?
    a. Mask only
    b. Mask and goggles when working within 3 feet of the patient
    c. Gown and gloves
    d. Gloves, gown, mask, and goggles
    e. Mask and goggles or respirator

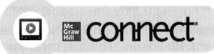

Go to CONNECT to see a video exercise about *Communicating Effectively with Patients from Other Cultures and Meeting Their Needs for Privacy.*

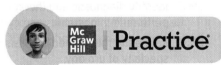

Go to CONNECT to complete the EHRclinic exercise: 38.01 Record a Patient's Physical Exam (PE) in an EHR.

SOFT SKILLS SUCCESS

A 59-year-old female patient who has generalized weakness in her extremities and is in a wheelchair has arrived at the office for her yearly physical. She is here for a pelvic exam, which will require her to be placed in the lithotomy position.

1. What would you say to the patient when you enter the room to prepare her for the examination?

2. Once you transfer her to the examination table, she blushes and does not seem willing to be placed in the correct position. What should you do?

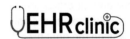

Go to PRACTICE MEDICAL OFFICE and complete the module Clinical: Interactions.

Menopause

Menopause, like menstruation, is a natural occurrence. It is the cessation (the end) of the menstrual cycle. Menopause usually occurs between ages 45 and 55. Several stages surround menopause. Premenopause is the time period before menopause, during which hormonal changes may be occurring but no changes are felt by the woman. The time just before and after menopause is called perimenopause. During perimenopause, a woman may experience irregular periods, hot flashes, and vaginal dryness, all caused by changing levels of estrogen. Because hormonal change is occurring, the woman may experience mood swings or other psychological changes. Menopause also can be brought on by the surgical removal of the uterus and ovaries, known as a hysterectomy and discussed in *section 39.3* of this chapter. The symptoms and treatment for menopause are the same for both surgical and naturally occurring menopause.

The Gynecologic Exam

The gynecologic exam is intended to provide an overview of a woman's health and to perform important cancer-screening exams and tests. The American College of Obstetricians and Gynecologists (ACOG) has specific recommendations regarding when a woman should have a gynecologic exam and tests related to the female reproductive system. These recommendations are outlined in Table 39-1.

During the exam, a female medical assistant should be in the exam room to assist a male licensed practitioner. In this case, the medical assistant can act as a witness to provide legal protection. Your role during the exam is similar to that for the general physical exam. In this role, you will complete the following:

TABLE 39-1	ACOG Examination and Screening Recommendations	
Age	**Exam(s) Needed**	**Frequency**
13–18	Chlamydia and gonorrhea screening	When sexually active
13–18	HIV screening	When sexually active (follow state's screening requirements)
21–29	Pelvic exam and cervical cytology	Every three years
<25	Chlamydia and gonorrhea screening	When sexually active
>30	Pelvic exam, cervical cytology and HPV	Co-test every 5 years; option screen with cytology every three years
>25	HIV screening	FDA-approved test alternative test to cytology
>40	Colorectal cancer and diabetes screening, lipid profile and mammography	Frequency and start year vary. See current guidelines at www.acog.org
>65	Bone mineral density screening	Every 2 years
>66	Pelvic exam, cervical cytology and HPV	Discontinue after 3 normal tests under certain conditions

- Ask the patient to empty her bladder; if a urine specimen is needed, it should be collected at this time.
- Provide the patient with a gown before the exam and give her privacy while she changes.
- During the interview, discuss her gynecologic and general health and inquire about any changes in appetite, weight, or emotional status.
- Observe for signs of problems such as substance abuse, sexually transmitted infections, or domestic violence. It is crucial that you bring to the licensed practitioner's attention any clues you notice during your interview. See the *Caution: Handle with Care* feature Detecting Domestic Violence.
- Determine the first day of her **last menstrual period (LMP).**
- Have the patient sit on the examining table while you check her vital signs. For accurate results, keep the patient's arm elevated during the blood pressure measurement. For example, you may have her rest her arm on your shoulder.

The Licensed Practitioner's Interview

The gynecologic physical exam is more than an internal pelvic exam. It is an evaluation of the patient's total health and a review of factors that could be an indication of possible cancer or sexually transmitted infections (STIs). STIs, previously known as STDs (sexually transmitted diseases), are discussed in *section 39.6* of this chapter and in the chapter *The Reproductive Systems*. The licensed practitioner asks questions about the patient's menstrual cycle and about any abnormal discharge or discomfort during sexual intercourse. These questions help the licensed practitioner determine what tests need to be ordered. The licensed practitioner also examines the breasts and listens to the patient's heart and lungs before beginning the gynecologic exam.

Breast Exam

While reviewing the patient's chart, the licensed practitioner checks to see when the last mammogram was performed. He also will ask the patient about any other concerns or changes in her breasts. Because the breast self-exam is now an optional screening tool for breast cancer, the physician may or may not ask whether she knows how to perform a breast self-exam (BSE) and how often she is performing this exam. The licensed practitioner will then perform a clinical breast exam (CBE) by examining the patient's breasts and underarm areas to check for abnormal lumps that could be cancerous.

Patients must understand the need for regular breast exams including mammograms (discussed in *section 39.3* of this chapter), clinical breast exams, optional breast self-exams, and additional tests, if needed. When interviewing the patient and after the exam, you should take a moment to emphasize the following breast cancer detection guidelines of the American Cancer Society and National Cancer Institute for women with average risk of breast cancer:

- A yearly screening mammogram is optional between ages 40 and 44.
- Women ages 45 to 54 should have screening mammograms every year.

Detecting Domestic Violence

Licensed practitioners and medical assistants are in a position to detect signs of domestic violence. These signs can be seen in unusual bruising or injuries that the patient may try to hide or excuse. You may hear signs in a patient's tone of voice or choice of words during a conversation in the office or over the telephone. Many times patients who are abused blame themselves. When the patient's injuries do not match his or her story, this may indicate the possibility of abuse. Observe the male or female who constantly answers questions for his or her partner. You play an important role in noticing these signs, and you must inform the licensed practitioner of any signs that you detect.

You also must create a supportive office environment in which the patient can seek help. Encourage the licensed practitioner to join the American Medical Association's National Coalition of Physicians Against Family Violence if not already a member. This organization provides posters—which often help patients feel encouraged to discuss domestic violence—in addition to pamphlets and other information. Reporting suspected domestic violence is mandatory in some states. You should have a folder that contains lists of the phone numbers for domestic violence hotlines, women's shelters, and other helpful resources. You can offer the following general guidelines to women:

- Ignoring the problem never works—silence does not help anyone.
- Understand that abusive family members may not be able to help themselves.
- Call for help if a physical threat exists.

- At age 55, women have the option to continue with yearly mammograms or to have one every other year. In either case, women should continue having mammograms as long as they are in good health.
- Women should know how their breasts normally look and feel and report any breast change promptly to their healthcare provider. A breast self-exam is an option for women starting in their 20s.
- Women with a family history of breast cancer, a genetic tendency for breast cancer, or certain other factors should be screened with an MRI in addition to mammograms. Less than 2% of all the women in the United States fall into this category.

For women who have above-average risk for breast cancer, screening should begin at age 30 with both a mammogram and a screening MRI and should continue as long as they are in good health. These women include those who have a BRCA1 or BRCA2 gene mutation or who have a close family member with this mutation, those who had radiation therapy to the chest between the ages of 10 and 30 years, or those who have certain health syndromes.

In some cases, you may be asked to instruct the patient in performing the BSE. Review the *Educating the Patient* feature How to Perform a Breast Self-Exam.

Pelvic Exam

During the pelvic exam, the licensed practitioner checks the external genitalia, cervix, vaginal wall, internal reproductive organs, and rectum. Exam methods include palpation and inspection. Inspection is done with a **speculum,** which is an instrument that expands the vaginal opening to permit viewing of the vagina and cervix (see Figure 39-1). The licensed practitioner wears gloves and may use a lubricant for patient comfort.

Your role is to assist the patient into position, with her feet in the stirrups of the examining table and her buttocks at the end of the table. Drape her so that only the area between the

---

How to Perform a Breast Self-Exam

The breast self-exam, although now considered an optional screening method for breast cancer, is still an important part of breast cancer prevention. As a medical assistant, you may be responsible for coaching the patient about the monthly breast self-exam. Check the office policy to see which of several methods it recommends for teaching BSE.

Consider the following when teaching the BSE:

1. Explain the purpose of the BSE. Make sure the patient knows that she should perform the BSE around the same date of each month after her period ends, if she is still menstruating. (At this time, the breasts are most normal and least swollen and lumpy.) Have the patient mark her calendar as a monthly reminder.

2. Emphasize that the BSE is not a substitute for mammograms or regular breast exams by a licensed practitioner.

3. Demonstrate the breast self-exam according to the method used at your facility. For example, the National Cancer Institute has established one method and provides the instructions on its Internet site.

4. Observe the patient's self-exam technique. (If the patient is reluctant to examine herself in front of you, have her repeat the highlights of the procedure or use the synthetic model.)

5. Review and reinforce teaching as needed. Provide patient educational materials that explain how to perform the BSE.

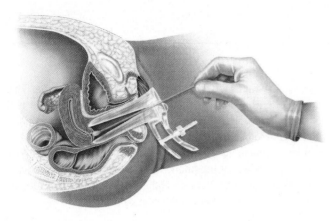

FIGURE 39-1 A speculum is used to expand the vaginal opening to help view the vagina and cervix and obtain specimens.

thighs is exposed. Assist the licensed practitioner by having gloves and instruments ready for use and by applying lubricant, if indicated, to the licensed practitioner's gloved fingers.

You also may warm the speculum for the patient's comfort. Be prepared to provide reassurance and explanation to a patient who appears to be uncomfortable or nervous. Encourage her to breathe deeply to help relax the pelvic muscles and reduce discomfort. After checking the vagina and cervix and while the speculum is still in place, the licensed practitioner obtains a specimen. The most common type of specimen the licensed practitioner will obtain is a Papanicolaou (Pap) smear. A specimen may also be taken to check for the human papillomavirus (HPV). These tests are discussed in *section 39.3* of this chapter.

Sometimes a sample is taken by the licensed practitioner to test for infections. These specimens are usually prepared by the medical assistant during the procedure and viewed by the licensed practitioner after the exam. To check for fungus, a sample may be mixed with potassium hydroxide (KOH) on a slide. The slide is viewed under a microscope. The KOH helps dissolve the cells and mucus in the sample so that the fungus

can be better visualized. A **wet mount** is prepared by mixing a sample with a saline solution. The slide is viewed to check for bacteria, yeast, and trichomoniasis. Trichomoniasis, commonly called "trich," is a vaginal infection caused by a microscopic organism and is transferred during sexual intercourse.

The licensed practitioner then removes the speculum and begins the bimanual phase of the exam. *Bimanual* means using two hands rather than the speculum. The practitioner may ask for your assistance in removing the examining gloves, putting on new gloves, and lubricating two fingers. Placing those fingers in the vagina and using the other hand to palpate the abdomen, the licensed practitioner assesses the position of the uterus. She may then place a lubricated finger in the rectum and palpate for abnormal growths with the other hand by pressing on the lower abdomen.

When the licensed practitioner completes the exam, she usually asks the patient if she has any questions or concerns. After the licensed practitioner leaves the exam room, be sure to ask the patient whether she has additional questions. You may need to provide written information in addition to answering the patient's questions orally. Materials are available from a variety of sources, including the AMA, government agencies, and pharmaceutical companies. The website of the National Women's Health Information Center is one excellent resource. See Procedure 39-1, at the end of this chapter, on how to assist with a gynecologic exam. The *Caution: Handle with Care* feature Guidelines for Cervical Specimen Collection and Submission provides information about how to ensure an adequate specimen for optimal screening.

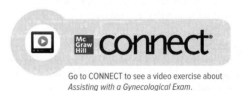

Go to CONNECT to see a video exercise about
Assisting with a Gynecological Exam.

CAUTION: HANDLE WITH CARE

Guidelines for Cervical Specimen Collection and Submission

In order to ensure that the cervical specimen collected is adequate for optimal screening, the American Society of Cytopathology has clinical guidelines for collecting patient information. As a medical assistant, you will be responsible for helping the licensed practitioner implement these guidelines, which include:

• Scheduling a patient appointment about 2 weeks after the patient's last menstrual period.

• Instructing patients not to douche; use tampons, foams, or jellies; or have sexual intercourse 48 hours prior to the test.

• Completing a lab requisition form, which includes the following information:

  • Patient name (note any recent name changes)

  • Date of birth

• Menstrual status (last menstrual period, hysterectomy, and so on)

• Any patient risk factors

• Specimen source

• Completing a specimen label, which includes the following materials and information:

  • Liquid samples

  • All requested information completed on the label and affixed to the vial

• Glass slide

  • Label the frosted end of the slide with the patient's first and last names.

Include an additional patient identifier, such as the patient record number.

Assisting with the Obstetric Patient

LO 39.2

When a woman discovers she is pregnant, one of the first things she wants to know is the baby's due date. One simple method to estimate the delivery date for a pregnant woman is called Nägele's rule. Begin with the first day of the patient's last menstrual period, subtract 3 months, and add 7 days plus 1 year. For example, if the first day of the last menstrual period was June 30, 2017, subtracting 3 months would give you March 30, 2017. After the addition of 7 days plus 1 year, April 6, 2018, would be the estimated delivery date.

Prenatal Care

Pregnant women should be attentive to nutrition, exercise, medical monitoring, and childbirth classes. They should avoid using tobacco, alcohol, and drugs. Normal changes occur during pregnancy, such as morning sickness (usually in the first trimester), weight gain, urinary frequency, fatigue, depression, constipation, and swollen hands and feet. Review Figure 39-2 and Table 39-2 regarding the trimesters of pregnancy and what changes may be expected.

You may perform or assist with routine tests for pregnant women, or you may send them to an outside laboratory. These tests include the complete blood count (CBC), Rh-antibody determination, blood typing, Pap smear, urinalysis, and hematocrit, as well as tests for syphilis (rapid plasma reagin, or RPR), hepatitis B antibodies, HIV, and chlamydia.

Encouraging the obstetric patient to have regular checkups and to take proper care of herself may be part of your job. Prenatal visits become more frequent as the pregnancy

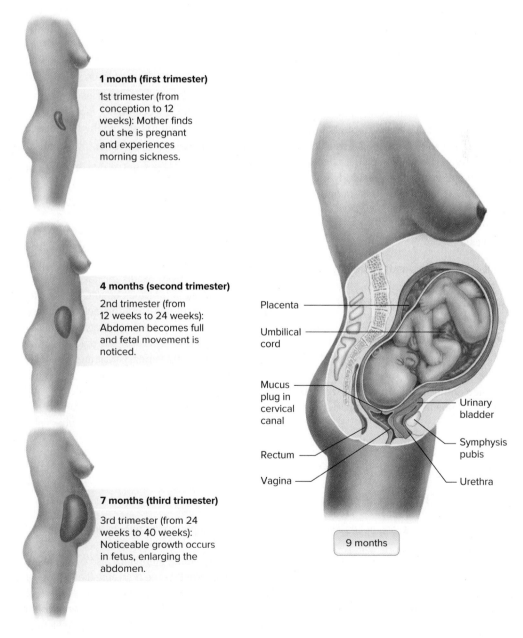

1 month (first trimester)

1st trimester (from conception to 12 weeks): Mother finds out she is pregnant and experiences morning sickness.

4 months (second trimester)

2nd trimester (from 12 weeks to 24 weeks): Abdomen becomes full and fetal movement is noticed.

7 months (third trimester)

3rd trimester (from 24 weeks to 40 weeks): Noticeable growth occurs in fetus, enlarging the abdomen.

Placenta
Umbilical cord
Mucus plug in cervical canal
Rectum
Vagina
Urinary bladder
Symphysis pubis
Urethra

9 months

FIGURE 39-2   The fetus develops over the course of three trimesters.

TABLE 39-2 Changes During Pregnancy

Stage of Pregnancy	Normal Changes	Possible Complications
1st trimester (weeks 1 to 12)	Missed period, fatigue, morning sickness, frequent urination, moodiness, heartburn, constipation, swollen and tender breasts	Ectopic pregnancy—severe dizziness with vaginal bleeding and abdominal pain
2nd trimester (weeks 12 to 24)	Weight gain up to 4 pounds a month; fetal movement around 16 weeks; stretched, enlarging breasts; back, pelvis, and hip pain; mild contractions known as Braxton Hicks or "false labor"	Deep vein thrombosis—blood clot in a leg vein causing pain and swelling Preterm labor—painful uterine contractions that have a regular pattern and don't go away with movement
3rd trimester (weeks 24 to 40)	Unable to sleep on back; leg cramps; frequent urination; strange dreams; nasal congestion; heartburn; constipation; hemorrhoids; varicose veins; puffiness, especially the feet	Pregnancy-induced hypertension—extreme swelling of the hands and face, headache, blurred vision

progresses. Unless complications occur, a typical schedule for prenatal visits includes:

- An initial prenatal visit.
- Monthly visits during the 2nd trimester.
- Visits every other week during the 3rd trimester up to 36 weeks' gestation.
- Once-a-week visits from 36 weeks until delivery.

In addition to assisting with prenatal examinations, you also may help teach and support both parents throughout the pregnancy. You must document all information given to or taken from the patient. Providing information on the effects of using drugs or alcohol during pregnancy is particularly important. See the *Caution: Handle with Care* feature Alcohol and Drugs During Pregnancy.

The following are your responsibilities when assisting with routine prenatal patient visits:

- Ask the patient about any problems and record any symptoms she reports.
- Ask the patient to empty her bladder and obtain a urine specimen in the cup you provide.
- Weigh the patient and note her weight in the chart.
- Perform the reagent urine test (chemical analysis) and note the results in her chart.
- Give the patient a drape and ask her to undress from the waist down if the licensed practitioner will be performing an internal exam.

- Assist the patient to the examining table. Some positions (such as the prone—on the stomach—and lithotomy—on the back with the feet up—positions) are not recommended for a pregnant patient, especially during late stages of pregnancy. Other positions also may be difficult or impossible for a pregnant woman to achieve.
- Take her vital signs. Record them in her chart.
- Assist the licensed practitioner as needed with the exam. Provide the flexible centimeter tape measure and Doppler, an instrument used to listen to the fetal heartbeat.
- Assist the patient from the examining table after the exam.

Procedure 39-2, at the end of this chapter, outlines steps to take that ensure that a pregnant woman's needs are addressed during an exam.

Prenatal Care by the Licensed Practitioner

The licensed practitioner carefully monitors the progress of a pregnancy. She monitors the patient's blood pressure, weight changes, and urinalysis results for possible signs of preeclampsia. Preeclampsia is a serious condition that can occur during pregnancy. Signs of this condition include increased blood pressure (hypertension), unusual weight gain because of edema, and protein in the urine. The licensed practitioner examines urine specimens for possible urinary tract infections (UTIs) and occasionally asks for other laboratory tests, such as a CBC. She may prescribe special vitamins and iron as dietary supplements.

During the prenatal period, the licensed practitioner will monitor for many conditions, including placenta previa,

CAUTION: HANDLE WITH CARE

Alcohol and Drugs During Pregnancy

Everything a pregnant woman eats, drinks, or smokes will affect her developing baby. Alcohol, for example, crosses the placental barrier and directly affects fetal development. Drinking alcohol during pregnancy can cause fetal alcohol syndrome (FAS). This syndrome may include fetal growth deficiencies, mental retardation or learning disabilities, heart defects, cleft palate, a small head, a small brain, and deformed limbs. Preventing FAS

by teaching all pregnant patients about the potential effects of alcohol on their unborn babies is crucial.

Drugs used during pregnancy also can pose problems for the unborn fetus. Whether the drugs are illegal, over-the-counter, or prescription, pregnant women should be aware of the potential effects. See the chapter *Principles of Pharmacology* for information about prescription drug pregnancy labeling.

abruptio placenta, and gestational diabetes. Placenta previa is indicated by bright red vaginal bleeding that is painless. Abruptio placenta is a more serious condition that includes vaginal bleeding and back and abdominal pain. Gestational diabetes is indicated by an increase in glucose in the blood or urine.

Labor

When working in an OB/GYN office, you will need to know the signs of labor and when to tell the patient to go to the hospital. Most practices provide patient instructions regarding when to seek medical care and procedures to follow if they believe they are in labor. For example, most patients will be told to go to the hospital if they are having regular contractions—six or more per hour for at least 2 hours. Also, a sudden surge of fluid from the uterus indicates that the "water broke," which signals impending labor and requires the patient to go to the delivering healthcare facility.

Delivery

Delivery of an infant is typically through the vagina. After the labor process and delivery, the licensed practitioner clamps, ties, and cuts the umbilical cord and presents the baby to the mother. Women either go into labor spontaneously or may need to have their labor induced. **Induction** of labor means that the patient is admitted to the delivering healthcare facility, then given medication to start uterine contractions. If labor is spontaneous, most women go to the delivering facility as directed by their licensed practitioner. However, the medical assistant may need to schedule inductions at the delivering healthcare facility.

If the pregnant woman cannot deliver the baby vaginally, the licensed practitioner may deliver the baby by performing an operation known as a cesarean section, or C-section. Several conditions may require a cesarean section, such as a large baby or a breech position. Again, the medical assistant may need to schedule C-sections with the delivering healthcare facility.

Deliveries can be an emergency. Although not a common occurrence or a typical job responsibility for a medical assistant, if you are working in a busy obstetric practice, knowing the steps of emergency childbirth may be appropriate. You could be called upon to assist a physician during an in-office emergency delivery.

Breastfeeding

Human milk is the preferred form of nutrition for an infant. Colostrum, the first milk the mother produces after delivery, is rich in antibodies that provide passive natural immunity to the baby. Breastfeeding is economical and convenient. There is no need to buy or make formula or wash bottles and nipples. Breast milk is always available to the baby at the correct temperature.

A woman's success at breastfeeding depends largely on her desire to breastfeed, her satisfaction with it, and her available support systems. You can support patients who choose to breastfeed by providing them with pamphlets and other written materials. Emphasize how essential the mother's nutritional intake is, and explain that she needs to follow a high-protein, high-calorie diet. Patients who need help can be referred to lactation consultants or support groups such as the La Leche League.

Bottle Feeding

Bottle feeding is an acceptable alternative for women who choose not to breastfeed or are unable to breastfeed. There are several acceptable formulas available, including milk-based, soy-based, and special formulas for low-birth-weight infants. The type of formula is recommended by the licensed practitioner. If an infant is to be bottle-fed, parents must be given instruction about the type of formula and how to prepare it correctly. Regular, full-fat cow's milk should not be given to a child until after his or her first birthday.

Postpartum

Postpartum is a period after the delivery of an infant. During this time, women experience many changes and challenges as their body is trying to get back to normal. These include:

- Shrinking of the uterus back to its prepregnancy size, which typically takes about 6 weeks.
- Sharp abdominal pains, known as afterpains, that occur while the uterus is shrinking. These usually subside about the third day.
- Sore muscles of the arms, neck, or jaw for women who have labored and/or delivered vaginally.
- Difficulty with urination and bowel movements.
- Postpartum bleeding (lochia), which may last up to 4 weeks and can come and go up to 2 months.
- Recovery from a vaginal tear, episiotomy (surgical incision for a vaginal delivery), or abdominal incision for C-section.
- Pain that may occur from pelvic bone separation during vaginal delivery.
- Emotional stress related to coping with the physical changes and the needs of the new family.

The postpartum patient returns to the licensed practitioner at least once after the delivery of her baby to be evaluated. As a medical assistant, you will need to ask questions regarding her recovery and document any complaints or concerns. You also may need to assist with a physical exam or provide information about birth control if asked to do so by the physician. Recall methods of birth control from the chapter *The Reproductive Systems*.

▶ OB/GYN Diagnostic and Therapeutic Tests and Procedures   LO 39.3

Many OB/GYN offices have their own small laboratories for immediate results, especially for pregnancy-related tests. Other diagnostic tests and procedures are sent to outside laboratories or performed at outpatient surgery centers or hospitals.

Pregnancy Test

Pregnancy tests are done on a specimen of blood or urine (the patient's first urine of the morning). These tests detect whether or not the hormone human chorionic gonadotropin (HCG)—produced during pregnancy—is present. A variety of testing kits are available, including over-the-counter urine self-test kits that the patient can use at home. These tests are not foolproof; false positives and false negatives do occur. For example, an abnormal pregnancy can result in a lower level of HCG that is not detectable by the tests. Urine specimens that contain blood, protein, or drugs also can give a false-positive result. False negatives may result from testing too early after getting pregnant or from a urine specimen that is too dilute. Dilute urine occurs when the woman has consumed too much fluid and the urine does not have enough HCG to cause the test to react as a positive. The tests also are subject to human error. The licensed practitioner confirms pregnancy after taking the patient's history, performing an exam, and ordering a pregnancy test. You can review and practice this procedure, presented in the *Collecting, Processing, and Testing Urine and Stool Specimens* chapter.

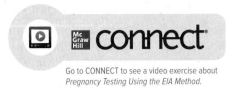

Go to CONNECT to see a video exercise about
Pregnancy Testing Using the EIA Method.

Tests for Sexually Transmitted Infections

The licensed practitioner diagnoses and treats sexually transmitted infections (STIs) by taking bacterial and tissue cultures, examining lesions, ordering blood tests, and discussing the patient's history, as appropriate for the specific disease. Some facilities do not permit the release of these results, even to the parents of a minor, without the patient's written consent. Be sure you are familiar with your state's regulations regarding the reporting of STIs to the state epidemiology department.

Radiologic Tests

Several radiologic tests are used in obstetrics and gynecology. The gynecologist uses X-ray, ultrasonography, CT scan, and MRI. X-rays are avoided when a patient is pregnant. If it is crucial for a pregnant woman to have an X-ray, a lead apron must cover her abdomen, and she must be made aware that the X-ray could cause an abnormality in the fetus. As a medical assistant, you will usually schedule the appointment for radiologic tests. Tell the patient when and where to go for the test and answer her questions about the procedure. Medical assistants need further training to assist with X-ray procedures.

Hysterosalpingography Hysterosalpingography is an X-ray exam of the fallopian or uterine tubes and the uterus that uses a contrast medium, such as dye or air. Because the procedure is quite uncomfortable, the licensed practitioner may prescribe a sedative.

Mammogram A mammogram is a picture of the breast on film or digital media. Digital mammograms are more easily stored and transported and require less radiation. Mammography can detect cancer about 2 years before it can be palpated

with a BSE. A baseline or first mammogram is done so that later mammograms can be compared. The mammogram procedure involves compressing the breast to obtain a clear X-ray (Figure 39-3). Recall our case study patient Raja Lautu, whose routine mammogram revealed an abnormality that was later found to be cancerous. Detailed information may need to be discussed with the patient before she has a mammogram. Review the *Educating the Patient* feature Checking for Breast Cancer to help you prepare the patient for a mammogram.

Fetal Screening

Fetal screening tests can indicate the presence of several types of birth defects, including Down syndrome and spina bifida. The licensed practitioner will consider the patient's age and medical history and the age of the unborn baby when ordering fetal screening tests. Tests for determining the health of an unborn child are performed on many women. Some, like an ultrasound, may be performed routinely. Other tests are used only for women whose unborn babies are at high risk of having birth defects. This includes women over 35, couples with a family history of genetic defects, and couples who have had a previous child with a birth defect.

Alpha Fetoprotein Alpha fetoprotein (AFP) is a protein produced by the unborn child that normally passes into the mother's blood. A blood test determines whether the AFP level in the blood is normal. Too little or too much AFP in the blood can indicate a fetal abnormality known as a neural tube defect. A neural tube defect is a developmental abnormality of the brain or spinal cord. AFP also is measured in amniotic fluid collected by amniocentesis. The licensed practitioner may order a blood test known as a triple screen or triple test. In addition to AFP, maternal levels of human chorionic gonadotropin and estriol are tested. These substances, like AFP, are only present during pregnancy. The triple test is used to detect neural tube defects and is a better indicator of Down

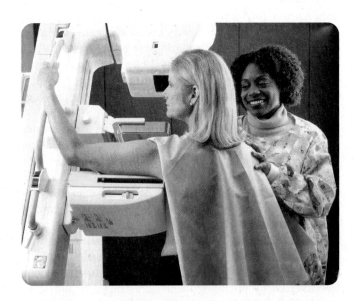

FIGURE 39-3 Mammography consists of two views of each breast and is achieved by compressing the breast between the radiography plates.
Source: Rhoda Baer/National Cancer Institute (NCI)

syndrome than AFP alone. This test is generally done between the 15th and 22nd weeks of pregnancy.

Ultrasound Ultrasound translates the echoes of sound waves into a picture of an internal part of the body. The picture, or image, is called a sonogram, and it can help identify and diagnose cysts and tumors in the abdominal cavity or obstructions of the urinary tract. Ultrasound is painless and safe to use on pregnant women to determine fetal size and position. It also is used to guide a licensed practitioner in performing amniocentesis as well as chorionic villus sampling (CVS) for chromosomal abnormalities and other inherited disorders. A patient who is going to have an ultrasound exam during early pregnancy should be instructed not to urinate before the test because a full bladder allows a better view of the uterus. The patient is asked to lie on an examining table and a gel or lotion is applied to the surface of her skin on the abdomen. This gel or lotion helps enhance sound wave conduction and reduce friction of the transducer on the skin (Figure 39-4).

Invasive Procedures

Many surgical OB/GYN procedures require the use of needles or other instruments to obtain tissue or amniotic fluid samples. Some procedures are used for obstetric reasons only; others may be used gynecologically and obstetrically.

Pap Smear A Pap smear is used to determine the presence of abnormal or precancerous cells. The HPV test, which may be done at the same time, looks for the human papillomavirus that can cause these cell changes. During a pelvic exam, cells from the cervix, endocervix, and vagina are smeared on a special, properly labeled slide. They are then sprayed with a fixative and sent to a laboratory for microscopic analysis. Obtaining accurate Pap smear results is an important tool in the successful treatment of cervical cancer. See the *Points on Practice* feature Pap Smear Technologies. The Pap test results are classified according to level of abnormality. The Bethesda system is used for interpreting the results. Review Table 39-3 to better understand Pap smear results.

Amniocentesis Amniocentesis is a procedure performed when a genetic or metabolic defect is suspected in a fetus. The test involves removing from the uterus a small amount of amniotic fluid, which surrounds the fetus. The licensed practitioner inserts a needle, which is guided with ultrasonography, through the anesthetized lower abdominal wall. Fetal skin cells obtained from the fluid are then grown in a culture and examined for chromosomal abnormalities. The level of AFP also may be measured in amniotic fluid.

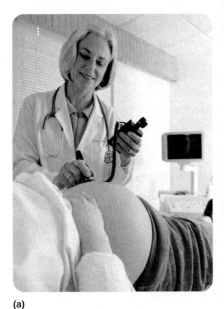

(a)

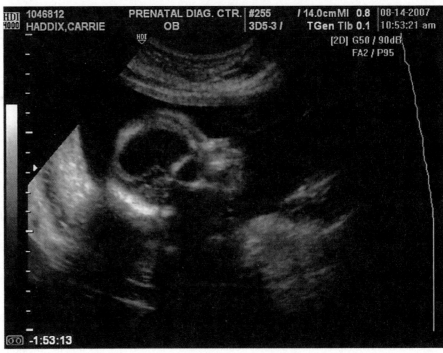

(b)

FIGURE 39-4 (a) An ultrasound technician lightly rubs the transducer over a pregnant woman's abdomen to reveal the anatomy of her fetus. (b) Routine ultrasounds are usually two-dimensional, as shown here; however, three-dimensional ultrasounds can be done.

©Andersen Ross/Getty Images; ©Total Care Programming, Inc.

POINTS ON PRACTICE
Pap Smear Technologies

During a Pap smear, a false-negative test occurs when abnormal cells are not detected. This can occur as a result of the following:

- Too many cells left on the sampling device (brush, broom, or spatula)
- Too many cells piled on top of one another on the slide
- Epithelial cells hidden by extraneous material (blood, mucus, and so on)

A false-negative result could cause a delay in treatment of a year or more, depending on the timing of the next Pap smear. Different types of tests have been developed to help reduce false negatives. The thin-layer preparation of cells is a liquid-based sampling technique. The licensed practitioner collects cervical cells in much the same way as for traditional Pap smears, using a brush- or broom-like device. Once collected, the cells are suspended in a liquid preserving medium rather than being smeared directly onto a glass slide. The cells are then sent to an outside laboratory, where they are filtered or centrifuged and placed on a slide in a thin layer. This method

has been shown to produce samples that are more accurately interpreted by cytotechnologists. A cytotechnologist is a healthcare professional who uses a microscope to examine cells for changes that might indicate the presence of cancer. The advantages of thin-layer preparation over conventional specimen preparation include the following:

- Artifacts caused by air-drying are reduced because cells are placed in a fixative solution immediately.
- The possibility of hidden cells is reduced because cells are placed on the slide in a single layer.
- Blood and cellular debris are removed from the field of view because they are washed away or filtered out.
- The fluid left over after the thin-layer slide preparation may be used for additional testing (for instance, DNA testing for human papillomavirus).

If your office uses a thin-layer cell preparation system, make sure you read and follow all instructions for handling specimens. These instructions can be found in the package inserts for the individual tests.

TABLE 39-3 Understanding Pap Smear Results*

Classification	What It Means	Tests and Treatments That May Be Indicated
Unsatisfactory	Inadequate sampling or other interfering substance	The test must be repeated.
Negative	Cells appear normal, and no identifiable infection is evident.	Continue routine Pap smears.
Benign	Cells are noncancerous, but smear shows infection, irritation, or normal cell repair.	Continue routine Pap smears.
Atypical cells of uncertain significance: either ASC-US or ASC-H	Abnormal cells are present, but it is uncertain what these cells may indicate.	Repeat the Pap smear; sometimes changes can go away without treatment. Estrogen cream may be prescribed for women who are at or near menopause. Do a follow-up test of cells for the presence of high-risk HPV (human papillomavirus). If HPV is present, a colposcopy is performed.
Low-grade changes (mild dysplasia)	Cells have changes that are not cancer but have the potential to be cancer. Cell changes may be caused by HPV infection.	HPV testing; repeat Pap test; colposcopy, and, if abnormal tissue is found, then endocervical curettage or biopsy
High-grade changes (moderate to severe dysplasia or carcinoma in situ, depending upon amount and location of cells)	Cells have more evident changes and look very different than normal cells.	Colposcopy and biopsy; LEEP procedure, cryotherapy, laser therapy, or conization
Squamous cell carcinoma	Cells invade deep into the cervix and other tissues or organs.	Immediate treatment including surgical removal; rare finding in well-screened populations such as the United States

Chorionic Villus Sampling Chorionic villus sampling (CVS) is a test done on patients over 35 or those with a history of genetic disorders to determine problems with the fetus. A sample of the chorionic villi (finger-shaped projections) of the placenta is collected either through amniocentesis or directly through the vagina. Collection through the vagina and cervix is done by using a small flexible tube with a long, thin needle. As in amniocentesis, an ultrasound is used as a guide to locate the correct spot for sampling. Unlike amniocentesis, which is usually done between 15 and 20 weeks, a sampling can be taken through the vagina as early as 10 to 12 weeks. This provides parents the results earlier in the pregnancy so a decision can be made whether to continue or end the pregnancy.

Biopsy Biopsy is the surgical removal of tissue for later microscopic exam. It is the most accurate and, in some cases, the only way to diagnose breast and other cancers. Biopsy of the endometrium, which is the mucous membrane lining the uterus, may help the licensed practitioner diagnose uterine cancer and show whether ovulation is occurring. It also may indicate whether infection, polyps, or abnormal cells are present. If a patient's Pap smear indicates abnormal cells, a cervical or endocervical biopsy may be performed to rule out or diagnose cervical cancer. Procedure 39-3, at the end of this chapter, explains how to assist with a cervical biopsy.

To assist with these biopsies, you must have knowledge of the female anatomy, the order of the procedure, and the instruments used. You also will need to instruct patients about having an escort, appropriate clothing, and any special dietary restrictions. A careful medical history must be obtained to screen for problems such as possible allergic reactions. The day before the biopsy, you might call the patient to confirm the appointment and address any concerns. A biopsy is considered minor surgery and consequently requires observance of standard precautions and sterile technique. Depending on the extent and site of the biopsy, the patient may receive sedation or local anesthesia. During the procedure, you may be responsible for clipping excess material from sutures (stitches) and any other special assistance the licensed practitioner requests. You must place the biopsy specimen in a sterile, solution-filled container provided by the laboratory. You also may assist with or perform the cleaning and bandaging of the site after the procedure. Because of the nature of the procedure, emotional support should be provided as needed during any biopsy.

Colposcopy Colposcopy is the exam of the vagina and cervix with an instrument called a colposcope. See Figure 39-5. The licensed practitioner first cleanses the cervix with saline solution. She then cleanses the cervix with acetic acid, which makes abnormal tissue appear white. The licensed practitioner inserts the colposcope into the vagina and uses the attached magnifying lens to identify abnormal cells, such as cancerous or precancerous cells. The abnormal cells may not be cancerous but may be caused by infection or medication.

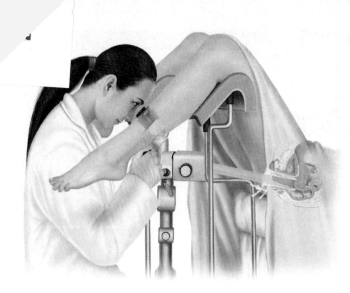

FIGURE 39-5 A colposcope is used to examine the vagina and cervix for abnormal cells.

This procedure is often performed prior to a biopsy or LEEP procedure after results of a Pap smear show the presence of abnormal cells. LEEP procedures are described later in this section.

Dilation and Curettage (D&C) A D&C consists of widening the opening of the cervix (dilation) and scraping the uterine lining (curettage). Reasons for the D&C procedure include assessing the size and shape of the uterus, removing polyps and fibroids from the endometrium, obtaining endometrial specimens for biopsy, performing an abortion, and completing an incomplete miscarriage. Other diagnoses for which a D&C may be performed include abnormal uterine bleeding, abnormal menstrual bleeding, **postcoital** bleeding, spotting between periods, postmenopausal bleeding, and an embedded intrauterine device (IUD).

The procedure is usually performed in a hospital or outpatient surgical facility. You must inform the patient that she will need to have someone take her to and from the facility and that she will have anesthesia before the licensed practitioner performs a routine pelvic exam. For the D&C procedure, the licensed practitioner swabs the vagina with an antiseptic and inserts a speculum. After dilating the cervix, the licensed practitioner uses a curette to remove a portion of the endometrium to assess the texture. Both cervical and endometrial tissue may be sent to a laboratory for examination. Exploration of the uterine cavity and removal of any abnormal growths complete the procedure. Instruct the patient not to have intercourse, take tub baths, or use tampons for 1 week after the procedure. She also should avoid strenuous activity.

Stereotactic Core Biopsy/Fine-Needle Aspiration In a fine-needle aspiration, the licensed practitioner uses a fine needle to remove by vacuum a sample of tissue from a cyst, lump, or tumor of the breast. The term *stereotactic* means that the licensed practitioner finds the target to aspirate using three-dimensional coordinates from a radiographic

mammogram, computed tomography, or MRI. This procedure may be used instead of mammography to diagnose breast disorders in pregnant patients, thus avoiding the use of radiation. Patients with fibrocystic breast disease (involving multiple cystic lumps within the breast tissue) may have needle aspiration of a cyst followed by replacement of the cystic fluid with a steroid to prevent recurrence.

Hysterectomy A hysterectomy is the surgical removal of the uterus. If surgery includes removal of one or both fallopian tubes, it is called a hysterosalpingectomy. Surgical removal of the uterus, the fallopian tubes, and the ovaries is called a hysterosalpingo-oophorectomy. A hysterectomy or a related surgery may be performed for the following reasons: cervical or endometrial cancer; severe endometriosis; unusual bleeding; a leiomyoma, or fibroid; defects of pelvic supports; pregnancy-related problems; and pelvic adhesions or other causes of uterine pain not controllable by other methods.

Inform the patient that an abdominal hysterectomy is major surgery that requires hospitalization. It also requires preadmission urine and blood tests, cleansing enemas, and shaving of the pelvic area. Normal activities, including sexual intercourse, can usually be resumed within a few weeks. Premenopausal women who have hysterectomies or hysterosalpingectomies may begin menopause sooner than they otherwise would have. Premenopausal women who have hysterosalpingo-oophorectomies will experience menopause immediately after the surgery.

Laparoscopy A laparoscope is a long, tubular instrument. It contains fiber-optic threads that illuminate the organs and a lens that resembles a small telescope. A licensed practitioner can use the laparoscope to view the internal female organs. Laparoscopy is used to help determine the cause of **infertility** (the inability to conceive), to obtain tissue samples, to remove abnormal growths, and to surgically sterilize a patient. It also is used in the treatment of ectopic pregnancies, endometriosis, and laparoscopy-assisted hysterectomy.

During laparoscopy the patient is anesthetized and the laparoscope tube is inserted through a small incision in or around the navel. Carbon dioxide or another gas is pumped into the abdomen to spread the organs apart, making them easier to see. The patient's body is then tilted with her head lower than her hips to allow the intestines to move away from the lower abdomen. This positioning permits a clearer view of the ovaries, uterus, and fallopian tubes.

Loop Electrosurgical Excision Procedure (LEEP) A **loop electrosurgical excision procedure (LEEP)** is when a thin wire loop electrode attached to the speculum is inserted in the vagina and used to cut away abnormal cervical tissue that was discovered during a Pap smear. The tissue is then sent to a lab for further testing. This procedure may last about 20 to 30 minutes and may be done as part of a colposcopy. A small amount of smoke may be seen during this procedure.

Cryosurgery Cryosurgery is using extremely cold temperatures to freeze and destroy abnormal tissues such as venereal

Testicular Self-Exam

Although testicular cancer is rare, it is currently the most common cancer in American males between the ages of 15 and 34. The American Cancer Society recommends that all men perform a monthly testicular self-exam starting at age 15 to increase the chances of early detection. Although testicular cancer is one of the most curable cancers, early detection is vital to its treatment. Warning signs of testicular cancer include a heavy or dragging feeling in the groin, enlargement of one testicle, and a dull ache in the groin.

A TSE should be performed in the following manner after a warm shower or bath, when scrotal skin is relaxed. A medical assistant may be responsible for coaching the patient through the steps of this technique. The steps of the technique are as follows:

1. The man first observes the testes for changes in appearance, such as swelling.

2. The man then manually examines each testicle, gently rolling it between the fingers and thumbs of both hands to feel for hard lumps (see Figure 39-6).

3. After examining each testicle, the man should locate the area of the epididymis and spermatic cord and know

these are normal structures. This area can be felt as a cord-like structure originating at the top back of each testicle.

4. A man who perceives an abnormality during a TSE should be examined by a physician right away.

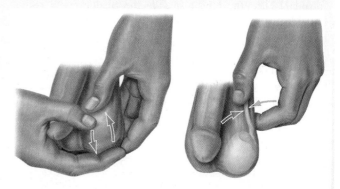

FIGURE 39-6 Males should perform a monthly testicular self-exam starting at age 15.

---

warts, to treat precancerous tumors, and to control bleeding. The procedure is done through the vagina using a vaginal speculum and a probe. Compressed gases flow through the probe, making it as low as −50°C. The extreme cold freezes and kills the tissues. A second treatment might be done after 3 minutes. Patients may experience slight cramping during the procedure. After the procedure, sexual intercourse and douching are avoided for up to 2 weeks, and discharge may be seen.

▸ Assisting in Urology
LO 39.4

The urologist focuses on the male and female urinary systems as well as the male reproductive system. Urologists perform surgical procedures such as hernia repairs and vasectomies. In a urologist's office, you will assist with general exams; collect and process urine, blood, and other specimens; and obtain cultures. You also may participate in patient education about conditions and about presurgical and postsurgical care, so you need to understand the urinary system and the diseases and disorders you are likely to encounter.

You must be thorough when you take a patient's history for a urologist. Much information about urinary problems is obtained by questioning the patient about changes in frequency or urgency of urination, difficulty or pain with urination (dysuria), and incontinence. The physical exam usually includes palpation of the kidneys and bladder and visual inspection of the external genitalia. Women are usually examined in the lithotomy position. Men are typically seated when the exam begins. During the examination of the male reproductive system, the urologist inspects and palpates the patient's penis and

scrotum. The genitalia are usually examined with the patient standing and the chest and abdomen draped. The physician usually examines the inguinal region for a hernia and, in men over 40, checks the prostate gland. This gland is examined by digital insertion into the rectum. The physician instructs the patient as needed in performing a regular testicular self-exam (TSE). This instruction, discussed in the *Educating the Patient* feature Testicular Self-Exam, also may be your responsibility.

▸ Urologic Diagnostic Tests and Procedures
LO 39.5

Urologists sometimes use imaging techniques such as CT scans and MRIs. Pyelography is an X-ray of the kidney area with an iodine-based contrast agent. It is used to diagnose renal (kidney-related) disorders. Urologists also use several other diagnostic techniques.

Urine and Blood Tests

Urinalysis (analysis of the urine) is the most commonly ordered test in a urology practice. Urine can be tested for the presence of bacteria, blood, and other substances. Blood testing also is done for a variety of reasons, including monitoring for dysfunctions of the prostate gland and for certain sexually transmitted infections (STIs). For example, a PSA (prostate-specific antigen) blood test is done to screen for prostate cancer.

Semen Analysis and Smears

Semen samples may be obtained to determine fertility. This test is done if a couple finds themselves unable to conceive or if the patient has had a vasectomy. A **vasectomy** is surgical sterilization by cutting the vas deferens. This is the tube that allows semen to pass outside the body. The patient usually collects these samples at home, but you may be required to provide the patient with a container, written instructions, and laboratory paperwork. Smears are used in diagnosing infections.

Cystometry

Cystometry is used to measure urinary bladder capacity and pressure. A catheter is passed through the urethra into the bladder. Then the physician fills the bladder with carbon dioxide gas. The test results are examined to diagnose bladder function disorders.

Cystoscopy

In cystoscopy, the physician examines the walls of the bladder and urethra by visualization and inspection. A viewing instrument called a cystoscope is used for this procedure. The cystoscope is inserted into the bladder through the urethra.

Testicular Biopsy

Testicular biopsy, an invasive procedure, involves obtaining a tissue sample of a mass for laboratory examination. The patient will need your emotional support because he will most likely be very anxious about the nature of the lump.

▶ Diseases and Disorders of the Reproductive and Urinary Systems   LO 39.6

Many of the diseases and disorders encountered in OB/GYN and urology practices have been mentioned in the context of the procedures in this chapter. Tables 39-4 and 39-5 outline common obstetric, gynecologic, and urologic diseases and disorders.

TABLE 39-4	Common Obstetric and Gynecologic Diseases and Disorders	
Condition	**Description**	**Treatment**
Cancer	Common occurrence in cervix, endometrium (uterus), and ovaries; cells divide uncontrollably, eventually forming a tumor or other growth of abnormal tissue; most often seen in women between the ages of 50 and 60; symptoms differ for each type of cancer	Surgery (hysterectomy), radiation, chemotherapy, hormones; for ovarian cancer, surgical removal of all reproductive organs, affected lymph nodes, appendix, and some muscle tissue, followed by chemotherapy (to extend survival time)
Ectopic pregnancy	Fertilized egg unable to move out of fallopian tube into uterus for implantation; patient experiences pain within a few weeks of conception; can be fatal	Surgery to remove the embryo from the fallopian tube before the tube ruptures
Endometriosis	Endometrial tissue present outside uterus, usually in pelvic area; not life-threatening but may cause sterility; symptoms include abnormal menstruation and pain (sometimes severe) in lower abdominal area and back	Hormone therapy, hysterectomy for severe cases, endometrial ablation (1-day surgery, alternative to hysterectomy), leuprolide acetate injection
Fibrocystic breast disease	Benign, fluid-filled cysts or nodules in breast; sometimes confused with malignant growths in breast until complete diagnostic tests are performed; symptoms include pain and tenderness	Depending on severity, vitamin E supplements, hormones, compresses, analgesics, aspiration, biopsy, restricted caffeine intake
Fibroids, or leiomyomas	Common, benign, smooth tumors of muscle cells (not fibrous tissue) grouped in uterus; symptoms include excessive menstruation and bloating; diagnosis by bimanual examination and ultrasound	Surgery for severe cases
Menstrual disturbances	May be (1) **amenorrhea** (absence of menstruation), (2) **dysmenorrhea** (painful menstruation), (3) **menorrhagia** (excessive amount of menstrual flow or prolonged period of menstruation), or (4) **metrorrhagia** (bleeding between menstrual periods)	Treatment according to symptoms; analgesics; possibly D&C or cryosurgery; for severe cases, hysterectomy
Ovarian cysts	Sacs of fluid or semisolid material, usually benign and without symptoms; occur anytime between puberty and menopause; extensive ovarian cysts may cause pelvic discomfort, lower back pain, and abnormal bleeding	Analgesics and bed rest if severe pain; hormone therapy; surgery is usually reserved for cysts that rupture or are large enough to put pressure on surrounding organs
Pelvic inflammatory disease (PID)	Acute, chronic infection of reproductive tract; causes include untreated STIs, such as gonorrhea and chlamydia, and organisms such as staphylococci and streptococci; symptoms include vaginal discharge, fever, and general discomfort	Antibiotics

(Continued)

TABLE 39-4 — Common Obstetric and Gynecologic Diseases and Disorders

Condition	Description	Treatment
Pelvic support problems (uterine prolapse, rectocele, cystocele)	Abnormal weakening of vaginal tissue, unusual increase in abdominal pressure, congenital weakness (weakness since birth); symptoms include urine leakage, pelvic heaviness ("bottom falling out"), pain or discomfort in pelvic area, pulling or aching feeling in lower back, abdomen, or groin	Kegel or perineal exercises to strengthen muscles, insertion of pessary (device to hold pelvic organs in place), surgery to repair muscles, physical therapy
Polyps	Red, soft, fragile growths, with slender stem attachment, sometimes found on mucous membranes of cervix or endometrium; may cause pain	Depending on size and shape, may be removed in office or hospital
Premenstrual dysphoric disorder (PMDD)	A severe form of premenstrual syndrome that affects 5% of women; symptoms have a very disrupting effect on the patient's life; screening tests and physician evaluation are necessary for diagnosis	Medications, including antidepressants, anti-anxiety drugs, analgesics, hormones, and diuretics; exercise, relaxation, diet modification, vitamins, minerals, and herbal preparations are also useful
Premenstrual syndrome (PMS)	Symptoms include swelling, bloating, weight gain, breast tenderness, headaches, and mood shifts 1 week to 10 days before menstruation	Vitamins, diuretics, hormones, oral contraceptives, tranquilizers, other medications; stress-reduction methods as needed; restricted intake of dietary sodium, alcohol, and caffeine
Sexual function disorders	Interruption or lack of sexual response cycle (excitement, plateau, orgasm, and resolution); unhealthy view of one's feelings about oneself as a woman and feelings toward sex; sometimes caused by painful intercourse, abusive partner, unrealistic demands on oneself, or menopause	Counseling (for both woman and partner) to teach relaxation, effective communication, and identification of cycle stages and natural responses
Vaginitis	Inflammation of vagina caused by bacteria, viruses, yeasts, or chemicals in sprays, douches, or tampons; symptoms include itching, redness, pain, swelling	Treatment prescribed according to cause; avoiding douches, tampons, tight pants; always wiping from front to back; sometimes avoiding sex during treatment

TABLE 39-5 — Common Urologic Diseases and Disorders

Condition	Description	Treatment
Epididymitis	Bacterial infection of the epididymis; causes pain, swelling, and sometimes fever	Rest and antibiotic medications
Hydrocele	Excess fluid in the scrotum; usually caused by infection of the epididymis or testes; also can result from a congenital defect or after injury	Aspiration of fluid to relieve discomfort
Impotence	Inability either to achieve or to maintain an erection; the cause may be physical, as when it results from cardiovascular or endocrine disease, or may be a side effect of a medication such as certain diuretics and chemotherapy agents; the cause also may be psychological or emotional	Depends on the cause or causes and may include medication, counseling, or surgical procedures
Incontinence	Loss of bladder control, which results in anything from mild urine leaking to uncontrollable wetting; most bladder-control problems happen when muscles are too weak or too active; stress incontinence occurs when the muscles that keep the bladder closed are too weak and urine leaks during a sneeze, when laughing, or when lifting a heavy object	Depends on the cause and severity of the problem; may include simple exercises, medicines, special devices or procedures prescribed by a licensed practitioner, or surgery
Kidney stones	Chemical substances in the urine form crystals in the kidney, ureter, or bladder; if kidney stones cannot pass through the ureter, they can cause excruciating pain	Some stones pass; however, large stones often must be removed surgically or broken up by means of sound waves (lithotripsy) or laser techniques
Prostate cancer	The most common type of cancer among men; often no symptoms are evident, but sometimes a nodule may be felt on palpation of the prostate; if the growth is large enough, problems with urination may occur; a blood test known as a prostate-specific antigen (PSA) is used for screening in men over 50 years of age; an abnormal elevation of the PSA could indicate prostate cancer	Radiation therapy, removal of the prostate, hormone therapy, chemotherapy, biologic therapy
Prostatic hypertrophy (hyperplasia)	Enlargement of the prostate gland; occurs most commonly in men over 50; may constrict the urethra, causing difficulty in urinating and repeated urinary infections	Medications to reduce the enlarged prostate, surgery

(Continued)

6. Using sterile method, open the sterile pack to create a sterile field on the tray or Mayo stand and arrange the instruments with transfer forceps. Add the vaginal speculum and sterile supplies to the sterile field.
   RATIONALE: *The instruments and supplies must stay sterile because this is an invasive procedure.*

7. When the physician arrives in the exam room, ask the patient to lie back, place her heels in the stirrups of the table, and move her buttocks to the edge of the table.
   RATIONALE: *Placing the patient in the lithotomy position too early can cause the patient's back and legs to cramp.*

8. Assist the physician by arranging the drape so that only the genitalia are exposed, and place the light so that the genitalia are illuminated.

9. Use transfer forceps to hand instruments and supplies to the physician as he requests them. You may don sterile gloves and hand the physician supplies and instruments directly.

10. When the licensed practitioner is ready to obtain the biopsy, tell the patient that it may hurt. If she seems particularly fearful, instruct her to take a deep breath and let it out slowly.

11. When the physician hands you the instrument with the tissue specimen, place the specimen in the specimen container and discard the instrument in the appropriate container.

12. Label the specimen container with the patient's name, the date and time, cervical or endocervical (as indicated by the physician), the physician's name, and your initials.

13. Place the container and the cytology laboratory requisition form in the envelope or bag provided by the laboratory.

14. When the physician has completed the procedure and removed the speculum, properly clean instruments as needed and dispose of used supplies and disposable instruments. Metal speculums, if used, should be placed in a clean basin for later sanitization, disinfection, and sterilization.

15. Remove the gloves and wash your hands.

16. Tell the patient that she may get dressed. Inform her that she may have some vaginal bleeding for a couple of days, and provide her with a sanitary napkin. Instruct her not to take tub baths or have intercourse and not to use tampons for 2 days. Encourage her to call the office if she experiences problems or has questions.

17. Document the procedure as appropriate (refer to Progress Note).

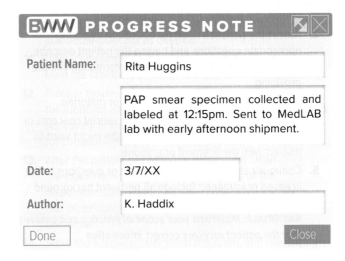

BWW PROGRESS NOTE

Patient Name:	Rita Huggins
	PAP smear specimen collected and labeled at 12:15pm. Sent to MedLAB lab with early afternoon shipment.
Date:	3/7/XX
Author:	K. Haddix

Done   Close

SUMMARY OF LEARNING OUTCOMES

OUTCOME	KEY POINTS
39.1 Carry out the role of the medical assistant in the medical specialty of gynecology.	Medical assistants assist with gynecologic exams, provide patient teaching for OB/GYN and breast health issues, and must handle cervical and other specimens correctly.
39.2 Carry out the role of the medical assistant in the medical specialty of obstetrics.	Medical assistants assist with examinations for pregnant females, providing for their needs, and provide education for the pregnant patient and new mother.
39.3 Identify diagnostic and therapeutic procedures performed in obstetrics and gynecology.	Diagnostic and therapeutic procedures performed in OB/GYN include pregnancy tests, tests for STIs, radiologic tests such as mammograms, fetal screening, Pap smears, D&C, and fine-needle aspiration.
39.4 Relate the role of medical assisting to the medical specialty of urology.	Medical assistants assist with urologic exams and diagnostic tests and provide patient education for urologic patients regarding TSE and other information.

OUTCOME	KEY POINTS
39.5 Identify diagnostic tests and procedures performed in urology.	Various urologic diagnostic tests and procedures are performed, including semen analysis, cystometry, cystoscopy, and testicular biopsy.
39.6 Recognize diseases and disorders of the reproductive and urinary systems.	Diseases and disorders of the reproductive and urinary systems are listed for review in Table 39-4, Common Obstetric and Gynecologic Diseases and Disorders, and Table 39-5, Common Urologic Diseases and Disorders.

CASE STUDY CRITICAL THINKING

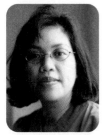

Recall Raja Lautu from the case study at the beginning of the chapter. Now that you have read the chapter, answer the following questions regarding her case.

1. How often should Raja Lautu have a pelvic exam, cervical cytology, HIV screen, and mammogram?

2. What should have been discussed with Raja Lautu before she had the mammogram?

3. How is stereotactic fine-needle biopsy performed?

©ERproductions Ltd/Blend Images LLC

EXAM PREPARATION QUESTIONS

1. (LO 39.2) A pregnant patient, Molly Holiday, has started feeling the movement of her baby. What is her current stage of pregnancy?
   a. 1st trimester
   b. Menarche
   c. 3rd trimester
   d. 2nd trimester
   e. 4th trimester

2. (LO 39.4) A TSE is
   a. Surgery that involves bypassing a blockage in the urethra
   b. An imaging procedure that uses magnets and radio waves
   c. An examination of the testicles by the patient
   d. A scan of blood flow and metabolic activity in the brain
   e. An examination of the testicles by the physician

3. (LO 39.2) A pregnant patient is monitoring her blood glucose level with a glucometer. She most likely has
   a. Type 2 diabetes
   b. Type 1 diabetes
   c. Gestational diabetes
   d. Hyperthyroidism
   e. Diabetes mellitus

4. (LO 39.1) Which of the following indicates the LMP?
   a. The last day of the last menstrual period
   b. The first day of the last menstrual period
   c. A late menstrual period
   d. A likely menopausal pregnancy
   e. The heaviest flow day of the last menstrual period

5. (LO 39.1) A speculum is used to
   a. Evaluate for a DVT
   b. Evaluate the LMP
   c. Perform a basic physical exam
   d. Perform a vaginal exam
   e. Examine the breasts

6. (LO 39.3) Which of the following patients would *most* likely have an alpha fetoprotein test?
   a. 28-year-old male patient with urinary frequency and urgency
   b. 36-year-old female in her 3rd trimester of pregnancy
   c. 27-year-old female with vaginal discharge
   d. 54-year-old female with urinary incontinence
   e. 35-year-old female in her 2nd trimester of pregnancy

7. (LO 39.5) Which of the following diagnostic tests would *least* likely be performed on a male urologic patient?

a. Colposcopy
b. Testicular biopsy
c. Semen analysis
d. Urinalysis
e. Cystoscopy

9. (LO 39.1) At what age should most women start having yearly mammograms, according to the American Cancer Society and National Cancer Institute?

a. 25
b. 35
c. 45
d. 55
e. 65

9. (LO 39.6) Your 27-year-old female patient has a menstrual disturbance. Which of the following does she *least* likely have?

a. Amenorrhea
b. Menorrhea
c. Dysmenorrhea
d. Metrorrhagia
e. Menorrhagia

10. (LO 39.6) Your male patient has an infection that is not an STI. Which of the following is most likely the problem?

a. Hydrocele
b. Vaginitis
c. Epididymitis
d. Gonorrhea
e. Prostatic hypertrophy

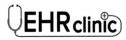

Go to CONNECT to complete the EHRclinic exercises: 39.01 Record a Gynecologic Exam in a Patient's EHR, 39.02 Add Test Results to a Patient's EHR, and 39.03 Document Patient Education for Testicular Self-Exam.

SOFT SKILLS SUCCESS

A young adult female patient begins asking you questions regarding birth control choices. She states she feels uncomfortable asking her physician, Dr. Buckwalter. Can you act as an "intermediary" for her with Dr. Buckwalter? Do you have any ideas to help her regarding her fears surrounding the need for this discussion?

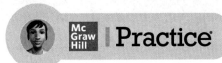

Go to PRACTICE MEDICAL OFFICE and complete the module Clinical: Interactions.

Assisting in Pediatrics

CASE STUDY

PATIENT INFORMATION	Patient Name	DOB	Allergies
	Christopher Matthews	11/19/2012	NKA
	Attending	**MRN**	**Other Information**
	Alexis N. Whalen, MD	00-AA-011	Home-schooled; parents refused immunizations

Christopher (Chris) Matthews' mother states he has had diarrhea for 3 days. He kept her up all night last night going to the bathroom at least three times. He says his stomach hurts, but he has not vomited, although he is eating very little. While you are preparing to weigh the patient,

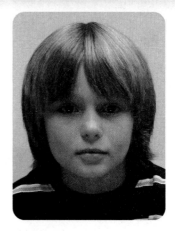

he initially does not want to get on the scale and begins to cry. After his mother has persuaded him to get on the scale and you have obtained all the measurements and vital signs, you check his immunization record. While doing so, you see a note on his chart indicating he is home-schooled and his parents have refused immunizations.

Keep Chris Matthews in mind as you study this chapter. There will be questions at the end of the chapter based on the case study. The information in the chapter will help you answer these questions.

LEARNING OUTCOMES

After completing Chapter 40, you will be able to:

40.1 Relate growth and development to pediatric patient care.

40.2 Identify the role of the medical assistant during pediatric examinations.

40.3 Discuss pediatric immunizations and the role of the medical assistant.

40.4 Explain variations of pediatric screening procedures and diagnostic tests.

40.5 Describe common pediatric diseases and disorders and their treatment.

40.6 Recognize special health concerns of pediatric patients.

KEY TERMS

addiction

bilirubin

contraindication

enuresis

fontanels

growth chart

immunization

jaundice

menarche

moro reflex

phenylketonuria (PKU)

puberty

substance abuse

CAAHEP

I.C.6 Compare structure and function of the human body across the life span

I.C.8 Identify common pathology related to each body system including:
(a) signs
(b) symptoms
(c) etiology

I.C.9 Analyze pathology for each body system including:
(a) diagnostic measures
(b) treatment modalities

I.P.1 Measure and record:
(a) blood pressure
(b) temperature
(c) pulse
(d) respirations
(e) height
(f) weight
(g) length (infant)
(h) head circumference (infant)

I.P.3 Perform patient screening using established protocols

I.P.7 Administer parenteral (excluding IV) medications

I.P.8 Instruct and prepare a patient for a procedure or a treatment

I.P.9 Assist provider with a patient exam

I.A.1 Incorporate critical thinking skills when performing patient assessment

I.A.2 Incorporate critical thinking skills when performing patient care

I.A.3 Show awareness of a patient's concerns related to the procedure being performed

II.C.6 Analyze healthcare results as reported in:
(a) graphs

II.P.4 Document on a growth chart

V.P.5. Coach patients appropriately considering:
(b) developmental life stage

X.C.12 Describe compliance with public health statutes:
(b) abuse, neglect, and exploitation
(c) wounds of violence

X.P.3 Document patient care accurately in the medical record

ABHES

2. Anatomy and Physiology
a. List all body systems and their structures and functions
b. Describe common diseases, symptoms and etiologies as they apply to each system
c. Identify diagnostic and treatment modalities as they relate to each body system

3. Medical Terminology
c. Apply medical terminology for each specialty

4. Medical Law and Ethics
a. Follow documentation guidelines

5. Human Relations
a. Respond appropriately to patients with abnormal behavior patterns
c. Assist the patient in navigating issues and concerns that may arise (i.e., insurance policy information, medical bills, and physician/provider orders)
d. Adapt care to address the developmental stages of life
e. Analyze the effect of hereditary and environmental influences on behavior

8. Clinical Procedures
b. Obtain vital signs, obtain patient history, and formulate chief complaint
c. Assist provider with general/physical examination
d. Assist provider with specialty examination including cardiac, respiratory, OB-GYN, neurological, and gastroenterology procedures
e. Perform specialty procedures including but not limited to minor surgery, cardiac, respiratory, OB-GYN, neurological, and gastroenterology procedures
f. Prepare and administer oral and parenteral medications and monitor intravenous (IV) infusions
j. Make adaptations for patients with special needs (psychological or physical limitations)
k. Make adaptations to care for patients across their lifespan

▶ Introduction

Pediatrics is a specialty area of medicine that involves the care of children up to the age of 18 and, in some cases, 21. To be a good pediatric medical assistant, you must first like children of all ages. If you do, you will be better able to relate to them and to communicate with them effectively. The pediatrician specializes in the healthcare of children, monitoring their development and diagnosing and treating their illnesses. Just as with other specialty fields, there are subspecialties of pediatrics, such as surgery and oncology.

As a medical assistant working in pediatrics, your primary areas of responsibility include parent or caregiver education, adherence to immunization schedules, and recognition of special health concerns. You also will assist with the pediatric patient's physical exam and treatment. Relating to the child, as well as being a liaison between the parent or caregiver and the physician, is essential to your job.

▶ Developmental Stages and Care LO 40.1

Different periods of childhood present different changes and challenges. As discussed in the *Interpersonal Communication* chapter, understanding lifespan development will, among other things, enhance your communication skills. This chapter focuses on the life stages from birth through the teenage years. Understanding the child's stages of growth and development will improve your skills as a medical assistant. During each stage of growth, the following developmental milestones occur:

- *Physical development* is the actual bodily changes that occur.
- *Intellectual-cognitive development* refers to the thinking skills the child is developing.
- *Psycho-emotional development* refers to the changes in feelings experienced during a particular period.
- *Social development* is the way a person relates to others.

The stages of growth and development for pediatric patients include neonate, infant, toddler, preschooler, elementary school child, middle school child, and adolescent. As you explore each stage, you also will review the related aspects of care to help you provide the necessary care and patient education.

Neonate: Birth to 1 Month

An infant is called a *neonate* from birth to 1 month of age. Many changes take place in this short time.

Physical Development The full-term infant usually weighs between 7 and 9 pounds and is 18 to 22 inches in length. The newborn infant's head seems large in comparison to the rest of her body. No wonder—the head is usually one-fourth of the infant's entire length! An adult head is usually only about one-ninth of the body length. An infant's head has two soft spots, or **fontanels,** which are tough, fibrous cartilage (Figure 40-1). The anterior, or front, fontanel is diamond-shaped. The baby's pulse can sometimes be seen here. The infant can move her head from side to side. However, because the neck muscles are not strong enough to hold the head up, the person holding the infant must provide support.

The newborn baby's skin is usually loose, wrinkled, and somewhat red in appearance. During the first week of life, this skin may start to peel. This is not harmful, and nothing needs to be done about it. The part of the umbilical cord still attached to the baby's body is a "stump" about 1 to 1½ inches in length. At birth it has a white, waxy appearance, then turns darker, and usually falls off around the tenth day of life (Figure 40-2).

Sometimes infants develop neonatal **jaundice**—a yellowish color of the skin—in the first few days of life. This is caused by an accumulation of **bilirubin,** the waste product from the normal breakdown of the red blood cells. Babies

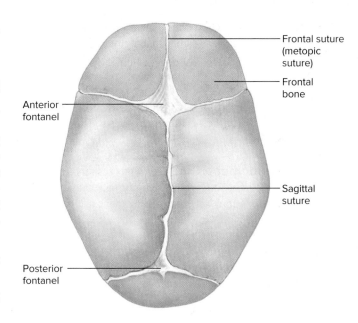

FIGURE 40-1 Be aware of the newborn's fontanels, or "soft spots." These areas are open at birth so that the brain can grow. They close as the infant ages.

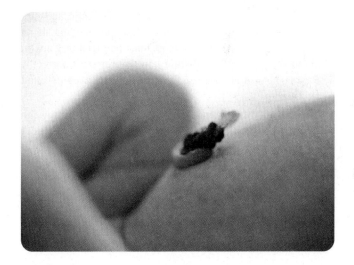

FIGURE 40-2 The umbilical cord usually falls off when the baby is about 10 days old.
©Ian Boddy/Science Source

have large numbers of red blood cells at birth. Their immature liver is unable to handle the breakdown of these cells. The waste product accumulates, giving the skin a yellowish tint. The whites of the eyes also may appear yellow, and the urine and feces may have a dark yellow color. This condition is rarely serious and usually goes away within a few weeks.

Certain reflexes can be observed in the newborn. Some are protective. For example, blinking is a reflex that protects the eyes. Everyone, including newborns, has this reflex. Other reflexes are due to the infant's immature nervous system. For example, the **moro reflex** is one in which the infant feels as if she is falling. The arms spread out and then back in and crying often occurs. The physician will check reflexes as part of an examination.

Infants can see objects within 8 inches of their eyes. They probably detect brightness rather than color. Their eyes tend to turn outward or even may cross. Infants seem to prefer high-pitched tones.

Intellectual-Cognitive Development Newborns will become calm when picked up and held firmly. They tune out disturbing stimulation by sleeping.

Social Development Early on, infants respond to stimulation and establish an individual activity pattern. Generally, an infant responds to a soft, gentle voice and tries to focus on the voice and face. Newborns can show excitement and distress.

Aspects of Care: Neonate Consider the following when caring for neonates or providing parent or caregiver education.

- Sponge baths with tepid water and limited amounts of mild infant cleansing soap are given until the cord has fallen off. The infant's face should be washed with tepid water. No oil should be rubbed on the baby. Lotions and powders also should be avoided.

- If an infant is to be breast-fed, parents are given instruction about frequency of feedings, duration of feedings, and care of the mother and her breasts while breast-feeding. If an infant is to be bottle-fed, parents must be given instruction about the type of formula and how to prepare it correctly. Parents also should be taught about bowel movements and spitting up.

- The treatment for jaundice in the newborn is keeping the infant well hydrated with breast milk or formula. If necessary, the infant is placed under ultraviolet light. These bright lights can damage the infant's eyes, so eye protection is necessary during this treatment. Some neonates may need to use a bili-blanket, which is a type of phototherapy device that helps the infant eliminate the bilirubin, thus improving the jaundice (Figure 40-3). Blood tests will

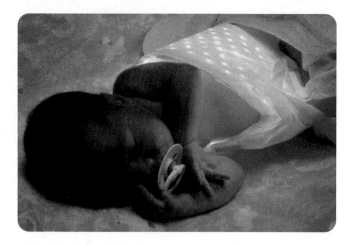

FIGURE 40-3 A newborn with excessive bilirubin may be sent home with an ultraviolet light bili-blanket to help reduce the jaundice.
©Aaron Haupt/Science Source

be performed fairly often to ensure that the bilirubin level does not become dangerously high.

- Other newborn blood tests also are performed, including screening tests for cystic fibrosis, galactosemia, hypothyroidism, sickle cell disease, and phenylketonuria (PKU). See the *Points on Practice* box Testing for Phenylketonuria (PKU) for more information about this important test.

The Infant: 1 Month to 1 Year

Many changes occur in an infant during the first year. Parents cherish the wonder of their growing, developing child during this period.

Physical Development Growth is rapid during the first year of life. Infants triple their birth weight by their first birthday. They develop in a cephalocaudal fashion, with the earliest development starting at the head and moving down. Infants first gain control of the head, neck, and shoulders, and then the arms, torso, and legs. This is why an infant

POINTS ON PRACTICE
Testing for Phenylketonuria (PKU)

Phenylketonuria (PKU) is a rare metabolic disorder. It is caused by a mutation in a gene that is responsible for creating an enzyme that breaks down phenylalanine, an amino acid found in protein-rich foods. If this amino acid is not broken down, it accumulates in the body and causes brain damage. Screening newborns for PKU is required in all states.

The screening test is a qualitative test for the presence of phenylalanine and related substances and is usually done 24–48 hours after birth. The newborn must ingest proteins prior to the test to ensure accuracy. Though this test is usually done in the hospital prior to discharge, there may be occasions when it is done in the physician's office.

To perform the test, a capillary puncture is done on the infant's heel. For more information about infant heel sticks, refer to the chapter *Collecting, Processing, and Testing Blood Specimens*. Three or four drops of blood are collected on a card or paper. Before the test is performed, the card must be filled out completely, including the following information:

- Mother's name and address.
- Ordering physician's name and contact information.
- Baby's name, date of birth, and weight.
- Gestational age.
- Date and time of the collection.

finds and uses his hands before he finds and uses his feet. Larger groups of muscles develop before the smaller groups of muscles develop. The nervous system develops rapidly. Changes are seen in reflexes and in the development of coordinated movement and eye-hand coordination. The following is a brief look at some specific types of physical development in infants.

- By about 3 weeks of age, infants can focus on objects.
- By about 4 weeks, infants can follow an object with their eyes and make eye-to-eye contact. The infant can lift his head when lying on his abdomen.
- At 2 months, infants can follow objects with their eyes from one side to the other, listen to sounds, bat at objects, and respond to sounds. At this age, the infant may string together vowel sounds.
- By 3 months, an infant may raise the head and shoulders while on the abdomen and may hold up the head (Figure 40-4). When the infant is pulled to a sitting position, the head remains in line with the backbone.
- By 4 months, the infant may roll from stomach to back and may begin to play with a rattle placed in the hand. Teething may begin at this time.
- By 5 months, the infant may transfer a rattle from one hand to the other.
- At 6 months, the infant rolls from back to stomach, may be able to sit up briefly, and can reach to retrieve a dropped object. The two bottom front teeth have probably erupted, or emerged, from the gums.
- At 9 months, the infant is able to sit and to creep on hands and knees. The infant is beginning to use the pincer grasp. The infant can put consonants with vowels and make repetitive sounds such as "mama" and "dada."
- At 12 months, the child can hold on to a piece of furniture and move around it, perhaps taking a step or two. With tooth development and the pincer grasp, the infant can pick up and eat small pieces of food.

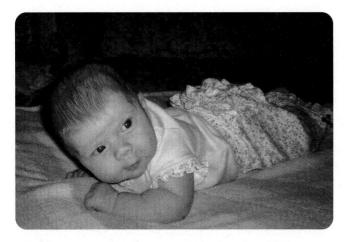

FIGURE 40-4   A 3-month-old infant should be able to hold up her head when lying on her stomach.
©Total Care Programming, Inc.

Intellectual-Cognitive Development   At 1 month of age, an infant can make eye contact. This progresses to recognition of familiar faces and then to "making faces" at 4 to 5 months. At around 6 months of age, the child is making babbling sounds and by 9 months is able to play games such as peek-a-boo. The infant begins to understand cause and effect. If the infant drops a toy and someone retrieves it, the infant will drop it again. This becomes a game. At 12 months, an infant can follow simple directions.

Psycho-Emotional Development   By the time a child is 1 month old, he or she can smile at another smiling face. By 3 months, the infant smiles spontaneously and displays pleasure in making sounds. At 4 months, the infant can vocalize a mood. At 6 months, there may be abrupt mood changes. At 9 months, the infant displays pleasure in playing simple games and by 1 year has learned to express many emotions. For infants to develop physically and emotionally, it is important that their physical needs be addressed quickly and calmly.

Social Development   Infants become social beings very quickly. By 1 month of age, infants are able to smile. At 3 months, the infant responds to voices. This can be seen when the infant pays attention and coos along with a person speaking in a quiet and gentle manner. At 6 months, the baby "babbles" and is interested in his or her own voice. Imitative play becomes an important part of the infant's interaction with others. At 9 months, the first development of words can be observed. This leads to increased interaction with family and others.

Aspects of Care: 1 Month to 1 Year   Consider the following when caring for infants or providing parent or caregiver education.

- Regular health checkups and immunizations should be followed. Immunizations will be discussed in *section 40.3* of this chapter.
- Infants need tactile stimulation for growth and development. Physical contact and cuddling, as well as prompt attention to their needs, help infants develop a sense of security and trust, which is necessary for them to thrive.
- In the first 4 to 6 months, the mother's breast milk or infant formula meets the growing infant's needs. The physician will provide guidance about the introduction of solid foods to the diet. You may be asked to assist the physician in guiding the parent or caregiver regarding the diet of a pediatric patient. Table 40-1 provides basic pediatric guidelines; however, always follow the policy of the facility where you are employed. In addition, be aware that dietary guidelines change with research.
- Ensure infant safety. See the *Educating the Patient* feature Keeping Infants and Toddlers Safe.

The Toddler: 1 to 3 Years

Children from the age of 1 to 3 years need constant attention from parents and others. Although they grow less

TABLE 40-1 Pediatric Dietary Guidelines*

AGE GROUP	RECOMMENDATIONS	SPECIFIC CONCERNS
Birth to 4 months	• Breast milk every 2 to 4 hours or formula six to eight times a day with 2 to 3 ounces per feeding.	• Never give infants honey; it may contain botulism spores. • Infants may need to be woken up at night if they are not eating enough during the day.
4 to 6 months	• Introduce 1 to 2 tablespoons of cereal mixed with formula or breast milk two times a day. Gradually increase to 3 to 4 tablespoons.	• Do not give cereal in a bottle unless directed by the physician. • Never put the infant to bed with a bottle in the mouth. This promotes tooth decay and can be a choking hazard.
6 to 8 months	• Introduce strained vegetables and fruits. Give 2 to 3 tablespoons and offer about four servings per day. • Teething foods such as toast strips, unsalted crackers, and teething biscuits also may be introduced.	• Introduce finger foods if recommended by the physician, but avoid things such as apple chunks or slices, grapes, hot dogs, sausages, peanut butter, popcorn, nuts, seeds, round candies, and hard chunks of uncooked vegetables.
8 to 12 months	• Introduce strained or finely chopped meats. • Increase vegetables and fruits to 3 to 4 tablespoons, four times a day. • Include egg yolks 3 to 4 times per week.	• Start breast-fed babies on meat at 8 months to improve iron intake. • Start weaning off the bottle. May introduce 2 to 4 ounces of water per day. • Do not give whole milk to infants under the age of 1.
1 to 2 years	• Whole milk can replace breast milk or formula. • Include fruits, vegetables, meats, breads, and grains.	• If a child does not like a food on the first attempt, try again later. • Offer one new food at a time.
2 years and older	• Balance dietary calories with physical activity to maintain normal growth. • Provide vegetables and fruits daily; limit juice intake. • Use vegetable oils and soft margarines low in saturated fat and trans fatty acids instead of butter or most other animal fats in the diet. • Provide whole-grain breads and cereals rather than refined-grain products. • Reduce the intake of sugar-sweetened beverages and foods. • Use nonfat (skim) or low-fat milk and dairy products daily. • Provide more fish, especially oily fish, broiled or baked. • Reduce salt intake, including salt from processed foods.	• Control when food is available and when it can be eaten. Regular meals and healthy snacks should be provided. • Have regular family meals that include social interaction with the family. • Teach about food and nutrition at the grocery store and when cooking meals. • Counteract inaccurate information from the media and other influences. • Teach other care providers (such as day care, babysitters) about what you want your children to eat. • Serve as role models and lead by example; "do as I do" rather than "do as I say." • Promote and participate in regular daily physical activity.

Source: Infants and children vary in growth and development; information intended as guidelines only. Adapted from Medline Plus http://www.nlm.hin.gov/medlineplus and American Academy of Pediatrics http://pediatrics.aappublications.org/.

rapidly during this period, their growth is still fast, and their communication skills begin to take shape in their use of language.

Physical Development Weight gain slows between 1 and 2 years. The arms and legs grow more than the trunk and head, and now seem to be in proportion to the child's overall size. Girls usually reach half of their adult height between 1½ and 2 years of age; boys reach half of their expected adult height between 2 and 2½ years.

Growth charts, as shown in Figure 40-6, are used to determine a child's growth in relation to average rates. The growth charts consist of percentile curves. Percentiles rank the position of an individual by indicating what percentage of the referenced population the individual would equal or exceed. Growth charts are available from the CDC for

both males and females of various ages. For example, on the weight-for-age growth charts, an 18-month boy whose weight is at the 90th percentile weighs the same or more than 90 percent of the reference population of 18-month boys and weighs less than 10 percent of the 18-month boys in the reference population. Pediatric growth charts are used as a clinical tool for health professionals to determine if a child's growth is adequate. Procedure 40-2, at the end of this chapter, provides more information about how to record height, weight, and head circumference on a growth chart.

Most toddlers will walk independently by 15 months of age. At 18 months, a toddler can squat to reach for a toy, kneel and remain upright, and precisely perform the pincer grasp. The toddler may use a spoon for self-feeding. By 2 years of age, the child can run, throw a ball, and scribble

Keeping Infants and Toddlers Safe

Teaching the parents or caregivers of infants and children about safety may be the responsibility of the medical assistant. Use the following points when teaching parents or caregivers:

- Keep emergency phone numbers close to the phone for the family and sitters.
- Make sure the crib meets federal safety standards.
- Never hold the infant or toddler on your lap in a car. Use an approved car seat placed in the back of the vehicle. Use the current recommendations from the American Academy of Pediatrics (http://www.aap.org) for forward-facing or rear-facing infant car seats. (See Figure 40-5.)
- Never leave the child unattended in the car.
- Do not put pillows, comforters, or plush toys in the infant's crib.
- Prevent falls. Place the baby on a low surface and use correctly installed gates across stairs.
- Prevent choking. Check toys for small objects that might come loose. Be sure that clothing does not have cords around the neck.
- Do not leave hanging toys over the crib once the child begins to reach, pull, and roll over.
- Keep all cords on window blinds, lamps, and electrical equipment out of reach.
- Never leave a child unattended around, near, or in any kind of water, including the water in toilets, mop buckets, or pools.

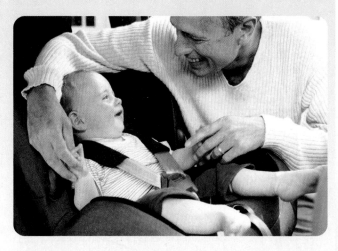

FIGURE 40-5 Infants and toddlers should be in approved car seats. Check the Internet site of the American Academy of Pediatrics for proper type and size.
©Lawrence Lawry/Getty Images

- Set the water temperature of the household hot water tank at 120°F. Turn pot handles inward, away from the edge of the stove, while cooking. Cover electrical outlets.
- Keep medicines and chemicals, including household cleaners, out of reach or in locked cabinets. Post the local poison control center's phone number in an accessible location.

---

with a pencil. The child may want to feed herself. At 3 years, the child is very active. Children of this age can dress themselves, ride a tricycle, draw simple shapes, and use a pair of child's scissors. Many children are toilet-trained between 2 and 3 years of age.

Intellectual-Cognitive Development During the toddler years, the child begins to learn about the world through play. Children enjoy imitating sweeping, raking, and making things they have seen adults make. A major task for the toddler is to develop independence. Toddlers are curious about their world, and their play may involve experimenting.

The toddler progresses with speech in the following ways:

- Speaks a few single words at 12 to 15 months.
- Speak up to 50 words by 2 years
- Repeats nursery rhymes at 3 years.

At 15 months, the child enjoys looking at books. Between 2 and 3 years of age, the toddler seems to be constantly asking, "Why?" By 3 years of age, the child may participate in the retelling of familiar stories and can draw and recognize simple shapes. During the toddler years, the child also enjoys playing with blocks.

Psycho-Emotional Development At 1 year of age, children are able to express many emotions. As children move from 1 year to 3 years, they gain some control over ways of expressing their feelings. Temper tantrums may become a problem between 18 months and 2 to 2½ years of age. A child of 15 months may respond to "No," but by the time the toddler approaches 18 to 21 months, he or she is resisting authority and is the one who is saying, "No!" Children of this age need consistent limits. If the child learns that a certain behavior will gain nothing, the behavior will stop fairly soon. As toddlers approach 3 years of age, they become sensitive to the feelings of others and may be characterized as affectionate.

Social Development Between 1 and 2 years, the toddler is unlikely to be able to truly play with another child. Play may involve taking toys from another child rather than sharing. Between 2 and 3 years, children become able to share and play with others. Adult guidance is necessary for the toddler to develop an awareness of what is appropriate when playing with other children.

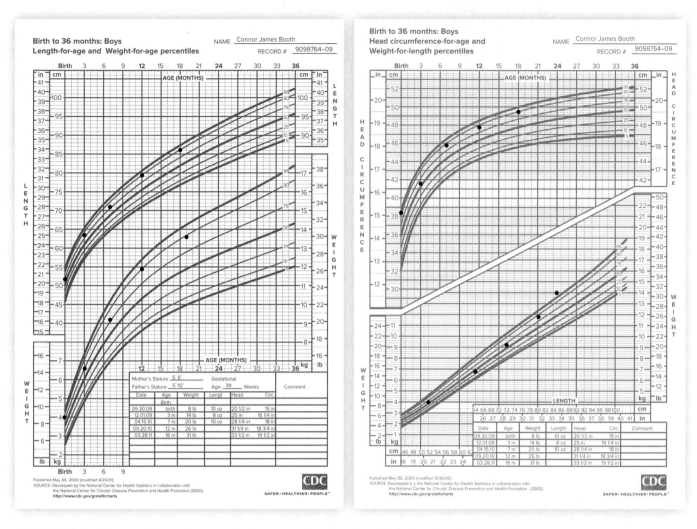

FIGURE 40-6 The curved lines on these growth charts are used to chart the growth for boys from birth to age 36 months. The child's length/height, weight, and head circumference are measured and recorded, then plotted on these graphs to show progress.

©Lawrence Lawry/Getty Images (a-b) Source: Developed by the National Center for Health Statistics in collaboration with the National Center for Chronic Disease Prevention and Health Promotion, 2000. http://www.cdc.gov/growcharts

Aspects of Care: 1 to 3 Years Consider the following when caring for toddlers or providing parent or caregiver education. Safety is of utmost importance. See the *Educating the Patient* feature Keeping Infants and Toddlers Safe. During the toddler years, it is also very important to allow a child to increase independence in a safe environment.

- Toddlers need opportunities to work on their fine-motor skills, such as those used in writing with crayons.
- Toddlers are developing their language skills, so simple explanations provide a positive environment for development.
- Setting limits helps the child to develop boundaries in relationships and behavior. At the same time, the environment should not be one in which the child is constantly told, "No."

The Preschooler: 3 to 5 Years

The child of 3 to 5 years is preparing to go out into the world.

Physical Development Individual differences, such as heredity, account for differences in height and weight among children between the ages of 3 and 5 years. During this time, it is best not to compare the preschooler's size to that of another preschooler. Each child's growth should be monitored and compared to the size documented on his or her ongoing growth chart. Girls progress more rapidly toward their adult height and weight than do boys. The respiratory rate and heart rate begin to slow down, coming closer to the adult range. Bones begin to ossify, or harden, between the ages of 2 and 7. During these years, it is important for children to be active in their play. They also need adequate calcium intake for the development of strong bones. Most children will have achieved nighttime bowel and bladder control by the time they are 3 or 4 years of age. If lack of bowel and/or bladder control persists beyond 4 or 5 years, this should be brought to the physician's attention.

During the 3- to 5-year period, many skills are achieved, including going up and down stairs using an alternating step approach, riding a tricycle, skipping, hopping on one foot, and throwing a ball with accuracy. Girls are usually about a year ahead of boys in small muscle coordination and fine-motor skills. A child of 3 can draw simple shapes and use a pencil to imitate the way an adult writes. At 4, the child can draw a simple human figure and can cut with blunt scissors, though not well at this age. A child of 5 can reproduce some shapes, letters, and numbers. By the age of 5, some children also may have learned how to tie their shoes.

Intellectual-Cognitive Development Language grows by leaps and bounds during these years. The imaginative child of 3 years has a vocabulary of about 900 words, forms simple sentences, and can tell simple stories that may be very "I"-oriented. At 4 years of age, the child's vocabulary is about 1,600 words, sentences are complete, and the favorite question is "Why?" Parents need to give very simple answers such as "Because it will keep you safe right now." The child's vocabulary at age 5 exceeds 2,000 words, and the stories the child tells involve more detail. At this age, the child has learned the difference between telling stories and lying.

Psycho-Emotional Development The 3-year-old child is very easy and pleasant. Children of this age usually enjoy music. A child at this age has an increasing sense of self, but imagination may lead the child to have unfounded worries and fears, especially at night. At 4 years of age, negativity may increase. Parents hear more of the "Nos" that they heard when the child was 2 years old. The 4-year-old child is testing limits and needs guided opportunities for freedom. Once a child reaches 5 years, life settles down a little. The child is more self-assured, well adjusted, and home-centered. At this age, the child likes to follow the rules, may want to "play by the rules," and is capable of accepting some responsibility.

Social Development Three-year-old children know what gender they are. The child knows how to take turns and may enjoy brief activities in a group with other children. A 3-year-old child likes to "help." Four-year-old children are very social and enjoy playing simple group games, such as tag and hide-and-seek. At 5 years, the child continues to be very social, enjoys playing with other children, and likes games in which the "rules" are observed.

Aspects of Care: 3 to 5 Years Consider the following when caring for children from 3 to 5 years or providing parent or caregiver education.

- The child of 5 years should receive a complete preschool developmental assessment and physical that includes an evaluation of hearing and vision.
- Immunizations, discussed in *section 40.3* of this chapter, must be up-to-date when the child enters kindergarten.
- Children of about 3 years may have night terrors. Parents should discuss these with the pediatrician if they are severe or persistent.

- Children may use delaying tactics at bedtime and may need to be shown repeatedly that there is nothing in the closet or under the bed. A nightlight is useful.
- Nighttime routines are important in helping a child feel secure.

The Elementary School Child: 6 to 10 Years

The following describes the stages of development of the 6- to 10-year-old child.

Physical Development During childhood, girls may be taller and heavier than boys. Bones continue to ossify in both boys and girls. Permanent teeth replace "baby teeth." Muscles continue to develop. Regular exercise is needed to encourage strength and coordination. At 9 and 10 years of age, the reproductive system also will be developing.

Intellectual-Cognitive Development Knowledge explosion happens once a child enters school. On entering school, the 6-year-old child has a brief attention span. By 10 years old, she is able to focus for longer periods of time. Most children of this age like to talk. As children move from 5 or 6 years of age toward 9 and 10 years, they are better able to separate fantasy from reality. They develop a sense of what is right and wrong, of honesty and fairness.

Psycho-Emotional Development When children approach 10 years of age, they may be more influenced by their peers than by their parents. During these years, children are beginning to develop a sense of self and learn gender-related roles. Children of 6 to 8 years of age may have trouble thinking about disasters that they hear about. As children approach 10 years of age, they are better able to grasp concepts of time and distance. A 9- to 10-year-old child may want to do something to help others. School-age children may be very sensitive to criticism and to what they see as failure.

Social Development School is central to the life of a child between 6 and 10 years of age. Although team sports and activities become important, parents need to avoid allowing the child to become overwhelmed with too many organized activities at this time. Children also need time to be quiet and alone. Outdoor activities help to use up some of the child's energy. Appropriate social behaviors are learned during this stage.

Aspects of Care: 6 to 10 Years Consider the following when caring for 6- to 10-year-olds or providing parent or caregiver education:

- Structure and a schedule help to maintain order and discipline.
- Monitor physical activities to prevent injury. The American Academy of Pediatrics advises against elementary-school-age children participating in contact sports.

- Consistency in daily activities and in discipline helps the child to develop intellectually, emotionally, and socially.
- Regular health and dental care and maintenance of immunizations are required.
- Communicable diseases are common.

The Middle School Child: 11 to 13 Years

The following sections will give you some insight into the stages of development of the 11- to 13-year-old child.

Physical Development **Puberty** refers to the physiological changes that make a person capable of sexual reproduction. In the United States and most other Western cultures, the onset of puberty occurs in females at around 12 or 13 years of age, but some may experience changes as early as 9. By the time a girl reaches middle school, a significant occurrence may be the onset of menstruation. It is important for everyone to remember that even though her body may be maturing, she is still only between 9 and 12 years old.

Males tend to go through the changes of puberty a little later than females (Figure 40-7). The average age for males to experience these changes is around 14 years, although some may begin noticing physical changes as early as age 9. Hormonal changes in both males and females may contribute to development of skin problems and acne.

Intellectual-Cognitive Development Grades may slip during this time. So much physical growth is taking place and so many physiological changes are occurring that less energy is available to concentrate on academics. Preadolescents may tend to exaggerate and "bend the truth."

Psycho-Emotional Development Although preadolescents crave independence, they are also very unsure of themselves. They are experiencing a wide range of physical changes and, at the same time, are learning the roles of sexuality. It is very important for preadolescents to receive accurate information about their changing bodies and feelings from appropriate and reliable sources. Middle-school-age students may not be comfortable asking parents questions about sexuality. Conflict may arise at this time. Parents may find that the preadolescent is easily annoyed and may be temperamental. Frequently, the preadolescent child will take on the behaviors of his or her peer group.

Social Development During the middle school years, children are learning about their own sexual identity and may not be comfortable in heterosexual relationships. Girls express an earlier interest in male-female relationships than do boys. Children of this age need to be able to turn to an adult with whom they are comfortable, so they can ask personal and intimate questions.

Aspects of Care: 11 to 13 Years Consider the following when caring for preadolescents or providing parent or caregiver education.

- A preadolescent needs to be assured that he or she is valued and loved.
- Consistency in discipline is very important.
- Parents should not be hypercritical or make too many demands.
- Friendships and associations should be monitored.
- Overscheduling of the child's time should be avoided.

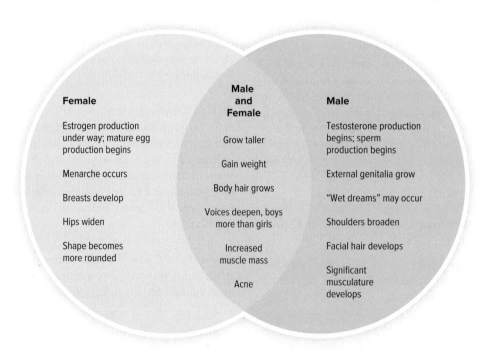

FIGURE 40-7 Some changes during puberty are the same for males and females. Others are unique to one sex.

The Adolescent: 14 to 19 Years

The teen years can be full of excitement for teenagers and their family and friends. They also can be difficult years. Tremendous physiological changes during this time may cause internal conflicts that can turn into external clashes. Parents may feel anxious about their child's quest for independence and about the child's upcoming departure from the home. The process of developing independence, a personal identity, and future plans is important during this stage.

Physical Development During the later teen years, females attain their adult height and weight. Males may continue to grow in height until 25 years of age. Physical growth and development in the teenage years are centered on normal sexual change. Girls usually have reached **menarche,** the onset of menstruation. Boys may have nocturnal emissions of seminal fluid (also called wet dreams). Weight control can be a concern. Some health problems of adulthood can be traced back to lifelong habits of poor dietary choices and lack of exercise begun in adolescence.

Intellectual-Cognitive Development During the early adolescent years, the child may have taken the word of an adult or a peer without question. Now, the teen asks questions and needs to work out answers that fit into his or her values. Adolescents often do not see the connection between behavior and consequences. This may lead to experimentation with drugs, alcohol, or sex.

Psycho-Emotional Development An adolescent knows the socially acceptable and appropriate ways to express feelings, but the pressures felt by adolescents may result in angry outbursts. Anger that is directed inward can be harmful. Anxiety and sometimes depression are part of adolescence.

Social Development Friendships are very important to adolescents. As teens get older, they become more comfortable with their parents and outgrow the attitude of "not wanting to be seen dead" with their parents. The teen years are wonderful and difficult at the same time. Problems faced by teens include eating disorders, substance abuse, sexually transmitted infection, suicide, and violence. You will examine these special concerns further in *section 40.6* of this chapter.

Aspects of Care: 14 to 19 Years Consider the following when caring for teens or providing education to the parents or caregiver:

- Teens need adequate amounts of calcium and weight-bearing exercise for strong bone development.
- Teens should know the risks of early, unplanned pregnancy and sexually transmitted infections when engaging in sexual activity.
- The adolescent needs to spend time enjoying friendships, sporting events, and social events.
- People who are caring for teens should:
  - Listen.
  - Give them the facts.

- Trust them.
- Provide them with firm and friendly discipline.
- Be consistent.
- Educate them with their independence in mind.
- Set limits and stick to them.
- Set examples of good behavior and good taste.
- Remember how it feels to be an adolescent.

▶ Pediatric Examinations LO 40.2

Many of the exam procedures for a pediatric patient are the same as those for an adult. While you prepare the child or adolescent for the exam, you may discuss with the parent, caregiver, or child topics such as eating habits, sleep patterns, daily activities, immunization schedules, and toilet training. Discussions should be appropriate for the child's developmental stage. This discussion will provide important clues to possible abnormal physical, cognitive-intellectual, psycho-emotional, and social development. Additional discussion topics such as sexually transmitted infections, drugs, and alcohol may be appropriate for an adolescent. Point out potential problems to the licensed practitioner.

Some children are afraid of going to the doctor's office. You can help relieve a child's fear by calmly explaining procedures before they occur, giving the reason for each procedure and being cheerful and mindful of a child's feelings. Allowing a child to examine some of the blunt instruments may also lessen fear (Figure 40-8). If a patient is physically

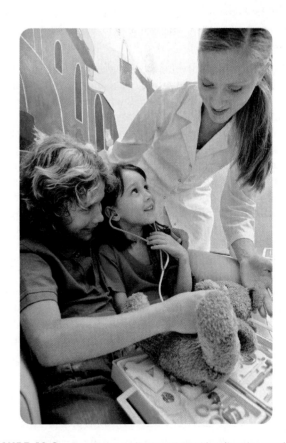

FIGURE 40-8 Providing a pediatric patient with a diversion may help lessen the child's fear.

©PhotoAlto/Laurence Mouton/Getty Images

resistant to the exam, you may need to call for assistance from the licensed practitioner or caregiver, or the child may need to be restrained.

Try to speak in terms aimed at the child's age level and kneel if necessary to make eye contact with the child. Treat the child with respect and provide positive reinforcement when a child is cooperative. Avoid making light of crying or pain. Make a game out of some aspect of a procedure and provide a small token reward at the end of a visit. For infants, a gentle approach, such as talking quietly and holding them comfortingly, is helpful.

Be mindful of adolescents' sensitivity toward rapid growth and physical, sexual, and social development when you prepare them for examination. Adolescents and preadolescents often feel awkward and self-conscious about being examined. They also may prefer to dress alone and to be alone with the licensed practitioner.

Well-Child Examination

Parents should bring their infants and children to the pediatrician for regular checkups and growth monitoring. The American Academy of Pediatrics (AAP) recommends the following frequency:

- Infants need seven well-baby exams during their first year, at these intervals: 3 to 5 days, 1 month, 2 months, 4 months, 6 months, 9 months, and 1 year.
- Children in the second and third years of life should have checkups at 15, 18, 24, and 30 months.
- From the age of 3, children should have checkups every year.

The AAP has developed recommendations for these examinations. See Table 40-2 for a summary of the components of the well-child examination based on the age of the child.

Follow standard precautions and prepare for the physical exam the same way you would for an adult, except for draping and positioning. Ask the parent of an infant or toddler to remove all the child's clothing except the diaper. Then keep the child covered until the physician enters the exam room. An infant or toddler may be crying during the exam. To assist the physician in hearing chest sounds with a stethoscope, ask the parent to allow the infant to suck on a pacifier, if used, to quiet the crying. Feeding the child during the exam is not encouraged because stomach sounds interfere with clear auscultation (listening to body sounds with a stethoscope). Distracting infants and toddlers with mobiles, shiny surfaces, or toys may help the exam go more smoothly. Review the *Points on Practice* feature Assisting with an Exam for an Infant or Child for additional information about the pediatric exam.

▶ Pediatric Immunizations　LO 40.3

An **immunization** is the administration of a vaccine to protect susceptible individuals from infectious diseases. As discussed in the *Infection Control Fundamentals* chapter, one of the

TABLE 40-2	Recommendations for Preventive Pediatric Healthcare
Developmental Stage	**Components of the Examination**
Infancy (birth to 12 months)	History and physical Length/height and weight Head circumference Weight for length Immunizations Newborn metabolic/hemoglobin screening Developmental surveillance Psychosocial/behavioral assessment
Early childhood (12 months to 4 years)	History and physical Length/height and weight Head circumference up to 24 months Body mass index starting at 24 months Weight for length up to 18 months Blood pressure and vision screening starting at 3 years Vision starting at 3 years Hearing starting at 4 years Immunizations Developmental surveillance Psychosocial/behavioral assessment
Middle childhood (5 years to 10 years)	History and physical Length/height and weight Body mass index Blood pressure Vision and hearing screening Oral health at 6 years Immunizations Developmental surveillance Psychosocial/behavioral assessment Ages 9–11 dyslipidemia screening
Adolescence (12 years to 21 years)	History and physical Length/height and weight Body mass index Blood pressure Vision and hearing screening Tobacco, alcohol, or drug use assessment Ages 15–18 HIV screening Ages 12–21 depression screening Ages 17–21 dyslipidemia screening Developmental surveillance Psychosocial/behavioral assessment

Source: Adapted from the American Academy of Pediatrics, Recommendations for Preventive Pediatric Health Care, copyright 2019.

necessary elements in the cycle of infection is the transmission of the pathogen to a susceptible host. To reduce the susceptibility of the host to infection, immunizations are given. When a healthy patient is vaccinated with a weakened strain of a virus, the patient's lymphocytes manufacture antibodies against that virus. These antibodies remain in the body, making it immune to that virus in the future. In general, there are two types of vaccines: live-attenuated and inactivated. Live-attenuated vaccines are a weakened form of the virus itself. Inactivated vaccines are either whole viruses, whole bacteria, or fractions of either. Inactivated vaccines usually require multiple doses for immunity to occur.

Assisting with an Exam for an Infant or Child

When assisting with an exam for an infant or child, you will need to take some special considerations. The techniques you use to prepare an infant or child emotionally and physically should be modified based on the patient's age and ability.

Emotional

Infants and toddlers are likely to be afraid of you because you are a stranger. Approach these children slowly, smile, and use a gentle voice. Children of preschool age are sometimes uncooperative and challenging. Remain calm, perform the procedures quickly, and restrain the child (with assistance from the parent) when appropriate. To prevent children from getting injured, watch them at all times.

Physical

Base your choice of an exam position for children on each child's age and ability to cooperate. Although young infants are usually examined on an examining table, older infants and toddlers may need to be examined while held on a parent's lap. Some toddlers may cooperate while standing on the examining table with a parent nearby. Some children may need to be restrained during parts of the examination or during an immunization. See Figure 40-9. Preschool children can usually be placed on the examining table if a parent is nearby. Regardless of their position, watch children at all times to prevent injury. When examining young children, licensed practitioners typically perform percussion (tapping on the surface to hear the underlying structures) and auscultation (listening) first because children are more likely to be calm and quiet at the outset. Practitioners always examine painful areas last. Practitioners may examine older children's genitalia last because, after a certain age, children tend to find such an exam embarrassing.

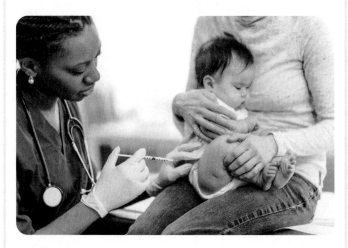

FIGURE 40-9   By fully immobilizing the child, you decrease the risk that his or her movement will result in injury.

©FatCamera/Getty Images

Immunizations are usually given during regular checkups (Figure 40-10). Immunizing children against diseases such as hepatitis B, diphtheria, tetanus, pertussis (whooping cough), poliomyelitis, measles, mumps, rubella (German measles), chickenpox, human papillomavirus (HPV), rotavirus, meningococcal disease, and *Haemophilus influenzae* type B (Hib) is recommended. Many vaccines have largely eliminated the threat of these once-prevalent, life-threatening diseases.

The first vaccine, for hepatitis B, is given to a newborn the day after birth. Some vaccines require a series of doses to give immunity. Booster doses may be required for a particular vaccine at a later age. The Centers for Disease Control and Prevention (CDC) recommends that physicians take every reasonable opportunity to vaccinate a child to ensure that the child receives the protection he needs. If a child gets behind on his immunizations, a catch-up schedule is available.

As a medical assistant, you will play a vital role in the immunization process. Your duties may include:

- Scheduling appointments and follow-up visits at the appropriate time based on the immunization schedule.
- Educating parents about the benefits and risks of vaccines and obtaining informed consent.
- Administering the vaccine correctly.
- Keeping careful immunization records, including the vaccine type, the date of vaccination, and the vaccine lot number.
- Ensuring proper vaccine storage and handling, including checking the temperature of the refrigerator and freezer daily.

Immunization Recommendations

The Advisory Committee on Immunization Practices, the American Academy of Pediatrics, and the American Academy of Family Physicians jointly publish immunization schedules for children. When working in a pediatrician's office, you should be familiar with the current vaccination schedule guidelines because they change occasionally. New guidelines, methods, and vaccines are constantly being developed. See Figure 40-11 for the birth to age 6 and the ages 7–18 immunization schedules. If you are

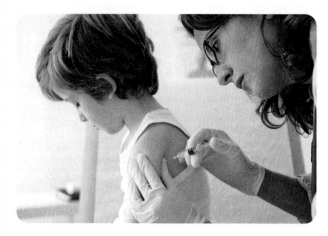

FIGURE 40-10   Immunizations are part of routine well-child visits in a pediatric practice.

©BSIP SA/Alamy Stock Photo

Figure 1. Recommended Immunization Schedule for Children and Adolescents Aged 18 Years or Younger—United States, 2017.

These recommendations must be read with the footnotes that follow. For those who fall behind or start late, provide catch-up vaccination at the earliest opportunity as indicated by the green bars in Figure 1. To determine minimum intervals between doses, see the catch-up schedule (Figure 2). School entry and adolescent vaccine age groups are shaded in gray.

Vaccine	Birth	1 mo	2 mos	4 mos	6 mos	9 mos	12 mos	15 mos	18 mos	19-23 mos	2-3 yrs	4-6 yrs	7-10 yrs	11-12 yrs	13-15 yrs	16 yrs	17-18 yrs
Hepatitis B[1] (HepB)	1st dose	◄----2nd dose----►			◄--------------------3rd dose----------------------►												
Rotavirus[2] (RV) RV1 (2-dose series); RV5 (3-dose series)			1st dose	2nd dose	See footnote 2												
Diphtheria, tetanus, & acellular pertussis[3] (DTaP: <7 yrs)			1st dose	2nd dose	3rd dose		◄----4th dose----►					5th dose					
Haemophilus influenzae type b[4] (Hib)			1st dose	2nd dose	See footnote 4		◄--3rd or 4th dose, --► See footnote 4										
Pneumococcal conjugate[5] (PCV13)			1st dose	2nd dose	3rd dose		◄------4th dose------►										
Inactivated poliovirus[6] (IPV: <18 yrs)			1st dose	2nd dose	◄----------------------3rd dose----------------------►							4th dose					
Influenza[7] (IIV)					Annual vaccination (IIV) 1 or 2 doses								Annual vaccination (IIV) 1 dose only				
Measles, mumps, rubella[8] (MMR)					See footnote 8		◄----- 1st dose -----►					2nd dose					
Varicella[8] (VAR)							◄----- 1st dose -----►					2nd dose					
Hepatitis A[10] (HepA)						◄--------2-dose series, See footnote 10 -------►											
Meningococcal[11] (Hib-MenCY ≥6 weeks; MenACWY-D ≥9 mos; MenACWY-CRM ≥2 mos)				See footnote 11										1st dose		2nd dose	
Tetanus, diphtheria, & acellular pertussis[12] (Tdap: ≥7 yrs)														Tdap			
Human papillomavirus[13] (HPV)														See footnote 13			
Meningococcal B[11]																See footnote 11	
Pneumococcal polysaccharide[5] (PPSV23)													See footnote 5				

| | Range of recommended ages for all children | | Range of recommended ages for catch-up immunization | | Range of recommended ages for certain high-risk groups | | Range of recommended ages for non-high-risk groups that may receive vaccine, subject to individual clinical decision making | | No recommendation |

NOTE: The above recommendations must be read along with the footnotes of this schedule.

This schedule includes recommendations in effect as of Januay 1, 2017. Any dose not administered at the recommended age should be administered at a subsequent visit, when indicated and feasible. The use of a combination vaccine generally is preferred over separate injections of its equivalent component vaccines. Vaccination providers should consult the relevant Advisory Committee on Immunization Practices (ACIP) statement for detailed recommendations, available online at www.cdc.gov/vaccines/hcp/acip-recs/index.html. Clinically significant adverse events that follow vaccination should be reported to the Vaccine Adverse Event reporting System (VAERS) online (www.vaers.hhs.gov) or by telephone (800-822-7967). Suspeded cases of vaccine-preventable diseases should be reported to the state or local health department. Additional information, including precautions and contraindications for vaccination, is available from CDC online (www.cdcgov/vaccines/hcp/admin/contraindications.html) or by telephone (800-CDC-INFO [800-232-4636]).

This schedule is approved by the Advisory Committee on Immunization Practices (www.cdc.gov/vaccines/acip), the American Academy of Pediatrics (www.aap.org), the American Academy of Family Physicians (www.aafp.org), and the American College of Obstetricians and Gynecologists (www.acog.org).

Footnotes—Recommended Immunization Schedule for Children and Adolescents Aged 18 Years or Younger, UNITED STATES, 2018

For further guidance on the use of the vaccines mentioned below, see: www.cdc.gov/vaccines/hcp/acip-recs/index.html.
For vaccine recommendations for persons 19 years of age and older, see the Adult Immunization Schedule.

Additional information

- For information on contraindications and precautions for the use of a vaccine, consult the *General Best Practice Guidelines for Immunization* and relevant ACIP statements, at www.cdc.gov/vaccines/hcp/acip-recs/index.html.
- For calculating intervals between doses, 4 weeks = 28 days. Intervals of ≥4 months are determined by calendar months.
- Within a number range (e.g., 12–18), a dash (–) should be read as "through."
- Vaccine doses administered ≤4 days before the minimum age or interval are considered valid. Doses of any vaccine administered ≥5 days earlier than the minimum interval or mininum age should not be counted as valid and should be repeated as age-appropriate. The repeat dose should be spaced after the invalid dose by the recommended minimum interval. For further detals, see Table 3-1, Recommended and minimum ages and intervals between vaccine doses, in *General Best Practice Guidelines for Immunization* at www.cdc.gov/vaccines/hcp/acip-recs/general-recs/timing.html.
- Information on travel vaccine requirements and recommendations is available at www.cdc.gov/travel/.
- For vaccination of persons with immunodeficiencies, see Table 8-1, *Vaccination of persons with primary and secondary immunodeficiencies*, in *General Best Practice Guidelines for Immunization* at www.cdc.gov/vaccines/hcp/acip-recs/general-recs/immunocompetence.html; and Immunization in Special Clinical Circumstances, (In: Kimberlin DW, Brady MT, Jackson MA, Long SS, eds. *Red Book: 2015 report of the Committee on Infectious Diseases, 30th ed.* Elk Grove Village, IL: American Academy of Pediatricss, 2015:68-107).
- The National Vaccine Injury Compensation Program (VICP) is a no-fault alternative to the traditional legal system for resolving vaccine injury claims. All routine child and adolescent vaccines are covered by VICP except for pneumococcal polysaccharide vaccine (PPSV23). For more information; see www.hrsa.gov/vaccinecompenstion/index.html.

FIGURE 40-11   Recommended immunization schedules for birth to 18 years. For more detail and the most current information, check the Centers for Disease Control and Prevention website.

Source: http://www.cdc.gov/vaccines/schedules/hcp/imz/child-adolescent.html.

responsible for administering immunizations, you should stay current with the most recent information, found online at https://www.cdc.gov/vaccines/schedules/downloads/child/0-18yrs-child-combined-schedule.pdf

You also should be aware that immunization schedules and requirements may be different for some pediatric patients. Some diseases, including some autoimmune diseases, may necessitate different guidelines. Refer to the CDC website listed above for more information.

Informed Consent

The licensed practitioner may ask you to explain the benefits and risks of an immunization to the parents. You will need to explain that the side effects of immunizations are usually mild, such as a slight fever or soreness, and of short duration. Review with the parent the vaccine information statement for the specific immunization you will be administering (Figure 40-12). Advise parents that the benefits of immunity greatly outweigh the risks. Then obtain informed consent for the child's immunization. Provide a copy of the vaccine information statement and then have the parent sign so the immunization can be given. Remember that religious or other personal beliefs may prevent parents from consenting to immunizations for their child. Some parents may want to delay or slow down the number of immunizations given at one time. Give immunizations as ordered, and record all appropriate information in the patient's chart.

DIPHTHERIA TETANUS & PERTUSSIS **VACCINES**

WHAT YOU NEED TO KNOW

Many Vaccine Information Statements are available in Spanish and other languages. See http://www.immunize.org/vis.

1. Why get vaccinated?

Diphtheria, tetanus, and pertussis are serious diseases caused by bacteria. Diphtheria and pertussis are spread from person to person. Tetanus enters the body through cuts or wounds.

DIPHTHERIA causes a thick covering in the back of the throat.
- It can lead to breathing problems, paralysis, heart failure, and even death.

TETANUS (Lockjaw) causes painful tightening of the muscles, usually all over the body.
- It can lead to "locking" of the jaw so the victim cannot open his mouth or swallow. Tetanus leads to death in up to 2 out of 10 cases.

PERTUSSIS (Whooping Cough) causes coughing spells so bad that it is hard for infants to eat, drink, or breathe. These spells can last for weeks.
- It can lead to pneumonia, seizures (jerking and staring spells), brain damage, and death.

Diphtheria, tetanus, and pertussis vaccine (DTaP) can help prevent these diseases. Most children who are vaccinated with DTaP will be protected throughout childhood. Many more children would get these diseases if we stopped vaccinating.

DTaP is a safer version of an older vaccine called DTP. DTP is no longer used in the United States.

2. Who should get DTaP vaccine and when?

Children should get 5 doses of DTaP vaccine, 1 dose at each of the following ages:
- 2 months
- 4 months
- 6 months
- 15–18 months
- 4–6 years

DTaP may be given at the same time as other vaccines.

3. Some children should not get DTaP vaccine or should wait.

- Children with minor illnesses, such as a cold, may be vaccinated. But children who are moderately or severely ill should usually wait until they recover before getting DTaP vaccine.

- Any child who had a life-threatening allergic reaction after a dose of DTaP should not get another dose.

- Any child who suffered a brain or nervous system disease within 7 days after a dose of DTaP should not get another dose.

- Talk with your doctor if your child:

  - had a seizure or collapsed after a dose of DTaP,
  - cried non-stop for 3 hours or more after a dose of DTaP,
  - had a fever over 105°F after a dose of DTaP.

Ask your healthcare provider for more information. Some of these children should not get another dose of pertussis vaccine but may get a vaccine without pertussis, called **DT**.

4. Older children and adults

DTaP is not licensed for adolescents, adults, or children 7 years of age and older.

But older people still need protection. A vaccine called **Tdap** is similar to DTaP. A single dose of Tdap is recommended for people 11 through 64 years of age. Another vaccine, called **Td**, protects against tetanus and diphtheria, but not pertussis. It is recommended every 10 years. There are separate Vaccine Information Statements for these vaccines.

| Diphtheria/Tetanus/Pertussis | 5/17/2007 |

FIGURE 40-12 Review the vaccine information sheet with the parent and obtain a signature before administering a vaccine.

Administering Immunizations

In many states, medical assistants may administer immunizations. Most immunizations are given as injections. You might be required to give more than two vaccinations in a single visit. Careful site selection is important when giving multiple injections. Refer to the *Medication Administration* chapter for information about administering various types of injections and selecting an appropriate injection site for pediatric patients. Some vaccines, such as live polio, are given orally. Most vaccinations may be administered even if the child has a mild illness. The physician will make the decision to vaccinate a child who is ill based on the disease and the severity of the symptoms. For the most part, if a child has a fever, the physician may postpone the immunization until the fever has subsided. However, do not postpone the visit if the child has an upper respiratory infection without a fever. Remember that the child does not need to restart a series of immunizations. He can simply receive the next scheduled immunization as soon as possible.

Before administering a childhood immunization, check for any contraindications to its use. A **contraindication** is a known risk or reason not to give the immunization. For example, pertussis vaccine must not be given to a child with a progressive neurologic disorder. It also must not be administered to a child who developed seizures, persistent crying, or a high fever after receiving a previous pertussis vaccine. In such a situation, the doctor would direct you to administer diphtheria and tetanus toxoids instead of the diphtheria and tetanus toxoid and pertussis vaccine (DTaP).

Immunization Records

Under the National Childhood Vaccine Injury Act of 1988, you must record certain information about immunizations in a child's permanent medical record. Required information includes:

- The vaccine's type, manufacturer, and lot number.
- The date on the vaccine information statement and the day and time the statement was given to the parent.
- The date of administration.
- The name, address, and title of the healthcare professional who administered the vaccine.

You also must document the vaccine type using standard abbreviations. For combination vaccines, such as Pediatrix™, you record the vaccine under all three components: DTaP, IPV, and hepatitis B. In addition, you must document:

- The administration site, route, and dosage.
- The vaccine's expiration date.

Parents should maintain an accurate, up-to-date immunization record for each child. They should be encouraged to bring this record with them to each healthcare visit. Each state and/or the CDC issues an immunization record form, which may be available in languages other than English. Complete a form after each child's first immunization. Instruct the parents to keep the form and bring it with the child for each subsequent immunization so that you can update the record. An example immunization record is shown in Figure 40-13. Advise parents that this record is important to keep because it acts as proof of immunization, which may be required by day care centers, schools, the military, and other organizations. This record also may be helpful when parents consult another doctor, in case of emergency, or when moving to a new location.

Vaccine Storage and Handling

Vaccines must be stored properly. As a medical assistant, in order to ensure vaccine safety and effectiveness, you are responsible for proper storage and handling from the time a vaccine arrives at your facility until it is administered to the patient. Follow these general guidelines:

- Store vaccines at the recommended temperatures immediately upon arrival at your facility. Check and record temperatures of refrigerators and freezers daily. If the correct temperature is not maintained, the vaccine will lose its effectiveness. Live-attenuated virus vaccines are especially sensitive to heat.
  - Store refrigerated vaccines between 35°F and 46°F (2°C and 8°C).
  - Store frozen vaccines between −58°F and +5°F (−50°C and −15°C).
- Rotate your supply of vaccines so those with the shortest expiration date are used first. Place the vaccine with the longest expiration date behind the vaccine that will expire the soonest. Remove expired vaccines from usable stock immediately.
- For disposal of vaccines that have expired or were drawn but not administered, follow the guidelines of your state health department.
- Prepare vaccines just prior to administration to the patient.
- Follow infection control guidelines when preparing and administering vaccines.

▶ Pediatric Screening and Diagnostic Tests LO 40.4

Pediatricians look for any sign of growth abnormality during routine well-child visits. Physicians compare a child's physical, cognitive-intellectual, psycho-emotional, and social signs to charts showing national averages. In general, physicians look for signs that the child is in the appropriate stage of growth for her age. The medical assistant's role in pediatric exams is similar to the role in adult patient exams. During the pediatric exam, the medical assistant may assist with or perform many tasks, including taking vital signs and body measurements, performing vision and hearing tests, collecting specimens, and administering medications and immunizations.

Vaccine (circle specific type given)	Date Given	Doctor or Clinic
1 Hep B	2/25/XX	BWW Assoc.
2 Hep B	3/21/XX	BWW Assoc.
3 Hep B	8/12/XX	BWW Assoc.
1 Hep A	5/12/XX	BWW Assoc.
2 Hep A		
Other		
Other		
Other		
Other		

Please fold on dotted line

1 *Flu (TIV/LAIV)		
2 *Flu (TIV/LAIV)		
Yearly *Flu (TIV/LAIV)		
Yearly *Flu (TIV/LAIV)		
Other		
Other		
Other		

All children ages 6 months through 8 years who receive seasonal influenza vaccine for the first time should be given 2 doses. Children who receive only one dose in the first year of vaccination should receive two doses in their second year of vaccination.

*Seasonal   Please fold on dotted line

Immunization Record

Name _____ Nelson, Isaiah _____
                         (Last, First, MI)

Date of Birth _____ 11/19/XX _____

Physician or Clinic _____ BWW Associates _____
        Alexis M. Whalen MD

Notice to Parents: Please take this card with you when you visit your doctor or clinic and have them fill in the information.

(a)

Vaccine (circle specific type given)	Date Given	Doctor or Clinic
1 DtaP/DT/Td	4/08/XX	BWW Assoc.
2 DtaP/DT/Td	6/10/XX	BWW Assoc.
3 DtaP/DT/Td	8/12/XX	BWW Assoc.
4 DtaP/DT/Td		
5 DtaP/DT/Td		
1 Tdap/Td		
1 Hib	4/08/XX	BWW Assoc.
2 Hib	6/10/XX	BWW Assoc.
3 Hib	8/12/XX	BWW Assoc.
4 Hib		
1 IPV	4/08/XX	BWW Assoc.
2 IPV	6/10/XX	BWW Assoc.
3 IPV	5/12/XX	BWW Assoc.
4 IPV		
5 IPV		
1 MMR/MMRV	5/12/XX	BWW Assoc.
2 MMR/MMRV		
1 Varicella	5/12/XX	BWW Assoc.
2 Varicella		
1 Rotavirus	4/08/XX	BWW Assoc.
2 Rotavirus	6/10/XX	BWW Assoc.
3 Rotavirus	8/12/XX	BWW Assoc.
1 PCV	4/08/XX	BWW Assoc.
2 PCV	6/10/XX	BWW Assoc.
3 PCV	8/12/XX	BWW Assoc.
4 PCV	5/12/XX	BWW Assoc.
1 MCV		
1 HPV		
2 HPV		
3 HPV		
other		

DH 686, 8/09 Stock Number 5740-000-0686-5

(b)

FIGURE 40-13   Example immunization record of Chris Matthews. (a) Front. (b) Back.

Vital Signs

Some variations in technique and results should be considered when performing vital signs on pediatric patients. In addition to the normal vital signs range variations (review Table 37-1 from the *Vital Signs and Measurements* chapter), some other things should be taken into account. Taking a child's or an infant's temperature can be a challenge. If the infant or child is likely to cry or become agitated, take the temperature last. Measure pulse, respiration, and blood pressure (if ordered) before you take the temperature to avoid having these measurements elevated because of the child's agitation. Oral thermometers are not appropriate for children younger than 5 years of age because these children are too young to safely hold the thermometer in their mouths. Instead, take axillary, rectal, tympanic, or temporal temperatures. If you use a rectal thermometer, hold it in place until the temperature registers to prevent the thermometer from being expelled or injuring the patient. Tympanic and temporal thermometers are especially useful in pediatric offices because of their speed and safety.

Blood pressure in children or infants is not routinely measured at each visit. Instead, the measurement is taken per the doctor's orders. The procedure is the same as that for taking blood pressure in adults, except for these modifications:

1. Ideally, take the patient's blood pressure before performing other tests or procedures that may cause anxiety. In this way, you can avoid a falsely high result.

2. Be sure to use the correct cuff size for the child or infant. The bladder width should not exceed two-thirds the length of the upper or lower arm. The bladder should cover three-fourths of the extremity's circumference.

3. Do not attempt to estimate an infant's blood pressure using the palpatory method (discussed in the *Vital Signs and Measurements* chapter). It is typically not used.

4. Inflate the pressure cuff to 20 mmHg above the point at which the radial pulse disappears.

5. Deflate the cuff at a rate of 2 mmHg per second.

6. You may continue to hear a heartbeat on a child or infant until the pressure reaches zero, so note when the strong heartbeat becomes muffled.

Body Measurements

Children and infants are weighed and measured at each office visit. Children who can stand may be weighed on an adult scale. If toddlers cannot remain still on an adult scale, weight may be determined by weighing an adult holding the toddler, then subtracting the adult's weight. Infants are weighed on infant scales, which typically measure pounds and ounces. Infant scales are sometimes built into a pediatric examining table.

The height of children and the length of infants are measured at each office visit. Measure children in the same manner as you measure an adult. Some offices are equipped with height bars or wall charts that are separate from a scale. Use these devices in the same way as those attached to a scale. Measure infants while they are lying down; in this instance, you are measuring length instead of height. Some pediatric examining tables have a built-in bar for measuring length. You also can use a tape measure or yardstick.

The circumference of an infant's head is an important measure of growth and development and is used to evaluate diseases such as hydrocephalus or excessive cerebrospinal fluid in the cranial cavity, which causes enlargement of the head. You may be asked to perform or assist with this measurement when you measure the infant's length. Measurement of head circumference may be performed at the same time as weight and length, or it may be part of the general physical exam (Figure 40-14). The steps for measuring infants are described in Procedure 40-1, at the end of this chapter. Review the

Vital Signs and Measurements chapter and the procedures for weighing and measuring children.

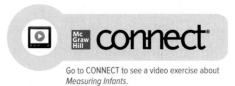

Go to CONNECT to see a video exercise about *Measuring Infants.*

General Eye and Vision Exam

As part of the general exam, the pediatrician examines the interior of the child's eyes with an instrument called an *ophthalmoscope*. You will probably perform the visual acuity test (Figure 40-15). Make a game of covering the child's eye if the child resists this part of the procedure. Use a pediatric vision chart as shown in Figure 40-16 for patients who cannot read. If the caregiver brought the child in specifically for a vision test, record in the child's chart whatever symptoms the caregiver mentions. Follow the procedure in the *Assisting with Eye and Ear Care* chapter, and use these modifications when performing vision screening on a pediatric patient:

- Watch for signs of visual difficulty during the test, such as tilting the head in a certain direction, blinking, squinting, or frowning. Observe the child for eyes that are misaligned or don't focus together. Keep in mind that some vision problems may have no warning signs. For example, amblyopia, or lazy eye, is a fairly common eye problem (affecting about 2 out of 100 children) that develops when a child has one eye that doesn't see well or is injured and he begins to use the other eye almost exclusively. The problem must be detected by the age of 3 in order to treat and restore normal vision in the affected eye by age 6. If this situation persists for too long (past 7 to 9 years of age), vision may be lost permanently in the unused eye.

- Use a pointer to select one symbol at a time in random order to prevent patients from memorizing the order.

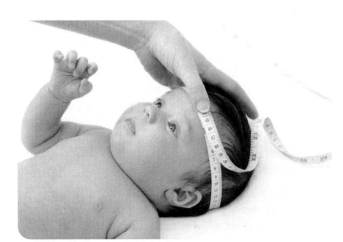

FIGURE 40-14 The medical assistant uses a flexible tape to measure the circumference of an infant's head.

©Science Photo Library/Ruth Jenkinson/Getty Images

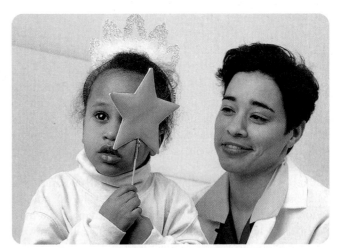

FIGURE 40-15 Making a game out of the visual acuity test helps put a child at ease.

©Ken Lax

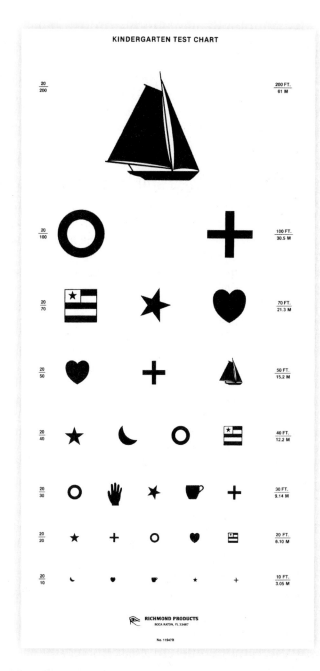

FIGURE 40-16 A kindergarten test chart is used to check the vision of a child who cannot read.

- It is common to start with children at the 40- or 30-foot line or larger if low vision is suspected and then proceed to the 20-foot line.
- Note the smallest line on which the child can identify three out of four or four out of six symbols correctly.

General Ear and Hearing Exam

A pediatric ear exam is important because so many children have ear infections or upper respiratory infections involving the ear. Because children's eustachian tubes are more horizontal than those of adults, fluid collects more easily in the tubes and can promote bacterial growth. The tubes are also short and connected to the throat, making it easy for any upper respiratory infections to travel to the ear.

You may be asked to perform a hearing test on a pediatric patient. Use the procedure *Measuring Auditory Acuity* found in the *Assisting with Eye and Ear Care* chapter.

Diagnostic Testing

Diagnostic procedures on adults, such as X-rays, blood and urine tests, and throat cultures, also are used for children. The pediatrician basically uses the same laboratory tests and radiologic tests. He performs some diagnostic tests in the office and needs the same types of specimens. Throat cultures, urine, and blood specimens are collected with a few extra considerations, explained in the following paragraphs.

Throat Culture Because streptococcal infection can be especially serious in a child, some pediatricians perform a rapid test for the presence of streptococcal bacteria so that they can immediately start the appropriate medical treatment. If the test is positive, the licensed practitioner begins treatment with antibiotics specifically for this type of bacterium. Whether the test is positive or negative, the practitioner also may do a throat culture. A throat culture can determine which of the streptococcal bacteria are present or whether other organisms are causing the symptoms. The results can indicate a possible change in medication. Review the method for obtaining a throat culture in the Obtaining a Throat Culture Specimen procedure in the chapter *Microbiology and Disease*. Having a small child lie down rather than sit may make the process easier. If the child refuses to open the mouth, gently squeeze the nostrils shut. The child will eventually open the mouth to breathe. Enlist the parent's help to restrain the child's hands if necessary.

Pediatric Urine Specimen When you collect a urine specimen from a pediatric patient, involve the child (if age-appropriate) and the parents or guardians. Explain the procedure thoroughly and ask specific questions, including the following:

- If the child is in diapers, ask whether there is a problem of persistent diaper rash. (Rash may indicate a change in urine composition because of renal dysfunction.)
- Is the child excessively thirsty? (In this case, the patient may not be taking in enough fluids for the amount of urine being excreted. Excessive thirst, combined with increased urinary frequency and volume, is symptomatic of diabetes.)
- Has the child experienced any difficulty urinating or a urine stream change? (These signs may suggest an obstruction in the urinary tract.)
- Does the child cry when urinating? (If so, the child may have pain or burning on urination, which can indicate a urinary tract infection.)
- If the child is in diapers, ask how many diapers are wet each day. Has the number changed recently? (Responses to these questions can rule out or confirm a urine volume

change. For example, a child with a fever and increased perspiration might experience decreased urine volume.)

- Has the child experienced deterioration in bladder control, such as bed-wetting (**enuresis**)? (The child may be under stress or may have a small bladder capacity or a urinary tract infection.)
- If the child is having problems with toilet training and is older than 4 years old, ask whether the child learned to sit, stand, and talk at the age-appropriate times. (If so, the child may have a urinary system dysfunction.)

When you collect a urine specimen from a child who is toilet-trained, follow the same procedures as for an adult. If the child is an infant or not toilet-trained, however, follow the steps outlined in Procedure 40-3, at the end of this chapter, and shown in Figure 40-17. The *Collecting, Processing, and Testing Urine and Stool Specimens* chapter provides additional information.

Blood-Drawing Procedures and Children Collecting blood may be part of your responsibility in a pediatric office. The *Collecting, Processing, and Testing Blood Specimens* chapter provides detailed information about this task. Note that when working with children, it is a challenge to explain blood-drawing procedures to them and that many children become visibly upset by the situation. If possible, it is best to talk with the parents or caregivers before working with the child. The adults can provide the best insight into how their child handles stressful situations.

Your primary concern when working with infants is to complete tests accurately. Because an infant's veins are too small for adequate blood collection, the best site for drawing blood is usually the heel, using a dermal puncture.

When working with children, address them directly. Speak clearly in a calm, soothing voice and explain the procedure briefly in terms they can understand. If they ask whether the process will hurt, be honest. A parent, guardian, or coworker should hold a very young child during a venipuncture or dermal puncture to prevent the child from moving. If a child is extremely distressed, it may be best to go on to another patient while the child calms down.

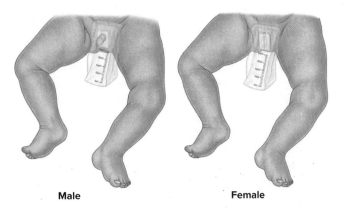

Male   **Female**

FIGURE 40-17   When you apply a pediatric urine bag, make sure there are no leaks. Follow the steps in Procedure 40-3, at the end of this chapter.

After you have begun the procedure, give the child status reports, such as "We're almost finished!" and make comments such as "You've been very brave." This also helps to calm nervous parents or caregivers. When the procedure is complete, offer a compliment on some aspect of the child's behavior. Gather your supplies and samples as quickly as possible to avoid alarming the child with the sight of blood-collection tubes. If parents or caregivers have questions, encourage them to discuss the tests with the child's physician.

▶ Pediatric Diseases and Disorders   LO 40.5

Many common disorders found in children are not specific diseases. Upper respiratory infections, including colds and viral influenza, occur frequently among children. Do not make assumptions regarding diagnosis or treatment. When reported symptoms include fever, sore throat, runny nose, and earache, any number of conditions could be the cause. Encourage the parent to bring the child to the office. You should, however, tell the doctor as soon as possible when a child has an extremely high fever. The doctor may want the child to go to an emergency room. Do not recommend aspirin for fever in children, as aspirin use in children has been associated with Reye syndrome, a potentially fatal disease of the central nervous system (CNS) and liver. Acetaminophen (Tylenol®) or ibuprofen (Motrin®) is preferred for treating fever in children. However, you should check with the doctor before recommending any fever-reducing medication such as Tylenol® or Motrin®.

Common Diseases and Disorders

When you work in a pediatric office, you should know the signs and symptoms of childhood diseases. These include infectious diseases such as chickenpox, influenza, croup, measles, mumps, pertussis, rubella, fever, and tetanus, which are discussed in the *Microbiology and Disease* chapter. In addition to infectious diseases, there are several other common diseases of childhood, which are outlined in Table 40-3.

Less Common Diseases and Disorders

Some less common diseases and disorders also can be found in children. You need to be aware of the basic symptoms and the treatments for these disorders.

AIDS Most childhood cases of human immunodeficiency virus (HIV) infection are transmitted from a mother to her infant. The transmission of HIV from an HIV-positive mother to her child during pregnancy, labor, delivery, or breast-feeding is called mother-to-child (*vertical*) transmission. In the absence of any interventions, transmission rates range from 15% to 45%. This rate can be reduced to levels below 5% with effective interventions. All babies born to HIV-positive mothers have HIV antibodies that are detectable through testing at birth. The antibodies persist for a period of 15 to 18 months, but not all of these babies remain permanently infected. AIDS has no cure, but treating the pregnant woman and newborn child with antiviral agents has been shown to lower the rate of HIV infection in the child.

TABLE 40-3	Common Pediatric Diseases and Disorders	
Condition	**Description**	**Treatment**
Asthma	Inflammation of the airways caused by triggers such as animals (hair or dander), dust, mold, pollen, tobacco smoke, exercise, strong emotions, and viral infection. Symptoms include tightness in the chest, chest retractions, shortness of breath, rapid breathing, and tiredness.	Avoidance of known triggers; measuring of peak flow to determine breathing function; inhaled medications for long-term treatment, including corticosteroids and leukotriene; for quick relief of symptoms, albuterol or Atrovent; allergy shots and oral medications
Head lice	Small insects easily spread among children by head-to-head contact and by sharing objects such as combs and hairbrushes. Lice live on the scalp and lay eggs strongly attached to hair shafts; symptoms include itchy scalp. Identify this condition by locating crawling lice or nits (eggs) attached to hair; examine parted hair carefully at the scalp and bottom of hair strands.	Anti-lice shampoo or 1% permethrin cream rinse; removal of eggs with fine-tooth comb; disinfection of clothing, bedding, and washable toys by machine washing and drying in hot cycles or by dry cleaning; tight bagging for 30 days of items that cannot be washed; disinfection of combs and brushes (used for hair) by washing in anti-lice shampoo
Herpes simplex virus (HSV)	The virus causes cold sore blisters on or near the mouth; diagnosis is made by inspecting lesions. The first stage (2–12 days before appearance of the blister) involves tingling and itching sensations; later, the blister ruptures and forms a yellow crust. An outbreak takes about 3 weeks to heal completely.	Application of ice cube to the blister, which may promote faster healing; ointments to alleviate cracking and discomfort; avoidance of sun exposure because it may trigger an outbreak
Impetigo	Highly contagious dermatologic disease caused by staphylococcal, or sometimes streptococcal, bacteria; transmitted by direct contact. Causes inflammation and pustules, which are small, lymph-filled bumps that rupture and become encrusted before healing; frequently seen around the mouth and nostrils.	Avoidance of scratching lesions and sharing utensils, towels, bed linens, or bath or pool water that could cause further transmission; careful washing of affected areas two or three times per day to keep lesions clean and dry; topical antibacterial cream
Infectious conjunctivitis ("pink eye")	Highly contagious streptococcal or staphylococcal bacterial infection of the conjunctiva of the eye; transmitted by direct contact. Causes redness, pain, swelling, and discharge; usually begins in one eye and spreads to the other.	Avoidance of scratching eyes and sharing utensils, towels, or bed linens that could cause further transmission; warm compresses to relieve discomfort; antibiotic drops or ointment
Pinworms	Parasites transmitted by swallowing worm eggs, by touching something that the infected person has touched, or by putting infested sand or dirt into the mouth. When the eggs hatch in the body, worms attach to the intestinal lining; mature females travel to areas just outside the rectum to lay eggs, which causes itching.	Medication given to the whole family to treat and prevent further infestation
Ringworm	Contagious fungal infection of the scalp, groin, feet, or other areas of body, causing flat, dry, and scaly or moist and crusty lesions; lesions develop into a clear center with an outer ring. When the scalp is affected, may cause bald patches.	Oral and topical antifungal medication; isolation to prevent spreading; frequent changing of towels and bedding, with no sharing with others in family; caution that the child should not use others' combs or brushes
Scabies	Contagious, itchy rash caused by mites that burrow under the skin.	Application of a medicated cream containing 5% permethrin or 10% crotamiton over the entire body surface, then washing it off after 8 to 14 hours; may be reapplied after 1 week
Scarlet fever ("scarlatina")	Red rash that starts as patches then turns to fine bumps. Occurs either before symptoms or up to 7 days after. Symptoms include fever, sore throat, chills, vomiting, and abdominal pain.	Antibiotics to clear up the symptoms and to prevent long-term health problems such as rheumatic fever or kidney disease
Streptococcal sore throat ("strep throat")	Contagious disease spread by droplet. Symptoms include headache, high fever, vomiting, and extremely painful, swollen, and red or white sore throat; causes difficulty swallowing. Complications include progression to rheumatic fever (with arthritis, nephritis, and inflammation of the inner lining of the heart).	Streptococci-specific antibiotics given as soon as possible; therapy based on the practitioner's experience is sometimes given without confirmed diagnosis; antibiotics are adjusted with confirmation of infecting organism; possible hospitalization in acute cases

Juvenile Rheumatoid Arthritis Juvenile rheumatoid arthritis (JRA) is an autoimmune disease of the joints that occurs in children aged 16 or younger. The symptoms of JRA include swelling, pain, and stiffness of the joints. The most common type of JRA affects four or fewer joints, typically the large joints such as the knees. A less common form of JRA affects five or more joints, most commonly the small joints of the hands and feet. The severity of the disease ranges from mild to severe and may affect the eyes and internal organs. A child with JRA will have periods of remission (a lessening of symptoms) and flare-up (a worsening of symptoms). JRA is diagnosed based on the severity of symptoms, specific laboratory tests, and X-rays. Treatment of this disease includes nonsteroidal anti-inflammatory drugs (NSAIDs), disease-modifying anti-rheumatic drugs (DMARDs), corticosteroids, biologic agents, and physical therapy.

As a medical assistant, your role in caring for children with JRA includes emphasizing the value of exercise and physical therapy, stressing the importance of taking medications as directed, and offering assistance by providing patient education brochures and information about local support groups and organizations.

Attention Deficit Hyperactivity Disorder and Learning Disabilities Attention deficit hyperactivity disorder (ADHD) and learning disabilities (LD) are found in children, adolescents, and adults. These disorders can cause gross motor disability, inability to read or write, hyperactivity, distractibility, impulsiveness, and generally disruptive behavior. ADHD encompasses all conditions formerly identified as hyperactivity, or hyperkinesis, and attention deficit. LD encompasses a wide range of conditions that interfere with learning, including dyslexia (reading problems), dysgraphia (writing problems), and dyscalculia (math problems).

ADHD is misunderstood, misdiagnosed, and overdiagnosed in children. Some physicians fail to recognize ADHD as a cause of academic, social, and emotional problems. Others are quick to attribute too many such problems to ADHD. When ADHD is the correct diagnosis, methylphenidate hydrochloride (Ritalin®) and other drugs may alleviate the symptoms, but not without risk of adverse effects, such as insomnia, increased heart rate and blood pressure, and interference with growth rate. Successful treatment usually requires a combination of drug and behavioral therapies and educational, psychological, and emotional support tailored to the child.

Cerebral Palsy Cerebral palsy, a birth-related disorder of the nerves and muscles, is the most common movement disorder in children. It is caused by brain damage that occurs before, during, or shortly after birth or in early childhood. Signs of spastic cerebral palsy (the most common form) include hyperactive tendon reflexes, rapid alteration between muscular contraction and relaxation, permanent muscle shortening, and underdevelopment of extremities. Among people who have this disease, 40% are mentally retarded, 25% have seizures, and 80% have impaired speech. There is no known cure, but the effects of the disorder can be alleviated with physical therapy, speech therapy, orthopedic surgery, splints, skeletal muscle relaxants, and anticonvulsant medication.

Congenital Heart Disease Congenital heart disease is caused by a cardiovascular malformation in the fetus before birth. If the fetus survives, the newborn is usually small. The defect may be so small, however, that it may not be recognized until days, months, or even years later. Some patients have such a mild case of the disease that no treatment is necessary. Others require only low-risk surgery. In still others, major high-risk surgery is necessary. Many patients diagnosed with the problem are treated with antibiotics to avoid secondary infections.

A cardiovascular defect can be caused by genetic mutations (changes in the genes), maternal infections (such as rubella or cytomegalovirus), maternal alcoholism, or maternal insulin-dependent diabetes. Blue lips and fingernails—signs of cyanosis in a newborn—are obvious indications of a cardiac defect.

Down Syndrome Down syndrome is a congenital disorder resulting from one extra chromosome in each of the millions of cells formed during development of the fetus. It is the most common chromosomal abnormality in humans, and it is not caused by any parental behavior, such as diet or activity. The estimated risk for a Down syndrome birth increases, however, as maternal age increases. Down syndrome is characterized by low muscle tone, which can be alleviated with physical therapy. Characteristic facial features are also evident (Figure 40-18). These include broad face, flattened nasal bridge, narrow nasal passages (increasing the risk of congestion), slanting eyes (vision problems are common), and small teeth and ears. Mild to severe impaired intellectual disability is also a characteristic of Down syndrome.

Hepatitis B Infection with the hepatitis B virus (HBV) can lead to a serious and chronic liver infection. A child can carry the virus for years and only later develop liver failure or liver cancer. The virus can be transmitted across the placenta or during birth if the mother is infected. The disease also may be transmitted sexually, by blood transfusion, or by direct contact. It is frequently seen among drug abusers who share needles. Immunization is available, and children should be immunized starting the day after birth. Children who have not been immunized should begin to receive the series of immunizations for protection from infection.

Respiratory Syncytial Virus The respiratory syncytial virus (RSV) is a major cause of lower respiratory disease in infants and young children. RSV is most often seen in the winter and spring as outbreaks of pneumonia, bronchiolitis, and tracheobronchitis. It is highly contagious, and reinfection is common. Treatment is difficult because the infection is viral rather than bacterial. Antibiotics are thus effective for treating only the possible secondary infections that develop during or after contracting RSV. You may be asked to obtain nasal smears to assist in the diagnosis of RSV. More information about collecting specimens is found in the *Microbiology and Disease* chapter.

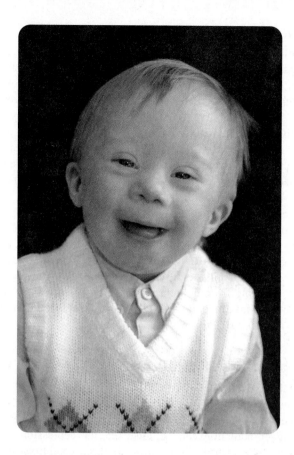

FIGURE 40-18 A child with Down syndrome usually has distinct facial features.
©JSCook/Getty Images

Sudden Infant Death Syndrome Sudden infant death syndrome (SIDS) is the sudden death of an infant, which occurs during sleep, that remains unexplained after all possible causes have been carefully ruled out. Most SIDS cases occur between 2 and 4 months of age. Victims appear to be healthy and are more likely to be male than female. When necessary, recommend and refer families to support groups that are helpful to the parents of a SIDS infant. The American SIDS Institute provides this advice as well as family support for victims of SIDS. Counseling and information are also available through local health organizations. Placing the infant on his back to sleep is highly recommended to help prevent SIDS. Other things that can be done to reduce the risk of SIDS include:

- Obtain good prenatal care.
- Do not smoke, drink, or take drugs when pregnant.
- Avoid pregnancy during the teenage years.
- Wait at least 1 year between pregnancies.
- Use a firm mattress and avoid covers, toys, pillows, and bumper pads.
- Keep the baby's crib in the parent's room until the baby is 6 months old, or use a monitor.
- Do not let babies sleep in adult beds.
- Do not overheat the infant with covers or clothing while sleeping.

- Avoid exposing the baby to smoke.
- Breast-feed whenever possible.
- Avoid exposure to people with respiratory infections; wash hands and clean anything that comes in contact with the baby.
- Offer the baby a pacifier.

Spina Bifida Spina bifida is a defect of spinal development that occurs during the first trimester of pregnancy. The tissues and bones around the spinal cord do not form correctly or close properly. Neurologic symptoms are common because the spinal cord is not fully protected by the spine's bony and connective tissues. These symptoms may vary with the defect's severity, ranging from foot weakness and bladder or bowel problems to paralysis of the lower extremities and mental retardation. In less severe cases, the skin over the spinal cord often has a depression, tuft of hair, or port wine stain. In more severe cases, the newborn has a sac sticking out of the mid to lower back (Figure 40-19).

The treatment and outcome of spina bifida are based on the extent of damage. Surgical closure or implants are sometimes required. Unfortunately, the neurologic conditions cannot be reversed. However, some research has indicated that taking folic acid while trying to get pregnant and during the first trimester of pregnancy may reduce the risk of spina bifida.

Viral Gastroenteritis Gastroenteritis is an inflammation of the stomach and intestines. Gastroenteritis caused by a virus may be called the flu, traveler's diarrhea, or food poisoning. Viral gastroenteritis usually subsides within 1 to 2 days. It can be serious in young children, however, because it can cause extreme fluid loss that results in dehydration and electrolyte imbalances.

Symptoms include fever, nausea, abdominal cramping, diarrhea, and vomiting. Gastroenteritis is treated with bed rest, increased fluid intake, dietary modifications (usually only clear liquids), and medication for vomiting and diarrhea, if necessary. Antibiotics may be prescribed if evidence of bacterial involvement is present.

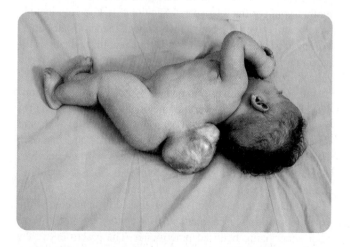

FIGURE 40-19 Spina bifida occurs when the tissue around the spinal cord does not develop completely. It can be mild, with no symptoms, or severe, causing neurologic symptoms such as paralysis of the lower extremities.
©Phototake

▶ Pediatric Patient Special Concerns

In addition to well-child exams, immunizations, and the diseases discussed in the previous sections, there are some special concerns for pediatric patients. Medical assistants should be aware of problems such as child abuse or neglect; eating disorders; depression, substance abuse, and addiction; violence; suicide; sexually transmitted infections; and unwanted pregnancies.

Detecting Child Abuse or Neglect

Child abuse is an all-too-common and potentially fatal problem. It frequently goes unnoticed. Whenever a child comes to the office, you should watch for any signs of serious problems in the relationship between the parent or caregiver and the child. Also notice any signs of physical injury, such as unexplained bruises or burns. Any suspicious lesion on a child's genitalia also should prompt an investigation of sexual abuse. Possible signs of neglect include a dirty or neglected appearance, hunger, extreme sadness or fear, and an inability to communicate. Note any suspicions in the chart and report them to the licensed practitioner before he sees the patient. The practitioner will respond to your information by examining the child for clues to indicate the following:

- Internal injuries: tenderness when palpated or auscultated.
- Malnutrition: tooth discoloration, unhealthy gums or skin color.
- Lack of cognitive ability: dulled neurologic responses.

Studies show that certain risk factors are usually present in parents who abuse their children. Risk factors for child abuse or neglect include stress, single parenthood, inadequate knowledge of normal developmental expectations, lack of family support, family hostility, financial problems, and mental health problems. Other risk factors include prolonged separation of parent and child, ambivalent feelings toward the child, and a mother younger than 16 years. Additional risk factors include an unhealthy or unsafe home environment, inappropriate supervision, substance abuse, a parental crime record, a negative attitude toward pregnancy, and a history of parents having been abused.

Intervention, such as home visits by healthcare professionals, can significantly lower the rate of child abuse. These professionals provide information on normal child growth and development and routine health needs, serve as informational support persons, and refer families to appropriate services when they require assistance. Keep in mind that according to the law, suspected child abuse and neglect must be reported. If you suspect that a child is being abused or neglected while you are working as a medical assistant, you must inform your supervising licensed practitioner. The practitioner may determine that a child protection agency should be contacted. Keep the child protection agency telephone number posted in your office.

Eating Disorders

Adolescents feel pressured to look good. Whether this pressure comes from modern media—magazines, television, movies, or the Internet—or from an adolescent's peer group, it's often focused on being slim and beautiful, which may include watching the scale and dieting, wearing stylish clothing, and having a certain hairstyle. This pressure may lead adolescents to develop abnormal eating behaviors such as anorexia nervosa. Although not limited to adolescents, patients with anorexia basically starve themselves by not eating. Males and females may suffer from anorexia, but it is more common in females.

Another eating disorder is bulimia nervosa—a pattern of binge eating and purging. Purging is done by vomiting, taking excessive doses of laxatives, abusing diuretics such as Diurex® water pills, or exercising excessively. However, a teen suffering from bulimia may still be of normal weight. Additional information about eating disorders is found in the *Nutrition and Health* chapter.

Depression, Substance Abuse, and Addiction

Signs of depression, addiction, and substance abuse in adolescents can be difficult to distinguish. Signs of substance abuse or addiction can be mistaken for depression. The reverse is also true. Sometimes all three conditions exist simultaneously. The use of alcohol, tobacco, club drugs, marijuana, cocaine, and heroin is an important concern with adolescents. Club drugs include GHB, a central nervous system (CNS) depressant; ecstasy, a mental stimulant that increases physical energy; and flunitrazepam, a sedative-hypnotic similar to Xanax®. The abuse of controlled prescription drugs, such as Ritalin® or Oxycontin®, is equally dangerous. Family members should be aware of and willing to discuss signs of adolescent depression, substance abuse, and addiction with the licensed practitioner. Although these signs are difficult to evaluate in a short office visit, as the medical assistant, you also should be alert to them. If the practitioner determines that a teen has a substance abuse problem, medical and health counseling services should be provided. Review the *Caution: Handle with Care* feature Signs of Depression, Substance Abuse, and Addiction in Adolescents for more information about this pediatric special concern.

Violence

Violence takes many forms. Teens of many cultures are exposed to violence in movies, television, video games, and music. Excessive exposure leads to insensitivity toward violence. Teens also may be victims of physical, emotional, psychological, or sexual violence at home. Bullying, browbeating, or abusing is recognized as a cause of violence at school. Many youths who have carried out homicidal acts of violence were deeply disturbed by repeated bullying experiences such as being teased, taunted, and rejected by peers. Most students

Signs of Depression, Substance Abuse, and Addiction in Adolescents

Signs of depression, substance abuse, and addiction are often hard to distinguish in adolescents, partly because adolescents are particularly skilled at hiding the signs of all three disorders. However, various signs may indicate depression in an adolescent. One teenager may lose interest in or be unable to enjoy everyday activities. Another may sleep for long periods and have difficulty getting up in the morning, whereas another may sleep very little. Chronic fatigue or aches and pains may signal depression, as may trouble with concentration or school absenteeism. These signs also may indicate substance abuse or addiction.

It is important to know the difference between substance abuse and addiction. **Substance abuse** refers to the use of a substance, even an over-the-counter drug, in a way that is not medically approved. Inappropriate use includes practices such as using diet pills to stay awake or consuming large quantities of cough syrup that contains codeine. It also includes taking larger-than-prescribed doses of a medication. Substance abusers are not necessarily addicts, however.

Addiction refers to a physical or psychological dependence on a substance. Addiction usually involves a pattern of behavior that includes an obsessive or compulsive preoccupation with a substance and the security of its supply, as well as a high rate of relapse after withdrawal.

As a medical assistant, you should not try to make a diagnosis. Quite probably, an adolescent with one or more of these disorders will be uncooperative and refuse to answer relevant questions. You must be aware, however, of physical signs and behaviors that may be associated with depression, substance abuse, or addiction in an adolescent patient. The following signs and behaviors are important clues that you should report immediately to the licensed practitioner:

- The patient complains of altered eating habits or disturbed sleep patterns (either too much or too little sleep).
- The patient's weight has changed drastically (either up or down) since the previous office visit.
- The patient appears lethargic or sullen or exhibits radical mood changes.
- The patient has slurred speech.
- The patient appears to have illogical thought patterns.
- The patient appears to have needle tracks (anywhere on the body, especially on the arms or legs).
- The patient has pinpoint (highly constricted) pupils.

---

are able to tolerate moderate amounts of teasing, but students who are depressed and harbor resentment and anger for a long time may explode in a violent way. In other cases, the teen may turn inward and commit suicide, which is discussed later. The medical assistant should be aware of the following warning signs of potential violence:

- Frequent physical fighting.
- Increased or serious use of drugs or alcohol.
- Increase in risk-taking behavior.
- Gang membership or strong desire to be in a gang.
- Trouble controlling feelings such as anger.
- Withdrawal from friends and usual activities.
- Feeling rejected or alone.
- Having been a victim of bullying.
- Feeling constantly disrespected.
- Failing to acknowledge the feelings or rights of others.

Suicide

According to the Centers for Disease Control and Prevention, suicide is the third leading cause of death for people aged 15 to 24. Unintentional or accidental injury and homicide are the first and second causes, respectively. The suicide rate among young people is greater for males than for females. Females are more likely to attempt suicide than males, but males are more likely to be successful in their first attempt at suicide. Be alert for warning signs:

- Depression
- Anger that is directed inward, toward the self
- Alcohol and/or other substance abuse
- Changes in habit—carelessness, sloppiness, and a lack of interest in personal appearance
- Giving away personal possessions
- Giving verbal hints about committing suicide

If you notice these signs or if you hear someone talking about committing suicide, you should listen and take the person seriously. Never assume that it's "just talk." Discuss your concerns with the licensed practitioner immediately.

Sexually Transmitted Infections and Pregnancy Prevention

Sexually transmitted infections (STIs) threaten long-term health and well-being. They are spread by bloodborne pathogens and require public education for teens as well as adults. Because teens may engage in sex, they should be aware of STIs and their effects. Teens also should know about pregnancy prevention. Information and education are available through schools, local and state departments of health, television ad campaigns, the Internet, and the Centers for Disease Control and Prevention. Further information about STIs is found in the chapter *The Reproductive Systems*. Additional information about birth control is found in the chapter *Assisting in Reproductive and Urinary Specialties*.

Respiratory System Changes in the respiratory system that occur with aging include:

- Some loss of elasticity of the lungs.
- Calcification of the intercostal cartilage (located between the ribs) and the development of **kyphosis** (curvature of the spine), making it difficult for the lungs to expand properly (Figure 41-3).
- Increased shortness of breath, caused by the physical changes listed above.

Immune System Changes in the immune system that occur with aging include:

- Susceptibility to infectious diseases.
- Susceptibility to autoimmune diseases such as cancer and rheumatoid arthritis.

Digestive System Changes in the digestive system that occur with aging include:

- Constipation, caused by lack of exercise and poor diet.
- Fecal incontinence, caused by lack of muscle tone.

Genitourinary System Changes in the genitourinary system that occur with aging include:

- Decreased number of nephrons, which are the functional units of the kidneys.

- The kidneys filtering blood more slowly, causing reduced tolerance to stress, medications, and illness.
- Loss of voluntary control of urination.

Endocrine System Changes in the endocrine system that occur with aging include:

- Decreased thyroid function.
- Loss of estrogen production in postmenopausal females.
- Decreasing levels of aldosterone, a hormone that has a role in regulating blood pressure.
- Increase in the time it takes for levels of the hormone cortisol to return to normal after stressful events.
- Deficiencies in response to insulin by various organs.

Cognitive-Intellectual Development

Age-related physical changes in geriatric patients in turn may cause changes in cognitive and intellectual development—how well the patients understand new concepts and learn new skills. Because of changes in the brain, geriatric individuals may take longer to process information. However, they can and do continue to learn. Long-term memory seems to remain intact. Short-term memory may be less acute. If they do not have a disease such as Alzheimer's, they can continue to perform the same functions as they always have. Their accumulated wealth of information and life experiences makes mature adults great teachers.

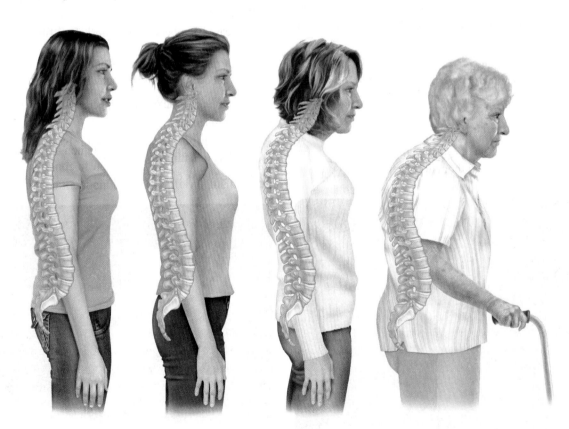

FIGURE 41-3 Kyphosis, a type of curvature of the spine also known as "humpback," occurs with age due to degeneration of the spine from a decrease in bone density.

Psycho-Emotional Development

Many changes may occur in the life of the mature adult. In Western cultures, people retire when they are about 65 to 70 years of age. Retirement is a major change that may have benefits or cause difficulties. For example, people who no longer have a career may feel an unexpected sense of loss and grief. Those who have developed interests outside of their careers may make a smoother transition to retirement. Today, however, many older adults keep working because of financial need.

The deaths of a spouse and of friends are more common life events as a person ages. These deaths may have a major effect on a person's emotional and psychological status. Dealing with the deaths of loved ones also may prompt mature adults to face the reality of their own eventual death. Sometimes, physical ailments and the inability to physically and mentally do what they used to do can lead to increasing dependence on other family members—frequently, middle-aged children. This may result in depression in the mature adult who does not want to "be a burden" to the family.

Social Development

Mature adults may experience an increased spirituality. Individuals who are financially and physically able may prefer to remain in their own home and familiar neighborhood. Others choose to move to their "dream" retirement home or community. Most mature adults in the United States live independently, contributing numerous volunteer hours to their communities. Frequently, relationships with grandchildren are a source of great pleasure.

Aspects of Care

Although patient needs vary, as a medical assistant working with mature adults, you should consider the following points when caring for and providing patient education to geriatric patients:

- Encourage regular weight-bearing and aerobic exercises to reduce and prevent bone loss.

- Provide patient education regarding a balanced nutritional plan. Specifics of a nutritional plan may need to be discussed with a nutritionist or other licensed healthcare practitioner, particularly if there are complicating medical conditions, such as cardiovascular disease or diabetes.

- Question mature adults about their sleeping patterns. As adults reach the age of maturity, their periods of extended sleep may decrease, but short periods of rest during the day may help to offset that loss. Adequate rest helps an individual to be alert and better able to perform the tasks of the day. Disturbances in sleep or excessive fatigue should be reported to a healthcare practitioner.

- Encourage socialization. Social contact persists throughout adult life and should be encouraged. As an adult matures, retires from the world of work, and maybe even loses a spouse, opportunities for socialization may decrease. It is essential that an individual join with other community members to maintain social contact. Frequently, this can be accomplished through volunteer activities.

- Encourage the patient to continue to get regular healthcare checkups, dental care checkups, and breast and prostate exams.

- Remember that the old adage "Use it or lose it!" applies. Keeping the brain active is necessary and sometimes can even prevent loss of function. Studies have shown that individuals who maintain active interests in the world around them maintain mental function better than those individuals who do not.

Diseases and Disorders of Geriatric Patients

LO 41.2

Aging-associated diseases, or diseases that increase in frequency as individuals age, include cardiovascular disease, hypertension, cancer, arthritis, cataracts, diabetes mellitus, and Alzheimer's disease. Other disorders, such as constipation, diarrhea, and osteoporosis—while not serious for young and middle-aged adults—can be major problems for the elderly. A complete discussion of diseases and disorders that commonly affect mature adults appears in Table 41-1.

Assisting with Geriatric Care

LO 41.3

Usually, examination, screening, diagnostic procedures, and treatments for geriatric patients are similar to those for younger adults. However, as a medical assistant, you should be aware of variations in the care and treatment of elderly patients. Notice the vast differences in the capabilities of people of this age group and do not stereotype all elderly patients as frail or confused (most are not). Each patient deserves to be treated according to her own individual abilities. Always treat geriatric patients with respect. Regardless of their physical or mental state, elderly patients are adults. Do not talk down to them. Good communication is necessary. To practice communicating with elderly patients, see Procedure 41-1 at the end of this chapter.

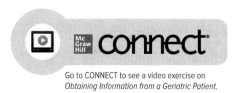

Go to CONNECT to see a video exercise on
Obtaining Information from a Geriatric Patient.

Patient Education

Patient education for elderly patients is especially valuable because it can help them prevent or manage health problems and remain independent. You may need to educate some older patients about the importance of taking measures to protect their health. You may work with elderly patients who have hearing or vision problems or physical limitations that restrict their ability to perform certain tasks.

TABLE 41-1   Diseases of the Elderly

Disease	Description	Treatment
Alzheimer's disease	Severely debilitating brain disorder, with warning signs that include changes in personality, mood, or behavior; recent memory loss and increased forgetfulness; decreased ability to perform familiar tasks; difficulty with use of language and abstract thinking; decreased powers of judgment; and disorientation to time or place	Because there is no cure, the primary role of caregivers is to provide comfort and safety to the patient. Medications such as Aricept® and Namenda® are available that can slow the symptoms of the disease.
Arthritis/osteoarthritis	Chronic inflammatory disease of joint tissues; symptoms include pain, swelling, and stiffness in joints (see Figure 41-2).	Anti-inflammatory medication for inflammation and pain; surgery, including joint replacement in severe cases
Cancer	Abnormal growth of cells that are able to invade other tissues	Surgery, chemotherapy, or radiation therapy; under-diagnosis and treatment as well as side effects of treatment are concerns for geriatric patients
Cardiovascular diseases	Dysrhythmias: abnormal heart rates	Medication or surgery to control the heart rate
	Coronary artery disease: blockages of the arteries surrounding the heart	Stop smoking, improve cholesterol levels with medication or diet and exercise, angioplasty and/or placement of stents, or coronary artery bypass surgery
	Valvular diseases: abnormalities of the heart valves	Most frequently, surgical repair of the affected valve
	Congestive heart failure	Medication to reduce excessive fluid and edema (diuretics) and to improve the beating of the heart (digoxin, beta blockers)
Cataracts	Lens of the eye becomes cloudy and opaque, causing decreased vision	Sunglasses, improved lighting, and changing of glasses; cataract surgery to replace the lens
Constipation-diarrhea cycle	The cycle of constipation followed by diarrhea occurs when people's diets lack the fiber and liquids to maintain healthy bowel function and they use harsh laxatives to treat their constipation. The patient then complains of diarrhea and asks for antidiarrheal medication, which in turn causes constipation again.	Encourage elderly patients to eat more high-fiber foods, such as cereals, fruits, and vegetables, and to increase their fluid intake, as well as increase their activity level if possible.
Diabetes mellitus Type 2	High levels of sugar (glucose) in the blood; symptoms include fatigue, hunger, increased thirst, increased urination, and blurred vision	Diet, exercise, and weight control; monitoring of blood sugar; oral medications such as metformin and, in rare cases, insulin
Hypertension	Elevation of blood pressure over 130 systolic and 80 diastolic; often, there are no symptoms or symptoms are mild	Dietary restrictions to reduce fat and sodium and lose weight; increased exercise to lose weight and strengthen the heart; medications to reduce blood pressure
Hyperlipidemia	A condition in which lipid (fat) levels are above normal. These include cholesterol and triglycerides. Although not just a disease of the elderly, it tends to be more common and serious with age. High cholesterol levels can lead to atherosclerosis, the accumulation of fatty deposits along the inner walls of arteries (Figure 41-4). These deposits, along with other substances in the blood, can form an atherosclerotic plaque. This plaque can narrow the opening in an artery to the point of obstructing blood flow. Atherosclerosis is a primary cause of cardiovascular disease and stroke.	Teach patients about eating foods with lower amounts of cholesterol and increasing exercise. Provide patients with printed materials about hyperlipidemia and cholesterol. The doctor may prescribe medication (statins) to lower cholesterol in patients when diet modification and exercise are not effective.
Osteomalacia	Softening of the bones due to vitamin D and calcium deficiency, especially in postmenopausal women	Teach patients about the need for proper nutrition; encourage postmenopausal women to take vitamin and mineral supplements as needed.
Osteoporosis	An endocrine and metabolic disorder of the musculoskeletal system. Thinning of bone tissue and loss of bone density occur over time, leading to fractures. More common in women than men, this disorder may be caused by inadequate calcium consumption, estrogen deficiency, or alcoholism.	Prevention methods include regular weight-bearing and strength exercises and a diet high in calcium (perhaps including supplemental calcium). Prescription medications, such as Fosamax® or Actonel®, and hormone replacement therapy also are used.

(Continued)

TABLE 41·1 Diseases of the Elderly

Disease	Description	Treatment
Sleep apnea	Sleep disorder in which the person stops breathing for several seconds at a time while sleeping; if not treated, can predispose the patient to other, more serious complications such as cardiovascular disease, depression, and even memory loss.	In mild cases, teach patients behavioral changes such as losing weight, avoiding alcohol, stopping smoking, avoiding sleeping pills, and avoiding sleeping on the back. In more severe cases, the licensed practitioner may recommend a continuous positive airway pressure (CPAP) machine, which provides the patient with a continuous flow of air into the nose to keep the airway open. Some practitioners also recommend dental devices to help keep the airway open. In very severe cases, surgery may be needed. See the *Educating the Patient* feature Sleep Disorders for more information about behavioral modification.

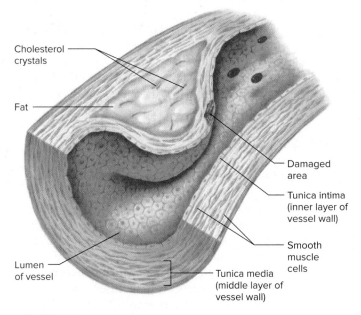

Cholesterol crystals

Fat

Damaged area

Tunica intima (inner layer of vessel wall)

Smooth muscle cells

Lumen of vessel

Tunica media (middle layer of vessel wall)

FIGURE 41·4 High cholesterol can lead to atherosclerosis. Help patients reduce their cholesterol through proper diet and exercise, along with medication, if prescribed.

Practice good communication in addition to keeping the following suggestions in mind when educating elderly patients.

- Speak in clear, low-pitched tones. High-pitched voices are more difficult for people with hearing impairments to understand. When asking questions, give the patient time to answer and confirm the response to prevent misunderstandings. Avoid both overly simple "yes" or "no" questions that the patient might answer without thinking and overly complex questions that might confuse the patient.

- Some older people have trouble understanding directions. Try to communicate with them at the highest level they can understand. Remember, never talk down to patients.

- Put instructions in writing. Because some elderly patients have problems with memory, detailed written instructions are an essential aspect of patient care. Patients can refer to the instructions as necessary or ask a relative to do so.

- Adjust procedures as needed. When demonstrating a procedure to elderly patients, keep in mind any physical limitations they have and adjust the procedure accordingly. Make sure patients understand the instructions by asking them to perform the procedure for you.

EDUCATING THE PATIENT

Sleep Disorders

Although some researchers believe that sleep requirements decline with age, according to the National Sleep Foundation, a person's need for sleep remains more or less constant throughout life. Seniors tend to have a harder time getting to sleep and the quality of their sleep is not as high as that of younger people.

Many sleep disorders can affect the sleep of geriatric patients, including sleep apnea, insomnia, restless leg syndrome, and lack of sleep due to symptoms of ongoing diseases such as chronic obstructive pulmonary disease (COPD), gastroesophageal reflux disease (GERD), or even pain associated with arthritis.

Medications may be prescribed for some sleep disorders, but most licensed practitioners prefer to try behavioral and lifestyle changes, referred to as "sleep hygiene," before prescribing medications.

Commonly recommended actions include:

- Go to bed at the same time every evening.
- Wake up at the same time every morning.
- Try not to take long naps during the day.
- Get regular exercise, but avoid exercising just before going to bed.
- Avoid consuming alcohol, caffeine, and nicotine before bedtime.
- Form routine habits for getting ready for bed, such as washing or brushing your teeth.
- Maintain a sleep environment that is conducive to sleep, such as a darkened, quiet room.
- Do not perform activities such as reading or watching television in bed.
- Do not eat heavy meals close to bedtime.

Denial or Confusion

Sometimes elderly patients, just like many other adult patients, deny that they are ill. A patient's perception of how he feels may be quite different from his actual state of health. The reverse situation also can occur. Elderly patients may over-react to a problem and consider themselves sicker than they really are. They may become dependent, passive, or anxious.

Elderly patients also may over- or underestimate their ability to perform certain tasks or to deal with certain limitations. Elderly patients may be confused if they have some impairment in memory, judgment, or other mental abilities. Signs of confusion can occur with Alzheimer's disease and other types of dementia, depression, head injury, or misuse of medications or alcohol. Elderly patients may or may not be aware of their condition. They may have difficulty understanding instructions. Mental health screenings are therefore an important part of healthcare for elderly patients.

The Importance of Touch

Therapeutic touch is based on an ancient therapy called the laying on of hands. It was reconceived in the early 1970s by a registered nurse. Essentially, the hands are used to direct human energies to help or heal someone who is ill. Although little scientific evidence exists about the effectiveness of this therapy, it is known that touch can improve health and well-being.

Because they often live alone, many elderly patients experience a lack of physical touch. Using touch—offering to hold a patient's hand or placing an arm around his shoulder—communicates that you care about the patient, and it may improve his health and well-being (Figure 41-5).

Incontinence

Elderly patients may suffer from urinary **incontinence,** or involuntary leakage of urine. Many people are too embarrassed to ask for help or are unaware of possible solutions. In general, if a patient has urinary incontinence that interferes

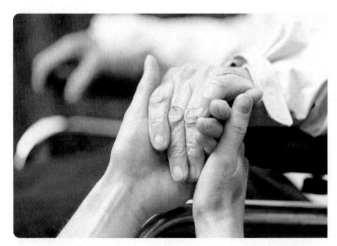

FIGURE 41-5 The importance of touch: Elderly patients may appreciate your touch as a sign of caring. Consider offering to hold their hand or placing an arm around their shoulder.
©Ocskay Bence/Shutterstock

with day-to-day life, the licensed practitioner should be notified of the problem. Incontinence will sometimes cause a patient to drink less, making her prone to urinary tract infections and other problems.

Preventive Medicine

Many elderly patients may not be aware of or do not practice the concept of **preventive medicine** (measures taken to prevent illness). They are from environments in which people went to a doctor only when they were very ill, so they do not realize the importance of preventive measures such as regular checkups, digital rectal exams, immunizations, and colonoscopy. Also, older women often do not recognize the need for regular mammograms and Pap smears to detect cancers of the breast and cervix.

As a medical assistant, you should use any educational tools available to you to make elderly patients more aware of the importance of preventive measures. If you reinforce the doctor's recommendations with education, you increase the chance that patients will heed the advice they are given.

Lack of Compliance When Taking Medications

Often, geriatric patients need several medications, and many of them find it difficult to keep track and take the right medication at the right time. Sometimes patients have difficulty swallowing or simply decide not to take a medication because they feel they do not need it. In your role as a medical assistant, you can help by telling geriatric patients about available medication reminder boxes, timers, and medication organizers. These devices can help ensure **patient compliance** (obedience in following the orders of the licensed practitioner). Patient compliance helps patients remain healthier and get well faster.

Collecting Urine Specimens

Consider the following when you are collecting urine from a geriatric patient: Bladder muscles weaken with age, often leading to incomplete bladder emptying and chronic urine retention, which can cause urinary tract infection, **nocturia** (excessive nighttime urination), and incontinence.

Weakening of the supports of the uterus may cause it to **prolapse** (work its way down the vaginal canal). The uterus pulls with it the vaginal walls, bladder, and rectum. This weakening—often the result of several childbirths—may not occur until a woman is postmenopausal. Symptoms include pressure, incontinence, and urinary retention. Normal activities, such as walking up stairs, can aggravate the problem.

Find out whether the patient ever loses bladder control. If so, ask whether it occurs suddenly or whether a feeling of intense pressure precedes it. These symptoms can be a sign of weakening of the bladder muscles.

Keep in mind that some elderly patients need assistance in providing a urine specimen. For example, you may have to accompany the patient to the bathroom and hold the specimen container. (Wash your hands before and after doing so, and wear gloves while providing this help.)

Conditions of the urinary system, especially the bladder, in the elderly can interfere with collecting urine specimens. This is especially true for 24-hour urine specimens. Careful and repeated explanations or reminders about the procedure or the specimens needed may be necessary to ensure accuracy.

Blood-Drawing Procedures

The challenges presented by elderly patients may test your technical skills as well as your interpersonal skills. Physically, some older adults are frail and may not withstand blood-drawing procedures as easily as younger patients. Changes in skin condition often make elderly patients more prone to bruising and other injuries. Decreased circulation may make it difficult to collect enough blood for testing. Be aware of these issues and take extra precautions when drawing blood on an elderly patient.

Hot and Cold Therapy

Elderly patients are usually more sensitive than others to cold and heat. As you may have noticed with elderly friends and relatives, there is a reduced ability to tolerate temperature changes. Sudoriferous (sweat-producing) glands of the skin decrease in number and, with less perspiration, high temperatures are more difficult to adjust to. At the same time, the loss of adipose tissue and decreased circulation result in a lessened ability to retain heat, which increases sensitivity to cold.

Along with possible poor circulation, geriatric patients also may have arthritis; impaired sensation; kidney, heart, or lung disease; or atherosclerosis. They also may have impaired skin integrity—thinning of the skin, resulting in increased risk of skin tearing, bruising, and burning. When administering cryotherapy (cold therapy) or thermotherapy (heat therapy), stay with an elderly patient during its application to check the patient's skin frequently for excessive paleness or redness.

Nutritional Guidelines

Universal nutritional guidelines for aging patients have not been developed. It is known, however, that energy and metabolic requirements usually decline with age, which calls for some dietary modification. The Food and Nutrition Board of the National Academy of Sciences recommends a 10% decrease in caloric intake for people over age 50 compared with that of young adults. Men and women older than age 75 should decrease their intake another 10% to 15%. The exact adjustment, however, depends on the individual patient's condition and needs.

Because protein requirements do not change, elderly patients should select foods that provide ample protein in a smaller quantity of food. To achieve daily nutritional goals, patients may require supplements for iron, calcium, and other minerals, such as phosphorus and magnesium.

Aging is often accompanied by decreased gastrointestinal muscle tone, so elderly patients should increase their intake of high-fiber foods and drink plenty of water. Of course, all people need to have an adequate amount of daily water. However, elderly patients sometimes restrict their fluid intake because they may need to urinate frequently, do not remember, or

do not understand the importance of keeping the body well hydrated by consuming enough fluid. See Procedure 41-2 at the end of this chapter. Poor fluid intake also can quickly lead to urinary tract infections in mature adults.

Although all people need a certain amount of fat in their diet to help the body absorb vitamins, too much may lead to atherosclerosis. Elderly individuals should keep fat intake to 20% of their total calories.

Certain factors can impair or impede eating in this age group and may even lead to malnutrition. If you recognize any of these factors, discuss them with the patient's doctor:

- Physical factors, such as chewing difficulty caused by tooth loss or poorly fitting dentures, swallowing difficulty, and lack of appetite caused by altered taste, smell, or sight.
- Medications, which may adversely affect food intake or nutrient use.
- Social factors, including apathy toward food caused by depression, grief, or loneliness.
- Economic factors, including homelessness or lack of money for food or transportation.

Many types of adaptations can be used to help ensure that the nutritional needs of mature adults are met. To overcome physical factors, seeing to the patient's dental needs can help. Assistive devices such as plates with high edges that help keep food from falling onto the table can help the patient scoop food onto serving utensils. Using nonskid placemats may help keep the dishes from sliding around.

To counteract social factors such as loneliness and depression, it may help to suggest eating frequently with friends or neighbors. Patients who live alone also may benefit from using tablecloths, cloth napkins, and attractive centerpieces to make dining a more pleasant experience. Other healthcare team members, such as social workers, may need to be consulted if economic factors are interfering with a patient's nutritional status.

Immunizations

Influenza and influenza-related pneumonia represent serious health risks for patients older than age 65. Although elderly patients can be immunized against influenza each year and against influenza-related pneumonia one time, they may have misconceptions about vaccinations. Another recommended vaccine for individuals over 60 is the shingles vaccine. No matter the vaccine, geriatric patients may worry about the expense, the possibility of getting the disease from the vaccine, or the need for a vaccination when they do not feel ill.

Explain to patients who are concerned about the cost of vaccinations that if they are not enrolled in one of the many insurance plans that cover immunization, Medicare Part B covers the cost. For those worried about the potential side effects of immunization, describe the mild symptoms they may encounter and emphasize that the symptoms are short-lived. You also might mention that compared to the potential dangers of contracting a serious infection, the symptoms are quite mild.

Because older patients are much more likely than younger patients to develop side effects as a result of immunizations, instruct older patients so that they recognize and immediately report any adverse reactions. That way, the licensed practitioner can treat elderly patients before their illness becomes severe.

▶ Geriatric Patient Special Concerns LO 41.4

As you can see, geriatric patients require a lot of special consideration. Four additional special concerns when working with the elderly are falls, depression, elder abuse, and polypharmacy.

Preventing Falls in the Elderly

Falls can occur at any age, but in the elderly, they can have especially serious consequences. Bones may become brittle with age due to osteoporosis and falls can cause breaks in major bones, such as those in the hip and wrist. Complications from falls and bone fractures can lead to death in individuals in this age group.

The elderly are prone to falling because of vision problems, slowing reflexes, quick position changes that can lower the blood pressure, and changes in the ear that cause equilibrium problems. In addition, medications can increase the risk of falls because they may make the patient less alert or cause dizziness.

As a medical assistant, you should discuss a safety checklist with elderly patients and their families. Point out that by taking precautions, elderly patients can reduce the risk of falling. Make sure patients and their families understand the following instructions:

- Remove reading glasses before getting up and walking around.
- Make sure that potentially hazardous areas, such as stairs and doorway entrances, are well lit.
- Use night-lights in the bedroom and bathroom to help prevent night falls.
- When getting up from a reclining or recumbent position, sit at the edge of the bed for a few minutes before trying to stand to allow blood flow and blood pressure to adjust.
- Wear well-fitting shoes with low heels and slippers with nonslip soles.
- Use a cane or walker if you are unsteady on your feet.
- Secure rugs and floor coverings to the floor to prevent slippage.
- Attach all electrical cords to the walls or floor moldings.
- Place sturdy banisters along all stairs inside and outside the home.
- Install secure handrails near the bathtub and toilet.
- Apply nonslip appliques to the bathtub and shower floor.
- Minimize clutter in the home.
- Store frequently used items within easy reach.

Depression

Depression is common in the elderly, but many of the symptoms of depression mimic those of other conditions. As a medical assistant, you can help elderly patients—and their families—recognize the signs of depression. Recall Peter Smith from our case study at the beginning of the chapter. What symptoms does he have? Do you think he has depression? Knowing what to look for may help patients seek help sooner than they otherwise would and receive prompt diagnosis and treatment. See the *Caution: Handle with Care* feature Helping Elderly Patients with Depression for a discussion of the symptoms and treatment of depression in the elderly.

Elder Abuse

Even though you may need to communicate verbally with an elderly patient's caregiver, always observe the elderly patient for nonverbal signs of problems such as grimacing, foul odors, or bruising even if the patient cannot speak to you verbally. Disabilities may make the elderly person defenseless against abuse, and a medical assistant should be alert to signs of abuse.

It is difficult to detect elder abuse. There is no uniform and comprehensive definition of this type of abuse, and bruises from falls and other accidents can be mistaken for abuse. Also, the signs of neglect can be similar to the signs of some chronic medical conditions. There are three basic categories of elder abuse: domestic elder abuse; institutional elder abuse; and self-neglect, or self-abuse. Elders can be abused physically, sexually, or psychologically. Elders also may be neglected, abandoned, or exploited materially or financially. Elders even may choose to neglect or abuse themselves. More than one type of abuse can occur simultaneously. Elder abuse occurs in all racial, socioeconomic, and religious groups. However, most victims are older women with chronic illness or disabilities. Risk factors and situations that increase the possibility of elder abuse include:

- History of alcoholism, drug abuse, or violence in the family.
- History of mental illness in the abuser or victim.
- Isolation of the victim from family members and friends other than the abuser.
- Recent stressful events affecting the abuser or victim.

  Signs of neglect include:

- Foul odor from the patient's body.
- Poor skin color.
- Inappropriate clothing for the season.
- Soiled clothing.
- Extreme concern about money.

You can assist the doctor by taking a careful history. Ask the patient about living arrangements, social contact, and emotional stress. Note the interaction between the caregiver and the patient. Be aware that a patient with dementia may be abused but is not able to report it and the caregiver may be able to cover it well. If you suspect abuse, inform the doctor. He will then be able to direct the physical exam toward possible internal injuries, malnutrition, or lack of cognitive ability. Most states require doctors who suspect elder abuse or neglect to report their concerns to a designated office. Early intervention usually results in better living arrangements for both the patient and the caregiver.

CAUTION: HANDLE WITH CARE

Helping Elderly Patients with Depression

The National Institutes of Health (NIH) considers depression in people age 65 and older to be a major public health concern. In fact, suicide is more common among the elderly than any other age group. The NIH also indicates that only about 10% of elderly people who need treatment for depression ever receive it.

One reason for the low rate of treatment is that many older people—and their families—believe that depression is a normal consequence of growing old. After all, older people may experience many difficult life changes, including enduring the deaths of a spouse and siblings, adjusting to retirement, being alone, dealing with a relocation, suffering economic hardship, and managing a variety of physical ailments. Because of these circumstances, doctors and family may miss the signs of depression.

Recognizing the Symptoms

There is, unfortunately, no specific diagnostic test for depression, so a diagnosis must be made on the basis of symptoms. The symptoms of depression in the elderly are similar to those in other age groups and include the following:

- Decreased ability to enjoy life or to show an interest in activities or people.
- Slow thinking, indecisiveness, or difficulty in concentrating.
- Increased or decreased appetite.
- Increased or decreased time spent sleeping.
- Recurrent feelings of worthlessness.
- Loss of energy and motivation.
- Exaggerated feelings of sadness, hopelessness, or anxiety.
- Recurrent thoughts of death or suicide.

The failure to realize that symptoms like these indicate an illness prevents many older people from seeking help. However, there is evidence that treatment for depression in the elderly can be highly effective.

Treatment for Depression

Depression has been linked to poor diet, lack of exercise, and reduced social contacts. Modification to these things may improve symptoms of mild depression. However, treatment for clinical depression generally combines a course of antidepressant drugs with psychotherapy. Older patients generally respond to antidepressants more slowly than younger patients, so older patients may not experience relief until more than 6 weeks after starting treatment. For this and other reasons, compliance in taking medications for depression is a problem with the elderly. Many elderly patients do not understand depression and the importance of taking medications as prescribed. They also may be frightened by the idea of taking medication for a mental problem. Psychotherapy aims to help older patients talk through their anxieties, develop coping skills, and improve the quality of their lives. Again, compliance is a problem. Many older adults are unwilling to admit that they have a mental health problem and refuse to follow up on referrals to mental health professionals.

Benefits of Treatment

Elderly patients who follow a course of treatment for depression benefit in several ways. They gain:

- Relief from many of the symptoms associated with depression.
- Relief from some of the pain and suffering associated with physical ailments.
- Improved physical, mental, and social well-being.

Healthcare providers, including you as the medical assistant, can play a significant role in recognizing symptoms of depression in elderly patients and in encouraging them to get the treatment they need.

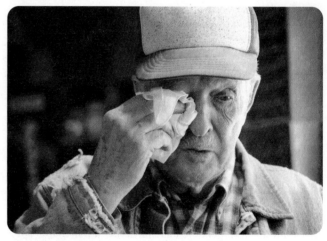

©Design Pics/Kristy-Anne Glubish

Polypharmacy

Age-related changes in the body can affect drug absorption, metabolism, distribution, and excretion. These normal changes can be exaggerated by various diseases or disorders. So as people age, they have an increased risk of drug toxicity, adverse reactions, or lack of therapeutic effects. Because of this risk, be especially alert when assessing an elderly patient who is on drug therapy.

Many elderly patients have complex, chronic diseases with unusual symptoms. This situation can make it difficult to tell whether a problem is caused by a drug. Listen closely to elderly patients and their family members; they are more likely to notice subtle changes than you are.

Patient and family education are important with elderly patients, particularly if they engage in **polypharmacy** (taking several medications concurrently). Polypharmacy is

CAUTION: HANDLE WITH CARE

Preventing Unsafe Polypharmacy

Before administering any drug by any route, you must know every drug, both prescription and nonprescription, that the patient is taking. Many patients, especially elderly ones, visit several doctors. It is possible that each doctor prescribes one or more drugs without being aware of other drugs the patient is taking. This practice can result in polypharmacy, which means taking several drugs at once. Polypharmacy can be safe, but if the doctor is unaware of the total drug profile, serious drug interactions can result.

When asking patients to identify *all* other drugs they are taking, including OTC drugs, keep in mind that patients may forget to mention all their medicines, OTC drugs, supplements, or herbal remedies to the doctor. Patients often forget to mention antacids (such as Tums® or Rolaids®), supplements that are part of a food or drink (such as flavored drinks with glucosamine-chondroitin), medicines that are used only as needed such as medicine for migraine headaches, vitamins, and herbal remedies such as ginkgo biloba or omega-3.

To help prompt patients about drugs they may have forgotten, ask patients who have seen an orthopedist or a cardiologist whether pain medication has been prescribed. Ask women who have seen a gynecologist if they are using a patch or other form of hormone replacement therapy. Ask all patients if they take any other dietary supplement, OTC medication, and/or herbal remedy. If a patient has been referred to any other doctor for any reason, ask whether that doctor has prescribed medication. After determining the total drug profile, you should:

- Update the patient's record (this should be done with every visit to your facility).
- Consider possible drug interactions, consulting online drug interaction checkers or other drug references, such as the *PDR*, if needed.
- Inform the licensed practitioner of your findings.

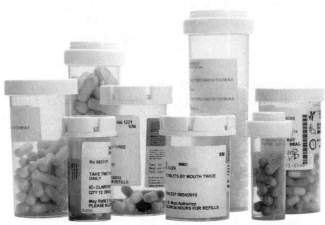
©Jeffrey Coolidge/Getty Images

common in elderly patients, and drug-drug interactions can be severe. See the *Caution: Handle with Care* feature Preventing Unsafe Polypharmacy.

If an elderly patient is forgetful or confused, talk to the licensed practitioner about simplifying the medication schedule to reduce the risk of drug administration errors or omissions. If the patient has vision problems, provide drug instruction sheets in large type. To do this, type instructions on a word processor in a large type size, enlarge the instructions on a photocopier, or clearly handwrite the instructions in large block letters. You also might contact a local association for the blind or visually impaired for devices and tips.

PROCEDURE 41-1 Coaching and Communicating with Geriatric Patients

Procedure Goal: To demonstrate techniques to effectively communicate with geriatric patients during a patient interview for a medical history

OSHA Guidelines: This procedure does not involve exposure to blood, body fluids, or tissues.

Materials: Patient's chart/progress note

Method:

1. Select a private setting for the patient interview.
   RATIONALE: *You must be mindful of HIPAA privacy rules when interviewing a patient.*

2. Show respect for the patient's age by addressing the patient with *Mr., Mrs., Ms.,* or *Miss,* unless the patient asks to be called by his or her first name.

3. Before you begin the interview, explain the type of questions you will ask and how the information will be used.

4. If the patient is hard of hearing, speak slightly more slowly than you normally would. Speak clearly and loudly, but do not shout. Shouting will insult and anger an older patient who does hear well. Enunciate well and use a lower tone of voice because elderly people lose the ability to hear high-frequency sounds first. If the

patient asks you to repeat a question, rephrase it instead of repeating it verbatim.

5. Look at the patient directly to let her know you care about what she has to say and so that you can make sure she understands what you tell or ask her.
   RATIONALE: *Most patients become more comfortable and communicative if they know someone is really listening to them and showing an interest in their emotions and needs.*

6. Be patient. Some older patients live alone or in relative isolation and may be out of practice with the two-way communication skills that make a conversation or interview go smoothly. The simple act of being interviewed, even for what may seem to you a straightforward medical history, may unsettle the older patient. For example, he may need to stop and think of a word here and there. Do not supply the word. Wait and let the patient think of it on his own. Also, do not rush through your questions. Rushing will only make the patient feel anxious and incompetent if he feels he cannot keep up with you.

7. Practice active listening skills. Pay attention to the patient's verbal and nonverbal cues. Do not interrupt the patient. After the patient finishes giving each answer,

repeat it to give her a chance to correct you if you misheard or misunderstood.

8. If you need to use medical terminology, also try to express the same information in lay terms. For example, you might ask, "Do you use a diuretic, or pill to help you eliminate fluids?"

9. Be cheerful and friendly but not sugary-sweet. Do not talk down to older patients; they are not stupid.

10. Avoid sounding surprised or excited by any answer to a question or to any information the patient gives.

11. Under no circumstances use endearments such as *dear, honey,* or *sweetie.*

12. Look for ways to make a connection so that the patient feels relaxed and comfortable. For example, in the course of taking a patient's history, you might find out that he enjoys swimming. Ask him to tell you about it.

13. Show an interest in the patient as a person. Ask about something she is interested in. For example, a patient might be wearing a piece of handmade jewelry. Ask where it came from. She might have a wonderful story to tell.

14. Document the interview and appropriate information in the patient's medical record.

PROCEDURE 41-2 Educating Adult Patients About Daily Water Requirements

WORK // DOC

Procedure Goal: To teach patients how much water their bodies need to maintain health

OSHA Guidelines: This procedure does not involve exposure to blood, body fluids, or tissues.

Materials: Patient education literature, patient's chart/progress note, and device to document education

Method:

1. Explain the importance of water to the body. Point out the water content of the body and the many functions of water in the body, including maintaining the body's fluid balance, lubricating the body's moving parts, and transporting nutrients and secretions.

2. Add any comments applicable to an individual patient's health status, such as issues related to medication use, physical activity, fluid limitation, or increased fluid needs. For example, geriatric patients have decreased gastrointestinal motility and require water to avoid constipation.
   RATIONALE: *Some elderly patients purposely limit their fluid intake because of incontinence or physical limitations that make getting to a bathroom difficult, so it is necessary to provide specific comments about their exact fluid needs.*

3. Explain that people obtain water by drinking water and other fluids and by eating foods that contain water. On average, an adult should drink six to eight glasses of water a day to maintain a healthy water balance in which intake equals excretion. People's daily need for water varies with size and age, the temperatures to which they are exposed, the degree of physical exertion, and the water content of foods eaten. Make sure you reinforce the physician's or dietitian's recommendations for a particular patient's water needs.

4. Caution patients that soft drinks, coffee, and tea are not good substitutes for water and that it would be wise to filter out any harmful chemicals contained in the local tap water or to purchase filtered water, if possible. A good rule of thumb is that for every soft drink, coffee, or tea, the patient should drink the same amount of water to ensure hydration.

5. Provide patients with tips about reminders to drink the requisite amount of water. Some patients may benefit from using a water bottle of a particular size, so that they know they have to drink, say, three full bottles of water each day. Another helpful tip is to make a habit of drinking a glass of water at certain points in the daily routine, such as first thing in the morning and after lunch or right before bedtime if it does not interrupt your sleep.

6. Provide patients with printed materials documenting the amount of water to drink and methods to ensure that their fluid intake is adequate.

7. Remind patients that you and the licensed practitioner are available to discuss any problems or questions.

8. Document any formal patient education sessions or significant exchanges with a patient in the patient's chart or on a progress note, noting whether the patient understood the information presented (refer to Progress Note).

   RATIONALE: *Many insurance companies require evidence of preventive health counseling, and documentation is an important aspect of patient insurance coverage.*

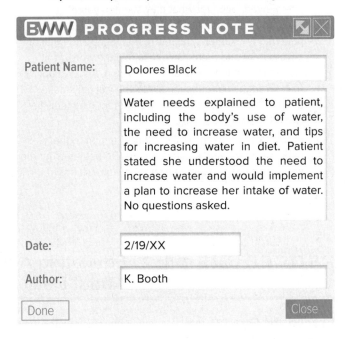

BWW PROGRESS NOTE

Patient Name: Dolores Black

Water needs explained to patient, including the body's use of water, the need to increase water, and tips for increasing water in diet. Patient stated she understood the need to increase water and would implement a plan to increase her intake of water. No questions asked.

Date: 2/19/XX

Author: K. Booth

Done   Close

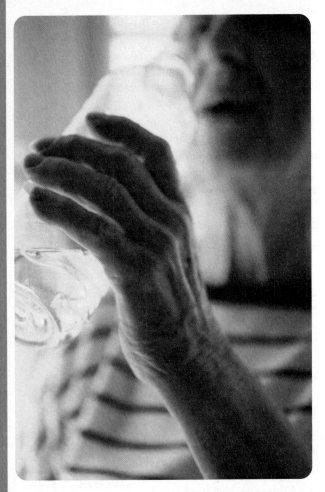

FIGURE Procedure 41-2 Step 5   Using a water bottle can help patients remember to drink a certain amount of water each day.

©Steven Puetzer/Getty Images

SUMMARY OF LEARNING OUTCOMES

OUTCOME	KEY POINTS
41.1 Relate developmental changes in geriatric patients to medical assisting practice.	Geriatrics is a subspecialty of internal medicine or family practice. Geriatricians typically care for patients over the age of 65. These patients have multiple physical changes as well as variations in psycho-emotional, cognitive-intellectual, and social development to consider when working with them as a medical assistant.
41.2 Describe common geriatric diseases and disorders and their treatment.	Common aging-associated diseases and disorders include cardiovascular disease, hypertension, cancer, arthritis, cataracts, diabetes mellitus, Alzheimer's disease, constipation, diarrhea, osteoporosis, osteomalacia, and sleep apnea. Understanding these will help you prepare to care for geriatric patients.
41.3 Identify variations of care for geriatric patients during examinations, screening procedures, diagnostic tests, and treatments.	When working with geriatric patients, you must treat them with respect and dignity. Be aware of their physical and mental changes so that you can adapt your care to meet their needs.
41.4 Explain special health concerns of geriatric patients.	Each of the following special concerns should be handled appropriately when caring for the elderly: falls, elder abuse, depression, and polypharmacy.

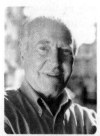
©Image Source/Getty Images

Recall Peter Smith from the case study at the beginning of the chapter. Now that you have completed this chapter, answer the following questions regarding his case.

1. Considering Peter Smith's age, what special aspects of care should you be aware of while caring for him?

2. Why would Peter Smith be prone to falls, and what can you do to help prevent them?

3. You need to collect a urine specimen from Peter Smith. What special considerations should you take?

4. What symptoms does Peter Smith have, and why is it important for you to recognize them?

EXAM PREPARATION QUESTIONS

1. (LO 41.1) Which of the following is the *least* likely to occur with a geriatric patient?
   a. Incontinence
   b. Kyphosis
   c. Hyperbilirubinemia
   d. Polypharmacy
   e. Lentigos

2. (LO 41.1) Your 68-year-old patient suffers from pain and swelling of his left knee. He also has poor vision and hearing. He needs education about how to care for his knee. Which of the following would be the best technique?
   a. Looking at your patient education sheet, give him simple directions at his level.
   b. Perform patient education in an open area of the clinic to prevent him from being uncomfortable.
   c. Have him go to a small class to teach him about his care.
   d. Speak in clear, high-pitched tones so that he can hear you.
   e. Look directly at the patient, speaking slightly slower in low-pitched tones.

3. (LO 41.3) Which of the following patients is *most* likely to suffer from urinary incontinence?
   a. A 78-year-old female patient with a prolapsed uterus
   b. A 65-year-old male patient with nocturia due to an enlarged prostate
   c. A 76-year-old female patient taking 12 different prescription medications and 2 over-the-counter supplements
   d. A 68-year-old male patient with a history of alcoholism
   e. An 82-year-old patient who uses a walker for ambulation

4. (LO 41.2) Your 68-year-old patient suffers from disorientation to time and place. Which of the following is the *most* likely problem?
   a. Cataracts
   b. Valvular disease
   c. Depression
   d. Alzheimer's disease
   e. Osteoporosis

5. (LO 41.3) When speaking to Peter Smith, which of the following is the best way to address him?
   a. Hi, Pete, how are you doing today?
   b. Mr. Smith, how are you feeling today?
   c. Sir, I would like to take your vital signs.
   d. What is your chief complaint today, mister?
   e. Hi there, honey, will you sit down right here so we can start the interview?

6. (LO 41.3) Your elderly patient refuses an immunization. Which of the following is the *least* likely reason?
   a. He is worried about the expense.
   b. He had a severe reaction to a previous immunization.
   c. He does not feel bad and does not want to feel bad.
   d. He does not have time to wait for the injection.
   e. He is afraid he will get the disease from the vaccine.

7. (LO 41.3) When providing nutritional education for an elderly patient, which of the following statements is *most* accurate?
   a. You will need to decrease the amount of protein in your diet.
   b. As you age, you will require more calories in your diet.
   c. High-fiber food and plenty of water should be included in your diet.
   d. Your daily intake of fat should be at least 30% or more.
   e. The medications you take will not affect your dietary intake.

8. (LO 41.2) Which medication would *most* likely be given to an elderly patient with congestive heart failure?
   a. Statin
   b. Glucophage®
   c. Actonel®
   d. Aricept®
   e. Digoxin

9. (LO 41.4) Which of following is *not* a practice of preventive medicine?

    a. Biopsy

    b. Colonoscopy

    c. Mammogram

    d. Immunization

    e. Pap smear

10. (LO 41.4) Which of the following patients is engaging in polypharmacy?

    a. A 78-year-old female patient with a prolapsed uterus

    b. A 65-year-old male patient with nocturia due to an enlarged prostate

    c. A 76-year-old female patient taking 12 different prescription medications and 2 over-the-counter supplements

    d. A 68-year-old male patient with a history of alcoholism

    e. An 82-year-old patient who uses a walker for ambulation

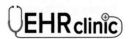

Go to CONNECT to complete the EHRclinic exercises: 41.01 Document Administration of Patient Education for Fall Prevention and 41.02 Document Administration of Patient Education for Daily Water Intake.

SOFT SKILLS SUCCESS

You are assisting with an examination of an 80-year-old female patient who is at the clinic with her daughter. When the daughter steps out of the room to speak to the licensed practitioner, the patient states, "You know, she pinches me all the time." You note that she has some bruises on her left forearm. What should you do or say?

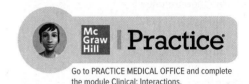

Go to PRACTICE MEDICAL OFFICE and complete the module Clinical: Interactions.

Assisting in Other Medical Specialties

42

C A S E   S T U D Y

PATIENT INFORMATION	Patient Name	DOB	Allergies
	Valarie Ramirez	08/04/1986	PCN
	Attending	**MRN**	**Other Information**
	Paul F. Buckwalter, MD	00-AA-006	According to her chart, this patient lost 5 pounds in the last month. She states that she has not been trying to diet.

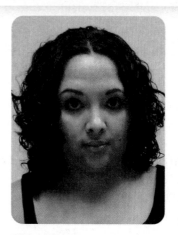

©McGraw-Hill Education

Valarie Ramirez arrives at the clinic for a follow-up check for the removal of a painful wart on her right hand. During the patient interview, she states she is not having trouble with her hand; however, she has noticed in the mirror that she has a lump on the front of her neck at the bottom. She is a little hoarse but denies any other symptoms. She thought she should tell the doctor. Her vital signs are BP 122/78, T 98.8, P 88, R 20, Ht. 5'2" and Wt. 135 lb. Dr. Buckwalter orders an ultrasound of the lump with needle biopsy if indicated. He also orders blood work, including TSH and CEA tests.

Keep Valarie Ramirez in mind as you study this chapter. There will be questions at the end of the chapter based on the case study. The information in the chapter will help you answer these questions.

L E A R N I N G   O U T C O M E S

After completing Chapter 42, you will be able to:

42.1 Describe the medical specialties of allergy, cardiology, dermatology, endocrinology, gastroenterology, neurology, oncology, and orthopedics.

42.2 Identify common diseases and disorders related to cardiology, dermatology, endocrinology, gastroenterology, neurology, oncology, and orthopedics.

42.3 Relate the role of the medical assistant in examinations and procedures performed in the medical specialties of allergy, cardiology, dermatology, endocrinology, gastroenterology, neurology, oncology, and orthopedics.

K E Y   T E R M S

angiography
arthroscopy
balloon angioplasty
benign
cardiac catheterization
colonoscopy
computed tomography
coronary artery bypass graft (CABG)
echocardiography
electroencephalography (EEG)
electromyography
endoscopy
intradermal test
magnetic resonance imaging (MRI)
malignant
patch test
positron emission tomography (PET)
RAST test
scratch test
sigmoidoscopy
stent
Wood's light examination

I.C.8 Identify common pathology related to each body system including:
(a) signs
(b) symptoms
(c) etiology

I.C.9 Analyze pathology for each body system including:
(a) diagnostic measures
(b) treatment modalities

I.C.11 Identify the classifications of medications including:
(a) indications for use

I.P.8 Instruct and prepare a patient for a procedure or a treatment

I.P.9 Assist provider with a patient exam

I.A.3 Show awareness of a patient's concerns related to the procedure being performed

V.P.4 Coach patients regarding:
(a) office policies
(b) health maintenance
(c) disease prevention
(d) treatment plan

V.A.3 Demonstrate respect for individual diversity including:
(a) gender
(b) race
(c) religion
(d) age
(e) economic status
(f) appearance

X.P.3 Document patient care accurately in the medical record

2. Anatomy and Physiology
a. List all body systems and their structures and functions
b. Describe common diseases, symptoms, and etiologies as they apply to each system
c. Identify diagnostic and treatment modalities as they relate to each body system

3. Medical Terminology
c. Apply medical terminology for each specialty

4. Medical Law and Ethics
a. Follow documentation guidelines

8. Clinical Procedures
a. Practice standard precautions and perform disinfection/sterilization techniques
d. Assist provider with specialty examination including cardiac, respiratory, OB-GYN, neurological, and gastroenterology procedures
e. Perform specialty procedures including but not limited to minor surgery, cardiac, respiratory, OB-GYN, neurological, and gastroenterology procedures
j. Make adaptations for patients with special needs (psychological or physical limitations)

▶ Introduction

As a medical assistant, you may choose employment in a medical specialty. This chapter introduces you to many of the specialties, their diseases and disorders, the types of exams involved, and how the medical assistant can assist with diagnostic testing. Certain specialized tests and the correct methods to administer them also are included in this chapter. As with any other practice, when working in a medical specialty, keep in mind that you also perform basic administrative and clinical skills and will have the responsibility of communicating with and educating patients. Certain concerns and questions are common to patients within a specialty area. Being prepared to address these concerns and questions will allow you to help patients effectively and fulfill a vital role on the healthcare team.

▶ Working in Other Medical Specialties
LO 42.1

Licensed practitioners working in medical specialties focus on one body system (such as the skin) or a single type of disease (such as cancer). The medical specialties discussed here include allergy, cardiology, dermatology, endocrinology, gastroenterology, neurology, oncology, and orthopedics.

Allergy

An allergist specializes in diagnosing and treating allergies. Allergies involve inappropriate immune system responses, or allergic reactions, to normally harmless substances called *allergens*. During an allergic reaction, inflammation and tissue damage occur. Common allergens include certain foods

Using an Epinephrine Autoinjector

When working in a medical office that treats people with allergies, you must be familiar with epinephrine so that you can teach patients how to self-administer it. Epinephrine is a drug used to treat allergies so severe that exposure to the allergen may be life-threatening. The following reactions indicate the possibility of anaphylaxis, or anaphylactic shock:

- Flushing
- Sharp drop in blood pressure
- Hives
- Difficulty breathing
- Difficulty swallowing
- Convulsions
- Vomiting
- Diarrhea and abdominal cramps

If a patient with a severe allergy experiences any or all of these symptoms, the reaction can be fatal unless emergency treatment is given immediately. Patients who cannot always control their exposure to an allergen—for example, bee or wasp venom—must have access to an epinephrine autoinjector for emergency intramuscular use. These prepackaged injectors (Figure 42-1) deliver either 0.3 mg of epinephrine—a single dose for an adult—or 0.15 mg of epinephrine—a single dose for a child. A patient who is exposed to the allergen should use the injector if the allergy is confirmed or if the allergy is suspected and signs of anaphylaxis appear. Teach the patient to follow these steps when using an autoinjector:

1. Remove the autoinjector from the packaging (box and/or plastic tube).
2. Pull back the gray cap.
3. Place the black tip of the injector on the outside of the upper thigh. (If needed, the injector can go through clothing.)
4. Press firmly into the thigh and hold for 10 seconds.
5. Remove the autoinjector and massage the injection site for a few minutes.
6. Call or have someone call 911 and go immediately to the nearest healthcare facility for follow-up care.

An autoinjector is for emergency supportive therapy only. It is not a replacement for immediate medical care. Make sure the patient is thoroughly familiar with the parts of the autoinjector, how to activate it, how to use it, and what to do next. Many injectors come packaged with a training injector for this task. If the patient is very young or otherwise unable to use the autoinjector reliably, teach a family member or companion how to use it. Additionally, "talking" autoinjectors are available and recommended for these patients.

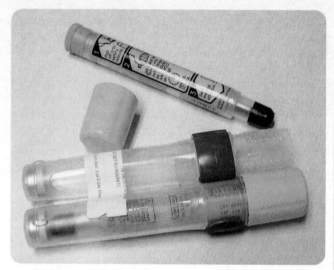

FIGURE 42-1 Epinephrine autoinjectors come prepackaged, containing the correct amount of the drug for an adult or a child.
©Leesa Whicker

(such as eggs and nuts), pollens, medications, insect venom, and animal saliva or dander.

Allergic reactions may show themselves locally—with a skin rash or nasal congestion—or may manifest themselves throughout the body. The most severe kind of allergic reaction is anaphylaxis, or anaphylactic shock, which is life-threatening. When anaphylaxis occurs, immediate medical intervention is needed to save the patient's life. You should know emergency medical intervention for anaphylaxis when preparing to work in an allergist's office. You may need to teach patients who have severe allergies how to use an epinephrine autoinjector. See the *Educating the Patient* feature Using an Epinephrine Autoinjector.

Cardiology

A cardiologist is a physician who specializes in heart diseases and disorders. To assist a cardiologist, you must be familiar with the structure of the cardiovascular system and the typical exams and measurements associated with it. You also need to know about common heart diseases and their treatments. Many diagnostic tests are performed in this specialty, including electrocardiography and stress testing. Imaging techniques, such as X-rays and **echocardiography** (see Figure 42-2), also may be employed. You will assist with or perform some of these tests. Because managing a heart condition often involves many lifestyle changes, educating the patient about topics such as diet and exercise will be especially important in this specialty. You also will provide emotional support to patients with serious illnesses.

Dermatology

Dermatologists diagnose and treat skin diseases and disorders such as acne, eczema, and skin cancer. Some skin conditions involve only the skin itself; others are a sign of disease elsewhere in the body. To assist in a dermatologist's office, you

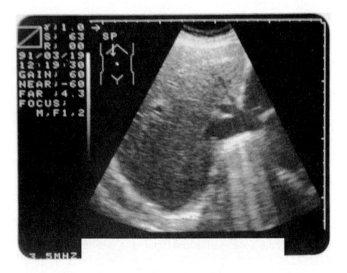

FIGURE 42-2 An echocardiograph shows the structures and function of the heart.

©Getty Images/Steve Allen

must understand the basic elements of dermatologic exams and procedures. In addition to developing familiarity with skin disorders and their treatments, you also need to understand the terminology used to describe skin lesions, as outlined in the chapter *The Integumentary System.* Assisting with positioning and draping during a skin examination and taking skin scrapings or wound cultures might be among your duties in a dermatologist's office. You might perform procedures such as administering sunlamp treatments and applying topical medications. You also will instruct patients about caring for a skin condition or wound site at home.

Endocrinology

Endocrinologists treat diseases and disorders of the endocrine system, which includes glands that regulate and coordinate the body's systems. Hormonal imbalances can affect the basic processes of growth, metabolism, and reproduction. Patients with thyroid imbalances, diabetes, or menopause frequently go to endocrinologists. In the endocrinologist's office, you will assist with exams and collect specimens for analysis.

Gastroenterology

Gastroenterologists diagnose and treat disorders of the entire gastrointestinal (GI) tract, from the mouth to the anus, as well as the liver and pancreas. Proctologists are another type of GI specialist. Unlike gastroenterologists, proctologists treat disorders of the rectum and anus only. A patient who sees a GI specialist has usually been referred by a family doctor, internist, or pediatrician who suspects a GI problem requiring additional expertise. You will need to understand the basic elements of GI exams and procedures to assist in a gastroenterologist's office. You also must be familiar with common GI disorders, their treatments, and the terminology used to describe them. In a gastroenterologist's office, you will tell patients how to prepare for a **colonoscopy** and other exams and procedures performed in the office, a radiology facility, or a hospital. Colonoscopy is discussed in *section 42.3* of this chapter.

Neurology

Neurologists diagnose and treat diseases and disorders of the central nervous system (CNS) and associated systems. Nervous system injuries or diseases can result in loss of sensation, loss or impairment of voluntary movement, seizures, or mental confusion. Your duties in a neurologist's office include assisting with exams by readying equipment for use, positioning the patient, and handing the physician tools and other items. You may be asked to perform parts of these exams. You also may assist with certain diagnostic tests, such as **electroencephalography (EEG)** (see Figure 42-3). Your responsibilities may include instructing and educating patients and their families about procedures, disorders, and treatments.

Oncology

An oncologist specializes in the detection and treatment of tumors and cancerous growths. The term *cancer* refers to a number of oncologic diseases that affect different body systems. All cancers are characterized by the uncontrolled growth and spread of abnormal cells. A tumor is a mass of abnormal cells. Tumors are classified as **benign** or **malignant.** Benign tumors contain abnormal cells, but the cells do not invade and actively destroy surrounding tissue. Malignant tumors contain cells that grow uncontrollably, invading and actively destroying the tissue around them. Malignant, or cancerous, growths are capable of *metastasis*—the spreading of abnormal cells to body sites far removed from the original tumor. When cells become malignant, the process is called *carcinogenesis.* You will encounter patients with a variety of medical conditions in an oncologist's office, so you must be aware of the common types of cancer, what their symptoms are, and how they are treated (Table 42-1). Part of your job may involve preparing patients for the side effects of cancer treatment and helping patients deal with them. Patient and family education and support are essential.

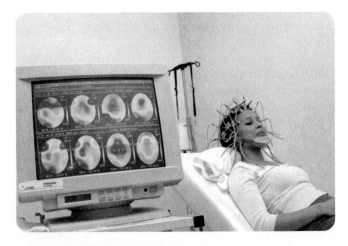

FIGURE 42-3 Electroencephalography (EEG) is performed by placing electrodes on the patient's forehead and scalp.

©AJ Photo/HOP Americain/SPL/Science Source

TABLE 42-1　Common Cancers by System

System	Cancer Type	Symptoms	Treatment
Reproductive (female)	Breast	Lump or thickening in breast, changed appearance, discharge	Surgery (lumpectomy or mastectomy), radiation, chemotherapy
	Endometrial	Postmenopausal bleeding	Surgery, radiation, chemotherapy
	Cervical	Usually none; possible painless vaginal bleeding and an abnormal Pap smear (Papanicolaou smear)	Surgery, radiation, chemotherapy
	Ovarian	Usually none; possible abdominal pain and bloating	Surgery, radiation, chemotherapy
Reproductive (male)	Prostate	Often none; possible difficult, frequent, or painful urination	Surgery, radiation, chemotherapy
	Testicular	Lump in testicle	Surgery, radiation, chemotherapy
Respiratory	Lung (including bronchus)	Often no early symptoms; later, new cough or cold that lingers; chest, shoulder, and/or back pain; wheezing and shortness of breath; hoarseness; coughing up blood; swelling in the face and neck; difficulty in swallowing; weight loss and anorexia; increased fatigue; recurrent respiratory infections	Surgery, radiation, chemotherapy
Digestive	Colorectal	Changes in bowel habits, blood in stools, rectal or abdominal pain	Surgery combined with radiation or chemotherapy
	Liver	Abdominal pain, fatigue, jaundice	Surgery, liver transplant
	Esophageal	Often no early symptoms; later, difficulty swallowing and/or regurgitation of food	Surgery, radiation, chemotherapy
	Oral (mouth and throat)	May begin with painless sore or mass; later, difficulty chewing or swallowing	Surgery, radiation, chemotherapy
	Stomach	Indigestion, weight loss, nausea	Surgery, chemotherapy
Circulatory	Leukemia (all types)	Fatigue, paleness, repeated infections	Chemotherapy, bone marrow transplants
	Non-Hodgkin's lymphoma	Enlarged lymph nodes, itching, fever, weight loss	Chemotherapy, radiation
Urinary	Kidney (renal cell)	Blood in urine; pain in side that does not go away; lump or mass in side or abdomen; weight loss for no known reason; fever; feeling very tired	Surgery, targeted therapy, radiation therapy
	Bladder	Blood in urine; urgent need to empty bladder; urinary frequency; feeling the need to empty the bladder without results; feeling pain when emptying the bladder	Surgery, chemotherapy, biological therapy, radiation therapy
Endocrine	Thyroid	A lump in the front of the neck; hoarseness or voice changes; swollen lymph nodes in the neck; trouble swallowing or breathing; pain in the throat or neck that does not go away	Surgery, thyroid hormone therapy, radioactive iodine therapy, external radiation therapy, chemotherapy
	Pancreatic	Dark urine, pale stools, and yellow skin and eyes from jaundice; pain in the upper part of the abdomen; pain in the middle part of the back that does not go away when shifting position; nausea and vomiting; stools that float in the toilet	Surgery, chemotherapy, targeted therapy, radiation therapy
Nervous	Malignant tumors of brain and brainstem	Headaches, nausea, and vomiting; changes in speech, vision, or hearing; problems balancing or walking; changes in mood, personality, or ability to concentrate; problems with memory; muscle jerking or twitching; numbness or tingling in the arms or legs	Surgery, radiation, chemotherapy
Skeletal	Osteosarcoma (most often in knee and upper arm)	Persistent, unusual pain or swelling in or near a bone	Surgery, chemotherapy, radiation therapy, immunotherapy, cryosurgery, vaccine therapy
	Chondrosarcomas: malignant tumors of cartilage (most often in hip, femur, humerus)	Usually no early symptoms; later, patients may feel a bony bump with pain, swelling, and limited movement of the affected bone	Surgery

Source: Adapted from American Cancer Society. http://www.cancer.org and National Cancer Institute. http://www.cancer.gov.

Orthopedics

Orthopedics is the medical specialty focusing on disorders, injuries, and diseases of the muscular and skeletal systems. The two systems are so interdependent they are sometimes referred to as the musculoskeletal system, especially by orthopedists. In an orthopedist's office, you will be asked to assist with general exams. Other responsibilities may include assisting with X-rays, helping with casting, applying hot or cold treatments, and educating patients about therapy regimens.

▶ Diseases and Disorders of Medical Specialties   LO 42.2

The medical assistant working in medical specialties should have a basic knowledge of the diseases and disorders related to these specialties. Understanding the conditions that commonly occur in certain medical specialties will improve your ability to assist the licensed practitioner and patients.

Cardiology Diseases and Disorders

Cardiology is a common specialty practice because of the prevalence of cardiovascular diseases and disorders. Every year since 1918, the number one cause of death in the United States has been cardiovascular disease, or a disease of the heart and blood vessels. Approximately 2,500 Americans die every day from coronary artery disease (CAD)—narrowing of the blood vessels surrounding the heart that causes a reduction of blood flow to the heart. Cardiovascular disease claims more lives than the next four leading causes of death combined. Unbelievably, one of every three American adults has some form of CAD. You may know someone who has hypertension (high blood pressure) or other heart conditions. Maybe someone you know has had a myocardial infarction (MI), or heart attack. Several factors put patients at risk for heart disease, including inactivity, obesity, high blood pressure, cigarette smoking, high cholesterol, and diabetes. As a medical

assistant working in a cardiology office, you should be able to teach patients about ways to reduce or prevent heart disease, stroke, and heart attack. See the *Educating the Patient* feature Ways to Reduce or Prevent Heart Disease, Stroke, and Heart Attack. Many of the diseases or disorders seen in a cardiology office are outlined in Table 42-2. Treatment for cardiovascular disease frequently includes medications, discussed in the *Principles of Pharmacology* chapter.

Dermatologic Conditions and Disorders

The condition of the skin plays a large part in a person's appearance. Patients with skin disorders, therefore, may worry about their attractiveness to and acceptance by others. Allow patients to express their anxieties; in return, provide encouragement about the course and outcome of their treatment. Table 42-3 discusses some of the most common dermatologic conditions and disorders. These and other diseases and disorders of the skin and accessory organs are discussed in the chapter *The Integumentary System*.

Endocrine Diseases and Disorders

The most common diseases and disorders seen in an endocrinologist's office are those related to the pancreas, thyroid, and reproductive organs. However, an endocrinologist treats any disorder related to the endocrine system. Diabetes occurs when the pancreas does not secrete enough insulin or the body is resistant to insulin. A deficiency of insulin or a resistance to it interferes with the metabolism of carbohydrates, proteins, and fats, raising the glucose level in the blood. This condition is known as *hyperglycemia*. The symptoms of diabetes are often subtle and include frequent urination, excessive thirst, extreme hunger, unexplained weight loss, fatigue, and blurry vision. Common types of diabetes are Type 1, Type 2, and gestational diabetes, discussed in the chapter *The Endocrine System*. No matter the type of diabetes, the goal is basically the same: Keep blood sugar levels within a normal range, eat a healthy diet, exercise regularly, and see a healthcare provider routinely (see Figure 42-4).

EDUCATING THE PATIENT

Ways to Reduce or Prevent Heart Disease, Stroke, and Heart Attack

As a medical assistant, you can help educate patients about ways to prevent or reduce their risk of cardiovascular disease. Explain to patients that the American Heart Association now recommends that you watch your ABCs:

Avoid Risky Behaviors

- Stop smoking. A smoker's risk is twice that of a nonsmoker. Even exposure to environmental tobacco smoke (secondhand smoke, passive smoking) may increase heart disease risk.
- Decrease stress.
- Maintain healthy blood pressure. Find ways to lower blood pressure and to keep the numbers down. The goal is a blood pressure of less than 120/80 mmHg.

- Maintain healthy blood cholesterol. Cholesterol will cause fat to lodge in your arteries, sooner or later causing a heart attack or stroke. Keep the total cholesterol less than 200 mg/dL.

Be More Active

- Increase physical activity. The goal is to increase physical activity to 30 to 60 minutes on most days of the week. Increasing activity can help decrease stress, blood pressure, blood cholesterol, and obesity.

Choose Good Nutrition

- Maintain a well-balanced diet, which helps decrease alcohol consumption, stress, blood cholesterol, diabetes, and obesity.

Source: Adapted from the American Heart Association's guidelines.

TABLE 42-2 Cardiovascular Diseases

Category of Disease/Disorder	Common Conditions*	Treatment
Arterial/vascular disorders	Aneurysm	Medication, surgery
	Arteriosclerosis	Medication, lifestyle and diet management, surgery
	Atherosclerosis	Medication, lifestyle and diet management, surgery
	Hypertension	Medication, lifestyle and diet management, stress management
	Varicose veins	Elastic stockings, weight loss, elevation of legs, surgery
Coronary artery disease	Angina pectoris	Medication, rest, lifestyle management
	Myocardial infarction	Medication, oxygen administration, rest, lifestyle management
Dysrhythmias	Atrial fibrillation	Medication, cardioversion (electric shock to the heart)
	Conduction delays or blocks (problems with electrical transmission within the heart)	Medication, pacemaker
	Tachycardia	Medication, diet management
Heart failure	Cardiomyopathy (weakening of the heart muscle)	Medication, heart transplant
	Congestive heart failure	Medication, diet management, rest
Inflammation of the heart tissue	Endocarditis (inflammation of heart lining and valves)	Medication, valve surgery
	Myocarditis	Specific treatment for underlying cause, medication, rest
	Pericarditis	Medication, rest
Valvular diseases	Aortic stenosis	Surgical replacement of valve
	Mitral stenosis	Medication, rest, valve surgery
	Mitral valve prolapse	Medication (usually antibiotic prophylaxis to prevent subacute bacterial endocarditis)

*Cardiovascular diseases and disorders are described in more detail in the chapter *The Cardiovascular System*.

Source: Adapted from the American Heart Association's guidelines.

TABLE 42-3 Common Dermatologic Conditions and Disorders

Condition	Description/Signs and Symptoms	Treatment/Prevention
Acne vulgaris (acne) ©Dr Harout Tanielian/Science Source	Inflammation of the follicles of the skin's sebaceous (oil) glands, causing skin eruptions. Pimples, blackheads, and cysts are seen on the face, back, and other areas.	Antibiotics, contraceptives, and retinoid are used to manage the outbreaks. Retinoid can damage a fetus, so it is not taken if a woman is pregnant or could get pregnant.
Contact dermatitis ©John Kaprielian/Science Source	Caused by irritants such as rough fabrics, cosmetics, pollen, or plants such as poison ivy or poison oak. Symptoms include redness, itching, edema, and lesions.	Treatment depends on the cause and type of lesions. Anti-inflammatory medications or antihistamines; oral corticosteroids are prescribed for severe inflammation.
Eczema ©Michel Jolyot/Science Source	Skin inflammation that may be an allergic response to allergens, such as chemicals or foods.	Combination of therapy and lifestyle changes to control flare-ups; oral or topical (applied to the skin) medication and phototherapy (light therapy)

(continued)

TABLE 42-3 Common Dermatologic Conditions and Disorders

Condition	Description/Signs and Symptoms	Treatment/Prevention
Mole 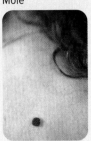 ©Lea Paterson/Science Source	Raised or unraised brown, black, or tan spot less than 6 mm in diameter. Has even coloring and a round or oval shape and clear borders. Monitor for bleeding, itching, or changes in color, size, shape, or texture.	May be surgically removed
Psoriasis  ©Biophoto Associates/Science Source	Patches of red, thickened skin with silver scales mostly found on the knees, elbows, scalp, face, palms, and soles of the feet. More common in adults than in children. Diagnosed through microscopic exam of skin scrapings.	Topical creams and ointments, light therapy, and systemic and combination therapies
Ringworm 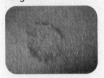 Source: CDC/Dr. Lucille K. Georg	Most often affects the feet (athlete's foot, or tinea pedis), groin (jock itch, or tinea cruris), and scalp (tinea capitis). Flat lesions are dry and scaly or moist and crusty, and develop a clear center with an outer ring. Creates scaly bald patches on scalp.	Topical antifungal medications; oral medications if severe. Contagious, so patient should not share bedding, combs, towels, or other personal items
Warts (verrucae) 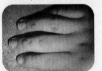 ©Biophoto Associates/Science Source	Benign skin tumors that result from a viral skin infection. If a wart is scratched open, the virus may spread by contact to another part of the body or to another person. Several kinds: • Common warts are raised, rounded, flesh-colored lesions that usually occur on the hands and fingers. • Plantar warts appear on the soles of the feet. • Venereal warts appear on the genitalia and anus and are transmitted through sexual contact.	Treatment depends on the type of wart. Some warts go away without treatment. May be removed by burning or freezing the wart tissue. Instruct the patient to keep the wart removal site clean and dry until a scab forms or the wart falls off.

Skin Cancer

Condition	Description/Signs and Symptoms	Treatment/Prevention
Basal cell carcinoma 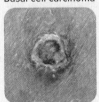 ©Dr P. Marazzi/Science Source	Risk factors: overexposure to the sun, X-rays, irritants, various chemical carcinogens, presence of premalignant lesions. Most common are malignant basal cell carcinomas on areas exposed to the sun, such as the face and neck. Higher-than-average risk of developing skin cancer: those who have had severe, blistering sunburns in their teens or 20s; those who have fair skin and hair and light-colored eyes; and those who work outdoors.	Treatments for skin cancer vary with the type of cancer and its extent. Treatments include surgery, electrosurgery, cryosurgery, radiation therapy, and chemotherapy.
Squamous cell carcinoma 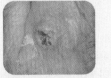 ©Biophoto Associates/Science Source	Appears on sun-exposed areas and looks ulcerated or has a crust. Invades deeper into the skin and has a greater tendency to spread to other body areas.	Treatments for skin cancer vary with the type of cancer and its extent. Treatments include surgery, electrosurgery, cryosurgery, radiation therapy, and chemotherapy.
Malignant melanoma  ©Tom Myers/Science Source	Originates in cells that produce the pigment melanin; this is the most dangerous type of skin cancer. Malignant cells may spread through the bloodstream or lymphatic system to the liver, lungs, and other parts of the body. A sudden or continuous change in the appearance of a mole may signal melanoma.	Treatments for skin cancer vary with the type of cancer and its extent. Treatments include surgery, electrosurgery, cryosurgery, radiation therapy, and chemotherapy.

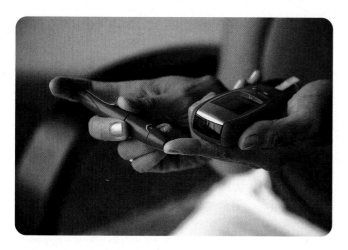

FIGURE 42-4 Patients with diabetes can use a glucometer to monitor their own blood glucose levels.
©Purestock/Getty Images

Disorders related to the thyroid gland include hypothyroidism and hyperthyroidism. Hypothyroidism is characterized by decreased activity of the thyroid gland and underproduction of the hormone thyroxine. This shortage can cause cretinism in children, with resulting mental and physical disabilities. Underproduction of thyroxine in adults results in myxedema.

Patients with this condition have fatigue, low blood pressure, dry skin and hair, facial puffiness, and goiter, or an enlarged thyroid gland. Treatment for hypothyroidism consists of thyroid hormone supplements.

Hyperthyroidism, also called Graves' disease, is characterized by increased thyroid gland activity. The patient has anxiety, irritability, elevated heart rate and blood pressure, tremors, and weight loss despite an increased appetite. Treatment includes the administration of radioactive iodine, antithyroid drugs, or surgery to remove part or all of the thyroid gland. Many patients require supplemental thyroid hormones following treatment for a hyperactive thyroid.

Gastrointestinal Diseases and Disorders

The level of discomfort from GI disorders can be misleading in relation to severity. There may be severe pain with intestinal gas, which is not serious, whereas there is virtually no pain in the initial stage of appendicitis, which is potentially life-threatening. Be sure your notes are accurate and complete when a patient reports GI symptoms. Note the level of the patient's pain, whether over-the-counter (OTC) drugs have been administered, and, if so, whether the OTC drugs provided any relief. Common diseases and disorders treated by a GI specialist are outlined in Table 42-4 and discussed in the chapter *The Digestive System.*

TABLE 42-4	Common Gastrointestinal Diseases and Disorders	
Condition*	**Description**	**Treatment**
Anal fissure	Ulcer in anal wall; may develop into fistula (an abnormal duct to the rectum)	Depends on extent; may require surgery to repair
Cholecystitis	Inflammation of the gallbladder caused by gallstones, tumor, or bile duct blockage; symptoms are pain, nausea, diarrhea	Avoidance of fatty foods if intolerant, lithotripsy to break up stones, antibiotic for bacterial infection
Cholelithiasis	Gallstones	Lithotripsy, antibiotics to prevent secondary infection, or a cholecystectomy (removal of the gallbladder)
Colitis	Inflammation of the colon caused by bacteria, food intolerance, anxiety, or emotional disorder	Diet modification (clear liquid for acute phase), medication, psychotherapy, fluid replacement, colostomy for severe cases
Constipation	Having fewer than three bowel movements a week along with hard feces that are difficult and painful to pass	Diet modification, stool-softener medication, enema, surgery if necessary for impaction
Diarrhea	Abnormally frequent, watery bowel movements	Diet modification, antibiotics for bacterial infection, fluids and medication to prevent dehydration
Diverticulitis	Inflammation of diverticulum	Diet modification, surgery for severe cases
Gastritis	Inflammation of stomach lining	Diet modification, drug therapy
Gastroesophageal reflux (GERD)	Gastric acid rising from stomach into esophagus	Diet modification, small meals, antacids, upright eating, remaining upright for several hours after eating, surgery (rarely)
Hemorrhoids	Enlargement of rectal or anal veins	Diet modification, surgery
Hernia	Organ pushes through a muscle or wall containing it; common abdominal hernias include hiatal hernia and inguinal hernia	Surgery to repair muscle
Stomatitis (canker sores)	Sore gums or other oral areas caused by herpes virus or acidic body chemistry; exacerbated by emotional distress, acidic foods; symptoms are ulcerations (canker sores) with burning, sometimes swelling	Bland diet, avoidance of stress, medicated mouth rinses, topical anesthetic

*Gastrointestinal diseases and disorders are described in more detail in the chapter *The Digestive System.*

Neurologic Diseases and Disorders

Common diseases of the neurologic system are described in Table 42-5. Trauma also can cause damage to the nervous system; such injuries can result in loss of sensation and voluntary motion. You should know the terms related to the various types of sensation loss:

- Hemiplegia: paralysis on one side of the body commonly caused by a stroke, brain injury, or tumor that occurs on the opposite side of the brain.
- Paraplegia: paralysis in the lower extremities.
- Quadriplegia: paralysis of the arms, legs, and all muscles below a cervical (neck) spinal injury.

Encephalopathy is a term for a disease of the brain that alters brain function or structure. Encephalopathy may be caused by an infectious agent, a metabolic dysfunction, a brain tumor, increased pressure in the skull, prolonged exposure to toxic elements, chronic progressive trauma, poor nutrition, or lack of oxygen or blood flow to the brain. The most prevalent sign of encephalopathy is an altered mental state. Common neurologic symptoms of encephalopathy are progressive loss of memory and cognitive ability, slight personality changes, inability to concentrate, lethargy, and progressive loss of consciousness.

Orthopedic Diseases and Disorders

Table 42-6 lists many of the diseases and disorders you will encounter in an orthopedic specialty. For example, back pain—especially lower back pain—is a common disorder. It can have many causes, including muscle strain, osteoarthritis, and the presence of a tumor. Treatments include the application of heat, the administration of analgesics or muscle relaxants, exercise therapy, special braces, traction, and surgery.

Another condition commonly encountered in the orthopedist's office is a fracture, or break in a bone. Fractures and their treatment are discussed in detail in the *Emergency Preparedness* chapter.

▶ Exams and Procedures in Medical Specialties
LO 42.3

As a medical assistant, understanding the anatomy and physiology of various body systems and the specific exam and procedural steps for each specialty area is key. Most specialists' offices have a procedure manual for you to use as a reference when learning new procedures. You will assist with exams and procedures and perform certain procedures on your own. This section will introduce you to basic exams and procedures performed in medical specialties.

Allergy Exams and Testing

An allergy exam involves a medical history and, usually, several diagnostic tests. You may assist with these tests or perform them yourself under a licensed practitioner's supervision. Skin tests, for example, involve introducing solutions containing suspected allergens onto or just below the skin. Any reaction is observed and assessed.

Allergy treatments include allergen avoidance, medications, and desensitization to a substance by means of injections. Part of your job will be to encourage patients to make necessary lifestyle changes to avoid allergens. See the *Educating the Patient* feature Creating a Dust-Free Environment.

TABLE 42-5	Common Diseases of the Neurologic System	
Condition*	**Description**	**Treatment**
Alzheimer's disease	Disabling disease that involves dementia and deterioration of physical function	Frequent stimulation to possibly help slow deterioration, medications that may slow progression of some symptoms
Bell's palsy	Disease that causes sudden weakness or paralysis on one side of the face because of damage to the facial nerve	Usually resolves without treatment in 1 to 8 weeks
Encephalitis	Inflammation of brain tissue usually caused by viral infection; symptoms: fever, headache, vomiting, stiff neck, drowsiness	Medication, rest
Epilepsy	Disease caused by misfiring of nerve groups in the brain, resulting in seizures	Medication
Herpes zoster (shingles)	Disease caused by the virus that causes chickenpox; symptoms: painful blisters that form along path of one or more nerves	Medication to relieve pain
Meningitis	Inflammation of the meninges	Antibiotics and drugs to reduce swelling
Migraine headaches	Severe headaches caused by vascular disturbance	Medication
Multiple sclerosis	Degenerative disease of the central nervous system	Anti-inflammatory medications
Neuritis	Inflammation of one or more nerves; symptoms: severe pain and discomfort or paralysis of the affected area	Medication and rest
Parkinson's disease	Progressive neurological disease	Medication to relieve symptoms
Sciatica	Inflammation of the sciatic nerve	Medication to relieve pain, rest, heat applications

*Neurologic diseases and disorders are described in more detail in the chapter *The Nervous System*.

TABLE 42-6	Common Diseases and Disorders of the Musculoskeletal System	
Condition*	**Description**	**Treatment**
Arthritis	Inflammation of joints	Anti-inflammatory medications, heat, rest, exercise, occupational and physical therapy, surgery (arthroplasty)
Bursitis	Inflammation of one or more bursae (sacs surrounding joints)	Anti-inflammatory medications
Carpal tunnel syndrome	Compression of the median nerve, causing wrist pain and numbness	Rest and occupational adjustments, splinting of wrist, injection of corticosteroids, surgical decompression of nerve
Dislocation	Displacement of bones at joint so that parts that are supposed to make contact no longer come together; occurs most often to fingers, shoulder, knee, and hip	Relocation, or shifting bones back into place; anti-inflammatory medications
Herniated intervertebral disk (HID)	Protruding contents of disk compress nerve roots, causing severe pain	Rest, traction, physical therapy, muscle relaxants, surgery
Osteomyelitis	Infection of bone; principal symptom is pain	Antibiotics and analgesics, surgery
Osteoporosis	Decreased bone mass, resulting in brittle, easily fractured bones	Exercise, dietary supplements, hormone therapy, drug therapy
Paget's disease	Chronic condition that causes bone deformities	Exercise, dietary supplements, hormone therapy, drug therapy
Scoliosis	Abnormal curving of spine	Back brace, surgery
Sprain	Injury to ligament caused by joint overextension	Rest, support, application of cold, anti-inflammatory medications
Tendonitis	Inflammation of tendon	Rest, support, anti-inflammatory medications

*Musculoskeletal diseases and disorders are described in more detail in the chapters *The Skeletal System* and *The Muscular System*.

You also will help patients adhere to regimens of injections or medication.

Three tests are commonly performed in the allergist's office: the **scratch test,** the **intradermal test,** and the **patch test.**

Patients with household dust allergies will need to reduce their dust exposure as much as possible. One way they can do this is to keep their environment, especially their bedroom, as clean as possible. Share these guidelines from the National Institute of Allergy and Infectious Diseases with your patients.

- Prepare the room by removing all contents, cleaning and scrubbing all woodwork, removing carpeting and drapery (if possible), and closing doors and windows. Maintain the room by cleaning it thoroughly once a week. This includes floors, the tops of doors, and windowsills and frames. Use a special vacuum filter, and wash any curtains often.

- Keep the bed and bedding as dust free as possible by encasing box springs and mattress in a dustproof cover and washing all pajamas in 130°F water.

- Keep furniture in the room to a minimum, use furnace air filters (high-efficiency particulate absorption [HEPA] filters are best), avoid stuffed animals, and keep pets out of the bedroom.

Prior to a scratch, patch, or intradermal test, patients are asked to stop taking antihistamines and steroids. These medications could interfere with the test results. Another test, the *radioallergosorbent (RAST)* test, is performed in a laboratory. The RAST test has the advantage of allowing patients to continue to take antihistamines to control their allergies while being tested.

Scratch Test A scratch test tests the patient for specific allergies. Extracts of suspected allergens are applied to the patient's skin, usually on the arms or back. One site is always a negative control—a solution like the one used to carry the allergens but containing no allergen is applied. Then the skin is scratched to allow the extracts to penetrate. A scratch test may be performed using sterile needles or lancets. Some allergists prefer to use applicators that allow the tester to apply allergens to and puncture the skin in several places at once, as shown in Figure 42-5. Be sure to let the patient know that the procedure may cause some discomfort and that itching afterward can be relieved with cold packs. See Procedure 42-1 at the end of this chapter. The licensed practitioner interprets the test results. Because a delayed reaction is possible, the practitioner may wish to recheck the scratch sites in 24 hours. When the results of the scratch test are inconclusive, another test, such as an intradermal test, may be ordered.

Intradermal Test This test introduces dilute solutions of allergens into the skin of the inner forearm or upper back with a fine-gauge needle. The intradermal test is more sensitive

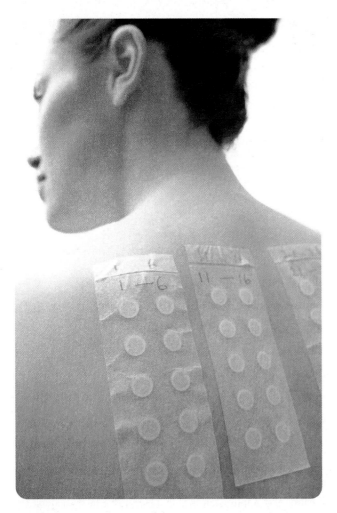

FIGURE 42-5 A multiple applicator allows the medical assistant to apply several allergens at one time.
©SCIENCE PHOTO LIBRARY/AGE Fotostock

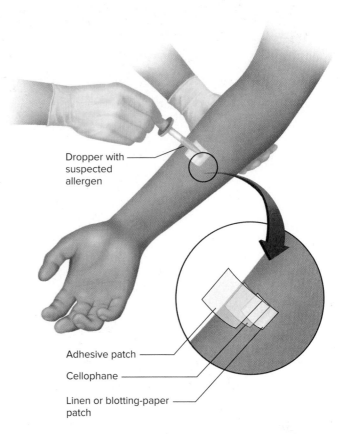

Dropper with suspected allergen

Adhesive patch

Cellophane

Linen or blotting-paper patch

FIGURE 42-6 A patch test is usually done on the arm and is read in 48 hours.

than the scratch test. A small blister, also known as a wheal, which is filled with the introduced fluid, appears on the skin over the injection site. The allergic reaction time is about 15 to 30 minutes, although some substances may cause delayed reactions. If no reaction appears, the test can be repeated with a more concentrated solution to confirm the result. If a severe reaction occurs, the licensed practitioner will order epinephrine to be administered.

The tuberculin test, or purified protein derivative (PPD) test, is another type of intradermal skin test. An extract from the tubercle bacillus is injected into the skin. The results are read in 48 to 72 hours. Raising and hardening of the skin around the area (induration), rather than redness alone, indicate a positive reaction. The procedure for administering an intradermal injection is found in the *Medication Administration* chapter.

Patch Test You perform a patch test by placing a linen or paper patch on uninvolved skin and then using a dropper to soak the patch with the suspected allergen (Figure 42-6). Cellophane or another occlusive material, usually covered with an adhesive patch, is then applied over the linen or paper

patch. Among other things, this test is used to discover the cause of contact dermatitis.

Radioallergosorbent Test (RAST) The RAST measures blood levels of antibodies to specific allergens. You obtain a blood sample from the patient and send it to a laboratory. There, the blood serum is exposed to suspected allergens and the levels of antibodies are measured. This test usually provides more information than skin testing but is more expensive.

Cardiology Exams

A general cardiovascular exam usually begins with a blood pressure reading and an evaluation of overall cardiac health. The cardiologist also palpates the chest wall and the vessels in the extremities to detect abnormal vibrations, pulses, swelling, or temperature. In addition, an electrocardiogram may be obtained.

Electrocardiogram An electrocardiogram (ECG or EKG) provides a measurement of the heart's electrical activity. Electrocardiography—a routine part of a cardiovascular exam—is a painless and safe diagnostic test. Electrodes are placed on the skin in particular areas of the chest and limbs. The heart's electrical activity is shown as a tracing on a strip of graph paper. Review the full procedure for performing an ECG in the *Electrocardiography and Pulmonary Function Testing* chapter.

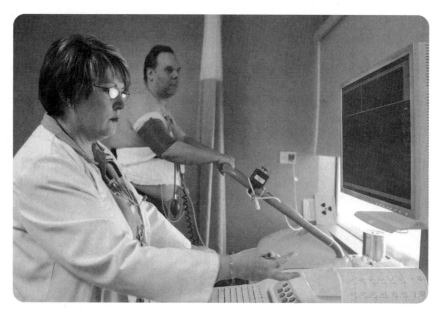

FIGURE 42-7 A stress test measures the electrical activity of the heart under a constant or increasing amount of exertion.
©BSIP/Newscom

Stress Test An exercise stress test involves recording an ECG while the patient is exercising on a stationary bicycle, treadmill, or stair-stepping ergometer (see Figure 42-7). This test measures the patient's response to a constant or increasing workload. Part of your job may involve keeping the equipment properly maintained and calibrated. You also may be responsible for administering the test itself, but a licensed practitioner always should be present because of the risk of cardiac crisis. Before the test, the patient has a screening appointment with the licensed practitioner, during which you take a careful medical history and explain pretest requirements. On the day of the test, be sure the patient has followed pretest directions, such as abstaining from smoking or consuming alcohol, and has signed the proper consent form. The patient is prepared as for an ECG by having electrodes attached to the skin. Show the patient how to use the exercise device. Review additional information regarding exercise electrocardiography (stress testing) in the *Electrocardiography and Pulmonary Function Testing* chapter.

Variations on the basic stress test are the chemical stress test and the nuclear stress test. Chemical stress tests are performed when a patient is unable to perform the physical exercise required by a basic stress test. A chemical that mimics the effect of exercise on the heart is injected through an IV line. A nuclear stress test is similar to a chemical stress test, except that radioactive tracers (radionuclides) are injected so that the licensed practitioner can trace the path of blood through the heart.

Holter Monitor An ambulatory monitor, often called a Holter monitor, is an ECG device that includes a digital recorder that allows readings to be taken over a period of time. Electrodes are attached to the patient's chest in the licensed practitioner's office. Lead wires are attached to the electrodes and to the portable recording device, which the patient wears on a belt or sling (Figure 42-8). The patient returns home,

and the device monitors heart activity for 24 or more hours. Review additional information regarding ambulatory electrocardiography (Holter monitoring) in the *Electrocardiography and Pulmonary Function Testing* chapter.

Radiography and Imaging Techniques

Various radiographic techniques are used in cardiology. Chest X-rays can reveal conditions such as cardiac enlargement. In radionuclide studies, the patient ingests or is injected with a

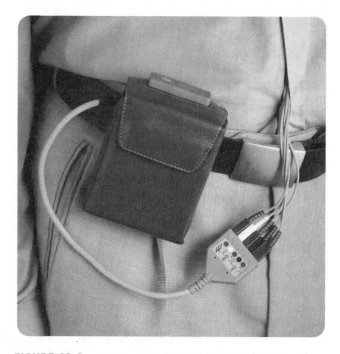

FIGURE 42-8 A Holter monitor allows the licensed practitioner to assess heart function during periods of normal activity.
©Sheila Terry/Science Source

radioactive contrast medium, often referred to as a dye. X-rays are then taken. For example, fluoroscopy studies are X-ray exams in which a contrast medium is injected and pictures of the heart in motion are projected onto a closed-circuit television screen. A venogram allows evaluation of the deep veins of the legs. **Angiography** is an X-ray examination of a blood vessel after the injection of a contrast medium. The test, performed in a hospital, evaluates the function and structure of one or more arteries.

Ultrasound, a noninvasive diagnostic method, also is used in cardiology. Doppler ultrasonography tests the body's main blood vessels for conditions such as weaknesses in vessel walls or blocked arteries. With the use of a handheld probe, sound waves are transmitted through the skin and are reflected by the blood cells moving through the blood vessels.

Echocardiography tests the structure and function of the heart through the use of reflected sound waves, or echoes. Sound waves of an extremely high frequency are projected through the chest wall into the heart and are reflected back through a mechanical device. The echoes, recorded on paper or video, can indicate conditions such as structural defects and fluid accumulation.

Heart magnetic resonance imaging (MRI) is a diagnostic procedure that uses strong magnets and radio waves to produce images of the heart. This procedure is noninvasive and does not use ionizing radiation, so it is safer than other imaging techniques. Detailed pictures of the heart and heart vessels can be obtained using heart MRI.

Cardiac catheterization is an invasive diagnostic method in which a catheter (a slender, hollow tube) is inserted into a vein or an artery in the right or left arm or leg and passed through the blood vessels into the heart. The cardiologist can use this method to take blood samples for analysis, measure the pressure in the heart's chambers, and view the heart's motions with the aid of fluoroscopy. During cardiac catheterization, the cardiologist may choose to perform a **balloon angioplasty** to open partially blocked coronary arteries. This procedure involves passing a slender, hollow tube through the artery at the blockage site. The balloon at the end of the tube is then inflated, compressing the blockage and widening the artery. A metal mesh tube known as a **stent** may be placed in the artery in order to keep it open. The stents are usually coated with medications that prevent the reclosure of the blood vessel.

If the blockage is extensive, the patient may need surgery known as **coronary artery bypass graft (CABG),** which involves bypassing the blockage with a vessel taken from another area. All of these procedures are performed in the hospital.

Dermatology Exams

During a whole-body skin examination, the dermatologist examines the visible top layer of the entire surface of the skin, including the scalp, the genital area, and the areas between the toes. The physician uses a magnifying lens and a bright light to look for lesions, especially suspicious moles or precancerous growths. Your role in this exam includes preparing patients and helping them into the proper position before examining each skin area. During the exam, drape patients to protect their privacy as much as possible while exposing the area to be examined. The physician also may ask you to take photographs or make sketches of lesions to aid in detecting future changes.

Another type of dermatologic exam is the **Wood's light examination,** in which the licensed practitioner inspects the patient's skin under an ultraviolet lamp in a darkened room. This examination highlights certain abnormal skin characteristics and aids in diagnosis. The dermatologist also may perform more limited, focused exams to evaluate specific skin conditions or disorders.

Endocrine Exams and Tests

Before an exam, you will take a thorough medical history. The licensed practitioner will assess the patient's skin condition, weight, and cardiac functioning for clues about illness. An endocrinologist will perform a complete physical exam, including palpation of glands. Most of the endocrine glands are located deep within the body; only the thyroid, the testes, and, to some extent, the ovaries can be examined with palpation or auscultation. Therefore, you may need to collect specimens for essential diagnostic urine and blood tests.

Other diagnostic tools used in endocrinology include radiologic tests such as X-rays and iodine scans. In a thyroid scan, the patient receives an oral or intravenous (IV) dose of radioactive iodine and the thyroid is X-rayed as the material is absorbed. Ultrasound also can be employed to view glands or detect tumors. Urine and blood may be tested for the presence of glucose or hormones.

Gastrointestinal Exams

The gastroenterologist's examination of the patient's GI tract covers the mouth (lips, oral cavity, and tongue), the abdomen and lower thorax, the lower sigmoid colon, the rectum, and the anus. Depending on the patient's symptoms, the physician may perform an invasive exam procedure during the patient's first visit. Formerly, such procedures were performed only in hospitals or special medical facilities. Now, many GI specialists' offices are equipped for these procedures and the management of possible resulting emergencies.

You must prepare the patient, provide reassurance during exams, and help patients be as comfortable as possible. Your duties during the procedures will vary according to your state's scope of practice and the physician for whom you work. Instruct patients in advance to arrange for someone to drive them to and from the exam. After a procedure in which patients have had a local anesthetic at the back of the throat, caution them to avoid eating until the drug has been eliminated from the body. Otherwise, they could choke or aspirate food particles into the trachea.

Endoscopy **Endoscopy** generally refers to any procedure in which a scope is used to visually inspect a canal or cavity within the body. Most endoscopic exams are performed with a flexible fiber-optic tube that has a lighted instrument on the end. These exams provide direct visualization of a body cavity and a means for collecting tissue biopsies and removing polyps, as in the colon. Endoscopy helps diagnose tumors, ulcers, structural abnormalities, and other problems. It is particularly useful in performing procedures that formerly would have required an incision, such as removing stones from the bile duct.

Peroral Endoscopy Peroral endoscopy involves inserting the scope by way of the mouth (Figure 42-9). The patient is sedated and the gag reflex is inhibited with a local anesthetic. The peroral endoscopic procedures include esophagoscopy (esophagus only); gastroscopy (stomach only); duodenoscopy (duodenum only); and panendoscopy (esophagus, stomach, and duodenum), also referred to as an EGD (esophagogastroduodenoscopy).

Colonoscopy Colonoscopy—performed by inserting a colonoscope through the anus—can provide direct visualization of the large intestine. The gastroenterologist uses this procedure to determine the cause of diarrhea, constipation, bleeding, or lower abdominal pain. A colonoscopy also is performed on patients over 50 to screen for abnormal growths called polyps that can lead to colon cancer.

Patient preparation is designed to clear the colon of fecal material so that the colon can be seen clearly. The type of preparation varies depending on the practice where you are working. For example, one regimen requires the patient to follow a liquid diet for 24 to 48 hours before the procedure, then take a cathartic on the two evenings prior to the colonoscopy. Patients also may need to use one or more prepackaged enema preparations the night before and the day of the procedure. Teach the patient the colon cleansing regimen and then tell him to expect diarrhea and possibly mild cramps.

Immediately before the procedure, instruct patients to empty the bladder. Patients should be given a sedative or an analgesic before undergoing the procedure. Patients lie in the Sims' position as the scope is guided through the large intestine. The licensed practitioner may manipulate the abdomen to facilitate passage of the scope.

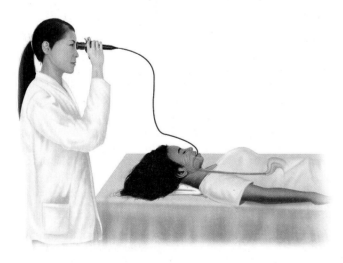

FIGURE 42-9 To perform a peroral endoscopy, the physician inserts a scope through the patient's mouth.

Proctoscopy Proctoscopy is an examination of the lower rectum and anal canal. After an initial digital exam, the proctoscopy is performed with a 3-inch instrument called a proctoscope. This exam can detect hemorrhoids, polyps, fissures, fistulas, and abscesses.

Sigmoidoscopy **Sigmoidoscopy** is similar to colonoscopy, except that only the sigmoid area of the large intestine (the S-shaped segment between the descending colon and the rectum) is examined. Sigmoidoscopy also aids in diagnosing colon cancer, ulcerations, polyps, tumors, bleeding, and other lower intestinal problems. Patient preparation involves using one or two prepackaged enemas either the night before or the morning of the procedure, depending on the physician's instructions. The method for assisting the physician during a sigmoidoscopy is described in Procedure 42-2 at the end of this chapter.

Diagnostic and Laboratory Testing A GI specialist may order laboratory tests to determine the presence of bacteria or bleeding in the stomach. GI specialists also may test the feces for occult, or hidden, bleeding from the intestinal tract. This is discussed in the *Collecting, Processing, and Testing Urine and Stool Specimens* chapter.

Gastroenterologists sometimes use imaging techniques such as X-rays, ultrasound, radionuclide imaging, computed tomography (CT), and magnetic resonance imaging. Most GI radiologic exams are not performed in an office, but you should know enough about them to answer patients' questions. Generally, these exams are performed in a hospital X-ray laboratory or an outpatient facility. You may be responsible for scheduling tests at such facilities for patients. You also may help prepare the patient for these exams. However, in some cases, the patient should discuss specific preparation with personnel from the other facility.

Gallbladder Function Test Cholecystography is an older gallbladder function test performed by X-ray with a contrast agent. The patient swallows tablets of the contrast agent the night before the test. X-rays taken 12 to 14 hours later should show the contrast agent in the gallbladder. The patient then swallows a substance high in fat, which should make the gallbladder contract and empty the contrast agent into the duodenum.

Cholescintigraphy, also known as a HIDA scan test, uses a radioactive chemical injected into a vein. The test chemical then disperses everywhere that the bile goes: into the bile ducts, the gallbladder, and the intestine. A special camera is used to visualize where the chemical is dispersed to determine the functioning of these organs. See the *Diagnostic Imaging* chapter for more information.

Ultrasound Ultrasound is used commonly for diagnosing problems in the gallbladder, pancreas, spleen, and liver. The patient should have nothing to eat or drink after midnight of the night before and on the morning of the exam. Some gastroenterologists perform ultrasound exams in the office.

Barium Swallow The barium swallow (also called an upper GI series) is used to detect abnormalities in the esophagus, stomach, and small intestine. The patient swallows a liquid containing barium—an insoluble contrast agent. This material is viewed using fluoroscopy (moving X-ray images) as the liquid is swallowed and passes into the stomach. X-ray films are taken at frequent intervals to record the diagnostic images. The patient is asked to move into various positions while the barium is tracked through the small intestine. To prepare for this test, the patient should have nothing to eat or drink after midnight the night before and on the morning of the procedure. Refer to the *Diagnostic Imaging* chapter for more information.

Barium Enema A barium enema (also called a lower GI series) is used to detect abnormalities in the large intestine. Barium is given as an enema in this test. A balloon-like tube is inflated in the rectum during the X-ray and the patient is asked to move into various positions to ensure that the barium is distributed completely (Figure 42-10). Patients must eat no meats or vegetables for 1 to 3 days before the test to avoid incorrect indications on the X-ray. For 24 hours before the test, they must also follow a liquid diet, which includes drinking special liquid laxative preparations and more than a quart of water. Specific steps vary depending on the facility, but the intent is to cleanse the colon completely. See the *Diagnostic Imaging* chapter for more information.

Radionuclide Imaging Radiology subspecialists trained in nuclear medicine perform nuclear medicine studies with radionuclide imaging. The patient is first injected with a radioactive substance, then waits a prescribed length of time for the radioactive substance to be taken up by the body part being imaged. The patient is scanned or photographed with a gamma camera, which can read the radioactive areas to determine abnormalities in their composition. This technique is commonly used for liver, spleen, thyroid, and bone scans.

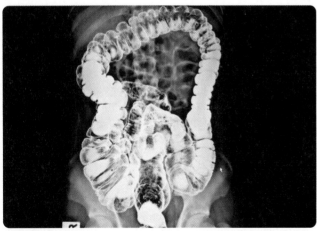

FIGURE 42-10   During a barium enema, the barium is tracked on X-rays.
©plepraisaeng/123RF

Neurologic Exams and Diagnostic Testing

The neurologist evaluates five categories of neurologic function in a complete exam:

- Cognitive function (mental status)
- Cranial nerves
- Motor system
- Reflexes
- Sensory system

Cognitive function can be assessed by observing general appearance and grooming as well as by asking patients specific questions. The neurologist also determines the status of the cranial nerves, which affect smell and taste, eye movements, hearing, voice quality, facial expression, and facial mobility. The physician may ask patients, for example, to close their eyes and then identify familiar smells. The neurologist observes patients' faces for symmetry of movement and tests visual and auditory acuity. The physician assesses motor ability by testing coordination, observing gait, and determining muscle strength. Finally, the neurologist tests patients' reflexes and examines the function of the sensory system in areas of tactile sensation, pain and temperature sensitivity, and awareness of vibration. You are likely to assist the physician in completing these exams, and you may perform certain components yourself.

Common diagnostic tests in neurology include electroencephalography and various radiologic tests. You may assist in performing these tests. Invasive tests may not be done at the physician's office. In such cases, you will need to schedule the procedures, instruct patients about pretest preparations, and educate them about the procedure and what to expect.

Electroencephalography Electroencephalography records the electrical activity of the brain on a strip of graph paper. The tracing is an electroencephalogram (EEG). Electrodes are attached to the patient's scalp and readings are taken while the patient is at rest and engaged in specific activities. An EEG can be used to detect or examine conditions such as tumors, seizure disorders, or brain injury. You may assist with electrode placement or, after training, obtain the EEG on your own.

Imaging Procedures Several imaging techniques are used as neurologic diagnostic tools. Types of procedures include angiograms, brain scans, computed tomography (CT), magnetic resonance imaging (MRI), positron emission tomography (PET), myelography, and skull X-rays.

Cerebral Angiography Cerebral angiography (or angiogram) is a radiologic study of the cerebral blood vessels. After a contrast medium is injected into an artery, X-rays are taken to visualize the cerebral blood vessels.

Brain Scan A brain scan is performed by injecting the patient with radioisotopes and, after a period of time, using a scanner to detect the material. The radioisotopes tend to gather in areas of abnormality, such as tumors or abscesses.

Computed Tomography Computed tomography, often called a CT scan, is a radiographic exam that produces a three-dimensional, cross-sectional view of the brain. Often one scan is done without a contrast medium. Then a contrast medium is injected for greater clarity. CT scans can help diagnose a wide range of conditions, including tumors, blood clots, and brain swelling.

Magnetic Resonance Imaging Magnetic resonance imaging (MRI) is a viewing technique that enables licensed practitioners to see areas inside the body without exposing the patient to X-rays or surgery. The procedure, which takes 30 to 60 minutes, requires the patient to lie still on a padded table that is moved into a tunnel-like structure. A powerful magnetic field produces an image of internal body structures. Patients who are unable to tolerate being inside a tunnel-like structure can be examined with an MRI scanner that has a more open structure (Figure 42-11).

Positron Emission Tomography Positron emission tomography, often called a **PET** scan, studies the blood flow and metabolic activity in the brain to help licensed practitioners identify certain neurologic and CNS disorders. These disorders include Parkinson's disease, multiple sclerosis, Alzheimer's disease, transient ischemic attack (TIA), amyotrophic lateral sclerosis (ALS), Huntington's disease, epilepsy, stroke, cancer, and schizophrenia.

Myelography Myelography is an X-ray visualization of the spinal cord after the injection of a radioactive contrast medium or air into the spinal subarachnoid space (the space between the second and innermost of three membranes covering the spinal cord). Although an MRI is used more frequently, myelography can reveal tumors, cysts, spinal stenosis, and herniated disks.

Skull X-Ray Skull X-rays may be used to detect fractures in the skull and to locate tumors.

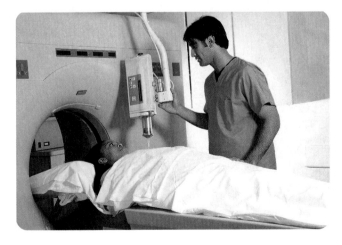

FIGURE 42-11 Magnetic resonance imaging is used to diagnose disorders in many specialties.
©Plush Studios/Blend Images LLC

Other Tests Other diagnostic tests—including lumbar puncture and electromyography—do not involve imaging techniques. A lumbar puncture, or spinal tap, involves collecting a sample of cerebrospinal fluid (CSF) to diagnose infection, measure CSF pressure, and check for blood cells and proteins in the fluid. A needle is inserted between two lumbar vertebrae and into the subarachnoid space. The collected fluid is sent to a laboratory for analysis. **Electromyography** is used to detect neuromuscular disorders or nerve damage. Needle electrodes are inserted into some of the patient's skeletal muscles. When the muscles contract, a monitor records the nerve impulses and measures conduction time.

Oncology Exams and Diagnostic Testing

An exam in an oncologist's office focuses on the area of the body where a problem is suspected. The oncologist's goal is to detect, diagnose, and treat cancer, which is done through a variety of procedures. You will schedule some of these tests and provide pretest instructions and explanations to patients.

A biopsy is a common procedure an oncologist may perform, and you may assist with the procedure. There are several types of biopsies. A physician performs an incisional, or open, biopsy by making an incision and removing a piece of tissue. A needle biopsy is performed by removing tissue with a needle inserted through the skin into the growth or area. Needle aspiration is performed by removing fluid from a lump or cyst with a needle. Procedure 42-3, at the end of this chapter, describes the steps in assisting with a needle biopsy. During a biopsy, standard precautions and sterile technique must be maintained. Always place the specimen in a prepared, labeled container provided by the laboratory. Transport it according to laboratory instructions, attaching the proper accompanying forms. After the biopsy, you might assist with or perform the cleaning and bandaging of the site.

In addition to a biopsy, you may obtain blood specimens for some tests and assist in other diagnostic procedures, such as the following:

- X-rays.
- CT scans.
- MRIs.
- Blood tests, especially those to detect tumor markers, such as carcinoembryonic antigen (CEA) (increased levels of CEA indicate a variety of cancers), CA125, and CA15-3.
- Ultrasonography.

Cancer Treatment

Cancer treatments fall into three general categories: surgery, radiation therapy, and chemotherapy. Often, a combination of these treatment methods is used. All methods damage healthy as well as cancerous cells. The success of treatment depends on many factors, and recovery varies greatly from patient to patient.

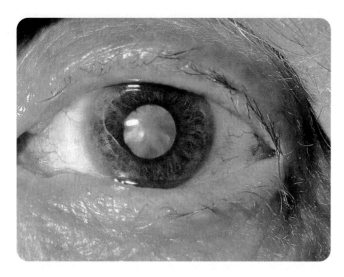

FIGURE 43-1 The lens of an eye with a cataract has a clouded appearance.
©Biophoto Associates/Science Source

Cataracts are more common in the elderly than in younger people because the lens deteriorates with aging. Cataracts also can be caused by iritis, injury, ultraviolet radiation, or diabetes. Some cataracts are congenital. Treatment includes surgically removing the lens and using an artificial lens in its place. The artificial lens may be in the form of special eyeglasses, contact lenses, or an intraocular lens inserted at the time of cataract surgery.

Glaucoma Glaucoma is a condition in which fluid pressure builds up inside the eye. This pressure damages the eye's internal structures and gradually destroys vision. Glaucoma is the second leading cause of blindness in the United States and the first cause among African Americans. According to Prevent Blindness America, 2.3 million Americans over age 40 have glaucoma.

Capillaries in the ciliary body produce aqueous humor—a sticky, watery fluid that circulates between the lens and the cornea. In a patient with healthy eyes, this fluid drains out of this area through the angle formed by the iris and the cornea. The aqueous humor then diffuses into a vascular channel (Schlemm's canal) that encircles the cornea where it meets the sclera—the white of the eye (see the *Special Senses* chapter). The aqueous humor then returns to the systemic circulation (the circulation of the blood to body tissues). However, in a patient with glaucoma, the fluid drains out of the eye too slowly or fails to drain at all. The result is a buildup of intraocular pressure. Retinal nerve fibers are damaged and blood vessels are destroyed, leading to loss of vision and possible blindness.

Glaucoma is treated with medication that reduces pressure in the eye. Drops, pills, or both may be prescribed to reduce the production of aqueous humor. Sometimes, an iridotomy—a type of laser surgery procedure in which a small hole is created in the iris to allow excess fluid to drain—is performed. If the surgery is not effective, an iridectomy (partial removal of the iris) is done to create a larger opening in the iris.

Uveitis Uveitis is inflammation of the uveal tract, which includes the iris, ciliary body, and choroid (refer to the *Special Senses* chapter). The most common type of uveitis is known as anterior uveitis. The term *iritis* is used sometimes to describe anterior uveitis, even though anterior uveitis involves other parts of the eye. The cause is often unknown but may be associated with eye trauma, infection, and some autoimmune diseases. White blood cells from the inflamed area and protein that leaks from small blood vessels float in the aqueous humor. The symptoms of uveitis are pain or discomfort in one or both eyes; pain may be worse in bright light. The eye is red and loss of vision may occur. Left untreated, uveitis can lead to other complications, such as glaucoma and cataracts. Anti-inflammatory drops or ointment is used to treat this condition.

Disorders of the Retina

Several serious disorders affect the retina—the internal layer of the back of the eye. These disorders include retinal detachment, diabetic retinopathy, and macular degeneration.

Retinal Detachment Retinal detachment occurs when the retina separates from the underlying choroid layer—the middle, vascular layer of the eye. When this separation occurs, vision is damaged.

Early symptoms of detachment include flashes of light or floating black shapes, both of which can occur as the hole in the retina forms. Patients occasionally describe their field of vision as being like a window shade that has been pulled down. Peripheral vision is lost as the retina detaches. Vision becomes progressively blurred as detachment continues.

A hole in the retina can be fixed with cryopexy—surgical fixation with cold. During the procedure, the physician places a freezing probe on the outside of the eye over the area of the retinal tear, freezing the area and creating a thin scar that seals the hole. If the retina has already detached, some vision often can be restored with surgical and laser treatments.

Diabetic Retinopathy Diabetic retinopathy is a complication of diabetes. People who have had diabetes for a long time or who do not keep their condition under control experience damage to small blood vessels that supply the retina. The vessels initially leak fluid, which distorts vision. As the disease progresses, fragile new blood vessels grow on the retina and bleed into the vitreous humor—the thick, jelly-like fluid that fills the posterior eye chamber. Scar tissue also may form on the retina. The result is loss of vision. The damage usually cannot be repaired, but the disorder can be controlled to prevent further loss of vision.

Macular Degeneration The macula is the area of the retina responsible for the central area of a person's visual field. For unknown reasons, the macula begins to deteriorate as some individuals age. Macular degeneration causes loss of vision in the center of an image; peripheral vision remains intact. Macular degeneration is the leading cause of blindness among the elderly in the United States. According to the National Eye Institute, 1.75 million Americans have age-related macular degeneration.

When an individual develops macular degeneration, the loss of sharp vision occurs very gradually and without pain.

One of the first signs is difficulty in reading. The loss of vision often appears as a dark spot in the center of the field of vision. If macular degeneration is detected early, laser surgery may restore some vision or prevent further loss.

Disorders Involving Eye Movement

Normally, both eyes move together when people look at objects. A deviation of one eye is called strabismus. In young children, misaligned or unbalanced eye muscles cause strabismus. This misalignment makes it appear as though the child is looking in two different directions. A condition called amblyopia may occur as the misaligned eye becomes "lazy." The brain tends to ignore what the lazy eye sees; if the condition is not treated, vision will be affected in this eye. Treatment involves putting a patch over the fully working eye to force the child to use the other eye. Eyeglasses may be used along with the patch. In some cases, surgery on the eye muscle is required.

Strabismus in adults usually results from problems with the nerves connecting the brain and the eye muscles or with the muscles themselves. Conditions that can cause such problems include diabetes, high blood pressure, brain injury, muscular dystrophy, and inflammation of certain cerebral arteries. Treatment depends on the cause of the condition.

Refractive Disorders

Refraction refers to the way light from objects is focused through the eye to form an image on the retina. The normal eye focuses light exactly at the retina, producing a clear image (Figure 43-2). In some people, the eye focuses light either in front of or behind the retina, so the image is not clear. The problem may be the result of an abnormal shape of the eye or abnormal focusing of the light by the cornea and lens. The most common refractive disorders are nearsightedness, farsightedness, presbyopia, and astigmatism.

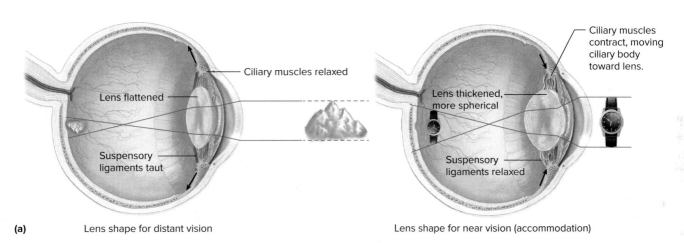

(a)   Lens shape for distant vision   Lens shape for near vision (accommodation)

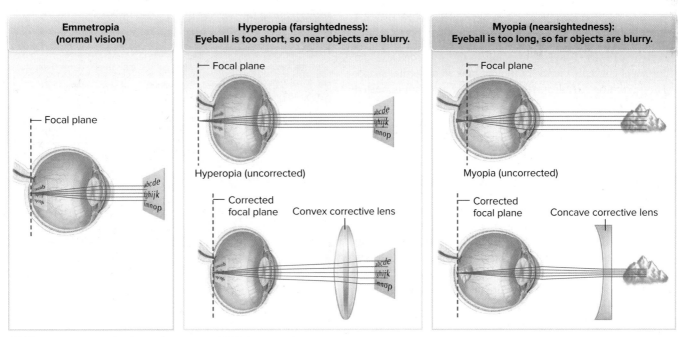

(b) Vision correction using (*center*) convex and (*right*) concave lenses

FIGURE 43-2   (a) Lens shape for distant vision and lens shape for near vision (accommodation). (b) Emmetropia, hyperopia, and myopia.

Myopia (Nearsightedness) Myopia is the condition in which images of distant objects come into focus in front of the retina and are blurred (Figure 43-2). This condition occurs if the eye is too long or if the cornea and lens bend light rays more than normally. Nearby objects are usually seen clearly, but objects far away are unclear.

Nearsightedness is corrected with eyeglasses or contact lenses that have inwardly curving (concave) lenses. The lenses correct the bending of light rays so that they focus on the retina. Surgical and laser techniques also are used to correct myopia by changing the shape of the cornea.

Hyperopia (Farsightedness) and Presbyopia Hyperopia, or hypermetropia, causes images to come into focus behind the retina (Figure 43-2). The eyeball may be too short or the cornea and lens may bend light rays less than normally. Far-away objects are usually seen clearly, but nearby objects are unclear. If the hyperopia is mild, young eyes can compensate for the problem by a process known as accommodation. The ciliary muscles contract during **accommodation,** thickening the lens and increasing its convexity. These changes allow the image to come into focus on the retina.

Patients with mild farsightedness may have no symptoms or may have blurred vision. They may have symptoms of eye strain (an aching in the eye) because the ciliary muscles are overworked. Farsightedness is corrected with eyeglasses or contact lenses that have outwardly turning (convex) lenses. Aging usually causes the ciliary muscles to weaken, so a person may need stronger eyeglasses over time.

Presbyopia is a condition that most commonly affects people starting in their mid-40s. Older eyes tend to lose the ability to accommodate because the lens becomes more rigid. As a result, images come into focus behind the retina, as they do with farsightedness. Individuals find they must hold reading materials farther away to see them clearly. Corrective lenses are used to treat this condition.

Astigmatism Sometimes vision is distorted because the cornea is unevenly curved or the lens has an abnormal shape. This condition is called **astigmatism.** Astigmatism is treated with lenses that correct the unevenness of the cornea or laser vision correction surgery known as LASIK. After surgery, patients may still need to wear glasses to correct presbyopia.

▶ Ophthalmic Exams   LO 43.3

An ophthalmologist performs an eye exam by inspecting the interior of the patient's eyes, including the retina, optic nerve, and blood vessels. The instrument used for this exam is an **ophthalmoscope,** a handheld instrument with a light to view the inner eye structures. You will maintain and prepare this instrument for the licensed practitioner's use, as described in Procedure 43-1, at the end of this chapter.

During the eye exam, the practitioner tests the patient's visual fields. The visual field is the entire area visible to the eye when the patient looks at an object straight ahead. Visual fields are assessed by the confrontation method. The practitioner stands or sits about 2 feet in front of the patient. The patient covers one eye, and the practitioner closes her own opposite eye. (This makes the visual fields of the two individuals roughly the same.) Then the practitioner moves a pencil or other object into the patient's horizontal or vertical visual field, asking the patient to say "Now" when the object comes into view. Defects in the field of vision are noted. The practitioner then tests the convergence of the eyes (or how the eyes come together) by bringing the handheld object to the patient's nose as the eyes focus on it.

The ophthalmologist also routinely tests for glaucoma with the aid of a **tonometer** (Figure 43-3). The tonometer measures intraocular pressure, shown by the eyeball's resistance to indentation by either direct pressure or pneumatic pressure. Your role is to explain the procedure to the patient, instill anesthetizing eye drops into the patient's eyes when required, assist the patient into position, and hand the instruments to the licensed practitioner.

Another instrument the ophthalmologist may use during the exam is the **slit lamp** (Figure 43-4). This instrument consists of a magnifying lens combined with a light source. It is used to examine the eye's anterior structures, including the eyelids, iris, lens, and cornea. Patients rest their chin

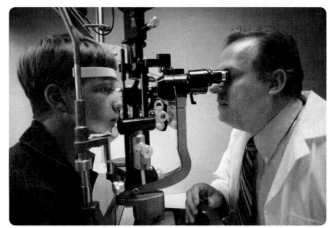

(a)

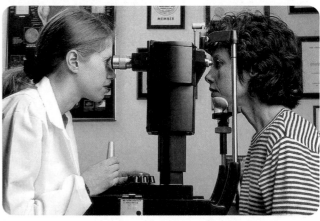

(b)

FIGURE 43-3   Two types of tonometers are (a) the applanation tonometer, which actually touches the eyeball during assessment, and (b) the noncontact, or airpuff, tonometer, which directs a puff of air at the cornea.

(a) ©Blend Images/ERproductions Ltd/Getty Images; (b) ©Ken Lax

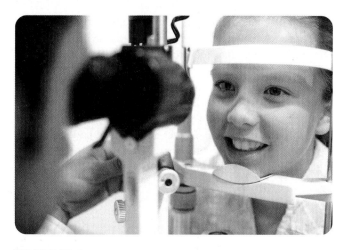

FIGURE 43-4 A slit lamp is used to examine the anterior structures of the eye.
©Ian Hooton/Science Source

on the device's chin rest and stare straight ahead while the practitioner shines a narrow beam (slit) of light into the eye and looks at the eye through the instrument's lens. A special dye—fluorescein—may be used to help visualize foreign bodies or problems with the cornea.

The eye exam also may include a **refraction examination** to verify the need for corrective lenses. Normally, the lens and other parts of the eye work together to focus images on the retina. When errors of refraction exist, images are focused incorrectly, causing conditions such as farsightedness and nearsightedness.

A refraction examination is performed with a retinoscope or a phoropter, a device that contains many different lenses. The practitioner has the patient look through a succession of lens combinations to find out which one creates the clearest image (Figure 43-5).

Types of Vision Screening Tests

Screening tests are used to detect a number of common visual problems, including hyperopia, presbyopia, and myopia. Others test the ability to distinguish shades of gray or colors.

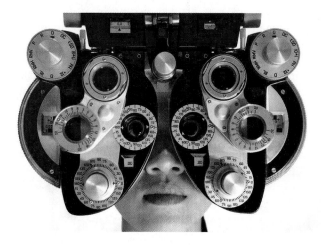

FIGURE 43-5 A phoropter helps the ophthalmologist assess errors of refraction.
©ERproductions Ltd/Getty Images

When you record the results of vision tests, be sure to document for which eye you are recording the results and note if the test was done with corrective lenses (glasses or contacts). If vision is tested with glasses or contacts, you will note this with the abbreviation (with correction). Details on how to perform various vision tests can be found in Procedure 43-2, at the end of this chapter.

Visual acuity screenings are procedures commonly performed by medical assistants either before or after the licensed practitioner's exam. These tests screen for distance vision, near vision, and color vision.

Distance Vision The Snellen chart is the most common screening tool for distance vision. You may be familiar with the Snellen letter chart used by many eye professionals. Snellen number charts and "tumbling E" charts are also available. (See Figure Procedure 43-2 Step 2a and b.) These charts and similar charts that use symbols instead of numbers or letters often are used to test the visual acuity of children.

Near Vision To test for near vision, a Jaeger chart is most common, although other charts are used (Figure Procedure 43-2 Step 21b and c). These handheld cards contain letters, numbers, or paragraphs in various print sizes. They may be held and read at a normal reading distance or mounted in a frame and read through optical lenses. As you may recall, presbyopia is an age-related loss of lens elasticity that affects a person's near vision. The combination of myopia and presbyopia is the reason many people require bifocal lenses as they age.

Color Vision Color vision is commonly tested using a system of colored dots. The two most frequently used testing systems are the Ishihara Color Test (Figure 43-6) and the Richmond pseudoisochromatic color test. Both contain letters, numbers, or symbols made up of colored dots that appear among dots of other colors. The patient is asked to identify what he sees. A patient who is color-blind will not be able to see the items. Color blindness may be inherited; it occurs more commonly in males. Changes in one's ability to see colors, however, may indicate a disease of the retina or optic nerve.

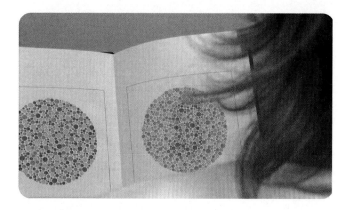

FIGURE 43-6 The Ishihara Color Test, one of the most common color vision tests, uses a system of colored dots to test for color blindness.
©McGraw-Hill Education

Contrast Sensitivity To test for the ability to distinguish shades of gray (contrast sensitivity), the Evans Letter Contrast Test (ELCT) and the CSV-1000E contrast sensitivity test are widely used. Some systems provide contrast variations in a projected image (Figure 43-7). These tests can detect cataracts or problems in the retina even before the sharpness of the patient's vision is impaired.

Patients with Special Needs Certain patients may need special attention when having vision tests. For example, children may be anxious, uncooperative, or unable to follow directions. A patient with Alzheimer's disease or another type of dementia also may require special attention during a vision test. Before the test, encourage a family member to stay with the patient so that she is more comfortable. During the test, use simple language to explain the procedure and demonstrate whenever possible. Proceed through the exam slowly, one step at a time. Because the patient's memory and language skills may be impaired, you may need to repeat directions many times and help her to name particular objects. If she appears to have trouble with one part of the exam, proceed to another part and return later to the part that was difficult for her.

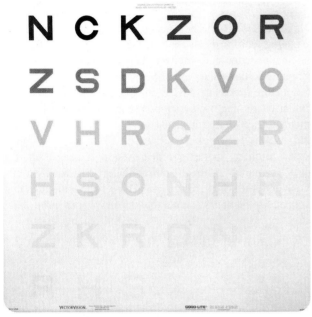

(a) Evans Letter Contrast Test (ELCT)

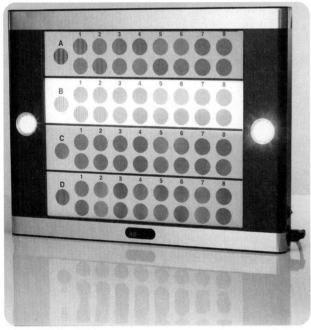

(b) CSV-1000E contrast sensitivity test

FIGURE 43-7 Contrast sensitivity, or the ability to distinguish between shades of gray, is most commonly tested with (a) the ELCT and (b) the CSV-1000E.

(a)-(b) Courtesy of Vector Vision

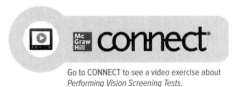

Go to CONNECT to see a video exercise about *Performing Vision Screening Tests.*

▶ Ophthalmologic Procedures and Treatments
LO 43.4

The eye is an extremely delicate organ. Even what seems to be a minor injury or infection can have lasting consequences. You must use the greatest caution as well as proper technique—including sterile technique—when treating a patient's eyes. You also should provide patients with information on how to routinely care for their eyes. See the *Educating the Patient* feature Preventive Eye Care Tips for specific guidelines to follow when presenting eye care information.

Administering Medications to the Eye

Licensed practitioners commonly administer eye medications or perform eye irrigations to assist patients in eye tests, reduce pressure in the eyes, relieve eye pain, and treat eye infections and inflammation. Your responsibility as a medical assistant may include dispensing medications and explaining their use. Some medications are used to diagnose conditions; others are used to treat conditions. Only medications for ophthalmic use should be used in the eye. If you administer eye medications as part of your job, avoid touching a dropper or ointment tube tip to the eye. Doing so can injure the eye, cause infection, and contaminate the medication. Teach patients how to check medication labels carefully before administering them at home. For example, optic medications for eye use could easily be confused for otic medications for the ear. Medications other than optic medications may be too concentrated or may contain substances that will injure sensitive eye tissue.

Although most eye medications are administered for local effect, some are absorbed systemically (affecting the whole body). To prevent systemic absorption, the practitioner may request that you apply pressure with one finger just below the inner corner of each eye after instilling medications.

Continue applying pressure for 2 to 3 minutes, as directed. Procedure 43-3, at the end of this chapter, provides information on administering eye medications.

Eye Irrigation

When foreign materials such as dust, sand, or chemicals enter the eye, they must be flushed out. Flushing—irrigation—should be done, whenever possible, with a sterile solution especially formulated for this purpose. Someone's eye also may need to be irrigated to relieve discomfort from irritating substances such as smog, pollen, chemicals, or chlorinated water. Procedure 43-4, at the end of this chapter, provides details about irrigating an eye. See the *Infection Control Fundamentals* chapter for more information on using an eyewash station.

▶ Otology   LO 43.5

An **otologist** treats diseases and disorders of the ears. Procedures common to this specialty are sometimes performed by other physicians as well, especially general practitioners, internists, and allergists. In your role as a medical assistant, you also may assist with or perform auditory screening, administer ear medications, perform ear irrigations, and help with diagnostic tests such as tympanometry. Otology specialists whose practices include problems affecting the nose and throat are called otorhinolaryngologists.

▶ Ear Diseases and Disorders   LO 43.6

When assisting licensed practitioners in administering various tests, treatments, and procedures, you may encounter a wide range of ear disease and disorder. Some—such as cerumen impaction and otitis externa—do not have lasting effects on hearing and may be treated by a general practitioner. Others affect the ear's middle or inner parts and may require a specialist's attention. Figure 43-8 shows the major parts of the ear. For more detailed information, refer to the *Special Senses* chapter.

Common Disorders of the Outer Ear

Several disorders affect the ear's external parts. These include cerumen impaction, otitis externa, and pruritus.

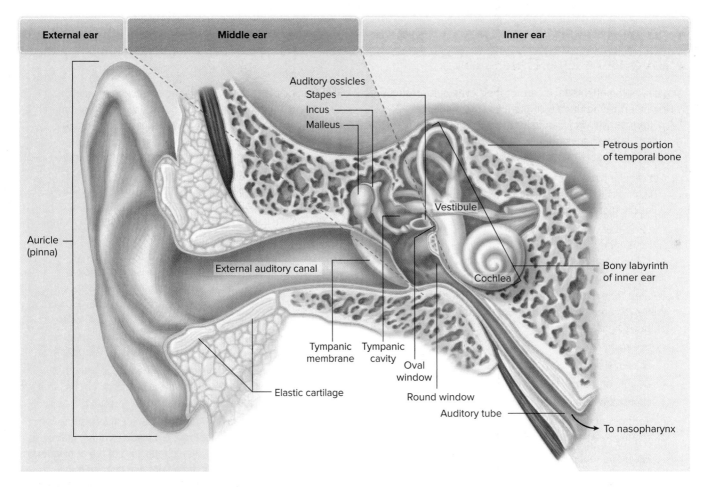

| External ear | Middle ear | Inner ear |

Auditory ossicles
Stapes
Incus
Malleus

Petrous portion
of temporal bone

Vestibule

Auricle
(pinna)

Cochlea

Bony labyrinth
of inner ear

External auditory canal

Tympanic
membrane

Tympanic
cavity

Oval
window

Elastic cartilage

Round window

Auditory tube

To nasopharynx

FIGURE 43-8 The major parts of the ear.

Cerumen Impaction A condition called cerumen impaction occurs when the ear canal becomes blocked by a buildup of cerumen (earwax). The wax can be softened with eardrops, and irrigation can be performed to remove the wax. Refer to Procedure 43-7, at the end of this chapter, for more information about ear irrigation.

Otitis Externa Otitis externa is an infection of the outer ear, usually caused by bacteria or fungi. Also known as swimmer's ear, fungal infections are common in swimmers due to persistent moisture in the ear canal. This infection is treated with a combination of antibiotic or antifungal eardrops and an anti-inflammatory medication.

Pruritus A common problem in the elderly is pruritus—or itching—of the ear canal. Because the sebaceous glands produce less wax with aging, the ear becomes dry and itchy. Dryness can be overcome by a regular routine of lubricating the ear canal with a few drops of mineral oil.

Common Disorders of the Middle Ear

Middle ear disorders involve the eardrum and the chamber behind it. They include otitis media, mastoiditis, otosclerosis, and ruptured eardrum.

Otitis Media Otitis media is an inflammation of the middle ear characterized by fluid buildup, most commonly referred to as an ear infection. For detailed information on otitis media, see the *Points on Practice* feature Otitis Media: The Common Ear Infection.

Mastoiditis The mastoid bone is located just behind the ear. It is connected to the middle ear by air cells, or sinuses, in the bone. Sometimes, if left untreated, an infection in the middle ear can spread to the mastoid bone through these air cells. Although mastoiditis is fairly rare, it may be serious because the mastoid air cells are close to the organs of hearing, important nerves, the covering of the brain, and the jugular vein. Severe cases of mastoiditis may require removal of the affected bone.

Otosclerosis Otosclerosis occurs when bone tissue grows abnormally around the stapes, or stirrup (the innermost of the three tiny bones that connect the eardrum and the inner ear). This overgrowth of tissue prevents the stapes from transmitting sound vibrations to the inner ear. The result is hearing loss in one or both ears. The condition is often hereditary.

POINTS ON PRACTICE

Otitis Media: The Common Ear Infection

Otitis media, commonly referred to as an ear infection, affects almost all children by age 6. This inflammation of the middle ear accounts for 22 million doctor visits each year—second only to routine well-child health exams.

Ear infections typically start when fluid becomes trapped in the middle ear. The lining of the middle ear and eustachian tube contains fluid similar to the mucus within the nasal passages. The normal flow of this fluid from the ear into the back of the nose where it joins the pharynx helps keep the middle ear and eustachian tube free of bacteria. When a child gets a cold or flu, the lining of the eustachian tube and middle ear can become inflamed and can trap the fluid, which becomes infected.

There are four distinct types of otitis media. One or both ears may be affected.

1. Acute otitis media typically is a bacterial infection of the middle ear that comes on suddenly. This type is common in children and typically follows an upper respiratory tract infection. The symptoms include pain, a feeling of fullness in the ear, some loss of hearing, and possibly fever. In severe cases, the eardrum may rupture because of the fluid pressure. Acute infections are not usually treated with oral antibiotics at first. Most infections will resolve on their own without treatment, so physicians usually wait 48–72 hours before prescribing antibiotic treatment for a patient with acute otitis media.

2. Recurrent otitis media is diagnosed when a child contracts acute otitis media repeatedly, perhaps once or twice every month.

3. Otitis media with effusion, also known as OME, involves an accumulation of fluid in the middle ear. Children with OME do not exhibit any symptoms, and they may not experience any discomfort.

4. Chronic otitis media is diagnosed when fluid is present in the ear and fails to clear up after 3 months or more. Infection may or may not be present. Without treatment, the undrained fluid thickens, possibly resulting in changes in the shape of the eardrum, erosion of the ossicles (tiny bones of hearing), and mastoiditis. Chronic otitis media left untreated for a sufficient amount of time can result in facial paralysis, brain infections, and balance problems. These changes may cause temporary or permanent hearing loss if not treated. Antibiotics and reconstructive surgery may be used to treat this condition.

If a child suffers from recurrent or chronic otitis media, myringotomy—surgical incision of the eardrum with insertion of tubes—may be recommended to keep the fluid draining continuously. This procedure usually removes enough fluid to clear up the infection. Depending on the type of tube, it falls out on its own within 3 to 18 months of insertion. See Figure 43-9.

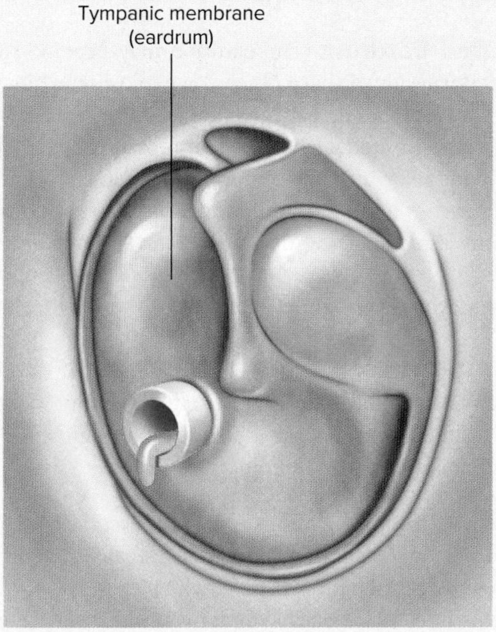

Tympanic membrane (eardrum)

FIGURE 43-9 A pressure-equalizing tube is inserted in the eardrum to help keep fluid from building up behind the eardrum.

Ear infections may be difficult to identify, especially in a young child who cannot talk. The following symptoms are indications of a possible ear infection, particularly if more than one is present:

- Tugging or rubbing of the ear
- Fever ranging from 100°F to 104°F
- Difficulty balancing
- Excessive crankiness
- Difficulty hearing or speaking
- An unwillingness to lie down (the pain may become more severe in a reclining position because of increased pressure against the eardrum)

Preventing ear infections is the best course of action. Several measures can be taken to reduce the likelihood of ear infections, including:

- Preventing colds by teaching children to wash their hands often and not share cups and other eating utensils.
- Limiting a child's exposure to secondhand smoke.
- Breastfeeding for at least 6 months.
- Bottle feeding in an upright position—*never* put a baby to bed with a bottle.
- Keeping immunizations such as flu shots and pneumococcal vaccines up to date.

Symptoms of otosclerosis include gradual loss of hearing and **tinnitus**—ringing in the ears. Surgery to replace the stapes—ossicular replacement prosthesis surgery—can restore or improve hearing in almost 90% of patients with otosclerosis. Alternatively, a hearing aid may improve hearing for some patients.

Ruptured Eardrum The eardrum may become ruptured in several ways: by a sharp object, an explosion, a blow to the ear, or a severe middle ear infection. Sometimes the eardrum is ruptured by a sudden change in air pressure, as might occur when flying in an airplane or diving. Symptoms include pain, partial hearing loss, and a slight discharge or bleeding. The symptoms typically last only a few hours. A ruptured eardrum usually heals on its own in 1 to 2 weeks, but the licensed practitioner may use a temporary patch to help close the defect.

Common Disorders of the Inner Ear

Disorders of the inner ear, or labyrinth, affect the cochlea and the semicircular canals. They include labyrinthitis, Ménière's disease, presbycusis, and tinnitus.

Labyrinthitis Labyrinthitis is an infection of the labyrinth, most commonly caused by a virus. Because the labyrinth includes the semicircular canals, which are involved in balance, this infection causes symptoms of dizziness or vertigo. The room may appear to spin and any movement exacerbates (worsens) the sensation, sometimes to the point of nausea and vomiting. Although disturbing, labyrinthitis disappears on its own within 1 to 3 weeks. The patient may need to rest in bed for a few days, and medication can be given for symptoms.

Ménière's Disease **Ménière's disease** is caused by increased fluid in the labyrinth. The pressure of the fluid disturbs the sense of balance and even may rupture the labyrinth wall or damage the cochlea with its hearing receptors. One or both ears may be affected. Symptoms of this disorder include vertigo, nausea, vomiting, distorted hearing, and tinnitus. Some people may suffer hearing loss ranging from mild to severe. Medications may be used to combat vertigo, nausea, and vomiting. Other treatments that help some people include using diuretics and following a low-sodium diet.

Presbycusis Presbycusis is a type of sensorineural hearing loss. It is the most common form of hearing loss in older adults, affecting about 25% of people by the age of 60 or 70. Men are affected more often than women. Hearing loss can be treated effectively, however, with a hearing aid.

Tinnitus Tinnitus is more commonly called a ringing in the ears. This "ringing" can take several forms, including a buzzing, whistling, or hissing sound. The most common causes of tinnitus are damage to the hearing receptors from noise or toxins, age-related changes in the ear's organs, and long-term use of nonsteroidal anti-inflammatory drugs (NSAIDs) such as aspirin and ibuprofen. Tinnitus can affect people at any age but is more common as people get older. If tinnitus becomes chronic, the patient may find relief by listening to quiet, soothing music or other distracting sounds or by using a device similar to a hearing aid that masks the noise with more pleasant sounds.

Hearing Loss

Hearing loss is actually a symptom of a disease, not a disease in itself. Contrary to what most people believe, hearing loss is not a normal part of the aging process and always should be evaluated for proper treatment. There are two types of hearing loss: conductive and sensorineural. The two types differ in the point at which the hearing process is interrupted.

A **conductive hearing loss** is caused by an interruption in the transmission of sound waves to the inner ear. Conditions that can cause conductive hearing loss include obstruction of the ear canal (cerumen impaction or a tumor), infection of the middle ear (otitis media), or otosclerosis (reduced movement of the bones of hearing known as the ossicles).

A **sensorineural hearing loss** occurs when there is damage to the inner ear, to the nerve that leads from the ear to the brain, or to the brain itself. In this kind of loss, sound waves reach the inner ear, but the brain does not perceive them as sound. This type of hearing loss can be hereditary, can be caused by repeated exposure to loud noises or viral infections, or can occur as a side effect of medications such as NSAIDs and some antibiotics. Tinnitus suggests damage to the auditory nerve.

Sensorineural hearing loss can be differentiated from conductive hearing loss by hearing tests. It is also possible for both types of hearing loss to occur together.

Noise Pollution Prolonged exposure to loud noises is a common cause of hearing loss because of damage to the sensitive cells in the cochlea. People who work around noisy equipment—such as construction workers, aircraft personnel, and machine operators—are likely to suffer from this type of hearing loss unless they protect their ears (Figure 43-10). Repeatedly listening to loud music from a personal stereo or car radio set at too high a volume also can damage the ears.

Working with Patients with a Hearing Impairment

You may come in contact with patients of all ages who have hearing impairments. Many patients wear hearing aids to amplify normal speech. Some patients, however, may not

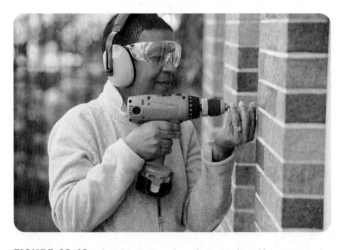

FIGURE 43-10 Loud noises, such as those produced by power tools, can damage hearing unless appropriate ear protectors are worn.
©Wave Royalty Free/AGE Fotostock

admit they have a problem—out of fear, vanity, or misinformation. It is estimated that one-third of patients between the ages of 65 and 74 and one-half of those between the ages of 75 and 79 suffer from some loss of hearing.

To improve communication with a patient whose hearing is impaired, you can do the following:

- Speak at a reasonable volume. Do not shout. Shouting can actually make your words harder to understand. A hearing aid filters out loud sounds, so the patient may not hear everything you say if you shout.
- Speak in clear, low-pitched tones. Elderly patients may lose the ability to hear high-pitched sounds.
- Avoid speaking directly into the patient's ear. Stand 3 to 6 feet away and face the patient so that she can see your lip movements and facial expressions. Avoid covering your mouth with your hands. Speak at a normal rate.
- Avoid overemphasizing your lip movements, which makes lip reading difficult.
- Avoid hand gestures unless they are appropriate.
- If the patient does not understand what you say, restate the message in short, simple sentences. Have the patient repeat the message to verify that your words were understood.
- Treat patients who have a hearing impairment with patience and respect.

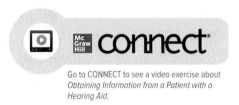

Go to CONNECT to see a video exercise about *Obtaining Information from a Patient with a Hearing Aid.*

▶ Hearing and Other Diagnostic Ear Tests

LO 43.7

Various tests are performed to find out whether a person hears normally. If the tests reveal a problem, follow-up tests are conducted to determine the cause of the problem. You may assist with the testing or educate the patient about caring for her ears.

Hearing Tests

As part of a general examination, licensed practitioners may perform simple hearing tests to determine whether a patient's stated hearing loss is conductive or sensorineural. The most common of these are the Weber test and the Rinne test. Both involve the use of tuning forks (see Figure 43-11).

In the Weber test, the licensed practitioner strikes a tuning fork against a hard surface to produce a sound and then places the tuning fork in the middle of the patient's head (Figure 43-12a). She then asks the patient whether the sound is coming from the right or the left, or both. In conductive hearing loss, the sound will be heard best through the ear with hearing loss. In sensorineural hearing loss, the sound travels toward the ear without hearing loss.

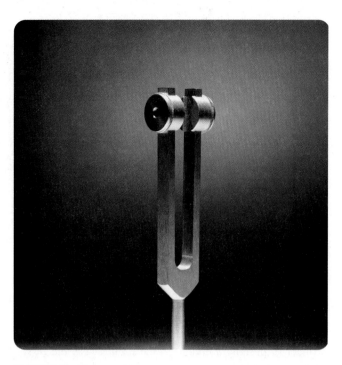

FIGURE 43-11 A tuning fork is used to perform simple hearing tests.
©Spike Mafford/Getty Images

To perform the Rinne test, the practitioner measures the amount of time the patient can hear the sound from a tuning fork placed near the mastoid bone (see Figure 43-12b). This measures sound conducted through the bone. She then measures the amount of time the patient can hear the sound when the tuning fork is placed near the ear canal to measure sound conducted through the air (see Figure 43-12c). The two times are then compared. A normal ear will hear the air-conducted sound twice as long as the bone-conducted sound. In a patient with conductive hearing loss, the bone-conducted sound will be at least as long as the air-conducted sound. In a patient with sensorineural hearing loss, the air-conducted sound will last slightly longer than the bone-conducted sound, but not twice as long.

If you have the necessary training, you may help perform a test that uses an audiometer to produce an audiogram. An **audiometer** is an electronic device that measures hearing acuity by producing sounds in specific frequencies and intensities. A **frequency** is the number of complete fluctuations—waves—of energy that pass a specific point in 1 second (Figure 43-13). Frequency is best described as the pitch of sound. High frequency is high-pitched and low frequency is low-pitched. The audiometer allows a licensed practitioner to test a person's hearing and to determine the nature and extent of hearing loss.

Many types of audiometers are available. Some machines automatically generate the various tones at different **decibels** (units for measuring the relative intensity—loudness—of sounds on a scale from 0 to 130) and print out the patient's responses. Others must be manually adjusted and the results charted by hand. During the test, the patient wears a headset to hear the sounds produced by the audiometer. Depending on the unit, the patient indicates hearing a sound by raising

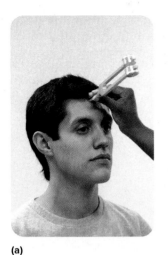
(a)

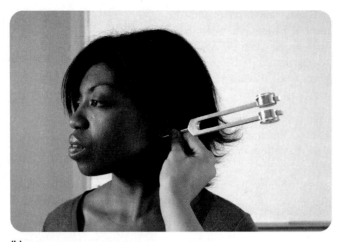
(b)

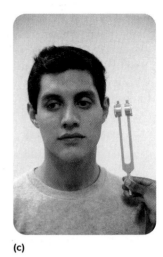
(c)

FIGURE 43-12 (a) During the Weber hearing test, the tuning fork is placed on the patient's forehead. (b) Place the tuning fork on the mastoid bone during the Rinne hearing test. (c) Place the tuning fork near the ear during the Rinne hearing test. Compare how long the patient can hear the sound during each step.

(a)-(c) ©McGraw-Hill Education/Jill Braaten, Photographer

a finger or pushing a button. In the former case, the person administering the test records the response. In the latter case, the response may be recorded automatically or by the test giver. Procedure 43-5, at the end of this chapter, provides additional information about measuring auditory acuity.

Adults and children who can understand directions and respond appropriately can be screened in this manner. If you work in a pediatrician's office, you also may help to check an infant's response to sounds. These tests require special techniques, as infants cannot understand directions. Refer to the general steps in the *Assisting in Pediatrics* chapter and procedure 43-5 to perform a hearing test on an infant.

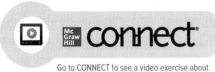

Go to CONNECT to see a video exercise about *Measuring Auditory Acuity.*

Tympanometry

A diagnostic test called tympanometry measures the eardrum's ability to move. This is an indication of the amount of pressure in the middle ear. Tympanometry is used to detect the following diseases and abnormalities of the middle ear or ear canal:

- Cerumen impaction
- Middle ear fluid
- Middle ear tumor
- Ossicular detachment
- Tympanic membrane perforation
- Tympanic membrane scars

To perform the test, a small, soft-rubber cuff is placed over the external ear canal, producing an airtight seal. The tympanometer then automatically measures air pressure against the tympanic membrane and prints a graph of the results. Let patients know that they will hear sounds during the test that may seem loud, but they need to remain as still as possible.

▶ Ear Treatments and Procedures LO 43.8

Licensed practitioners use various approaches, devices, and techniques with each type of ear problem to improve patients' hearing and maintain or improve their ear health. As a medical assistant, you can provide patients with information on

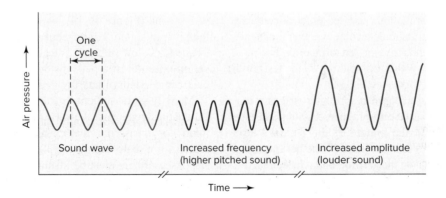

FIGURE 43-13 Sound frequency is determined by the number of waves per second that pass a specified point.

preventive ear care techniques, as described in the *Educating the Patient* feature Preventive Ear Care Tips.

You also may administer ear medications, perform ear irrigations, and assist the physician in earwax removal.

Administering Medications to the Ear

Licensed practitioners often administer eardrops or perform ear irrigations to treat patients' ear infections or inflammation, relieve ear pain, or loosen earwax. Like eye medications, eardrops are used primarily for their local effects. They are not usually absorbed systemically, nor do they cause systemic effects. It is important that you warm the eardrops slightly before administration to avoid making the patient dizzy. Holding them in your hand for a minute or two will usually warm them enough. Procedure 43-6, at the end of this chapter, provides instructions for this procedure.

Earwax and Foreign Body Removal

Cerumen, or earwax, may build up in the ear canal, causing a full feeling in the ear, ear pain, partial hearing loss, and tinnitus. Cerumen normally protects the ear, but if a person produces too much, it can harden and block the ear canal. Also, cleaning your ear with cotton-tipped swabs can push the cerumen down into the ear canal. There are several treatments for removing earwax. In some cases, if the wax is close enough to reach, the licensed practitioner may be able to remove the wax with an ear curette, a small instrument with a scoop or loop on one end. Home remedies include over-the-counter wax softening drops, mineral oil, and glycerin. These may work if the impaction is not too severe. But if the wax is extremely hard or is stuck to the ear canal, irrigation may be the best treatment.

Ear Irrigation Irrigating the ear may relieve inflammation or irritation of the ear canal and help loosen and remove impacted earwax or a foreign body. This procedure is performed in the licensed practitioner's office. Irrigation is contraindicated in (inadvisable for) patients who:

- Currently have or have had a ruptured eardrum.
- Have pressure equalizing tubes in their eardrum.
- Have an ear infection.
- Have had ear surgery, including mastoidectomy.

Always ask the patient about ear surgeries and other conditions before beginning the irrigation and make sure the irrigation solution is at body temperature before starting. This helps reduce the possibility of the patient becoming dizzy during the procedure. Procedure 43-7, at the end of this chapter, provides instructions for ear irrigation.

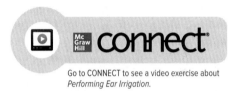

Go to CONNECT to see a video exercise about *Performing Ear Irrigation.*

Microscopic Earwax and Foreign Body Removal

Occasionally, irrigation does not work to remove a cerumen impaction. With the help of a microscope, an otologist can use suction or an instrument to remove the wax. Foreign bodies in the ear also are removed with the aid of a microscope. During the procedure, the licensed practitioner looks through the microscope into the patient's ear canal. This gives her a better view of the ear, allowing her to get deeper into the ear canal without damaging the delicate structures within the ear. The patient must remain extremely still during this procedure. Your role as a medical assistant is to help keep the patient at ease and comfortable and to make sure the practitioner has the necessary instruments.

Hearing Aids

Hearing aids may be worn inside or outside the ear (Figure 43-14). If worn outside, they may be located behind the ear, mounted on eyeglasses, or worn on the body. Hearing aids consist of the following parts:

- A tiny microphone to pick up sounds.
- An amplifier to increase the volume of sounds.
- A tiny speaker to transmit sounds to the ear.

You may need to teach patients how to obtain a hearing aid. You also can pass along tips to help them take proper care of their hearing aids and to troubleshoot problems.

Obtaining a Hearing Aid A patient with signs of hearing loss should be referred to an otologist, a medical doctor specializing in the health of the ear, or an **audiologist,** a specialist who focuses on evaluating and correcting hearing problems. Audiologists are not medical doctors and do not treat diseases of the ear. Instead, they evaluate the patient's hearing, fit hearing aids, give instruction in the use of hearing aids, and provide service for hearing aids if necessary. It is important for hearing aids to fit properly. If they do not, sounds may not be transmitted well into the ear.

Care and Use of Hearing Aids Hearing aids run on batteries that typically last about 2 weeks. So the patient must keep a fresh supply of batteries on hand. The hearing aid itself must be routinely cleaned or the microphone, switches, or dials may not work properly. Moisture can damage the aid, so it must not get wet. Hair sprays can clog hearing aid openings or interfere with the operation of moving parts. For these reasons, spray should be applied before a hearing aid is inserted. Cerumen often builds up behind hearing aids that are worn in the ear, reducing sound transmission. If buildup does occur, the cerumen plug should be removed by ear irrigation.

Other Devices and Strategies

People whose hearing cannot be substantially improved by hearing aids may need to use other devices or strategies to

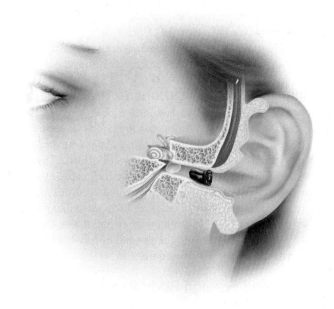

FIGURE 43-14 A hearing aid can be so small that it is inserted inside the ear canal.

overcome the problem. These devices include appliances that light up as well as ring—such as telephones, doorbells, smoke detectors, alarm clocks, and burglar alarms. Patients can purchase amplifiers for the telephone, television, and radio. Many closed-captioned television programs are also available. To benefit from closed captioning, the patient must have a television with a decoder that translates the captioning and displays the captions on the screen.

Cochlear Implants

A person who is profoundly deaf and cannot benefit from using a hearing aid may be a candidate for a **cochlear implant,** an electronic device that stimulates the auditory nerve. A cochlear implant has an external and an internal component. The external portion sits just behind the ear and the internal portion has an array of electrodes implanted directly into the cochlea. Cochlear implants do not amplify sound like a hearing aid but send signals through the auditory nerve to the brain. This gives patients the ability to detect warning signals such as smoke alarms and recognize speech patterns so that they can be better understood. Hearing with a cochlear implant is not the same as normal hearing; patients have to learn to recognize sounds. Adults with cochlear implants often can learn to understand speech without using visual cues such as lip reading. Children can learn to speak with extensive speech therapy. More than 42,000 adults and 28,000 children in the United States have cochlear implants.

PROCEDURE 43-1 Preparing the Ophthalmoscope for Use

Procedure Goal: To ensure that the ophthalmoscope is ready for use during an eye exam

OSHA Guidelines: This procedure does not involve exposure to blood, body fluids, or tissues.

Materials: Ophthalmoscope, lens, spare bulb, spare battery

Method:

1. Wash your hands.
2. Take the ophthalmoscope out of its battery charger. In a darkened room, turn on the ophthalmoscope light.
3. Shine the large beam of white light on the back of your hand to check that the instrument's tiny lightbulb is providing strong enough light.
4. Replace the bulb or battery if necessary. (The battery is located in the ophthalmoscope's handle.)
5. Make sure the instrument's lens is screwed into the handle. If it is not, attach the lens.

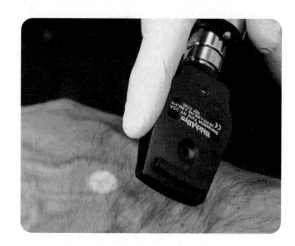

FIGURE Procedure 43-1 Step 3 Shine the ophthalmoscope light on your hand to check the strength of the beam.
©McGraw-Hill Education/Aaron Roeth, photographer

PROCEDURE 43-2 Performing Vision Screening Tests [WORK // DOC]

Procedure Goal: To screen a patient's ability to see distant or close objects, to determine contrast sensitivity, or to detect color blindness

OSHA Guidelines:

Materials: Eye occluder or card to block vision in one eye; alcohol; gauze squares; appropriate vision charts to test for distance vision, near vision, and color blindness; patient chart/progress note

Method:

Distance Vision

1. Wash your hands, clean the occluder with a gauze square dampened in alcohol, identify the patient, introduce yourself, and explain the procedure.
2. Mount one of the following eye charts at eye level: Snellen letter or similar chart (for patients who can read) or Snellen tumbling E, Landolt C, pictorial, or similar chart (for patients who cannot read).

   If using the Snellen letter chart, verify that the patient knows the letters of the alphabet. With children or nonreading adults, use demonstration cards to verify that they can identify the pictures or direction of the letters.
   RATIONALE: *If the patient cannot identify the letters or does not understand the instructions, the results will not be accurate.*

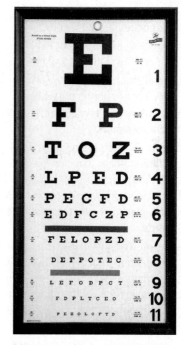

(a)

FIGURE Procedure 43-2 Step 2 (a) The Snellen letter chart is used to test the vision of people who can read.
©McGraw-Hill Education/Rick Brady, Photographer

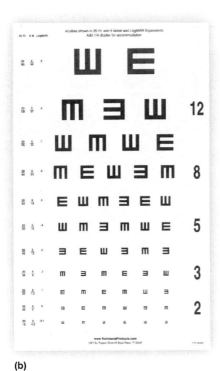

(b)

FIGURE Procedure 43-2 Step 2 (b) The Snellen "tumbling E" chart is used to test the vision of children and nonreading adults.

Reprinted with permission of Richmond Products, Inc.

3. Make a mark on the floor 20 feet away from the chart.

4. Have the patient stand with his or her heels at the 20-foot mark or sit with the back of the chair at the mark.

5. Instruct the patient to keep both eyes open and not to squint or lean forward during the test.
   RATIONALE: *Closing one eye, squinting, or leaning will lead to inaccurate results.*

6. Test both eyes first, then the right eye, and then the left eye. (Different offices may test in a different order. Follow your office policy.)
   RATIONALE: *Following a specific testing order based on office policy leads to consistency in the results of all medical records.*

7. Have the patient read the lines on the chart (or identify the picture/direction), beginning with the 20-foot line. If the patient cannot read this line, begin with the smallest line the patient can read. (Some offices use a pointer to select one symbol at a time in random order to prevent patients from memorizing the order.)

8. Note the smallest line the patient can read or identify with no more than two errors. (Some offices only allow one error per line. Follow office policy when performing this test.)

9. Record the results as a fraction (for example, Both Eyes 20/40 −1 if the patient misses one letter on a line or Both Eyes 20/40 −2 if the patient misses two letters on a line).

10. Show the patient how to cover the left eye with the occluder or card. Again, instruct the patient to keep both eyes open and not to squint or lean forward during the test.

11. Have the patient read the lines on the chart.

12. Record the results of the right eye (for example, Right Eye 20/30).

13. Have the patient cover the right eye and read the lines on the chart.

14. Record the results of the left eye (for example, Left Eye 20/20).

15. If the patient wears corrective lenses, record the results using $\overline{cc}$ (if your office uses this abbreviation for "with correction") in front of the abbreviation (for example, $\overline{cc}$ Both Eyes 20/20).
    RATIONALE: *For charting accuracy, vision correction must be noted using your office format.*

16. Note and record any observations of squinting, head tilting, excessive blinking, or tearing.

17. Ask the patient to keep both eyes open and to identify the color of the two colored bars on the Snellen chart, and record the results in the patient's chart.
    RATIONALE: *This step is sometimes done as a basic color vision screening.*

18. Clean the occluder with a gauze square dampened with alcohol.

19. Properly dispose of the gauze square and wash your hands.
    RATIONALE: *Maintain principles of aseptic technique at all times.*

Near Vision

20. Wash your hands, identify the patient, introduce yourself, and explain the procedure.

21. Have the patient hold one of the following at normal reading distance (approximately 14 to 16 inches): Jaeger, Richmond pocket, or similar chart or card.

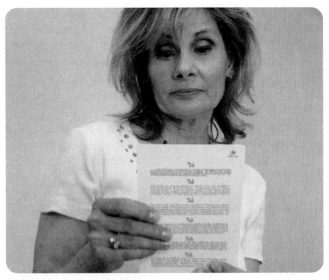

(a)

FIGURE Procedure 43-2 Step 21 (a) Have the patient hold the card at a comfortable reading distance.

©McGraw-Hill Education.

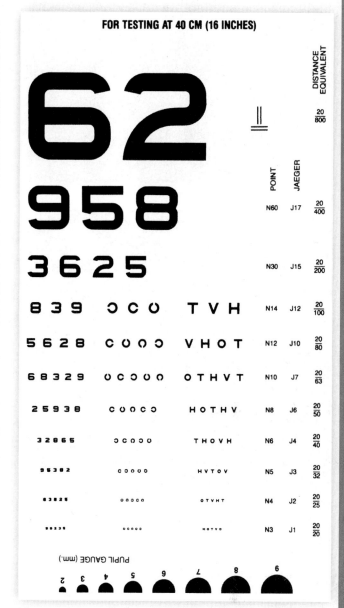

FOR TESTING AT 40 CM (16 INCHES)

		DISTANCE EQUIVALENT
		20/800
POINT	JAEGER	
N60	J17	20/400
N30	J15	20/200
N14	J12	20/100
N12	J10	20/80
N10	J7	20/63
N8	J6	20/50
N6	J4	20/40
N5	J3	20/32
N4	J2	20/25
N3	J1	20/20

PUPIL GAUGE (mm.)

(c)

FIGURE Procedure 43-2 Step 21   (c) The Richmond pocket vision screener also is used to test near vision.

V = .50 D.

The fourteenth of August was the day fixed upon for the sailing of the brig Pilgrim, on her voyage from Boston round Cape Horn, to the western coast of North America. As she was to get under way early in the afternoon, I made my appearance on board at twelve o'clock in full sea-rig, and with my chest, containing an outfit for a two or three years' voyage,

which I had undertaken from a determination to cure, if possible, by an entire change of life, and by a long absence from books and study, a weakness of the eyes which had obliged me to give up my pursuits, and which no medical aid seemed likely to cure. The change from the tight dress coat, silk cap and kid gloves of an undergraduate at Cambridge, to the

V = .75 D.

loose duck trousers, checked shirt and tarpaulin hat of a sailor, though somewhat of a transformation, was soon made, and I supposed that I should pass very well for a Jack tar. But it is impossible to deceive the practiced eye in these matters; and while I supposed myself to be looking as salt as Neptune himself, I was, no doubt, known for a landsman by every one on board, as soon as I hove in sight. A sailor has a peculiar cut to his clothes, and a way of wear-

V = 1.   D.

ing them which a green hand can never get. The trousers, tight around the hips, and thence hanging long and loose around the feet, a superabundance of checked shirt, a low-crowned, well-varnished black hat, worn on the back of the head, with half a fathom of black ribbon hanging over the left eye, and a peculiar tie to the black silk neckerchief, with sundry other *details*, are signs the want of which betray the beginner at once.

V = 1.25 D.

Beside the points in my dress which were out of the way, doubtless my complexion and hands would distinguish me from the regular *salt*, who, with a sun-browned cheek, wide step and rolling gait, swings his bronzed and toughened hands athwartships half open, as though just to ready to grasp a rope. "With all my imperfections

V = 1.50 D.

on my head," I joined the crew, and we hauled out into the stream and came to anchor for the night. The next day we were employed in preparation for sea, reeving and studding-sail gear, crossing royal yards, putting on chafing gear, and taking on board our powder. On the

V = 1.75 D.

following night I stood my first watch. I remained awake nearly all the first part of the night, from fear that I might not hear when I was called; and when I went on deck, so great were my ideas of the importance of my trust, that I

V = 2.   D.

walked regularly fore and aft the whole length of the vessel, looking out over the bows and taffrail at each turn, and was not a little surprised at the unconcerned manner in which the billows turned up their

Your glasses are of value to you only as they accurately interpret your prescription and this only as they are fitted and serviced in accordance with these needs. They are a therapeutic device.

(b)

FIGURE Procedure 43-2 Step 21   (b) This near vision chart is used to test the ability to see objects at a normal reading distance.

---

22. Ask the patient to keep both eyes open and to read or identify the letters, symbols, or paragraphs.
    RATIONALE: *If both eyes are not open, results may not be accurate.*

23. Record the smallest line read without error.

24. If the card is laminated, clean it with a gauze square dampened with alcohol.

25. Properly dispose of the gauze square and wash your hands.
    RATIONALE: *Maintain principles of aseptic technique at all times.*

Color Vision

26. Wash your hands, identify the patient, introduce yourself, and explain the procedure.

27. Hold one of the following color charts or books at the patient's normal reading distance (approximately 14 to 16 inches): Ishihara, Richmond pseudoisochromatic, or similar color-testing system.

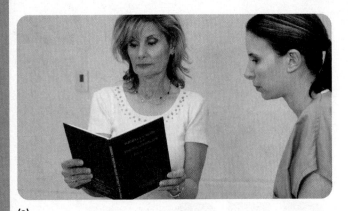

(a)

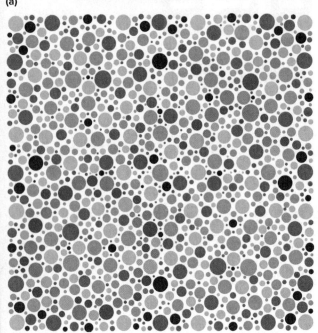

(b)

FIGURE Procedure 43-2 Step 27 (a) Have the patient hold the chart at a comfortable reading distance. (b) The Richmond pseudoisochromatic color chart is used to test a person's ability to see colors.

©McGraw-Hill Education

28. Ask the patient to tell you the number or symbol within the colored dots on each chart or page.

29. Proceed through all the charts or pages, usually totaling 24.

30. Record the number correctly identified and failed with a slash between them (for example, 23 passed/1 failed).

31. If the charts are laminated, clean them with a gauze square dampened with alcohol.

32. Properly dispose of the gauze square and wash your hands.
    RATIONALE: *Maintain principles of aseptic technique at all times.*

33. Document the results after you have completed the procedure (refer to Progress Note).

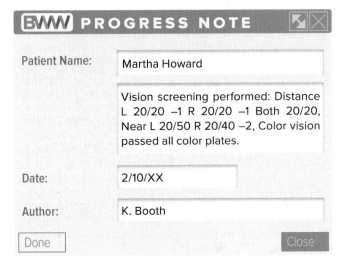

BWW PROGRESS NOTE

Patient Name:	Martha Howard
	Vision screening performed: Distance L 20/20 −1 R 20/20 −1 Both 20/20, Near L 20/50 R 20/40 −2, Color vision passed all color plates.
Date:	2/10/XX
Author:	K. Booth

Done   Close

PROCEDURE **43-3** Administering Eye Medications   `WORK // DOC`

Procedure Goal: To instill (introduce) medication into the eye for treatment of certain eye disorders

OSHA Guidelines:

Materials: Medication (drops, cream, or ointment), tissues, eye patch (if applicable), progress note/patient chart

Method:

1. Identify the patient, introduce yourself, and explain the procedure.

2. Review the licensed practitioner's medication order. This should include the patient's name, drug name, concentration, number of drops (if a liquid), into which eye(s) the medication is to be administered, and the frequency of administration.
   RATIONALE: *The licensed practitioner's order must be followed exactly.*

3. Compare the drug with the medication order three times and complete a check of the rights of medication administration, including the right patient, medication, doses, route, time, and documentation.
   RATIONALE: *To ensure necessary accuracy.*

4. Ask whether the patient has any known allergies to substances contained in the medication.

5. Wash your hands and put on gloves.

6. Assemble the supplies.

7. Ask the patient to lie down or to sit back in a chair with the head tilted back.

8. Give the patient a tissue to blot excess medication as needed.

9. Remove an eye patch, if present.

10. Instruct the patient to look at the ceiling and to keep both eyes open during the procedure.

11. With a tissue, gently pull the lower eyelid down by pressing downward on the patient's cheekbone just below the eyelid with your nondominant hand. This pressure will open a pocket of space between the eyelid and the eye.

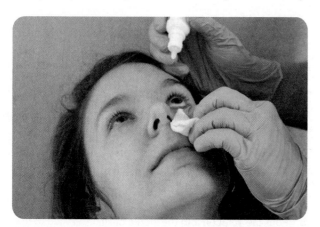

FIGURE Procedure 43-3 Step 11 Use a tissue to press down on the patient's cheekbone just below the eyelid, opening up a pocket of space between the eyelid and the eye.
©McGraw-Hill Education/Pam Buckwalter, photographer

Eyedrops

12. Resting your dominant hand on the patient's forehead, hold the filled eyedropper or bottle approximately ½ inch from the conjunctiva.
RATIONALE: *Touching the patient's skin with the dropper or bottle tip will cause contamination.*

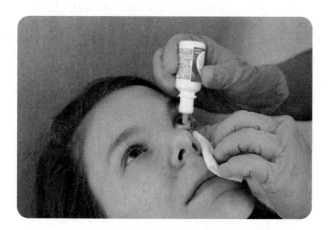

FIGURE Procedure 43-3 Step 12 The medication container should be approximately ½ inch from the conjunctiva as you prepare to instill drops into the patient's eye.
©McGraw-Hill Education/Pam Buckwalter, photographer

13. Drop the prescribed number of drops into the pocket. If any drops land outside the eye, repeat instilling the drops that missed the eye.

Creams or Ointments

14. Rest your dominant hand on the patient's forehead and hold the tube or applicator above the conjunctiva.

15. Without touching the eyelid or conjunctiva with the applicator, evenly apply a thin ribbon of cream or ointment along the inside edge of the lower eyelid on the conjunctiva, working from the medial (inner) to the lateral (outer) side.
RATIONALE: *Touching the patient's skin with the applicator will cause contamination.*

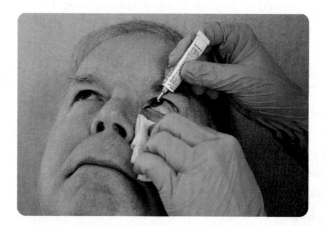

FIGURE Procedure 43-3 Step 15 Apply a thin ribbon of cream or ointment along the inside of the lower eyelid on the conjunctiva.
©McGraw-Hill Education/Pam Buckwalter, photographer

All Medications

16. Release the lower lid and instruct the patient to gently close the eyes.

17. Repeat the procedure for the other eye as necessary.

18. Remove any excess medication by wiping each eyelid gently with a fresh tissue from the medial to the lateral side.

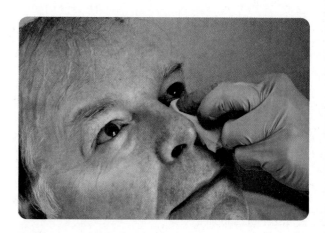

FIGURE Procedure 43-3 Step 18 Use a tissue to remove excess medication from the eyelid.
©McGraw-Hill Education/Pam Buckwalter, photographer

19. Apply a clean eye patch to cover the entire eye, if ordered.

20. Ask whether the patient felt any discomfort and observe for any adverse reactions. Notify the licensed practitioner as necessary.

21. Instruct the patient on self-administration of medication and patch application, if ordered.

22. Ask the patient to repeat the instructions.

23. Provide written instructions.

24. Properly dispose of used disposable materials.

25. Remove gloves and wash your hands.

26. Document administration in the patient's chart. Include the drug, the concentration, the number of drops or amount, the time of administration, and the eye(s) that received the medication (refer to Progress Note).

BWW PROGRESS NOTE

Patient Name:	Ken Carter
	Instilled Latanoprost 0.005% ophthalmic solution 1 drop both eyes at 4:30 pm.
Date:	10/01/XX
Author:	K. White

Done   Close

PROCEDURE 43-4 Performing Eye Irrigation

WORK // DOC

Procedure Goal: To flush the eye to remove foreign particles or relieve eye irritation

OSHA Guidelines:

Materials: Patient chart/progress note, sterile irrigating solution, sterile basin, sterile irrigating syringe and kidney-shaped basin, tissues

Method:

1. Identify the patient, introduce yourself, and explain the procedure.

2. Review the licensed practitioner's order. This should include the patient's name, the irrigating solution, the volume of solution, and for which eye the irrigation is to be performed.

3. Compare the solution with the instructions three times and complete a check of the rights of medication administration, including the right patient, medication, doses, route, time, and documentation.
   RATIONALE: *To ensure necessary accuracy.*

4. Wash your hands and put on gloves, a gown, and a face shield.
   RATIONALE: *Splashing is possible when a syringe is used.*

5. Assemble supplies.

6. Ask the patient to lie down or to sit with the head tilted back and to the side that is being irrigated. The solution should not spill over into the other eye.

RATIONALE: *Cross-contamination between the eyes must be avoided.*

7. Place a towel or a disposable waterproof underpad over the patient's shoulder. Have the patient hold the kidney-shaped basin at the side of the head next to the eye to be irrigated.

8. Pour the solution into the sterile basin.

9. Fill the irrigating syringe with solution (approximately 50 mL).

10. Hold a tissue on the patient's cheekbone below the lower eyelid with your nondominant hand and press downward to expose the eye socket.

11. Holding the tip of the syringe ½ inch away from the eye, direct the solution onto the lower conjunctiva from the inner to the outer aspect of the eye. (Avoid directing the solution against the cornea because it is sensitive; do not use excessive force.)
    RATIONALE: *To avoid contamination, do not let the tip touch the eye or skin. Excessive force could damage the cornea.*

12. Refill the syringe and continue irrigation until the prescribed volume of solution is used.

13. Dry the area around the eye with tissues or gauze squares.

14. Properly dispose of used disposable materials.

15. Remove your gloves, gown, and face shield and wash your hands.

16. Record the following in the patient's chart: procedure, type of solution, amount of solution used, time of administration, and eye(s) irrigated.

17. Put on gloves and clean the equipment and room according to OSHA guidelines.

Procedure Goal: To determine how well a patient hears

OSHA Guidelines:

Materials: Patient chart/progress note, audiometer, headset, graph pad (if applicable), alcohol, gauze squares

Method:

Infants and Toddlers

1. Identify the patient and introduce yourself.
2. Wash your hands.
3. Pick a quiet location.
4. The patient can be sitting, lying down, or held by the parent.
5. Instruct the parent to be silent during the procedure.
6. Position yourself so that your hands are behind the child's right ear and out of sight.
   RATIONALE: *You want the child to respond to sound, not to sight.*
7. Clap your hands loudly. Observe the child's response. (Never clap directly in front of the ear because this can damage the eardrum. As an alternative to clapping, use devices such as rattles or clickers (which may be available in the office) to generate sounds of varying loudness.)
8. Record the child's response as positive or negative for loud noise.
9. Position one hand behind the child's right ear, as before.
10. Snap your fingers. Observe the child's response.
11. Record the response as positive or negative for moderate noise.
12. Repeat steps 6 through 11 for the left ear.
13. Document the information (refer to Progress Note).

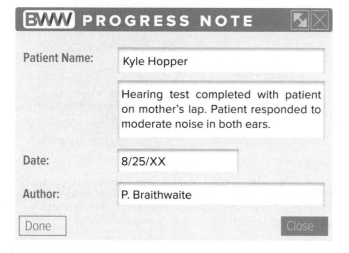

BWW PROGRESS NOTE

Patient Name:	Kyle Hopper
	Hearing test completed with patient on mother's lap. Patient responded to moderate noise in both ears.
Date:	8/25/XX
Author:	P. Braithwaite

Done   Close

Adults and Children

1. Wash your hands, identify the patient, introduce yourself, and explain the procedure.
2. Clean the earpieces of the headset with a sanitizing wipe according to the manufacturer's instructions.
   RATIONALE: *Maintain aseptic technique at all times.*
3. Have the patient sit with his back to you.
   RATIONALE: *To prevent the patient from using visual clues to pass the hearing test.*
4. Assist the patient in putting on the headset and adjust it until it is comfortable.
5. Tell the patient he will hear tones in the right ear.
6. Tell the patient to raise his finger or press the indicator button when he hears a tone.
7. Set the audiometer for the right ear.
8. Set the audiometer for the lowest range of frequencies and the first degree of loudness (usually 15 decibels). (When using automated audiometers, follow the instructions printed in the user's manual.)
9. Press the tone button or switch and observe the patient.
10. If the patient does not hear the first degree of loudness, raise it two or three times to greater degrees, up to 50 or 60 decibels.
11. If the patient indicates that he has heard the tone, record the setting on the graph.
12. Change the setting to the next frequency. Repeat steps 9, 10, and 11.
13. Proceed to the midrange frequencies. Repeat steps 9, 10, and 11.
14. Proceed to the high-range frequencies. Repeat steps 9, 10, and 11.
15. Set the audiometer for the left ear.
16. Tell the patient that he will hear tones in the left ear and ask him to raise his finger or press the indicator button when he hears a tone.
17. Repeat steps 8 through 14.
18. Have the patient remove the headset.
19. Clean the earpieces with a sanitizing wipe.

20. Properly dispose of the used sanitizing wipe and wash your hands.

RATIONALE: *Maintain aseptic technique at all times.*

21. Document the following information after you have completed the procedure (refer to Progress Note).

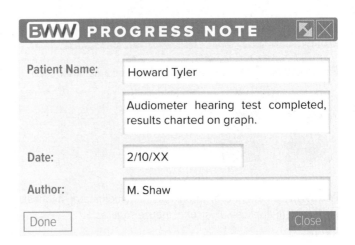

BWW PROGRESS NOTE

Patient Name:	Howard Tyler
	Audiometer hearing test completed, results charted on graph.
Date:	2/10/XX
Author:	M. Shaw

Done   Close

PROCEDURE 43-6 Administering Eardrops

WORK // DOC

Procedure Goal: To instill medication into the ear to treat certain ear disorders

OSHA Guidelines:

Materials: Patient chart/progress note, liquid medication, cotton balls

Method:

1. Identify the patient, introduce yourself, and explain the procedure.

2. Check the licensed practitioner's medication order. It should include the patient's name, drug name, concentration, number of drops, into which ear(s) the medication is to be administered, and frequency of administration.

3. Compare the drug with the instructions three times and complete a check of the rights of medication administration, including the right patient, medication, doses, route, time, and documentation.

   RATIONALE: *To ensure necessary accuracy.*

4. Ask whether the patient has any allergies to ear medications.

5. Wash your hands and put on gloves.

6. Assemble supplies.

7. Warm the medication with your hands or by placing the bottle in a pan of warm water.

   RATIONALE: *Internal ear structures are very sensitive to extreme heat or cold. Administering cold medications can result in severe vertigo (dizziness) or nausea.*

8. Have the patient lie on his or her side with the ear to be treated facing up.

9. Straighten the ear canal by pulling the auricle upward and outward for adults, down and back for infants and children.

   RATIONALE: *Straightening the ear canal ensures that the medication reaches its destination.*

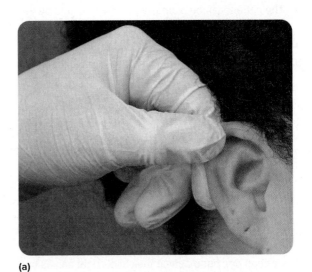

(a)

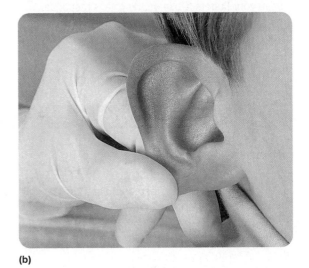

(b)

FIGURE Procedure 43-6 Step 9   (a) Straighten an adult's ear canal by pulling the auricle upward and outward. (b) Straighten an infant's or child's ear canal by pulling the auricle downward and back.

(a) ©McGraw-Hill Education/Aaron Roeth, photographer; (b) ©Terry Wild Studio

10. Hold the dropper ½ inch above the ear canal.
RATIONALE: *The dropper must not be contaminated by touching the patient's skin or any other surface.*

11. Gently squeeze the bottle or dropper bulb to administer the correct number of drops.

12. Have the patient remain in this position for 10 minutes.

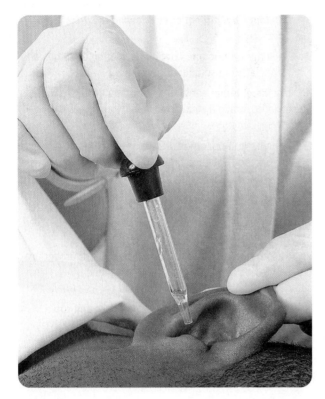

FIGURE Procedure 43-6 Step 11   Apply slow, gentle pressure to the dropper bulb so that you can count the drops and administer the prescribed number.
©Terry Wild Studio

13. If ordered, loosely place a small wad of cotton in the outermost part of the ear canal.

14. Note any adverse reaction, notifying the licensed practitioner as necessary.

15. Repeat the procedure for the other ear, if ordered.

16. Instruct the patient on how to administer the drops at home.

17. Ask the patient to repeat the instructions.
RATIONALE: *For maximum effectiveness, it is important that the patient understand how to correctly continue treatment at home.*

18. Provide written instructions.

19. Remove the cotton after 15 minutes.

20. Properly dispose of used disposable materials.

21. Remove gloves and wash your hands.

22. Record in the patient's chart the medication, the concentration, the number of drops, the time of administration, and which ear(s) received the medication (refer to Progress Note).

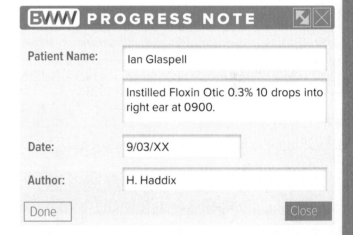

BWW PROGRESS NOTE

Patient Name:	Ian Glaspell
	Instilled Floxin Otic 0.3% 10 drops into right ear at 0900.
Date:	9/03/XX
Author:	H. Haddix

Done   Close

PROCEDURE 43-7 Performing Ear Irrigation   WORK // DOC

Procedure Goal: To wash out the ear canal to remove impacted cerumen or remove a foreign body

OSHA Guidelines:

Materials: Patient chart/progress note, fresh irrigating solution, clean basin, clean irrigating syringe, towel or absorbent pad, kidney-shaped basin, cotton balls

Method:

1. Identify the patient, introduce yourself, and explain the procedure.

2. Check the licensed practitioner's order. It should include the patient's name, the irrigating solution, the volume of solution, and for which ear(s) the irrigation is to be performed. If the practitioner has not specified the volume of solution, use only the amount needed to remove the wax or foreign body.

3. Compare the solution with the instructions three times and complete a check of the rights of medication administration, including the right patient, medication, doses, route, time, and documentation.
RATIONALE: *To ensure necessary accuracy.*

4. Wash your hands and put on gloves, a gown, and a face shield.
RATIONALE: *Splashing is possible when a syringe is used.*

5. Look into the patient's ear to identify cerumen or a foreign body needing to be removed. You will know you have completed the irrigation when the cerumen or foreign body is removed.
RATIONALE: *Identifying the cerumen or foreign body visually will help you assess when you have successfully completed the irrigation.*

6. Assemble the supplies.

7. If the solution is cold, warm it to body temperature by placing the bottle in a pan of warm water.
RATIONALE: *Internal ear structures are very sensitive to extreme heat or cold. Administering cold liquids can result in severe vertigo or nausea.*

8. Have the patient sit or lie on his or her back with the ear to be treated facing you.

9. Place a towel or disposable waterproof underpad over the patient's shoulder (or under the head and over the shoulder if the patient is lying down) and have the patient hold the kidney-shaped basin under the ear.

10. Pour the solution into the other basin.

11. If necessary, gently clean the external ear with cotton moistened with the solution.

12. Fill the irrigating syringe with solution (approximately 50 mL).

13. Straighten the ear canal by pulling the auricle upward and outward for adults or downward and back for infants and children.

RATIONALE: *Straightening the ear canal allows the solution to reach its destination.*

14. Holding the tip of the syringe ½ inch from the opening of the ear and tilted toward the top of the ear canal, slowly instill the solution into the ear. Allow the fluid to drain out during the process.
RATIONALE: *Do not contaminate the syringe by allowing it to touch the patient or by allowing the draining fluid to touch it.*

15. Refill the syringe and continue irrigation until the canal is cleaned or the solution is used up.

16. Dry the external ear with a cotton ball and, if ordered, leave a clean cotton ball loosely in place for 5–10 minutes.

17. If the patient becomes dizzy or nauseated, allow him or her time to regain balance before standing up. Assist the patient as needed.

18. Properly dispose of used disposable materials.

19. Remove your gloves, gown, and face shield and wash your hands.

20. Record the following in the patient's chart: procedure and result, amount of solution used, time of administration, and ear(s) irrigated.

21. Put on gloves and clean the equipment and room according to OSHA guidelines.

SUMMARY OF LEARNING OUTCOMES

OUTCOME	KEY POINTS
43.1 Describe the medical assistant's role in eye exams and procedures performed in a medical office.	The medical assistant may assist or perform some of the procedures that involve measuring various aspects and functions of the eye, such as visual acuity, color vision, and intraocular pressure.
43.2 Discuss various eye disorders encountered in a medical office.	Disorders of the eye include those of the external eye structures, such as blepharitis, ptosis, and sty; disorders of the anterior eye structures, such as conjunctivitis and corneal abrasions; disorders involving internal eye structures, such as cataracts, glaucoma, iritis, and retinal disorders; and refractive disorders, such as myopia, hyperopia, astigmatism, and presbyopia.
43.3 Identify ophthalmic exams performed in the licensed practitioner's office.	Ophthalmic exams performed in the licensed practitioner's office include inspecting internal eye structures; testing visual fields; glaucoma testing; inspecting external eye structures; and refraction exams.
43.4 Summarize ophthalmologic procedures and treatments.	Ophthalmologic procedures and treatments include administering eye medications such as eyedrops and ointments and performing eye irrigation.
43.5 Describe the medical assistant's role in otology.	Medical assistants in an otology office may assist with or perform auditory screening, administer ear medications, perform ear irrigations, and help with diagnostic tests such as tympanometry.

OUTCOME	KEY POINTS
43.6 Describe disorders of the ear encountered in the medical office.	Ear diseases and disorders include those of the outer ear, such as cerumen impaction, otitis externa, and pruritus; middle ear disorders, such as otitis media, mastoiditis, otosclerosis, and ruptured eardrum; and those of the inner ear, such as labyrinthitis, Ménière's disease, presbycusis, tinnitus, and hearing loss.
43.7 Recall various hearing and other diagnostic ear tests.	Hearing and other diagnostic ear tests include audiometry and tympanometry.
43.8 Summarize ear procedures and treatments.	Ear treatments and procedures include administration of ear medications, ear irrigation, microscope-aided earwax or foreign body removal, hearing aid fitting, and cochlear implants.

CASE STUDY CRITICAL THINKING

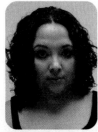

©McGraw-Hill Education

Recall Valarie from the case study at the beginning of the chapter. Now that you have completed the chapter, answer the following questions regarding her case.

1. What is the medical assistant's role during the eye irrigation?

2. What are some of the reasons a licensed practitioner might order an eye irrigation procedure?

EXAM PREPARATION QUESTIONS

1. (LO 43.2) Which of the following is the common name for an inflammation of the conjunctiva?
   a. Pruritus
   b. Pinkeye
   c. Blepharitis
   d. Iritis
   e. Hordeolum

2. (LO 43.2) Drooping of the upper eyelid is known as
   a. Astigmatism
   b. Sty
   c. Ptosis
   d. Amblyopia
   e. Conjunctivitis

3. (LO 43.5) An otologist treats which of the following disorders?
   a. Glaucoma
   b. Refractive disorders
   c. Mastoiditis
   d. Cataracts
   e. Strabismus

4. (LO 43.6) Ringing in the ears is known as
   a. Presbycusis
   b. Tinnitus
   c. Ménière's disease
   d. Labyrinthitis
   e. Otitis media

5. (LO 43.2) The buildup of which fluid causes glaucoma?
   a. Aqueous humor
   b. Lacrimal fluid
   c. Vitreous humor
   d. Cerumen
   e. Perilymph

6. (LO 43.2) Which of the following is *not* a visual disturbance?
   a. Presbyopia
   b. Astigmatism
   c. Refractive error
   d. Presbycusis
   e. Hyperopia

7. (LO 43.3) Which of the following would be determined by a refraction exam?
   a. Astigmatism
   b. Blepharitis
   c. Corneal ulcers
   d. Diabetic retinopathy
   e. Strabismus

8. (LO 43.6) Which of the following would improve communication with a hearing-impaired patient?
   a. Speak very loudly.
   b. Speak in clear, low-pitched tones.
   c. Speak directly into the patient's ear.
   d. Overemphasize your lip movements so that the patient can read your lips.
   e. Write everything down for the patient to read.

9. (LO 43.7) The units for measuring the relative intensity of sounds on a scale from 0 to 130 are
   a. Frequencies
   b. Waves
   c. Audiometers
   d. Periods
   e. Decibels

10. (LO 43.6) Sensorineural hearing loss is caused by
   a. Damage to the inner ear
   b. Impacted cerumen
   c. Otitis media
   d. Tinnitus
   e. Otosclerosis

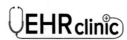

Go to CONNECT to complete the EHRclinic exercises: 43.01 Record Vision Test (Snellen) Results and 43.02 Document Results of an Auditory Acuity Test.

SOFT SKILLS SUCCESS

You are assigned to assist with an audiogram on a patient. You have not yet used the new machine that the office just purchased for the audiogram. When you enter the room to introduce yourself to the patient, he looks at you blankly and does not appear to understand.

   1. How should you proceed with the new equipment?
   2. How should you interact with the patient?

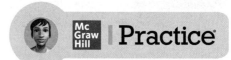

Go to PRACTICE MEDICAL OFFICE and complete the modules Clinical: Work Task Proficiencies and Clinical: Interactions.

Assisting with Minor Surgery

CASE STUDY

PATIENT INFORMATION		
Patient Name	**DOB**	**Allergies**
Peter Smith	03/28/1946	NKA
Attending	**MRN**	**Other Information**
Paul F. Buckwalter, MD	00-AA-003	Started swimming last week

Peter Smith, a patient with a history of mild depression, arrives at the clinic holding a bloody towel over his left forearm. He is taken immediately back to the treatment area. He states that he cut himself with a large knife while cutting a pineapple. You take his vital signs while waiting for the physician. You notice the blood is leaking through the towel. You need to control the bleeding.

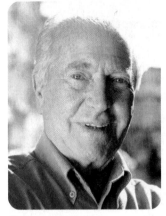
©Image Source/Getty Images

You put on PPE, most importantly gloves, and apply a large dressing over the area, holding firm pressure. The physician arrives, examines the patient, and determines that the patient will need sutures. While you are preparing Peter Smith for his wound repair procedure, he tells you that he recently started swimming for exercise and is going to the Bahamas for a snorkeling trip in 2 weeks. He wants to know if this will ruin his trip.

Keep Peter Smith in mind as you study this chapter. There will be questions at the end of the chapter based on the case study. The information in the chapter will help you answer these questions.

LEARNING OUTCOMES

After completing Chapter 44, you will be able to:

44.1 Define the medical assistant's role in minor surgical procedures.

44.2 Describe surgical procedures performed in an office setting.

44.3 Identify the instruments used in minor surgery and describe their functions.

44.4 Describe the procedures for medical and sterile asepsis in minor surgery.

44.5 Summarize the medical assistant's duties in preoperative procedures.

44.6 Describe the medical assistant's intraoperative duties.

44.7 Implement the medical assistant's duties in the postoperative period.

KEY TERMS

abscess	ligature
anesthesia	maturation phase
anesthetic	medical asepsis
approximate	needle biopsy
cryosurgery	postoperative
debridement	preoperative
electrocauterization	proliferation phase
formalin	puncture wound
incision	sterile field
inflammatory phase	surgical asepsis
intraoperative	suture
laceration	swaged needle

CAAHEP

I.P.8 Instruct and prepare a patient for a procedure or a treatment

I.P.9 Assist provider with a patient exam

III.C.3 Define the following as practiced within an ambulatory care setting:
(a) medical asepsis
(b) surgical asepsis

III.P.2 Select appropriate barrier/personal protective equipment (PPE)

III.P.3 Perform handwashing

III.P.6 Prepare a sterile field

III.P.7 Perform within a sterile field

III.P.8 Perform wound care

III.P.9 Perform dressing change

III.P.10 Demonstrate proper disposal of biohazardous material
(a) sharps
(b) regulated wastes

V.P.4 Coach patients regarding:
(b) health maintenance
(c) disease prevention
(d) treatment plan

X.P.3 Document patient care accurately in the medical record

ABHES

2. Anatomy and Physiology
c. Identify diagnostic and treatment modalities as they relate to each body system

8. Clinical Procedures
a. Practice standard precautions and perform disinfection/sterilization techniques
e. Perform specialty procedures including but not limited to minor surgery, cardiac, respiratory, OB-GYN, neurological, and gastroenterology

9. Medical Laboratory Procedures
c. Dispose of biohazardous materials

▶ Introduction

Minor surgical procedures are frequently performed in ambulatory care settings and office practices. Assisting with minor surgery requires a variety of duties and skills. As a medical assistant, you must be knowledgeable of the types of procedures performed where you are employed. You need to know how to prepare the patient for surgery, assist the practitioner during surgery, and care for the patient after surgery. Because all types of surgery require surgical asepsis, a working knowledge of this technique is mandatory.

▶ The Medical Assistant's Role in Minor Surgery   LO 44.1

Medical assistants play an important role in all aspects of minor surgical procedures. You will perform administrative tasks prior to the patient's surgery, including completing forms for insurance and obtaining signed informed consent from the patient. You will explain basic aspects of the surgical procedure and answer the patient's questions. Informing the doctor of all current prescription and over-the-counter (OTC) medications that the patient is currently taking is also an administrative task. Finally, you will make sure the patient knows how to follow the appropriate presurgical instructions.

In addition to presurgical administrative tasks, you also will perform many tasks directly related to the surgical procedure. You will make sure the surgical room is clean, neat, and properly lit. You will see that all the equipment, instruments, and supplies the doctor will use are clean, disinfected or sterilized, and properly arranged. You also may function as an unsterile assistant, ensuring the safety and comfort of the patient during the procedure and performing other duties. At other times, you may directly assist with the surgical procedure in a sterile capacity.

Following the surgical procedure, you will help dress the wound and perform other postoperative patient care, making sure the patient is not experiencing ill effects from the surgery or local anesthetic. You will educate the patient about wound care and proper procedures to follow after surgery and make sure the patient has safe transportation home. You also will clean the room and prepare it for the next patient.

▶ Surgery in the Physician's Office   LO 44.2

Minor surgical procedures are those that can be safely performed in the physician's office or clinic without general anesthesia. **Anesthesia** is a loss of sensation, particularly the feeling of pain. An **anesthetic** is a medication that causes anesthesia. A general anesthetic affects the entire body, whereas a local anesthetic affects only a particular area. Minor surgical procedures typically involve the use of a local anesthetic in the form of an injection or a cream applied to the skin.

Minor surgery is performed for many reasons, whether it be to diagnose an illness or repair an injury. Other procedures may be elective, or optional. Removal of a wart, skin tag (a small outgrowth of skin, occurring frequently on the neck as people get older), or other small growth for cosmetic reasons is an elective procedure. Some of the common minor surgical procedures you may assist the doctor with include the following:

- Repair of a laceration.
- Irrigation and cleaning of a puncture wound.
- Wound debridement.
- Removal of foreign bodies.
- Removal of small growths.
- Removal of a nail or part of a nail.
- Drainage of an abscess.
- Collection of a biopsy specimen.
- Cryosurgery.
- Laser surgery.
- Electrocauterization.

Common Surgical Procedures

Many surgical procedures are routinely performed in a doctor's office. You may perform some of these procedures on your own. For example, you may change dressings for surgical wounds, and under a doctor's orders, you may remove sutures (commonly called stitches) or staples after wounds have healed. Any procedure that requires an **incision** (a surgical wound made by cutting into body tissue) must be performed by a doctor.

Draining an Abscess An **abscess** is a collection of pus (white blood cells [WBCs], bacteria, and dead skin cells) that forms as a result of infection. A protective lining can form around an abscess and prevent it from healing. In such a case, the physician may make an incision in the lining of the abscess. This procedure is known as an incision and drainage (I&D). The physician may allow the abscess to drain on its own or insert a drainage tube.

Obtaining a Biopsy Specimen A biopsy specimen is a small amount of tissue removed from the body for examination under a microscope. Most biopsies involve cutting the tissue. For a **needle biopsy,** the doctor uses a needle and syringe to aspirate (withdraw by suction) fluid or tissue cells. (The procedure in the *Assisting in Other Medical Specialties* chapter describes how to assist with a needle biopsy.) All specimens must be placed in a preservative, most commonly a 10% **formalin** solution (a dilute solution of formaldehyde), to prevent changes in the tissue.

Mole Removal A mole, also called a *nevus,* is a small, discolored area of the skin. It may be raised or flat. Any mole that changes shape, size, or color should be evaluated for possible removal. Moles are typically removed by excision or by slicing flush with the skin. If the mole is excised, sutures are usually necessary. Moles that are removed by slicing flush with the skin do not require sutures but may need to be cauterized.

Caring for Wounds A wound is any break in the skin. The break may be accidental or intentional, as from a surgical procedure. There are several types of accidental wounds. A **laceration** is a jagged, open wound in the skin that can extend down into the underlying tissue. The jagged edges may have to be cut away before the wound is closed. A **puncture wound** is a deep wound caused by a sharp object. (See the *Emergency Preparedness* chapter for further information on types and care of accidental wounds.) Both surgical and accidental wounds require special care to prevent infection. Proper wound care that promotes healing without infection is discussed in the *Caution: Handle with Care* feature.

Cleaning a Wound The first step in preventing a nonsurgical wound from becoming infected is careful cleansing. First, clean around the wound with soap and water. Then, it must be irrigated with sterile saline solution or sterile water, applied with a syringe and needle.

Debridement is the removal of debris or dead tissue from a wound. This special type of cleaning may be required for a wound that has dead or sloughing tissue. This procedure helps to expose healthy tissue and promote healing. The doctor may use one of a number of wound debridement methods:

- Surgical—cutting away tissue with scalpel and scissors.
- Chemical—using special compounds to dissolve tissue.
- Mechanical—applying a dressing that sticks to the wound, removing dead tissue when the dressing is removed, or irrigating the wound with sterile saline.
- Autolytic—applying a dressing that helps the body's natural fluids dissolve dead tissue.

Wound Healing It is important to know how a wound heals so that you can care for it properly. A wound heals in three phases: inflammatory phase, proliferation phase, and maturation phase. The time it takes for a wound to heal depends on several factors, including the patient's age, nutritional status, and overall health. During the initial phase, or **inflammatory phase,** bleeding is reduced as blood vessels in the affected area constrict. Platelets, clotting factors, and WBCs play an important role in this phase. They seal the wound, clot the blood that has seeped into the area, and remove bacteria and debris from the wound. The wound contracts under the clot or scab that forms.

During the second phase, or **proliferation phase,** new tissue forms. Skin cells at the edges of the wound begin to move together to close off the wound. The scab that often forms over a wound actually slows down this movement of skin cells. The edges of the wound eventually come together and form a continuous layer, closing off the wound.

The proliferation phase speeds up if the edges of an incision or a nonsurgical wound are **approximated,** or brought

Conditions That Interfere with Fast, Effective Wound Healing

The goals for treating both surgical and nonsurgical wounds are similar: to heal the wound without infection and to preserve normal skin function and appearance. Nonsurgical wounds often involve conditions that do not promote fast, effective healing. In these cases, the wounds require special attention to ensure good results.

Many types of nonsurgical wounds contain foreign material that can lead to infection. For example, a child may have a deep laceration from landing on a dirty, broken bottle when falling off a bicycle. These types of wounds always need vigorous cleaning. Some may need debridement.

Wounds heal better when the edges are brought closely together, or approximated. Jagged edges in a laceration make approximation harder. It is also difficult to approximate crushed tissue, as you would see with fingers closed in a car door. Crushing disrupts a tissue's blood supply by rupturing blood vessels throughout the affected area. A physician might debride this type of wound with a scalpel to remove severely damaged tissue and achieve a clean wound edge before suturing.

After a surgical or nonsurgical wound is closed and sutured, it is essential to keep the wound clean and dry to help prevent infection. Infection delays the healing process and can have other serious consequences.

A sutured wound heals more quickly and smoothly when no scab forms because the migrating skin cells encounter no barrier to their movement. Proper postoperative care, including daily cleaning with soap and water or a mild antiseptic, keeps a wound scab-free. Although skin cells migrate across the space of a wound more easily in a somewhat moist environment, a wet wound offers the ideal conditions for bacteria to grow and cause infection. Covering a wound with a clean, dry dressing helps prevent infection.

Wound healing may be delayed in a number of instances not directly related to the surgery or injury. The presence of any of the following conditions can put a patient at risk for wound healing problems. Wounds in such patients may require extra attention and care.

- Poor circulation. This condition results in inadequate supplies of nutrients, blood cells, and oxygen to the wound, all of which delay the healing process.
- Aging. Physiologic changes that occur with age can decrease a person's resistance to infection.
- Diabetes. Patients with diabetes experience changes in their artery walls that result in poor circulation to peripheral tissues. These patients also may have a decreased resistance to infection.
- Poor nutrition. Patients who are undernourished, particularly those who are deficient in protein or vitamin C, do not have the physiologic resources for vigorous healing.
- High levels of stress. An increase in stress-related hormones can decrease resistance to infection.
- Weakened immune system. Patients who are on certain medications or who have certain chronic diseases may have weakened immune systems, putting them at increased risk of infection.
- Obesity. When someone is obese, the circulation directly under the skin is often poor, leading to slow healing.
- Smoking. Nicotine constricts the blood vessels in the skin, reducing circulation to the wound area and slowing healing.

together so that the tissue surfaces are close. This intervention protects the area from further contamination and minimizes scab and scar formation. Small wounds can be held together with butterfly closures, sterile strips, or adhesive. Skin adhesive is a special type of glue used for closing small wounds. Larger wounds or those subject to strain may require suturing or stapling.

The **maturation phase** (the third phase) involves the formation of scar tissue. Scar tissue is important for closing large, gaping, or jagged wounds. The continuous layer of skin cells formed during the second phase becomes thicker and pushes off the scab, leaving a scar. Scar tissue contains no nerves or blood vessels and lacks the resilience of skin.

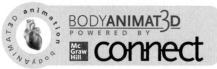

Go to CONNECT to see an animation exercise about *Wound Healing.*

Closing a Wound Sutures are surgical stitches a physician uses to close a wound. Suture materials, or **ligatures,** can be either absorbable or nonabsorbable. The type and location of the wound will determine the type of suture material the healthcare practitioner chooses. The body breaks down absorbable sutures, so they do not require removal after the wound has healed. If a wound is particularly deep, the healthcare practitioner may need to suture in layers, from inside to outside. In this case, absorbable sutures are used for the inner suturing. Removable (nonabsorbable) sutures are generally used for the outside layer. Nonabsorbable ligatures must be removed after wound healing is well under way. Sutures are discussed in greater detail in *section 44.3* of this chapter.

Staples may be used to bring the edges of a wound together if there is considerable stress on the incision. For example, a long and deep surgical wound or a wound across the leg would have a strong tendency to gape open if not firmly secured. Surgical staples look somewhat like ordinary staples. They are inserted into the skin with a disposable staple unit.

Special Minor Surgical Procedures

Some types of minor surgical procedures require special surgical instruments. These procedures include laser surgery, cryosurgery, and electrocauterization. They all remove excess or abnormal tissue, as in the case of warts or skin lesions, and usually require surgical aseptic technique because they break the integrity of the skin.

Laser Surgery A laser emits an intense beam of light that is used to cut away tissue. Laser surgery is sometimes preferred over conventional surgery because it causes less damage to surrounding healthy tissue than does conventional surgery. Laser surgery also promotes quick healing and helps prevent infection.

When a laser is used in an office setting, close blinds and shades to keep out stray light. Remove any items—such as the paper from wrapped sterile instruments or syringes—that could catch fire if they came in contact with the laser beam. Cover any shiny or reflective surfaces or use nonshiny instruments. Make sure that everyone in the room, including the patient, wears special safety goggles to protect the eyes. You should have a fire extinguisher in the room where it is out of the way but easily accessible. Post a standard laser warning placard in the room's entryway, per Occupational Safety and Health Administration (OSHA) regulations.

Position, drape, and prepare the patient as you would for conventional surgery. Place gauze around the surgical site and assist the physician with administration of a local anesthetic if requested. The physician uses the laser to vaporize the unwanted tissue; vaporized tissue is cleared away by the vacuum hose portion of the unit (see Figure 44-1). You may be asked to apply pressure to control any bleeding. Clean the wound with an antiseptic and apply a sterile dressing. Give the patient the normal instructions on wound care, including the recommendation to protect the site from sun exposure.

Cryosurgery The use of extreme cold to destroy unwanted tissue is called **cryosurgery.** Cryosurgery is often used to remove skin lesions and lesions on the cervix. Before cryosurgery, inform the patient that an initial sensation of cold will be followed by a burning sensation. Instruct the patient to remain as still as possible to prevent damage to nearby tissue.

The doctor may freeze the tissue by touching it with a cotton-tipped applicator dipped in liquid nitrogen or by spraying it with liquid nitrogen from a pressurized can. Sometimes, a special cryosurgical instrument is used, most often during surgery on the cervix.

Make the patient aware that more than one freezing cycle may be necessary. A local anesthetic is usually not required because the cold itself reduces sensation in the area. After the procedure, the area is cleaned with an antiseptic and a sterile dressing may be applied. An ice pack may be applied to reduce swelling and pain relievers given for pain.

Reassure the patient that some pain, swelling, or redness is normal after a cryosurgical procedure. Encourage the patient to use ice and pain relievers as necessary. Let the patient know that a large, painful, bloody blister may form. Left undisturbed, the blister usually ruptures in about 2 weeks. It should be left intact to promote healing and prevent infection. The patient should call the doctor if a blister becomes too painful. Be sure to provide the patient with complete wound care instructions.

Electrocauterization This is a technique whereby a needle, probe, or loop heated by electric current destroys the target tissue. A physician may use **electrocauterization** to remove growths such as warts, to stop bleeding, and to control nosebleeds that either will not subside or continually recur.

Several types of electrocautery units are in use. Some are small, handheld units powered by battery or by ordinary household electric current. Other, larger units are designed for countertop placement or wall mounting. Some units use disposable probes, and others employ reusable ones.

With certain units, a grounding pad or plate is placed on or under the patient's body during the procedure. This grounding completes the circuit and prevents electric shock to the patient, the physician, and staff members. Reassure the patient that grounding causes no discomfort.

A local anesthetic may be administered before the procedure. After electrocauterization, a scab or crust generally forms over the area. Healing may take 2 to 3 weeks. General wound care instructions are appropriate for this procedure, except that a dressing may be omitted to keep the area drier.

▶ Instruments Used in Minor Surgery   LO 44.3

The type of minor surgical procedure determines which surgical instruments are used. Surgical instruments have specific purposes and may be classified by function.

Cutting and Dissecting Instruments

Cutting and dissecting instruments have sharp edges and are used to cut (incise) skin and tissue. Figure 44-2 illustrates some of the basic cutting and dissecting instruments you will

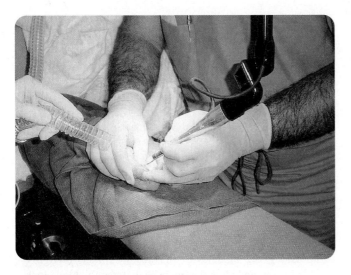

FIGURE 44-1 Suction eliminates vaporized tissue as a physician uses a laser to remove a wart from a patient's hand.
©Barry Slaven Photography

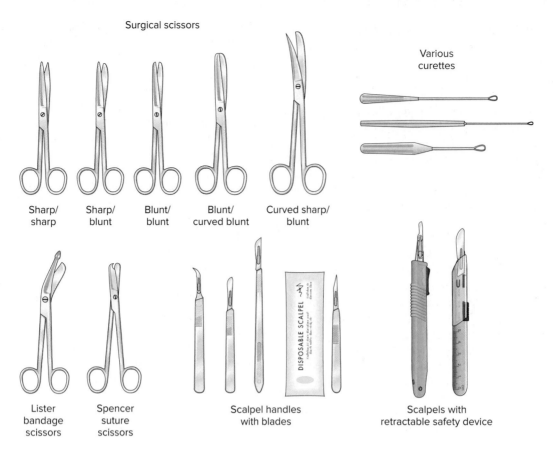

Surgical scissors

Various curettes

Sharp/ sharp | Sharp/ blunt | Blunt/ blunt | Blunt/ curved blunt | Curved sharp/ blunt

Lister bandage scissors | Spencer suture scissors | Scalpel handles with blades | Scalpels with retractable safety device

FIGURE 44-2 These are typical cutting and dissecting instruments used in minor surgical procedures.

encounter. You must be careful when cleaning, sterilizing, and storing these instruments to avoid injuring yourself and to protect the instruments' sharp edges.

Scalpels A scalpel consists of a handle that holds a disposable blade. Scalpel handles are either reusable or disposable and vary in width and length. A scalpel's specific use determines the shape and size of its blade. General-purpose scalpels have wide blades and a straight cutting surface (Figure 44-3). A no. 15 blade is the most common one for performing minor procedures.

Take special care when handling a scalpel. If the physician requests a reusable scalpel handle, it is essential that you load and unload the blade correctly on the handle. Carefully follow these steps when loading and unloading a scalpel blade:

Steps for Loading a Scalpel Handle

1. Carefully grasp the blade with a needle holder, staying away from the sharp edge.
2. Ensure that the blade edge is pointed away from you and you are gripping the blade just above the blade slot.
3. Firmly hold the scalpel handle in your nondominant hand. Hold the handle in the center, not close to the blade lock.
4. Carefully slide the blade over the grooves of the blade lock until it snaps into place.
5. The blade should slide smoothly down the groove. If it jams, carefully slide it back up the blade lock while

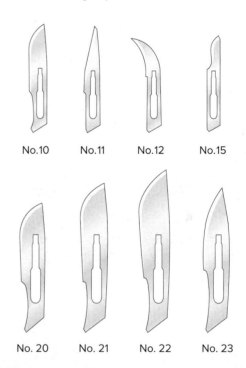

No.10   No.11   No.12   No.15

No. 20   No. 21   No. 22   No. 23

FIGURE 44-3 Scalpel blades come in various sizes and shapes, some of which are represented here.

grasping the blade with the needle holder, realign the blade slot, and slide the blade back down the blade lock.

6. Never use your fingers to load a blade on a scalpel handle. The blade is very sharp and may slip, causing serious injury.

Steps for Unloading a Scalpel Handle

1. Using your nondominant hand, hold the scalpel handle in the center.

2. With the blade lock facing up, point the blade and handle downward over a sharps container (make sure the sharps container is well below the blade and the blade is not pointed toward anyone in the room).

3. Using the needle holder, grasp the angled edge of the blade near the blade lock.

4. Lift the blade slightly over the blade lock and slide it up to disengage the blade from the blade lock.

5. Immediately drop the blade into the sharps container.

6. Do not touch the blade with your fingers.

7. The blade handle is now ready for sanitization and sterilization.

A number of special blade removal devices are also available. These devices contain the blade in a case or box before removal. Follow the manufacturer's instructions for safe scalpel blade removal.

Scissors Surgical scissors come in various sizes. They may be straight or curved and have either blunt or pointed tips. Tissue scissors must be sharp enough to cut without damaging or ripping surrounding tissue. Suture scissors have blunt points and a curved lower blade. The lower blade is inserted under the suture material to cut it. Bandage scissors are used to remove dressings. They have a blunt lower blade to prevent injuring the skin next to the dressing. Clippers are scissor-like instruments used for cutting nails or thick materials.

Curettes The doctor uses a curette for scraping tissue. Curettes come in a variety of shapes and sizes and consist of a circular blade—actually a loop—attached to a rod-shaped handle. The blade is blunt on the outside and sharp on the inside. The inner part of the blade also may be serrated. Serrated blades may be used to take Pap (Papanicolaou) smears. Blunt curettes, known as Buck ear curettes, are used to remove wax from the ear canal when a large amount of cerumen has accumulated.

Grasping and Clamping Instruments

Special instruments are used for grasping and clamping tissue. Grasping instruments are used to hold surgical materials or to remove foreign objects, such as splinters, from the body. Clamping instruments are used to apply pressure and close off blood vessels. They also are used to hold tissue and other materials in position. Figure 44-4 shows some common grasping and clamping instruments.

Forceps Forceps are instruments that are commonly used to grasp or hold objects. Grasping types are usually shaped like tweezers and include thumb forceps and tissue forceps.

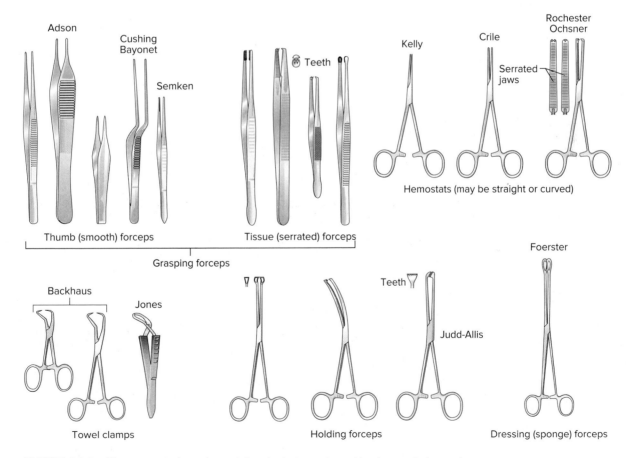

FIGURE 44-4 These are typical grasping and clamping instruments used in minor surgical procedures.

Thumb forceps, also called smooth forceps, vary in shape and size. The blades of thumb forceps are tapered to a point and have small grooves at the tip. Tissue forceps (serrated forceps) have one or more fine teeth at the tips of the blades. When closed, these forceps hold tissue firmly. Holding forceps have handles with ratchets that lock the teeth in a closed position. Dressing, or sponge, forceps have ridges to hold a sponge or gauze when it is used to absorb body fluids.

Hemostats The most commonly used surgical instruments are hemostats. These surgical clamps vary in size and shape and are typically used to close off blood vessels. The serrated jaws of hemostats taper to a point. Like holding forceps, hemostats have handles that lock on ratchets, holding the jaws securely closed.

Towel Clamps Towel clamps are used to keep towels used for draping the surgical site in place during a surgical procedure. This stability is important in maintaining a sterile field.

Retracting, Dilating, and Probing Instruments

Retracting instruments are used to hold back the sides of a wound or an incision. Dilating and probing instruments may be used to enlarge, examine, or clear body openings, body cavities, or wounds. The shapes of these instruments vary with their functions. Some typical retracting, dilating, and probing instruments are shown in Figure 44-5.

Retractors The use of retractors allows greater access to and a better view of a surgical site. Some retractors must be held open by hand, while others have ratchets or locks to keep them open.

Dilators Dilators are slender, pointed instruments used to enlarge a body opening, such as a tear duct.

Probes A surgical probe is a slender rod with a blunt, bulb-shaped tip. Probes are used to explore wounds or body cavities and to locate or clear blockages.

Suture Materials and Suturing Instruments

Suturing instruments are used to introduce suture materials into and retrieve them from a wound. Some carry the suture material, whereas others manipulate the suture carriers. Examples of suturing instruments are shown in Figure 44-6.

Suture Materials As a medical assistant, you need to be familiar with the various types of sutures. The healthcare practitioner will ask for a specific suture type based on

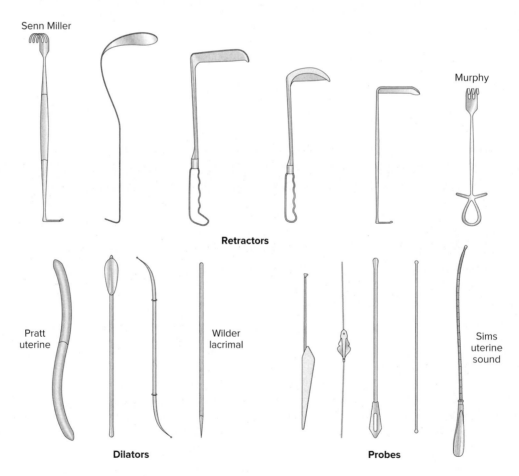

Senn Miller

Murphy

Retractors

Pratt uterine

Wilder lacrimal

Sims uterine sound

Dilators

Probes

FIGURE 44-5 These are typical retracting, dilating, and probing instruments used in minor surgical procedures.

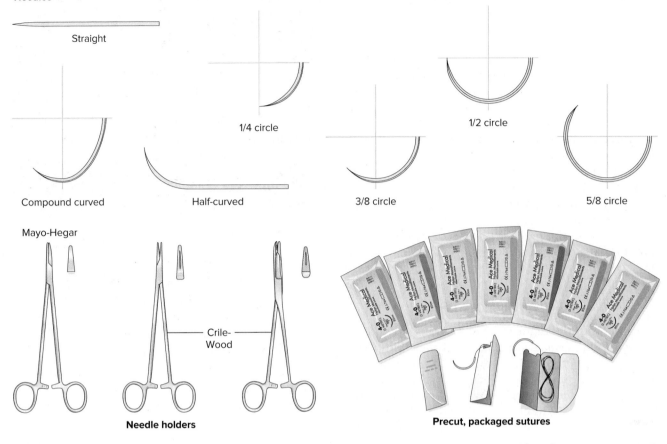

Needles

Straight

1/4 circle

Compound curved

Half-curved

1/2 circle

3/8 circle

5/8 circle

Mayo-Hegar

Crile-
Wood

Needle holders

Precut, packaged sutures

FIGURE 44-6 These are typical suturing instruments.

several considerations, including the type and location of the wound. Sutures may be natural or synthetic, absorbable or nonabsorbable. The healthcare practitioner will choose a needle that causes the least possible trauma to the tissues. The needle may be curved or straight, cutting, blunt, or tapered. A **swaged needle** has the suture material permanently attached to the needle. The needle also may have an eye where the suture material is manually threaded. It is important that you be able to quickly find information about the type of suture material in a package. Figure 44-7 illustrates the most common information found on a suture package.

General Features of Suture Materials Regardless of the type, suture materials have some general qualities in common:

- Sterility.
- Uniform diameter.
- Tensile strength (resistance to breaking under tension or pull).
- Flexibility.
- Ability to retain or hold a knot.
- Low incidence of tissue reactivity.

Suture Size Suture size is determined by the diameter or thickness of the strand. Sizes range from 11-0 (smallest) to 7

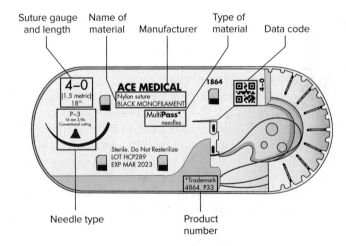

Suture gauge and length Name of material Manufacturer Type of material Data code

Needle type Product number

FIGURE 44-7 Information about the suture material can be found on the package.

(largest). The number in front of the "0" determines the number of zeros. Remember, the more zeros in the size, the smaller the suture. For example, a 6-0 suture is smaller in diameter than a 3-0 suture. The sizes you most often will see used for minor surgical procedures are 6-0 to 3-0. Sutures sized 6-0 and 5-0 are used most often to close wounds of the face, lips, and eyebrow. Wounds of the sole of the foot generally require a suture that is thicker in diameter. These wounds are usually repaired with a 3-0 or 4-0 suture.

Suture Needles Surgical suture needles carry suture material, or ligature, through the tissue being sutured. They are either pointed or blunt at one end and may have an eye at the other end to hold suture material. Ligature often comes prepackaged with the needle already connected. Prepackaged suture needles with attached ligature (swaged) have no eye and produce less trauma to the tissue being sutured than do suture needles with eyes.

Suture needles may be straight, or they may be curved to allow deeper suture placement. Taper point needles (needles that taper into a sharp point) are used to suture tissues that are easily penetrated. They create only very small holes, thus minimizing tissue fluid leakage. Cutting needles (needles that have at least two sharpened edges) are used on tough tissues that are not easily penetrated, such as skin.

Several measurements are used to determine the size of a surgical needle. Needle length is the distance from the tip to the end, measuring along the body of the needle. Chord length is the straight-line distance from the tip to the end of the needle. (Chord length is not the same as needle length in curved needles.) The radius of a curved needle is determined by mentally continuing the curve of the needle into a full circle and finding the distance from the center of the circle to the needle body. The diameter is the thickness of the needle. Needle size generally corresponds to the size of suture material used. Smaller needles are used for delicate procedures, such as eye surgery or repair of a facial laceration. Larger needles are used for suturing wounds of less delicate parts of the body, such as the hands or legs.

Needle Holders Curved suture needles require special instruments to hold, insert, and retrieve them during suturing. Most needle holders look like hemostats with short, sturdy jaws.

Syringes and Needles

Sterile syringes and needles are used to inject anesthetic solutions, withdraw fluids, and obtain biopsy specimens. The size of the syringe and needle varies with the intended use. For example, a needle used to perform a biopsy is generally larger than needles used for most injections. (Syringes and needles used for injections are discussed and illustrated in the *Medication Administration* chapter.) Both syringes and needles are provided in individual sterile envelopes.

Instrument Trays and Packs

All the surgical instruments needed for a specific procedure are usually assembled beforehand. They are then sterilized together in a pack. Certain surgical supplies necessary for the procedure (such as gauze) are included in the pack because they, too, must be sterile. Surgical trays can be quickly set up with these instrument packs. Individually wrapped items also may be added as needed.

These are the common types of instrument trays:

- Laceration repair tray (see Figure 44-8).
- Laceration repair with debridement tray.

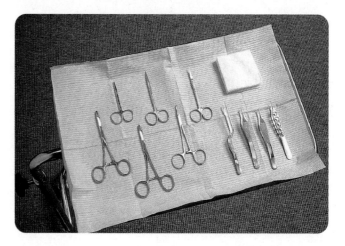

FIGURE 44-8 This laceration repair tray contains scissors, several pairs of forceps, a needle holder, and sterile gauze. Suture material must be added for the procedure.
©David Kelly Crow

- Incision and drainage tray.
- Foreign body or growth removal tray.
- Onychectomy (nail removal) tray.
- Vasectomy (male sterilization procedure) tray.
- Suture removal tray.
- Staple removal tray.

▶ Asepsis   LO 44.4

Maintaining asepsis during surgical procedures is always a priority. It is critical to the health and safety of both the patient and the healthcare professional. The two levels of aseptic technique are **medical asepsis** (clean technique) and **surgical asepsis** (sterile technique). Medical asepsis is discussed in detail in the *Infection Control Fundamentals* chapter. You will use both levels of asepsis when assisting with minor surgery.

Personal Protective Equipment

Personal protective equipment, or PPE, includes all items used as a barrier between the wearer and potentially infectious or hazardous medical materials. PPE includes gloves, gowns, and masks and protective eyewear or face shields. OSHA regulations regarding PPE are discussed in detail in the *Infection Control Fundamentals* and *Infection Control Practices* chapters.

Gloves are of particular importance during surgical procedures. You should wear properly sized latex, nitrile, or vinyl gloves during any procedure that might expose you to potentially infectious or hazardous materials. (Gloves that are too big can catch on instruments or equipment and cause accidents.) When you wear gloves, you also protect the patient from any infectious organisms on your hands.

Vinyl, nitrile, and latex gloves can all prevent contamination of the hands with bacteria. Although latex gloves were the preference of healthcare professionals for many years, the incidence of latex allergy among healthcare professionals has grown. Allergic reactions to latex can range from a skin rash to shock and even death. Many healthcare institutions are switching to less allergenic low-powder or powderless non-latex gloves. The powder in latex gloves, which makes them easier to put on, is one of the primary sources of latex allergy. The latex protein that causes the allergy mixes with the powder. When the gloves are removed, the powder containing the latex protein becomes airborne and is inhaled.

If you work in a facility that uses latex gloves, take these steps to prevent latex allergy:

- If possible, use powder-free gloves only.
- Thoroughly dry hands after washing.
- Frequently apply non-oil-based lotion to the hands.
- Clean areas and equipment contaminated with latex-containing dust frequently.

If you notice latex allergy symptoms, consider consulting an allergist. You also should discuss your symptoms with your supervisor, who will recommend that you switch to hypoallergenic or vinyl gloves. If you have an allergy, the healthcare facility is required to provide nonlatex gloves for your use.

Sharps and Biohazardous Waste Handling and Disposal

Sharp medical and surgical instruments have great potential for transmitting infection through cuts and puncture wounds. Used scalpels, needles, syringes, and other sharp objects should be disposed of in a puncture-resistant sharps container.

All items other than sharps that have come in contact with tissue, blood, or body fluids must be disposed of in a leakproof plastic bag or container. The container must be either red or labeled with the orange-red biohazard symbol. The proper procedure for handling and disposing of sharps and biohazardous waste is discussed in detail in the *Infection Control Fundamentals* and *Infection Control Practices* chapters.

Surgical Asepsis

Surgical asepsis completely eliminates microorganisms. The goal of surgical asepsis is to control microorganisms before they enter the body. To accomplish this goal, the items used in healthcare must be sterile (completely free of microorganisms). Surgical instruments are sterilized before use and sterile technique procedures must be followed.

You will be expected to perform the following common procedures involving sterile technique:

- Creating a sterile field.
- Adding sterile items to the sterile field.
- Performing a surgical scrub.
- Putting on sterile gloves.
- Sanitizing, disinfecting, and sterilizing equipment.

Creating a Sterile Field A **sterile field** is an area free of microorganisms that is used as a work area during a surgical procedure. Always be aware that the sterile field is understood to become contaminated and must be redone in the following circumstances:

- An unsterile item touches the field.
- Someone reaches across the field.
- The field becomes wet.
- The field is left unattended and uncovered.
- You turn your back on the field.

For more rules of sterile technique, see the *Caution: Handle with Care* feature.

The sterile field is often set up on a Mayo stand—a movable, stainless steel instrument tray on a stand. Adjust the stand so that the tray is slightly above waist level. Remember, items placed below waist level are considered contaminated. Before beginning, disinfect the Mayo stand with 70% isopropyl alcohol and allow it to dry.

To create the sterile field, cover the stand with two layers of sterile material. This material can be sterile disposable drapes, separately sterilized muslin towels, or the muslin towels that the surgical instruments are wrapped in before autoclaving to produce office-sterilized sterile instrument packs.

CAUTION: HANDLE WITH CARE

Rules for Sterile Technique

A sterile field is a microorganism-free area used during a surgical procedure. To maintain sterility throughout the procedure, follow surgical technique and adhere to these rules:

1. Do not touch a nonsterile article to a sterile article or area. This will cause the sterile area or article to be considered nonsterile.
2. If you are unsure about the sterility of an article or area, consider it nonsterile.
3. Unused, opened sterile supplies must be discarded or resterilized.
4. Packages must be wrapped or sealed in such a way that they can be opened without contamination.

5. The edges of wrappers (1-inch margin) covering sterile supplies and the outer lips of bottles and flasks containing sterile solutions are not considered sterile.
6. If a sterile surface or package becomes wet, it is considered contaminated and should not be used.
7. Do not reach over a sterile field when you are not wearing sterile clothing. This action contaminates the sterile field.
8. Keep your hands between your shoulders and your waist when wearing sterile gloves to maintain sterility.
9. Do not turn your back on a sterile field even if you are in a sterile gown. Your back is always considered contaminated.

Commercially prepared sterile instrument packs, usually with disposable paper wrappings, are also used to create a sterile field. Procedure 44-1, at the end of this chapter, describes how to prepare a sterile field and how to open sterile packages.

When assembling the necessary supplies, place all unsterile items that may be used during the procedure outside the sterile field. Unsterile items include items that are sterile on the inside but not on the outside, such as a sterile gauze pack or a sterile liquid such as alcohol, saline, or peroxide inside an unsterile bottle. Unsterile supplies should be arranged on a counter away from the sterile field. A typical arrangement of unsterile items used in surgery is shown in Figure 44-9. If you place an unsterile item within the sterile field, the field is no longer sterile and you must repeat the entire process.

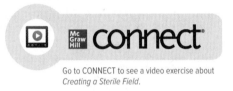

Go to CONNECT to see a video exercise about *Creating a Sterile Field*.

Adding Sterile Items to the Sterile Field The outer 1 inch of the sterile field is considered contaminated. So before you add sterile items to the sterile field, carefully plan where you will place the instruments so that they are within the sterile field.

Instruments and Supplies If you have used sterile disposable drapes or separately sterilized muslin towels to create the sterile field, you will need to add the necessary instruments. Stand away from the sterile field and open the sterile instrument pack in the manner described in Procedure 44-1. Place the pack on a counter or hold it open in your hand. Transfer and arrange the instruments on the sterile field with sterile transfer forceps. Never reach across the sterile field.

Some instruments are sterilized individually in autoclave bags and many sterile supplies are prepackaged. Stand away from the sterile field as you open an individual bag or package.

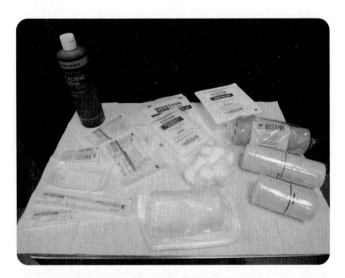

FIGURE 44-9 For each surgical procedure, unsterile surgical supplies must be gathered and arranged in an area separate from the sterile field.
©McGraw-Hill Education/David Moyer, photographer

You can pull the flaps of the packaging partway apart, then snap (remove from position by a sudden movement) the item onto the sterile field from a distance of 8 to 12 inches. Alternatively, you can use sterile forceps to grasp and place the items in the sterile field.

Pouring Sterile Solutions Sterile solutions are often required during the surgical procedure to rinse or wash the wound. These can be added to the sterile field after the sterile instruments. Several sterile solutions are commonly used during minor surgical procedures, including sterile water and normal saline (0.9% sodium chloride).

Bottles of these sterile solutions come in a variety of sizes. Choose the smallest size that will supply the amount of solution needed during the procedure to help minimize cost because unused solutions are typically discarded.

When pouring a solution, cover the label on the bottle with the palm of your hand to keep the label dry. Pour a small amount of the liquid into a liquid waste receptacle to clean the lip of the bottle. As you pour the solution into a sterile bowl on the field, hold the bottle at an angle to avoid reaching over the sterile area. Hold the bottle fairly close to the bowl without touching it. Pour the contents slowly to avoid splashing the drape, which would contaminate the field (see Figure 44-10).

When a sterile solution bottle is opened and may be used again during the procedure, do not let any unsterile object touch the inside of its cap. To accomplish this, place the cap on a clean location with the sterile inside of the cap facing up.

Performing a Surgical Scrub and Donning Sterile Gloves If you assist in a surgical procedure, you must perform a surgical scrub and wear sterile surgical gloves. Surgical scrub procedures are similar to those for aseptic handwashing, but there are several distinctions:

- A sterile scrub brush is used instead of a disposable nailbrush.
- Both the hands and the forearms are washed.
- The hands are kept above the elbows to prevent water from running from the arms onto washed areas.

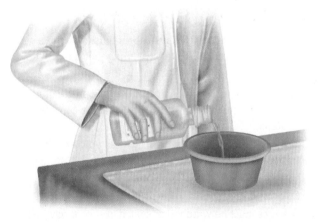

FIGURE 44-10 When pouring a sterile solution for use on a sterile field, be careful not to splash the solution.

- Sterile towels are used instead of paper towels.
- Sterile gloves are put on immediately after the hands are dried.

You may wonder why a surgical scrub is necessary if you are planning to wear sterile gloves. The answer is that there is always the possibility that a glove may be punctured. If the skin is as clean as possible, the risk of contamination from a punctured glove is minimized. Nevertheless, if a glove is damaged during a sterile procedure, you must consider anything touched by that glove after it is damaged to be contaminated. Contaminated items must be resterilized or replaced before you continue.

A surgical scrub removes microorganisms more effectively than does routine handwashing. Routine handwashing removes bacteria present on the skin's surface, whereas the surgical scrub removes bacteria in deeper layers of the skin—where the hair follicles and oil-producing glands exist. Procedure 44-2, at the end of this chapter, describes the process for performing a sterile scrub.

Sterile gloves are required for many procedures. You don sterile gloves after you perform the surgical scrub. The process for donning sterile gloves is described in Procedure 44-3 at the end of this chapter.

Remember, once you are wearing sterile gloves, you may touch only the items in the sterile field. So you must remove any drape covering the sterile instrument tray before you glove. Sterile gloves provide a small margin of safety in preventing contamination; your movements must be controlled and precise to work within this margin to protect the sterile area.

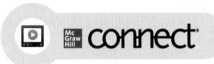

Go to CONNECT to see video exercises about *Performing a Surgical Scrub and Donning Sterile Gloves.*

Sanitizing, Disinfecting, and Sterilizing Equipment

Many supplies used in a doctor's office are disposable. Many surgical instruments, however, are made of steel and are reusable. Preparing surgical instruments for reuse involves cleaning them with germicidal soap and water (a process called *sanitization*), then disinfecting and/or sterilizing them, depending on how the equipment will be used. These procedures are described more fully in the *Examination and Treatment Areas* and *Infection Control Practices* chapters.

▶ Preoperative Procedures LO 44.5

You must complete a number of steps before a surgical procedure, including performing various preliminary duties, preparing the surgical room, and physically preparing the patient for surgery.

Preliminary Duties

The first tasks you will perform before the surgery include providing **preoperative** (prior to surgery, or "pre-op")

instructions to the patient, completing various administrative tasks, and easing the patient's fears.

Preoperative Instructions When a patient is scheduled for a minor surgical procedure in the doctor's office, you must explain the preoperative instructions. Be prepared to answer the patient's questions about the procedure and possible risks. The patient may ask you, rather than the doctor, such questions or may need clarification of information provided by the doctor.

A patient may need to follow certain dietary and fluid restrictions before a minor surgical procedure. Not eating or drinking for a specific period of time is a common restriction. The patient's medications also may be restricted because of anesthetic administration during the procedure. Non-English-speaking patients may need an interpreter who can help them understand the forms they must sign and their instructions.

Instruct the patient to wear either comfortable, loose-fitting clothes that will not interfere with the procedure or clothing that can be removed easily. In most cases, patients also need to arrange for someone to drive them home and stay with them for 24 hours after the procedure.

Administrative and Legal Tasks You must ensure that all the necessary paperwork is completed before surgery. Routine administrative tasks include completing the required insurance forms and obtaining prior authorization from the patient's insurance company.

Make absolutely certain the patient reads, understands, and signs the surgical consent form. The patient needs a clear understanding of what to expect during and after the surgery to give informed consent as required by law. Sometimes surgery is performed on a child or a patient with limited understanding of legal documents. In such cases, the consent form must be signed by the patient's parent or legal guardian.

Failure to obtain the necessary paperwork prior to a surgical procedure can cause serious legal problems. The doctor and other staff members could be held legally liable if problems were to develop during or after the procedure.

It is common practice to call the patient the day before the surgery to confirm the appointment. This call also provides a chance to ensure that the patient follows the preoperative instructions. You may be responsible for making this call.

Easing the Patient's Fears Knowing what to expect during and after a surgical procedure will ease the patient's fears. This information allows him or her to plan daily activities and, if necessary, to arrange for help at home during the recovery period.

Some offices have educational materials such as brochures, fact sheets, or videos about the procedure the patient will undergo. You may assist in preparing or acquiring these materials if your office's policy includes such participation for medical assistants. This type of information may increase patient compliance with pre- and postoperative instructions.

Much of a patient's fear about a surgical procedure can be overcome if you spend sufficient time before the procedure explaining what to expect. Be prepared to answer the patient's questions honestly, calmly, and confidently. Your calm and knowledgeable manner will reassure the patient. If the answer to a question requires experience or knowledge beyond your own, pass the question on to the healthcare practitioner.

Preparing the Surgical Room

Prior to surgery, the doctor should inform you of specific instructions concerning patient preparation. He also will tell you what special equipment or supplies are necessary for the procedure.

Because patients are likely to feel anxious before a procedure, it is best to have everything ready in the surgical room before you escort the patient into the room. Make sure the room is clean, neat, and free of waste from previous procedures. The examining table should have been cleaned and disinfected, and surface barriers (table paper and pillow covers) should have been changed.

Check to see that there is adequate lighting. Make sure that all equipment and supplies necessary for the procedure are available. Check the date and sterilization indicator on sterilized packs and supplies.

You will then wash your hands and prepare the sterile field as outlined in Procedure 44-1 at the end of this chapter. The sterile field and the instruments should be draped with a sterile towel.

Preparing the Patient

Just before the surgery, various concerns must be addressed and procedures completed in sequence. The initial tasks are followed by gowning and positioning the patient and preparing the patient's skin for surgery.

Initial Tasks Before leading the patient into the surgical room, give the patient an opportunity to use the bathroom. You also must find out whether she has followed the presurgical instructions. Restrictions on food and fluid intake are of particular concern. Also, ask what medications the patient is taking and whether she has taken that day's dosage.

Measure the patient's vital signs. Ask if there are any symptoms or problems the doctor should know about before the surgery. If any unusual signs or symptoms are present, notify the doctor. The doctor will want to examine the patient before proceeding.

Check the chart for medication orders, such as pain medication or a tranquilizer to calm the patient. Medications should be administered at this time so that they can take effect before surgery.

Gowning and Positioning the Patient Some procedures require the patient to disrobe and put on a gown to expose the surgical site. If this is the case, you should offer to assist, if appropriate, or leave the room while the patient changes. You should then help the patient onto the table and into the position required for the procedure. You may use one or more small pillows to make the patient as comfortable as possible. Then adequately drape the patient to retain body heat and preserve personal dignity.

Sterile drapes also are used to create a sterile field on a patient's body around the surgical site. Drapes come in a variety of sizes and styles. A fenestrated drape has a round or slit-like opening cut out in the center to provide access to the surgical site.

Surgical Skin Preparation Prior to surgery, the patient's skin must be prepared to reduce the number of microorganisms and the risk of surgical site infection. Preparation includes cleaning the area, removing the hair, and applying antiseptic. The area prepared should be 2 inches larger than the intended surgical field. The surgical field is the area exposed in the center of the fenestrated drape. The extra prepared skin area allows for draping without contaminating the surgical field.

Cleaning the Area Before proceeding with the surgical skin preparation, wash your hands and don exam gloves. Confirm that the patient is not allergic to iodine or iodine-based products. Place a plastic-backed drape under the surgical site to absorb any liquids. Clean the site first with an iodine-based solution, using forceps and gauze sponges dipped in the solution. Begin at the center of the surgical site and work outward in a firm, circular motion (Figure 44-11). Discard the gauze sponge after each complete pass. Clean in concentric circles until you cover the full preparation area. Continue the process, repeating as necessary, for at least 2 minutes or the amount of time specified in the office's procedure manual. Cleaning takes more time if a wound is dirty or contains foreign materials. When procedures are performed on a hand or foot, clean the entire hand or foot. The skin and body openings, particularly the nose, mouth, and perineum, cannot be considered sterile. Nevertheless, the principles of aseptic technique require that you try to keep the area as contamination-free as possible.

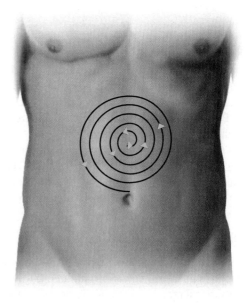

FIGURE 44-11 Clean the surgical site with an iodine-based solution. Begin at the center of the surgical site and work outward in a firm, circular motion. Clean in a circular, outward pattern 2 inches larger than the surgical field.

Removing Hair from the Area Depending on office policy, you may be required to remove hair from the surgical site. Shaving often causes many small wounds on the skin, which increases the risk of infection, and is not recommended. Some experts feel that hair should not be removed unless it is thick enough to interfere with surgery. If this is the case, hair may be trimmed with scissors or electric trimmers or smoothed out of the way. This should be done with care—to avoid damaging the skin—immediately before surgery.

Applying the Antiseptic Antiseptics are agents applied to the skin to limit the growth of microorganisms and to help prevent infection. Povidone iodine (Betadine®) is most commonly used, but chlorhexidine gluconate (Hibiclens®) or benzalkonium chloride (Zephiran®) also may be used, particularly if the patient is allergic to iodine. After cleaning or removing the hair when needed, swab an area 2 inches larger than the surgical field with the antiseptic solution in a circular, outward motion, starting at the surgical site. This is the same motion used for cleaning the surgical site. For surgery on a hand or foot, swab the entire hand or foot. Allow the antiseptic to air-dry; do not pat it dry—that would remove some of the solution's antiseptic properties.

When the area is dry, treat it as a sterile field. Instruct the patient not to touch the area. Cover the area with a sterile fenestrated drape, from front to back. Avoid reaching over the field. At this point, notify the physician that the patient is ready. Then prepare yourself to assist with the surgery.

▶ Intraoperative Procedures LO 44.6

Intraoperative procedures are procedures that take place during surgery. You may be asked to perform a wide variety of unsterile and sterile tasks during surgery, such as preparing a local anesthetic, monitoring the patient, processing specimens, and handing instruments to the doctor. The doctor also may ask you to explain to the patient step by step what will be done next during the procedure.

Administering a Local Anesthetic

Before beginning the surgical procedure, the physician will administer a local anesthetic. Some local anesthetics are injected. An injected anesthetic is packaged in a sterile vial (a small glass bottle with a self-sealing rubber stopper). Other local anesthetics come in a cream, gel, or spray form. These anesthetics are topical (applied directly to the skin) and affect only the area to which they are applied. The choice of administration method depends on how invasive or painful the procedure is likely to be.

Lidocaine (Xylocaine®) is the most commonly used anesthetic, used as an injectable or a topical gel anesthetic. Tetracaine hydrochloride (Pontocaine®), a long-acting anesthetic, is injected or topical.

Topical Application A topical anesthetic is useful when the pain will be mild or when only the skin's upper layers are affected. It is common to use such agents to anesthetize the area of a small laceration prior to suturing. Sometimes an anesthetic cream is applied before a local anesthetic is injected to reduce or eliminate the pain caused by the injection. A topical anesthetic must usually remain on the skin for 10 to 15 minutes for the area to become sufficiently anesthetized.

Injections If a local anesthetic is to be injected, it is typically administered after the skin is prepared but before the patient is draped. In some cases, however, the anesthetic is injected prior to skin preparation to allow time for it to take effect. In either case, it is important to note the time of anesthetic administration in the patient's chart.

If the doctor is already wearing sterile gloves, you may be asked to assist in administering the anesthetic. Because administering an anesthetic is an unsterile task (the outside of the vial is unsterile), when performing it, follow proper procedure to protect the sterility of the doctor's gloves and the anesthetic solution.

First, check the label of the anesthetic vial two times to confirm that it is the correct solution. Then, clean the vial's rubber stopper with a 70% isopropyl alcohol solution and leave the alcohol pad on top of the stopper. Present the requested needle and syringe to the doctor by peeling half the outer wrapper away and allowing the doctor to remove them from the wrapper.

Remove the pad from the rubber stopper and hold the vial so that the doctor can verify it is the proper medication. Turn the vial upside down and hold it securely around the base, without touching the sterile stopper. Be sure to hold the vial in front of you at shoulder height. Because significant force will be necessary to push the needle through the rubber stopper, brace the wrist of the hand holding the vial with your free hand. Hold the vial firmly so that the doctor can withdraw the anesthetic from it (Figure 44-12). Check the vial a third time to confirm that it is the correct solution.

Potential Side Effects of the Anesthetic Patients sometimes have reactions to anesthetic medications and should be informed of this prior to the procedure. Although

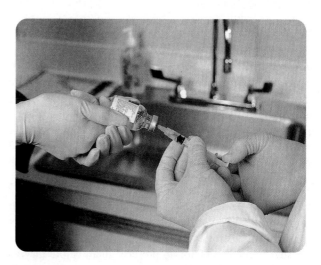

FIGURE 44-12 You must hold the anesthetic vial firmly to allow the physician to puncture the rubber stopper with the needle.
©Cliff Moore

rare, reactions may include dizziness, loss of consciousness, seizures, or cardiac arrest. Adverse reactions can occur if the anesthetic dose is too high or if it is absorbed too quickly. Reactions also can occur if the patient is taking other medications that should not be mixed with the anesthetic. All medications (including over-the-counter medications) that a patient is taking at the time of surgery must be documented to avoid possible reactions.

Use of Epinephrine Epinephrine is a sterile solution that is sometimes injected along with an anesthetic. It constricts the blood vessels, making them narrower, which reduces bleeding and prolongs the action of the local anesthetic. Epinephrine is used if the surgery site is an area with many small blood vessels that are expected to bleed profusely (such as the head). Reducing bleeding makes it easier to see and to repair the wound.

Epinephrine should be used with caution, however, in patients with heart disease or respiratory disease. Epinephrine also prolongs the anesthesia because epinephrine slows the rate at which the anesthetic spreads into the tissue. This effect may or may not be desirable. There is some concern that epinephrine may increase wound infection rates. If the wound is highly contaminated, the physician may choose to use anesthetic without epinephrine.

Assisting the Physician During Surgery

Your role in surgical assisting depends on the type of surgery and the physician's preference. You may assist the physician in one of two capacities with different duties: as a floater—an unsterile assistant who is free to move about the room and attend to unsterile needs—or as a sterile scrub assistant—who assists in handling sterile equipment during the procedure.

The Floater If you are assisting as a floater (sometimes called a circulator), you will perform a routine handwash and don exam gloves. Remember, you cannot touch sterile items in the sterile field because you have not performed a surgical scrub and are not wearing sterile gloves. Procedure 44-4, at the end of this chapter, outlines the tasks performed by a floater (unsterile assistant).

Monitoring and Recording One of a floater's most important duties is to monitor the patient during the procedure. You must measure vital signs regularly and observe the patient for reactions to the anesthetic. Record all observations in the patient's chart. Also, record any information or notes the doctor requests. You must keep a record of time, including when the anesthetic is administered, when the procedure begins, and when the procedure is completed.

Processing Specimens When you serve as a floater during surgery, the doctor may ask you to receive and process specimens for laboratory examination. Most tissues are placed in a 10% formalin solution to preserve them before they are sent to the laboratory. If the container is not prefilled, half-fill the specimen container with the formalin solution ahead of time. Remove the lid of the specimen container without

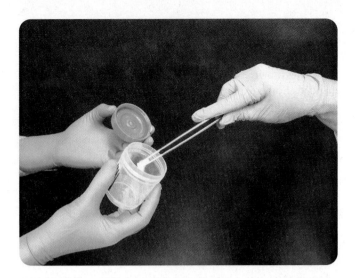

FIGURE 44-13 Be sure to hold the specimen container so that the doctor can place the tissue in it without touching the rim or outside of the container with the tissue.
©McGraw-Hill Education/David Moyer, photographer

touching the rim. Hold the container out toward the doctor so that she can place the tissue directly into it without contaminating the sample (Figure 44-13).

The container should be labeled with the following information:

- The patient's name and the doctor's name.
- The date and time of collection.
- The body site from which the specimen was obtained.
- Your initials.

If more than one specimen is obtained from a patient, place each specimen in a separate container. Label each container with the necessary information, along with a number to indicate the order in which the specimens are obtained (no. 1, no. 2, and so on). The physician will usually tell you the exact location of each specimen taken. You also will fill out a laboratory requisition slip to send along with the specimen(s). Specimen containers should be placed in a special transport bag labeled with the biohazard symbol. Most transport bags have an outside pouch for the lab requisition form. The form should accompany the sample but not be placed in contact with the specimen container. This protects lab personnel when they handle the requisition form.

Other Duties As a floater, you also may be asked to perform a number of other duties, including:

- Assisting with the injection of additional anesthetic.
- Adding additional sterile items to the sterile tray.
- Pouring sterile solutions.
- Keeping the surgical area clean and neat during the procedure.
- Repositioning the patient as necessary.
- Adjusting lighting.

The Sterile Scrub Assistant When serving as a sterile scrub assistant, you must perform a surgical scrub and wear sterile gloves. You may be asked to perform a variety of tasks under sterile conditions. Follow the rules of sterile technique listed earlier in this chapter and remember not to touch unsterile items after putting on sterile gloves. Procedure 44-5, at the end of this chapter, and the sections that follow outline the tasks performed by a sterile scrub assistant.

Handling Instruments Your first duty as a sterile scrub assistant is, typically, to close the instruments on the sterile tray because they are left in the open position during sterilization. Your next duty is to rearrange the instruments on the tray in the order in which they will be used or according to the doctor's preference. Instruments are generally used in the following sequence:

- Cutting instruments
- Grasping instruments
- Retractors
- Probes
- Suture materials
- Needle holders and scissors

Prepare for swabbing by placing several sterile gauze squares in the dressing forceps, to be ready when needed. As the sterile scrub assistant, you will be asked to pass instruments to the doctor during the procedure. You must hold instruments so that the doctor can grasp them safely and securely, without needing to reposition them in her hands. At the same time, the instruments must be handled properly to maintain their sterility.

When passing scissors and clamps, hold them by the hinge (Figure 44-14). You will have a clear view of the instrument's tip and the doctor will have full use of the handles. Firmly slap the instrument handles into the doctor's extended palm. The doctor's hand will close around the handles as a reflex action to the slapping. This technique reduces the risk of dropping an instrument. If the scissors or clamp is curved, the curve should follow the same curve as the doctor's hand.

When passing a scalpel, hold it above and just behind the cutting edge of the blade with the blade facing away from your palm so that the doctor can grasp the entire handle (Figure 44-15). You should wait until the doctor has fully grasped the handle before taking your hand away. The doctor will wait until your hand is fully out of the way before moving the scalpel. This requires good communication between you and the doctor and helps avoid any injury while passing the scalpel. Pass a needle holder with suture material so that the needle is pointing up, and hold the end of the suture material with your other hand to prevent the material from becoming tangled in the handles. You also may use a sterile tray called a passing tray when passing sharp instruments to the doctor. Using a passing tray reduces the likelihood of having an exposure incident while passing instruments (Figure 44-16).

Other Duties As a sterile scrub assistant, you also may be asked to swab fluids from a wound or to retract the edges of a wound to help the doctor view the area. While the doctor is closing the wound, you may be required to cut the suture material after each stitch. The doctor may not verbalize every request to you. With practice and after experience with a particular doctor, you will learn how to respond to the doctor's actions.

When cutting suture materials, leave ⅛ inch of the material above the knot. This length prevents the suture from coming untied but is short enough that it does not bother the patient.

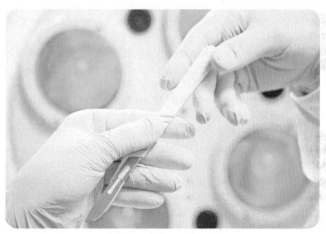

FIGURE 44-15 Hold a scalpel above and just behind the cutting edge as you pass the handle into the palm of the doctor's hand.
©Poprotskiy Alexey/Shutterstock

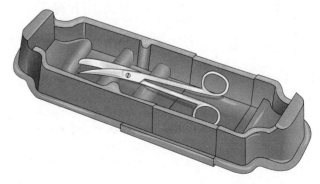

FIGURE 44-16 A passing tray may be used to safely pass sharp instruments during a surgical procedure.

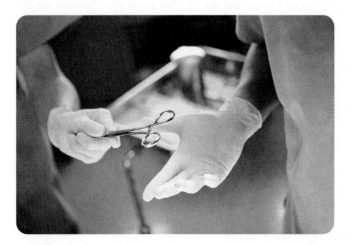

FIGURE 44-14 Holding the scissors by the hinge, slap the handles into the doctor's hand.
©MIXA/Getty Images

▶ Postoperative Procedures   LO 44.7

You will be responsible for the patient's **postoperative** ("post-op") follow-up after the surgical procedure. Your duties may include immediate care of the patient, proper cleaning of the surgical room, and follow-up care of the patient. Procedure 44-6, at the end of this chapter, outlines the tasks performed after a minor surgical procedure.

Immediate Patient Care

Patient care is your top priority as a medical assistant. Except for intravenous medications, you will administer postoperative medications the physician requests for the patient. You also will ensure that the patient remains lying down on the examining table for the prescribed length of time after the procedure. During this period, continue to monitor the patient's vital signs and watch for adverse reactions. Document your observations in the patient's chart.

Dressing the Wound You also may dress the wound during the monitoring period. Dressings are sterile materials used to cover an incision. They serve a number of functions. They protect the wound from further injury and keep the wound clean, thus preventing infection. Dressings also reduce bleeding, absorb fluid drainage, reduce discomfort to the patient, speed healing, and reduce the possibility of scarring. Gauze dressings are the most common type and come in a variety of sizes and shapes.

Before dressing the wound, don clean exam gloves. Place the sterile dressing over the site and secure it appropriately.

Bandaging the Wound It may be necessary to apply a bandage (a clean strip of gauze or elastic material) over the dressing to help hold it in place. Tube gauze may be needed for bandaging wounds on fingers or other extremities. Application of this type of gauze requires an applicator. The applicator is a wire cage on which the gauze is loaded. Bandages also may be used to improve circulation, to provide support or reduce tension on a wound or suture and prevent it from reopening, or to prevent movement of that area of the body. Adhesive tape also may be used for these purposes. Some patients are allergic to the adhesive, but most tapes are now hypoallergenic. The patient is usually more comfortable after a bandage or adhesive tape has been applied.

Postoperative Instructions After the procedure, provide oral postoperative instructions to the patient. You may do this during the monitoring part of the postoperative period or afterward. These instructions include guidelines for pain management and instructions for wound care. Postoperative information also includes dietary or activity restrictions, if any, and when to come in for a follow-up appointment. It is a good idea to ask patients to repeat what you have said so that you know they understand the information.

Instructions should be provided in writing as part of a complete postoperative information packet. You may be asked to help prepare or update packet materials, especially if you routinely assist patients as they recover from minor surgery. A postoperative information packet might include the following information:

- Proper wound care instructions.
- Suggestions for pain relief and reduction of swelling, such as medications and hot or cold packs.
- Dietary restrictions.
- Activity restrictions.
- Timing for a follow-up appointment or an appointment card.

Wound care instructions include details on changing the dressing, keeping the wound clean, recognizing signs of infection, and protecting the wound. The instructions may vary depending on the depth and size of the wound. In general, the bandage should be removed after the first 24 hours or if it becomes soaked with blood, wet, or dirty. A wet dressing allows bacteria and other contaminants to enter the wound. In most cases, the wound may be cleaned with soap and water after 24 to 48 hours. Once cleaned, the incision should be gently dried and covered with a clean, dry bandage.

You should teach the patient about the signs of infection. For more information, see the *Educating the Patient* feature When to Call the Doctor About a Wound. Encourage the patient to protect the incision from sun exposure for the first 6 months; doing so helps prevent the incision line from becoming darker than the surrounding skin.

EDUCATING THE PATIENT

When to Call the Doctor About a Wound

Whether a wound is postsurgical or from an accident, it is important for patients to know when they should call the doctor. Understanding when a wound needs medical attention can reduce the instances of scarring and infection. You can help by teaching them what to look for when they have a wound. Patients with any wounds should call the office if they have any of the following:

- Jagged or gaping edges.
- A face wound.

- Limited movement in the area of the wound.
- Tenderness or inflammation at the wound site.
- Purulent drainage.
- A fever greater than 100°F.
- Red streaks near the wound.
- A puncture wound.
- Bleeding that does not stop after 10 minutes of pressure.
- Sutures coming out on their own or too early.

The length of time it takes for a wound to heal varies with the site, the patient's age and health status, and the severity of the wound. So each patient needs specific instructions on how long to continue with the dressings and when to return for suture or staple removal. He or she also may need specific information about limiting activities.

Patient Release Notify the doctor when the patient is stabilized and ready to leave. The doctor may want to further observe and instruct the patient. Be sure to offer assistance if the patient needs help getting dressed.

Then help the patient check out. Schedule the next appointment for the patient. Make sure the patient has the correct discharge packet. Confirm arrangements to transport the patient home. Finally, assist the patient to the car or other transport if this is part of office procedure.

If a patient insists on driving himself home, enter this information on the chart. Indicate the time and have the patient initial the entry. This documentation is important for legal reasons. It would clarify liability, should an accident occur as a result of a reaction to the surgery or the anesthetic.

Surgical Room Cleanup

If there is time during the monitoring period, begin to clean up the surgical area. If time is not available then, perform the cleanup routine after the patient has been released. Refer to the *Examination and Treatment Areas* chapter for sanitization and disinfection guidelines.

Follow-Up Care

During a follow-up appointment, the physician examines the patient's surgical wound. The healthcare practitioner may ask you to change the dressing or remove the wound closures. Typically, suture or staple removal takes place 5 to 10 days after minor surgery. The sutures or staples are ready for removal when a clean, unbroken suture line is observed. There should be no scabs, no seepage from the wound, and no visible opening. Any of these signs may indicate unhealed areas. Suture removal is described in Procedure 44-7, at the end of this chapter. Staple removal is similar, except that staple removal forceps, rather than thumb forceps and scissors, are used to remove the staples.

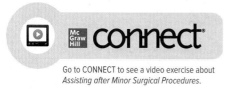

Go to CONNECT to see a video exercise about *Assisting after Minor Surgical Procedures.*

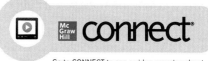

Go to CONNECT to see a video exercise about *Suture Removal.*

PROCEDURE 44-1 Creating a Sterile Field

WORK // DOC

Procedure Goal: To create a sterile field for a minor surgical procedure

OSHA Guidelines: This procedure does not involve exposure to blood, body fluids, or tissues.

Materials: Tray or Mayo stand, sterile instrument pack, sterile transfer forceps, cleaning solution, sterile drape, and additional packaged sterile items as required

Method:

1. Clean and disinfect the tray or Mayo stand.
2. Wash your hands and assemble the necessary materials.
3. Check the label on the instrument pack to make sure it is the correct pack for the procedure.
4. Check the date and sterilization indicator on the instrument pack to make sure the pack is still sterile.
   RATIONALE: *Using an out-of-date pack puts the patient at risk for surgical site infection.*
5. Place the sterile pack on the tray or stand and unfold the outermost fold away from yourself.
6. Unfold the sides of the pack outward, touching only the areas that will become the underside of the sterile field.
   RATIONALE: *Touching the inside of the pack will contaminate the sterile field.*
7. Open the final flap toward yourself, stepping back and away from the sterile field.

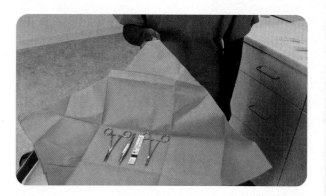

FIGURE Procedure 44-1 Step 7   Open the flap toward yourself last to avoid reaching over the sterile field.
©McGraw-Hill Education

8. Place additional packaged sterile items on the sterile field.
   - Ensure that you have the correct item or instrument and that the package is still sterile.
   - Stand away from the sterile field.
   - Grasp the package flaps and pull apart about halfway.
   - Bring the corners of the wrapping beneath the package, paying attention not to contaminate the inner package or item.
   - Hold the package at the edge of the sterile field with the opening down. Do not reach over the sterile field.

With a quick movement, pull the flap completely open and snap the sterile item onto the field.

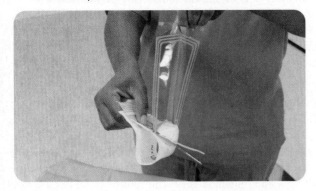

FIGURE Procedure 44-1 Step 8   Hold the package over the sterile field with the opening down. Pulling the flap open, snap the instrument onto the field.
©McGraw-Hill Education

9. Place basins and bowls near the edge of the sterile field so that you can pour liquids without reaching over the field.
    RATIONALE: *Reaching over the field may drop contaminants into the field.*

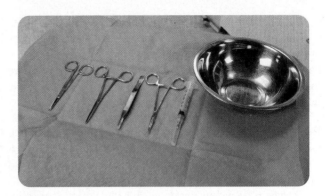

FIGURE Procedure 44-1 Step 9   Placing the bowl at the edge of the sterile field keeps you from reaching over the sterile field when you pour liquids into the bowl.
©McGraw-Hill Education

10. Use sterile transfer forceps to add any additional items to the sterile field.

11. If necessary, don sterile gloves after a sterile scrub to arrange items on the sterile field.

PROCEDURE **44-2** Performing a Surgical Scrub

Procedure Goal: To remove dirt and microorganisms from under the fingernails and from the surface of the skin, hair follicles, and oil glands of the hands and forearms

OSHA Guidelines: This procedure does not involve exposure to blood, body fluids, or tissues.

Materials: Dispenser with surgical soap, sterile surgical scrub brush or sponge, and sterile towels

Method:

1. Remove all jewelry and roll up your sleeves to above the elbow.

2. Assemble the necessary materials.

3. Turn on the faucet using the foot or knee pedal.

4. Wet your hands from fingertips to elbows, keeping your hands higher than your elbows.
    RATIONALE: *This prevents water from running down your arms and contaminating the washed area.*

5. Under running water, use a sterile brush to clean under your fingernails.

6. Apply surgical soap and scrub your hands, fingers, areas between the fingers, wrists, and forearms with the scrub sponge, using a firm, circular motion. Follow the manufacturer's recommendations to determine appropriate length of time (usually 2 to 6 minutes).
    RATIONALE: *Scrubbing all surfaces dislodges microorganisms so that they can be rinsed away.*

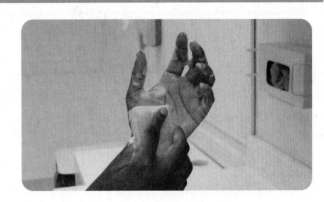

FIGURE Procedure 44-2 Step 6   With a sterile scrub brush, use a circular motion to scrub every surface of your hands and forearms.
©McGraw-Hill Education

7. Rinse from fingers to elbows, always keeping your hands higher than your elbows.

8. Thoroughly dry your hands and forearms with sterile towels, working from the hands to the elbows.
    RATIONALE: *Using sterile towels prevents recontaminating your hands.*

9. Turn off the faucet with the foot or knee pedal. Use a sterile paper towel if a foot or knee pedal is not available.

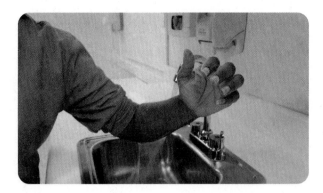

FIGURE Procedure 44-2 Step 7 Keep your hands higher than your elbows when rinsing after a surgical scrub so that water runs away from the fingertips.
©McGraw-Hill Education

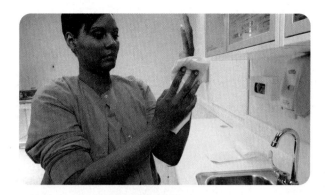

FIGURE Procedure 44-2 Step 8 Dry your hands with sterile towels, working from the hands to the elbows.
©McGraw-Hill Education

PROCEDURE **44-3** Donning Sterile Gloves

Procedure Goal: To don sterile gloves without compromising the sterility of the gloves' outer surface

OSHA Guidelines: This procedure does not involve exposure to blood, body fluids, or tissues.

Materials: Correctly sized, prepackaged, double-wrapped sterile gloves

Method:

1. Obtain the correct size gloves.
2. Check the package for tears and ensure that the expiration date has not passed.
   RATIONALE: *A torn or expired package should be considered unsterile.*
3. Perform a surgical scrub.
4. Peel the outer wrap from the gloves and place the inner wrapper on a clean surface above waist level.

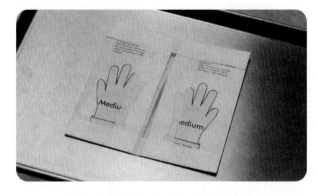

FIGURE Procedure 44-3 Step 4 Place the inner wrap on a clean surface, above waist level, with the cuff end closest to your body.
©McGraw-Hill Education

5. Position gloves so that the cuff end is closest to your body.
6. Touch only the flaps as you open the package.
   RATIONALE: *Touching the inside of the package could contaminate the gloves.*

7. Use instructions provided on the inner package, if available.
8. Do not reach over the sterile inside of the inner package.
9. Follow these steps if there are no instructions:
   a. Open the package so that the first flap is opened away from you.
   b. Pinch the corner and pull to one side.
   c. Put your fingertips under the side flaps and gently pull until the package is completely open.
10. Use your nondominant hand to grasp the inside cuff of the opposite glove (the folded edge). Do not touch the outside of the glove. If you are right-handed, use your left hand to put on the right glove first, and vice versa.
    RATIONALE: *Grabbing the inside of the glove allows you to put it on without contaminating its outside.*
11. Holding the glove at arm's length and waist level, insert the dominant hand into the glove, palm facing up. Do not let the outside of the glove touch any other surface.

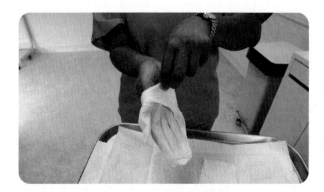

FIGURE Procedure 44-3 Step 11 When donning the glove, do not let the outside of the glove touch any other surface.
©McGraw-Hill Education

12. With your sterile gloved hand, slip the gloved fingers into the cuff of the other glove.

13. Pick up the other glove, touching only the outside. Do not touch any other surfaces.

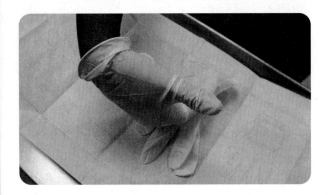

FIGURE Procedure 44-3 Step 13   Slip the fingers of your gloved hand into the other glove's cuff, touching only the outside.
©McGraw-Hill Education

14. Pull the glove up and onto your hand, ensuring that the sterile gloved hand does not touch your skin.

15. Adjust your fingers as necessary, touching only glove to glove.

16. Do not adjust the cuffs because your forearms may contaminate the gloves.

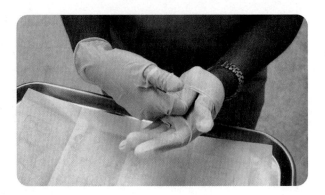

FIGURE Procedure 44-3 Step 14   Pull the glove up and onto your hand without touching the sterile gloved hand to your skin.
©McGraw-Hill Education

17. Keep your hands in front of you, between your shoulders and waist. If you move your hands out of this area, they are considered contaminated.

18. If contamination or the possibility of contamination occurs, change gloves.

19. Remove these gloves the same way you remove clean gloves, by touching only the inside.
RATIONALE: *Touching only the inside of the gloves reduces exposure to the patient's blood and body fluids.*

PROCEDURE 44-4   Assisting as a Floater (Unsterile Assistant) During Minor Surgical Procedures

WORK // DOC

Procedure Goal: To provide assistance to the doctor during minor surgery while maintaining clean or sterile technique as appropriate

OSHA Guidelines:

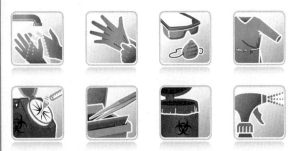

Materials: Sterile towel, tray or Mayo stand, appropriate instrument pack(s), needles and syringes, anesthetic, antiseptic, sterile water or normal saline, small sterile bowl, sterile gauze squares or cotton balls, specimen containers half-filled with preservative, suture materials, sterile dressings, tape, patient's chart/progress note, laboratory requisition form

Method:

1. Perform routine handwashing and don exam gloves.

2. Monitor the patient during the procedure; record the results in the patient's chart.

3. During the surgery, assist as needed.

4. Add sterile items to the tray as necessary.

5. Pour sterile solution into a sterile bowl as needed.

6. Assist in administering additional anesthetic.
   a. Check the medication vial two times.
   b. Clean the rubber stopper with an alcohol pad (write the date opened when using a new bottle); leave the pad on top.
   c. Present the needle and syringe to the doctor.
   d. Remove the alcohol pad from the vial and show the label to the doctor.
   e. Hold the vial upside down and grasp the lower edge firmly; brace your wrist with your free hand.
   RATIONALE: *This firmly supports the vial to sustain the force of the needle being inserted into the rubber stopper.*
   f. Allow the doctor to fill the syringe.
   g. Check the medication vial a final time.

7. Receive specimens for laboratory examination.
   a. Uncap the specimen container; present it to the doctor for the specimen's introduction.
   b. Replace the cap and label the container.
   c. Treat all specimens as infectious.
   d. Place the specimen container in a transport bag or other container.
   e. Complete the requisition form to send the specimen to the laboratory.

PROCEDURE 44-5 Assisting as a Sterile Scrub Assistant During Minor Surgical Procedures

Procedure Goal: To provide assistance to the doctor during minor surgery while maintaining clean or sterile technique as appropriate

OSHA Guidelines:

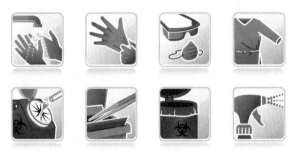

Materials: Sterile towel, tray or Mayo stand, appropriate instrument pack(s), needles and syringes, anesthetic, antiseptic, sterile water or normal saline, small sterile bowl, sterile gauze squares or cotton balls, specimen containers half-filled with preservative, suture materials, sterile dressings, and tape

Method:

1. Perform a surgical scrub and don sterile gloves. (Remember, remove the sterile towel covering the sterile field and instruments before gloving.)
   RATIONALE: *You will be handling sterile instruments.*
2. Close and arrange the surgical instruments on the tray.
   RATIONALE: *They should be quickly and easily located.*
3. Prepare for swabbing by inserting gauze squares into the sterile dressing forceps.
4. Pass the instruments as necessary.
5. Swab the wound as requested.
6. Retract the wound as requested.
7. Cut the sutures as requested.

PROCEDURE 44-6 Assisting After Minor Surgical Procedures

Procedure Goal: To provide assistance to the doctor during and the patient after minor surgery while maintaining clean or sterile technique as appropriate

OSHA Guidelines:

Materials: Examination gloves, antiseptic, tray or Mayo stand, sterile dressings, and tape

Method:

1. Monitor the patient.
2. Don clean exam gloves and clean the wound with antiseptic.
3. Dress the wound.
   RATIONALE: *To protect the wound.*
4. Remove the gloves and wash your hands.
5. Give the patient oral postoperative instructions in addition to the release packet.
   RATIONALE: *The patient will need to understand wound care, medication use, and dietary instructions for proper healing.*
6. Discharge the patient.
7. Put on clean exam gloves.
8. Properly dispose of used materials and disposable instruments.
9. Sanitize reusable instruments and prepare them for disinfection and/or sterilization as needed.
10. Clean equipment and the exam room according to OSHA guidelines.
11. Remove the gloves and wash your hands.

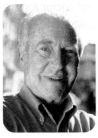

Recall Peter Smith from the case study at the beginning of the chapter. Now that you have completed the chapter, answer the following questions regarding his case.

1. What is the medical assistant's role before, during, and after this minor surgical procedure?

2. Why is it important to document the number of sutures Dr. Buckwalter uses to close Peter Smith's wound?

3. How should you answer Peter Smith's question about his trip to the Bahamas?

4. Knowing that Peter Smith started swimming last week, what should you tell him about protecting his sutures?

©Image Source/Getty Images

EXAM PREPARATION QUESTIONS

1. (LO 44.2) The removal of dead tissue from a wound is known as
   a. Incision
   b. Debridement
   c. Ligature
   d. Cauterization
   e. Approximation

2. (LO 44.3) An instrument used to clear a blockage is a
   a. Probe
   b. Scalpel
   c. Retractor
   d. Syringe
   e. Forceps

3. (LO 44.4) Why is it important to keep your hands higher than your elbows when performing a surgical scrub?
   a. To avoid touching the sink
   b. So that the soap reaches the elbows
   c. To prevent water from contaminating the washed area
   d. It is not important to keep the hands higher than the elbows.
   e. Your hands should be lower than your elbows.

4. (LO 44.2) Another name for a mole is a
   a. Wart
   b. Hemangioma
   c. Ligature
   d. Birthmark
   e. Nevus

5. (LO 44.3) Which of the following is the suture with the smallest diameter?
   a. 2
   b. 2-0
   c. 3
   d. 3-0
   e. 4-0

6. (LO 44.2) A jagged, open wound of the skin is a(n)
   a. Incision
   b. Avulsion
   c. Laceration
   d. Puncture
   e. Abrasion

7. (LO 44.4) When adding solutions to a sterile field, you should cover the label with your palm to keep it
   a. Sterile
   b. Dry
   c. From pouring too quickly
   d. From dripping
   e. Visible

8. (LO 44.5) A medical assistant is working in the preoperative area. Which of the following duties would he most likely perform?
   a. Prepare the surgical room
   b. Perform a surgical scrub
   c. Clean the surgical room
   d. Work as a floater
   e. Work as a surgical scrub assistant

9. (LO 44.7) Sterile materials used to cover an incision are
   a. Bandages
   b. Sterile strips
   c. Sutures
   d. Drapes
   e. Dressings
10. (LO 44.3) What type of instrument is a curette?
   a. Probing and dilating
   b. Cutting and dissecting
   c. Grasping
   d. Retracting
   e. Clamping

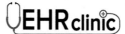

Go to CONNECT to complete the EHRclinic exercises: 44.01 Document a Patient's Informed Consent and 44.02 Document Patient Education - Wound Care after Mole Removal.

SOFT SKILLS SUCCESS

You are assisting Dr. Sanford with a mole removal. You have already set up the surgical tray and are handing Dr. Sanford her sterile gloves. She tells you that she prefers a no. 11 scalpel blade for this procedure. You know you set up the tray with a no. 10 scalpel blade. How should you respond to Dr. Sanford, and what action should you take?

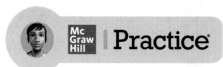

Go to PRACTICE MEDICAL OFFICE and complete the module Clinical: Work Task Proficiencies.

Orientation to the Lab

	Patient Name	DOB	Allergies
PATIENT INFORMATION	Sylvia Gonzales	09/01/1968	PCN
	Attending	**MRN**	**Other Information**
	Alexis N. Whalen, MD	00-AA-004	Last Hemoglobin A1C 6.3%

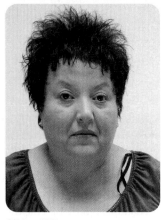
©McGraw-Hill Education

Sylvia Gonzales is at the office for a 3-month return check for her newly diagnosed Type 2 diabetes. She states that she has taken the medication she received for her "sugar," and she knows the doctor wants to a do a special "sugar test" this time. Her medication list includes Januvia® 100 mg daily.

The physician has ordered a fasting blood sugar (FBS) and a hemo-globin A1C blood test. You will need to perform both of these waived tests in your office lab.

Keep Sylvia Gonzales in mind as you study this chapter. There will be questions at the end of the chapter based on the case study. The information in the chapter will help you answer these questions.

LEARNING OUTCOMES

After completing Chapter 45, you will be able to:

45.1 Describe the purpose of the physician's office laboratory.

45.2 Identify the medical assistant's duties in the physician's office laboratory.

45.3 Identify important pieces of laboratory equipment.

45.4 Illustrate measures to prevent accidents.

45.5 Explain the goal of a quality assurance program in a physician's office laboratory.

45.6 Carry out communication with patients regarding test preparation and follow-up.

45.7 Carry out accurate documentation, including patient results, specimen tracking, laboratory requests, and inventory control.

KEY TERMS

artifact
centrifuge
Certificate of Waiver tests
compound microscope
control sample
objectives
ocular
oil-immersion objective
optical microscope
photometer
physician's office laboratory (POL)

point of care tests (POCT)
proficiency testing program
qualitative test response
quality assurance program
quality control program
quantitative test result
reagent
reference laboratory
standard
10× lens

I.C.10 Identify CLIA waived tests associated with common diseases

I.C.12 Identify quality assurance practices in healthcare

I.P.10 Perform a quality control measure

I.A.3 Show awareness of a patient's concerns related to the procedure being performed

III.C.5 Define the principles of standard precautions

X.P.7 Complete an incident report related to an error in patient care

II.A. 1. Reassure a patient of the accuracy of the test results

3. Medical Terminology
   c. Apply medical terminology for each specialty
   d. Define and use medical abbreviations when appropriate and acceptable

4. Medical Law and Ethics
   a. Follow documentation guidelines

8. Clinical Procedures
   a. Practice standard precautions and perform disinfection/sterilization techniques

9. Medical Laboratory Procedures
   a. Practice quality control
   b. Perform selected CLIA-waived tests that assist with diagnosis and treatment
      (1) Urinalysis
      (6) Kit testing
   c. Dispose of biohazardous materials

▶ Introduction

Laboratory testing of patients' specimens is an integral component of patient care. Medical assistants often perform a role in the clinical laboratory setting in the physician's office. This chapter will introduce you to the various types and uses of common laboratory equipment. You will learn about safety in the laboratory and steps to aid in preventing accidents. A discussion of the Clinical Laboratory Improvement Amendments of 1988 (CLIA '88) and this law's impact on the laboratory setting is included in this chapter to help you understand quality assurance, quality control procedures, and required recordkeeping.

▶ The Role of Laboratory Testing in Patient Care
LO 45.1

Laboratory analysis of blood, urine, or other body fluids and substances provides three kinds of information about a patient. First, regular monitoring through laboratory tests, such as those that are part of an annual exam, can help a physician identify possible diseases or other problems. Second, specific tests can help confirm or contradict a physician's initial diagnosis. Third, laboratory testing can help a physician determine and monitor the proper dosage of a patient's medication.

Kinds of Laboratories

Some physicians prefer to have all laboratory tests performed by a **reference laboratory,** a laboratory owned and operated by an organization outside the practice. Other physicians choose to have some tests completed by the reference laboratory and some completed in the office in the **physician's office laboratory (POL).**

Each method of managing laboratory analyses has advantages and disadvantages. Reference laboratories often have more technological resources than those available in the POL. A reference laboratory offers a complete range of tests in all specialties and subspecialties, including:

- Cytology—microscopic examination of cells to make a diagnosis; Pap smears (tests for detecting cervical cancer) are evaluated in the cytology department.
- Toxicology—testing to identify poisons or other chemicals in the body; workplace drug testing is a type of toxicology test.
- Immunology—testing to identify disorders and diseases of the immune system; tests for autoimmune diseases are performed in the immunology department.
- Blood banking—the laboratory department responsible for processing and storing blood and blood products for transfusion and blood disorder treatments; this department would provide blood to someone with severe anemia who needs a transfusion.
- Urinalysis—testing urine for kidney diseases and disorders and certain metabolic disorders; testing for glucose in the urine (a test done on people with diabetes) is part of a urinalysis.
- Histology—microscopic evaluation of tissues to make a diagnosis; a biopsy of a skin lesion is sent to the histology department to examine the tissue for signs of cancer.
- Serology—testing the liquid part of the blood for antibodies against specific microorganisms; testing for malaria and viral hepatitis are serologic tests.

- Chemistry—testing for certain substances in the blood, urine, or other body fluids; substances tested for include cholesterol, electrolytes, glucose, calcium, and potassium; a lipid panel for cholesterol and triglycerides is a blood chemistry test.
- Microbiology—testing for the presence of pathogenic microorganisms such as bacteria, viruses, fungi, protozoans, and parasites in blood, urine, sputum, reproductive fluids, and fluids from wounds; a nasal culture for MRSA is a microbiology test.
- Hematology—testing of blood to identify problems with count, size, or number of blood cells to diagnose diseases and disorders; testing for anemia and leukemia are hematology tests.

Using a reference laboratory frees a physician's staff from testing duties and allows more time for patient care. It also reduces or eliminates the cost of running an in-house lab. Furthermore, some managed care companies have contracts with laboratory companies that require their subscribers to use a specific reference laboratory. An advantage of a POL is that processing tests produces a quicker turnaround and eliminates the need for the patient to travel to other test locations.

The Purpose of the Physician's Office Laboratory

Office policy determines which tests, if any, will be performed at your location and which tests will be performed by a reference laboratory. A POL, like the one shown in Figure 45-1, is responsible for accurate and timely processing of routine tests and for reporting test results to the physician. Tests most often performed in the POL include chemical analyses, hematologic tests, microbiologic tests, and urinalysis.

Point-of-Care Testing

Over the last few decades, there has been a growing trend to bring laboratory testing closer to the patient's location. To this end, point-of-care tests are increasingly being utilized in healthcare. **Point-of-care tests (POCT)** are tests performed at or near the patient, normally where the patient is being treated. POCTs are not meant to replace large reference labs or POLs; instead, they are meant to be used in conjunction with these facilities. In general, reference labs and POLs are involved in preliminary patient diagnosis, and POCTs are used to monitor the patient's condition after the diagnosis is made. POCTs may be used by healthcare practitioners in the facility or by the patient at home. Think about a patient who has diabetes. Most likely, she has a glucometer—a handheld device used to check blood sugar—that she uses on a regular basis. Glucometers were some of the first POCT devices available.

There are a variety of other POCTs available today. These include but are not limited to:

- Pregnancy tests.
- Urine dipstick tests.
- Hemoglobin concentration tests.

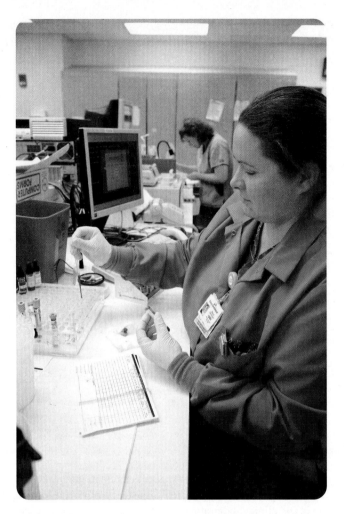

FIGURE 45-1 A physician's office laboratory (POL) may be simple or elaborate, depending on the tests the office performs.
©Jim West/Alamy Stock Photo

- Fecal occult blood detection tests.
- Rapid strep tests.
- Rapid influenza tests.
- Blood clotting tests.

POCTs are used in emergency departments, radiology departments, and ambulances; during natural disaster recovery (hurricanes, earthquakes, etc.); on cruise ships; and even on the International Space Station.

The benefits of these tests include:

- Shorter waiting times for test results.
- Earlier treatment for diseases and conditions.
- Decreased number of follow-up appointments to get lab results.
- Increased patient involvement in his or her own care.
- Test results in remote areas that do not have comprehensive labs.

As a medical assistant, you should be aware of certain cautions or challenges associated with POCTs. The tests are relatively simple but are not completely error proof. Make sure you follow the instructions that come with the test. Different instruments may have slightly different instructions, including sample size or waiting times. Patients should be trained in the use of a POCT device before they are sent home to perform the test on their own. Any questionable results should be reported to the healthcare practitioner so that additional testing at a reference lab or POL can be ordered.

Remember, even though the tests are easy to perform and give the patient nearly immediate results, point-of-care tests must be treated like any other lab tests. This means the results must be documented in the patient's medical record. No matter how simple the test, if it is not documented, it is not done! Point-of-care testing is a valuable resource for patient care. It is fast, convenient, simple, and, if done correctly, reliable, but it should be used in conjunction with more comprehensive testing at a reference lab or POL.

▶ The Medical Assistant's Role   LO 45.2

As a medical assistant, you may be responsible for processing tests done in the POL, including preparing the patient for the test, collecting the sample, completing the test, reporting the results to the physician, and communicating information about the test from the physician to the patient. Your role in the POL requires you to integrate a great deal of information to serve both the physician and the patient effectively. You will need to master the following subjects:

- Use of laboratory equipment.
- Regulations governing laboratory practices and procedures.
- Precautions for accident prevention.
- Waste disposal requirements.
- Housekeeping and maintenance routines.
- Quality assurance and control procedures.
- Technical aspects of specimen collection and test processing, including expected results.
- Communication with patients.
- Reporting of test results to the physician.
- Recordkeeping of test specimens, procedures, and results.
- Inventory and ordering of equipment and supplies.
- Use of reference materials in the POL.
- Screening and follow-up of test results.

▶ Use of Laboratory Equipment   LO 45.3

As a medical assistant, you must be familiar with the operation of common laboratory equipment. Learning to use a specific piece of equipment may take the form of on-the-job training or attending training programs conducted by manufacturers' representatives. You may routinely use the following equipment:

- Autoclave.
- Centrifuge.
- Microscope.
- Electronic equipment and software.
- Equipment used for measurement.

Autoclave

A steam autoclave is used to sterilize, or eradicate, all organisms on the surfaces of instruments and equipment before they are used on a patient or in testing procedures. Use of the autoclave is discussed in the *Infection Control Practices* chapter.

Centrifuge

A **centrifuge** is a device for spinning a specimen at high speed until it separates into its component parts. The centrifuge in a POL is generally used to separate whole blood samples into blood components or to prepare urine samples for examination. Use of a centrifuge is described in greater detail in the *Collecting, Processing, and Testing Urine and Stool Specimens* chapter.

Microscope

An instrument often used in a POL is the microscope, commonly used for the examination of blood smears and identification of microorganisms in body fluid samples. Although on-site blood smear evaluation is convenient and fast for both patient and physician, it is important to know which procedures are routinely covered. Only CLIA-approved microscopy procedures are eligible for payment by Medicare and Medicaid. Table 45-1 lists CLIA-approved provider-performed microscopy procedures.

The **optical microscope,** also called the light microscope, is the type most often found in the POL (Figure 45-2). With this type of microscope, light is concentrated (condensed) through a condenser and then focused through the object being examined. This produces an image of the object. **Compound microscopes** use two lenses to magnify the image. The effect of the two lenses is compounded—added together—giving greater magnification than one lens can provide. Compound microscopes are the most common type of optical microscope used in the medical office.

TABLE 45-1	CLIA-Approved Provider-Performed Microscopy Procedures
Wet mounts—vaginal, cervical, or skin specimens	
Potassium hydroxide preparations	
Pinworm examinations	
Fern test (for the presence of amniotic fluid in vaginal secretions)	
Urinalysis by dipstick with microscopy	
Urinalysis; two or three glass test (for the presence of blood 1—at the beginning of the urine stream, 2—midstream, and/or 3—at the termination of urination)	
Fecal leukocyte examination	
Semen analysis (for presence or motility of sperm)	
Nasal smears for eosinophils	

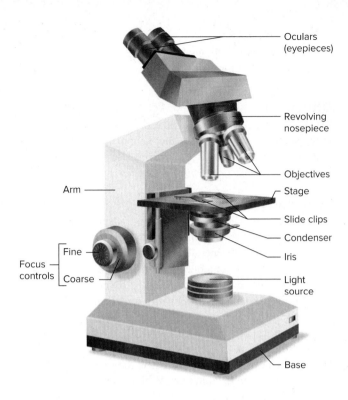

FIGURE 45-2 The microscope is an often-used piece of equipment in a POL.

You must be able to operate an optical microscope correctly. First, you need to become familiar with the component parts, described in the following paragraphs.

Oculars The **oculars** are the eyepieces through which you view the image. A microscope is either monocular, with a single eyepiece, or binocular, with two eyepieces. You can adjust the oculars on a binocular microscope to compensate for differences in visual acuity between your right and left eyes. You also can adjust the distance between oculars to match the distance between your eyes. The ocular contains a magnifying lens—called a **10× lens**—that usually magnifies an image 10 times.

Objectives Just below the ocular or oculars, the **objectives** are mounted on a swivel or rotating base called the *nosepiece*. These are known as objectives because they are closest to the object being magnified. An objective contains another magnifying lens. Generally, microscopes used in the POL have a three-piece objective system with three different magnifications. An objective is moved into position directly under the ocular by rotating the nosepiece.

Two of the objectives are dry objectives; this means there is air space between the specimen under examination and the objective. Condensed (concentrated) light passes through the specimen and the air space above the specimen and then travels toward the objective lens. These dry objectives are low- and high-power lenses, usually 10× and 40×, respectively. When the low-power objective lens is combined with the ocular lenses, the total magnification

factor is 100× (10× times 10×). The high-power lens and ocular lenses yield a magnification factor of 400× (10× times 40×).

The third objective is an **oil-immersion objective,** which is used for specimens that need extreme magnification, such as blood smears and bacteriologic slides. It is designed to be lowered into a drop of immersion oil placed directly on the slide above the prepared specimen under examination. This design eliminates the air space between the microscope slide and the objective, where some of the light scatters beyond the objective. Placing the end of the objective in oil reduces the loss of light by creating a column of oil that tightly focuses the light, keeping it from scattering. This results in a much sharper, brighter image, allowing for greater magnification. An oil-immersion objective has a magnification factor of 100×. Combined with the ocular lenses, the total magnification factor is 1,000×.

Arm and Focus Controls The ocular(s) and objectives, collectively referred to as the body tube, are attached to the base of the microscope by the arm. The microscope arm is also the location of the focus controls. The two focus controls—coarse and fine—move the body tube up and down to bring into focus the object being examined.

Stage and Substage The objectives and oculars are focused on a specimen placed on the microscope's stage. The stage is the platform on which the specimen slide rests, held in place by metal clips. Located directly under the stage is the substage. This is where the condenser, which concentrates the light and focuses it through the sample on the slide, is located. Also located on the substage is the iris. The iris is a diaphragm that opens and closes like the shutter of a camera to increase or decrease the amount of light illuminating the specimen. The stage is controlled by the stage mechanisms, which control left-right and forward-backward movements of the stage, allowing you to examine different areas of the specimen without reseating the slide.

Light Source Under the stage and substage assemblies is the light source. Most POL microscopes use a built-in electric light source, and most of these are equipped with controls that allow you to adjust the light intensity. In place of a built-in light source, older microscopes use a mirror, which gathers and focuses light from a microscope lamp onto the specimen.

Specimen Slides and Coverslip Although the specimen slide is not technically part of the microscope assembly, it is necessary for using the microscope. All specimens must be placed on slides. Many specimens also require a coverslip, or cover glass. The slide and coverslip support and position the specimen. They also prevent contamination of the microscope by the specimen. Specimens that are to be stained or immersed in oil, such as blood smears, do not require coverslips.

Using an Optical Microscope To use an optical microscope, you must be able to focus it using each of the

Care and Maintenance of the Microscope

The microscope is the workhorse of the POL. For it to provide trouble-free service, however, it must be well cared for. Dust, oil, and other contaminants cause major problems with microscopes. Careless cleaning and haphazard storage also will eventually cause problems. These problems may include mechanical difficulties with the microscope or contamination of the specimen being examined. Foreign objects visible through a microscope but unrelated to the specimen are called **artifacts** and may be misinterpreted when the specimen is examined.

Clean the microscope after each use. Inspect the body tube, arm, and stage to make sure they are dust- and contaminant-free. Clean the ocular and objective lenses with lens paper, not tissue or other products. Tissue fibers are a common artifact. The eyepiece is an area in which skin oil, dust, and eye makeup may collect, posing a risk of disease transmission and making images difficult to see. Use lens-cleaning products according to the manufacturer's guidelines. Excess amounts of these products may dissolve the cement holding the lenses in place, rendering the microscope useless.

When not in use, the microscope should be stored under its plastic cover. If there is a power cord, wrap it loosely around the base and secure it with a twist-tie or elastic band. Lower the low-power objective close to the stage and center the stage.

If the microscope must be moved, hold it by the arm and support it under the base. Never carry a microscope with one hand or by just the arm. Carry the cord so that it does not dangle and pose a tripping hazard. Place the microscope on a sturdy table or bench, away from the edge.

---

three objectives. Procedure 45-1, at the end of this chapter, describes how to operate an optical microscope correctly.

You also will be responsible for the proper care and maintenance of the optical microscope in your office. Related concerns and techniques are described in the *Caution: Handle with Care* feature Care and Maintenance of the Microscope.

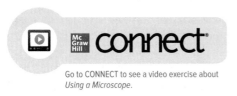

Go to CONNECT to see a video exercise about *Using a Microscope.*

Electronic Equipment and Software

Electronic equipment is used in the POL because it is safer, more accurate, and more efficient than manual methods; generally requires little maintenance; and does not require extensive training prior to its use. A wide variety of tasks, such as cell counting and complex chemical analyses, are performed with electronic equipment. A range of clinical laboratory software systems are available, which are used to create and maintain clinical data, making remote access and tracking between facilities easier. Manufacturers' instructions for operation and maintenance of these systems must be followed to ensure safety, efficiency, and reliable results.

A **photometer,** which measures light intensity, is a basic electronic component of many pieces of analytic laboratory equipment. A handheld glucometer (Figure 45-3), for example, may contain a photometer that measures reflected light. Patients with diabetes and clinical personnel use a glucometer to monitor blood glucose levels.

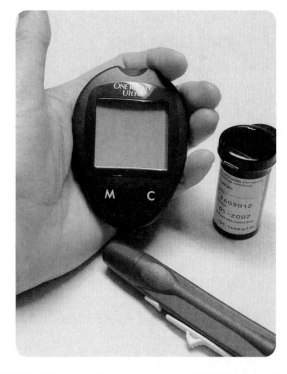

FIGURE 45-3 A handheld glucometer translates the amount of reflected light into the level of glucose in a blood sample.
©Leesa Whicker

Equipment Used for Measurement

Precise measurement is critical in the POL because it produces accurate test results. Much of this measurement is built into the electronic equipment or premeasured kits you will use. However, you still will need to perform various measurements manually when blood, semen, urine, and other body fluids are analyzed using manual tests. Some reagents also require measuring.

Metric system units are commonly used in the POL. For information on metric system weight, height, and temperature measurements, see the *Vital Signs and Measurements* chapter. To learn how to convert between measurement systems, see the *Dosage Calculations* chapter.

A variety of equipment are used to provide accurate measurements. You must take these measurements carefully for them to be of value in the final test results. Other types of measuring equipment include:

- Pipettes (mechanical or manual)—used to measure small amounts of liquids.
- Volumetric or graduated flasks or beakers—used to measure the relatively large amounts (volumes) of liquids necessary for reagents and solutions.
- A hemocytometer—a specialized slide calibrated to the exact measurements needed to count blood cells and sperm under a microscope.
- Thermometers (generally in degrees centigrade)—used to provide legal documentation that refrigerators, bacterial incubators, and other appliances maintain the precise temperature range required for accurate laboratory work.

▶ Safety in the Laboratory LO 45.4

Safety is a primary concern in any laboratory environment, and it is especially important in a physician's office laboratory because patients and laboratory workers may be at risk. For your own protection, as well as that of patients and coworkers, you always must be aware of and observe laboratory safety guidelines.

Use standard precautions when handling all body fluids, excretions, and secretions. If you have any doubt about whether you need to take precautions, take them. Even though some substances do not present a risk of transmitting blood-borne pathogens, they may present a high risk of transmitting other bacteria, viruses, or parasites. Follow these guidelines:

- Wear gloves when handling all body fluids, secretions, and excretions.
- Change gloves every time you move from patient to patient as you collect specimens for testing.
- Wash your hands immediately after removing used gloves.
- Wear other protective gear such as eye protection and face masks during procedures in which there is a risk that droplets or spray may come in contact with your eyes, nose, or mouth.
- Take special care to avoid injury from sharp or pointed instruments or equipment. Although gloves protect you from surface exposure to potentially infected substances, they offer little protection against exposure from needlesticks or cuts. Never use needles or other sharp instruments unnecessarily.
- Use only recommended instruments and equipment. A once-common laboratory technique that has been discontinued

is the use of a mouth pipette (a type of calibrated glass or plastic straw) to transfer specimens. Under no circumstances should you use a mouth pipette to transfer blood from one collection device to another; doing so puts you at risk for getting blood or other hazardous fluids in your mouth.

- Take care to prevent spills and splashes when transporting specimens to the laboratory and when moving specimens in the laboratory.
- If a work surface becomes contaminated because of spilling or splashing, disinfect the area completely, using an approved solution such as 10% bleach, before beginning any other procedure.
- Dispose of waste products carefully and correctly.
- Be sure to remove protective gear before leaving the laboratory.

Biologic Safety

You will work with test specimens that may be contaminated with bloodborne or other pathogens. Treat every specimen as if it were contaminated. Additional information regarding OSHA's Bloodborne Pathogens Standard may be found in the *Infection Control Fundamentals* chapter. Follow standard precautions.

- If you have any cuts, lesions, or sores, do not expose yourself to potentially contaminated material. Consult your supervisor if you have any doubt about whether you can safely perform test procedures.
- Wash your hands before and after every procedure and whenever you come in contact with a potentially contaminated substance.
- Wear gloves at all times. Use other protective gear as appropriate to prevent exposing your eyes, nose, and mouth to potentially contaminated material.
- Mouth pipetting is prohibited at all times. Use specially made rubber suction bulbs to draw specimens mechanically.
- Work in a biologic safety cabinet (similar to a fume hood) when completing procedures that are likely to generate droplet sprays or splashes of potentially contaminated material.
- When transferring a blood specimen from a collection tube to another container, wear appropriate PPE (including a mask and goggles or a face shield) and cover the tube stopper with an absorbent pad or a commercial stopper remover to prevent spray or splatter from the tube. Do not rock the stopper back and forth because this could cause the tube to break. Always remove the stopper by opening it away from your face so that the vapor pressure flows away from you. Place the stopper on a sterile gauze pad while you work with the collection tube. Do not allow the stopper to come in contact with other work surfaces. Keep the collection tube stoppered unless you are actively using it.
- Establish clean and dirty areas in the laboratory. Place all used instruments and equipment in the dirty area for sanitization, disinfection, and sterilization.

- Disinfect your work area at least once a day with a 10% bleach solution or a germ-killing solution approved by the Environmental Protection Agency (EPA). If a spill occurs, immediately disinfect the work area.
- Dispose of waste products immediately.
- Dispose of needles in the appropriate sharps container.
- If an instrument or piece of equipment must be serviced, be sure it has been decontaminated first.
- If you use a bleach solution for disinfection, change it daily.

Accident Reporting

Despite all precautions, laboratory accidents still occur. Armed with an understanding of the materials with which you are working and basic first-aid procedures, you should be able to deal with most emergencies. Your office also should have written procedures to follow in the event of an accident. Familiarize yourself with the procedures beforehand so that you will know what to do if an accident occurs.

If the accident involves exposure to blood or blood products, OSHA regulations require that several steps be followed:

1. Immediate cleaning of the area, including disinfection of contaminated surfaces and sterilization of contaminated instruments and equipment.
2. Notification of a designated emergency contact, as identified in your office's safety manual.
3. Documentation of the incident on a form similar to that shown in Figure 45-4, including the names of all parties involved, the names of witnesses, a description of the incident, and a record of medical treatments given to those involved.
4. Medical evaluation and follow-up exam of the employees involved.
5. Written evaluation of the medical condition of the involved individuals and testing for infection, provided that such testing does not violate confidentiality regulations.

Housekeeping

There is a high risk of serious contamination in the laboratory, and housekeeping duties are designed to reduce this risk. Great care must be taken by following these guidelines to ensure good operating procedures and to reduce the risk of infection:

- Refer to your office's written policies and procedures to ensure that you are performing housekeeping duties correctly and according to schedule.
- Immediately clean up spills or splashes of potentially contaminated material. Depending on the material, you may need to use special hazardous waste control products, such as those shown in Figure 45-5. Be sure to dry the area, if appropriate, or clearly indicate that the area is still wet.
- Clean laboratory equipment immediately after use. Contaminants often become hard to remove if they are left on for a long time.

- Dispose of waste products carefully and correctly.
- Use extreme caution when handling and disposing of sharps.

▶ Quality Assurance Programs   LO 45.5

The operation of a POL can have a significant impact on the health of the patients who depend on the medical practice for care. Accurate patient specimen testing is a primary concern. A **quality assurance program** is designed to monitor the quality of the patient care a medical laboratory provides. It also helps to ensure laboratory worker safety. An effective quality assurance program should be a written plan that includes both internal and external reviews of procedures. It assesses the quality of the tests performed in a clinical laboratory based on a set of written standards and procedures.

Clinical Laboratory Improvement Amendments

In response to public concern over the accuracy of laboratory tests, Congress enacted the Clinical Laboratory Improvement Amendments of 1988 (CLIA '88). This law placed all laboratory facilities that conduct tests for diagnosing, preventing, or treating human disease or for assessing human health under federal regulations administered by the Centers for Medicare and Medicaid Services (CMS) and the CDC. State governments may implement their own standards, which must be at least as stringent as federal standards. If your state has its own standards, your office will operate under those standards. The state health department provides information about which standards to follow in a given locale.

CLIA '88 has had a major impact on office laboratories. Because of the complexity of the regulations and the expense required to meet them, many doctors have closed their laboratories or sharply reduced the number of tests they perform. Several attempts have been made to change the federal legislation, including an effort to exempt POLs from the regulations. As the healthcare debate continues, you may see changes in laboratory operations as a result of changes in CLIA '88 regulations.

CLIA '88 standards apply to four areas of laboratory operation:

- Standards—requirements for maintaining a laboratory; specific standards are determined by the complexity of the test.
- Fees—charges for maintaining a laboratory.
- Enforcement—penalties imposed for violating CLIA standards.
- Proficiency testing programs—for laboratories that perform moderate- to high-complexity testing; labs in this category must go through a special inspection and assessment to perform tests that are moderately or highly complex.

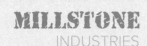

Central State Division
Incident Report

Name of Injured Employee ....

Department .... Job Title ....

Supervisor ....

Date of Accident .... Time ....

Nature of Injury ....

Was injured acting in a regular line of duty? ....

Was first aid given? .... By whom? ....

Was designated emergency contact notified? ....

Did injured receive medical treatment? ....

Was injured tested for infection? .... If no, why not? ....

Did injured go to ER? .... Other? ....

Did injured leave work? .... Date .... Hour .... A.M. P.M.

Did injured return to work? .... Date .... Hour .... A.M. P.M.

Other Parties Involved ....

Names of Witnesses ....

Describe where and how accident occurred. ....

What, in your opinion, caused the accident? ....

Has anything been done to prevent a similar accident? ....

Has the hazard causing the injury been reported by telephone or in writing? ....

Date	Employee's Signature
Date	Supervisor's Signature

IF TREATMENT IS NEEDED, TAKE THE ORIGINAL AND DUPLICATE OF THIS FORM TO
THE EMERGENCY ROOM.

This part for Employee Health Office use only

Was incident investigated? ....

Has injured had follow-up medical care? ....

Comments ....

Original copy to Employee Health Office   Duplicate copy to supervisor

FIGURE 45-4   In the event of an accident or exposure incident in the POL, OSHA regulations require completion of an incident report form.

Source: Millstone Industries

Most of the regulations relate to laboratory standards. Tests have been divided into these three categories, based on complexity: Certificate of Waiver tests, tests of moderate complexity, and tests of high complexity.

Certificate of Waiver Tests The **Certificate of Waiver tests,** as listed in Table 45-2, are simple laboratory examinations and procedures that have an insignificant risk of an erroneous result. These tests are often performed in a POL but

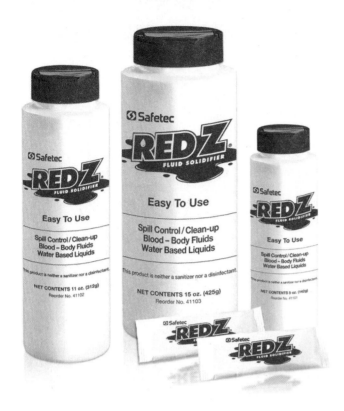

FIGURE 45-5 Certain substances require cleanup with specially formulated products such as these.
Courtesy of Safetec of America

also may be performed as point-of-care tests at the patient's bedside or home. In order for a test to be classified as a waived test, it must:

- Pose an insignificant risk to the patient if it is performed or interpreted incorrectly.
- Involve procedures that are simple and accurate so that the risk of obtaining incorrect results is minimal.
- Be approved by the Food and Drug Administration (FDA) for use by patients at home.

If laboratory management decides to perform these tests only, the office may apply for a Certificate of Waiver. When the certificate is granted, the laboratory is exempt from meeting various CLIA '88 standards that apply to the other two test categories. Such laboratories, however, are subject to the following: (1) random inspections to ensure that laboratories operating under a Certificate of Waiver are performing only those tests that qualify for the waiver and (2) investigation of the laboratory if there is any reason to believe the laboratory is not operating safely or if there have been complaints against the laboratory. See the *Caution: Handle with Care* feature Operating a Reliable Certificate of Waiver Laboratory for more information about good lab practice.

Tests of Moderate Complexity Tests of moderate complexity make up approximately 75% of all tests performed in the laboratory. Among these tests are blood cell counts and cholesterol screening. Test procedures falling into this category include studies involving bacteriology, mycobacteriology, mycology, parasitology, virology, immunology, chemistry, hematology, and immunohematology.

A laboratory that performs moderate-complexity testing must be run by a pathologist who has an MD or PhD degree. Technicians performing the tests must have training beyond the high school level as defined by CLIA '88 regulations. All personnel must participate in a quality assurance program for laboratory procedures, and the laboratory is subject to periodic unannounced inspections and proficiency testing.

Tests of High Complexity Tests of high complexity include more complicated tests in the specialties and subspecialties, including tests in clinical cytogenics, histopathology, histocompatibility, cytology, and any test not yet categorized by the CMS. Manufacturers' guidelines for testing products are often the best source for discovering a test's CMS determination. The CMS publishes a directory of all moderate- and high-complexity tests.

Like a laboratory that conducts moderate-complexity tests, a laboratory that conducts high-complexity tests is subject to inspection, proficiency testing, and participation in a quality assurance program, and it must be headed by a medical doctor or a scientist who has a PhD degree. Testing procedures can be performed only by qualified laboratory personnel whose training exceeds that provided by high schools and meets the requirements of CLIA '88 regulations. Medical assistants will

TABLE 45-2	**Certificate of Waiver Tests**
Urine Tests	Urinalysis by dipstick (reagent strip) or tablet reagent (nonautomated) for bilirubin, glucose, hemoglobin, ketone, leukocytes, nitrite, pH, protein, specific gravity, and urobilinogen
	Ovulation (visual color comparison tests)
	Pregnancy (visual color comparison tests)
	Home-screening tests for drugs (opioids, cocaine, methamphetamines, cannabinoids, phencyclidine, methadone, benzodiazepines, barbiturates, oxycodone)
	Nicotine detection tests
	Urine chemistry analyzer for microalbumin and creatinine (semi-quantitative)
	Tumor-associated antigen for bladder cancer (using devices approved by the FDA for home use)
	Catalase
	Ascorbic acid

(Continued)

TABLE 45-2   Certificate of Waiver Tests

Blood Tests	Erythrocyte sedimentation rate (ESR), nonautomated
	Hemoglobin by copper sulfate, nonautomated
	Spun microhematocrit
	Blood glucose (using devices approved by the FDA for home use)
	Hemoglobin by single analyte instruments, automated
	Prothrombin time
	Platelet aggregation
	Ketones in whole blood, over-the-counter test only
	Total cholesterol, high-density lipoprotein (HDL), low-density lipoprotein (LDL), and triglycerides
	Hemoglobin A1C
	Liver panel (alanine aminotransferase, alkaline phosphatase, amylase, gamma-glutamyl transferase, aspartate aminotransferase, total bilirubin)
	Lactate in whole blood
	Chloride
	Carbon dioxide
	Calcium
	Sodium
	Potassium
	Urea
	Uric acid
	Creatinine
	Lead in whole blood
	Thyroid-stimulating hormone, rapid test
	Mononucleosis rapid test
	Helicobacter pylori rapid antibody test
	Lyme disease antibodies
	HIV antibody test
Fecal Tests	Fecal occult blood
Saliva Tests	Alcohol in saliva
Nasal Smear Tests	Adenovirus
	Influenza A and B antigens
	Respiratory syncytial virus
Vaginal Smear Tests	*Trichomonas vaginalis* antigens
	Vaginal pH
Throat Swab Tests	Strep A antigens
	Influenza A and B
Semen	Sperm concentration, home screening

need additional training and education to perform moderate- and high-complexity tests.

Components of Quality Assurance

Every quality assurance program must include the following components, in a measurable and structured system, to satisfy CLIA '88 requirements:

- Quality control.
- Instrument and equipment maintenance.
- Proficiency testing.
- Training and continuing education.
- Standard operating procedures documentation.

Quality Control and Maintenance

A **quality control program** is one component of a quality assurance program. The focus of the quality control program is to ensure accuracy in test results through careful monitoring of test procedures. To be in compliance with quality control standards, a laboratory must follow certain procedures.

Calibration Medical equipment used for testing patient specimens must be calibrated regularly in accordance with manufacturers' guidelines. Calibration ensures that the equipment is operating correctly and is producing accurate results. To calibrate a medical instrument, you must have a set of known standards. A **standard** is a specimen, like the patient specimens you would normally process with the equipment, except that the value for each standard is already known. When you calibrate medical equipment, you run the standard with the known value. If the results do not match the known value, then the equipment is not in calibration. If the equipment does not yield the expected results during the calibration procedure, it must be adjusted until the expected results

Operating a Reliable Certificate of Waiver Laboratory

CLIA requires that Certificate of Waiver laboratories obtain a certificate of waiver, pay biennial certificate fees, and follow manufacturers' test instructions. It also requires that Certificate of Waiver laboratories submit to random inspections and investigation if indicated. CLIA does not require laboratory personnel to have any specific qualifications or training, nor does it require quality control procedures or routine quality assessment, except as recommended by the manufacturer of each waived test. Although waived tests are simple to perform and interpret, they may have serious consequences if done incorrectly. Patient care decisions often are made based on the outcome of waived tests.

In order to help ensure quality testing procedures and reduce patient error, the Clinical Laboratory Improvement Advisory Committee (CLIAC) has made several recommendations for good practice in a Certificate of Waiver laboratory. These include laboratory management considerations and testing procedures before, during, and after the test. To ensure that you are operating a reliable laboratory, follow these recommendations:

Laboratory Management and Personnel

- Designate the person who will be responsible for laboratory supervision—usually a physician or someone with enough laboratory experience to make decisions about testing.
- Follow all applicable federal, state, and local regulations.
- Perform waived tests only.
- Follow the manufacturer's instructions in the package insert.
- Do not make modifications to the instructions.
- Allow random inspections by authorized agencies such as the Centers for Medicare and Medicaid Services (CMS).
- Establish a laboratory safety plan that follows OSHA guidelines.
- Have a designated area that has adequate space and conditions.

- Have enough personnel in the lab and train them appropriately.
- Have written documentation of each test performed.

Before the Test

- Confirm written test orders.
- Establish a procedure for patient identification.
- Give patients pretest instructions and determine whether they have followed them.
- Collect specimens according to package insert instructions.
- Label specimens appropriately.
- Never use expired reagents of test kits.

During the Test

- Perform quality control testing as indicated in the package insert.
- Correct any problem discovered during quality control testing before testing patient samples.
- Establish a policy for control testing frequency.
- Carefully follow all test-timing recommendations.
- Interpret test results using product inserts as a guide.
- Record test results according to your office policy.

After the Test

- Report test results to the physician in a timely manner.
- Follow package insert recommendations for follow-up or confirmatory testing.
- Follow OSHA regulations for disposing of biohazardous waste.
- Participate in quality assurance assessment programs:
  - Internal assessment—routine, in-house testing to ensure a test's accuracy
  - External assessment—voluntary inspection of your facility by an outside agency

---

are obtained. Each calibration must be recorded in a quality control log like the one shown in Figure 45-6. Calibration routines are run on the standards alone, never with patient samples. They are used exclusively to ensure that the equipment is performing according to manufacturers' specifications. Check the manufacturer's instructions to determine how often the equipment should be calibrated. Calibration of some equipment must be performed by trained service personnel.

Control Samples **Control samples** are similar to standards in that they are specimens like those taken from a patient and have known values. Unlike standards, however, control samples are used before each patient sample is processed. Using a control sample serves as a check on the accuracy of the test. If the control

tests do not fall within the manufacturer's prescribed ranges, patient samples should not be analyzed until the equipment is calibrated. This helps prevent erroneous patient test results.

The control samples for certain laboratory procedures show both normal (negative) and abnormal (positive) results. Generally, positive and negative control samples are used with tests that yield that **qualitative test response.** A qualitative test is testing to see if the substance is present in the specimen. It is not testing for the amount of a substance in the specimen, only if it is there or not.

Tests that yield **quantitative test results** require different control samples. Quantitative tests give the concentration or amount of a substance in a tested specimen. Control samples are formulated to show when results fall within a

QUALITY CONTROL DAILY LOG

Name of Unit	Glucose Control Solution	Strip Lot No./ Exp. Date	Low Control Value 35–65 mg/dL	High Control Value 75–235 mg/dL	Analyzed By	Date	Remedial Action Taken If Control Values Abnormal	Retest After Remedial Action Taken
XYZ Glucometer	Check-strip control solution	Lot 851 10/15/XX	39 mg/dL	230 mg/dL	MSM	1/17/XX		
Mitchell Drugs Glucometer	Check-strip control solution	Lot 851 10/15/XX	50 mg/dL	267 mg/dL	MSM	1/17/XX	Machine cleaned	220 mg/dL high value
XYZ Glucometer	Check-strip control solution	Lot 851 10/15/XX	Unable to read	Unable to read	LMC	1/18/XX	Battery changed	38 mg/dL low 198 mg/dL high
Mitchell Drugs Glucometer	Check-strip control solution	Lot 851 10/15/XX	45 mg/dL	226 mg/dL	LMC	1/18/XX		

FIGURE 45-6 The quality control log shows the completion of every quality control check conducted on a piece of equipment.

normal range. At least two control samples containing different concentrations—usually a high and a low value—of the test substance should be run for quantitative tests.

Reagent Control Control samples or standards also are run every time you open a new supply of testing products, such as staining materials, culture media, and reagents. **Reagents** are chemicals or chemically treated substances used in test procedures. A reagent is formulated to react in specific ways when exposed under specific conditions. One example of a reagent is the chemically coated strip used in urine glucose and ketone monitoring. A visual change on the reagent strip (also called a dipstick) occurs in the presence of glucose and ketones in a urine sample.

To ensure the quality of reagents, you should keep a reagent control log. If a defective reagent test is identified, it can be tracked to its source. A sample reagent control log is shown in Figure 45-7. Running controls on a routine basis gives you information about the equipment and the reagents used during the test. If a control consistently yields unexpected results (for example, a positive control yields a negative result), you should check the reagents first and then the equipment calibration.

Maintenance Testing instruments and equipment must be properly maintained, and all maintenance procedures must be documented. Follow manufacturers' guidelines for performing instrument and equipment maintenance. A maintenance log provides a complete record of all work performed on an instrument or a piece of equipment (Figure 45-8).

Troubleshooting You may need to investigate the cause of a problem with a piece of equipment or a test. To do this, you should take a systematic approach to rule out the cause of the problem. For more information regarding investigating equipment and test malfunctions, see the *Caution: Handle*

with Care feature Troubleshooting Problems in a Physician's Office Laboratory.

Documentation A quality control program depends first on careful adherence to procedures designed to identify problems with equipment calibration, errors in testing procedures, and defective testing supplies. The second component of a quality control program is the careful documentation of all procedures. Besides maintaining the quality control log, the reagent control log, and the equipment maintenance log, you also will complete the following records as part of a quality control program:

- Reference laboratory log, which lists specimens sent to another laboratory for testing.
- Daily workload log, which shows all procedures completed during the workday.

Proficiency Testing

All laboratories that perform moderate- and high-complexity tests as identified by CLIA '88 must participate in a proficiency testing program. **Proficiency testing programs** measure test result accuracy and adherence to standard operating procedures. Generally, proficiency tests include two parts: (1) an unknown (testing) sample supplied by the proficiency testing organization contracted by your laboratory and (2) forms that must be completed to record the steps in the testing procedure. The unknown sample is processed normally, under the same conditions as any patient sample. The results, the forms, and sometimes the unknown samples are returned to the proficiency testing organization, which then informs your office whether it has passed or failed the test. A passing mark means that your laboratory can continue to perform that particular test. A failing mark can mean that your laboratory must discontinue that test and possibly other tests, too.

URINE REAGENT STRIP CONTROL LOG

Control Solution _____ Exp. Date _____ Lot # _____

Reagent Strip / Lot # & Exp. Date	Test	Specific Gravity	pH	Protein	Glucose	Ketone	Bilirubin	Blood	Nitrite	Urobi-linogen	Control Test Date	Remedial Action Taken If Reading Is Abnormal	Retest Date	Technician Initials
	Reagent Strip Expected Range													
	Test Results													
	Reagent Strip Expected Range													
	Test Results													

FIGURE 45-7 The reagent control log shows the quality testing performed on every batch or lot of reagent products.

ACME MEDICAL SUPPLIES
Equipment Maintenance Record

Date 6/1/20XX

Practice	BWW Medical Associates
Name of Equipment	Acme Microscope Model ABC-123
Location	Lab Purchased 12/1/20XX

Date	Cleaning	Maintenance/Repair	Technician Initials
6/5	Microscope	Cleaned	CJC
6/11	Microscope high objective	Cleaned	DWM
6/14	Microscope	Changed bulb	CJC
6/16	Microscope eyepiece	Lens cover replaced	CJC
6/17	Microscope high objective	Cleaned	CJC

FIGURE 45-8 A maintenance log must be kept for every piece of laboratory equipment. All work done on the equipment must be recorded in the log.
Source: ACME Medical Supplies

Training, Continuing Education, and Documentation

One of your employer's responsibilities is to provide opportunities for employee training and continuing education. Another is to provide written reference materials and documentation for all procedures conducted in the POL. Your responsibility is to consult reference materials and take part in available training to keep your skills sharpened and up to date.

It may seem unnecessary to refer to written instructions for procedures you perform many times a day. Changes can be made in a procedure for many reasons, however, and you must be aware of these changes. Here are some reference materials with which you should be familiar:

- Safety Data Sheets.
- Standard operating procedures.
- Safety manuals.
- Equipment manufacturers' user or reference guides.
- Clinical Laboratory Technical Procedure Manuals.
- Regulatory documentation (OSHA standards, CLIA '88 requirements).
- Maintenance and housekeeping schedules.

▶ Communicating with the Patient LO 45.6

In your job as a medical assistant, you will be involved with patients before they submit samples for laboratory testing, during the specimen collection procedure, and after the physician has interpreted the test results. It is your responsibility to ensure that patients understand what is expected of them every step of the way.

Before the Test

Certain tests require patients to prepare by fasting or restricting fluid intake. It is your duty to explain test preparations. Use simple, nontechnical language and check with patients to be sure they understand the information. In some cases, providing a written instruction sheet may be helpful.

Explaining the reason for the preparation can help ensure compliance or unearth potential problems. For example, if you explain to a patient that he is to refrain from drinking anything for a particular period, he might ask whether that includes the water he uses to take a certain medication. You can then make sure the patient receives the answers he will need for carrying out the physician's orders.

If you are the person who collects specimens, you need to determine whether patients have correctly completed the required test preparations. Test results are invalid in some cases if patients fail to follow test preparation guidelines. When preparations have not been completed correctly, discuss the situation with the physician or other appropriate staff member as required by your office to determine whether the specimen still should be collected. If the specimen is not collected, document the reason the test was not carried out as requested. Review the guidelines for specimen collection with the patient and schedule another appointment if appropriate.

During Specimen Collection

Before collecting a specimen, you first must be sure you have the right patient. You do not want to collect a blood sample from someone who only needs a urinalysis. Patients do not always understand the tests they are having. It is up to you to make sure you have the right patient and are performing the test as it is ordered.

The instructions you deliver to patients during specimen collection vary with the nature of the specimen. Always deliver instructions clearly and in language patients can understand. Do not assume that patients do not need to hear the instructions, even if they have had the test before. Explain what you must do and what patients must do before moving to each new step in the process.

Patients are understandably nervous during many collection procedures. In addition to communicating technical information, you should provide any helpful advice that may make the test easier. Also provide reassurance as appropriate. For example, if a patient asks whether the blood-drawing procedure is painful, explain that a sharp stick or stinging sensation may be experienced when the needle is inserted but that no pain should be felt after that. Let the patient be your guide in determining how much information to provide. Some people want to know every detail, whereas others prefer to know as little as possible.

One important aspect of communicating with patients about testing procedures is your nonverbal communication skills. Even if you deliver accurate technical information and answer every question patients have, there still can be a breakdown in communication if your nonverbal signals do not support your verbal message. Follow these guidelines to ensure that your nonverbal actions are helping, not hindering, the communication process:

- Strike a balance between a strict, business-like attitude and overly familiar friendliness. Your actions must impress on the patient that you are well informed about the procedure and that you care about the patient's understanding of it.
- Treat the patient with respect. Address the patient by name, using the appropriate courtesy title unless you have been invited to use the patient's first name or the patient is a child. Provide privacy during specimen collection. Privacy needs may be met by using a separate room or contained area for drawing blood; for example; a private bathroom is best for collecting urine specimens.
- Recognize that the patient may be under stress because of the test procedure or the pending results. Some patients may be familiar with the test procedures, but others may not know what to expect. You may need to repeat instructions or explain what you are doing more than one time. Remain calm and patient. Never be abrupt or condescending.
- Direct your attention to the patient, particularly during a procedure that might be uncomfortable, such as drawing blood. Unless an emergency develops, pay attention to nothing else at that time.

After Specimen Collection

If the patient must follow particular guidelines after you collect the specimen, explain them. Commonly, post-test instructions deal with the care of venipuncture sites, signs and symptoms of infection, additional or continuing dietary restrictions, and the schedule for further testing if it is necessary.

When the Test Results Return

When you receive the test results, communicate them not to the patient but to the doctor. Only the doctor is qualified to interpret test results for the patient. Your role in reporting results comes after the doctor examines the test information and prepares a report. Sometimes, the doctor discusses the results with the patient. Other times, you will be asked to convey the test results to the patient along with instructions from the doctor. Answer only those patient questions that are within the range of your knowledge and experience. If the patient needs more information than you can provide, refer the patient to the doctor.

▶ Recordkeeping   LO 45.7

The importance of accurate and complete recordkeeping can be summed up in one statement: If it is not written down, it was not done. This motto applies to all your duties as a medical assistant. Besides recording information about quality control and equipment maintenance, you must keep track of every specimen that passes through your hands, or you may be called on to handle inventory control and record test results in patient records. You may need to use standard abbreviations for measures when recording test results. Table 45-3 provides a list of common abbreviations used in the laboratory.

Filling Out a Laboratory Requisition Form

As a medical assistant, it is your responsibility to ensure that the laboratory requisition form is properly completed. Missing information can lead to improper testing or lost results. The completed form should be included with the specimen collected or sent with the patient to the laboratory. Be sure to include the following information on all requisitions:

- Patient's full name, sex, date of birth, and address.
- Patient's insurance information.
- Physician's name, address, and phone number.
- Source of the specimen.
- Date and time of the specimen collection.
- Test(s) requested.
- Preliminary diagnosis.
- Any current treatment that might affect the results.

See Figure 45-9 for a sample laboratory requisition form.

Specimen Identification

All specimens must immediately be clearly identified with the patient's name, the patient's identification code (if your office uses one), the date and time the specimen was collected, the initials of the person who collected the specimen, the physician's name, and other information as required by the test procedure or your office. If you encounter an unidentified or

TABLE 45-3	Abbreviations for Common Laboratory Measures
cm	centimeter
cm³	cubic centimeter
dL	deciliter
fl oz	fluid ounce
g	gram
L	liter
lb	pound
m	meter
mcg	microgram
mg	milligram
mL	milliliter
mm	millimeter
mmHg	millimeters of mercury
oz	ounce
pt	pint
QNS	quantity not sufficient
QS	quantity sufficient
qt	quart
wt	weight

Laboratory Requisition

BWW
BWW Medical Associates, PC
305 Main Street, Port Snead YZ 12345-9876
Tel: 555-654-3210, Fax: 555-987-6543
Web: BWWAssociates.com

Laboratory Name and Address
_____
_____
_____
_____

Requesting Provider
Paul F. Buckwalter, MD
Alexis N. Whalen, MD
Elizabeth H. Williams, MD

Please Indicate Bill Type Below
Attach Copy of Insurance Card

Patient Data (Please Print)

Last Name	First Name	Maiden Name
Address		Apt No.
City	State	Zip
SS#	Phone #	
Date of Birth (Month, Day, Year) ☐ Male ☐ Female	Date Collected	Time Collected : ☐ a.m. ☐ p.m.
Physician 1	Physician 2	

Billing Information (Please Print Clearly)

Please Bill to: ☐ Dr. Account (Client) ☐ Patient Self Pay ☐ Insurance Co

Responsible Party (Last, First) Relationship to Subscriber ☐ Self ☐ Child ☐ Spouse ☐ Other

Primary Insurance Co. Name ☐ HMO ☐ PPO

Insurance Policy # Insurance Group #

Primary Insurance Co: Address (Street, City, State, Zip)

Insured Date of Birth Insured SS#

PLEASE PROVIDE MANDATORY ICD 10 CODE BELOW

1 _____ 2 _____ 3 _____ 4 _____ 5 _____

CALL TEST RESULTS TO:	FAX RESULTS TO:
Test: _____	To: _____
To: _____	Fax: ( ) _____
Phone: ( ) _____	

☐ Veni   Tech Code _____   Tubes Received _____

Please (X) desired Panel(s)/Profile(s)/Tests. See back of requisition for profile components.

PANELS/PROFILES	
Hepatitis Panel, Acute	**2S**
Basic Metabolic Panel	MT
Comp Metabolic Panel	MT
Electrolyte Panel (Lytes)	MT
Hepatic Function Panel	MT
General Health Panel	MTL
Lipid Panel	**MT**
Obstetric Panel AMH	P2SL
Renal Panel	MT

MICROBIOLOGY	
Source of Specimen:	
Culture, Anaerobe	
Chlamydia/GC Amp Probe	
Culture, Ear	
Culture, Eye	
Leukocytes Stool	
Culture, Fungal	
Culture, Genital	
Culture, Herpes	
Occult Blood Screen	
Ova & Parasites	
Rapid Strep Throat	
Culture, Stool	
Culture, GROUP A BetaStrep Screen	
Culture GROUP B Screen	
Culture, Throat	
Culture, Urine	
Culture, Wound / Abscess	
Culture, Viral	
C. Difficile Toxin A&B AMH	

INDIVIDUAL TESTS	
ABO Group/RH	P
Acid Phosphatase, Prostatic	**S**
Albumin	MT
Alkaline Phosphatase	MT
Amylase	MT
Antinuclear Antibodies (ANA Send)	S
HCG, Beta Quant	**MT**
Bilirubin T / D Neonate	A
Bilirubin T / D Adult	MT
BNP Screen	**L**
BUN	MT
CA-125	**S**
CA-125 to Dianon	**S**
CRP	MT
CRP Cardio	MT
Calcium	**MT**
Carbamazepine/Tegretol	R
CBC & PLT w/o Diff	**L**
CBC & PLT w Diff	**L**
Carcino Embryonic Antigen (CEA)	**S**
Cholesterol Total	**MT**
Cortisol Level	MT
Creatine Kinase, Total (CK)	MT
CPK total w CKMB	MT
Creatinine Clearance	U
Creatinine	MT
D Dimer Quant	B
DNA AB Double Strand	S
Digoxin Level	**R**

INDIVIDUAL TESTS (cont.)	
Drug Screen Urine	**U**
Drug Screen Urine c Confirm	**U**
Estradiol Level	MT
Ferritin Level	**MT**
Fetal Fibronectin (FFN)	SWAB
Folic Acid (PROTECT)	MT
Follicle Stimulating Hormone	MT
GGT (Gamma Glut Trans)	**MT**
Glucose	**MT**
Glucose Fasting	**MT**
Glucose Challenge 1° Preg	MT
Glycosylated Hemoglobin (HA1C)	**L**
Hepatitis B Surface AG	**S**
Hepatitis B Surface AB	**S**
Hepatitis C Antibody	S
Herpes Simplex 1 & 2 IgG AB	S
Herpes Simplex 1 & 2 IgM AB	S
HIV I & II Abs	**S**
Homocysteine	L
Iron/TIBC	**MT**
Lactate Dehydrogenase (LDH)	MT
Lipase	MT
Lithium	R
Luteinizing Hormone	MT
Microalbumin Random/24 Hr.	U
Magnesium	**MT**
MONO test heterophile	S
Phenobarbital	R
Phenytoin/Dilantin	R
Phosphorous	**MT**
Potassium	MT
Progesterone	S
Prolactin	MT
PSA Free and Total	**S**
PSA Screen (Medicare)	**S**
PSA Diagnostic	**S**
Prothrombin Time	**B**
aPTT	**B**
PTH Intact	**S**
Reticulocyte Count	L
Rheumatoid Factor (RF)	MT
RPR QUAL	**S**
Rubella, IgG	S
ESR (Sed Rate)	**L**
SGOT (AST)	MT

SGPT (ALT)	MT
Testosterone	S
Testosterone Free & Total	S
TSH	**MT**
Total T3	**MT**
T3 Uptake	S
Free T3	**MT**
Free Thyroxine (FT4)	**MT**
Total T4	**S**
Free Thyroxine index (FTI)	**S**
Thyroid Antibodies	S
Troponin/Quant	**MT**
Triglycerides	**MT**
Uric Acid	MT
Urinalysis	U
Valproic Acid / Depakote	R
Vitamin B12 (PROTECT)	MT
Vitamin D 25 Hydroxy	S

ADDITIONAL ORDERS

FIGURE 45-9 The laboratory requisition form must be accurately completed.

incorrectly identified specimen, you must make an effort to track it to its source. The specimen probably will be discarded or destroyed, however, because there is no guarantee that it was identified correctly. Even if you do manage to identify it, it may have been compromised in some way.

Inventory Control

You will be responsible for taking inventory of equipment and supplies to ensure that the POL never runs out of them. To do so, you will keep a list of items that are used routinely and reordered systematically. Establish a regular schedule—perhaps weekly—for counting items in the POL. Then estimate when

you will probably need to reorder an item—based on how quickly you use the item or material—and put the date on your calendar.

Patient Records

When recording test results, it may be your responsibility to identify unusual findings. Many offices require out-of-range test results to be circled or underlined in red. Follow the procedure established by your office. The physician usually initials or otherwise marks the records after examining them. Electronic health records automatically identify out-of-range tests when the results are entered.

PROCEDURE 45-1 Using a Microscope

WORK // DOC

Procedure Goal: To correctly focus the microscope using each of the three objectives for examination of a prepared specimen slide

OSHA Guidelines:

Materials: Microscope, lens paper, lens cleaner, prepared specimen slide, immersion oil, and tissues

Method:

1. Wash your hands and don exam gloves.

2. Remove the protective cover from the microscope. Examine the microscope to make sure it is clean and that all parts are intact.

3. Plug in the microscope and make sure the light is working. If you need to replace the bulb, refer to the manufacturer's guidelines. (Be sure to note bulb replacements in the maintenance log for the microscope.) Turn the light off before cleaning the lenses.

4. Clean the lenses and oculars with lens paper. Avoid touching the lenses with anything except lens paper. Pay careful attention to the oculars, as they are easily dirtied by dust and eye makeup. If a lens is particularly dirty, use a small amount of lens cleaner. Oil-immersion lenses are prone to oil buildup if not cleaned properly. Too much lens cleaner, however, can loosen the cement that holds the lens in place.
   RATIONALE: *The lenses must be clean to reduce artifacts.*

5. Place the specimen slide on the stage. Slide the edges of the slide under the slide clips to secure the slide to the stage. ·

6. Adjust the distance between the oculars to a position of comfort.

7. Adjust the objectives so the low-power (10×) objective points directly at the specimen slide, as shown. Before

swiveling the objective assembly, be sure you have sufficient space for the objective. Recheck the distance between the oculars, making sure the field you see through the eyepieces is a merged field, not separate left and right fields. Raise the body tube by using the coarse adjustment control and lower the stage as needed.
RATIONALE: *If the objective assembly is too close to the stage, you may hit the specimen slide and crack it. The specimen is then contaminated and cannot be used. The objective also may be damaged.*

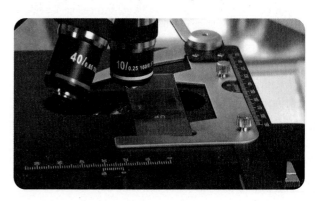

FIGURE Procedure 45-1 Step 5   Carefully secure the specimen slide on the stage of the microscope.
©McGraw-Hill Education

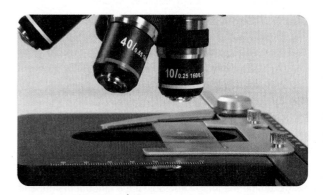

FIGURE Procedure 45-1 Step 7   Move the low-power objective into position above the specimen slide.
©McGraw-Hill Education

8. Turn on the light and, using the iris controls, adjust the amount of light illuminating the specimen so that the light fills the field but does not wash out the image. (At this point, you are not examining the specimen image for focus but adjusting the overall light level.)

9. Observe the microscope from one side and slowly lower the body tube to move the objective closer to the stage and specimen slide. This adjustment is shown below. If you used the stage controls to lower the stage away from the objectives, you also may need to adjust those controls. Again, take care not to strike the stage with the objective. The objective should almost meet the specimen slide but not touch it.

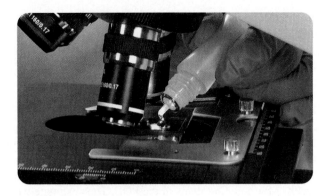

FIGURE Procedure 45-1 Step 14   Place a small drop of immersion oil directly on the dry specimen.
©McGraw-Hill Education

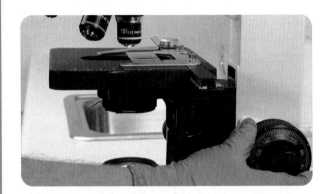

FIGURE Procedure 45-1 Step 9   When lowering the objective toward the stage and specimen slide, observe the microscope from the side to be sure you do not hit the stage with the objective and crack the slide.
©McGraw-Hill Education

10. Look through the oculars and use the coarse focus control to slowly adjust the image. If necessary, adjust the amount of light coming through the iris.

11. Continue using the fine focus control to adjust the image. When the image is correctly focused, the specimen will be clearly visible and the field illumination will be bright enough to show details but not so bright that it is uncomfortable to view or washed out.

12. Switch to the high-power (40×) objective. Only use the fine focus controls to view the specimen clearly.
    RATIONALE: *Using the coarse adjustment could cause lens damage if the lens touches the slide.*

13. Rotate the objective assembly so that no objective points directly at the stage and specimen slide. You will now have enough room to apply a drop of immersion oil to the slide. (Only dry slides, without coverslips, are used with the oil-immersion objective.)

14. Apply a small drop of immersion oil to the specimen slide, as shown.

15. Gently swing the oil-immersion (100×) objective over the stage and specimen slide so that it is surrounded by the immersion oil.

16. Examine the image and adjust the amount of light and focus as needed. Only use the fine focus adjustment with this objective. To eliminate air bubbles in the immersion oil, gently move the stage left and right.

17. After you have examined the specimen as required by the testing procedure, lower the stage and raise the objectives.

18. Remove the slide. Dispose of it or store it as required by the testing procedure. If you must dispose of the slide, be sure to use the appropriate biohazardous waste container. If you must store the slide, remove the immersion oil with a tissue.

19. Turn off the light. Unplug the microscope if that is your laboratory's standard operating procedure.

20. Clean the microscope stage, ocular lenses, and objectives. Be careful to remove all traces of immersion oil from the stage and oil-immersion objective. Clean the oil-immersion lens last.
    RATIONALE: *So that you do not get oil from the oil-immersion lens on the other lenses*

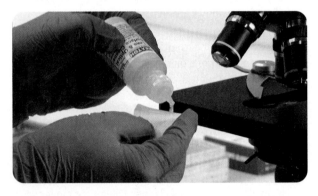

FIGURE Procedure 45-1 Step 20   Clean the oil-immersion lens last using a small amount of lens cleaner.
©McGraw-Hill Education

21. Rotate the objective assembly so that the low-power objective points toward the stage. Lower the objective so that it comes close to but does not rest on the stage.

22. Cover the microscope with its protective cover. Check the work area to be sure you have cleaned everything correctly and disposed of all waste material.

23. Remove the gloves and wash your hands.

OUTCOME	KEY POINTS
45.1 Describe the purpose of the physician's office laboratory.	The physician's office laboratory (POL) is responsible for accurate and timely processing of routine tests, usually involving blood or urine, and for reporting test results to the physician.
45.2 Identify the medical assistant's duties in the physician's office laboratory.	The medical assistant's duties in a physician's office laboratory include preparing the patient for the test, collecting the sample, completing the test, reporting the results to the physician, and communicating information about the test from the physician to the patient.
45.3 Identify important pieces of laboratory equipment.	Common laboratory equipment includes autoclaves, centrifuges, microscopes, electronic equipment and software, and equipment used for measurement.
45.4 Illustrate measures to prevent accidents.	Preventing accidents in the physician's office laboratory begins by observing all safety guidelines, including standard precautions, reporting all laboratory accidents in a timely manner, and maintaining appropriate housekeeping in the lab setting.
45.5 Explain the goal of a quality assurance program in a physician's office laboratory.	The goal of a quality assurance program in a physician's office laboratory is to monitor the quality of the patient care that a medical laboratory provides.
45.6 Carry out communication with patients regarding test preparation and follow-up.	It is the medical assistant's responsibility to ensure that patients understand what is expected of them before a test. Providing clear pretest instructions in both oral and written form is an essential part of the test procedure.
45.7 Carry out accurate documentation, including patient results, specimen tracking, laboratory requests, and inventory control.	Accurate documentation in a physician's office laboratory is an essential step in quality patient care and includes recording patient results, tracking specimens that come through the lab, completing laboratory requests forms, and inventory control.

CASE STUDY CRITICAL THINKING

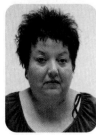

©McGraw-Hill Education

Recall Sylvia Gonzales from the case study at the beginning of the chapter. Now that you have completed the chapter, answer the following questions regarding her case.

1. Identify equipment used by a medical assistant in an office laboratory.
2. You will be measuring Sylvia Gonzales's fasting blood glucose using a glucometer. You know this is classified as a waived test. What does the classification of waived test mean?
3. The glucometer contains an instrument called a photometer. How is blood glucose measured using a photometer?
4. Measuring blood glucose is a quantitative test. What does this mean?
5. What type of controls do you expect to use when measuring Sylvia Gonzales's blood glucose?
6. When should you run the controls?

1. (LO 45.1) A laboratory owned by a company other than the physician's practice is a
   a. Physician's office laboratory
   b. Reference laboratory
   c. Pathology department
   d. Waived testing center
   e. High-complexity testing center

2. (LO 45.3) The eyepieces on a microscope also are called
   a. Objectives
   b. Condensers
   c. Oculars
   d. Irises
   e. Stages

3. (LO 45.3) An object visible through a microscope but unrelated to the specimen is a(n)
   a. Iris
   b. Aperture
   c. Artifact
   d. Speck
   e. Inclusion

4. (LO 45.5) A simple laboratory examination or procedure that has an insignificant risk of an erroneous result is a
   a. Waived test
   b. Moderate-complexity test
   c. High-complexity test
   d. Quality assurance test
   e. Reference test

5. (LO 45.5) Which of the following is a test to determine the amount of a substance in a specimen?
   a. Qualitative
   b. Waived
   c. Complex
   d. Quantitative
   e. Assurance

6. (LO 45.3) A device for spinning a specimen at high speed until it separates into its component parts is a
   a. Refractometer
   b. Photometer
   c. Concentrator
   d. Condenser
   e. Centrifuge

7. (LO 45.4) The most common disinfectant used in a physician's office laboratory is
   a. Germicidal soap
   b. 10% bleach
   c. Hydrogen peroxide
   d. Betadine®
   e. 70% alcohol

8. (LO 45.5) A laboratory that performs moderate-complexity testing must be run by a
   a. Pathologist
   b. Medical technologist
   c. Medical assistant
   d. Medical lab specialist
   e. CLIA-trained employee

9. (LO 45.5) Chemicals or chemically treated substances used in test procedures are known as
   a. Controls
   b. Standards
   c. Reagents
   d. Strips
   e. Negatives

10. (LO 45.3) An instrument used in a medical laboratory to measure light intensity is called a(n)
    a. Photometer
    b. Microscope
    c. Condenser
    d. Analyte
    e. Reflector

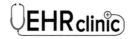

Go to CONNECT to complete the EHRclinic exercises: 45.01 Order a Patient's Labs and 45.02 Record a Patient's Lab Results.

SOFT SKILLS SUCCESS

You are working in the lab today for Heather, who is out sick. Taylor brings you two tubes of blood and asks you to perform a blood glucose test for Sylvia Gonzales. After Taylor leaves the lab, you notice that one of the tubes is not labeled and the other tube has only the letter *S* written on it. What action should you take?

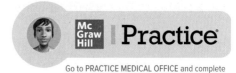

Go to PRACTICE MEDICAL OFFICE and complete the module Clinical: Privacy and Liability.

Microbiology and Disease

CASE STUDY

Patient Name	DOB	Allergies
Cindy Chen	07/15/1993	NKA

Attending	MRN	Other Information
Alexis N. Whalen, MD	00-AA-001	Last CD4 count 250 cells/mm^3

PATIENT INFORMATION

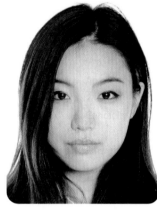
©excentric_01/iStock/Getty Images

Cindy Chen arrives at the clinic complaining of the inability to sleep and nervousness. She tested positive for HIV in 2014. Currently, she lives with her aunt and is going to school to become a phlebotomist. She has lost 20 pounds since her last visit to the clinic. She also has had a persistent cough and sore throat for the last 3 months. The physician orders a series of blood tests, including the helper T-cell test and a throat culture. Dr. Whalen asks you to send the throat culture to the reference lab for culture instead of doing a rapid strep test in the office.

Keep Cindy Chen in mind as you study the chapter. There will be questions at the end of the chapter based on the case study. The information in the chapter will help you answer these questions.

LEARNING OUTCOMES

After completing Chapter 46, you will be able to:

46.1 Explain the medical assistant's role in microbiology.

46.2 Summarize how microorganisms cause disease.

46.3 Describe how microorganisms are classified and named.

46.4 Discuss the role of viruses in human disease.

46.5 Discuss the role of bacteria in human disease.

46.6 Discuss the role of protozoans in human disease.

46.7 Discuss the role of fungi in human disease.

46.8 Discuss the role of multicellular parasites in human disease.

46.9 Describe the process involved in diagnosing an infection.

46.10 Identify general guidelines for obtaining specimens.

46.11 Carry out the procedure for transporting specimens to outside laboratories.

46.12 Compare two techniques used in the direct examination of culture specimens.

46.13 Carry out the procedure for preparing and examining stained specimens.

46.14 Carry out the procedure for culturing specimens in the medical office.

KEY TERMS

acid-fast stain	facultative
aerobe	Gram-negative
agar	Gram-positive
anaerobe	Gram stain
bacillus	KOH mount
coccus	mordant
colony	spirillum
culture	stain
culture and sensitivity (C&S)	vibrio
etiologic agent	

These types may be further divided into groups that share certain characteristics. For example, within the bacteria classification are the mycobacteria and rickettsiae groups.

Specific microorganisms are named in a standard way, using two words. The first word refers to the *genus* (a category of biologic classification between the *family* and the *species*) to which the microorganism belongs. The second word refers to the particular species of the organism. Each species represents a distinct kind of microorganism. For example, within the bacteria classification is the *Staphylococcus* genus. Then within that genus are various species such as *Staphylococcus aureus* and *Staphylococcus epidermidis*. Although the two bacteria belong to the same genus, they differ greatly in their ability to cause disease. The first letter of the genus is always capitalized, and the species name is always written in all lowercase letters.

▶ Viruses   LO 46.4

Viruses, which are among the smallest known infectious agents and cannot be seen with a regular microscope, are the cause of many common illnesses and conditions seen frequently in the medical office. Table 46-3 lists common viral pathogens. Because viruses are a simpler life form than the cell (see Figure 46-1), they can live and grow only within the living cells of other organisms.

Significant Viral Bloodborne Pathogens

In the medical office, you will likely encounter patients who are living with HIV and hepatitis. As you learned in the *Infection Control Fundamentals* chapter, proper technique is essential when handling blood and body fluids. You also must understand how HIV and hepatitis cause infection and how to recognize the symptoms of each disease.

AIDS/HIV Infection HIV is a virus that infects and gradually destroys components of the immune system. There are three stages of HIV infection. The first stage is acute HIV infection and the second stage is chronic HIV infection. AIDS, the third stage, is the condition that results from the advanced stages of this viral infection and is the most severe stage.

Over a period of time and in most cases, HIV infection develops into AIDS, which results in death. The pathogen gradually destroys helper T cells (CD4 cells). *Helper T cells* are white blood cells that are a key component of the body's immune system, working in coordination with other white blood cells (B cells, macrophages, and so on) to combat infection.

The virus also attacks neurons, causing demyelination (destruction of the myelin sheath of a nerve), which results in neurologic problems, including dementia. Unlike a person with a properly functioning immune system, most AIDS patients are prone to various opportunistic infections—infections caused by microorganisms that do not ordinarily cause disease in people with properly functioning immune systems. Virtually everyone is at risk for contracting HIV. Although its initial outbreak in the United States appeared in the male homosexual population, and currently homosexual and bisexual men make up a large percentage of AIDS cases, the disease knows no limits.

Symptoms HIV infection can cause a variety of problems as it progresses to AIDS. Patients with AIDS may complain of any of the following symptoms:

- Systemic complaints, such as weight loss, fatigue, fever, chills, and night sweats.
- Respiratory complaints, such as sinus fullness, dry cough, shortness of breath, difficulty swallowing, and sinus drainage.
- Oral complaints, such as gingivitis, oral lesions, and hairy leukoplakia, which is a white lesion on the tongue.
- Gastrointestinal complaints, such as diarrhea and bloody stool.
- Central nervous system (CNS) complaints, such as depression, personality changes, concentration difficulties, and confusion or memory loss.
- Peripheral nervous system complaints, such as tingling, numbness, pain, and weakness in the extremities.
- Skin-related complaints, such as rashes, dry skin, and changes in the nail bed.
- Kaposi sarcoma, an unusual malignancy occurring in the skin and sometimes in the lymph nodes and organs and manifested by reddish purple to dark blue patches or spots on the skin.

Because many other diseases can cause these symptoms, the occurrence of any one symptom is not necessarily indicative of AIDS. Be aware, however, that patients exhibiting a combination of symptoms should be tested. The two symptoms most indicative of AIDS are hairy leukoplakia and Kaposi sarcoma.

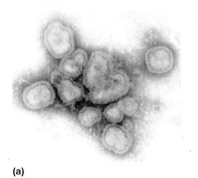 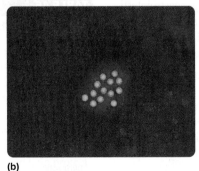 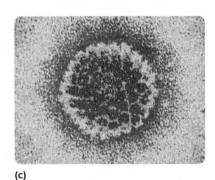

(a)   (b)   (c)

FIGURE 46-1 The three types of viral diseases often seen in medical offices are (a) influenza, (b) hepatitis, and (c) warts.

Source: (a) CDC/F.A. Murphy (b) ©BSIP/Getty Images (c) ©Science Photo Library - PASIEKA./Getty Images

TABLE 46-3	Viral Pathogens		
Disease	**Causative Organism**	**Route of Transmission**	**Signs and Symptoms**
Viral pharyngitis	Adenovirus	Direct person-to-person contact and respiratory droplet contact	Colds, pharyngitis, bronchitis, pneumonia, diarrhea, pinkeye, fever, cystitis, gastroenteritis, and/or neurologic disease
Infectious mononucleosis	Epstein-Barr virus	Direct contact with saliva from an infected person	Fever, sore throat, and swollen lymph glands
Hepatitis	Hepatitis A virus	Fecal-oral	Fever, fatigue, loss of appetite, nausea, vomiting, abdominal pain, dark urine, clay-colored bowel movements, joint pain, and jaundice
	Hepatitis B virus	Bloodborne, sexually transmitted infection (STI)	
	Hepatitis C virus	Bloodborne	
Cold sores	Herpes simplex virus, type 1	Direct contact with someone infected with Herpes simplex, type 1 (sharing eating utensils or drinking glasses, kissing)	Pain; tingling; small, painful, fluid-filled blisters on a raised, red area of the skin, typically around the mouth
Genital herpes	Herpes simplex virus, type 2	STI	Pain, itching, small red bumps, blisters, and ulcers
CMV	Cytomegalovirus	Direct contact, maternal-fetal transmission	Healthy adults: usually asymptomatic but may have mild hepatitis and prolonged fever Congenital: premature birth, liver problems, lung problems, spleen problems, small size at birth, small head size, seizures, hearing loss, vision loss, lack of coordination, and/or mental disability
AIDS	HIV	Bloodborne, STI	Initial: flu-like symptoms Untreated or advanced: heart, kidney, and liver disease; cancer; and opportunistic infections
Influenza	Influenza virus	Airborne, respiratory droplets	Fever, cough, sore throat, runny or stuffy nose, muscle or body aches, headaches, and fatigue
Measles	Measles virus	Airborne, respiratory droplets	Blotchy rash, fever, cough, runny nose, conjunctivitis, malaise, and tiny white spots with bluish-white centers inside the mouth
Mumps	Mumps virus	Airborne, respiratory droplets	Fever, headache, muscle aches, fatigue, loss of appetite, and swollen and tender salivary (parotid) glands
HPV infection	Human papillomavirus	STI	The majority of cases are asymptomatic; some strains cause genital warts; others are associated with cervical cancer.
Upper respiratory infections, viral	Parainfluenza virus	Direct contact with respiratory secretions (droplets)	HPV1: croup HPV3: bronchiolitis and pneumonia
Polio	Poliovirus	Direct person-to-person contact	Fever, fatigue, nausea, headache, flu-like symptoms, back and neck stiffness, limb pain, and/or paralysis
Rabies	Rabies virus	Direct contact with saliva of rabid animal, usually through the bite of an infected animal	Initially: weakness, fever, and headache Untreated: cerebral dysfunction, anxiety, confusion, agitation, delirium, abnormal behavior, hallucinations, insomnia, and death

(Continued)

TABLE 46-3	Viral Pathogens		
Disease	**Causative Organism**	**Route of Transmission**	**Signs and Symptoms**
Norovirus infection, acute gastroenteritis	Norovirus	Fecal-oral; foodborne (most common cause of foodborne illness in the United States)	Diarrhea, nausea, stomach pain, vomiting, fever, headache, and body aches
Rotavirus infection	Rotavirus	Fecal-oral	Fever, diarrhea, abdominal pain, and vomiting
Fifth disease	Parvovirus B19	Direct contact with respiratory secretions (droplets); can be spread through blood or blood products	Fever, runny nose, headache, rash on face (slapped cheek appearance) and body, and arthralgia
RSV	Respiratory syncytial virus	Airborne, respiratory secretions (droplets)	Cough, sneezing, runny nose, fever, loss of appetite, wheezing, and dyspnea
German measles (3-day measles)	Rubella virus	Airborne, respiratory secretions (droplets)	Fever and rash; if acquired during pregnancy, fetal symptoms may include deafness, cataracts, heart defects, mental retardation, and liver and spleen damage
Chickenpox	Varicella-zoster virus	Direct contact with respiratory secretions (droplets); airborne, respiratory secretions (droplets)	High fever, fatigue, loss of appetite, headache, and itchy rash that becomes blistered, then scabs over

Chronic Disorders of the AIDS Patient The impaired immune system of the AIDS patient permits opportunistic infections, which further reduce the body's ability to fight off infection. These infections attack many different parts of the body.

One of the cornerstones of the care of patients who have AIDS is to prevent opportunistic infections and identify such infections as quickly as possible when they occur. Identifying malignancies, if they occur, is also of utmost importance. If you are familiar with the common disorders an AIDS patient faces, you will be better able to identify early signs of infection or malignancy and point them out to the doctor, in turn initiating early treatment, which is usually most effective. You can help patients who have been diagnosed with HIV to understand the risks they face and the measures best suited to preventing particular infections. Opportunistic infections and chronic disorders include:

- *Pneumocystis carinii* pneumonia
- Kaposi sarcoma
- Non-Hodgkin's lymphoma
- Tuberculosis
- *Mycobacterium avium* complex (MAC) infection
- Meningitis
- Oral candidiasis
- Vaginal candidiasis
- Herpes simplex
- Herpes zoster

Hepatitis Hepatitis is a viral infection of the liver that can lead to cirrhosis and death. Hepatitis virus variants differ in their means of transmission and in their presenting symptoms

of infection. Those variations commonly transmitted through the bloodborne route include the following:

- Hepatitis B is the most common bloodborne hazard heathcare workers face. It is spread through contact with contaminated blood or body fluids and through sexual contact. Most patients recover fully from hepatitis B virus (HBV) infection, but some patients develop chronic infection or remain carriers of the pathogen for the rest of their lives. Adults and children with hepatitis B who develop lifelong infections may experience serious health problems, including cirrhosis (scarring of the liver), liver cancer, liver failure, and death. Preventing the spread of the infection is the most effective means of combating the disease. Following standard precautions and receiving HBV vaccinations are the most effective ways to control the spread of the infection.

- Hepatitis C also is spread through contact with contaminated blood or body fluids and through sexual contact. There is no vaccine for this variant, which has resulted in more deaths than hepatitis A and hepatitis B combined. Many people become carriers of hepatitis C without knowing it because they do not experience any symptoms. If the infection causes immediate symptoms, they often resemble the flu. There are several drugs used to treat acute and chronic hepatitis C currently available. If left untreated, over time, hepatitis C is likely to damage the liver, causing cirrhosis, liver failure, and cancer. As with hepatitis B, preventing the spread of the infection is the best way to combat the disease.

- Hepatitis D (delta agent hepatitis) occurs only in people infected with HBV. Delta agent infection may make hepatitis B symptoms more severe, and it is associated with liver cancer. The HBV vaccine also prevents delta agent infection.

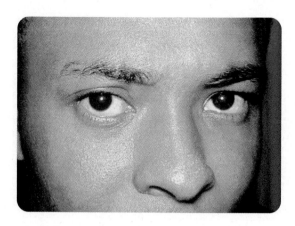

FIGURE 46-2 Jaundice is caused by excess bilirubin, which is produced in the liver and deposited throughout the body, resulting in the yellow appearance of the patient's eyes and skin.

Source: Center for Disease Control (CDC) - PHIL

Symptoms People infected with hepatitis may show no symptoms, may experience such mild or subtle symptoms that they do not realize they are seriously ill, or may experience severe symptoms. When you treat patients with hepatitis, any of these signs and symptoms may be present:

- Jaundice (Figure 46-2)
- Diminished appetite
- Fatigue
- Nausea
- Vomiting
- Joint pain or tenderness
- Stomach pain
- General malaise

▶ Bacteria

LO 46.5

Bacteria are single-celled prokaryotic (without a nucleus) organisms that reproduce very quickly and are one of the major causes of disease. Under the right conditions—the right temperature, the right nutrients, and moisture—bacterial cells can double in number in 15 to 30 minutes. This rapid reproduction is one reason that untreated infections can be dangerous.

Classification and Identification

Bacteria can be classified according to their shape, their ability to retain certain dyes, their ability to grow with or without air, and certain biochemical reactions.

Shape The most common way to classify bacteria is according to their shape. The four common shape classifications are the coccus, bacillus, spirillum, and vibrio (see Figure 46-3).

A **coccus** (plural, *cocci*) is spherical, round, or ovoid. Cocci can be further divided into three types:

- *Staphylococci* are grape-like clusters of cocci commonly found on the skin (*staphylo-* means "cluster of grapes"). One species of this microorganism causes a variety of infections, including boils, acne, abscesses, food poisoning, and a type

of pneumonia. When viewed under a microscope, stained staphylococci look like clusters of purple grapes.

- *Diplococci* are pairs of cocci (*diplo-* means "double"). The causative agents for gonorrhea and some forms of meningitis are diplococci. When viewed under a microscope, stained diplococci are said to look like little boxing gloves.
- *Streptococci* are cocci that grow in chains (*strepto-* means "twisted chain"). These microorganisms are responsible for infections such as strep throat, certain types of pneumonia, and rheumatic fever. When viewed under the microscope, stained streptococci look like long chains of round beads.

A **bacillus** (plural, *bacilli*) is rod-shaped (*bacillo-* is derived from the Latin word meaning "stick"). Bacilli are responsible for a wide variety of infections, including gastroenteritis, tuberculosis, pneumonia, whooping cough, urinary tract infections (UTIs), botulism, and tetanus. When viewed under the microscope, stained bacilli look like little rods or rounded sticks.

A **spirillum** (plural, *spirilla*) is spiral-shaped (*spira-* means "coil"). Spirilla are responsible for infections such as syphilis and Lyme disease. When viewed under a microscope, stained spirilla look like stretched-out springs or coils.

A **vibrio** (plural, *vibrios*) is comma-shaped (*vibrio* means "vibrate"). Most vibrio bacteria are found in water and are motile, meaning that they move. Vibrios are responsible for diseases such as cholera and some cases of food poisoning. When viewed under a microscope, stained vibrios look like commas or hooked structures.

Ability to Retain Certain Dyes In addition to their shape, bacteria are commonly classified by how they react to certain stains. A **stain** is a specific dye or group of dyes that imparts a color to microorganisms. The most common staining procedure in use today is the **Gram stain.** This method of staining uses a group of dyes and decolorizers to differentiate bacteria according to the chemical composition of their cell walls. Gram staining techniques separate bacteria into two groups: **Gram-positive** and **Gram-negative.** Gram-positive bacteria retain the crystal violet stain during the staining process, causing them to appear blue when viewed under the microscope. Gram-negative bacteria do not retain the crystal violet stain during the staining process; however, they do take up the red counter stain. This causes them to appear red when viewed under the microscope. The **acid-fast stain** is a staining procedure for identifying bacteria with a waxy cell wall. The bacteria that cause tuberculosis have waxy cell walls and can be stained with this procedure.

Ability to Grow in the Presence or Absence of Air Bacteria that grow best in the presence of oxygen are referred to as **aerobes.** Those that grow best in the absence of oxygen are referred to as **anaerobes.** Organisms that can grow in either environment are referred to as **facultative.** Although most common bacteria are aerobes, many of the bacteria that make up the body's resident normal flora are anaerobes. Not surprisingly, anaerobes are often responsible for infections within the body.

Biochemical Reactions Many closely related bacteria can be differentiated from one another only by certain

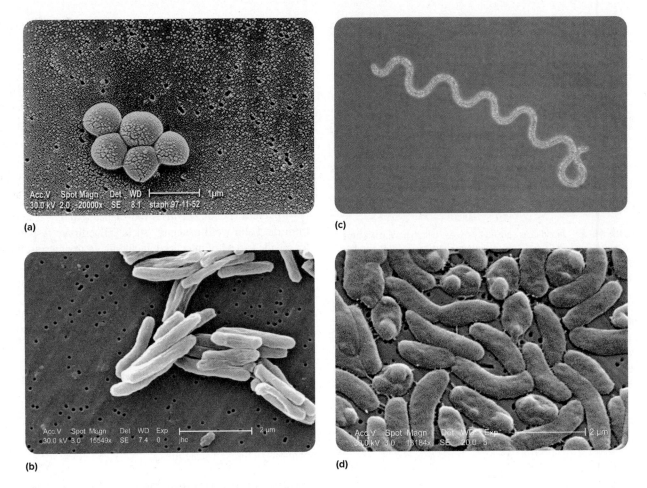

FIGURE 46-3 The four bacterial classifications by shape are (a) coccus, (b) bacillus, (c) spirillum, and (d) vibrio.

(a-b) Source: CDC/Janice Carr; (c) ©MELBA PHOTO AGENCY/Alamy Stock Photo; (d) Source: CDC/Janice Haney Carr

biochemical reactions that occur within the bacterial cell. For example, one way to identify a particular bacterial strain is to look at what types of sugars the bacteria can grow on.

Special Groups of Bacteria

Several groups of bacteria have certain characteristics that set them apart from most other bacteria. These include the mycobacteria, rickettsiae, chlamydiae, and mycoplasmas.

Mycobacteria Mycobacteria are rod-shaped bacilli with a waxy cell wall, making them acid-fast. Certain types of mycobacteria cause disease in humans. For example, *Mycobacterium tuberculosis* causes the respiratory disease tuberculosis and *Mycobacterium leprae* causes leprosy, also known as Hansen's disease.

Rickettsiae Rickettsiae are unusually small bacteria that can live and grow only within other living cells. Rickettsiae are commonly found in insects such as ticks and mites but may be transmitted to humans through bites. Rickettsiae are responsible for diseases such as Rocky Mountain spotted fever and typhus.

Chlamydiae Chlamydiae differ from other bacteria in the structure of their cell walls. Like rickettsiae, they can live and grow only within other living cells. In humans, chlamydiae

can cause sexually transmitted infections (STIs), eye disease, certain types of pneumonia, and certain types of heart disease.

Mycoplasmas Mycoplasmas are unusually small bacteria that completely lack the rigid cell wall of other bacteria. These bacteria cause a variety of human diseases, including STIs and a form of pneumonia.

Bacterial Pathogens

In spite of our efforts to eradicate disease-causing bacteria through the use of antibiotics, bacterial pathogens are still with us. Table 46-4 lists some of these pathogens and the diseases they cause.

Drug-Resistant Microorganisms

Drug-resistant pathogens are the cause of many infections. Drug resistance has been linked to overuse of antibiotics. It is the responsibility of physicians, medical staff, and patients to use antibiotics wisely, as resistance to antimicrobial agents is a severe problem. Bacteria and other microorganisms that have developed resistance to antimicrobial drugs include but are not limited to the following:

- MRSA—methicillin/oxacillin-resistant *S. aureus*.
- VRE—vancomycin-resistant enterococci

TABLE 46-4 Bacterial Pathogens

Disease	Causative Organism	Characteristics	Route of Transmission	Signs and Symptoms
Anthrax	*Bacillus anthracis*	Aerobic, Gram-positive, spore-forming bacillus	Contact with animals infected with or inhalation of *B. anthracis* spores, or consumption of raw or undercooked meat from infected animals	Cutaneous: raised, blistered skin lesion with development of black eschar (dead tissue) Inhalation: high fever, dyspnea, stridor, cyanosis, and shock
Whooping cough	*Bordetella pertussis*	Gram-negative bacterium	Airborne	Stage 1: runny nose, low-grade fever, and mild cough Stage 2: bursts of rapid, uncontrollable coughs with characteristic "whoops" at the end of the cough; cyanosis; and exhaustion Stage 3: recovery and less persistent cough
Lyme disease	*Borrelia burgdorferi*	Spirochete that does not have typical Gram stain characteristics	Tick-borne (*Ixodes* tick)	Red, expanding, "bull's-eye" rash; fatigue; fever; chills; headache; muscle and joint aches; and swollen lymph nodes
Campylobacteriosis	*Campylobacter jejuni*	Gram-negative, microaerophilic, spiral-shaped	Fecal-oral, foodborne	Diarrhea, sometimes bloody; abdominal cramps; and fever
Chlamydia	*Chlamydia trachomatis*	Coccus; does not have typical Gram stain characteristics but is considered Gram-negative; obligate, intracellular bacteria (must live within an animal cell)	STI	Women: often "silent"; possible vaginal discharge and dysuria Men: penile discharge and dysuria
Botulism	*Clostridium botulinum*	Anaerobic, Gram-positive, spore-forming bacillus	Foodborne	Double vision, blurred vision, drooping eyelids, slurred speech, difficulty swallowing, dry mouth, and muscle weakness
Pseudomembranous colitis	*Clostridium difficile*	Anaerobic, Gram-positive, spore-forming bacillus	Fecal-oral (healthcare-associated infection)	Watery diarrhea, fever, loss of appetite, nausea, and abdominal pain/tenderness
Tetanus	*Clostridium tetani*	Anaerobic, Gram-positive bacillus (sometimes forms spores)	Direct contact through a deep cut	Early: lockjaw, neck and abdomen stiffness, and difficulty swallowing Late: severe muscle spasms and generalized tonic-seizure-like activity
Diphtheria	*Corynebacterium diphtheria*	Gram-positive bacillus	Direct person-to-person contact with respiratory droplets or cutaneous lesions	Sore throat; low-grade fever; and presence of a pseudomembrane over the tonsils, throat, and nose
E. coli diarrhea	*Escherichia coli*	Gram-negative bacillus	Foodborne (some strains do not cause disease)	Diarrhea, severe abdominal cramps, and vomiting
Haemophilus influenzae Serotype b (Hib) disease (epiglottitis, pneumonia)	*Haemophilus influenzae*	Gram-negative coccobacillus	Direct contact with respiratory droplets	Epiglottitis: sore throat and difficulty breathing Pneumonia: difficulty breathing and fever
Peptic ulcer	*Helicobacter pylori*	Microaerophilic, Gram-negative bacillus	Not well understood; may be fecal-oral or oral-oral	Gnawing or burning stomach pain, nausea, bloating, and burping
Legionnaire's disease	*Legionella pneumophila*	Gram-negative bacillus	Water aerosol	High fever, chills, cough, chest pain, and pneumonia

(Continued)

TABLE 46-4 Bacterial Pathogens

Disease	Causative Organism	Characteristics	Route of Transmission	Signs and Symptoms
Leprosy	*Mycobacterium leprae*	Acid-fast bacillus	Airborne, respiratory droplets	Skin lesions, nodules, plaques, and thickened dermis
Tuberculosis	*Mycobacterium tuberculosis*	Acid-fast bacillus	Airborne, respiratory droplets	Bad cough lasting 3 weeks or longer, pain in the chest, coughing up blood or sputum, weakness or fatigue, weight loss, no appetite, chills, fever, and night sweats
Mycoplasma pneumonia	*Mycoplasma pneumoniae*	Wall-less bacteria, usually coccoid in shape with polar extensions	Direct contact with respiratory droplets	Fever, nonproductive cough, malaise, and headache
Gonorrhea	*Neisseria gonorrhoeae*	Gram-negative diplococcus	STI	Women: most have no symptoms; some have dysuria and vaginal discharge Men: dysuria and green, yellow, or white penile discharge Left untreated can cause complications in both women and men
Meningitis	*Neisseria meningitidis*	Gram-negative diplococcus	Direct contact with respiratory droplets	Stiff neck, fever, confusion, light sensitivity, nausea, and vomiting
	Haemophilus influenzae	Gram-negative coccobacillus		
	Group B *Streptococcus* (*Streptococcus agalactiae*)	Gram-positive coccus		
	Listeria monocytogenes	Gram-positive, flagellated bacillus		
Pseudomonas infection (hot tub rash)	*Pseudomonas aeruginosa*	Gram-negative bacillus	Direct contact with water contaminated with *P. aeruginosa*	Itchy, red rash and pustules around hair follicles
Rocky Mountain spotted fever	*Rickettsia rickettsi*	Gram-negative coccobacillus	Tick-borne (wood or dog tick)	Fever, rash (occurs 2–5 days after fever), headache, nausea, vomiting, abdominal pain, muscle pain, lack of appetite, and conjunctival inflammation
Shigellosis	*Shigella sonnei*	Gram-negative bacillus	Fecal-oral	Diarrhea, fever, and stomach cramps
Methicillin-resistant *Staphylococcus aureus* (MRSA) infection	*Staphylococcus aureus*	Gram-positive coccus	Direct contact	Red, swollen, painful pustules
Bacterial pneumonia	*Streptococcus pneumonia*	Gram-positive diplococcus	Direct person-to-person contact	Cough, chest pain, shortness of breath, malaise, and poor appetite
Strep throat	*Streptococcus pyogenes*	Gram-positive coccus	Direct contact with respiratory droplets	Sore throat and fever
Syphilis	*Treponema pallidum*	Gram-negative spirochete	STI	Primary stage: single sore (chancre) at site of the organism's entry into the body Secondary stage: skin rash and mucous membrane lesions Late stage: uncoordinated muscle movements, paralysis, numbness, gradual blindness, and dementia
Cholera	*Vibrio cholerae*	Gram-negative curved rod	Fecal-oral from contaminated water	Profuse watery diarrhea ("rice-water stools"), vomiting, rapid heart rate, loss of skin elasticity, dry mucous membranes, low blood pressure, thirst, muscle cramps, and restlessness or irritability

- VISA—vancomycin-intermediate *S. aureus.*
- VRSA—vancomycin-resistant *S. aureus.*
- ESBLs—extended-spectrum beta-lactamases, which are resistant to cephalosporins and monobactams.
- PRSP—penicillin-resistant *Streptococcus pneumoniae.*

MRSA and VRE are the most common multidrug-resistant organisms in patients who reside in nonhospital healthcare facilities (for example, nursing homes and other long-term care facilities). People outside of healthcare facilities are increasingly at risk for MRSA, as community-associated MRSA, an infection found in otherwise healthy individuals, is on the rise in the United States. PRSP is more common in patients seeking care in physicians' offices and clinics, especially in pediatric settings. This is thought to be because penicillin is the most commonly prescribed antibiotic in outpatient settings.

Risk Factors

There are a number of risk factors for both the development of and infection with drug-resistant organisms. These risk factors include:

- Advanced age.
- Invasive procedures, which include dialysis, the presence of invasive devices, and urinary catheterization.
- Previous use of antimicrobial agents.
- Repeated contact with the healthcare system.
- Severity of the illness.
- Underlying diseases or conditions, especially chronic renal disease, insulin-dependent diabetes mellitus, peripheral vascular disease, and dermatitis or skin lesions.

Preventing Antibiotic Resistance in Healthcare Settings

In response to a growing concern over the emergence of antibiotic-resistant infections, the CDC began the Be Antibiotics Aware program. This program has several strategies to reduce the incidence of antibiotic-resistant microorganisms, including:

- Avoiding infection.
- Improving antibiotic prescribing and use.
- Improving diagnostic testing to determine if antibiotics are appropriate.

- Educating patients about appropriate antibiotic use.
- Reducing antibiotic use in long-term care facilities.
- Limiting antibiotic use in food animals.

▶ Protozoans
LO 46.6

Protozoans are single-celled eukaryotic (with a nucleus) organisms that are generally much larger than bacteria. Found in soil and water, most do not cause disease in people. Certain protozoans are pathogenic, however, and cause diseases such as malaria, amebic dysentery (a type of diarrhea), and trichomoniasis vaginitis (a type of STI; see Figure 46-4). Protozoal diseases are a leading cause of death in developing countries because the lack of proper sanitation in some areas promotes their spread. These diseases are also common in patients with depressed immune systems. Table 46-5 lists some of the parasitic protozoans and multicellular parasites that affect humans.

▶ Fungi
LO 46.7

A *fungus* (plural, *fungi*) is a eukaryotic organism that has a rigid cell wall at some stage in the life cycle. Fungi that grow mainly as single-celled organisms and reproduce by budding are referred to as *yeasts,* whereas fungi that grow into large, fuzzy, multicelled organisms that produce spores are called *molds.* Figure 46-5 shows the differences between these two types of fungi.

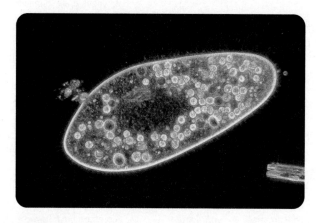

FIGURE 46-4   The protozoan *Trichomonas vaginalis* causes a common STI in humans.
©MELBA PHOTO AGENCY/Alamy Stock Photo

TABLE 46-5	Human Protozoal and Multicellular Parasites			
Disease	**Causative Organism**	**Notable Features**	**Route of Transmission**	**Signs and Symptoms**
Intestinal				
Amebiasis	*Entamoeba histolytica*	Can become invasive and cause liver abscess	Fecal-oral	Loose stool, abdominal pain, abdominal cramping, bloody diarrhea, and fever
Intestinal hookworm	*Necator americanus* and *Ancylostoma duodenale*	Larvae migrate to the intestinal tract.	Larvae in soil contaminated with feces from an infected person penetrate bare feet and cause infection.	Itching at the site of entry, abdominal pain, diarrhea, anorexia, and anemia due to loss of blood at the site of attachment in the intestine

(Continued)

TABLE 46-5   Human Protozoal and Multicellular Parasites

Disease	Causative Organism	Notable Features	Route of Transmission	Signs and Symptoms
Round worm	*Ascaris lumbricoides*	Most common helminthic (worm) infection in the world	Contact with contaminated soil	Can be asymptomatic; symptoms include abdominal discomfort and intestinal blockage
Cryptosporidiosis	*Cryptosporidium parvum* and *C. hominis*	Can be found in recreational water such as swimming pools and hot tubs contaminated with *Cryptosporidium*	Waterborne	Abdominal cramps and pain, dehydration, nausea, vomiting, fever, and weight loss
Cyclosporiasis	*Cyclospora cayetanensis*	Outbreaks in the United States have been linked to imported fresh produce.	Fecal-oral	Frequent, explosive, watery diarrhea; abdominal cramps; loss of appetite; weight loss; bloating; excessive gas; and fatigue
Fish or broad tapeworm	*Diphyllobothrium latum*	Longest human tapeworm, reaching up to 30 feet in length	Foodborne from eating raw or undercooked fish infected with *D. latum*	Abdominal discomfort, diarrhea, vomiting, weight loss, and vitamin B$_{12}$ deficiency
Pinworm	*Enterobius vermicularis*	While the infected person is sleeping, female pinworms leave the intestine and lay their eggs on the skin surrounding the anus.	Fecal-oral	Anal itching, and nighttime restlessness due to anal itching
Giardiasis	*Giardia intestinalis* (formerly *G. lamblia*)	Once outside the body, can live in soil or water for weeks or months	Fecal-oral	Greasy, floating stool; gas; diarrhea; abdominal pain and cramping; nausea; and dehydration
Lung fluke (Paragonimiasis)	*Paragonimus kellicotti*	Linked to eating raw or undercooked crab or crayfish infected with *P. kellicotti;* ingested larvae migrate to the lungs	Foodborne	Initially diarrhea and abdominal pain, followed by fever, chest pain, fatigue, and cough
Bloodborne/Vector-borne				
Chagas disease	*Trypanosome cruzi*	Found only in the Americas (mostly Latin America but also the United States)	Vector-borne (triatomine bug)	Acute phase: fever, fatigue, body aches, headache, and diarrhea Chronic phase: cardiomyopathy, heart failure, heart arrhythmia, enlarged esophagus, enlarged colon, and difficulty eating or passing stool
Malaria	*Plasmodium falciparum, P. vivax, P. ovale, P. malariae*	Fifth most common cause of death worldwide from infectious disease	Vector-borne (mosquito)	Fever, chills, sweats, headache, nausea, body aches, and general malaise
Skin				
Swimmer's itch (cercarial dermatitis)	*Austrobilharzia variglandis*	Ducks and geese are the most common host; however, the larvae will burrow into a human swimmer's skin.	Contact with larvae in water	Tingling, burning, or itching of the skin; small, reddish pimples; and small blisters
Head lice (pediculosis)	*Pediculus humanus capitis*	Can be transmitted by contact with clothing, combs, or brushes used by an infested individual	Direct contact with the hair of infested individual	Feeling that something is moving in your hair, itching, difficulty sleeping because of louse activity, and scalp sores
Pubic lice (pthiriasis)	*Phthirus pubis*	Can be transmitted through contact with bed linens or towels used by an infested individual	Direct contact with an infested individual (usually sexual contact)	Genital itching, visible nits (eggs), or crawling adult lice
Scabies	*Sarcoptes scabiei*	Symptoms worse at night	Prolonged, direct contact with an infested individual	Intense itching and papular rash
Bed bugs	*Cimex lectularius* and *C. hemipterus*	Not known to carry any disease and not considered a public health threat	Exposure to bedding or furniture infested with *C. lectularius* or *C. hemipterus*	Bite marks on the head, neck, face, hands, or other body parts occurring at night while sleeping

(Continued)

TABLE 46-5   Human Protozoal and Multicellular Parasites

Disease	Causative Organism	Notable Features	Route of Transmission	Signs and Symptoms
Muscle				
Trichinellosis	*Trichinella spiralis*	Currently uncommon in commercial pork; more cases in the United States are now associated with wild game.	Foodborne from eating raw or undercooked pork or wild animals	Nausea, diarrhea, vomiting, fatigue, fever, abdominal pain, headache, chills, coughing, eye swelling, and joint pain
Toxoplasmosis	*Toxoplasma gondii*	Forms cysts that may be found in skeletal muscle, myocardium, brain, and eyes	Foodborne, animal-to-human, mother-to-child (congenital)	Some have no or very mild symptoms; swollen lymph glands and muscle aches
Vagina, Vulva, Urethra				
Trichomoniasis	*Trichomonas vaginalis*	Considered the most common and most curable STI	Sexual contact	Women: itching, burning, redness or soreness of the genitals, dysuria, and watery discharge with an unusual smell Men: itching or irritation inside the penis, burning after urination or ejaculation, and some penile discharge

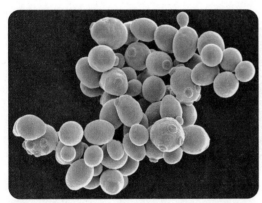

(a)

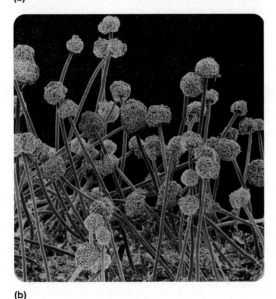

(b)

FIGURE 46-5   Because fungi lack the ability to make their own food, they depend on other life forms. (a) Single-celled fungi are called yeasts. (b) Multicelled fungi are called molds.

(a) ©Science Photo Library - STEVE GSCHMEISSNER./Getty Images; (b) ©David Scharf/Science Source

Most fungi do not cause disease in humans. Of those that do, the majority produce superficial infections such as athlete's foot (tinea pedis), ringworm, thrush, and vaginal yeast infections. Fungi can produce serious, life-threatening illness, however, when they infect the internal tissues. This kind of infection can occur when patients have a depressed immune system, as in patients who are undergoing cancer treatment and patients with AIDS. Table 46-6 lists some of the most common fungal diseases and the organisms that cause them.

▶ Multicellular Parasites   LO 46.8

A *parasite* is an organism that lives on or in another organism and uses that other organism for food or for some other advantage to the detriment of the host organism. For example, a leech is a type of parasite that lives off of the host's blood. Viruses, rickettsiae, chlamydiae, and some protozoans are parasitic. Multicellular organisms also can be parasitic, and some of these organisms are microscopic during all or part of their lives. An infection caused by a parasite is called an *infestation*. Multicellular parasites that cause human disease include certain worms and insects, as illustrated in Figure 46-6 and listed in Table 46-5.

Parasitic Worms

People can be infested with a parasitic worm by ingesting its eggs or an immature form of the worm or by having the parasite penetrate the skin. As with the protozoans, infestation by these parasites is more common in developing nations with poor sanitation.

Worms that infect people include roundworms, flatworms, and tapeworms. Roundworms can occur in the intestines, as in the case of pinworms, a common infection in children. Other roundworms, such as *Trichinella,* are found in muscle tissue. *Trichinella spiralis,* which causes the infection trichinosis, enters the human body in infected meat eaten raw or insufficiently cooked. People also may get flatworms and tapeworms by eating undercooked meats.

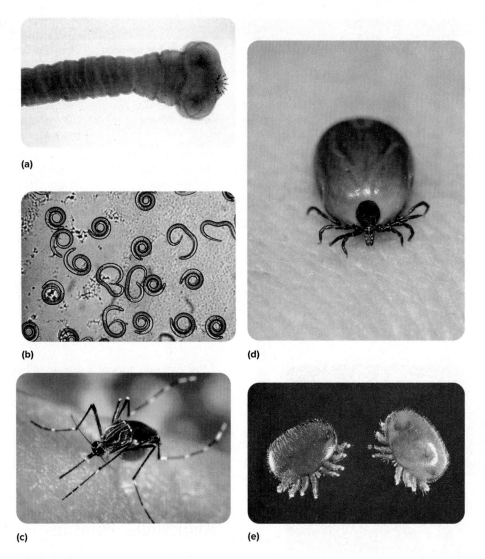

FIGURE 46-6 Parasitic worms, such as (a) tapeworms (Cestoda) and (b) *Trichinella,* cause disease in humans when they are ingested. Parasitic insects, such as (c) mosquitoes, (d) deer ticks, and (e) mites, cause disease by biting or burrowing into the skin.

(a) Source: Centers for Disease Control; (b) ©Dickson Despommier/Science Source; (c) Source: CDC/James Gathany; (d) ©Jay Ondreicka/Shutterstock; (e) Source: Photo by Scott Bauer/USDA

TABLE 46-6	Pathogenic Fungi		
Disease	**Causative Organism**	**Route of Transmission**	**Signs and Symptoms**
Aspergillosis	*Aspergillus fumigatus* and *A. flavus*	Airborne (inhalation of spores)	Wheezing, coughing, fever, chest pain, shortness of breath, and aspergilloma (fungus ball)
Blastomycosis	*Blastomyces dermatitidis*	Airborne (inhalation of spores)	Fever, chills, cough, muscle aches, joint pain, and chest pain
Candidiasis • Oropharyngeal (thrush) • Vaginal • Invasive	*Candida albicans*	*C. albicans* is part of the body's resident normal flora; conditions that cause an imbalance in the resident normal flora cause an overgrowth of the fungus.	• Oropharyngeal—white patches on the tongue and other oral mucous membranes, redness or soreness in the affected areas, difficulty swallowing, and cracking at the corners of the mouth • Vaginal—genital itching; burning; and thick, white vaginal discharge • Invasive—fever and chills

(Continued)

TABLE 46-6 Pathogenic Fungi

Disease	Causative Organism	Route of Transmission	Signs and Symptoms
Coccidioidomycosis (valley fever)	*Coccidioides*	Airborne (inhalation of spores)	Fever, cough, headache, rash on upper trunk or extremities, muscle aches, joint pain in the knees or ankles, skin lesions, chronic pneumonia, meningitis, and bone or joint infection
Ringworm	Dermatophytes *(Trichophyton rubrum* and *T. tonsurans)*	Direct contact with an infected person	Redness, scaling, cracking of the skin, or a ring-shaped rash; loss of hair at the site of infection
Cryptococcosis	*Cryptococcus neoformans* and *C. gattii*	Airborne; *C. neoformans* is usually associated with large amounts of bird droppings.	Shortness of breath, cough, fatigue, fever, headache, and meningitis
Histoplasmosis	*Histoplasma capsulatum*	Airborne, usually associated with large amounts of bird or bat droppings	Fever, chest pains, and nonproductive cough
Pneumocystis pneumonia (PCP)	*Pneumocystis jirovecii*	Airborne, inhalation of spores; most common opportunistic infection in people with HIV/AIDS	Fever, dry cough, shortness of breath, and fatigue
Sporotrichosis	*Sporothrix schenckii*	Direct contact with spores	Small, painless nodule at contact site; lesion becomes larger over time and may ulcerate

A trained medical professional must inspect a patient's stool for the presence of the parasite or its eggs to diagnose an intestinal infection with a parasitic worm.

Parasitic Insects

Insects that can bite or burrow under the skin include mosquitoes, ticks, lice, and mites. These insects spread many viral, bacterial (including rickettsial), and protozoal diseases. The causative organisms can live in the insects' bodies and enter people's bodies when they are bitten by the insects. Such diseases include Lyme disease, malaria, Rocky Mountain spotted fever, and encephalitis. Lice are small insects that live on hair and skin and feed on blood. Scabies infestations are caused by mites that burrow under the skin.

▶ How Infections Are Diagnosed   LO 46.9

To assist with the diagnosis and treatment of an infection, a medical assistant must work closely with other medical team members. The basic steps in diagnosis and treatment are summarized in Figure 46-7.

Step 1. Examine the Patient

When a patient comes in to the office with signs or symptoms that suggest an infection, begin by taking the patient's vital signs and noting the patient's complaints. On the basis of these findings and the patient examination, the doctor can make a presumptive, or tentative, clinical diagnosis.

In many cases, signs and symptoms of a particular infection are so characteristic of the disease that the doctor need

not perform additional tests to reach a diagnosis. An example is a case of chickenpox or mumps. At other times, however, the doctor needs to gather additional information to confirm a diagnosis and determine the cause.

Step 2. Obtain One or More Specimens

To determine the cause of an infection, you may need to obtain specimens from one or more areas of the patient's body. Label each specimen properly and include with it the physician's presumptive diagnosis. If the sample is to be transported to an outside laboratory, ensure that it is transported in such a way that any pathogenic organisms remain alive (and safely contained) during transit.

Step 3. Examine the Specimen Directly

You must sometimes obtain more than one specimen from each site. The doctor or specially trained laboratory or microbiology personnel will then directly examine one specimen under the microscope. The specimen may be viewed in one of two ways:

- As a wet mount, a preparation of a specimen in a liquid that allows the organisms to remain alive and mobile while they are being identified.
- As a smear, in which a specimen is spread thinly and evenly across a slide.

If you make a smear, allow it to dry and then treat or stain it as ordered before it is examined microscopically. In some cases, direct examination allows the doctor to make a presumptive diagnosis of the microorganism.

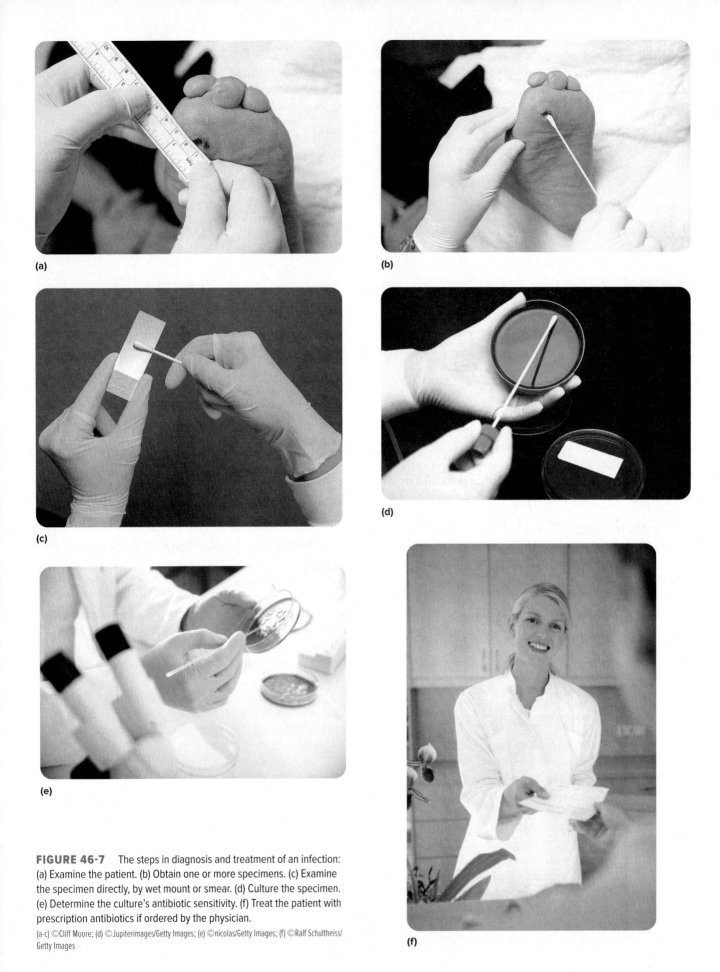

FIGURE 46-7 The steps in diagnosis and treatment of an infection: (a) Examine the patient. (b) Obtain one or more specimens. (c) Examine the specimen directly, by wet mount or smear. (d) Culture the specimen. (e) Determine the culture's antibiotic sensitivity. (f) Treat the patient with prescription antibiotics if ordered by the physician.

(a-c) ©Cliff Moore; (d) ©Jupiterimages/Getty Images; (e) ©nicolas/Getty Images; (f) ©Ralf Schultheiss/Getty Images

Step 4. Culture the Specimen

If the physician still needs a more definitive identification of the microorganism, you may perform a **culture,** in which a sample of the specimen is placed in or on a substance that allows microorganisms to grow. A *culture medium* is a substance that contains all the nutrients a particular type of microorganism needs. Most media come in the form of a semisolid gel. After it has been inoculated (by placing a sample of the specimen in or on) the medium, it is placed in an incubator (a chamber that can be set to a specific temperature and humidity) to allow the microorganism to grow. This is most often done by a laboratory technologist.

The culture is examined visually and microscopically after a specified time and a preliminary identification is made. The physician sets up additional tests to confirm the identification of the microorganism that has been isolated from the specimen. Most microbiology laboratories and some physicians' office laboratories are equipped to grow routine bacterial cultures and some fungal cultures. Physicians' office laboratories, in particular, may have to send other types of cultures, such as virus cultures, to a specialized laboratory for identification.

Step 5. Determine the Culture's Antibiotic Sensitivity

In many cases of bacterial infection, a **culture and sensitivity (C&S)** is performed. This procedure involves culturing a specimen and then testing the isolated bacterium's susceptibility (sensitivity) to certain antibiotics. The results help the doctor determine which antibiotics might be most effective in treating the infection.

Step 6. Treat the Patient as Ordered by the Physician

On the basis of identification of the microorganism and antibiotic sensitivity, if determined, the physician can prescribe an *antimicrobial.* This agent, which kills microorganisms or suppresses their growth, should help clear up the patient's infection.

▶ Specimen Collection   LO 46.10

Perhaps the most important step in isolating and identifying a microorganism as the cause of an infection is collecting the specimen. If this is done incorrectly, the organism may not grow in the culture in a way that it can be identified, resulting in an untreated infection. Furthermore, if the specimen becomes contaminated during collection and the contaminant is mistakenly identified as the cause of the infection, the patient may receive incorrect or even harmful therapy.

In addition to vaginal specimens (discussed in detail in the *Assisting in Reproductive and Urinary Specialties* chapter), the most common types of culture specimens involve the following:

- Throat
- Urine
- Sputum

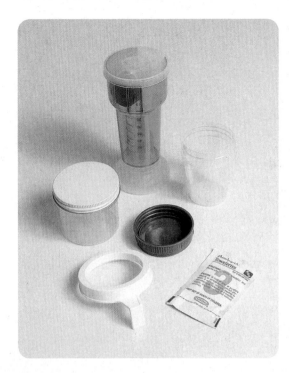

FIGURE 46-8   You may use specially designed collection containers to collect sputum, urine, and stool specimens.
©Cliff Moore

- Wound
- Stool

Specimen-Collection Devices

To help ensure optimal recovery of microorganisms, you must use the appropriate collection device and specimen container. Specimen-collection devices are available for the collection of sputum, urine, and stool specimens, as shown in Figure 46-8. These containers are designed with large openings to allow specimen collection with minimal chance of contamination. They also have tight-fitting caps to prevent leakage and contamination.

Sterile Swabs   The most common device for obtaining cultures is the sterile swab. Sterile swabs vary in the absorbent material at the tip and in the composition of the shaft (Figure 46-9).

Although cotton is absorbent, it is no longer used for culture swabs because natural chemicals in cotton inhibit the growth of certain microorganisms. Polyester, rayon, or calcium alginate fibers are preferred. Most swabs used to collect routine specimens have a wooden or plastic shaft for rigidity. Swabs with a small tip and a flexible wire shaft are made especially for culturing hard-to-reach areas and obtaining pediatric specimens. Some collection containers contain two swabs—one for a culture and one for a smear.

Collection and Transport Systems

Sterile, self-contained systems for obtaining and transporting specimens are commercially available from many suppliers. The CULTURETTE Collection and Transport System, manufactured by Becton Dickinson Microbiology Systems of Sparks, Maryland, is a well-known example. The unit, shown

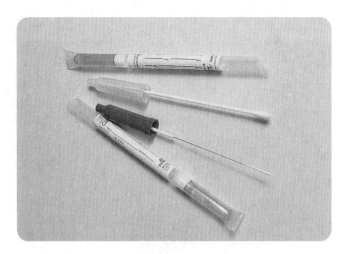

FIGURE 46-9 Sterile swabs vary in size and material.
©Cliff Moore

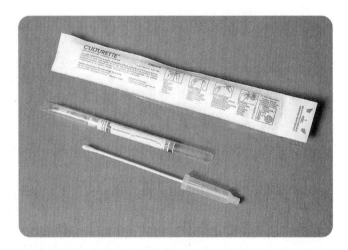

FIGURE 46-10 The CULTURETTE is used to obtain and transport microbiologic specimens to outside laboratories.
Source: Courtesy of Becton Dickinson Microbiology Systems. ©Cliff Moore

in Figure 46-10, contains a polyester swab and a small, thin-walled vial of transport medium in a plastic sleeve. If a specimen will not be tested within 30 minutes after it is obtained, the swab is replaced in the sleeve and the vial is crushed between the thumb and the index finger. The moisture and nutrients provided by the transport medium help keep the bacteria alive during transport to the laboratory.

Several collection systems are also available for culturing anaerobic organisms. These systems provide a means of generating an oxygen-free environment so the anaerobic organisms remain viable (alive and able to reproduce) during transport.

Specimen-Collection Guidelines

To collect specimens properly, you should follow a number of general guidelines.

- Obtain the specimen with great care to avoid causing the patient harm, discomfort, or undue embarrassment. If patients are to collect specimens on their own, give them clear, detailed instructions along with the proper container.

- Collect the material from a site where the organism is most likely to be found and where contamination is least likely to occur. For example, the best location to obtain a specimen for diagnosing strep throat is at the back of the throat in the area of the tonsils. A properly collected sputum specimen should contain mucus coughed up from the respiratory tract but should not contain saliva, which is a contaminant.

- Obtain the specimen at a time that allows optimal chance of recovery of the microorganism. Knowledge of the infectious disease process allows the doctor to determine the best time to collect a specimen. For example, certain viruses are more readily isolated during the early, symptomatic stage of an illness.

- Use appropriate collection devices, specimen containers, transport systems, and culture media to ensure optimal microorganism recovery. The purpose of such equipment and materials is to preserve the viability of any microorganisms so that they will grow in culture. Special collection devices are available for certain body areas or suspected pathogens.

- Obtain a sufficient quantity of the specimen for performing the requested procedures. If, for example, both a culture and a direct examination of a swabbed specimen will be done, you must collect two specimens. Each procedure requires its own sample.

- Obtain the specimen before antimicrobial therapy begins. If the patient is already taking an antibiotic, note this fact on the laboratory request form or ask the doctor whether you should obtain the specimen.

After correctly collecting the specimen, you must label the container and include the appropriate requisition form. The label should contain the following information:

- Patient's name and identification number (if appropriate).
- Source (collection site) of the specimen.
- Date and time of collection.
- Doctor's name.
- Your initials (if you obtained the specimen).

The requisition form should include the following information:

- Patient's name, address, and identification number.
- Patient's age and gender.
- Patient's insurance billing information.
- Type and source of the microbiologic specimen (for example, discharge from wound, big toe).
- Date and time of microbiologic specimen collection.
- Test requested.
- Medications the patient is currently receiving.
- Doctor's presumptive diagnosis.
- Doctor's name, address, and phone number.
- Special instructions or orders.

Throat Culture Specimens

The doctor may request a throat culture on patients with signs or symptoms of an upper respiratory, throat, or sinus infection. In most cases, the doctor wants to determine whether the patient has strep throat, an infection caused by the bacterium *Streptococcus pyogenes,* a group A streptococcus. It is particularly important to diagnose and treat this infection because, left untreated, strep throat can lead to complications such as rheumatic fever. Rheumatic fever is an inflammation of the heart tissue that occurs most frequently in school-age children.

When you obtain a throat culture specimen, avoid touching any structures inside the mouth, as this will contaminate the specimen. The correct technique for obtaining a throat culture specimen is outlined in Procedure 46-1 at the end of this chapter.

Many doctors order rapid strep tests if strep is suspected. Antigen-antibody test kits for strep are available in a variety of brands and provide immediate indications of the strep antigen's presence on a throat swab, sparing the patient the expense and waiting period associated with having a culture done. The correct technique for performing a rapid strep test is outlined in Procedure 46-2 at the end of this chapter.

If your office does not culture microbiologic specimens, use a sterile collection system to obtain the specimen. If your office has the equipment to perform its own cultures, use a sterile swab and inoculate a culture plate directly with the swab. Specimens to be evaluated in the office should be cultured immediately after collection.

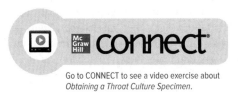

Go to CONNECT to see a video exercise about *Obtaining a Throat Culture Specimen.*

Urine Specimens

To minimize contaminants in urine specimens, it is important to obtain a clean-catch mid-stream specimen. You must process urine specimens within an hour of collection or refrigerate them to prevent continued bacterial growth. (Collection of urine specimens for culturing is discussed in detail in the *Collecting, Processing, and Testing Urine and Stool Specimens* chapter.)

Sputum Specimens

To obtain sputum specimens, have the patient expectorate (cough up) mucus from the lungs into a wide-mouthed specimen container. Beforehand, instruct the patient to avoid contaminating the specimen with saliva. If sputum specimens are not cultured right away, they should be refrigerated.

Observe standard precautions whenever you handle sputum samples and wear a face shield or mask and goggles when collecting such specimens, especially if the patient is coughing. Even when tuberculosis is not suspected, the potential for its transmission always exists.

Wound Specimens

You usually obtain specimens from infected wounds and lesions by swabbing. The procedure is similar to that of a throat culture. Be sure you obtain representative material from a deep area and a surface area of the wound without contaminating the swab by touching areas outside the site.

Transporting Specimens to an Outside Laboratory   LO 46.11

Many physicians' offices do not perform microbiologic testing on-site, choosing instead to send their culture specimens to an outside laboratory. This is particularly true for many specialized microbiologic procedures such as virus cultures and bacteria cultures (including chlamydia) that require special techniques and equipment rarely found in a physician's office laboratory.

Your Main Objectives

When you collect and transport a microbiologic specimen to an outside laboratory, you have three main objectives:

1. Making sure proper collection procedures are followed, including using the proper collection device. Improperly handled specimens will not be processed at the lab.
2. Maintaining the samples in a state as close to their original as possible. You must take specific steps to prevent them from deteriorating.
3. Protecting anyone who handles a specimen container from exposure to potentially infectious material. To do so, ensure that the specimen container has a tight-fitting lid. As extra protection against leakage, place the specimen container in a secondary container or zipper-type plastic bag (usually provided by the laboratory).

Methods of Transportation

Specimens to be tested by an outside laboratory may be transported in one of three ways:

- During regularly scheduled daily pickups by the laboratory.
- During an as-needed pickup by the laboratory.
- Through the mail.

Pickup by the laboratory is the most reliable and timely method of transporting microbiologic specimens. Although each laboratory has its own procedure, the general steps for preparing specimens for transport to a laboratory are outlined in Procedure 46-3 at the end of this chapter.

Sending Specimens by Mail

There may be times when you must send a specimen through the mail to a special reference laboratory for a test not normally done by a local laboratory. The US Postal Service accepts a package containing microbiologic specimens as long as the total volume of specimen material is less than 50 milliliters and it is packaged under strict regulations specified by the US Public Health Service.

When sending specimens through the mail, pack them securely with adequate cushioning material to prevent breakage and leakage. Leakage can contaminate the package, putting mail handlers at risk of contamination with infectious materials. The proper technique for packaging and labeling microbiologic specimens is outlined by the Centers for Disease Control and Prevention (CDC) and is shown in Figure 46-11.

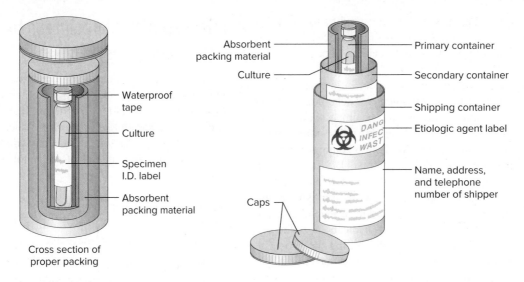

FIGURE 46-11 When packaging and labeling a specimen for mail delivery, you must follow the procedures set by the CDC, based on US Public Health Service regulations.

Securely close the primary culture container and surround it with enough absorbent packing material to absorb the entire fluid contents if the container were to leak. Place these items together in a secondary container, commonly a metal container with a screw-top or snap-on lid. Then place the secondary container in an outer shipping carton made of cardboard or Styrofoam®.

In addition to the address label, microbiologic specimens sent through the mail must have an etiologic agent label affixed to the package, as shown in Figure 46-11. This label uses the biohazard symbol to alert the mail carrier as to the nature of the contents. The term **etiologic agent** refers to a living microorganism or its toxin that may cause human disease.

▶ Direct Examination of Specimens LO 46.12

At times, the physician may directly examine the specimen under a microscope to detect the presence of microorganisms or to identify them. Two types of procedures that allow direct examination of microbiologic specimens are preparing wet mounts and preparing potassium hydroxide (KOH) mounts. You may be required to perform these procedures as part of your duties.

Wet Mounts
A wet mount permits quick identification of many microorganisms and is easy to prepare.

1. Wearing examination gloves, mix a small amount of the specimen with a drop of normal saline (0.9% sodium chloride [NaCl] solution) on a glass slide.
2. Apply a coverslip over the mixture.
3. Give the slide to the doctor for direct examination under the microscope.

If you obtain a specimen from a body site that is normally sterile, detection of microorganisms on a wet mount immediately tells the doctor whether there is infection. Wet mounts are also useful in determining whether a microorganism is motile, which helps in identifying the microorganisms.

Potassium Hydroxide (KOH) Mounts
A **KOH mount** is a type of wet mount used when a physician suspects that a patient has a fungal infection of the skin, nails, hair, or vagina. It is difficult to visualize a fungus directly in these types of specimens because the body produces a tough, hard protein called keratin, which often masks any fungus present. The chemical potassium hydroxide (KOH) is added to the specimen to dissolve the keratin and allow visualization of any fungus.

To prepare a KOH mount, follow these steps:

1. Wearing examination gloves, suspend the specimen in a drop of 10% KOH on a glass slide.
2. Apply a coverslip.
3. Allow the specimen to sit at room temperature for 30 minutes to dissolve the keratin.
4. Provide the physician with the slide to examine for microscopic evidence of fungal structures.

▶ Preparation and Examination of Stained Specimens LO 46.13

Although wet mounts are a useful tool for detecting microorganisms, microorganisms and their structures can be seen more clearly when you stain them with a dye or group of dyes. As with wet mounts and KOH mounts, the doctor can make a quick, tentative diagnosis with stained specimens. A stained specimen also enables the doctor to differentiate between types of infections, such as bacterial and yeast infections, or between bacterial infections of one type and another. Stains also help doctors identify microorganisms that have grown on culture plates.

Preparation of Smears
The first step in staining a microbiologic specimen is to prepare a smear. To do so, simply apply a small amount of the specimen in a thin layer on a glass slide. Allow the sample to dry and then briefly heat the slide to "fix" the sample to the slide so that it does not wash off during the staining process.

The steps are described in detail in Procedure 46-4 at the end of this chapter.

Gram Stain

The Gram stain is the most frequently used stain for microscopic examination of bacteriologic specimens. This stain is a moderate-complexity test that you may assist with in the medical office if you have additional training. The steps for performing a Gram stain are outlined in Procedure 46-5 at the end of this chapter.

A Gram stain involves performing a series of staining and washing steps on the heat-fixed smear. First, apply a purple stain called crystal violet (also known as gentian violet) to the smear. After washing the slide in water, apply iodine. The iodine acts as a **mordant**, a substance that fixes a stain, keeping it from being washed away. Iodine helps bind the dye to the bacterial cell wall.

After washing the slide again in water, apply a decolorizing solution (alcohol or acetone-alcohol). As you learned in *section 46.5* of this chapter, certain bacterial species retain the purple dye even after the decolorizer is added. These bacteria appear blue or violet and are Gram-positive (positive because they retained the purple dye).

Other bacteria lose their purple color when the decolorizer is added. To allow the physician to visualize these bacteria, apply a red counterstain (safranin) to the smear. Bacteria that lose the purple color and pick up the red color of the safranin are Gram-negative. Figure 46-12 illustrates Gram-positive and Gram-negative bacteria. It is important that you follow each step in the Gram stain process carefully to reduce the likelihood of misidentifying the microorganisms.

On the basis of a bacterium's staining characteristics and the shape and arrangement of cells, the physician can make a presumptive identification of an organism. For example, clusters of cocci that appear Gram-positive typically suggest an infection with staphylococci.

▶ Culturing Specimens in the Medical Office   LO 46.14

If your medical office is equipped with a laboratory and if you have had the necessary on-the-job training or additional courses, you may be required to culture certain specimens. It is, however, becoming more common for doctors' offices to send specimens to outside laboratories because of Clinical Laboratory Improvement Amendments of 1988 (CLIA '88) guidelines and the additional requirements concerning personnel and administrative work.

Culturing involves placing a sample of the specimen on or in a specialized culture medium, which contains nutrients that enable microorganisms such as bacteria and fungi to grow. The medium is placed in an incubator set at 37°C (body temperature), the optimal temperature for growth. As the microorganism multiplies, a **colony**—a distinct group of the organisms—can be seen on the culture medium's surface. The microorganism is identified according to the colony appearance, its staining characteristics, and certain

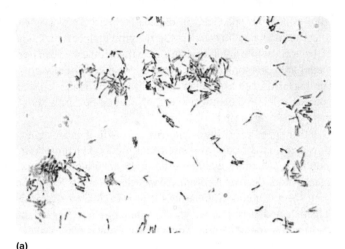

(a)

(b)

FIGURE 46-12 (a) Gram-positive organisms appear blue or violet after staining. (b) Gram-negative organisms appear red.

(a-b) Source: Centers for Disease Control and Prevention, Dr. PB Smith.

biochemical reactions. A microorganism's biochemical reactions are determined by their growth on specific types of culture media.

Culture Media

Culture media come in liquid, semisolid, and solid forms. In the medical office, you will most likely work with a semisolid. The medium contains **agar**, a gelatin-like substance derived from seaweed that gives the medium its consistency. This form of medium comes commercially prepared in culture plates—round, covered, glass or plastic dishes called *petri dishes.*

Handle petri dishes on the outside only, so that they do not become contaminated. You can avoid introducing contaminants by storing the petri dishes with the agar side up. Use the palm of your hand to pick up the agar-containing part of the dish when you are ready to inoculate it with a specimen.

Types of Media Many different types of semisolid media are commercially available. The type of medium used for culturing depends on the type of suspected organism and the site from which the specimen is obtained. Some types—called selective media—allow (select for) the growth of certain kinds of bacteria while inhibiting the growth of others. Selective media are commonly used for specimens that normally contain bacteria, such as stool or vaginal samples. This is so that you can select for pathogenic organisms and not grow those that you expect to find.

Other types of media support the growth of most organisms and are referred to as nonselective media. The most common type of culture medium used in the laboratory is blood agar, a nonselective medium. Blood agar gets its red color from sheep's blood. Comparing the growth of a specimen on selective and nonselective media often provides important information about the microorganisms present.

You will typically use a blood agar plate when you culture a throat swab specimen. The organism that causes strep throat (*Streptococcus pyogenes*) can be identified when it grows on blood agar because it destroys the blood cells (hemolysis) in the agar, leaving a clear zone surrounding each colony.

Special Culture Units Small physicians' office laboratories often use commercial culture units with specific culturing purposes. Units for performing rapid urine culture, such as Uricult® (manufactured by Orion Diagnostica, Somerset, New Jersey), are typical. Uricult® consists of a small vial with a double-sided paddle attached to a screw-on top (Figure 46-13). Each side of the paddle contains a different type of medium on its surface. To culture a urine specimen, simply dip the media paddle into the clean-catch mid-stream urine specimen or catheterized specimen, coating both sides of the paddle. Then remove the paddle from the specimen, screw it into the vial, and place it upright in the incubator for 18 to 24 hours. If bacteria are present, they will grow on the surfaces of the media. Other units for culturing urine, throat specimens, vaginal specimens, and blood also are simple to use. These units usually enable you to obtain an estimate of

the number of bacteria in the sample in addition to identifying the bacteria.

Inoculating a Culture Plate

Inoculating a culture plate involves transferring some or all of the specimen onto the plate. Before inoculating a plate, label it on the bottom (agar side) rather than the lid because the lid can be lost or switched. Write close to the edge to avoid obscuring colony identification. Label the plate with the patient's name, doctor's name, source of the sample, date and time of inoculation, and your initials. You can apply a label or write the information with a grease pencil or permanent marker.

In the case of a specimen swab, inoculate the plate by streaking the swab across the plate. Bacterial colonies can be identified by their appearance. This determination of the type of pathogen is referred to as a qualitative analysis of the specimen.

To perform a qualitative analysis of a specimen such as urine, introduce only a small portion of the specimen onto the plate. A calibrated inoculating loop is used for this purpose. A loop is a small circle of wire or plastic attached to a long handle. When this loop is dipped into the specimen, a small, specific amount of liquid can be transferred to the plate. Different sizes of calibrated loops deliver different volumes of fluid. For example, calibrated loops may allow you to pick up either 0.01 or 0.001 milliliter of liquid.

In addition, a quantitative analysis—of the number of bacteria present in specimens such as urine—may be ordered by the physician. A quantitative analysis is important with such a specimen because a few bacteria may contaminate a urine sample during collection. A true infection is confirmed by the presence of a specified number of bacteria; any number beneath this level is typically considered contamination.

Inoculating for Qualitative Analysis To inoculate an agar plate for qualitative analysis, perform the first pass with a culture swab (as with a throat culture) or an inoculating loop (as with a urine culture). If you use a culture swab, roll and streak it back and forth across an area, covering roughly one-third of the culture plate to deposit the microorganisms. When using an inoculating loop, spread the material by streaking the loop across one-third of the plate in the same back-and-forth pattern. Figure 46-14 shows the correct pattern for inoculating a plate.

Because there may be several microorganisms in the specimen, you need to streak the inoculated (first pass) area with a sterile loop to separate out individual colonies that can be identified on the remaining areas of the culture plate. Unless you use a sterile disposable loop, first sterilize the loop by heating it in a bacterial loop incinerator until it glows red. Allow the loop to cool and then pass it once across the inoculated area of the plate to pick up a small number of microorganisms. Then streak it in a back-and-forth pattern over the second one-third of the plate. Next, sterilize the loop again, pass it once across the second inoculated area of the plate,

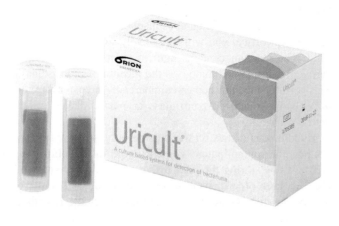

FIGURE 46-13 The Uricult® is one type of urine culture device that consists of a lid and attached, double-sided paddle that screws into a vial. ©Orion Diagnostica

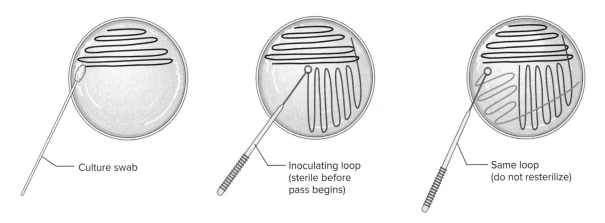

FIGURE 46-14   When inoculating a plate for qualitative analysis, roll and streak the culture swab or streak the inoculating loop of specimen material across one-third of the surface of the culture plate. Begin the next pass with a sterile loop.

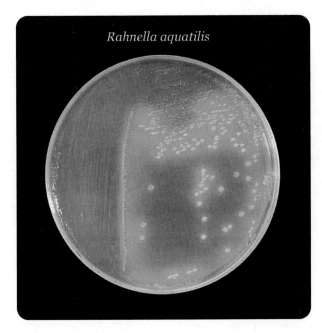

FIGURE 46-15   You can see individual colony-forming units in the last third of an inoculated culture plate.

Source: Center for Disease Control (CDC) - PHIL

and then streak it back and forth over the last one-third of the plate. Each successive pass reduces the microorganism concentration. This procedure allows isolated colonies, or colony-forming units, to be observed in the area of the last pass of the loop, as Figure 46-15 shows.

For throat cultures, the physician may simply want you to screen the sample for the presence of streptococcal organisms. You may not need to use a loop to spread the microorganisms; the swab will be sufficient, as described in Procedure 46-1, at the end of this chapter, when preparing the specimen for screening.

Inoculating for Quantitative Analysis   To perform a quantitative analysis of a urine specimen, the laboratory technician will use a calibrated loop to withdraw a portion of

urine from the sample. She will sterilize, cool, and dip the calibrated loop into the well-mixed sample. She will transfer the entire volume to the surface of an agar plate by making a single streak down the center of the plate. Next, she spreads the specimen evenly across the plate at a right angle to the initial streak, using the same loop (without sterilizing it). She will then turn the plate and spread the material again, at a right angle to the last streak, over the entire surface. Figure 46-16 illustrates this technique.

After the microorganisms are allowed to grow for 24 hours, the laboratory technician will estimate the number of microorganisms by counting the number of colonies that appear on the surface of the plate. For example, if she uses a 0.001 milliliter calibrated loop to streak the plate and 50 colonies grow, she will multiply the 50 colonies by 1,000 to obtain the number of colonies per milliliter. In this case, the estimated number would be 50,000 colony-forming units per milliliter of urine. Care must be taken that the counts and calculations are correct so that the doctor has accurate information on which to base a diagnosis.

Incubating Culture Plates

After inoculation, the technician will place the plate in an incubator set at 35°C (95°F) to 37°C (98.6°F) (human body temperature) to allow the bacteria to grow. Plates are always incubated with the agar side up, so that any moisture that collects in the plate will fall on the inside of the lid and not on the microbes growing on the surface of the agar. How long plates are allowed to incubate varies with the type of culture. Most bacteria grow sufficiently within 24 hours, but some require 48 hours. Fungi typically take longer to grow than bacteria and may grow at a slightly lower temperature (95°F to 96.8°F).

Interpreting Cultures

After incubation, cultures are assessed for growth and are interpreted. This process requires considerable skill and practice because pathogens must often be differentiated from resident normal flora. This step may be performed by the physician, a microbiologist, or a technician who has been properly trained to do so through on-the-job training or additional coursework.

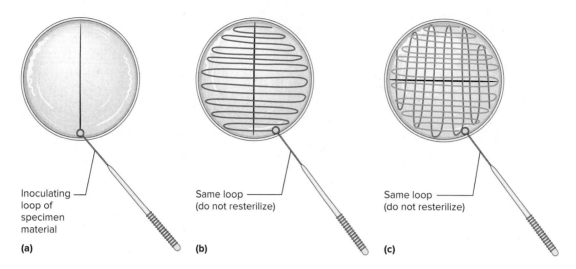

FIGURE 46-16 When inoculating a plate for quantitative analysis, (a) streak the loop down the center of the plate. Next, (b) streak the loop at right angles to the first inoculation. Then, (c) turn the plate 90° and streak the entire surface once more.

The process of interpreting a culture typically involves several determinations. The characteristics of the colonies growing on the agar are noted, along with their relative numbers. In addition, any changes in the media surrounding the colonies are noted because changes may reflect certain characteristics of the microorganism.

The physician decides at this point whether additional procedures are required. In the case of a throat culture, the presence of colonies of a characteristic shape, size, and color, surrounded by areas of hemolysis, suggests strep throat, as shown in Figure 46-17. A Gram stain and determination of bacterial shape may be all that is necessary for a confirmed diagnosis. Many cultures, however, require additional biochemical and, in some cases, serologic tests for definitive pathogen identification. Because this is an advanced skill, either the physician or an outside microbiology laboratory will make the final interpretation of the cultured microorganism.

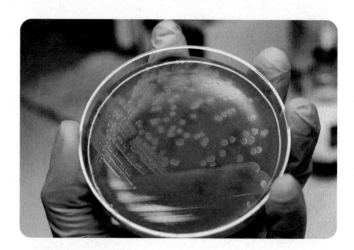

FIGURE 46-17 A positive strep throat culture contains distinctive colonies surrounded by areas of hemolysis.
©By R Parulan Jr./Getty Images

PROCEDURE 46-1 Obtaining a Throat Culture Specimen WORK // DOC

Procedure Goal: To isolate a pathogenic microorganism from the throat or to rule out strep throat

OSHA Guidelines:

Materials: Patient chart/progress note, tongue depressor, sterile collection system or sterile swab plus blood agar culture plate

Method:

1. Identify the patient, introduce yourself, and explain the procedure.

2. Assemble the necessary supplies; label the culture plate if used.

3. Wash your hands and don examination gloves, goggles, and a mask or face shield.
   RATIONALE: *The patient may cough while you swab the throat.*

4. Have the patient assume a sitting position. (Having a small child lie down rather than sit may make the process easier. If the child refuses to open the mouth, gently squeeze the nostrils shut. The child will eventually open the mouth to breathe. Enlist the help of the parent to restrain the child's hands if necessary.)

5. Open the collection system or sterile swab package by peeling the wrapper halfway down; remove the swab with your dominant hand.

6. Ask the patient to tilt back her head and open her mouth as wide as possible.

7. With your other hand, depress the patient's tongue with the tongue depressor.

8. Ask the patient to say "Ah."

9. Insert the swab and quickly swab the back of the throat in the area of the tonsils, twirling the swab over representative areas on both sides of the throat. Avoid touching the uvula (the soft tissue hanging from the roof of the mouth), the cheeks, or the tongue.
RATIONALE: *Touching these areas will contaminate the specimen.*

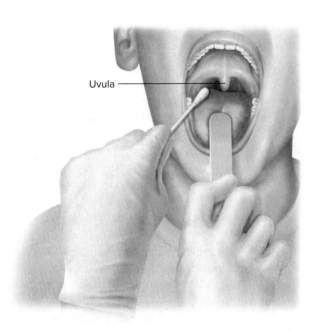

Uvula

FIGURE Procedure 46-1 Step 9   When obtaining a throat culture specimen, swab the back of the throat in the area of the tonsils on each side, taking care to avoid touching the uvula.

10. Remove the swab and then the tongue depressor from the patient's mouth.

11. Discard the tongue depressor in a biohazardous waste container.

To Transport the Specimen to a Reference Laboratory

12. Immediately insert the swab back into the plastic sleeve, being careful not to touch the outside of the sleeve with the swab.

13. Crush the vial of transport medium to moisten the tip of the swab.
RATIONALE: *To keep the microorganisms alive during transport.*

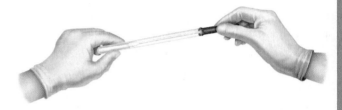

FIGURE Procedure 46-1 Step 13   The transport medium released from the crushed capsule keeps microorganisms alive while in transit to the laboratory for culturing.

14. Label the collection system and arrange for transport to the laboratory.

To Prepare the Specimen for Evaluation in the Physician's Office Laboratory

12. Immediately inoculate the culture plate with the swab, using a back-and-forth motion.

13. Discard the swab in a biohazardous waste container.

14. Place the culture plate in the incubator.

When Finished with All Specimens

15. Remove the gloves and wash your hands.

16. Document the procedure in the patient's chart.

PROCEDURE 46-2 Performing a Quick Strep A Test on a Throat Specimen

WORK // DOC

Procedure Goal: To determine the presence of strep A antigen in a throat specimen

OSHA Guidelines:

Materials: Patient chart/progress note, strep A testing kit, throat swab specimen, and a timer or watch

Method:

1. Review the laboratory requisition form and gather the supplies.

2. Confirm the patient's identity, introduce yourself, and explain the procedure.

3. Wash your hands and don gloves, goggles, and a mask or face shield.

4. Open the strep A testing kit and check the expiration date on the kit.

5. Obtain a throat specimen with a sterile swab, being careful not to touch the tongue, teeth, or cheeks.
RATIONALE: *Swabbing only the throat reduces the likelihood of getting a false positive test result.*

6. Complete the quality control tests provided with the testing kit.
RATIONALE: *To ensure the test is working correctly*

7. Put the required amount of the first reagent in the test tube or testing device provided in the kit.

8. Place the swab into the test tube or testing device. Following the manufacturer's instructions, swirl the swab and press it against the sides of the tube or device.

9. Add the second reagent as directed.

10. Read the results at the required time.

11. Dispose of testing supplies in the appropriate waste container according to OSHA requirements.

12. Remove your gloves and wash your hands.

13. Document the results in the patient's chart.

PROCEDURE 46-3 Preparing Microbiologic Specimens for Transport to an Outside Laboratory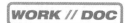

Procedure Goal: To properly prepare a microbiologic specimen for transport to an outside laboratory

OSHA Guidelines:

Materials:
Specimen-collection device, requisition form, secondary container or a zipper-type plastic bag

Method:

1. Wash your hands and don examination gloves (and goggles and a mask or face shield if you are collecting a microbiologic throat culture specimen).

2. Obtain the microbiologic culture specimen.

   a. Use the collection system specified by the outside laboratory for the test requested.

   b. Label the microbiologic specimen-collection device at the time of collection.

   c. Collect the microbiologic specimen according to the guidelines provided by the laboratory and office procedure.

RATIONALE: To ensure the specimen is correctly collected and handled.

3. Remove the gloves and wash your hands.

4. Complete the test requisition form.

5. Place the microbiologic specimen container in a secondary container or zipper-type plastic bag.
   RATIONALE: To prevent contaminating anyone who handles the specimen during transport.

6. Attach the test requisition form to the outside of the secondary container or bag, per laboratory policy.

7. Log the microbiologic specimen in the list of outgoing specimens.
   RATIONALE: So that you can follow up on lab tests sent to outside laboratories.

8. Store the microbiologic specimen according to guidelines provided by the laboratory for that type of specimen (for example, refrigerated, frozen, or 37°C).

9. Call the laboratory for pickup of the microbiologic specimen, or hold it until the next scheduled pickup.

10. At the time of pickup, ensure that the carrier takes all microbiologic specimens that are logged and scheduled to be picked up.

11. If you are ever unsure about collection or transportation details, call the laboratory.

PROCEDURE 46-4 Preparing a Microbiologic Specimen Smear

Procedure Goal: To prepare a smear of a microbiologic specimen for staining

OSHA Guidelines:

Materials: Glass slide with frosted end, pencil, specimen swab, Bunsen burner, and forceps

Method:

1. Wash your hands and don exam gloves.

2. Assemble all the necessary items.

3. Use a pencil to label the frosted end of the slide with the patient's name.

4. Roll the specimen swab evenly over the smooth part of the slide, making sure all areas of the swab touch the slide.
   RATIONALE: To make sure a representative specimen is transferred to the slide.

5. Discard the swab in a biohazardous waste container.

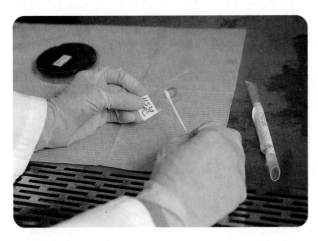

FIGURE Procedure 46-4 Step 4   Rolling the swab ensures that representative microorganisms collected on it are deposited on the slide.
©Cliff Moore

6. Allow the smear to air-dry. Do not wave the slide to dry it.
   RATIONALE: *Waving the slide may spread pathogens or contaminate the slide.*

7. Heat-fix the slide by holding the frosted end with forceps and passing the clear part of the slide, with the smear side up, through the flame of a Bunsen burner three or four times. (Your office may use an alternate procedure for fixing the slide, such as flooding the smear with alcohol, allowing it to sit for a few minutes, and either pouring off the remaining liquid or allowing the smear to air-dry. Chlamydia slides come with their own fixative.)
   RATIONALE: *The specimen must be fixed to the slide to prevent washing the microorganism off during staining or handling.*

8. Allow the slide to cool before the smear is stained.

9. Return the materials to their proper location.

10. Remove the gloves and wash your hands.

PROCEDURE 46-5 Performing a Gram Stain

Procedure Goal: To make bacteria present in a specimen smear visible for microscopic identification

OSHA Guidelines:

Materials: Heat-fixed smear, slide staining rack and tray, crystal violet dye, iodine solution, alcohol or acetone-alcohol decolorizer, safranin dye, wash bottle filled with water, forceps, and blotting paper or paper towels (optional)

Method:

1. Assemble all the necessary supplies.

2. Wash your hands and don examination gloves.

3. Place the heat-fixed smear on a level staining rack and tray, smear side up.

4. Completely cover the specimen area of the slide with the crystal violet stain. (Many commercially available Gram stain solutions have flip-up bottle caps that allow you to dispense stain by the drop. If the stain bottle you are using does not have an attached dropper cap, use an eyedropper.)

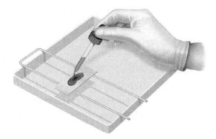

FIGURE Procedure 46-5 Step 4   Apply crystal violet. Wait 1 minute.

5. Allow the stain to sit for 1 minute; rinse the slide thoroughly with water from the wash bottle.
   RATIONALE: *Rinsing the slide after 1 minute stops the staining process and prevents overstaining.*

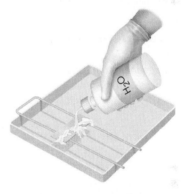

FIGURE Procedure 46-5 Step 5   Wash the slide with water.

6. Use the forceps to hold the slide at the frosted end, tilting the slide to remove excess water.

7. Place the slide flat on the rack again and completely cover the specimen area with iodine solution.

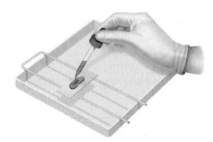

FIGURE Procedure 46-5 Step 7   Apply iodine solution. Wait 1 minute.

8. Allow the iodine to remain for 1 minute; rinse the slide thoroughly with water.
   RATIONALE: *The iodine helps increase cell staining.*

9. Use the forceps or a gloved hand to hold and tilt the slide to remove excess water.

10. While still tilting the slide, apply the alcohol or decolorizer until no more purple color washes off. (This step usually takes no more than 10 seconds to 30 seconds.)
    RATIONALE: *The decolorizing step is essential for differentiation between Gram-positive and Gram-negative bacteria.*

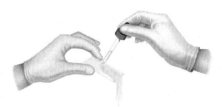

FIGURE Procedure 46-5 Step 10   Apply decolorizing solution.

11. Rinse the slide thoroughly with water; use the forceps to hold and tip the slide to remove excess water.

12. Completely cover the specimen with safranin dye.

13. Allow the safranin to remain for 1 minute; rinse the slide thoroughly with water.
    RATIONALE: *To counterstain the specimen so that Gram-negative organisms can be visualized.*

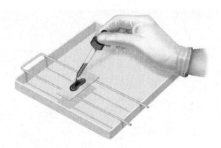

FIGURE Procedure 46-5 Step 12   Apply safranin dye to the slide. Wait 1 minute.

14. Use the forceps to hold the stained smear by the frosted end and carefully wipe the back of the slide to remove excess stain.

15. Place the smear in a vertical position and allow it to air-dry or blot it lightly between blotting paper to hasten drying. Take care not to rub the slide or the specimen may be damaged.

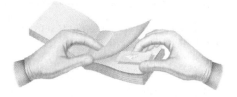

FIGURE Procedure 46-5 Step 15   Blot and allow the slide to air-dry.

16. Sanitize and disinfect the work area.

17. Remove the gloves and wash your hands.

SUMMARY OF LEARNING OUTCOMES

OUTCOME	KEY POINTS
46.1 Explain the medical assistant's role in microbiology.	As an office medical assistant, you may assist the physician with several microbiologic procedures that aid in diagnosing and treating infectious diseases, including obtaining specimens or assisting the physician in doing so; preparing specimens for direct examination by the physician; and preparing specimens for transportation to a microbiology laboratory for identification.
46.2 Summarize how microorganisms cause disease.	Microorganisms can cause disease by using up nutrients or other materials needed by the cells and tissues they invade, damaging body cells, and producing toxins.
46.3 Describe how microorganisms are classified and named.	Microorganisms are classified on the basis of their structure. Specific microorganisms are named in a standard way, using the genus (a category of biologic classification between the family and the species) to which the microorganism belongs and the particular species of the organism.

OUTCOME	KEY POINTS
46.4 Discuss the role of viruses in human disease.	Viruses are among the smallest known infectious agents causing common diseases, including the common cold, influenza, chickenpox, croup, hepatitis, and warts.
46.5 Discuss the role of bacteria in human disease.	Bacteria are single-celled, prokaryotic organisms that reproduce very quickly and cause diseases such as pneumonia, tuberculosis, meningitis, boils, urinary tract infections, Lyme disease, cholera, and tetanus.
46.6 Discuss the role of protozoans in human disease.	Protozoans are single-celled, eukaryotic organisms found in soil and water. They can cause malaria, amebic dysentery, and trichomoniasis vaginitis.
46.7 Discuss the role of fungi in human disease.	Fungi are eukaryotic organisms, including molds and yeasts. Diseases caused by fungi include athlete's foot, thrush, ringworm, and vaginal yeast infections.
46.8 Discuss the role of multicellular parasites in human disease.	Multicellular parasites include roundworms, tapeworms, flatworms, ticks, lice, and mites.
46.9 Describe the process involved in diagnosing an infection.	The steps involved in diagnosing an infection are to examine the patient, obtain one or more specimens, examine the specimen directly by either wet mount or smear, culture the specimen, and determine the culture's antibiotic sensitivity.
46.10 Identify general guidelines for obtaining specimens.	The general guidelines for obtaining specimens are to obtain the specimen with great care to avoid causing the patient harm, discomfort, or undue embarrassment; collect the material from a site; obtain the specimen at the proper time; use appropriate collection devices; obtain a sufficient quantity of the specimen; and obtain the specimen before antimicrobial therapy begins.
46.11 Carry out the procedure for transporting specimens to outside laboratories.	When transporting specimens to outside laboratories, the medical assistant should follow proper collection techniques using specific containers provided by the laboratory, maintain the samples in a state as close to their original as possible, and protect anyone who handles a specimen container from exposure to potentially infectious material.
46.12 Compare two techniques used in the direct examination of culture specimens.	Direct examination of culture specimens is accomplished in two ways: wet mounts and KOH mounts.
46.13 Carry out the procedure for preparing and examining stained specimens.	To prepare a stained specimen, the medical assistant must first prepare a smear, fix the sample to the slide so that it does not wash off during the staining process, and follow a specific staining procedure. The sample is then observed under a microscope for certain characteristics.
46.14 Carry out the procedure for culturing specimens in the medical office.	To culture a specimen, the medical assistant should place a sample of the specimen on or in a specialized culture medium and allow it to grow in an incubator for 24 to 48 hours.

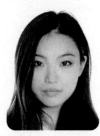

©excentric_01/iStock/Getty Images

Recall Cindy Chen from the case study at the beginning of the chapter. Now that you have completed the chapter, answer the following questions regarding her case.

1. Why are Cindy Chen's helper T cells being tested?

2. Why might Cindy Chen be more susceptible to other diseases than the general population?

3. As Cindy Chen's HIV infection progresses, what symptoms might she exhibit?

4. If Cindy Chen is HIV positive, does that mean she has visible symptoms? Why or why not?

5. What special precautions should you take when drawing Cindy Chen's blood?

6. Why do you think Dr. Whalen asked you to send the throat culture to the reference lab instead of doing a rapid strep test in the POL?

EXAM PREPARATION QUESTIONS

1. (LO 46.1) Microorganisms normally found on the skin and other body tissues are known as
   a. Tissue pathogens
   b. Viruses
   c. Resident normal flora
   d. Colonies
   e. Infections

2. (LO 46.3) Which of the following is an example of a subcellular microorganism?
   a. Bacterium
   b. Virus
   c. Fungus
   d. Helminth
   e. Multicellular organism

3. (LO 46.9) A specimen that is spread thinly and evenly across a slide is a
   a. Smear
   b. Wet prep
   c. Culture
   d. Medium
   e. Streak

4. (LO 46.12) A KOH mount is used to detect which of the following?
   a. Gonococci
   b. Fungi
   c. Viruses
   d. Pinworms
   e. HIV

5. (LO 46.10) Which of the following is an appropriate guideline for collecting specimens?
   a. The specimen label includes the patient's name and number, source of specimen, date and time, doctor's name, and your initials.
   b. The best location to obtain a throat culture to diagnose strep throat is from the sides of the throat.
   c. When a patient is collecting a specimen on her own, you should trust that she knows how to do it without an explanation.
   d. When a patient is taking an antibiotic, you should never obtain a specimen.
   e. Allow the patient to use a container from home to collect a sputum specimen.

6. (LO 46.2) Organisms capable of causing disease are known as
   a. Commensals
   b. Flora
   c. Pathogens
   d. Facultative
   e. Aerobes

7. (LO 46.4) Infectious mononucleosis is caused by which of the following?
   a. Adenovirus
   b. Parvovirus
   c. Norovirus
   d. Epstein-Barr virus
   e. Rotavirus

8. (LO 46.7) Athlete's foot, thrush, and ringworm are all caused by types of
   a. Prions
   b. Parasites
   c. Bacteria
   d. Viruses
   e. Fungi

9. (LO 46.13) A substance that fixes a stain, keeping it from being washed away, is a
   a. Mordant
   b. Substrate
   c. Wash
   d. Dye
   e. Counterstain

10. (LO 46.8) An organism that lives on or in another organism and uses that other organism for its own nourishment is a(n)
    a. Obligate
    b. Eukaryote
    c. Resident
    d. Parasite
    e. Prokaryote

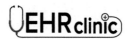

Go to CONNECT to complete the EHRclinic exercises: 46.01 Order a Strep Test for a Patient and 46.02 Record Strep Test Results for a Patient.

S O F T   S K I L L S   S U C C E S S

Recall Cindy Chen from the case study at the beginning of the chapter. After drawing Cindy Chen's blood, you leave her lab requisition on the counter at the front of the lab while you escort her to the front office. When you return, Charlie Goodpasture is waiting to have his blood drawn for routine lab work. You notice he is glancing at the lab requisition you left on the counter. He asks you if that was Cindy Chen he saw. He also tells you that he knew Cindy Chen in phlebotomy school and she has lost a lot of weight. Charlie Goodpasture asks if Cindy Chen is sick. How should you handle this situation? What should you have done differently?

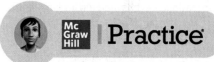

Go to PRACTICE MEDICAL OFFICE and complete the module Admin Check Out: Privacy and Liability.

Collecting, Processing, and Testing Urine and Stool Specimens

CASE STUDY

<table>
<tr><td rowspan="5">PATIENT INFORMATION</td><td>Patient Name</td><td>DOB</td><td>Allergies</td></tr>
<tr><td>Ken Washington</td><td>12/01/1958</td><td>Sulfa</td></tr>
<tr><td colspan="3"></td></tr>
<tr><td>Attending</td><td>MRN</td><td>Other Information</td></tr>
<tr><td>Paul F. Buckwalter, MD</td><td>00-AA-008</td><td>Vital Signs: BP 142/88, T 99.2, P 76, R 16</td></tr>
</table>

Ken Washington arrived today for a follow-up visit from a recent hospitalization for a stroke. Up until this hospitalization, he has had no major health issues. He now has weakness in his left arm, and his speech is difficult to

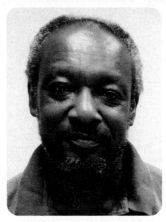
©McGraw-Hill Education

understand. His wife tells you that she has noticed some blood in the toilet after he urinates. She also tells you that he has had some pain when he urinates and often only urinates a small amount. Dr. Buckwalter would like for you to obtain a urine sample for a reagent test and have Ken Washington collect a 24-hour urine sample for analysis.

Keep Ken Washington in mind as you study this chapter. There will be questions at the end of the chapter based on the case study. The information in the chapter will help you answer these questions.

LEARNING OUTCOMES

After completing Chapter 47, you will be able to:

47.1 Discuss the role of the medical assistant in collecting, processing, and testing urine and stool samples.

47.2 Carry out procedures for collecting urine specimens according to guidelines.

47.3 Describe the process of urinalysis and its purpose.

47.4 Carry out the proper procedure for collecting and processing a stool sample for fecal occult blood testing.

KEY TERMS

anuria
cast
catheterization
clean-catch midstream urine specimen
crystal
fecal occult blood test (FOBT)
first morning urine specimen
glycosuria
hematuria

O&P specimen
oliguria
proteinuria
refractometer
supernatant
turbidity
24-hour urine specimen
urinalysis
urinary pH
urine culture
urine specific gravity
urobilinogen

I.C.10	Identify CLIA waived tests associated with common diseases
I.C.12	Identify quality assurance practices in healthcare
I.P.8	Instruct and prepare a patient for a procedure or a treatment
I.P.11	Obtain specimens and perform: (c) CLIA waived urinalysis
I.A.3	Show awareness of a patient's concerns related to the procedure being performed
II.P.2	Differentiate between normal and abnormal test results
II.A.1	Reassure a patient of the accuracy of the test results
III.P.2	Select appropriate barrier/personal protective equipment (PPE)
III.A.1	Recognize the implications for failure to comply with Centers for Disease Control (CDC) regulations in healthcare settings
V.A.4	Explain to a patient the rationale for performance of a procedure
X.P.3	Document patient care accurately in the medical record

3. **Medical Terminology**
   d. Define and use medical abbreviations when appropriate and acceptable

4. **Medical Law and Ethics**
   f. Comply with federal, state, and local health laws and regulations as they relate to healthcare settings

8. **Clinical Procedures**
   a. Practice standard precautions and perform disinfection/sterilization techniques
   e. Perform specialty procedures including but not limited to minor surgery, cardiac, respiratory, OB-GYN, neurological, and gastroenterology
   j. Make adaptations for patients with special needs (psychological or physical limitations)

9. **Medical Laboratory Procedures**
   a. Practice quality control
   b. Perform selected CLIA-waived tests that assist with diagnosis and treatment
      (1) Urinalysis
      (6) Kit testing
   c. Dispose of biohazardous materials
   e. Instruct patients in the collection of
      (1) Clean-catch mid-stream urine specimen
      (2) Collection of fecal specimen

▶ Introduction

Proper collection and testing of urine and stool (fecal) samples is a crucial step in the diagnostic process. The routine analysis of a urine specimen is a simple, noninvasive diagnostic test that provides a healthcare provider with a window to a patient's health. Many significant conditions may be noted as a result of the physical, chemical, and microscopic examinations of a patient's urine.

In this chapter, you will learn about various types of urine specimens and how to properly instruct or assist patients with their collection. Additionally, you will learn how to correctly process a specimen, including a random specimen and a chain-of-custody drug screen. You will learn to identify normal and abnormal constituents of urine samples and what may cause these abnormal elements to be present in a specimen.

You also will learn about stool samples, which are collected for a variety of reasons, including detecting bacterial infections, detecting parasites, and screening for cancer. Teaching patients proper techniques for collecting stool samples is key to getting accurate test results.

▶ The Role of the Medical Assistant LO 47.1

In your role as a medical assistant, you will help collect, process, and test urine and stool specimens. To perform your duties, you need to know about the anatomy and physiology of the kidneys, how urine is formed, and what its normal contents are. You also will need to understand the anatomy and physiology of the digestive system and common medical abbreviations used in testing. Be sure to review the anatomy and physiology of the urinary system and the digestive system in chapters *The Urinary System* and *The Digestive System*. Also, see Table 47-1 for a list of abbreviations commonly used in urine analysis and stool testing. Dealing with a variety of special patient groups, including elderly and pediatric patients, will be an important part of your job.

When obtaining and processing urine and stool specimens, you will deal with potentially infectious body waste. For this reason, you must take precautions to protect yourself, the patient, and others in the environment from exposure to disease-causing microorganisms. Most medical offices use standard precautions when dealing with urine. (See the *Infection Control Fundamentals* chapter for detailed information on

TABLE 47-1 Abbreviations Common to Urine Analysis and Stool Testing

BIL; bili; BR	bilirubin	RBCs	red blood cells
Ca	calcium	SPG; sp gr; sp.gr.	specific gravity
CC	clean-catch (urine)	U/A	urinalysis
CCMS	clean-catch, midstream (urine)	UBG	urobilinogen
CL VOID	clean voided specimen (urine)	U/C	urine culture
CrCl	creatinine clearance	UC	urinary catheter
CSU	catheter specimen (urine)	UC&S	urine culture and sensitivity
Cys	cysteine	UcaV	urinary calcium volume
CYS	cystoscopy	UCRE	urine creatinine
EMU	early morning urine(s)	UFC	urinary free cortisol
FOBT	Fecal occult blood test	UK	urine potassium
HCG; hcg; hCG	human chorionic gonadotropin	UNa	urinary sodium
IVP	intravenous pyelogram	Uosm	urine osmolarity
K	potassium	UTI	urinary tract infection
Na	sodium	UUN	urinary urea nitrogen
O&P	Ova and parasites	UV	urinary volume
pH	hydrogen ion concentration	Vol	volume
PKD	polycystic kidney disease	WBCs	white blood cells
PKU	phenylketonuria		

these precautions.) During all procedures, you must be sure to wear adequate personal protective equipment (PPE); handle and dispose of specimens properly; dispose of used supplies and equipment properly; and sanitize, disinfect, and/or sterilize all reusable equipment according to facility policy.

▶ Obtaining Urine Specimens LO 47.2

It is essential to collect, store, and preserve urine specimens in ways that do not alter their physical, chemical, or microscopic properties. You must follow guidelines each time you obtain specimens and instruct patients in the proper guidelines to follow.

General Collection Guidelines

When you collect urine specimens from patients, follow these guidelines:

- Follow the procedure specified for the urine test that will be performed.
- Use the type of specimen container indicated by the laboratory. If a patient must bring in a specimen, be sure the container is provided by the licensed practitioner's office or that it's appropriate for the testing protocol. If you provide the patient with a container that contains a preservative, make sure the appropriate warning labels are attached. You also should warn patients that the additive may contain acid and they should take care not to spill the acid on themselves.
- Label the specimen container before giving it to the patient or on receipt of a container the patient provides. Include the patient's name, the licensed practitioner's name, the date and time of collection, and your initials. Label the side of the specimen container, not the lid, because lids may be lost or switched.

- If the patient is having an invasive test, such as catheterization, always explain the procedure to the patient completely, using simple, clear language.
- If you are assisting in the collection process, wash your hands before and after the procedure and wear gloves during the procedure.
- If the urine specimen needs to be transferred to another container or if it is to be sent to a reference lab for testing, use a urine transfer straw or provide the patient with a container that has a transfer straw integrated into the collection cup. Label the container.
- Complete all necessary paperwork, recording the collection in the patient's chart and making sure you use the correct laboratory request slip for the ordered test.

In many instances, patients need to collect a urine specimen at home. It is your responsibility to give patients instructions for obtaining the specific type of specimen. In addition, provide them with the following general instructions:

- Urinate into the container indicated by the laboratory. In most instances, urinate into a wide-mouthed, throw-away, spouted specimen container as instructed. Do not add anything to the container except the urine.
- If the collection container contains liquid or powdered preservative, do not pour it out.
- If any of the preservative spills on you, wash the area immediately and contact the licensed practitioner's office.
- Always refrigerate the labeled collection container or keep it in a cooler or pail filled with ice.
- Be sure to keep the lid on the container.

Specimen Types

Many different tests are performed on urine. You may need to obtain different types of specimens for different tests, such as quantitative analysis or qualitative analysis. A quantitative analysis is a test that measures the amount or how much of a specific substance is in the urine. A qualitative analysis simply indicates that a substance is present or absent in the urine. Specimens also vary in two other ways: in the method used to collect them and in the time frame in which they are collected.

Quality assurance is essential in the licensed practitioner's office laboratory. As discussed in the *Orientation to the Lab* chapter, control samples must be used every time you test patient specimens. These are the types of urine specimens:

- Random
- First morning
- Clean-catch midstream
- Timed
- 24-hour

Random Urine Specimen The random urine specimen is the most common type of sample. It is a single urine specimen taken at any time of the day and collected in a clean, dry container.

If a random urine specimen collection is to be done at the licensed practitioner's office, supply the patient with a labeled urine specimen container. Show the patient to the bathroom and ask the patient to void a few ounces of urine into the specimen cup and leave the cup in the specimen door or on the sink. Retrieve the specimen when the patient leaves the bathroom and add the time of collection to the label. Transport the specimen to the laboratory immediately. Urine specimens should be processed within 1 hour of collection. If this is not possible, refrigerate the specimen. Before processing refrigerated specimens, however, allow them to come to room temperature. If specimens will be shipped to an outside laboratory, chemical preservatives are added or the specimens are transferred to a suitable container containing preservatives.

If patients are to collect a random urine specimen at home, have them use the container indicated by the laboratory. Either provide patients with a urine specimen container or instruct them to use a clean, wide-mouthed glass jar with a tight-fitting lid. Explain that a household dishwasher provides hot enough water to disinfect a jar adequately. Tell patients to refrigerate specimens until they bring them to the licensed practitioner's office and to keep them cool during transport.

First Morning Urine Specimen The **first morning urine specimen** is collected after a night's sleep. This type of specimen contains greater concentrations of substances that collect over time than do specimens taken during the day. A urine specimen container or clean, dry jar is used to collect the urine according to the laboratory's request.

Clean-Catch Midstream Urine Specimen The **clean-catch midstream urine specimen**, sometimes referred to as midvoid, may be collected and submitted for culturing to identify the number and types of pathogens present. A clean-catch midstream urine specimen may be collected at random or first thing in the morning. The presence of clinical symptoms or unexplained bacteria in a urinalysis specimen is an indication for urine culture.

The clean-catch midstream specimen method is not like other urine tests in which urine is simply voided into a specimen container. Instead, the clean-catch midstream method requires special cleansing of the external genitalia to avoid contamination by organisms residing near the urethral meatus (the external opening of the urethra). Voiding a small amount of urine into the toilet prior to collecting the midstream specimen flushes the normal flora out of the distal urethra to prevent possible contamination of the specimen. Procedure 47-1, at the end of this chapter, describes how to collect a clean-catch midstream urine specimen and how to instruct patients to perform this technique.

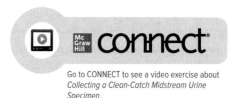

Go to CONNECT to see a video exercise about *Collecting a Clean-Catch Midstream Urine Specimen.*

Timed Urine Specimen A licensed practitioner may order a timed urine specimen to measure a patient's urinary output or to analyze substances. First, determine whether the required time period means that the patient must collect the specimen at home. If so, provide the patient with the proper collection container; written instructions on the process, including specimen preservation; and the following instructions:

- Discard the first specimen.
- Then collect *all* urine for the specified time (2 to 24 hours).
- Be sure the urine does not mix with stool or toilet paper.
- Keep the sample refrigerated until returning it to the licensed practitioner's office or laboratory.

24-Hour Urine Specimen A **24-hour urine specimen** is collected over a 24-hour period and is used to complete a quantitative and qualitative analysis of one or more substances, such as sodium, chloride, and calcium. You need to instruct the patient in the proper collection process. If an outside laboratory will be testing the specimen, the laboratory will provide specific protocols for collection, preservation, and transport. Procedure 47-2, at the end of this chapter, outlines the steps in collecting a 24-hour urine specimen.

Catheterization

A urinary catheter is a sterile plastic tube inserted into the kidney, ureter, or bladder to provide urinary drainage. **Catheterization** is the procedure during which the catheter is inserted, and it is performed for various reasons, including to:

- Relieve urinary retention.
- Obtain a sterile urine specimen from a patient.
- Measure the amount of residual urine in the bladder to determine how much urine remains after normal voiding

(patient voids and is then catheterized; more than 50 milliliters is considered abnormal).

- Obtain a urine specimen if the patient cannot void naturally.
- Instill chemotherapy as a treatment for bladder cancer.
- Empty the bladder before and during surgery and before some diagnostic exams.

The two primary types of urinary catheters are splinting catheters and drainage catheters. Splinting catheters are inserted after plastic repair of the ureter and must remain in place for at least a week after surgery. Drainage catheters are used to withdraw fluids. Types of drainage catheters include:

- Indwelling urethral (Foley) catheters placed in the bladder.
- Retention catheter placed in the renal pelvis.
- Ureteral catheter.
- Cystostomy tube, which is a catheter for drainage through a wound that leads to the bladder.
- Straight catheter to collect specimens or instill medications.

Catheterization is not routinely recommended because it can introduce infection. Some states do not permit medical assistants to perform catheterization, and in most healthcare institutions, only a physician or nurse can insert or withdraw a catheter. Check the protocol in your state. Even if you are not permitted to perform the procedure, you may be asked to assemble the necessary supplies and to assist the licensed practitioner during the procedure.

Catheterization performed in a licensed practitioner's office is usually done for diagnostic purposes using a specially prepared catheterization kit. This kit contains all necessary instruments and supplies, including a sterile instrument pack that is used to create a sterile field for the procedure.

If a patient has **incontinence**, the licensed practitioner may use a bladder-drainage catheter to help drain the bladder and keep the patient dry. Another type of drainage catheter, a ureteral catheter, is inserted into the ureter to help drain urine.

The indwelling urethral (Foley) catheter is designed to stay in place within the bladder (Figure 47-1). It consists of two tubes, one inside the other. The outside tube is connected to a balloon, which is filled with water or air to keep the catheter from slipping out of the bladder. Urine travels through the bladder and drains from the inside tube into a soft plastic container. The licensed practitioner may order a leg bag to attach to the patient's thigh. The bag is anchored to the leg by two bands placed around the thigh. Make sure the bag is positioned so that there is no tension on the catheter tube. To prevent backflow into the patient's bladder, the container must always be lower than the bladder.

Special Considerations

When you obtain a urine specimen from a patient or take a history of a patient who may have a urinary problem, you need to consider the patient's sex, condition, and age. Some patients require special care during collection procedures.

Special Considerations in Male and Female Patients

Depending on the test, you may need to alter guidelines for collecting urine specimens from a male or female patient. Procedure 47-1, at the end of this chapter, describes how to assist in collecting a clean-catch urine specimen from a female patient and from a male patient. In addition, when you take a medical history on a male or female patient, you will need to ask gender-specific questions as part of your assessment. For example, if a female patient leaks urine when laughing or coughing, she may have bladder dysfunction, which would affect the collection of a 24-hour urine specimen.

Special Considerations in Pregnant Patients Pregnant women normally have increased urinary frequency. They also may be prone to urinary tract infections. When a woman is

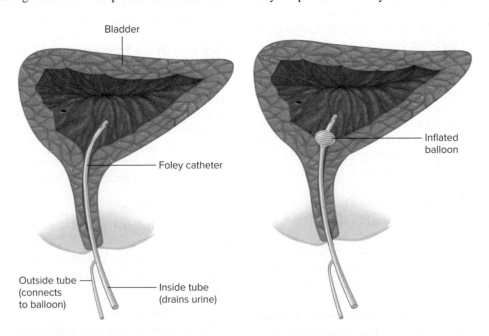

Bladder

Foley catheter

Outside tube (connects to balloon)

Inside tube (drains urine)

Inflated balloon

FIGURE 47-1 A Foley catheter stays in place within the bladder and has a collection container, which is emptied periodically.

pregnant, urine testing is done to screen for pregnancy-related issues. A pregnant woman's urine is checked for glucose. If this test shows elevated glucose (sugar) in the urine, it may indicate the possibility of gestational diabetes. When the urine tests positive for glucose, additional testing is performed. The woman's urine also is checked for abnormal levels of protein. Excess protein in her urine may indicate renal problems or preeclampsia, a condition brought on by pregnancy in which the blood pressure rises and other organs, such as the kidneys, may be damaged.

Ask a pregnant patient whether she has any pain during urination or in the kidney area. A positive response may indicate a urinary tract infection or kidney stones. Also ask about urine leakage and whether she has previously been pregnant. Leakage may occur in a woman who has had multiple births because the pressure of the fetus on the bladder or the delivery of the baby may have weakened the patient's bladder control. Additionally, ask whether any of the babies were delivered by forceps, which can injure urinary and genital structures.

Establishing Chain of Custody

Occasionally, you may need to obtain urine specimens for drug and alcohol analysis. These are considered legal specimens because they may be used in a court of law and must be handled carefully. The specimen must be placed in a specimen transfer bag that permanently seals the specimen bag until it is cut open for analysis. The seal ensures that there has been no tampering with the bag's contents prior to reaching the lab for testing. A chain of custody must be established to document the handling of this specimen.

The specific steps to establish a chain of custody are described in Procedure 47-3 at the end of this chapter. Because medicolegal issues are involved when handling a legal specimen, it is important to follow the procedure exactly to avoid breaking the chain. Also, because supplying a specimen for drug or alcohol testing could be incriminating to the patient, it is important to thoroughly explain the procedure to the donor and have him or her sign a consent form (Figure 47-2). The consent form may be a part of the chain-of-custody form (CCF) (Figure 47-3), or it may be a separate form. The consent form states the purpose of the test and gives you permission to collect the specimen, prepare it for transport to the laboratory for analysis, and release the results to the agency requesting the test. Distribute copies of the CCF to the medical review officer, laboratory, patient, collector, and employer or other requesting party.

Inform the patient that medication (both prescription and nonprescription), drugs, and alcohol will show up in the test results. Encourage the patient to list on the consent form or CCF all substances consumed in the last 30 days, including what was taken and how much.

The CCF indicates the source of the specimen. It verifies through signatures that the patient whose name is on the CCF and consent form is the same person who provided the sealed specimen sent to the laboratory. Follow Procedure 47-3, at the end of this chapter, when collecting a urine sample for drug or alcohol testing.

BWW

BWW Medical Associates, PC
305 Main Street, Port Snead YZ 12345-9876
Tel: 555-654-3210, Fax: 555-987-6543
Web: BWWAssociates.com

DRUG SCREEN CONSENT FORM

A urine drug test is required by _____ as part of your pre-employment screening. Please provide us with a list of all medications that you are presently taking.

_____

_____

_____

_____

I understand that my prospective or continued employment is contingent on a successful screening.

Date: _____   Signature: _____

Witness: _____

FIGURE 47-2 A consent form is a legal requirement when urine is collected for drug testing.

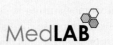

Morris A. Turner, MD

C.L.I.A #21.1862

266 Line Road
Montelair, Delaware 00956
800-555-1567

CHAIN-OF-CUSTODY FORM
SPECIMEN I.D.NO:

| STEP 1—TO BE COMPLETED BY COLLECTOR OR EMPLOYER REPRESENTATIVE. |

Employer Name, Address, and I.D. No.:   OR   Medical Review Officer Name and Address:

_____   _____

_____   _____

_____

Donor Social Security No. or Employee I.D. No.: _____

Donor I.D. verified: ☐ Photo I.D.   ☐ Employer Representative _____
                                                                          Signature

Reason for test: (check one)   ☐ Preemployment   ☐ Random   ☐ Postaccident
                                    ☐ Periodic   ☐ Reasonable suspicion/cause
                                    ☐ Return to duty   ☐ Other (specify)

Test(s) to be performed: _____   Total tests ordered: ☐

Type of specimen obtained: ☐ Urine   ☐ Blood   ☐ Semen   ☐ Other (specify)
                               Submit only one specimen with each requisition.

| STEP 2—TO BE COMPLETED BY COLLECTOR. |

For urine specimens, read temperature within 4 minutes of collection.
Check here if specimen temperature is within range. ☐ Yes, 90°–100°F/32°–38°C
Or record actual temperature here: _____

| STEP 3—TO BE COMPLETED BY COLLECTOR. |

Collection site _____   Address _____
City _____   State _____   Zip _____   Phone _____
Collection date: _____   Time: _____   ☐ a.m.   ☐ p.m.

I certify that the specimen identified on this form is the specimen presented to me by the donor identified in step 1
above, and that it was collected, labeled, and sealed in the donor's presence.

Collector's name: _____   Signature of collector: _____

| STEP 4—TO BE INITIATED BY DONOR AND COMPLETED AS NECESSARY THEREAFTER. |

Purpose of change	Released by Signature	Received by Signature	Date
A. Provide specimen for testing			
B. Shipment to Laboratory			
C.			

Comments:

| STEP 5—TO BE COMPLETED BY THE LABORATORY. |

Specimen package seal(s) intact when received in lab?   ☐ Yes   ☐ No   If no, explain.
Laboratory receiver's initials _____

Copy 1 - Original - Must accompany specimen to laboratory.

FIGURE 47-3 The chain-of-custody form provides documentation that specific specimen collection safeguards
have been followed.

Preservation and Storage

Proper specimen preservation and storage are essential. Changes that can affect the physical, chemical, and microscopic properties of urine, and invalidate certain test results occur in urine kept at room temperature for more than 1 hour.

Refrigeration is the most common method for storing and preserving urine. It prevents bacterial growth in a specimen for at least 24 hours. Refrigeration can cause other changes in the urine, however, that may affect the physical characteristics of sediment and specific gravity. Bringing the specimen back to room temperature before testing will correct these problems. You also can use chemical preservatives to preserve specimens, especially 24-hour specimens or those that must be sent a long distance to a laboratory.

▶ Urinalysis

LO 47.3

Urinalysis is the evaluation of urine by various types of testing methods to obtain information about body health and disease. Urinalysis consists of three types of testing:

- Physical
- Chemical
- Microscopic

There are normal values for all tests done on urine. The normal value for a specific substance may be negative or none or "normal". This result is from a qualitative analysis. A quantitative analysis shows a range in concentration of a substance. Urine test results within normal ranges indicate health and normality. Table 47-2 identifies normal values for a variety of urine tests. Urinalysis is done as part of a general physical exam to screen for certain substances or to diagnose various medical conditions (Table 47-3).

TABLE 47-2 Standard Urine Values

Physical Characteristics		Microscopic Examination	
Test	**Normal Values***	**Test**	**Normal Values***
Color	Pale yellow to yellow	***Crystals***	
Clarity	Clear to slightly turbid	Sulfonamide	Negative
Reagent Strip Test		Triple phosphate	Normal
Bilirubin	Negative	Tyrosine	Negative
Blood	Negative	Uric acid	Normal
Glucose	Negative	***Epithelial cells***	
Ketone bodies (acetone)	Negative	Renal	Negative
Leukocytes	Negative	Squamous, adult females	Moderate
Nitrites	Negative	Squamous, adult males	Few
pH	4.5–8.0	Transitional	Rare
Protein	Negative to trace	***24-Hour***	
Specific gravity	1.002–1.028**	5-HIAA	2–8 mg
Urobilinogen	0.3–1.0 E.U.	Albumin (quantitative)	10–140 mg/L
Microscopic Examination		Ammonia	140–1,500 mg
Bacteria	Negative	Calcium (quantitative)	100–300 mg
Mucus	Rare–few	Catecholamines, total	<100 mcg
Protozoa	Negative	Chloride	110–120 mEq
Red blood cells	0–3/high-powered field	Cortisol	10–100 mcg
White blood cells	0–8/high-powered field	Creatine, nonpregnant women/men	<100 mg
Yeast	Few	Creatine, pregnant women	≤12% of creatinine
Casts		Creatinine, men	1.0–1.9 g
Epithelial cell	Negative	Creatinine, women	0.8–1.7 g
Granular	Negative	Cystine and cysteine	<38.1 mg
Hyaline	Few	Glucose, quantitative	50–500 mg
Red blood cell	Negative	Phosphorus	0.4–1.3 g
Waxy	Negative	Potassium	25–120 mEq/L
White blood cell	Negative	Protein (Bence Jones)	Negative
Crystals		Sodium	80–180 mEq
Amorphous phosphates	Normal	Urea nitrogen	6–17 g
Calcium carbonate	Normal	Uric acid	0.25–0.75 g
Calcium oxalate	Normal	Urobilinogen, quantitative	1.0–4.0 mg
Cholesterol	Negative	Volume, adult females	600–1,600 mL
Cystine	Negative	Volume, adult males	800–1,800 mL
Leucine	Negative	Volume, children	3–4 times adult rate/kg

*Individual laboratories may have slightly different reference values. Consult the reference values provided by the lab performing the test.

**Specific gravity is a physical property of urine.

TABLE 47-3 Common Urine Tests According to Clinical Condition

Clinical Condition or Suspected Disease	Types of Urine Testing
Acidosis	Reagent strip* for pH
	Specific gravity
Alkalosis (metabolic, respiratory)	Reagent strip* for pH
	Specific gravity
Diabetes mellitus	Odor (fruity)
	Microscopic examination for fatty, waxy casts
	Reagent strip* for ketonuria and glycosuria
	Specific gravity
Drug abuse	Gas chromatography
	Mass spectrometry**
Genitourinary infections (prostatitis, urethritis, vaginitis)	Cultures for bacteria, yeasts, and parasites
	Microscopic examination for bacteria and RBCs
Human immunodeficiency virus (HIV)	Culture for virus (antibiotic added to kill bacteria)
	Other tests as indicated by specific symptoms
Hypercalcemia	Microscopic examination for calcium oxalate crystals
	Specific gravity
Hypertension	Microscopic examination for casts (hyaline, RBC)
	Specific gravity
Infectious diseases (bacteria) or other inflammatory diseases	Color and odor
	Cultures for bacteria, yeasts, and viruses
	Microscopic examination for bacteria and WBCs
	RBC casts (in severe cases)
	Reagent strip* for bacteria
	Turbidity (cloudiness)
Metabolic disorders (except diabetes mellitus)	Color
	Microscopic examination for cystine crystals
	Reagent strip* for ketonuria, fructosuria, galactosuria, pentosuria, and pH
Nephron disorders (nephrotic syndrome, glomerulonephritis, nephrosis, nephrolithiasis, pyelonephritis)	Color
	Microscopic examination for casts (epithelial, fatty, waxy, RBC) and RBCs
	Reagent strip* for proteinuria
	Specific gravity
	Turbidity
Phenylketonuria	Color
	Reagent strip* for pH
Poisoning (arsenic, cadmium, lead, mercury)	Color
	Mass spectrometry**
Polycystic kidney disease	Proteinuria
	Urinary volume
Pregnancy	Reagent strip* for human chorionic gonadotropin (HCG)

(Continued)

TABLE 47-3   Common Urine Tests According to Clinical Condition

Clinical Condition or Suspected Disease	Types of Urine Testing
Renal infections (acute glomerulonephritis, nephrotic syndrome, pyelonephritis, pyogenic infection)	Color
	Microscopic examination for epithelial cells (especially with tubular degeneration), numerous casts (granular, hyaline, WBC), RBCs, and WBCs
	Radioimmunoassay (RIA)**
	Reagent strip* for bacteria, albumin
	Specific gravity
	Turbidity
	Urinary volume
Renal disease, renal failure, severe renal damage, acute renal failure, renal tubular degeneration	Microscopic examination for epithelial cells (especially with tubular degeneration) and numerous casts (hyaline, fatty, waxy, RBC)
	Reagent strip* for proteinuria (albumin), pH
	Specific gravity
	Turbidity
	Urinary volume
Sickle cell anemia	RBC casts
Starvation, dietary imbalance, extreme change in diet, dehydration	Color
	Odor (fruity)
	Reagent strip* for ketonuria
	Specific gravity
Urinary tract infection or mild inflammation (cystitis, pyelonephritis)	Color and odor
	Cultures for bacteria, yeasts, and viruses
	Microscopic examination for bacteria, WBC casts, RBCs, and WBCs
	Reagent strip* for bacteria, albumin, and pH
	Specific gravity
	Turbidity
Urinary obstruction (tumor, trauma, inflammation)	Color
	Microscopic examination for RBCs
	Specific gravity
	Urinary volume

*Federal listings of waived tests refer to these as *dipstick* tests.

**Drug screening and some other common urine tests must be performed by a forensic laboratory or other laboratory capable of performing gas chromatography, mass spectrometry, and radioimmunoassay.

For example, daily urine output provides a picture of renal function. With adequate fluid intake, the average adult daily urine output is 1,250 milliliters, or approximately 5 cups per 24 hours. When total intake and output measurements are not approximately equal, urinary tract dysfunction may be the cause.

The urinary system works with other body systems to help the body function normally. So a disorder in another body system can affect urinary function. For example, the kidneys interact with the nervous system to help regulate blood pressure and control urination. Thus, a nervous system disorder can affect the circulatory and urinary systems. The cardiovascular system delivers blood to the kidneys for filtration, and the kidneys regulate fluid balance, which helps maintain circulation of blood and myocardial function. A cardiovascular system disorder can allow blood to be delivered to the kidneys at a pressure inadequate for filtration, which would affect urinary system function.

Physical Examination and Testing of Urine Specimens

After confirming that the specimen is properly labeled, the first step in urinalysis is the visual examination of physical characteristics. As part of quality assurance, examine it to make sure there is no visible contamination and that no more than 1 hour has passed since collection (or since a refrigerated sample was brought back to room temperature). You will examine these physical characteristics:

- Color and turbidity
- Volume

- Odor
- Specific gravity

Color and Turbidity Normal urine ranges from pale yellow (straw-colored) to dark amber. The color, which comes from a yellow pigment called *urochrome,* depends on food and fluid intake, medications (including vitamin supplements), and waste products present in the urine. In general, a pale color indicates dilute urine and a dark color indicates concentrated urine.

Assess urine for turbidity, or cloudiness, by noting whether the urine is clear, slightly cloudy, cloudy, or very cloudy. Typically, urine is clear, although cloudy urine does not always indicate an abnormal condition.

The color of urine and any turbidity present can reveal medical conditions that require treatment. Table 47-4 provides more information on variations in urine color and turbidity and the possible causes or sources of these variations. Both pathologic (resulting from disease) and nonpathologic causes are noted.

Volume Normal urine volume, or output, varies according to the patient's age. Normal adult urine volume is 600 to 1,800 milliliters per 24 hours (average of 1,250 milliliters per 24 hours). Infants and children have smaller total urine volumes, although they produce more urine per unit of body weight. Urine volume is typically measured on a timed specimen (such as a 24-hour urine specimen) rather than a random specimen.

Oliguria, insufficient production (or volume) of urine, occurs in conditions such as dehydration, decreased fluid intake, shock, and renal disease. The absence of urine production is called **anuria.** Renal or urethral obstruction and renal failure can cause anuria.

Odor Although urine odor is not typically recorded or considered a significant indicator of disease, it can provide clues about the body's condition. The odor of normal, freshly voided urine is distinct but not unpleasant and is sometimes characterized as aromatic. After urine has been standing for a while, bacteria in the specimen decompose the urea, which causes an odor similar to ammonia.

Diseases, the presence of bacteria, and particular foods (such as asparagus and garlic) can cause changes in urine odor. For example, in the presence of urinary tract infections, urine is foul-smelling, and in patients with uncontrolled diabetes, the smell is characterized as fruity (because of the

TABLE 47-4 Urine Color and Turbidity: Possible Causes

Color and Turbidity	Pathologic Causes	Other Causes
Colorless or pale straw color (dilute)	Diabetes, anxiety, chronic renal disease	Diuretic therapy, excessive fluid intake (water, beer, and/or coffee)
Cloudy	Infection, inflammation, glomerular nephritis	Vegetarian diet
Milky white	Fats, pus	Amorphous phosphates, spermatozoa
Dark yellow, dark amber (concentrated)	Acute febrile disease, vomiting or diarrhea (fluid loss or dehydration)	Low fluid intake, excessive sweating
Yellow-brown	Excessive RBC destruction, bile duct obstruction, diminished liver cell function, bilirubin	Drugs (primaquine)
Orange-yellow, orange-red, orange-brown	Excessive RBC destruction, diminished liver cell function, bile, hepatitis, urobilinuria, obstructive jaundice, hematuria	Drugs (such as pyridium, rifampin), dyes
Salmon pink	No pathologic cause	Amorphous urates
Cloudy red	RBCs, excessive destruction of skeletal or cardiac muscle	None
Bright yellow or red	RBCs (hemorrhage, myoglobin, hemoglobin), excessive destruction of skeletal or cardiac muscle, porphyria	Beets, drugs (such as phenazopyridine hydrochloride), dyes (such as food coloring and contrast media)
Dark red, red-brown	Porphyria, RBCs (menstrual contamination, hemorrhage, hemoglobin), blood from previous hemorrhage	Menstrual contamination
Green, blue-green	Biliverdin, *Pseudomonas* organisms, oxidation of bilirubin	Vitamin B, methylene blue, asparagus (for green)
Green-brown	Bile duct obstruction	Drugs (cascara)
Brownish black	Methemoglobin, melanin	Drugs (levodopa)
Dark brown or black	Acute glomerulonephritis	Drugs (nitrofurantoin, chlorpromazine, iron preparations)

presence of ketones). Phenylketonuria, a congenital metabolic disease, produces a strange, "mousy" or "musty" odor in an infant's wet diaper.

Specific Gravity Urine **specific gravity** is a measure of the concentration or amount of substances dissolved in urine. Because the kidneys remove metabolic wastes and other substances from the blood, the specific gravity of the urine they produce is an indicator of the body's water balance and/or kidney function. The physician's office laboratory uses one of these two methods to determine specific gravity:

1. Refractometer
2. Reagent strip (dipstick)

Specific gravity is a relative measure that is always compared to a standard. The standard for liquids is distilled water, which contains no dissolved substances.

$$\text{Specific gravity} = \frac{\text{Weight of sample}}{\text{Weight of distilled water}}$$

The specific gravity of distilled water is 1.000. You may use special equipment to test for specific gravity (Figure 47-4).

The normal range of urine specific gravity is 1.002 to 1.028. Specific gravity fluctuates throughout the day in response to fluid intake. For example, a first morning urine specimen normally has a higher specific gravity than a specimen provided later in the day. An increase in urine specific gravity may indicate that the kidneys cannot properly dilute the urine. The urine then becomes more concentrated, causing it to darken. Increased specific gravity may indicate conditions such as a urinary tract infection (UTI), dehydration (for example, from fever, vomiting, or diarrhea), adrenal insufficiency, hepatic disease, or congestive heart failure (CHF).

A decrease in the specific gravity of urine causes a lighter-than-normal urine color, may indicate that the kidneys cannot properly concentrate the urine, and may suggest conditions such as overhydration (excess fluid in the body), diabetes insipidus, chronic renal disease, or systemic lupus erythematosus.

Refractometer Measurement A **refractometer** is an optical instrument that measures the refraction, or bending, of light as it passes through a liquid. The degree of refraction, or refractive index, is proportional to the amount of dissolved material in the liquid. You must calibrate a refractometer each

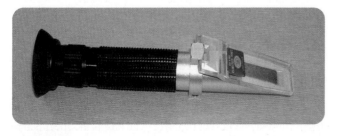

FIGURE 47-4 Specific gravity is commonly determined using a refractometer or reagent strips.
©Leesa Whicker

day with distilled water by setting the instrument at 1.000 with the set screw. Two standard solutions (solutions of known specific gravity) also are used to ensure accuracy. Advantages of using a refractometer to measure urine specific gravity are that the process takes little time and requires little urine. Only a drop of urine is used for this determination. Procedure 47-4, at the end of this chapter, describes how to measure specific gravity with a refractometer.

Reagent Strip Measurement You may use special reagent strips, or dipsticks, to test for specific gravity. Test pads along these plastic strips contain chemicals that react with substances in the urine and change color in precise ways. The reagent strip container includes a color chart for interpreting color changes on the test pads. When you evaluate urine specific gravity in this way, keep in mind that this type of test depends on precisely timed intervals identified by the manufacturer. Follow all directions exactly. Procedure 47-5, at the end of this chapter, describes how to perform a reagent strip test.

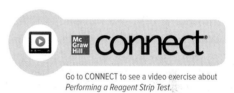

Go to CONNECT to see a video exercise about *Performing a Reagent Strip Test.*

Chemical Testing of Urine Specimens

As a medical assistant, you may be asked to perform chemical tests on urine. Prior to performing chemical tests, always check for proper identification on the urine specimen to be tested. Chemical testing is usually done with reagent strips. It also can be performed with certain automated machines that use photometry.

The licensed practitioner orders chemical testing of urine to determine the status of body processes such as carbohydrate metabolism, liver or kidney function, or acid-base balance. Other reasons for chemical testing include determining the presence of drugs, toxic environmental substances, or infections.

Testing with Reagent Strips As described earlier, reagents (on plastic strips) are chemicals that react with a particular substance in urine and change color in precise ways. These changes indicate the presence of that substance and its amount or concentration in the urine specimen. For example, when a reagent strip is used to test for ketones, the reacted color on the strip will correspond either to a specific concentration of ketone bodies, such as acetoacetic acid, or to the absence of ketones.

Reagent strips are used to test urine for a number of substances. In addition to ketones, reagent strips test for nitrite, pH, blood, bilirubin, glucose, specific gravity, protein, and leukocytes.

There are numerous trade names for urine reagent strips (for example, Multistix® and Chemstrip®). Because not all reagents are reactive for the same chemicals, you must choose the appropriate strip according to the chemical test requested. All reagent strips are used once and discarded.

Follow the exact directions that come with the reagent strips to ensure accurate results. For quality assurance, take these basic precautions: Keep strips in tightly closed containers in a cool, dry area. Never remove them from the container until immediately before testing. Never touch the pads on the strip with your fingers or gloved hands. Examine strips for discoloration before use; discard discolored strips. Check the expiration date on the bottle; do not use strips that have expired. Use strips within 6 months of opening the container. Every time you open a new supply of reagents, run control samples to check for proper operation. Write the date opened on the bottle.

Although the process is essentially the same for all reagent strip tests, there are variations in time intervals before reading results. Some reagent strips are designed to test for several substances at once. The basic procedure for using reagent strips for chemical tests can be found in Procedure 47-5 at the end of this chapter. In some cases, if the reagent strip test is positive, a confirmatory test is performed to ensure the accuracy of the results.

Ketone Bodies

Ketone bodies (or ketones) are produced by the liver from fatty acids during fat metabolism. They include acetone, acetoacetic acid, and betahydroxybutyric acid. Only the first two substances can be determined using a reagent strip test. Normally, there are no ketones in urine. The presence of ketones in the urine may indicate that a patient is following a low-carbohydrate diet, or it may indicate that the patient has a condition such as starvation, excessive vomiting, or diabetes mellitus. Because ketones evaporate at room temperature, be sure to test urine immediately or cover the specimen tightly and refrigerate it until testing can be done.

pH

Urinary pH is a measure of the urine's degree of acidity or alkalinity. Determination of pH can provide information about a patient's metabolic status and diet, the medications being taken, and several conditions. The normal pH of freshly voided urine ranges from 4.5 to 8.0. The average urine pH is 6.0, which is slightly acidic. A pH of 7.0 is neutral, a lower pH is acidic, and a higher one is alkaline. Patients with excessively alkaline urine may have conditions such as urinary tract infection (UTI) or metabolic or respiratory alkalosis. Those with excessively acidic urine may have conditions such as phenylketonuria or acidosis. Reagent strip tests on both urine and blood are used to measure pH in the body. (See the *Collecting, Processing, and Testing Blood Specimens* chapter for information on blood tests for pH.)

Blood

A patient who has blood in the urine may be menstruating, have a urinary tract infection, or have trauma or bleeding in the kidneys. To test for blood in urine, use a reagent strip that reacts with hemoglobin. There are two indicators on the strip: One is for nonhemolyzed blood, the other for hemolyzed blood.

Colors on the strip range from orange through green to dark blue and may indicate **hematuria** (the presence of blood in the urine) caused by cystitis; kidney stones; menstruation; or ureteral, bladder, or urethral irritation. The presence of free hemoglobin in the urine is known as *hemoglobinuria,* a rare condition caused by transfusion reactions, malaria, drug reactions, snakebites, or severe burns. Injured or damaged muscle tissue—as occurs in crushing injuries, myocardial infarction, muscular dystrophy, or contact sports injuries—can cause *myoglobinuria* (the presence of myoglobin in the urine). Reagent strip testing does not distinguish between these two conditions.

Bilirubin and Urobilinogen

When hemoglobin breaks down, it converts into conjugated bilirubin in the liver and then to urobilinogen in the intestines. Presence of the bile pigment bilirubin in the urine (*bilirubinuria*) is one of the first signs of liver disease or conditions that involve the liver. When bilirubin is present, urine turns yellow-brown to greenish orange. You usually use a reagent strip to test for bilirubin. If the reagent strip test is positive, a confirmatory test called an Ictotest® is usually performed. The Ictotest® is a reagent tablet test that is more sensitive than the reagent strip test.

Although **urobilinogen** is normally present in the urine in small amounts, elevated levels may indicate increased *hemolysis* (red blood cell destruction) or liver disease. A total bile obstruction is suggested by lack of urobilinogen. When this occurs, urobilinogen stops being formed in the intestines or reabsorbed in the circulation. To test for urobilinogen, you use reagent strips.

Testing for either bilirubin or urobilinogen must be performed on a fresh urine specimen. Bilirubin decomposes rapidly in bright light to form biliverdin, which is not detected by the reagent strip test for bilirubin. Urobilinogen breaks down to urobilin on standing.

Glucose

Glucose is normally present in urine, but only in small quantities not detectable by the reagent strip test for glucose. **Glycosuria** (the presence of significant glucose in the urine) is common in patients with diabetes. Blood is more commonly tested for glucose than urine is because reagent strip tests may show false-negative results when used for testing urine.

Protein

Although a small amount of protein is excreted in the urine every day, an excess of protein in the urine (**proteinuria**) usually indicates renal disease. Proteinuria is also common in pregnant patients and after heavy exercise.

Nitrites

Bacteria in urine makes an enzyme that changes urine nitrates to nitrites. If nitrites are found in the urine, it suggests a bacterial infection of the urinary tract. The test is not definitive, however. If an insufficient number of bacteria are present in the urine or if the urine has not incubated long enough in the bladder for a reaction to take place, the nitrite test result may be falsely negative. The best urine specimen to test for nitrites is the first morning specimen.

When testing for urinary nitrites, you must test the urine immediately or refrigerate the specimen. Bacteria can multiply in a specimen allowed to sit at room temperature, causing a false-positive test result. Bacteria also can further metabolize the nitrites already produced, causing a false-negative result.

Leukocytes Leukocytes (white blood cells) appear in the urine in urinary tract or renal infections. Use strip tests for leukocyte esterase, a chemical seen when leukocytes are present, to test for leukocytes.

Other Types of Chemical Testing Other types of chemical tests—such as those that test for electrolytes and osmolality—may be performed on urine specimens. Because these tests are performed in an outside laboratory rather than in a physician's office laboratory, you do not need to know the steps in each procedure.

Phenylketones The presence of phenylketones in a patient's urine indicates phenylketonuria (PKU), a genetically inherited disorder in which the body cannot properly metabolize the nutrient phenylalanine. This rare disorder causes phenylalanine to build up in the body, resulting in mental retardation. PKU can be treated successfully by limiting the dietary intake of phenylalanine, which makes up 5% of all natural protein, from early infancy. Although urine can be tested for the presence of phenylketones, blood testing is routine for newborns before discharge, at least 24 hours after birth.

Pregnancy Tests Pregnancy testing is based on detecting the hormone—called *human chorionic gonadotropin*, or *HCG*—secreted by the placenta. HCG levels vary throughout pregnancy: They usually peak at about 8 weeks, drop to lower levels in the second trimester, and then rise to detectable levels in the last trimester. Many commercial pregnancy tests are manufactured for use both in the clinical setting and at home. These tests are sensitive, are easy to perform and interpret, and give quick results. Most tests are now designed as an enzyme immunoassay (EIA) test usually a *membrane* EIA. These tests involve an antigen, an antibody specific for the antigen, and a second antibody conjugated to an enzyme. The reagents are typically incorporated into an absorbent membrane in a plastic case. A sample of either urine or serum is added through a chamber window, where it migrates through the membrane and combines with the reagents to produce a reaction. Although the technology used in the design of these tests is quite complex, the test itself is easy to set up and interpret (see Procedure 47-6 at the end of this chapter). The tests are all designed with a control feature incorporated into the reagent pack for quality assurance of the test results.

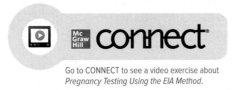

Go to CONNECT to see a video exercise about *Pregnancy Testing Using the EIA Method.*

Urine Tests for the Presence of STIs In response to increasing numbers of sexually transmitted infections, the CDC recommends that all sexually active females between the ages of 15 and 25 be screened annually for chlamydia. To accomplish this, several tests called *nucleic acid amplification tests* (*NAATs*) have recently been developed. These tests utilize urine samples to detect the presence of nucleic acid. Patients infected with either *Chlamydia trachomatis* or *Neisseria gonorrhoeae* will have nucleic acid in their urine. By amplifying nucleic acids specific to chlamydia and gonorrhea, the test can detect the presence of very small numbers of bacteria.

These tests have several advantages:

- Sample collection is noninvasive and the sample is easily collected.
- The tests are highly specific.
- The tests are highly sensitive. As little as one copy of bacterial nucleic acid can be detected in a urine specimen.
- Organisms do not have to be living to be detected.
- The tests are good screening tools for asymptomatic patients.

The tests also have some disadvantages:

- The tests are expensive.
- No living organisms remain for use in a follow-up culture, so positive tests must be confirmed by culture from an endocervical or urethral swab.

Microscopic Examination of Urine Specimens

The licensed practitioner performs a microscopic examination of urine sediment to view elements visible only with a microscope. You will use a centrifuge to obtain sediment for analysis. A centrifuge spins test tubes containing fluid at speeds that cause heavier substances in the fluid to settle to the bottom of the tubes.

The substances in urine that form sediment (precipitate) when urine is centrifuged include cells, casts, crystals, yeast, bacteria, and parasites. These elements are categorized and counted during microscopic examination. You may use the KOVA System®, manufactured by Hycor Biomedical, Irvine, California, to prepare urine sediment for microscopic examination. When you use the KOVA System®, the sediment is evenly distributed to four calibrated chambers before the microscopic elements are counted. Procedure 47-7, at the end of this chapter, describes how to process a urine specimen for microscopic examination of sediment.

Cells High-power magnification is used to classify and count cells. Three types of cells may be found in urine:

- Red blood cells.
- White blood cells.
- Epithelial cells.

Red Blood Cells Red blood cells (RBCs) are typically pale, round, nongranular, and flat or biconcave (Figure 47-5). They have no nucleus and enter the urinary tract during

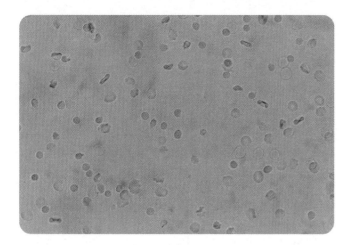

FIGURE 47-5 A large number of red blood cells in the urine may indicate injury, inflammation, or disease.
©plenoy m/Shutterstock

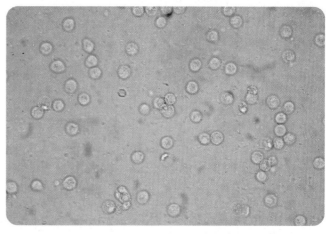

FIGURE 47-6 Unlike RBCs, WBCs have nuclei. The multilobed nuclei are visible as irregularly shaped darker areas in these cells.
©toeytoey/Shutterstock

inflammation or injury. From zero to three RBCs per high-power field in urine are normal. However, numerous RBCs may indicate a variety of problems, including urinary infection, obstruction, inflammation, trauma, or tumor.

White Blood Cells White blood cells (WBCs) are larger than red blood cells. They have a granular appearance and usually contain a multilobed nucleus (Figure 47-6). They are typically found in large numbers in the urine (greater than the normal zero to eight per high-power field) if inflammation is present or if the specimen was contaminated during collection.

Epithelial Cells Epithelial cells are classified as squamous, transitional, or renal. Squamous epithelial cells—large, flat, irregular cells with a small, round, centrally located nucleus—line the genitourinary tract's lower portion (Figure 47-7). They often occur in sheets or clumps and can be easily recognized under low-power magnification.

Transitional epithelial cells line the urinary tract from the renal pelvis (the beginning of the ureter) to the upper portion of the urethra. They can be round to oval and may have a tail and, occasionally, two nuclei. Often, however, they appear similar to squamous cells, but smaller. A few transitional cells appear normally in urine, but the presence of several may indicate tubular damage.

Renal epithelial cells can be round to oval and have a large, oval, and sometimes eccentric nucleus. Although a few of these cells appear normally in urine, several may indicate tubular damage in the kidneys. Damage in the renal tubules causes epithelial cells to die and slough off, or shed. These shed cells can then be seen in a urine sample.

Casts Casts—cylinder-shaped elements with flat or rounded ends—form when protein from the breakdown of cells accumulates and precipitates in the kidney tubules and is washed into the urine. The protein then assumes the size and shape of the tubules. Think of a clogged drain in your bathroom sink. The drain may start out just slow at

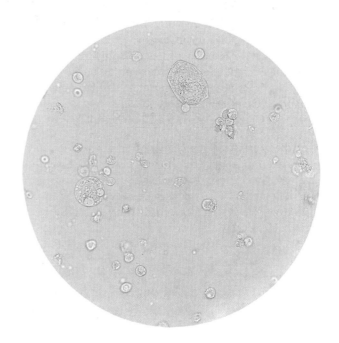

FIGURE 47-7 A squamous epithelial cell in a field that shows multiple WBCs. Notice the size difference.
©Chamaiporn Naprom/Shutterstock

first but, after a while, very little water will pass through. If you remove the drain pipe, you will find that the material plugging up the drain has taken on the shape of the pipe. It works the same in the kidney tubules, but with different materials.

Casts differ in composition and size, as described in Table 47-5. Classified according to their appearance and composition, casts can indicate renal pathologic conditions or can be caused by strenuous exercise.

Crystals Crystals, naturally produced solids of definite form, are commonly seen in urine specimens, especially those permitted to cool. They usually do not indicate a significant disorder, except when found in large numbers in

TABLE 47-5 Types of Urine Casts

Cast Type	Appearance	Description
Hyaline casts	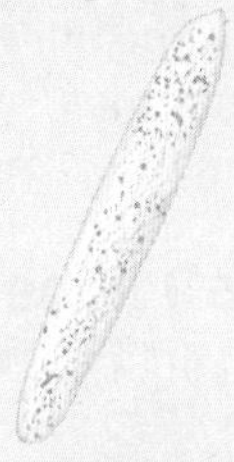 ©McGraw-Hill Education	Pale, transparent, and cylinder-shaped with rounded ends and parallel sides. Composed of protein, they form because of diminished urine flow through individual nephrons. They are present in patients with kidney disease or in people who have exercised strenuously. A few hyaline casts observed in the urine is normal.
Granular casts	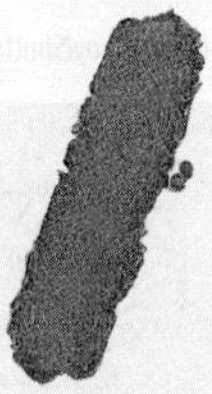	Resemble hyaline casts and can result from kidney disease or strenuous exercise.
Red blood cell casts	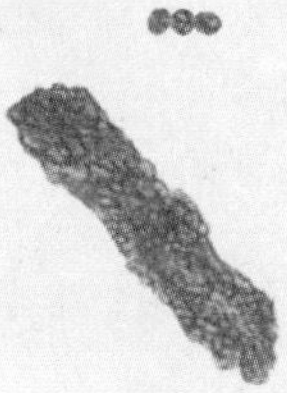 ©McGraw-Hill Education	Hyaline casts with embedded red blood cells. Because of the RBCs, these casts sometimes appear brown. Red blood cell casts always indicate an abnormality.
White blood cell casts	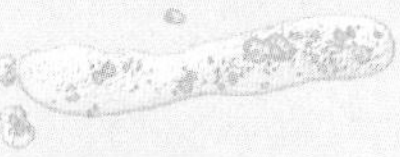 ©McGraw-Hill Education	Hyaline casts with leukocytes. These casts typically have a multilobed nucleus and may indicate pyelonephritis—an inflammation of the kidney and renal pelvis.
Epithelial cell casts	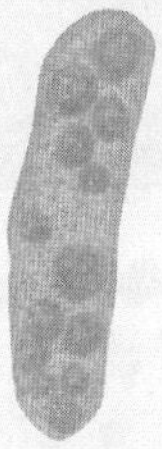	Casts that contain embedded renal tubular epithelial cells and indicate excessive kidney damage. Causes include shock, renal ischemia, heavy-metal poisoning, certain allergic reactions, and nephrotoxic drugs. These casts are often confused with white blood cell casts.
Waxy casts	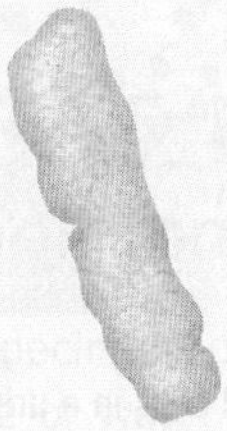	Yellow, glassy, brittle, smooth, and homogeneous casts with cracks or fissures and squared or broken ends. Although rare, these casts may occur with severe renal disease.

patients with kidney stones and in a few pathologic conditions (such as hypercalcemia and some inborn errors of metabolism). Figure 47-8 shows crystals commonly found in urine specimens. Because different substances tend to crystallize in acidic and alkaline urine, it is important to determine the pH of a patient's urine before you try to identify any present crystals.

Yeast Cells Yeast cells, which are usually oval and may show budding, may be confused with RBCs (Figure 47-9). Yeast cells in urine sediment are associated with genitourinary tract infection, external genitalia contamination, vaginitis,

urethritis, and prostatitis. These cells also are commonly seen in the urine of patients with diabetes.

Bacteria Although a few bacteria are normally found in urine, urinary tract infection may be indicated if the urine has bacteria along with a putrid odor and numerous white blood cells. Bacteria under high-power magnification appear rod- or cocci-shaped (spherical). See Figure 47-10.

Parasites The presence of parasites in sediment may signal genitourinary tract infection or external genitalia contamination. The most common urinary parasite, *Trichomonas vaginalis*

Successful recovery of these pathogenic bacteria from a stool specimen depends on timely inoculation of special culture media. The licensed practitioner may ask the patient to provide a sample in the office whenever possible to avoid delay in processing the specimen. Several types of culture media promote the growth of intestinal pathogens while suppressing the growth of other microorganisms.

Suspected Protozoal or Parasitic Infection

In cases of a suspected protozoal or parasitic infection, the licensed practitioner may request an **O&P specimen**, short for *ova and parasites specimen*. This type of stool sample is examined for the presence of certain forms of protozoans or parasites, including their eggs (ova).

When a practitioner requests an O&P test, obtain both a fresh and a preserved stool specimen. A fresh specimen is examined both macroscopically and microscopically for the presence of microorganisms. A preserved specimen is also necessary because certain forms of these organisms are destroyed within a short time after leaving the body and may

not be detected in the fresh specimen. You must always obtain a preserved specimen when stool samples are sent to an outside laboratory.

Special stool collection kits are available. They contain a specimen container for a fresh sample along with vials of two types of preservatives: formalin (a dilute solution of formaldehyde) and polyvinyl alcohol (PVA). Instruct the patient to place the stool sample in the specimen container and to mix portions of the specimen in each of the preservative vials. The laboratory will examine all specimens for the presence of microorganisms.

When a licensed practitioner suspects that a patient has a protozoal or parasitic infection, he will request that a series of at least three stool specimens be examined. Three specimens are required because different forms of the microorganism may be present in the stool at different times, and some could be missed with only one sample. Because certain medications can interfere with detecting these microorganisms, the patient may be asked to refrain from using medications such as antidiarrheal compounds, antacids, and mineral oil laxatives for at least a week before samples are obtained.

PROCEDURE 47-1 Collecting a Clean-Catch Midstream Urine Specimen

WORK // DOC

Procedure Goal: To collect a urine specimen that is free from contamination

OSHA Guidelines:

Materials: Dry, sterile urine container with lid; label; written instructions (if the patient is to perform procedure independently); antiseptic towelettes; laboratory requisition form; patient chart/progress note

Method:

1. Confirm the patient's identity and be sure all forms are correctly completed.

2. Label the sterile urine specimen container with the patient's name, ID number, and date of birth; the licensed practitioner's name; the date and time of collection; and the initials of the person collecting the specimen.

When the Patient Will Be Completing the Procedure Independently

3. Explain the procedure in detail. Provide the patient with written instructions, antiseptic towelettes, and the labeled sterile specimen container.

4. Confirm that the patient understands the instructions, especially not to touch the inside of the specimen

container and to refrigerate the specimen until bringing it to the licensed practitioner's office.
RATIONALE: *Touching the inside of the container will introduce microorganisms into the container and can interfere with the test results. The specimen should be refrigerated to keep bacteria from growing and causing a false-positive result.*

When You Are Assisting a Patient

3. Explain the procedure and how you will be assisting in the collection.

4. Wash your hands and don exam gloves.

When You Are Assisting in the Collection for Female Patients

5. Remove the lid from the specimen container and place the lid upside down on a flat surface.

6. Use three antiseptic towelettes to clean the perineal area by spreading the labia and wiping from front to back. Wipe with the first towelette on one side and discard it. Wipe with the second towelette on the other side and discard it. Wipe with the third towelette down the middle and discard it. To remove soap residue that could cause a higher pH and affect chemical test results, rinse the area once from front to back with water.
RATIONALE: *The area must be thoroughly cleaned so that microorganisms from the vulva do not contaminate the specimen.*

PROCEDURE 47-4 Measuring Specific Gravity with a Refractometer

Procedure Goal: To measure the specific gravity of a urine specimen with a refractometer

OSHA Guidelines:

Materials: Urine specimen, refractometer, dropper, laboratory report form, and patient chart/progress note

Method:

1. Wash your hands and don exam gloves.
2. Check the specimen for proper labeling and examine it to make sure there is no visible contamination and that no more than 1 hour has passed since collection (or since the specimen was removed from the refrigerator and brought back to room temperature).
3. Swirl the specimen.
   RATIONALE: *To mix the specimen thoroughly.*
4. Confirm that the refractometer has been calibrated that day. If not, you must calibrate it with distilled water. You also must use two standard solutions as controls to check the refractometer's accuracy. Follow Steps 6 through 11, using each of the three samples in place of the specimen. Clean the refractometer and the dropper after each use, and record the calibration values in the quality control log.
   RATIONALE: *To ensure that the refractometer is standardized prior to testing the specimen.*
5. Open the hinged lid of the refractometer.
6. Draw up a small amount of the specimen into the dropper.
7. Place one drop of the specimen under the cover.
8. Close the lid.
9. Turn on the light and look into the refractometer's eyepiece. As the light passes through the specimen, the refractometer measures the refraction of the light and displays the refractive index on a scale on the right, with corresponding specific gravity values on the left.

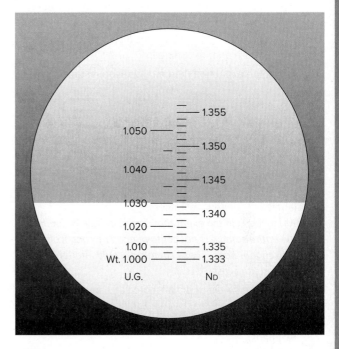

FIGURE Procedure 47-4 Step 9 A refractometer uses light refraction to measure specific gravity.

10. Read the specific gravity value at the line where light and dark meet.
11. Record the value on the laboratory report form.
12. Sanitize and disinfect the refractometer and the dropper. Put them away when they are dry.
13. Clean and disinfect the work area.
14. Remove the gloves and wash your hands.
15. Record the value in the patient's chart/progress note.

PROCEDURE 47-5 Performing a Reagent Strip Test

Procedure Goal: To perform chemical testing on urine specimens to screen for the presence of various elements, including leukocytes, nitrites, urobilinogen, protein, pH, blood, specific gravity, ketones, bilirubin, and glucose

OSHA Guidelines:

Materials: Urine specimen, laboratory report form, pipette or urinalysis transfer straw, reagent strips, paper towel, timer, and patient chart/progress note

Method:

1. Wash your hands and don personal protective equipment.

2. Check the specimen for proper labeling and examine it to make sure there is no visible contamination. Perform the test as soon as possible after collection. Refrigerate the specimen if testing will take place more than 1 hour later. Bring the refrigerated specimen back to room temperature prior to testing.

3. Check the expiration date on the reagent strip container and check the strip for damaged or discolored pads.
   RATIONALE: *To ensure that the reagent strip is still valid.*

4. Swirl the specimen.
   RATIONALE: *To mix the specimen thoroughly.*

5. Remove a small amount (aliquot) of the urine with a pipette or a urinalysis transfer straw and place it into a labeled secondary container.
   RATIONALE: *In the event that a urine culture is needed, the entire sample is not contaminated by chemicals on the reagent pads. These chemicals could interfere with a urine culture test.*

   Dip a urine strip into the aliquoted specimen, making sure each pad is completely covered. Briefly tap the strip sideways on a paper towel. *Do not blot* the test pads.
   RATIONALE: *Excess urine could migrate to the other pads and alter the test results.*

6. Read each test pad against the chart on the bottle at the designated time.
   Note: It is important to read each pad at the appropriate time. Most reagent strip results are invalid after 2 minutes.
   RATIONALE: *Test pads read at inappropriate times will yield inaccurate results.*

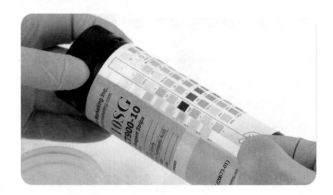

FIGURE Procedure 47-5 Step 6 Read the reagent strip by the time indicated in the manufacturer's instructions.
©McGraw-Hill Education

7. Record the values on the laboratory report form.

8. Discard the used disposable supplies.

9. Clean and disinfect the work area.

10. Remove your gloves and wash your hands.

11. Record the result in the patient's chart/progress note.

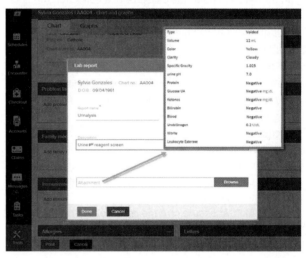
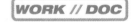

FIGURE Procedure 47-5 Step 11 Always document the results of the reagent strip test in the EHR immediately and accurately.
©McGraw-Hill Education

PROCEDURE 47-6 Pregnancy Testing Using the EIA Method

WORK // DOC

Procedure Goal: To perform the enzyme immunoassay in order to detect HCG in the urine (or serum) and to interpret results as positive or negative

OSHA Guidelines:

Materials: Gloves, urine specimen, urinalysis transfer straw, timing device, surface disinfectant, pregnancy control solutions, pregnancy test kits, quality control log, and patient chart/progress note

Method:

1. Wash your hands and don exam gloves.

2. Gather the necessary supplies and equipment.

3. If materials have been refrigerated, allow all materials to reach room temperature prior to conducting the testing.

4. Label the test chamber with the patient's name or identification number; label one test chamber for a negative and positive control.

5. Apply the urine (or serum) to the test chamber per the manufacturer's instructions. A urine transfer straw may be used.
  RATIONALE: *Different tests may have slightly different instructions.*

6. At the appropriate time, read and interpret the results.
  RATIONALE: *Most tests are invalid after 10 minutes.*

7. Document the patient's results in the patient chart/progress note; document the quality control results in the appropriate quality control log book.

8. Dispose of used reagents in a biohazard container.

9. Clean the work area with a disinfectant solution.

10. Remove your gloves and wash your hands.

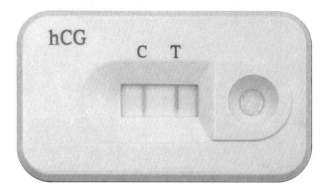

(a)

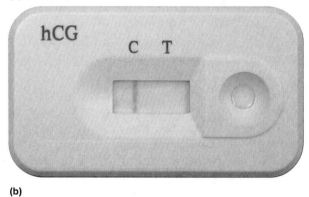

(b)

FIGURE Procedure 47-6 Step 6   A positive pregnancy test (a) and a negative pregnancy test (b). Note that if the line does not appear in the C (Control) area, the test is invalid.

(a-b) ©McGraw-Hill Education

PROCEDURE 47-7 Processing a Urine Specimen for Microscopic Examination of Sediment [WORK // DOC]

Procedure Goal: To prepare a slide for microscopic examination of urine sediment

OSHA Guidelines:

Materials: Fresh urine specimen, two glass or plastic test tubes, water, centrifuge, tapered pipette or urinalysis transfer straw, glass slide with coverslip, microscope with light source, laboratory report form, and patient chart/progress note

Method:

1. Wash your hands and don exam gloves.

2. Check the specimen for proper labeling and examine it to make sure there is no visible contamination and that no more than 1 hour has passed since collection (or since the specimen was removed from the refrigerator and brought back to room temperature).

3. Swirl the urine specimen.
  RATIONALE: *To mix the specimen thoroughly.*

4. Use a urinalysis transfer device to place approximately 10 mL of urine into a labeled test tube. Pour 10 mL of plain water into the balance tube.

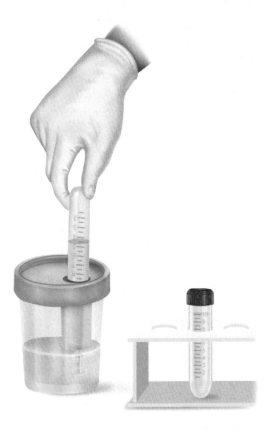

FIGURE Procedure 47-7 Step 4   Fill one test tube with approximately 10 mL of urine and the other with 10 mL of water.

5. Balance the centrifuge by placing the test tubes on opposite sides of the centrifuge.
   RATIONALE: *An unbalanced tube could cause the centrifuge to "walk" or wobble off the table.*

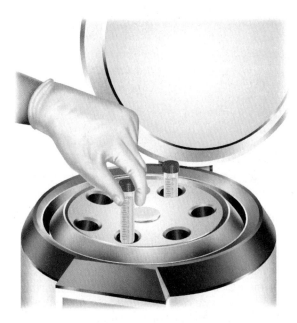

FIGURE Procedure 47-7 Step 5   The centrifuge must be balanced by placing one test tube on each side.

6. Make sure the lid is secure and set the centrifuge timer for 5 to 10 minutes.

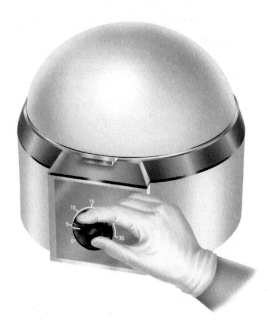

FIGURE Procedure 47-7 Step 6   Set the centrifuge timer for 5 to 10 minutes.

7. Set the speed as prescribed by your office's protocol (usually 1,500 to 2,000 revolutions per minute) and start the centrifuge.
   RATIONALE: *Spinning the urine will force the solids (cells, casts, and crystals) to the bottom of the tube.*

8. After the centrifuge stops, lift out the tube containing the urine and carefully pour most of the liquid portion—called the **supernatant**—down the sink drain, washing it down the drain with water.

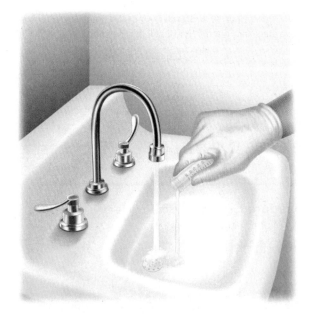

FIGURE Procedure 47-7 Step 8   Make sure you do not lose any sediment when you pour off the urine.

9. A few drops of urine should remain in the bottom of the test tube with any sediment. Mix the urine and sediment

together by gently tapping the bottom of the tube on the palm of your hand.

RATIONALE: *To resuspend the solid material.*

10. Use the tapered pipette or transfer straw to obtain a drop or two of urine sediment. Place the drops in the center of a clean, labeled glass slide.

11. Place the coverslip over the specimen, allow it to settle, and place it on the stage of the microscope.

12. Correctly focus the microscope as directed in the *Orientation to the Lab* chapter.

Note: Most medical assistants are trained to perform this procedure only up to this point. After this, the licensed practitioner usually examines the specimen. However, you may be asked to clean the items after the examination is completed. The remaining steps are provided for your information.

13. Use a dim light and view the slide under the low-power objective. Observe the slide for casts (found mainly around the coverslip's edges) and count the casts viewed.

14. Switch to the high-power objective. Identify the casts. Identify any epithelial cells, mucus, protozoans, yeasts, and crystals. Adjust the slide position so that you can view and count the cells, protozoans, yeasts, and crystals from at least 10 different fields. Turn off the light after the examination is completed.

15. Record the observations on the laboratory report form.

16. Properly dispose of used disposable materials.

17. Sanitize and disinfect nondisposable items; put them away when they are dry.

18. Clean and disinfect the work area.

19. Remove the gloves and wash your hands.

20. Record the observations in the patient's chart/progress note.

PROCEDURE 47-8 Fecal Occult Blood Testing Using the Guaiac Testing Method

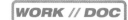

Procedure Goal: To test for the presence of blood in a fecal sample

OSHA Guidelines:

Materials: Fecal occult blood testing cards or slides, fecal collection spoon or other device, written patient instructions, testing reagents, and patient chart/progress note

Method:

1. Confirm the patient's identity and ensure that all forms are completed correctly.

2. Label the occult blood testing card or slide with the patient's name and date of birth. Give the patient the test card or slide and collecting spoon or applicator.

3. Give the patient pretest and collection instructions:

   a. Do not collect a sample if you are menstruating or if visible blood is seen in the feces or toilet.

   b. For 3 days prior to collecting the sample, avoid red meats (beef, veal, and lamb); horseradish; vitamin C supplements; certain fruits and vegetables, such as cabbage, cucumbers, broccoli, carrots, beets, radishes, mushrooms, and citrus fruits; aspirin or other nonsteroidal anti-inflammatory drugs; and other medications, including corticosteroids. (Consult the specific test instructions for dietary and medication restrictions because these may vary from test to test.)

   RATIONALE: *Some foods and medications may cause a false-positive or a false-negative test result.*

   c. Collect the samples (depending on the specific test) on 2 or 3 different days.

   d. Collect the specimen before it comes into contact with the toilet water. (The patient may use a clean container or a specimen collection hat.)

   RATIONALE: *Chemicals in the toilet could interfere with the test.*

   e. Place a small amount of fecal material on each slide or test card window with the applicator. The sample should be thinly smeared in the sample area.

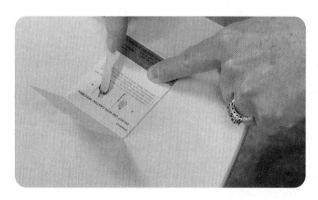

FIGURE Procedure 47-8 Step 3e   The patient should apply a thin smear of fecal material on each window of the test card.
©McGraw-Hill Education

   f. Close the card window or place the slide in the provided container and write the collection date on the card or slide.

   g. Return the card or slide to the office.

Processing the Test

4. Wash your hands and don gloves.

5. Open the back of the card. Add the recommended amount of developing reagent directly over the smeared area on the back side of the paper and over the positive and negative controls, if present, on the card.

RATIONALE: *To ensure that the test is working correctly.*

6. Read the test results at the appropriate time according to the manufacturer's instructions (usually within 60 seconds). There will be a blue color on the guaiac paper if blood is present.

7. Dispose of the testing card according to OSHA regulations.

8. Remove your gloves and wash your hands.

9. Document the results in the patient's chart.

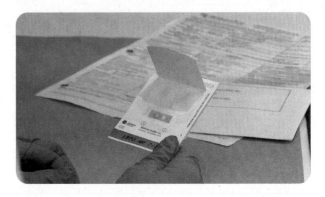

FIGURE Procedure 47-8 Step 6   Read the card by the time indicated in the manufacturer's instructions.
©McGraw-Hill Education

SUMMARY OF LEARNING OUTCOMES

OUTCOME	KEY POINTS
47.1 Discuss the role of the medical assistant in collecting, processing, and testing urine and stool samples.	Your role as a medical assistant includes collecting, processing, and testing urine samples and processing and testing stool samples. You also will be responsible for teaching patients proper collection methods for urine and stool samples.
47.2 Carry out procedures for collecting urine specimens according to guidelines.	The general guidelines for collecting a urine specimen include following the procedure specified for the urine test that will be performed; using the type of specimen container indicated by the laboratory; properly labeling the specimen container; explaining the procedure to the patient when assisting in the collection process; washing your hands before and after the procedure and wearing gloves during the procedure; and completing all necessary paperwork.
47.3 Describe the process of urinalysis and its purpose.	Urinalysis is the evaluation of urine by various types of testing methods to obtain information about body health and disease. A typical urinalysis includes physical examination and testing, chemical testing, microscopic examination, and, if necessary, urine culture and sensitivity testing.
47.4 Carry out the proper procedure for collecting and processing a stool sample for fecal occult blood testing.	The general guidelines for collecting a stool specimen include instructing the patient about the need to follow all collection procedures, including when to collect, how to collect, and how to return the specimen to the office; following the testing procedure for fecal occult blood testing; using standard precautions when performing the test; and documenting the test and results in the patient's chart.

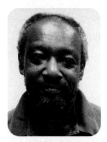

©McGraw-Hill Education

Recall Ken Washington from the case study at the beginning of the chapter. Now that you have completed the chapter, answer the following questions regarding his case.

1. What instructions will you give Ken Washington for collecting the urine specimen for reagent testing?
2. What tests are included in a reagent test?
3. Describe the instructions you will need to give Ken Washington regarding his 24-hour urine collection.

EXAM PREPARATION QUESTIONS

1. (LO 47.2) Which of the following catheters is used after plastic repair of the ureter?
   a. Indwelling
   b. Urinary
   c. Drainage
   d. Splinting
   e. Permanent

2. (LO 47.3) The average adult urinary output is
   a. 650 mL
   b. 1,000 mL
   c. 1,250 mL
   d. 1,500 mL
   e. 2,000 mL

3. (LO 47.3) A urine sample that is turbid is said to be
   a. Cloudy
   b. Clear
   c. Odorous
   d. Dark
   e. Dilute

4. (LO 47.3) What is the specific gravity of distilled water?
   a. 0.00
   b. 1.000
   c. 1.001
   d. 1.010
   e. 1.100

5. (LO 47.3) Which of the following is (are) normally found in a urine sample?
   a. Cholesterol
   b. Tyrosine
   c. Ketone bodies
   d. Amorphous phosphates
   e. Glucose

6. (LO 47.4) A test for the presence of hidden blood in a stool sample is which of the following?
   a. SGOT
   b. FOBT
   c. Bilirubin
   d. EIA
   e. Urobilinogen

7. (LO 47.3) Calcium carbonate, calcium oxalate, and triple phosphate are types of which kind of structure sometimes present in urine?
   a. Casts
   b. Blood cell components
   c. Bence Jones proteins
   d. Vitamins
   e. Crystals

8. (LO 47.3) Which of the following is a chemical component of urine?
   a. Color
   b. Volume
   c. Blood
   d. Ketones
   e. Clarity

9. (LO 47.2) The most common type of urine sample is
   a. First morning
   b. 24-hour
   c. Timed
   d. Random
   e. Midstream

10. (LO 47.3) The term meaning insufficient production of urine is
   a. Anuria
   b. Oliguria
   c. Polyuria
   d. Proteinuria
   e. Hematuria

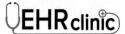

Go to CONNECT to complete the EHRclinic exercises: 47.01 Record Urine Dipstick Results and 47.02 Document Release of Urine Specimen for Chain of Custody.

SOFT SKILLS SUCCESS

The licensed practitioner has ordered a test of stool for blood on a patient. The patient is given a home testing kit, and he will need to take three samples of stool, one on each of 3 separate days. You are teaching the patient about the procedure when, in a rough and hostile voice, he states, "There is no way I am going to collect my own s***! You can tell that doctor to forget it!" What should you do?

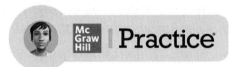

Go to PRACTICE MEDICAL OFFICE and complete the module Clinical: Interactions.

CASE STUDY

<table>
<tr><td rowspan="5">PATIENT INFORMATION</td><td colspan="3"></td></tr>
<tr><td>Patient Name</td><td>DOB</td><td>Allergies</td></tr>
<tr><td>Sylvia Gonzales</td><td>09/01/1968</td><td>PCN</td></tr>
<tr><td>Attending</td><td>MRN</td><td>Other Information</td></tr>
<tr><td>Alexis N. Whalen, MD</td><td>00-AA-004</td><td>Vital Signs: BP 136/86, T 97.6, P 92, R 20</td></tr>
</table>

Sylvia Gonzales is at the office for a 3-month return check for her newly diagnosed Type 2 diabetes. She states that she has taken the medication she received for her "sugar," and she knows the doctor wants to do a special "sugar test" this time. Her medication list includes Januvia® 100 mg

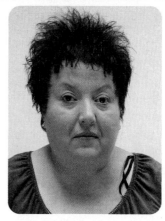
©McGraw-Hill Education

daily. The physician has ordered a fasting blood sugar (FBS), electrolytes, and a CBC. You will need to collect a venipuncture blood specimen to send the lab. During the exam, Sylvia Gonzales states she is feeling light-headed, so the licensed practitioner asks you to perform a waived blood sugar and hemoglobin A1C immediately.

Keep Sylvia Gonzales in mind as you study this chapter. There will be questions at the end of the chapter based on the case study. The information in the chapter will help you answer these questions.

LEARNING OUTCOMES

After completing Chapter 48, you will be able to:

48.1 Discuss the role of the medical assistant when collecting, processing, and testing blood specimens.

48.2 Describe the equipment needed to collect a blood specimen.

48.3 Summarize ways to communicate with patients and to respond to their needs when collecting blood.

48.4 Carry out the procedure for collecting a blood specimen.

48.5 Carry out the procedure for performing blood tests.

KEY TERMS

anticoagulants
automatic puncturing devices
buffy coat
butterfly system
capillary puncture
complete blood (cell) count (CBC)
erythrocyte sedimentation rate (ESR)
ethylenediaminetetraacetic acid (EDTA)
formed elements
hematoma

hemolysis
lancet
micropipette
morphology
packed red blood cells
phlebotomy
requisition
serum separators
tourniquet
venipuncture
venoscope
whole blood

CAAHEP		ABHES
I.C.10	Identify CLIA waived tests associated with common diseases	**3. Medical Terminology** d. Define and use medical abbreviations when appropriate and acceptable
I.C.12	Identify quality assurance practices in healthcare	**8. Clinical Procedures** a. Practice standard precautions and perform disinfection/sterilization techniques

I.P.2	Perform:
	  (b) venipuncture
	  (c) capillary puncture
		j. Make adaptations for patients with special needs (psychological or physical limitations)

I.P.8	Instruct and prepare a patient for a procedure or a treatment	**9. Medical Laboratory Procedures** a. Practice quality control
I.P.10	Perform a quality control measure	b. Perform selected CLIA-waived tests that assist with diagnosis and treatment

I.P.11	Obtain specimens and perform:
	  (a) CLIA waived hematology test
	  (b) CLIA waived chemistry test
	  (d) CLIA waived immunology test
		(2) Hematology testing
		     (3) Chemistry testing
		     (4) Immunology testing

I.A.3	Show awareness of a patient's concerns related to the procedure being performed	c. Dispose of biohazardous materials

II.P.2	Differentiate between normal and abnormal test results	d. Collect, label, and process specimens
		     (1) Perform venipuncture
		     (2) Perform capillary puncture

II.P.3	Maintain laboratory test results using flow sheets	
II.A.1	Reassure a patient of the accuracy of the test results	
III.P.2	Select appropriate barrier/personal protective equipment (PPE)	
III.A.1	Recognize the implications for failure to comply with Centers for Disease Control (CDC) regulations in healthcare settings	
X.P.3	Document patient care accurately in the medical record	

▶ Introduction

In many healthcare settings, the medical assistant is responsible for collecting blood specimens from patients and sometimes performing waived testing. In this chapter, you will be introduced to venipuncture and capillary collection procedures, and you will learn the appropriate supplies and equipment needed to perform these procedures. You also will learn techniques for dealing with different types of patients and how to obtain blood specimens efficiently and effectively. Additionally, you will receive instruction on performing common blood tests.

▶ The Role of the Medical Assistant LO 48.1

The examination of blood can provide extensive information about a patient's condition. You may be asked to collect and process blood specimens for examination in your work as a medical assistant. A basic understanding of the anatomy and physiology of the circulatory system will help you properly perform these tasks. You also will need a working knowledge of the functions of blood and the kinds of cells that make up blood tissue. (See the chapters *The Cardiovascular System* and *The Blood* for more information.)

You will use several techniques to obtain blood specimens. **Phlebotomy** is the withdrawal of blood from a vein. This is done using a procedure called **venipuncture;** the puncture of a vein with a needle for the purpose of drawing blood. Phlebotomists receive special training in phlebotomy; drawing blood is the main task in their work. Smaller blood specimens may be obtained by using a small, disposable instrument to pierce the surface of the skin and collect blood from the capillaries there. This is known as **capillary puncture.** It is sometimes referred to as *dermal puncture* because the puncture is made through the dermis of the skin. You must be able to perform such procedures correctly so that the specimen is appropriate for the ordered tests and the results are accurate. You also must be skilled in putting the patient at ease during this procedure. Your reassuring manner, ability to handle technical problems, and careful preparation for answering many kinds of questions will be important to your success in this area.

In addition to your many duties as a medical assistant, you should understand how to process certain blood specimens and conduct various blood tests, particularly if you work in a laboratory. You also must be able to complete the necessary paperwork to ensure that test results are handled efficiently and accurately. All of these skills may be required, regardless of whether you collect blood specimens in a physician's office laboratory (POL), hospital, a patient's home, or a laboratory drawing station.

▶ Preparation for Collecting Blood Specimens
LO 48.2

Following the steps in the standard process for drawing blood specimens will enable you to perform the procedure smoothly, accurately, and safely while ensuring properly completed documentation.

Reading and Interpreting the Test Order

The first steps in preparing to draw blood for testing are to review the written testing request and to assemble the equipment and supplies. The patient should arrive with a laboratory **requisition** form and/or the patient's EHR will reflect the licensed practitioner's order for the laboratory tests.

Your first step is to review this blood-collection order to determine what tests will be run. See Figure 48-1. Many tests require expedited or special handling to ensure accurate results.

Your office will have specific collection procedures for each type of test. If you will be sending the blood specimen to a reference laboratory for testing, make sure you know its requirements. The cost of reprocessing a test far surpasses the extra time needed to be sure of the process requirements.

When reviewing the test order, you will need to know the meaning of certain abbreviations in order to understand the requisition and to collect the correct amount of blood using the correct technique. See Table 48-1. If you are ever in doubt and the resources in your facility do not provide the answers, you should ask your supervisor or supervising practitioner.

Equipment for Drawing Blood

Specific blood-drawing equipment and collection devices vary with the type of test. Make sure you have the appropriate equipment to collect all necessary specimens if more than one test is ordered. All specimen-collection tubes, slides, and other containers should be labeled immediately after collection with the patient's name, the date and time of collection, the initials of the person collecting the specimen, and other information as required by the test procedure or your office (see Figure 48-2a). Some offices use an identification code for each patient.

Alcohol wipes, sterile gauze, and adhesive bandages are standard supplies for procedures during which blood is drawn from a vein or capillaries. However, alcohol can cause inaccurate results for certain tests, so for these tests, povidone-iodine or benzalkonium chloride may be used to clean the puncture site. You will need a disposable **tourniquet** (a flat, broad length of vinyl or rubber) for venipuncture (see Figure 48-2b).

All blood collection requires the use of a needle or other sharps device. Needles are discussed in more detail in the chapter *Infection Control Practices*. Recall also from that chapter that you must follow safe injection practices and use safety-engineered devices. In addition, personal protective equipment (PPE) must be used. See the *Caution: Handle with Care* feature Phlebotomy and Personal Protective Equipment.

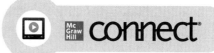

Go to CONNECT to see a video exercise about *Quality Control Procedures for Blood Specimen Collection.*

Venipuncture requires puncturing a vein with a needle and collecting blood into either a tube or, in some cases, a syringe. Capillary puncture requires a superficial puncture of the skin with a sharp point. Capillary puncture releases a smaller amount of blood.

Various instruments are used to perform venipuncture and capillary puncture. See Figure 48-3. Be familiar with and practice using the devices so that your technique is smooth, steady, and competent.

Evacuated Systems Evacuated systems—the most common is the Vacutainer® system (manufactured by Becton Dickinson)—use a double-pointed needle, a plastic needle holder/adapter, and collection tubes (Figure 48-4). The collection tubes are sealed to create a slight vacuum and are called evacuated tubes. You insert the covered inner point of the needle into one end of the holder/adapter and the first collection tube into the other end.

An evacuated system has several advantages over other methods of blood collection. It is easy to collect several specimens from one venipuncture site using the interchangeable collection tubes, which are calibrated by vacuum to collect the exact amount of blood required. Some collection tubes are prepared with additives, such as anticoagulants, that are needed to correctly process the blood specimen for testing. Finally, because there is no need to transfer blood from a collection syringe to a specimen tube, the potential for exposure to contaminated blood is reduced.

Butterfly Systems You may use a **butterfly system,** or winged infusion set, when you work with patients who have small or fragile veins. Flexible wings attached to the needle simplify needle insertion. A length of flexible tubing (either 5 or 12 inches, approximately) connects the needle to the collection device. The inserted needle remains completely undisturbed while the collection device is manipulated. Because it is motionless, the needle causes less trauma to the vein and surrounding tissue than other venipuncture systems. A butterfly system also generally uses a smaller needle (23-gauge) than other venipuncture techniques and can be used with an evacuated collection tube or a syringe (Figure 48-5).

Laboratory Requisition

BWW
BWW Medical Associates, PC
305 Main Street, Port Snead YZ 12345-9876
Tel: 555-654-3210, Fax: 555-987-6543
Web: BWWAssociates.com

Laboratory Name and Address

Requesting Provider
Paul F. Buckwalter, MD
Alexis N. Whalen, MD
Elizabeth H. Williams, MD

Please Indicate Bill Type Below
Attach Copy of Insurance Card

Patient Data (Please Print)

Last Name	First Name	Maiden Name
Gonzales	Sylvia	

Address		Apt No.
84 Denham Blvd, Bldg. 2		21C

City	State	Zip
Sneadsville	VZ	12345-9876

SS#	Phone #
101-01-0000	123-555-8901

Date of Birth (Month, Day, Year)	Male	Date Collected	Time Collected	a.m.
09 01 19XX	X Female		:	p.m.

Physician 1	Physician 2
Alexis N. Whalen, MD	

Billing Information (Please Print Clearly)

Please Bill to: ☐ Dr. Account (Client) ☒ Patient Self Pay ☐ Insurance Co

Responsible Party (Last, First)	Relationship to Subscriber	☒ Self ☐ Child ☐ Spouse ☐ Other
Gonzales, Sylvia		

Primary Insurance Co. Name ☐ HMO ☐ PPO

Insurance Policy #	Insurance Group #

Primary Insurance Co: Address (Street, City, State, Zip)

Insured Date of Birth	Insured SS#

PLEASE PROVIDE MANDATORY ICD 10 CODE BELOW

1 E11.9	2	3	4	5

CALL TEST RESULTS TO:

Test: CBC, Lytes FBS
To: Alexis N. Whalen, MD
Phone: (555) 654-3210

FAX RESULTS TO:

To:
Fax: (   )

☐ Veni   Tech Code   Tubes Received

Please (X) desired Panel(s)/Profile(s)/Tests. See back of requisition for profile components.

PANELS/PROFILES	
Hepatitis Panel, Acute	2S
Basic Metabolic Panel	MT
Comp Metabolic Panel	MT
X Electrolyte Panel (Lytes)	MT
Hepatic Function Panel	MT
General Health Panel	MTL
Lipid Panel	MT
Obstetric Panel AMH	P2SL
Renal Panel	MT

MICROBIOLOGY	
Source of Specimen:	
Culture, Anaerobe	
Chlamydia/GC Amp Probe	
Culture, Ear	
Culture, Eye	
Leukocytes Stool	
Culture, Fungal	
Culture, Genital	
Culture, Herpes	
Occult Blood Screen	
Ova & Parasites	
Rapid Strep Throat	
Culture, Stool	
Culture, GROUP A BetaStrep Screen	
Culture GROUP B Screen	
Culture, Throat	
Culture, Urine	
Culture, Wound / Abscess	
Culture, Viral	
C. Difficile Toxin A&B AMH	

INDIVIDUAL TESTS	
ABO Group/RH	P
Acid Phosphatase, Prostatic	S
Albumin	MT
Alkaline Phosphatase	MT
Amylase	MT
Antinuclear Antibodies (ANA Send)	S
HCG, Beta Quant	MT
Bilirubin T / D Neonate	A
Bilirubin T / D Adult	MT
BNP Screen	L
BUN	MT
CA-125	S
CA-125 to Dianon	S
CRP	MT
CRP Cardio	MT
Calcium	MT
Carbamazepine/Tegretol	R
X **CBC & PLT w/o Diff**	L
CBC & PLT w Diff	L
Carcino Embryonic Antigen (CEA)	S
Cholesterol Total	MT
Cortisol Level	MT
Creatine Kinase, Total (CK)	MT
CPK total w CKMB	MT
Creatinine Clearance	U
Creatinine	MT
D Dimer Quant	B
DNA AB Double Strand	S
Digoxin Level	R

INDIVIDUAL TESTS (cont.)	
Drug Screen Urine	U
Drug Screen Urine c Confirm	U
Estradiol Level	MT
Ferritin Level	MT
Fetal Fibronectin (FFN)	SWAB
Folic Acid (PROTECT)	MT
Follicle Stimulating Hormone	MT
GGT (Gamma Glut Trans)	MT
Glucose	MT
X **Glucose Fasting**	MT
Glucose Challenge 1° Preg	
Glycosylated Hemoglobin (HA1C)	L
Hepatitis B Surface AG	S
Hepatitis B Surface AB	S
Hepatitis C Antibody	S
Herpes Simplex 1 & 2 IgG AB	S
Herpes Simplex 1 & 2 IgM AB	S
HIV I & II Abs	S
Homocysteine	L
Iron/TIBC	MT
Lactate Dehydrogenase (LDH)	MT
Lipase	MT
Lithium	R
Luteinizing Hormone	MT
Microalumin Random/24 Hr.	U
Magnesium	MT
MONO test heterophile	S
Phenobarbital	R
Phenytoin/Dilantin	R
Phosphorous	MT
Potassium	MT
Progesterone	S
Prolactin	MT
PSA Free and Total	S
PSA Screen (Medicare)	S
PSA Diagnostic	S
Prothrombin Time	B
aPTT	B
PTH Intact	S
Reticulocyte Count	L
Rheumatoid Factor (RF)	MT
RPR QUAL	S
Rubella, IgG	S
ESR (Sed Rate)	L
SGOT (AST)	MT

INDIVIDUAL TESTS (cont.)	
SGPT (ALT)	MT
Testosterone	S
Testosterone Free & Total	S
TSH	MT
Total T3	MT
T3 Uptake	S
Free T3	MT
Free Thyroxine (FT4)	MT
Total T4	S
Free Thyroxine index (FTI)	S
Thyroid Antibodies	S
Troponin/Quant	MT
Triglycerides	MT
Uric Acid	MT
Urinalysis	U
Valproic Acid / Depakote	R
Vitamin B12 (PROTECT)	MT
Vitamin D 25 Hydroxy	S

ADDITIONAL ORDERS

FIGURE 48-1a   Include all patient, specimen, and billing information on a laboratory requisition form (written laboratory requisition form for Sylvia Gonzales).

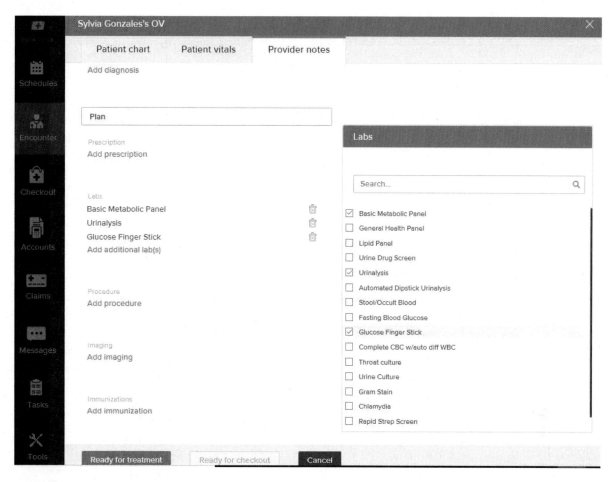

FIGURE 48-1b The laboratory requisition and/or the EHR order must be reviewed before any specimen is collected (EHRclinic laboratory order for Sylvia Gonzales).

©McGraw-Hill Education

TABLE 48-1	Abbreviations Routinely Used in Blood Tests		
Abbreviation	**Meaning**	**Abbreviation**	**Meaning**
Ab	Antibody	BT	Bleeding time
ABO	Classification system for four blood groups	BUN	Blood urea nitrogen
AcAc	Acetoacetate	Ca; Ca^{++}	Calcium
ACE	Angiotensin-converting enzyme	CA	Cancer antigen
ACT	Activated coagulation time	CBC	Complete blood (cell) count
ACTH	Adrenocorticotropic hormone	CEA	Carcinoembryonic antigen
ADH	Antidiuretic hormone	CHS	Cholinesterase test
AFB	Acid-fast bacillus	CMV	Cytomegalovirus
AFP	Alpha-fetoprotein	CO	Carbon monoxide
Ag	Antigen	CO$_2$	Carbon dioxide
AG	Anion gap	COHb	Carboxyhemoglobin
A/G R	Albumin-globulin ratio	CPK	Creatine phosphokinase
ALB	Albumin	CRCL	Creatinine clearance
ALP; alk phos	Alkaline phosphatase	Cre	Creatinine
ALT	Alanine aminotransferase	DHEA-SO4	Dehydroepiandrosterone sulfate
ANA	Antinuclear antibody	Dif, Diff	Differential (blood cell count)
APAP	Acetaminophen	EBNA-IgG	Epstein-Barr virus nuclear antigen
APTT	Activated partial thromboplastin time	EBV	Epstein-Barr virus
ASA	Acetylsalicylic acid (aspirin)	EDTA	Ethylenediaminetetraacetic acid

(Continued)

TABLE 48-1   Abbreviations Routinely Used in Blood Tests

Abbreviation	Meaning	Abbreviation	Meaning
AST	Aspartate aminotransferase	ELP	Electrophoresis, protein
AT-III	Antithrombin III	Eos	Eosinophil
B	Blood (whole blood)	Eq	Equivalent
Baso	Basophil	ESR	Erythrocyte sedimentation rate
BCA; BRCA	Breast cancer antigen	ETOH	Alcohol
BJP	Bence Jones protein	FBS	Fasting blood sugar
Free T_4	Free thyroxine	MPV	Mean platelet volume
FSH	Follicle-stimulating hormone (follitropin)	msAFP	Maternal serum alpha-fetoprotein
FTI	Free thyroxine index	NE	Norepinephrine
GFR	Glomerular filtration rate	OGTT	Oral glucose tolerance test
GH	Growth hormone	P	Plasma
GHRH	Growth hormone-releasing hormone	PBG	Porphobilinogen
GnRH	Gonadotropin-releasing hormone	PCT	Prothrombin consumption time
GTT	Glucose tolerance test	PCV	Packed cell volume (hematocrit)
HA	Hemagglutination	Pi	Inorganic phosphate
HA1C, HgbA1c	Glycosylated hemoglobin	PKU	Phenylketonuria
HAI	Hemagglutination inhibition test	PLT	Platelet
HAV	Hepatitis A virus	PMN	Polymorphonuclear (leukocyte; neutrophil)
Hb; Hgb	Hemoglobin	PRL	Prolactin
HbCO	Carboxyhemoglobin	PSA	Prostate-specific antigen
HBV	Hepatitis B virus	PT	Prothrombin time
HCG; hCG	Human chorionic gonadotropin	PTH	Parathyroid hormone
Hct	Hematocrit	PTT	Partial thromboplastin time
HCV	Hepatitis C virus	PZP	Pregnancy zone protein
HDL	High-density lipoprotein	RAIU	Thyroid uptake of radioactive iodine
HDV	Hepatitis delta virus	RBC	Red blood cell; red blood (cell) count
HGH; hGH	Human growth hormone	RBP	Retinol-binding protein
HIV	Human immunodeficiency virus	RDW	Red cell distribution of width
HLA	Human leukocyte antigen	Retic	Reticulocyte
HPV	Human papillomavirus	RF	Rheumatoid factor; relative fluorescence unit
HSV	Herpes simplex virus	Rh	Rhesus factor
HTLV	Human T-cell lymphotrophic virus	RIA	Radioimmunoassay
Ig	Immunoglobulin	rT_3 or $REVT_3$	Reverse triiodothyronine
IgE	Immunoglobulin E	S	Serum
INH	Inhibitor	Segs	Segmented polymorphonuclear leukocyte
IV	Intravenous	SPE	Serum protein electrophoresis
L	Liver	T_3	Triiodothyronine
LD; LDH	Lactate dehydrogenase	T_4	Thyroxine
LDL	Low-density lipoprotein	TBG	Thyroxine-binding globulin
LH	Luteinizing hormone	TBV	Total blood volume
LMWH	Low-molecular-weight heparin	TG	Triglyceride
Lytes	Electrolytes	TRH	Thyrotropin-releasing hormone
MCH	Mean corpuscular hemoglobin	TSH	Thyroid-stimulating hormone
MCHC	Mean corpuscular hemoglobin concentration	VDRL	Venereal Disease Research Laboratory (test for syphilis)
MCV	Mean corpuscular volume	VLDL	Very low-density lipoprotein
MHb	Methemoglobin	WB	Western blot
MONO	Monocyte	WBC	White blood cell; white blood (cell) count

Source: http://labtestsonline.org/.

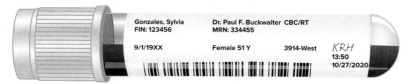

(a) Specimen collection tubes must be labeled with all required information immediately after collection.

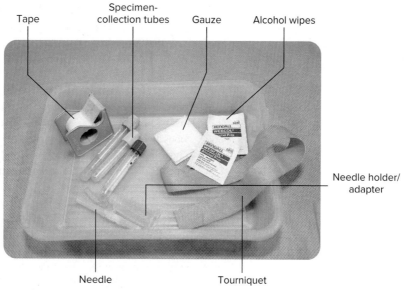

(b) Common blood collection equipment.

FIGURE 48-2 A variety of equipment is needed to perform routine blood collection.

©McGraw-Hill Education/Sandra Mesrine, Photographer

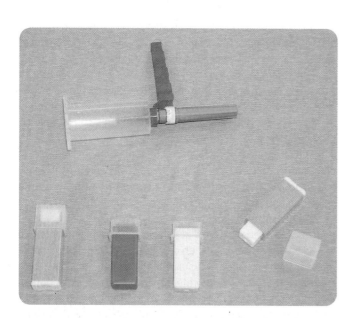

FIGURE 48-3 Venipuncture and capillary puncture safety devices.

©Leesa Whicker

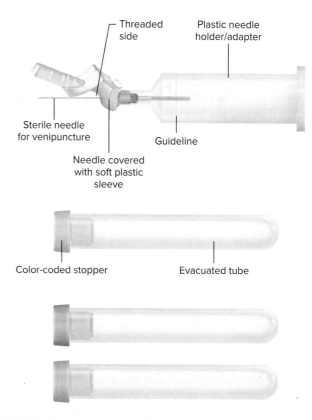

FIGURE 48-4 The Vacutainer® system uses interchangeable collection tubes that allow you to draw several blood specimens from the same venipuncture site.

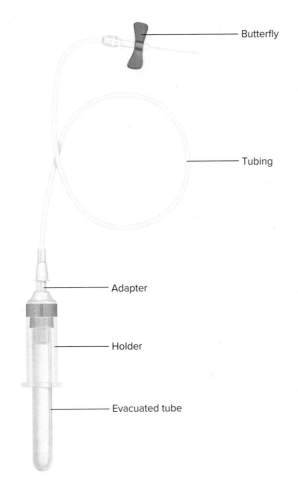

Butterfly

Tubing

Adapter

Holder

Evacuated tube

FIGURE 48-5 Once inserted, the needle of a butterfly system remains undisturbed during specimen collection.

Needle and Syringe Systems When a patient has small or fragile veins, the vacuum created when the collection tube is pressed over the needle point can cause the veins to collapse. Although it is the least desirable method of collection, in rare cases you may need to collect blood using a sterile needle and syringe assembly when an evacuated system is not suitable. You can use a smaller needle—no smaller than 23-gauge to avoid hemolyzing the blood—and control the vacuum in the syringe by pulling the plunger back slowly. Other aspects of the procedure are essentially the same, except that the blood specimen is collected in the syringe and must immediately be transferred to a collection tube using a transfer device.

Collection Tubes No matter which method is used to collect blood, the specimens must immediately be mixed by gentle inversion with the appropriate additives in the correct collection tubes before they are transported to the laboratory for testing. The tube stoppers are different colors, each color identifying the type of additives (if any) a collection tube contains (Figure 48-6).

These additives must be compatible with the laboratory process the specimen will undergo. Each laboratory may choose which tubes to use for a particular test.

Additives include anticoagulants, such as **ethylenediaminetetraacetic acid (EDTA),** and other materials that help preserve or process a specimen for particular types of testing. When you collect a blood specimen, double-check that you are using the appropriate collection tubes for the tests ordered. You also must fill the tubes in a specific order to preserve the integrity of each blood specimen. The order of draw prevents carryover of tube additives from one tube to the next. Each laboratory requires a specific order of draw for collection

CAUTION: HANDLE WITH CARE

Phlebotomy and Personal Protective Equipment

The Centers for Disease Control and Prevention (CDC) has classified all phlebotomy procedures as a risk for exposure to contaminated blood or blood products. You must use appropriate personal protective equipment (PPE) during all phlebotomy procedures. Remember, it is up to you to protect yourself and the patient.

Gloves
Gloves—which protect against spills and splashing of contaminated blood—are the first line of defense during a phlebotomy procedure. Wash your hands and don clean exam gloves that fit snugly before you work with each patient. Remove the gloves, dispose of them in a biohazardous waste container, and wash your hands after working with each patient.

Garments
Garments such as laboratory coats and aprons can protect your clothing from spills and splashes and provide a measure of protection from contaminated materials. Some garments are designed to resist penetration by blood or blood products. You may find it necessary to wear such garments when drawing blood or performing blood tests.

Masks and Protective Eyewear
Mucous membranes are especially vulnerable to invasion by infectious agents. Use masks and protective eyewear to help safeguard mucous membranes in your mouth, nose, and eyes from infection.

Masks help protect your mouth and nose from splashes or sprays of blood or blood products. You cannot predict when exposure to blood may occur. Accidental puncture of an artery during a phlebotomy procedure could result in a spray of blood, or blood may spray or splash accidentally during testing protocols. Most medical assistants do not routinely wear masks for phlebotomy procedures once they have achieved proficiency in performing them. Goggles also can protect your eyes from splashing and spraying during blood drawing or testing.

Clear plastic face shields combine the protection of masks and goggles and often are used during major surgical procedures. You may use a face shield if you do extensive testing on blood specimens, but face shields are not usually worn when drawing blood.

PPE works two ways: It protects you from a patient's contaminated blood, and it protects the patient from infectious agents you may be carrying. By using PPE correctly, you will make your workplace a safer place for you and the patients.

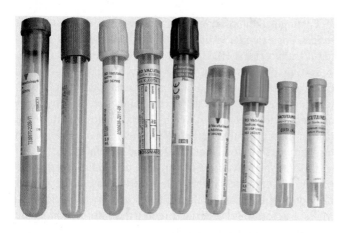

FIGURE 48-6 Special color-coded stoppers on collection tubes indicate which additives are present and, therefore, which types of laboratory tests may be performed on each blood specimen.
©Lillian Mundt

tubes. The Clinical and Laboratory Standards Institute (CLSI) also publishes its recommended order of draw. Table 48-2 identifies collection tube stopper colors, additives present in the tubes, and types of tests, in a typical order of draw.

Capillary Puncture Blood from a capillary puncture may be collected in small, calibrated glass tubes; collected on glass microscope slides; or applied directly to reagent strips (or dipsticks), which are specially treated paper or plastic strips used in specific diagnostic tests. Blood also may be collected on special cards or paper and sent to an outside laboratory for special screening tests such as PKU. PKU and other newborn screen testing is discussed in the *Assisting in Pediatrics* chapter.

Lancets Lancets are used in the capillary puncture technique. This technique is employed when the amount of blood required for a specific procedure is not very large or when technical difficulties prevent the use of the venipuncture technique. A **lancet** is a small, disposable instrument with a sharp point used to puncture the skin and make a shallow incision (between 2.0 and 3.0 mm deep for an adult and no deeper than 2.4 mm for an infant). The blood welling up from the incision is then collected.

Automatic Puncturing Devices **Automatic puncturing devices** are loaded with a lancet. Because the depth to which they puncture the skin is mechanically controlled, they are more accurate and comfortable than the traditional lancet method. These spring-loaded devices have disposable platforms that rest on the finger. Different platforms are used, depending on the desired depth of the puncture. Both the lancet and the platform should be discarded after use. Pen-like devices also can hold a lancet inside. They are held against the skin and activated by pushing a button. The advantages of these devices are that they are easy to use, the puncture depth can be adjusted easily, and there is an automatic ejection button for lancet disposal. Some companies also manufacture completely disposable devices, which come individually wrapped and are used only once.

Micropipettes A pipette is a calibrated glass tube for measuring fluids. A **micropipette** is a small pipette that holds a small, precise volume of fluid. You will use micropipettes to collect capillary blood for some tests. Capillary tubes, with a single calibration mark, also are used to collect capillary blood for certain tests.

TABLE 48-2	Blood-Collection Tubes		
Stopper Color		**Additive**	**Test Types and Treatment**
Yellow	○	Two types: 1. SPS (Sodium polyanethol sulfonate) 2. ACD (Acid citrate dextrose)	SPS - Blood cultures, invert tube to prevent clotting ACD - blood bank studies, DNA, and paternity testing
Light blue	●	Sodium citrate	Coagulation studies Fill tube completely and invert tube immediately after filling to activate anticoagulant.
Red	●	Clot activator	Blood chemistries, HIV/AIDS antibody, viral studies, and serologic tests
Gold or red/gray	○ ○	Clot activator Silicone serum separator	Tests requiring blood serum, routine blood donor screening, and infectious disease testing
Green	●	Sodium Heparin OR Lithium Heparin	Electrolyte studies (Lithium heparin only) and arterial blood gases Invert tube immediately after filling to prevent coagulation.
Lavender	○	Ethylenediaminetetraacetic acid (EDTA) (anticoagulant)	Hematology and blood chemistry Invert tube immediately after filling to prevent coagulation.
Gray	○	Potassium oxalate (anticoagulant) or sodium fluoride (preservative)	Blood glucose Invert tube immediately after filling to prevent coagulation.
Royal blue**	●	Two types: 1. EDTA (anticoagulant) 2. none	Trace element analysis Determine tube based upon metals being tested.

Note: Tubes are listed in the order they should be collected (order of draw). **Royal blue tubes are generally recommended by the manufacturers to be drawn first or through a separate draw, to avoid contamination.

Microtainer® Tubes Microtainer® tubes (manufactured by Becton Dickinson Vacutainer® Systems) are small plastic tubes with a wide-mouthed collector, similar to a funnel, that allows blood to flow quickly and freely into the tube. Like collection tubes in an evacuated system, Microtainer® tubes have different colored tops indicating the additives, if any, they contain.

Reagent Products Several common tests do not require processing of blood specimens. For these tests, you may apply droplets of freshly collected blood to chemically treated paper or plastic reagent strips (dipsticks) or add freshly collected blood droplets to small containers holding chemicals that react in the presence of specific substances or microorganisms. Some of the blood tests performed in this way detect blood glucose levels, sickle cell anemia, infectious mononucleosis, and rheumatoid arthritis.

Smear Slides You may need to apply a drop of freshly collected blood to a prepared microscope slide for some tests. More commonly, a smear slide is prepared in the laboratory from a blood specimen containing an anticoagulant for examination under a microscope.

▶ Patient Preparation and Communication
LO 48.3

After you review the test order and assemble the necessary equipment and supplies, take a moment to relax, gather your thoughts, and consider the patient and your purpose. You need to greet the patient and explain the procedure, as well as ensure patient compliance. In addition, the patient may be anxious about the blood test, and some patients have special needs or present special problems that make drawing blood challenging. Being aware of possible sources of patient anxiety and understanding a wide range of special concerns can help you respond to patient needs with sensitivity and competence.

Greeting and Identifying Patients
Greet patients pleasantly, introduce yourself, and explain that you will be drawing some blood. It is essential to identify patients correctly before you begin the procedure. Ask patients to state their full name and be sure you hear both the first and last names correctly. Verify that the name the patient gives is the name on the order by asking the patient to spell the name. In most facilities, the phlebotomist should ask for a date of birth and verify the patient ID or chart number against the order to further identify the patient as mandated by The Joint Commission (TJC).

Confirming Pretest Preparation
The presence and level of certain substances in blood are affected by food and fluid intake or by other daily life activities. Some tests require the patient to follow certain pretest restrictions to minimize the influence of the restricted food on the blood or to stress the body to see how it responds, as indicated by the blood.

Fasting is the most common requirement for pretest preparation. For example, a lipid profile, which measures cholesterol, triglycerides, HDL, LDL, and VLDL, requires fasting. A fasting blood sugar (FBS) requires fasting, as do other types of glucose testing. For example, the glucose tolerance test measures a patient's ability to metabolize carbohydrates and is used to detect hypoglycemia and diabetes mellitus. The patient must eat a high-carbohydrate diet for 3 days before the test and fast for 8 to 12 hours before the appointment.

Before you draw blood for any test, determine whether the patient has complied with pretest instructions. If the patient has not complied, explain that the test cannot be performed. Make a note on the order and report the information to the licensed practitioner or your supervisor.

Explaining the Procedure and Safety Precautions
Explain to the patient the procedure you will use to obtain the blood specimen for testing. Be clear and brief when you describe what you will do; too much detail leaves some patients queasy. Explain the need for each of the preventive measures, such as the use of PPE, in language the patient can understand. Assure the patient that these measures protect against exposure to infection.

Establishing a Chain of Custody
You will need to follow specific guidelines to establish a chain of custody for blood specimens drawn for drug and alcohol analysis. Because donating a specimen for drug and alcohol testing is potentially self-incriminating, the patient must sign a consent form for the testing. The *Collecting, Processing, and Testing Urine and Stool Specimens* chapter explains general chain-of-custody procedures.

Patient Fears and Concerns
Some patients express their fears or concerns directly. Other patients ask questions that highlight their fears. Providing more information or a complete understanding is reassuring to many patients. For others, the information serves only to confuse, overwhelm, or create more fear. You must decide how much information to give each patient and be prepared to answer questions.

Patients sometimes ask questions that are not appropriate for you to answer. A patient may ask you about his prognosis, medical condition, blood type, or other medical information. It is not appropriate for you to discuss these topics with the patient. Encourage the patient to discuss these issues with the licensed practitioner. Some commonly expressed fears and concerns to which you should respond, however, are covered in the following paragraphs.

Pain The question medical assistants performing phlebotomy probably hear most often is "Will this hurt?" Never lie to a patient who asks this question. Inform the patient that he will feel a stick just as the lancet or point of the needle is inserted but that this pain goes away almost immediately. Tell a patient who seems particularly nervous to take a deep breath and let it out slowly. Also suggest that the patient focus on something else in the room or close his eyes and relax during the procedure.

A patient may express concern and report a previous unpleasant experience with blood testing. Listen to the patient's concerns. Describe what you will do to reduce discomfort and what the patient can do to be more at ease. Let the patient know you will help him sit comfortably or lie down while the blood specimen is being obtained. Tell the patient to let you know if he begins to feel light-headed. You also might ask the patient whether one arm is better to use than the other. Many patients have had blood drawn before and can tell you which sites were successful. Consulting the patient helps the patient feel more in control and provides you with important information.

Scars Some patients may express fear of getting a bruise or scar from a blood collection procedure. Explain that some bruising is possible but that it will fade within a few days. Most bruising is caused by a hematoma, which occurs when blood leaks out of the vein and collects under the skin. Hematomas can be prevented by releasing the tourniquet before withdrawing the needle and applying proper pressure over the puncture site after the needle has been withdrawn. Bruising is common with fair-skinned patients. Scars, on the other hand, are unlikely.

Serious Diagnosis Patient fears are not always rational. One fear patients express is that the more tubes of blood you require, the more serious their condition must be. Patients also may fear that a blood test is being done to help the practitioner diagnose an extremely serious disease.

You can help relieve a patient's fears by explaining that a blood test is one of the best ways to obtain an overall picture of health (emphasize health, not disease). Note that blood tests show what is normal about the blood as well as any abnormalities. You also might explain that several specimens are being taken because the blood used in blood tests is processed in different ways; the blood collected for one test cannot be used in another.

Blood testing also may be done to determine how well and at what levels medications are acting in the blood. Explain that the practitioner may want to see how much medication is in the blood to better manage the prescribed dosage. When a patient needs repeated tests for drug levels, explain that the tests show how the body is using the medication.

Contracting a Disease from the Procedure Probably the greatest fear of patients undergoing blood tests is contracting HIV/AIDS or hepatitis B virus (HBV). Although many people are now well informed about how HIV/AIDS and other serious diseases are contracted, it is understandable for a patient to worry about bloodborne pathogens. Do not dismiss the patient's concerns, and do not downplay the importance of following standard precautions.

Explain the precautions you will take to prevent the spread of infection. Allow the patient to see you wash your hands and put on new gloves before you begin to take the blood specimen. Stress that the needle is sterile. Explain that you have not touched the needle and that it will be discarded when you finish. Let the patient see you put the needle in the sharps container.

Use this opportunity to educate the patient about the transmission of HIV/AIDS. Emphasize that HIV/AIDS and other infections transmitted by blood can be transmitted only when there is direct contact with contaminated blood or other body fluids. Explain that your gloves protect both you and the patient by providing a barrier to infection transmission from one person to another. Explain that your other protective equipment, such as goggles or a mask, also helps prevent the spread of infection.

Special Considerations

As you collect blood specimens, you will encounter a variety of patients, some of whom have special needs. You will find yourself in many different situations, some of them problematic. Some of these situations are fairly common, and you must be prepared to deal with them.

Patients at Risk for Uncontrolled Bleeding Patients who have hemophilia or are taking blood-thinning medications are at risk for uncontrolled bleeding at the collection site. (Hemophilia is a disorder in which the blood does not coagulate at a wound or puncture site.) Be especially careful and alert as you follow the standard procedures for collecting a blood specimen. In addition, hold pressure with several gauze squares over the puncture site for at least 5 minutes to make sure bleeding has stopped completely. If uncontrollable bleeding does occur, call the licensed practitioner immediately.

Difficult Patients You may encounter a particular challenge in working with a patient either because of technical problems or because of personality issues. Being prepared for these situations is the best method for coping with them.

The Difficult Venipuncture There will be times when you simply cannot get a good blood specimen. If your first attempt at drawing blood fails, try again at another site. Give the patient (and yourself) a short break and make an attempt on the other arm, for instance. Sometimes the veins in one arm are easier to work with than the veins in the other arm. Some facilities may have available an instrument, such as a **venoscope,** to visualize the vein. The battery-operated venoscope uses light-emitting diode (LED) lights to illuminate the subcutaneous tissue and highlight the veins, making the veins easier to locate. If you cannot get a good specimen on the second try, stop. Ask for assistance from your supervisor or the licensed practitioner.

Fainting Patients It is impossible to predict which patients will have a reaction to a blood-drawing procedure. Generally, however, an ill patient is more likely to experience a reaction than a well patient. The best way to deal with this potential problem is to position every patient so that, if fainting does occur, no injury will result. Have patients sit in a

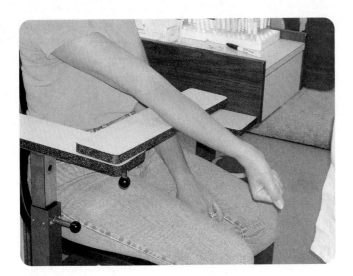

FIGURE 48-7 Venipuncture chairs are designed to make blood drawing easier and to prevent patients from falling if they should faint.
©Leesa Whicker

special venipuncture chair (Figure 48-7), designed to help prevent patients from sliding to the floor in the event of fainting. If your office is not equipped with a venipuncture chair, have patients lie down on an examining table. A patient who has a history of fainting or feels ill should lie down with feet elevated or knees drawn up while you complete the procedure. Sometimes just talking with the patient, asking her simple questions, will help keep her from fainting.

If a patient does faint and the needle is still in the vein, release the tourniquet and withdraw the needle quickly and steadily. Apply pressure to the site. Most people revive promptly and no other action is required. Do not leave the patient alone. Notify the licensed practitioner that the patient has fainted and ask the practitioner whether you should continue with the procedure.

If there is a more severe reaction, notify the appropriate staff member and remain with the patient. If the patient is in a chair and begins to slide out, raise the safety arm and gently lower the patient to the floor. Protect the patient's head at all times, and make sure the patient is breathing. The licensed practitioner should examine the patient before the patient is moved. Follow the practitioner's instructions.

When the patient begins to recover, assist the patient into a sitting position and then to a chair or couch. The patient should rest until feeling strong enough to walk—usually about 15 minutes. When the patient feels steady, take the patient to another area of the office, such as the patient reception area. At this point, another staff member usually becomes responsible for the patient's care and determines when it is safe for the patient to leave.

Angry or Violent Patients Some patients are extremely resistant to having blood drawn. Although their objections may seem illogical, remember, people often do not think as clearly in moments of high emotion as they normally do.

Encourage a patient who is mildly upset and wants to argue about the need for the blood test to let you take the specimen and then discuss the situation with the licensed practitioner. If you convince the patient to submit to the test, complete the procedure quickly and accurately. Avoid arguing with the patient.

Do not force the issue with a patient who becomes violent or refuses outright to submit to the procedure. A patient does have the right to refuse testing or treatment. Under no circumstances should you attempt to physically force a patient to give a blood specimen. Never endanger yourself, other patients, or your colleagues by refusing to back down from an angry or violent patient. Report the problem to the appropriate staff, make a note on the order, and follow other established procedures as determined by your facility.

▶ Performing Blood Collection   LO 48.4

Venipuncture

Some states permit medical assistants to obtain blood specimens. Your health care facility will clarify which phlebotomy-related duties, if any, you may perform. If your duties include collecting blood specimens, you will obtain them through either venipuncture or capillary puncture. You must understand when these techniques are used and know how to perform them. Procedure 48-1, at the end of this chapter, details quality control procedures for collecting blood specimens.

The most common sites for venipuncture are the median cubital and cephalic veins of the forearm. Other sites may be used if a primary site is unavailable. Figure 48-8 shows the veins in the antecubital fossa (the small depression inside the bend of the elbow) and the forearm.

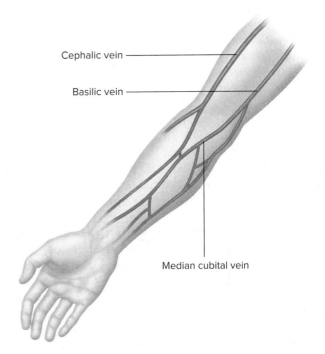

FIGURE 48-8 Shown here are the veins commonly used for venipuncture. In recommended order they include the median cubital vein, the cephalic vein, and the basilic vein.

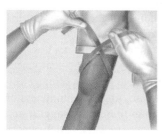
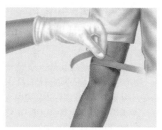
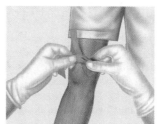
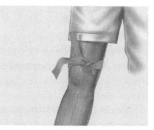

(a) Position the tourniquet under the arm while grasping the ends above the arm and venipuncture area. The tourniquet should be 3 to 4 inches above the site.

(b) Cross the left end over the right end and apply a small amount of tension to the tourniquet.

(c) Using the right middle finger or index finger, tuck the left end under the right end.

(d) A loose end of the tourniquet will be pointing toward the shoulder and the loop will be pointed toward the hand.

FIGURE 48-9 Follow these steps for proper tourniquet application.

In order to locate the correct site and perform the venipuncture, you will need to apply a tourniquet. The tourniquet is applied to the arm 3 to 4 inches above the venipuncture site. Follow the steps shown in Figure 48-9 for proper application of the tourniquet. Procedure 48-2, at the end of this chapter, provides step-by-step instructions for performing the venipuncture using an evacuated system.

Capillary Puncture

Capillary puncture requires a superficial puncture of the skin with either a lancet or an automatic puncture device. Capillary puncture in adults and children is usually performed on the great (middle) finger or the ring finger. Use the patient's nondominant hand for this procedure if possible. The puncture should be made slightly off-center on the pad of the fingertip because the pad's center is usually more sensitive. Capillary puncture in infants is usually performed on one of the outer edges of the underside of the heel (Figure 48-10). Procedure 48-3, at the end of this chapter, explains how to perform a capillary puncture and collect a sample of capillary blood.

Blood Cultures

Blood culture specimens are collected to test for the presence of bacteria in the blood. When collecting blood for a culture, it is important that no skin organisms contaminate the specimen. Skin organisms such as staphylococci and streptococci can cause a false-positive blood culture test result. For this reason, proper aseptic technique is essential. Pay special attention to keeping the collection bottle, syringe, and needle sterile and properly cleansing the skin. If you are drawing additional specimens for other tests, always draw the blood culture first. This eliminates the possibility of contaminating the culture with additives from other tubes. When collecting a blood culture specimen, you should follow these steps:

1. Select an appropriate site for venipuncture.
2. Cleanse the skin with isopropyl alcohol.
3. Cleanse the skin again with an iodine or chlorhexidine solution applied in an outward, circular pattern (cleansing from inside to outside).
4. Allow the iodine solution to air-dry.

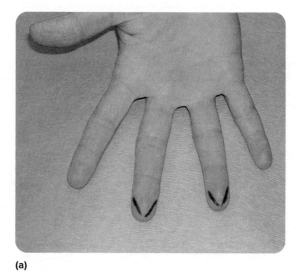
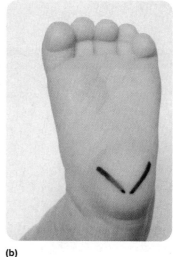

(a)   (b)

FIGURE 48-10 Capillary puncture sites for (a) an adult and (b) an infant.
©Leesa Whicker

5. Remove the plastic top from the collection bottle and wipe with a sterile alcohol pad.

6. Allow the alcohol to air-dry.

7. Draw the blood from the selected site.

8. Properly label the specimens.

Separate blood specimens are put into two collection bottles, one for aerobic and one for anaerobic culture. Practitioners often order two sets of blood cultures from two different sites, such as from both of the patient's arms. Use the same technique for each specimen, and make sure all specimens are properly identified, including the site from which each specimen was taken.

Venipuncture Complications

Venipuncture is, in general, a safe procedure. Most of the complications you encounter are mild and simply a nuisance. Serious complications are rare. You must be aware of complications, ways to avoid them, and understand how to deal with them if they occur.

- **Hematoma.** A collection of blood will sometimes form under the skin. This is especially a problem in patients who have bleeding disorders, are elderly, or are taking anticoagulants. In some cases, you may need to use a butterfly collection device. If a hematoma forms during collection, remove the needle and apply immediate pressure. To avoid hematomas, hold the needle as still as possible while filling and changing the tubes and remove the tourniquet and the tube from the holder before removing the needle. Before bandaging make sure the site is sealed. If a hematoma does form apply extra gauze to the puncture site and wrap with stretch bandage. Watch the patient and alert the licensed practitioner if necessary.

- *Accidental arterial puncture.* If an artery is accidentally punctured the site will rapidly form a hematoma or the tube will fill too rapidly. When this occurs remove the needle and apply direct forceful pressure for at least 5 minutes and until active bleeding stops. The licensed practitioner should be notified when this occurs.

- *Nerve injury.* Know the anatomy of the antecubital fossa because accidentally inserting a needle into a nerve can cause nerve damage. Permanent sensory and/or motor damage to the arm and hand can occur if the venipuncture is done incorrectly. If the patient has shooting, electrical pain, severe or unusual pain, tingling, numbness or a a new onset tremor in the limb these may suggest nerve damage. If you suspect you have stuck the patient's nerve, withdraw the needle immediately and alert the licensed practitioner.

- **Hemolysis.** When hemolysis occurs a blood specimen cannot be used and the specimen must be collected again. To avoid hemolysis you should *avoid* mixing the specimen too vigorously; shaking the specimen during transport; leaving the tourniquet on for more than a minute; collecting the specimen from an IV start; and collecting the specimen using a 25-gauge needle.

- *Infections.* Though quite rare, infections after venipuncture do occur and can be very serious. Use only approved single-use venipuncture equipment. Cleanse the venipuncture site well before the procedure. An infection at the venipuncture site may not be evident for several days after the procedure. If the patient calls, complaining of redness, heat, or drainage at the site, have her return to the office to see the licensed practitioner. A more serious blood infection (sepsis) may at first seem like the patient has the flu, as fever and chills are the first symptoms. A patient with a blood infection can go into shock if left untreated. If you suspect that the patient has a blood infection, have her see the licensed practitioner immediately.

▶ Performing Common Blood Tests LO 48.5

Many blood tests are routinely ordered as part of a complete general exam to determine a patient's overall health. The results of individual tests can provide information that aids in the diagnosis of specific conditions, diseases, and disorders, as noted in Table 48-3.

TABLE 48-3 Common Blood Tests and the Conditions They Help Identify

Substance Identified or Quantified	Stopper Color and Additive	Part of Blood Tested	Indication, Disease, or Disorder
Alanine aminotransferase (ALT)	Clot activator Silicone serum separator	Serum	Liver disorders
Alpha-fetoprotein (AFP)	Clot activator Silicone serum separator	Fetal serum	Fetal liver and gastrointestinal tract status, and hepatitis

(Continued)

TABLE 48-3 Common Blood Tests and the Conditions They Help Identify

Substance Identified or Quantified	Stopper Color and Additive		Part of Blood Tested	Indication, Disease, or Disorder
Amylase		Clot activator Silicone serum separator	Serum	Drug toxicity and parotid or pancreas disorders
Angiotensin-converting enzyme (ACE)		Clot activator Silicone serum separator	Serum	Lung cancer, sarcoidosis, and acute or chronic bronchitis
Antidiuretic hormone (ADH)		EDTA	Plasma	Syndrome of inappropriate ADH, Guillain-Barré syndrome, and brain tumor
Aspartate aminotransferase (AST)		Clot activator Silicone serum separator	Serum	Liver disease (including viral hepatitis), infectious mononucleosis, and damaged heart or skeletal muscle
Bilirubin		Clot activator Silicone serum separator	Serum	Liver disease, fructose intolerance, and hypothyroidism
Blood urea nitrogen (BUN)		Clot activator Silicone serum separator	Serum	Kidney disorders
Calcium, total (fasting)		Clot activator Silicone serum separator	Serum	Hyperparathyroidism and malignant disease with bone involvement
Cancer antigens (numbers 125, 15-3, 549, 72-4), tumor-associated glycoprotein (TAG)		Clot activator Silicone serum separator	Serum	Specific cancers identified, depending on antigen tested
Carbon dioxide, total		Clot activator Silicone serum separator	Venous serum	Acidosis or alkalosis (acid-base balance)
Cholesterol, total		Clot activator Silicone serum separator	Serum	Hyperlipoproteinemia, coronary artery disease, and atherosclerosis
Creatine kinase (CK)		Clot activator Silicone serum separator	Serum	Muscular dystrophies, Reye's syndrome, heart disease, shock, and some neoplasms

(Continued)

TABLE 48-3 Common Blood Tests and the Conditions They Help Identify

Substance Identified or Quantified	Stopper Color and Additive	Part of Blood Tested	Indication, Disease, or Disorder
Erythrocyte count (RBC)	EDTA	Whole blood	Anemia
Erythrocyte sedimentation rate (ESR)	EDTA	Whole blood	Inflammation, infectious diseases, malignant neoplasms, and sickle cell anemia
Glucose (fasting)	Potassium oxalate or sodium fluoride	Whole blood	Pancreatic function and ability of intravenous insulin to offset diet in diabetes mellitus
Glucose (fasting—tolerance test)	Potassium oxalate or sodium fluoride	Serum	Diabetes mellitus and hypoglycemia
Lactate dehydrogenase (LD)	Clot activator Silicone serum separator	Serum	Anemia, viral hepatitis, shock, hypoxia, and hyperthermia
Leukocyte count (WBC)	EDTA	Whole blood	Leukemia, infection, and leukocytosis
Phenylalanine	Heparin or newborn screening card	Plasma	Hyperphenylalaninemia, obesity, and phenylketonuria
Potassium (K^+) and sodium (Na^+)	Clot activator Silicone serum separator	Serum	Fluid-electrolyte balance
Prostate-specific antigen (PSA)	Clot activator Silicone serum separator	Serum	Prostate cancer and BPH
Sickle cells	EDTA	Whole blood	Sickle cell anemia
Thyroid-stimulating hormone (TSH), triiodothyronine (T_3), thyroxine (T_4)	Clot activator Silicone serum separator	Serum	Thyroid function
Trace elements (lead, cadmium, mercury, arsenic, molybdenum, chromium, manganese, nickel, silver, zinc, copper, selenium, aluminium)	EDTA or none	Whole blood	Deficiency or excess amounts
Uric acid	Clot activator Silicone serum separator	Serum	Gout and leukemia

Note: Different laboratories may have different testing protocols and may require other tube tops than those represented in this table. Consult your laboratory procedures manual for additional information regarding required collection tubes.

The number of blood tests routinely performed in POLs has declined since the implementation of Clinical Laboratory Improvement Amendments of 1988 (CLIA '88) regulations. Many POLs now perform only waived tests. Each POL is different, however, and regulations do change. Check with your employer about what tests your office performs regularly. You should be familiar with a wide range of tests and the steps involved with each, even if you do not anticipate performing them.

Because some testing can occur in the POL, you may encounter several chemical substances while performing your responsibilities in the laboratory. These chemicals include

- **Anticoagulants,** which cause the blood to remain in a liquid, uncoagulated state.
- **Serum separators,** which form a gel-like barrier between serum and the clot in a coagulated blood specimen.
- Stains, which color specific types of cells, making microscopic studies easier to complete.

Anticoagulants or serum separators are already present in blood-collection tubes and do not need to be added to the specimen.

You must be absolutely clear about which chemicals are used for which tests and the precise amounts involved. It is also important to understand the purpose of blood tests so that you can educate patients. You must know, in addition, the range of normal test values so that you can be aware of potential problems and note them for the licensed practitioner's attention. Table 48-4 shows the normal ranges for a variety of blood tests.

Hematologic Tests

Hematologic tests—including blood cell counts, morphologic studies, coagulation tests, and the nonautomated erythrocyte sedimentation rate test—are commonly performed in routine blood testing. These tests can be performed on venous or capillary whole blood specimens.

TABLE 48-4 Normal Ranges for Blood Tests*				
Blood Test	**Stopper Color and Additive****		**Blood Component Tested**	**Normal Range***
Blood Counts				
Red blood cells (erythrocytes)		EDTA	Whole blood	
Men			Whole blood	$4.7–6.1 \times 10^6$ cells/mcL
Women				$4.2–5.4 \times 10^6$ cells/mcL
White blood cells (leukocytes)		EDTA	Whole blood	$4.5–11.0 \times 10^3$ cells/mcL
Platelets			Whole blood	$150–400 \times 10^3$ cells/mcL
Differential				
Neutrophils			Whole blood	40%–60%
Eosinophils			Whole blood	1%–4%
Basophils			Whole blood	0.5%–1%
Lymphocytes			Whole blood	20%–40%
Monocytes			Whole blood	2%–8%
Hematocrit (Hct)		EDTA	Whole blood	
Men				40.7%–50.3%
Women				36.1–44.3%
Hemoglobin (Hb, Hgb)		EDTA	Whole blood	
Men				13.8–17.2 g/dL
Women				12.1–15.1 g/dL
Erythrocyte Sedimentation Rate (ESR)				
Wintrobe		EDTA	Whole blood	
Men				0–5 mm/hour
Women				0–15 mm/hour
Westergren		EDTA	Whole blood	
Men				0–15 mm/hour
Women				0–20 mm/hour
Coagulation Tests				
Prothrombin time (PT)		Sodium citrate	Plasma	11–15 seconds
Bleeding time		Sodium citrate	Whole blood	2–7 minutes
INR (International Normalized Ratio)		Sodium citrate	Plasma	< 1.1 is normal 2.0 to 3.0 is therapeutic for patients on blood thinners

(Continued)

TABLE 48-4 Normal Ranges for Blood Tests*

Blood Test	Stopper Color and Additive**	Blood Component Tested	Normal Range***
Electrolytes			
Bicarbonate (HCO$_3$$^-$)	Clot activator	Arterial plasma	21–28 mEq/L
	Silicone serum	Venous plasma	27–29 mEq/L
Calcium (Ca^{++})	separator	Serum	8.6–10.0 mEq/L
Chloride (Cl$^-$)	Heparin	Serum, plasma	98–108 mEq/L
Potassium (K$^+$)		Serum	3.5–5.1 mEq/L
Sodium (Na$^+$)		Serum	136–145 mEq/L
Chemical and Serologic Tests			
Alanine aminotransferase (ALT)	Clot activator	Serum	
Men	Silicone		10–40 U/L
Women	serum		7–35 U/L
	separator		
Alpha-fetoprotein (AFP)	Clot activator	Serum	
Fetal, first trimester	Silicone		20–400 mg/dL
Adult	serum		<15 ng/mL
	separator		
Aspartate aminotransferase (AST, formerly SGOT)	Clot activator	Serum	
	Silicone		
Men	serum		11–26 U/L
Women	separator		10–20 U/L
Bilirubin, total direct	Clot activator	Serum	0.3–1.2 mg/dL
	Silicone		
	serum		
	separator		
Blood urea nitrogen (BUN)	Clot activator	Serum, plasma	6–20 mg/dL
	Silicone		
	serum		
	separator		
Carcinoembryonic antigen (CEA)	Clot activator	Serum	<5.0 ng/mL
	Silicone		
	serum		
	separator		
Cholesterol, total	Clot activator	Serum, plasma	Desirable: Less than 200 mg/dL (5.18 mmol/L) Borderline high: 200–239 mg/dL (5.18 to 6.18 mmol/L)High: 240 mg/dL (6.22 mmol/L) or higher
	Silicone		
	serum		
	separator		
High-density lipoproteins (HDLs)	Clot activator	Serum, plasma	Low level, increased risk: Less than 40 mg/dL (1.0 mmol/L) for men and less than 50 mg/dL (1.3 mmol/L) for women Average level, average risk: 40-50 mg/dL (1.0–1.3 mmol/L) for men and between 50–59 mg/dl (1.3–1.5 mmol/L) for women High level, less than average risk: 60 mg/dL (1.55 mmol/L) or higher for both men and women
	Silicone		
	serum		
	separator		

(Continued)

TABLE 48-4   Normal Ranges for Blood Tests*

Blood Test	Stopper Color and Additive**	Blood Component Tested	Normal Range***
Low-density lipoproteins (LDLs) Men Women	Clot activator Silicone serum separator	Serum, plasma	Optimal: Less than 100 mg/dL (2.59 mmol/L); for those with known disease (ASCVD or diabetes), less than 70 mg/dL (1.81 mmol/L) is optimal Near/above optimal: 100–129 mg/dL (2.59–3.34 mmol/L)Borderline high: 130–159 mg/dL (3.37–4.12 mmol/L) High: 160–189 mg/dL (4.15–4.90 mmol/L) Very high: Greater than 190 mg/dL (4.90 mmol/L)
Non-HDL cholesterol	Clot activator Silicone serum separator	Serum, plasma	Optimal: Less than 130 mg/dL (3.37 mmol/L) Near/above optimal: 130–159 mg/dL (3.37–4.12mmol/L) Borderline high: 160–189 mg/dL (4.15–4.90 mmol/L) High: 190–219 mg/dL (4.9–5.7 mmol/L) Very high: Greater than 220 mg/dL (5.7 mmol/L)
Fasting Triglycerides	Clot activator Silicone serum separator	Serum, plasma	Desirable: Less than 150 mg/dL (1.70 mmol/L) Borderline high: 150–199 mg/dL(1.7–2.2 mmol/L) High: 200–499 mg/dL (2.3–5.6 mmol/L) Very high: Greater than 500 mg/dL (5.6 mmol/L)
Creatine kinase (CK) Men Women	EDTA	Serum, plasma	 38–174 U/L 26–140 U/L
Creatinine Men Women	Clot activator Silicone serum separator	Serum, plasma	 0.9–1.3 mg/dL 0.6–1.2 mg/dL
Cytomegalovirus (CMV)	Clot activator Silicone serum separator	Serum	Negative
Epstein-Barr virus (EBV)	Clot activator Silicone serum separator	Whole blood	Negative
Fibrinogen	Sodium citrate	Plasma	200–400 mg/dL
Glucose (fasting blood sugar, FBS)	Potassium oxalate or sodium fluoride	Serum	74–120 mg/dL
Group A beta-hemolytic streptococci	Clot activator Silicone serum separator	Serum	Negative

(Continued)

TABLE 48-4 Normal Ranges for Blood Tests*

Blood Test	Stopper Color and Additive**	Blood Component Tested	Normal Range***
Human immunodeficiency virus (HIV) antibodies	EDTA	Serum, plasma	Negative
Insulin	Clot activator Silicone serum separator	Serum	<17 micro U/mL
Iron, total	Clot activator Silicone serum separator	Serum	
Men			65–175 micrograms/dL
Women			50–170 micrograms/dL
Lactate dehydrogenase (LD)	Clot activator Silicone serum separator	Serum, plasma	140–280 U/L
pH	Clot activator Silicone serum separator	Arterial blood	7.35–7.45
		Venous blood	7.32–7.43
Proteins	Clot activator Silicone serum separator	Serum	
Total			6.2–8.0 g/dL
Albumin			3.4–4.8 g/dL
Uric acid	Clot activator Silicone serum separator	Serum	
Men			4.4–7.6 mg/dL
Women			2.3–6.6 mg/dL

*Laboratory test results vary. Check the laboratory results at the facility where you are employed

**Different laboratories may have different testing protocols and may require other tube tops than those represented in this table. Consult your laboratory procedures manual for additional information regarding required collection tubes.

***Reference ranges for normal values may be slightly different in different labs. Consult the reference ranges provided by your individual lab for each test.

Blood Counts **Whole blood** contains **formed elements** (RBCs, WBCs, and platelets) and a fluid portion (plasma). The total number of blood cells and the percentage of the whole specimen each type represents can tell the licensed practitioner a great deal about a patient's condition. A practitioner can order an individual test or a **complete blood (cell) count (CBC),** which includes the following tests:

- Red blood (cell) count—the total number of RBCs in a specimen and the red cell morphology.
- White blood (cell) count—the total number of WBCs in a specimen.
- Differential WBC count—the percentage of each type of WBC (basophils, eosinophils, neutrophils, lymphocytes, and monocytes) in the first 100 leukocytes of a specimen.
- Platelet count (automated)—the number of platelets in a specimen, or a platelet estimate, which indicates whether the number of platelets is adequate.
- Hematocrit determination—identifies how much of a specimen's volume (expressed as a percentage) is made up of RBCs after the specimen has spun in a centrifuge.
- Hemoglobin determination—measures the amount of hemoglobin by weight per volume in the specimen.

Most POLs use automated equipment to perform blood cell counts. Automated equipment performs a differential by counting and classifying all of the WBCs in the sample. You may need to understand how to perform blood counts manually. All manual counts are estimates. The types of blood cell counts differ in specimen preparation and in the equipment and methods used. Check your state regulations and office policy to find out if you are allowed to perform differential blood cell counts.

Differential Cell Counts A medical assistant may be trained to prepare a blood smear slide and stain the smear for a manual differential cell count. Procedure 48-4, at the end of this chapter, details preparation of a blood smear slide. When you carry out this process correctly, there will be a region of the slide where blood cells are dense but lie in a single plane (not stacked or bunched together). This is the region where the cells are counted.

A polychromatic (multicolored) stain like Wright's stain simplifies a differential cell count. The blue and red-orange dyes (methylene blue and eosin, respectively) stain cell structures in ways that identify each of the five WBC types. Table 48-5 identifies the staining characteristics of each WBC type.

TABLE 48-5   Characteristics of Stained White Blood Cells

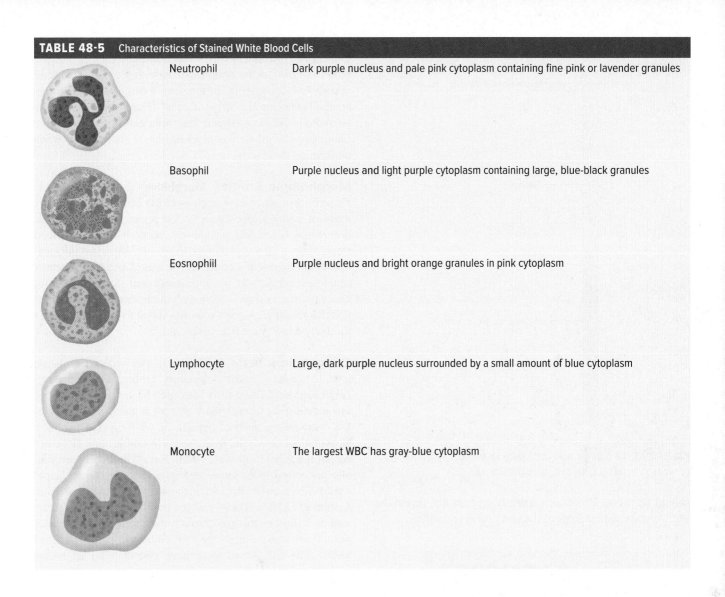

	Neutrophil	Dark purple nucleus and pale pink cytoplasm containing fine pink or lavender granules
	Basophil	Purple nucleus and light purple cytoplasm containing large, blue-black granules
	Eosnophiil	Purple nucleus and bright orange granules in pink cytoplasm
	Lymphocyte	Large, dark purple nucleus surrounded by a small amount of blue cytoplasm
	Monocyte	The largest WBC has gray-blue cytoplasm

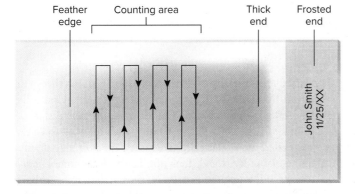

FIGURE 48-11   Follow this pattern when counting leukocytes visible in the field under the oil-immersion objective of the microscope.

There are several types of blood staining kits. Follow the manufacturer's instructions when performing this procedure.

Figure 48-11 shows the zigzag pattern for counting leukocytes visible in the field when using the microscope's oil-immersion objective. A total of 100 leukocytes are counted and recorded on a differential counter. Each cell type is expressed as a percentage of the 100 leukocytes counted.

This process is repeated in 10 to 15 fields and the results are averaged.

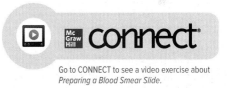

Go to CONNECT to see a video exercise about *Preparing a Blood Smear Slide*.

Hematocrit You measure a patient's hematocrit percentage by collecting a small specimen of the patient's blood in a microhematocrit tube, sealing the tube, and spinning it in a centrifuge. This process is described in Procedure 48-5 at the end of this chapter. During this process, heavier RBCs move to one end of the tube and lighter plasma moves to the other end. Between the RBCs, or **packed red blood cells,** and the plasma is the buffy coat (Figure 48-12). The **buffy coat** contains the WBCs and platelets.

Always process two specimens of the patient's blood. After removing the specimens from the centrifuge, compare the column of packed RBCs in each specimen with a standard hematocrit gauge. Read on the gauge the percentage of total blood volume represented by the RBCs. The specimens

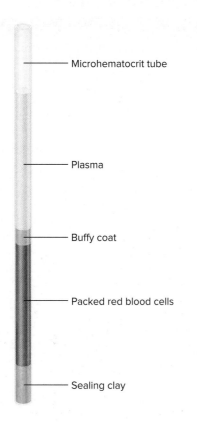

Microhematocrit tube

Plasma

Buffy coat

Packed red blood cells

Sealing clay

FIGURE 48-12   Blood in a centrifuged capillary tube separates into packed red blood cells, the buffy coat, and plasma.

should be within 2% of each other. If they are not, repeat the test. Average the readings of the two patient specimens.

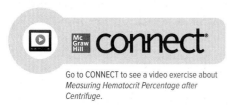

Go to CONNECT to see a video exercise about *Measuring Hematocrit Percentage after Centrifuge.*

Automated Hematocrit Readers You also may use a handheld device to obtain hematocrit readings. Devices such as the UltraCrit® are CLIA-waived testing devices for rapid and accurate measurement of hematocrit. The test may be completed on venous or capillary blood, and results are obtained in less than 1 minute. These devices often are used by blood banks to rapidly screen donors for eligibility to donate.

Hemoglobin RBCs contain hemoglobin. You will determine the concentration of hemoglobin in the blood by lysing (rupturing) the RBCs (hemolysis) and evaluating the color of the specimen. This procedure may be done with a hemoglobinometer—a handheld device that makes color evaluation. Blood specimens mixed with a reagent, such as Drabkin's reagent, undergo a color reaction that can be quantified by reading color intensity in a photoelectric colorimeter (an instrument that uses light to read color).

Several automated hemoglobin analyzers are now included on the CLIA '88 waived list. These analyzers measure the amount of hemoglobin in a whole blood sample using a photometer (an instrument used to measure absorbed light). The blood sample can be obtained from either a finger stick or venous blood. Examples of automated hemoglobin analyzers are the HemoCue HB 301 Analyzer® (HemoCue AB) and the HemoPoint H2 Hemoglobin Measurement System® (Stanbio Laboratory). Follow the manufacturer's instructions when performing these tests.

Morphologic Studies   **Morphology** is the study of the shape or form of objects, such as blood cells. A morphologic study of a blood specimen is often performed just after the differential count and platelet estimate on the same blood smear slide. Cell morphology can provide important information about a patient's condition. It examines a blood smear specimen and records the appearance and shape of cells for abnormal size, shape, or content and abnormal cell organization. Morphologic studies require special training and are not routinely done by medical assistants.

Coagulation Tests   A physician may order coagulation tests to identify potential bleeding problems before surgical procedures. These tests also may be ordered to monitor therapeutic drug levels when a patient is receiving anticoagulant medications such as heparin or warfarin (Coumadin®). Coagulation studies include the prothrombin time (PT) and partial thromboplastin time (PTT) tests. These tests are usually performed using automated devices such as the Coaguchek XS System™ (Roche Diagnostics) or the Alere INRatio System™ (Alere). These systems monitor the changing pattern of light transmission through the specimen as coagulation occurs and calculate the INR (International Normalized Ratio). The INR—used to evaluate patients who are taking blood thinners such as warfarin—measures the amount of time it takes for the test specimen to clot and compares it to a reference average. The World Health Organization (WHO) developed the INR method so that specimens from different labs can be compared. Medical assistants sometimes perform these studies.

Erythrocyte Sedimentation Rate   The **erythrocyte sedimentation rate (ESR)** is the rate at which red blood cells (RBCs) settle in whole blood. The test measures the distance, in millimeters, the cells fall in 1 hour when allowed to settle in a calibrated tube. The ESR screens for the presence of any inflammatory process and does not diagnose any one condition. When inflammation is present, plasma proteins, such as albumin and globulin, are increased. An increase in these substances causes red blood cells to come closer together, which may result in the red blood cells sticking together. Several cells sticking together settle faster than a single RBC does. This results in an elevated sedimentation rate. See Figure 48-13 and these general guidelines:

- Use only a fresh sample of blood.
- Draw the blood into a tube with anticoagulant additives.
- Temperature, either too hot or too cold, will affect the test. Maintain laboratory temperatures near 70°F.

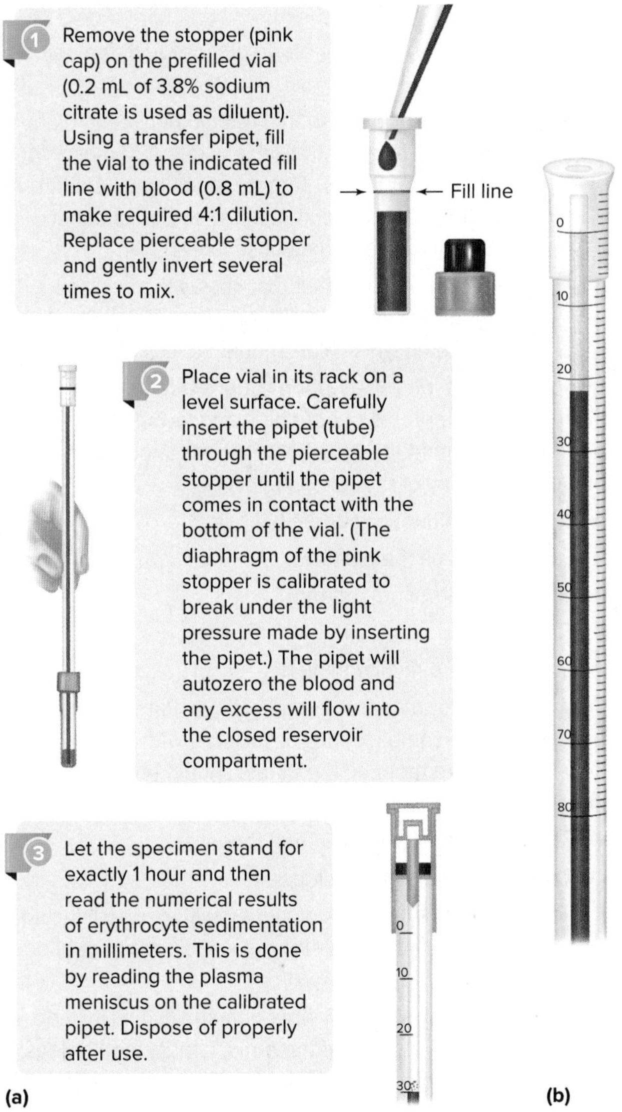

① Remove the stopper (pink cap) on the prefilled vial (0.2 mL of 3.8% sodium citrate is used as diluent). Using a transfer pipet, fill the vial to the indicated fill line with blood (0.8 mL) to make required 4:1 dilution. Replace pierceable stopper and gently invert several times to mix.

← Fill line

② Place vial in its rack on a level surface. Carefully insert the pipet (tube) through the pierceable stopper until the pipet comes in contact with the bottom of the vial. (The diaphragm of the pink stopper is calibrated to break under the light pressure made by inserting the pipet.) The pipet will autozero the blood and any excess will flow into the closed reservoir compartment.

③ Let the specimen stand for exactly 1 hour and then read the numerical results of erythrocyte sedimentation in millimeters. This is done by reading the plasma meniscus on the calibrated pipet. Dispose of properly after use.

(a)

(b)

FIGURE 48-13 Erythrocyte sedimentation rate. (a) An example of one manufacturer's method for Westergren erythrocyte sedimentation rate (Sediplast ESR system). (b) An example of an erythrocyte sedimentation after 1 hour. The reading in this example is 22 millimeters.

- Precisely position the specimen tubes vertically in the rack. They must not be leaning.
- Avoid vibrating or bumping the rack during the test.
- Avoid introducing bubbles into the specimen when transferring blood into the tube.
- Carefully watch the time and read the results at exactly 1 hour.

Chemical Tests

Blood chemistry analysis examines several dozen chemicals found in human blood. Tables 48-3 and 48-4 include many of these chemical tests. Highly detailed studies are rarely performed in the POL because they require expensive, sophisticated equipment and techniques. Complex testing also is subject to strict CLIA '88 regulations that increase the administrative work and the need for more highly trained personnel. So these types of tests are commonly performed at an independent reference laboratory. Automated equipment for analyzing blood chemistry is becoming more available, less expensive, and simpler to operate than it was in the past. Waived tests for an increasing array of chemicals in the blood are developed each year, making it more likely that you may use automated equipment to perform some blood chemistry tests. Keeping abreast of new developments will help prepare you for possible changes in your laboratory duties.

Blood Glucose Monitoring One of the blood chemistry tests routinely conducted in the POL is blood glucose monitoring, which often is performed by a medical assistant or by a patient. Glucose monitoring systems require sterile lancets to perform a capillary puncture. You will collect the blood on reagent strips that change color in accordance with glucose levels present in the blood. The level is determined either by comparing the color on the strip with color standards provided with the reagent strips or by feeding the strip into a handheld reading device. You will teach patients to perform this kind of test at home.

EDUCATING THE PATIENT

Managing Diabetes

Diabetes affects an estimated 9% of the US population, with more than 1 million newly diagnosed cases each year. In order to reduce the complications associated with diabetes, patients need to maintain stable blood sugar. Proper patient education and medical care will help patients achieve this goal. As a medical assistant, you can assist patients and their families by providing them with the following information about diabetes:

1. The risks and consequences associated with uncontrolled blood sugar. Patients whose blood sugar is unstable are at greater risk of developing the following conditions:
   - Loss of vision
   - Kidney failure

- Heart disease
- Nerve damage
- Stroke

2. The patient's type of diabetes. Patients need to know the type of diabetes they have so that they can understand the type of treatment prescribed. The types of diabetes are:
   - Type 1 diabetes—an autoimmune disorder characterized by the body's inability to make enough insulin. Insulin is required for glucose utilization. Patients with Type 1 diabetes need to take insulin daily.
   - Type 2 diabetes—the most common type of diabetes. Insulin is still being produced at normal levels but

can no longer be utilized by the body's cells. This causes a buildup of unused glucose in the blood. This type of diabetes is often controlled with careful diet management and increased exercise. A number of oral medications also can be used.

- Gestational diabetes—develops only during pregnancy. This type of diabetes is generally managed through proper diet and exercise. Careful monitoring is important to reduce the risk of fetal complications. Women who have had gestational diabetes have an increased risk of developing Type 2 diabetes.

3. Maintaining proper diet and exercise, including:
- Making proper food choices.
- Keeping a food diary.
- Reading food labels.
- Choosing proper food exchanges.
- Creating and implementing a routine exercise program.

4. Routine self-monitoring of blood sugar and hemoglobin A1C levels. Information should include:
- The types of blood glucose monitors available. Figure 48-14 illustrates one type—a glucometer.
- Instructions on obtaining monitoring supplies.
- The number of times and the specific intervals at which blood sugar should be checked, based on individual needs and the physician's recommendations.
- Instructions on performing blood glucose testing.
- Guidelines on how to maintain a chart of blood glucose levels, including the time of day, associated meals and activities, and actual blood sugar values.
- Hemoglobin A1C monitoring. The patient should understand what hemoglobin A1C is and why it is important to monitor these values.

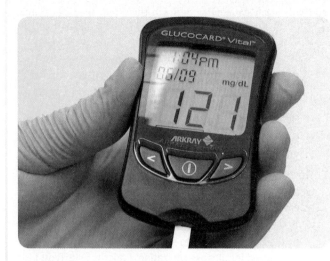

FIGURE 48-14 A handheld glucometer is an important tool in helping patients manage diabetes.
©McGraw-Hill Education

- Normal (target) values for blood glucose and hemoglobin A1C:
  - Blood glucose levels should remain between 70 and 130 mg/dL before meals and less than 180 mg/dL for 1 to 2 hours after meals. Target ranges may be different for each patient. Consult the licensed practitioner about individual blood glucose levels.
  - Hemoglobin A1C is a test that shows the average amount of glucose in the blood over a 3-month period. Ideally, this value should be less than 7%.

5. Symptoms of uncontrolled blood sugar. Patients need to be aware of the symptoms of both high and low blood sugar—both require immediate attention. Patients should test their blood sugar if any of the following occur:
- Nausea, vomiting, or abdominal pain.
- Feeling tired all the time.
- Excessive thirst or dry mouth.
- Flushed skin.
- Confusion or difficulty thinking.

6. Self-screening for diabetes complications. Patients should be aware of the complications associated with diabetes and how to recognize them, and patients should be instructed to do the following:
- Perform a daily foot inspection for sores.
- Recognize changes in vision.
- Recognize the symptoms of kidney failure, which include nausea, vomiting, yellow skin, and swelling of the hands and feet.
- Recognize early signs of nerve damage, which include numbness and tingling of the arms, hands, feet, or legs; dizziness; double vision; and drooping of the eyelid or lip.

7. Additional sources of information. Encourage patients to continue their education about diabetes. Providing patients with additional information encourages them to take an active role in controlling their diabetes. The following are additional information sources:

- American Association of Diabetes Educators 1-800-338-DMED; https://www.diabeteseducator.org/
- American Diabetes Association 1-800-DIABETES; www.diabetes.org
- American Dietetic Association 1-800-366-1665; www.eatright.org
- Centers for Disease Control and Prevention Diabetes Public Health Resource 1-800-CDC-INFO (232-4636); https://www.cdc.gov/diabetes/home/index.html
- Juvenile Diabetes Research Foundation International 1-800-223-1138; https://www.jdrf.org/
- National Institute of Diabetes and Digestive and Kidney Diseases: National Diabetes Information Clearinghouse 1-800-860-8747; https://www.niddk.nih.gov/

Be sure to stress the importance of following the manufacturer's guidelines for correct operation. Procedure 48-6, at the end of this chapter, outlines the general steps for measuring blood glucose using a handheld glucometer.

You also will teach patients and their families how to manage diabetes. This will include performing the blood glucose test, managing diet and exercise, and self-monitoring for complications associated with diabetes. You also may provide additional resources for further education. See the *Educating the Patient* feature Managing Diabetes.

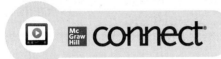

Go to CONNECT to see a video exercise about *Measuring Blood Glucose Using a Handheld Glucometer.*

Hemoglobin A1C Another test used to monitor the health of diabetic patients is the hemoglobin A1C test. This test measures the amount of glycosylated hemoglobin (hemoglobin with glycosal groups attached) in the blood. When blood glucose levels are elevated, the glucose molecules bind with hemoglobin to form hemoglobin A1C (HgbA1c). Once HgbA1c is formed, it remains for the RBC's life (90 to 120 days). For this reason, the test results provide an idea of the average blood sugar for 2 to 3 months.

Large fluctuations in blood sugar are problematic in patients with diabetes and can cause complications such as eye disease, stroke, renal failure, and cardiovascular disease. The HgbA1c test gives the physician a good overall picture of the patient's compliance with and the effectiveness of diabetes treatment.

Several options for performing this test include:

- Sending it to an outside reference laboratory. Results are available in 1 to 7 days.

- Performing it in the office laboratory if the necessary equipment is available. Results are usually available in less than 10 minutes.

- Taking the test at home. Several home tests are available, allowing patients to monitor their own HgbA1c levels and, therefore, the efficiency of their diabetes treatment.

Testing of HgbA1c should always be done in conjunction with routine blood glucose monitoring. Daily monitoring of blood glucose helps the patient with insulin therapy and diet maintenance. HgbA1c monitoring is important in assessing the patient's overall glucose levels. The advantages of this testing include:

- No pretesting preparation. The test may be done without regard to meals.

- Better overall assessment of long-term blood glucose control. Blood glucose testing gives information about glucose levels at one point in time. HgbA1c gives information over a period of 2 to 3 months.

Patients should have their HgbA1c levels checked two to four times per year. The target range for HgbA1c levels is less than 7%. Patients whose HgbA1c levels exceed 8% are at a greater risk for diabetes-associated complications.

Cholesterol Tests Blood cholesterol tests are performed on a routine basis in the POL. Several automated devices can be used for metabolic chemistry testing both in the POL and at home. These analyzers test a variety of blood chemicals, including glucose, total cholesterol, HDL cholesterol, and triglycerides. The sample required is minimal and can be obtained with a capillary puncture.

FDA-approved waived tests include the following:

- Polymer Technology Systems CardioChek™ Analyzer (Polymer Technology Systems, Inc.)
- SpotChem™ HDL, Total Cholesterol, and Triglyceride (Arkray, Inc.)
- Piccolo® Lipid Panel Plus Reagent Disc (Abaxis, Inc.)

Serologic Tests

Serologic tests detect the presence of specific substances in a blood specimen. The terms *serologic test* and *immunoassay* refer to the introduction of an antigen or antibody into the specimen and the detection of a specific reaction to the antigen or antibody. Serologic testing methods can be used to detect disease antibodies, drugs, hormones, and vitamins in the blood and to determine blood types. They also are used to test urine and other body fluids.

Immunoassays Although medical assistants usually do not perform immunoassays, you should be familiar with several immunoassay methods that have common applications. These methods include:

- Western blot, in which antigens are blotted onto special filter paper for examination. Western blot tests are generally used to confirm HIV infection diagnosis.

- Radioimmunoassay (RIA), in which radioisotopes are used to "tag" antibodies. RIA tests are extremely sensitive and are generally performed in a reference laboratory.

- Enzyme-linked immunosorbent assay (ELISA), in which enzyme-labeled antigens and substances that can absorb antigens generate reactions to specific antibodies. These reactions are identified through visual or photoelectric color detection. HIV infection is diagnosed using an ELISA test.

- Immunofluorescent antibody (IFA) test, in which dye, visible when the specimen is examined under a fluorescent microscope, colors specific antibodies.

Rapid Screening Tests Several serologic tests have been developed for quick processing. Some, such as early pregnancy tests performed on urine, are available for home use. There are also rapid screening tests for detecting antibodies to certain infections:

- Infectious mononucleosis
  - LifeSign Status Mono (Princeton Boimeditech Corp.)
  - BioStar Acceava Mono II (Acon Laboratories, Inc.)
- HIV
  - Clearview HIV—Stat-Pak (Chembio Diagnostic Systems, Inc.)
  - Uni-gold Recombigen HIV Test (Trinity Biotech plc)

- *Helicobacter pylori*
  - Rapid Response *H. pylori* Rapid Test Device (Acon Laboratories, Inc.)
  - Beckman Coulter ICON HP Test (Princeton Biomedtech Corp.)

When you use tests of these types or explain their use to a patient, keep in mind that the manufacturer's guidelines must be carefully followed to ensure accurate results. Procedure 48-7, at the end of this chapter, outlines the steps for performing a rapid mononucleosis test.

PROCEDURE 48-1 Quality Control Procedures for Blood Specimen Collection

WORK // DOC

Procedure Goal: To follow proper quality control procedures when collecting a blood specimen

OSHA Guidelines:

Materials: Necessary sterile equipment, specimen-collection container, paperwork related to the type of blood test the specimen is being drawn for, requisition form (chemistry request form), marker, and proper packing materials for transport

Method:

1. Review the request form for the test ordered, verify the procedure, prepare the necessary equipment and paperwork, and prepare the work area.

2. Identify the patient and confirm the patient's identification. Ask the patient to spell her name. Explain the procedure to be performed and make sure the patient understands it, even if she has had it done before.

3. Confirm that the patient has followed any pretest preparation requirements such as fasting, taking any necessary medication, or stopping a medication. For example, if a fasting specimen is being taken, the patient should not have eaten anything after midnight of the day before. Some practitioners' offices will let the patient drink water or black coffee, however. It often depends on the type of specimen being taken.
   RATIONALE: *The test may be invalid if the patient did not follow the pretest instructions.*

4. Collect the specimen properly. Collect it at the right time intervals if that applies. Use sterile equipment and proper technique.

5. Use the correct specimen-collection containers and the right preservatives, if required. For example, blood collected into a test tube with additives should be mixed immediately.
   RATIONALE: *To prevent clotting.*

6. Immediately label the specimens. The label should include the patient name, the date and time of collection, the test name, and the name of the person collecting the specimen. Do not label the containers before collecting the specimen.
   RATIONALE: *To keep from wasting tubes if there is a problem drawing the blood.*

7. Follow correct procedures for disposing of hazardous specimen waste and decontaminating the work area. Used needles, for instance, should immediately be placed in a biohazard sharps container.

8. Thank the patient. Keep the patient in the office if any follow-up observation is necessary.

9. If the specimen is to be transported to an outside laboratory, prepare it for transport in the proper container for that type of specimen, according to OSHA regulations. Place the container in a clear plastic bag with a zip closure and dual pockets with the international biohazard label imprinted in red or orange. The requisition form should be placed in the bag's outside pocket. This ensures protection from contamination if the specimen leaks. Have a courier pick up the specimen and place it in an appropriate carrier (such as an insulated cooler) with the biohazard label. Place specimens to be sent by mail in appropriate plastic containers, and then place the containers inside a heavy-duty plastic container with a screw-down, nonleaking lid. Then place this container in either a heavy-duty cardboard box or a nylon bag. The words *Human Specimen* or *Body Fluids* should be imprinted on the box or bag. Seal with a strong tape strip.
   RATIONALE: *To protect the courier and anyone else who handles the package from exposure to bloodborne pathogens.*

PROCEDURE 48-2 Performing Venipuncture Using an Evacuated System

Procedure Goal: To collect a venous blood specimen using an evacuated system

OSHA Guidelines:

Materials: Patient chart/progress note, requisition form, blood collection components (safety needle, needle holder/adapter, collection tubes), antiseptic wipes, tourniquet, sterile gauze squares, and sterile adhesive bandages

Method:

1. Review the laboratory requisition form and make sure you have the necessary supplies.

2. Greet the patient, confirm the patient's identity, and introduce yourself.

3. Explain the purpose of the procedure and confirm that the patient has followed the pretest instructions.
   RATIONALE: *To ensure that the test will be valid.*

4. Make sure the patient is sitting in a venipuncture chair or is lying down.

5. Wash your hands. Don exam gloves.

6. Prepare the safety needle holder/adapter assembly by inserting the threaded side of the needle into the adapter and twisting the adapter in a clockwise direction. Push the first collection tube into the other end of the needle holder/adapter until the outer edge of the collection tube stopper meets the guideline.
   RATIONALE: *So that the tube is stabilized but not completely punctured.*

7. Ask the patient whether one arm is better than the other for the venipuncture. The chosen arm should be positioned slightly downward.

8. Apply the tourniquet to the patient's upper arm 3 to 4 inches above the intended venipuncture site. Wrap the tourniquet around the patient's arm and cross the ends. Holding one end of the tourniquet against the patient's arm, stretch the other end to apply pressure against the patient's skin. Pull a loop of the stretched end under the end held tightly against the patient's skin, as shown in the figure. The tourniquet should be tight enough to cause the veins to stand out but should not stop the flow of blood. You should still be able to feel the patient's radial pulse.
   RATIONALE: *To make the veins in the forearm stand out more prominently.*

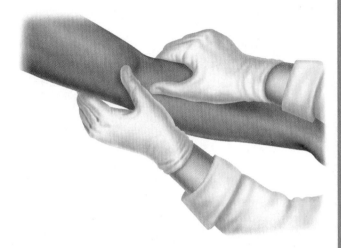

FIGURE Procedure 48-2 Step 7   The patient's arm should be positioned slightly downward for a venipuncture.

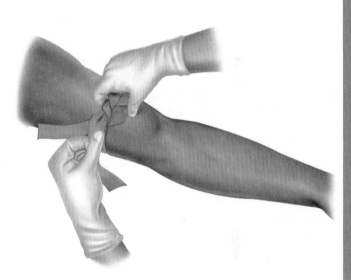

FIGURE Procedure 48-2 Step 8   Applying a tourniquet makes it easier to find a patient's vein when you are drawing blood.

9. Palpate the proposed site and use your index finger to locate the vein, as shown in the figure. The vein will feel like a small tube with some elasticity. If you feel a pulsing beat, you have located an artery. Do not draw blood from an artery. If you cannot locate the vein within 1 minute, release the tourniquet and allow blood to flow freely for 1 to 2 minutes. Then reapply the tourniquet and try again to locate the vein.

10. After locating the vein, cleanse the site with friction using an antiseptic wipe or commercially prepared alcohol pad. Allow the site to air-dry.
    RATIONALE: *The alcohol, when wet, could interfere with some of the tests and takes 30 seconds to kill the bacteria.*

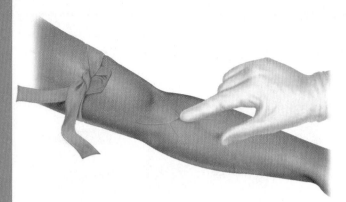

FIGURE Procedure 48-2 Step 9   Use your index finger to locate the vein.

11. Remove the plastic cap from the outer point of the needle cover and ask the patient to tighten the fist. Hold the patient's skin taut below the insertion site.
RATIONALE: *To anchor the vein so that it does not roll.*

12. With a steady and quick motion, insert the needle—held at an angle of 30° or less, bevel side up, and aligned parallel to the vein—into the vein. You will feel a slight resistance as the needle tip penetrates the vein wall. Penetrate to a depth of ¼ to ½ inch. Grasp the holder/adapter between your index and great (middle) fingers. Using your thumb, seat the collection tube firmly into place over the needle point, puncturing the rubber stopper. Blood will begin to flow into the collection tube.

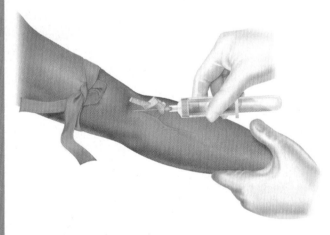

FIGURE Procedure 48-2 Step 12   When performing venipuncture, hold the needle at a 15-degree angle.

13. Fill each tube until the blood stops running to ensure the correct proportion of blood to additives. Switch tubes as needed by pulling one tube out of the adapter and inserting the next in a smooth and steady motion. (The soft plastic cover on the inner point of the needle retracts as each tube is inserted and recovers the needle point as each tube is removed.)

14. Once blood is flowing steadily in the last tube, ask the patient to release the fist and untie the tourniquet by pulling the end of the tucked-in loop. The tourniquet should, in general, be left on no longer than 1 minute.
RATIONALE: *Longer periods may cause hemoconcentration, an increase in the blood-cell-to-plasma ratio, and invalidate test results.*
You must remove the tourniquet before you withdraw the needle from the vein.
RATIONALE: *Removing the tourniquet releases pressure on the vein.*

15. Remove the last tube, then withdraw the needle in a smooth and steady motion, while placing a sterile gauze square over the insertion site. Immediately activate the safety device on the needle if it is not self-activating. Properly dispose of the needle immediately. Instruct the patient to hold the gauze pad in place with slight pressure. The patient should keep the arm straight and slightly elevated for several minutes.
RATIONALE: *To reduce the possibility of a hematoma.*

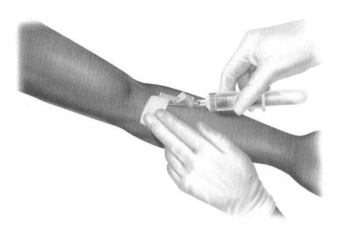

FIGURE Procedure 48-2 Step 15   Place a sterile gauze square over the insertion site as you withdraw the needle.

16. If the collection tubes contain additives, you will need to invert them slowly several times.
RATIONALE: *To mix the chemical agent and the blood specimen.*

17. Label specimens and complete the paperwork.

18. Check the patient's condition and the puncture site for bleeding. Replace the sterile gauze square with a pressure dressing.

19. Properly dispose of used supplies and disposable instruments and disinfect the work area.

20. Remove the gloves and wash your hands.

21. Instruct the patient about when to remove the pressure dressing.

22. Document the procedure in the patient's chart/progress note.

PROCEDURE 48-3 Performing Capillary Puncture

Procedure Goal: To collect a capillary blood specimen using the finger puncture method

OSHA Guidelines:

Materials: Patient chart/progress note, laboratory requisition form, capillary puncture device (safety lancet or automatic puncture device such as an Autolet® or Glucolet®), antiseptic wipes, sterile gauze squares, sterile adhesive bandages, reagent strips, micropipettes, and smear slides

Method:

1. Review the laboratory requisition form and make sure you have the necessary supplies.

2. Greet the patient, confirm the patient's identity, and introduce yourself.

3. Explain the purpose of the procedure and confirm that the patient has followed the pretest instructions, if indicated.
   RATIONALE: *The test may be invalid if the patient did not follow the pretest instructions.*

4. Make sure the patient is sitting in the venipuncture chair or is lying down.

5. Wash your hands. Don exam gloves.

6. Examine the patient's hands to determine which finger to use for the procedure. Avoid fingers that are swollen, bruised, scarred, or calloused. Generally, the ring and great (middle) fingers are the best choices. If you notice that the patient's hands are cold, you may want to warm them between your own, wrap them in a warm cloth, or have the patient put them in a warm basin of water or under warm running water.
   RATIONALE: *Warming the patient's hands improves circulation.*

7. Prepare the patient's finger with a gentle "massaging" or rubbing motion toward the fingertip. Keep the patient's hand below heart level so that gravity helps the blood flow.

8. Clean the area with an antiseptic wipe or a cotton ball moistened with antiseptic. Allow the site to air-dry.
   RATIONALE: *The alcohol may interfere with some tests.*

9. Hold the patient's finger between your thumb and forefinger. Hold the safety lancet or automatic puncture device at a right angle to the patient's fingerprint, as shown in the figure. Puncture the skin on the pad of the fingertip with a quick, sharp motion. The depth to which you puncture the skin is generally determined by the length of the lancet point. Most automatic puncturing devices are designed to penetrate to the correct depth.

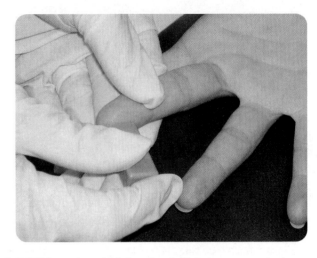

FIGURE Procedure 48-3 Step 9   Hold the lancet or automatic puncture device at a right angle to the patient's fingerprint.
©Leesa Whicker

10. Allow a drop of blood to form at the end of the patient's finger. If the blood droplet is slow in forming, apply steady pressure. Avoid milking the patient's finger.
    RATIONALE: *It dilutes the blood specimen with tissue fluid and causes hemolysis.*

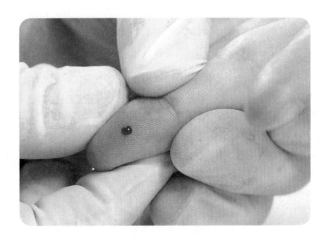

FIGURE Procedure 48-3 Step 10   Apply steady pressure to the patient's finger, but do not milk it.
©Terry Wild Studio

11. Wipe away the first droplet of blood. (This droplet is usually contaminated with tissue fluids released when the skin is punctured.) Then fill the collection devices, as described.
    Micropipettes: Hold the tip of the tube just to the edge of the blood droplet. Make sure the drop of blood is

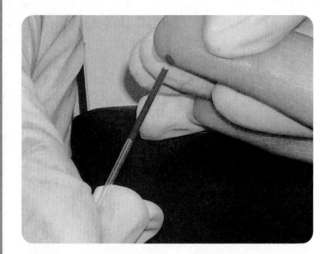

FIGURE Procedure 48-3 Step 11 Touch the tube to the drop of blood to fill it.
©Leesa Whicker

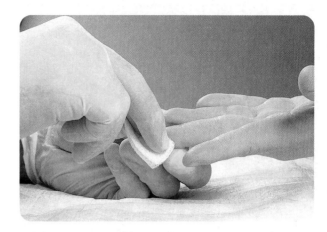

the patient's finger with a sterile gauze square. Instruct the patient to apply pressure to stop the bleeding.

FIGURE Procedure 48-3 Step 12 Use a sterile gauze square to wipe remaining blood from the patient's finger.
©Terry Wild Studio

well-rounded and do not touch the finger to the tube. The tube will fill through capillary action. If you are preparing microhematocrit tubes, you need to seal one end of each tube with clay sealant. (See Procedure 48-5 for this process.)

Reagent strips: With some reagent strips (dipsticks), you must touch the strip to the blood drop but not smear it; with other strips, you must smear it. Follow the manufacturer's guidelines.

Smear slides: Gently touch the blood droplet to the smear slide. Make sure the drop of blood is well-rounded and do not touch the finger to the strip, then process the slide as described in Procedure 48-4.

12. After you have collected the required specimens, dispose of the lancet immediately in a sharps container. Then wipe

13. Label specimens and complete the paperwork. Some tests, such as glucose monitoring, must be completed immediately.

14. Check the puncture site for bleeding. If necessary, replace the sterile gauze square with a sterile adhesive bandage.

15. Properly dispose of used supplies and disposable instruments and disinfect the work area.

16. Remove the gloves and wash your hands.

17. Instruct the patient about care of the puncture site.

18. Document the procedure in the patient's chart/progress note. (If the test has been completed, include the results.)

PROCEDURE 48-4 Preparing a Blood Smear Slide

[WORK // DOC]

Procedure Goal: To prepare a blood specimen to be used in a morphologic or other study

OSHA Guidelines:

Materials: Blood specimen (from either a capillary puncture or a specimen tube containing anticoagulated blood), capillary tubes, sterile gauze squares, slide with frosted end, and wooden applicator sticks

Method:

1. Wash your hands and don exam gloves.

2. If using blood from a capillary puncture, follow the steps in Procedure 48-3 to express a drop of blood from the patient's finger. If using a venous specimen, check the specimen for proper labeling, carefully uncap the specimen tube, and use wooden applicator sticks to remove any coagulated blood from the inside rim of the tube. You may use a safety transfer device if available.
   RATIONALE: *Uncapping the specimen tube puts you at risk of exposure to bloodborne pathogens. The blood can spray or splatter or the tube could break. The safety device decreases the likelihood of exposure.*

3. Touch the tip of the capillary tube to the blood specimen from either the patient's finger or the specimen tube. Make sure the drop of blood is well-rounded and do not

touch the finger to the tube. The tube will take up the correct amount through capillary action.

4. Pull the capillary tube away from the specimen, holding it carefully to prevent spillage. Wipe the outside of the capillary tube with a sterile gauze square.
RATIONALE: *To remove excess blood.*

5. With the slide on the work surface, hold the capillary tube in one hand and the frosted end of the slide against the work surface with the other.

6. Apply a drop of blood to the slide, about ¾ inch from the frosted end, as shown in the figure below. Place the capillary tube in the sharps container.

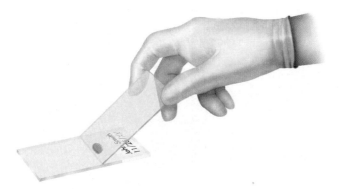

FIGURE Procedure 48-4 Step 6   Apply a drop of blood to the slide about ¾ inch from the frosted end.

7. Pick up the spreader slide with your dominant hand. Hold the slide at approximately a 30- to 35-degree angle. Place the edge of the spreader slide on the smear slide close to the unfrosted end. Pull the spreader slide toward the frosted end until the spreader slide touches the blood drop. Capillary action will spread the droplet along the edge of the spreader slide.
RATIONALE: *So that the specimen can be thinly spread on the slide.*

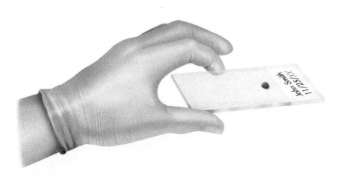

FIGURE Procedure 48-4 Step 7   Hold the spreader slide at a 30- to 35-degree angle. Pull the spreader slide toward the frosted end until it touches the drop of blood.

8. As soon as the drop spreads out to cover most of the spreader slide edge, push the spreader slide back toward the unfrosted end of the smear slide, pulling the specimen across the slide behind it, as shown in the figure below. Maintain the 30- to 35-degree angle.

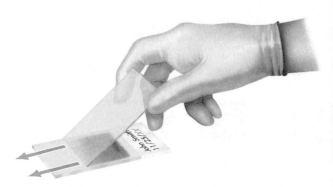

FIGURE Procedure 48-4 Step 8   When the drop covers most of the spreader slide edge, push the spreader slide back toward the unfrosted end of the smear slide.

9. Continue pushing until the spreader slide comes off the end, still maintaining the angle, as shown in the figure below. The resulting smear should be approximately 1½ inches long, preferably with a margin of empty slide on all sides. The smear should be thicker on the frosted end of the slide.

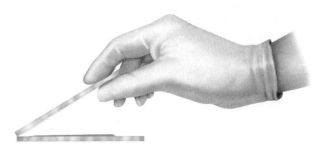

FIGURE Procedure 48-4 Step 9   Push the spreader slide off the end of the smear slide, maintaining a 30- to 35-degree angle. The smear should be thicker on the frosted end of the slide.

10. Properly label the slide, allow it to dry, and follow the manufacturer's directions for staining it for the required tests.

11. Properly dispose of used supplies and disinfect the work area.

12. Remove the gloves and wash your hands.

Procedure Goal: To identify the percentage of a blood specimen represented by RBCs after the specimen has been spun in a centrifuge

OSHA Guidelines:

Materials: Blood specimen (from either a capillary puncture or a specimen tube containing anticoagulated blood), microhematocrit tube, sealant tray containing sealing clay, centrifuge, hematocrit gauge, wooden applicator sticks, gauze squares, patient chart/progress note, and laboratory report form

Method:

1. Wash your hands and don exam gloves.

2. If using blood from a capillary puncture, follow the steps in Procedure 48-3 to express a drop of blood from the patient's finger. If using a venous blood specimen, check the specimen for proper labeling, carefully uncap the specimen tube, and use wooden applicator sticks to remove any coagulated blood from the inside rim of the tube. Alternately, use a safety transfer device if available.

   RATIONALE: *The safety device decreases the likelihood of exposure to bloodborne pathogens.*

3. Touch the tip of one of the microhematocrit tubes to the blood specimen, as shown in the figure below. The tube will take up the correct amount through capillary action.

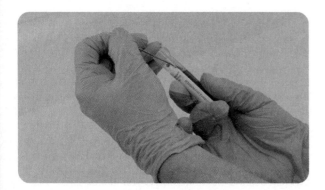

FIGURE Procedure 48-5 Step 3   Touch the tip of one of the microhematocrit tubes to the blood specimen.
©McGraw-Hill Education

4. Pull the microhematocrit tube away from the specimen, holding it carefully to prevent spillage. Wipe the outside of the microhematocrit tube with a gauze square.

   RATIONALE: *To remove excess blood so that it is not splashed or splattered on the inside of the centrifuge.*

5. Hold the microhematocrit tube in one hand and press the other end of the tube gently into the clay in the sealant tray. You may need to place a gloved finger over the other end of the tube to prevent leakage. The clay plug must completely seal the end of the tube.

   RATIONALE: *The tube must be sealed to prevent the specimen from being forced out of the tube during the spinning process.*

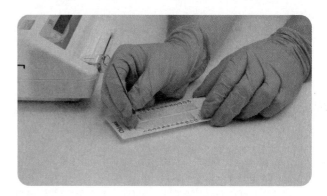

FIGURE Procedure 48-5 Step 5   Press the end of the tube into the clay in the sealant tray.
©McGraw-Hill Education

6. Repeat the process to fill another microhematocrit tube. Tubes must be processed in pairs.

   RATIONALE: *To maintain a balance in the centrifuge.*

7. Place the tubes in the centrifuge, with the sealed ends pointing outward. If you are processing more than one specimen, record the position identification number in the patient's chart to track the specimen.

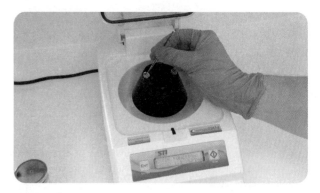

FIGURE Procedure 48-5 Step 7   Be sure to place the tubes in the centrifuge so that the sealed ends are pointing outward or downward.
©McGraw-Hill Education

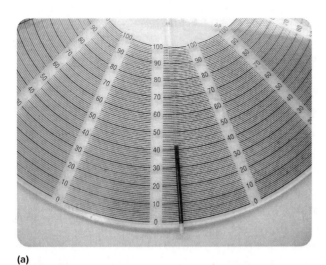

(a)

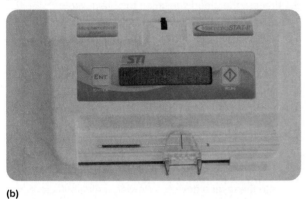

(b)

FIGURE Procedure 48-5 Step 10   Read the column of packed red blood cells using the microhematocrit gauge (a) or reader (b) to determine the hematocrit percentage.

(a) ©Total Care Programming, Inc.; (b) ©McGraw-Hill Education

8. Seal the centrifuge chamber.

9. Run the centrifuge for the required time, usually between 3 and 5 minutes. Allow the centrifuge to come to a complete stop before unsealing it.

10. Determine the hematocrit percentage by comparing the column of packed RBCs in the microhematocrit tubes with the hematocrit gauge, as shown in the figure. Position each tube so that the boundary between sealing clay and RBCs is at zero on the gauge. Some centrifuges are equipped with gauges, but others require separate handheld gauges.

11. Record the percentage value on the gauge that corresponds to the top of the column of RBCs for each tube. Compare the two results. They should not vary by more than 2%. If you record a greater variance, at least one of the tubes was filled incorrectly and you must repeat the test.

12. Calculate the average result by adding the two tube figures and dividing that number by 2.

13. Properly dispose of used supplies and clean and disinfect the equipment and the area.

14. Remove the gloves and wash your hands.

15. Record the test result in the patient's chart/progress note and/or the laboratory report form as required. Be sure to identify abnormal results.

PROCEDURE 48-6 Measuring Blood Glucose Using a Handheld Glucometer

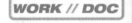

Procedure Goal: To measure the amount of glucose present in a blood specimen

OSHA Guidelines:

Materials: Safety-engineered capillary puncture device (automatic puncture device or other safety lancet), antiseptic and cotton balls or antiseptic wipes, sterile gauze squares, sterile adhesive bandages, handheld glucometer, reagent strips

appropriate for the device, patient's chart/progress note, and quality control log

Method:

1. Wash your hands and don exam gloves.

2. Review the manufacturer's instructions for the specific device used.

3. Check the expiration date on the reagent strips.
   RATIONALE: *To make sure they are not outdated.*

4. Code the meter to the reagent strips if required.
   RATIONALE: *Some machines will need to be coded to account for small differences in the strips that occur during the manufacturing process.*

5. Turn the device on according to the manufacturer's instructions.

6. Perform the required quality control procedures.
   RATIONALE: *To ensure that the machine is working as expected.*

7. Insert the strip into the meter, following the manufacturer's instructions.

8. Perform a capillary puncture, following the steps outlined in Procedure 48-3.

9. Touch the drop of blood to the reagent strip, allowing it to be taken up by the strip. Make sure the drop of blood is well-rounded and do not touch the finger to the strip.

10. Read the digital result after the required amount of time.

11. Discard the reagent strip and used supplies according to OSHA standards.

12. Record the time of the test and the result on the laboratory slip.

13. Disinfect the equipment and area.

14. Remove the gloves and wash your hands.

15. Document the test results in the patient's chart/progress note. Record the quality control tests in the quality control log.

PROCEDURE 48-7 Performing a Rapid Infectious Mononucleosis Test

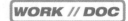

Procedure Goal: To determine the presence of antibodies associated with infectious mononucleosis using whole blood, serum, or plasma

OSHA Guidelines:

Materials: Infectious mononucleosis test kit, patient blood specimen, a watch or timer, patient's chart/progress note, and/or laboratory report form, quality control log

Method:

1. Review the laboratory requisition form and gather the necessary supplies.

2. Greet the patient, confirm the patient's identity, and introduce yourself.

3. Explain the procedure.

4. Wash your hands and don required PPE.

5. Obtain a specimen of the patient's blood using appropriate venipuncture technique.

6. Process the blood specimen to obtain whole blood, plasma, or serum as required by the testing procedure.

7. Open the test kit and check the expiration date.

8. Run the recommended controls according to the manufacturer's instructions and record in the quality control log.
   RATIONALE: *To ensure that the test is working correctly, and that the procedure was properly followed.*

9. Place the required amount of blood, serum, or plasma onto the testing device, following the manufacturer's instructions.

10. Add testing reagent or reagents to the testing device, according to the manufacturer's instructions.

11. Wait the required amount of time. Do not go over the recommended time.
    RATIONALE: *Reading the test too early can result in a false negative, and reading the test too long after the recommended time can result in a false positive.*

12. Read the results and record them in the patient's chart/progress note and/or the laboratory report form.

13. Discard the testing supplies according to OSHA regulations.

14. Disinfect the work area.

15. Remove your PPE and wash your hands.

SUMMARY OF LEARNING OUTCOMES

OUTCOME	KEY POINTS
48.1 Discuss the role of the medical assistant when collecting, processing, and testing blood specimens.	As a medical assistant, you will collect and process blood specimens for examination, make sure the test results are handled efficiently and accurately, and complete the necessary paperwork before and after each test.

OUTCOME	KEY POINTS
48.2 Describe the equipment needed to collect a blood specimen.	Preparation for collecting blood specimens includes reading and interpreting the test order and collecting the necessary equipment for the type of specimen to be collected. General equipment includes alcohol wipes, sterile gauze, and adhesive bandages. For venipuncture, you will need a tourniquet, specimen-collection tubes, and a needle system such as Vacutainer®. For capillary puncture, you will need a puncture device and capillary tubes.
48.3 Summarize ways to communicate with patients and to respond to their needs when collecting blood.	Patients are often concerned about pain, bruising, and scarring when having blood drawn. They are sometimes afraid they may have a serious disease, especially if large amounts of blood are drawn. Good communication by the medical assistant is the key to easing these fears. Many patients will have special needs, including children, the elderly, patients who have bleeding disorders, and difficult patients. Each patient will present a special set of challenges and should be treated with the utmost care and concern.
48.4 Carry out the procedure for collecting a blood specimen.	Blood is collected by one of two means: venipuncture or capillary puncture. Venipuncture is the process of obtaining a blood specimen from a vein. Capillary puncture is the process of obtaining blood from a superficial skin puncture. When collecting blood specimens, it is essential that you confirm the patient's identity before the specimen is collected, cleanse the skin prior to collection, follow standard precautions, collect the specimen needed in the appropriate tube or container, and ensure the patient's safety at all times.
48.5 Carry out the procedure for performing blood tests.	Performing hematologic, chemical, and serologic tests requires special care. The medical assistant should review the manufacturer's instructions carefully for important information about correctly performing each test.

CASE STUDY CRITICAL THINKING

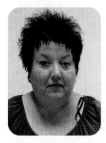

©McGraw-Hill Education

Recall Sylvia Gonzales from the case study at the beginning of the chapter. Now that you have completed the chapter, answer the following questions regarding her case.

1. What blood tube(s) would you fill to collect a specimen for the CBC and electrolytes? Which tube would you fill first?
2. Compare a fasting blood sugar test to a hemoglobin A1C test.
3. What steps will you take to perform a dermal puncture?
4. If Sylvia Gonzales tells you that she ate breakfast before coming in for the test, what should you do?

1. (LO 48.4) The small depression inside the bend of the elbow is the
   a. Cephalic space
   b. Median cubital depression
   c. Basilic area
   d. Axillary depression
   e. Antecubital fossa

2. (LO 48.5) The rupturing of erythrocytes is known as
   a. Hemolysis
   b. Hemoglobin
   c. Hematopoiesis
   d. Hemorrhage
   e. Erythrocytosis

3. (LO 48.2) A lavender-topped venipuncture collection tube contains which of the following additives?
   a. Sodium citrate
   b. Heparin
   c. EDTA
   d. SST
   e. Potassium oxalate

4. (LO 48.5) What is contained within the buffy coat?
   a. Plasma
   b. White blood cells
   c. Red blood cells
   d. Fibrinogen
   e. Serum

5. (LO 48.5) Which of the following tests gives the licensed practitioner an overall picture of a patient's compliance with diabetes diet and treatment?
   a. Blood glucose
   b. Hemoglobin A1C
   c. Cholesterol
   d. CBC
   e. Fasting blood sugar

6. (LO 48.2) A flat, broad length of vinyl or rubber used to apply pressure to the forearm so that the underlying veins stick out is a
   a. Drain
   b. Velcro® closure
   c. Butterfly
   d. Tubing
   e. Tourniquet

7. (LO 48.3) A patient arrives at the clinic for a FBS. He tells you he just ate his breakfast. What is your best course of action?
   a. Draw the blood immediately.
   b. Tell the patient to come back later in the day.
   c. Ask another medical assistant to assist you with the test.
   d. Do not draw a fasting blood sugar because the patient is not fasting.
   e. Encourage the patient to drink a lot of water before you draw the blood.

8. (LO 48.5) Which of the following keeps blood from clotting?
   a. Serum separator
   b. Anticoagulant
   c. Antibody
   d. Silicone
   e. Clot activator

9. (LO 48.5) Which of the following tests is *most* likely used to test for inflammation, infectious diseases, and malignant neoplasms?
   a. Erythrocyte sedimentation rate
   b. RBC count
   c. AST
   d. Amylase
   e. FBS

10. (LO 48.2) Which of the following represents the correct "order of draw" from first venipuncture collection tube to last?
    a. Gold, light blue, green, lavender, yellow
    b. Light blue, green, gold, yellow, lavender
    c. Yellow, light blue, gold, green, lavender
    d. Green, yellow, lavender, gold, light blue
    e. Yellow, lavender, gold, light blue, green

EHRclinic

Go to CONNECT to complete the EHRclinic exercises: 48.01 Order Bloodwork for a Patient and 48.02 Record Glucose Test Results.

You are asked to collect a capillary blood specimen on a 3-year-old child. He is crying and kicking. How should you handle this situation?

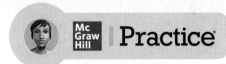

Go to PRACTICE MEDICAL OFFICE and complete the module Clinical: Work Task Proficiencies.

Electrocardiography and Pulmonary Function Testing

CASE STUDY

<table>
<tr><th colspan="3">PATIENT INFORMATION</th></tr>
<tr><td>**Patient Name**
John Miller</td><td>**DOB**
02/05/1954</td><td>**Allergies**
Bee stings</td></tr>
<tr><td>**Attending**
Paul F. Buckwalter, MD</td><td>**MRN**
00-AA-005</td><td>**Other Information**
PFT scheduled for next week.</td></tr>
</table>

John Miller arrives at the clinic complaining of his shoes not fitting and feeling like he cannot take a deep breath. During the patient interview, he also states that he is having intermittent pain in his chest. He is taking glyburide 2.5 mg daily, captopril 25 mg twice a day, and HCTZ 25 mg daily.

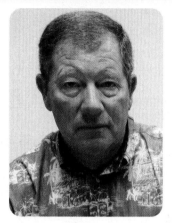
©McGraw-Hill Education

He has not taken the HCTZ for 2 weeks and is hoping to get this medication refilled. The physician wants to evaluate his congestive heart failure. He orders an ECG and a stress echocardiogram. The patient has not previously had a stress echocardiogram, and you need to explain it to him before the test begins.

Keep John Miller in mind as you study this chapter. There will be questions at the end of the chapter based on the case study. The information in the chapter will help you answer these questions.

LEARNING OUTCOMES

After completing Chapter 49, you will be able to:

49.1 Discuss the medical assistant's role in electrocardiography and pulmonary function testing.

49.2 Explain the basic principles of electrocardiography and how it relates to the conduction system of the heart.

49.3 Identify the components of an electrocardiograph and what each does.

49.4 Carry out the steps necessary to obtain an ECG.

49.5 Summarize exercise electrocardiography and echocardiography.

49.6 Explain the procedure of ambulatory (Holter) monitoring.

49.7 Carry out the various types of pulmonary function tests.

KEY TERMS

artifact
calibration syringe
cardiac cycle
deflection
depolarization
dysrhythmia
echocardiography
electrocardiogram (ECG)
electrocardiograph
electrocardiography
electrode
forced vital capacity (FVC)

Holter monitor
lead
peak expiratory flow rate (PEFR)
polarity
pulmonary function test (PFT)
repolarization
rhythm strip
spirometer
spirometry
stress test

I.C.9 Analyze pathology for each body system including:
(a) diagnostic measures
(b) treatment modalities

I.P.2 Perform:
(a) electrocardiography
(d) pulmonary function testing

I.P.3 Perform patient screening using established protocols

I.P.8 Instruct and prepare a patient for a procedure or a treatment

I.A.3 Show awareness of a patient's concerns related to the procedure being performed

2. Anatomy and Physiology

c. Identify diagnostic and treatment modalities as they relate to each body system

8. Clinical Procedures

a. Practice standard precautions and perform disinfection/sterilization techniques

e. Perform specialty procedures including but not limited to minor surgery, cardiac, respiratory, OB-GYN, neurological, and gastroenterology

▶ Introduction

As a medical assistant, you may be responsible for performing screening and/or diagnostic testing in the physician's office for patients with cardiovascular or respiratory problems. To correctly perform cardiac and respiratory testing, you need to review the anatomy and physiology of the heart and the respiratory system. (Refer to the chapters *The Cardiovascular System* and *The Respiratory System.*) This chapter introduces you to the electrocardiograph instrument and how to administer an electrocardiogram. You also will learn how to apply electrocardiograph electrodes and wires, operate the instrument, and troubleshoot problems that can occur while recording the heart's electrical activity. Because many physicians perform more complex cardiac diagnostic testing, you also will learn about Holter monitors and stress testing. Pulmonary function testing is a procedure performed in physicians' offices, and this chapter introduces you to the basics of performing respiratory procedures such as spirometry and peak flow.

▶ The Medical Assistant's Role in Electrocardiography and Pulmonary Function Testing   LO 49.1

Electrocardiography and pulmonary function testing are two procedures you may be required to perform in a medical office. **Electrocardiography** is the process by which a graphic pattern is created from the electrical impulses generated within the heart as it pumps. This procedure is often performed as part of a general examination or physical. It also may be performed to evaluate symptoms of heart disease, to detect abnormal heart rhythms, to evaluate a patient's progress after a myocardial infarction (MI), or to check the effectiveness or side effects of certain medications.

Pulmonary function tests (PFTs) measure and evaluate a patient's lung capacity and volume. Such tests are commonly performed when a person suffers from shortness of breath, but they also may be performed as part of a general examination. Pulmonary function tests can help detect and diagnose pulmonary problems. They also are used to monitor certain respiratory disorders and to evaluate the effectiveness of treatment.

▶ Basic Principles of Electrocardiography   LO 49.2

Weak or strong, fast or slow, each heartbeat produces an electrical current. Electrical currents in the heart cause the heart to beat. This electrical activity can be measured with an electrocardiograph. Measuring and recording this current gives the physician a "picture" of how the heart's electrical system is working. Understanding the basics of the conduction system and how it appears on an ECG tracing is essential when performing electrocardiography.

Conduction and Electrocardiography

Electrocardiography records the transmission, magnitude (size), and duration of the heart's various electrical impulses. Before you can understand how electrocardiography works, you must understand **polarity,** the condition of having two separate poles, one of which is positive and the other negative. Similar to a bar magnet with one end north and one south, a resting cardiac cell is polarized; that is, it has a negative charge inside and a positive charge outside. When the cardiac cell loses its polarity (a natural occurrence), depolarization occurs. **Depolarization** is the release of electrical energy within the cells of the heart, much like the flash of a camera. This wave of electrical activity results in a contraction. This wave of depolarization flows from the SA node through the electrical conduction system to the ventricles and can be detected by **electrodes,** or electrical impulse sensors, placed on specific areas on the surface of the body. During electrocardiography, electrodes detect the heart's electrical activity, including abnormalities in its rhythm. The signal is relayed through the cables to the galvanometer in the ECG machine which converts the signals into a tracing with waveforms.

Depolarization is always followed by a period of electrical recovery called **repolarization.** During repolarization, the cardiac *myocytes* are resting and rebuilding the electrical energy that was just released during depolarization. During this relaxation period the chambers in that part of the heart are refilling with blood. Once the cells have completed repolarization, they reach a state referred to as *polarization*. This is the peak resting energy state of the cells. The cells are now ready to respond to the next electrical impulse for the next contraction. The electrical cycle is then repeated, leading to another **cardiac cycle**—the sequence of contraction and relaxation. See Table 49-1 and Figure 49-1.

The Basic Pattern of the Electrocardiogram

The waves of electrical impulses responsible for the cardiac cycle produce a series of waves and lines on an **electrocardiogram** (abbreviated **ECG** or **EKG**), which is the tracing made by an **electrocardiograph,** an instrument that measures and displays these impulses (Figure 49-2). These peaks and valleys, called waves or **deflections,** are labeled with the letters P, Q, R, S, T, and U. Each letter represents a specific part of the pattern, as explained in Table 49-2. The recognition of abnormalities in the size of the waves or the various time intervals can aid in the diagnosis of certain types of heart problems.

Each type of electrocardiograph works in the same way. The electrical impulses produced by the heart can be detected through the skin; these impulses are measured, amplified, and recorded on the ECG. Detection begins with electrodes that conduct and transmit the electrical impulses to the electrocardiograph through insulated wires. An amplifier increases the signal, making the cardiac complex (PQRST) visible. The impulses received through various combinations of electrodes constitute different **leads,** or views of the electrical activity of the heart, that are recorded on the ECG. Keep in mind that the

TABLE 49-1	Parts of the Conduction System
Part	**Function**
Sinoatrial (SA) node (pacemaker)	Electrical impulses occur at a rate of 60 to 100 beats per minute, initiating the heartbeat with an electrical impulse that causes depolarization
Atrioventricular (AV) node	Delays the electrical impulse to allow for the atria to complete their contraction and ventricles to fill before the next contraction; also serves as a secondary pacemaker if the SA node fails
Bundle of His (AV bundle)	Conducts electrical impulses from the atria to the ventricles
Bundle branches	Conduct impulses down both sides of the interventricular septum
Purkinje fibers (network)	Distribute the electrical impulses throughout the right and left ventricles

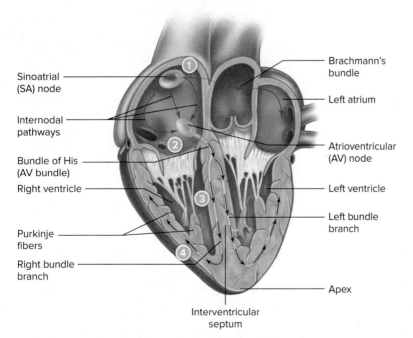

1. The heartbeat originates in the sinoatrial (SA) node; it travels across the wall of the atrium through the internodal pathways to the atrioventricular (AV) node and Bachmann's bundle to the left atrium.

2. The impulse passes through the AV node into the bundle of His (AV bundle) to the interventricular septum.

3. The impulse is divided between the right and left bundle branches and travels to the apex of the heart through the interventricular septum via the bundle branches.

4. The Purkinje fibers carry the impulse throughout the right and left ventricles, causing them to contract.

FIGURE 49-1 Conduction pathways.

TABLE 49-2 ECG Components

Component	Appearance	Heart Activity
P wave	Upward, small curve	Atrial depolarization with resulting atrial contraction
QRS complex	Q, R, and S waves	Ventricular depolarization and resulting ventricular contraction (larger than the P wave); atrial repolarization occurs (not seen)
T wave	Small, upward-sloping curve	Ventricular repolarization
U wave	Small, upward curve	Repolarization of the bundle of His and Purkinje fibers (not always seen); may be seen in instances of electrolyte imbalance
PR interval	P wave and baseline prior to QRS complex	Beginning of atrial depolarization to the beginning of ventricular depolarization
QT interval	QRS complex, ST segment, and T wave	Period of time from the start of ventricular depolarization to the end of ventricular repolarization
ST segment	End of QRS complex to beginning of T wave	Time between ventricular depolarization and the beginning of ventricular repolarization

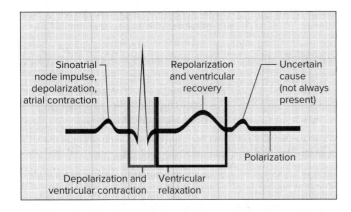

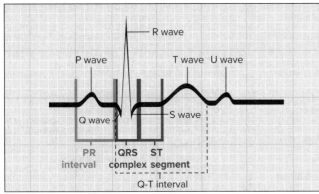

FIGURE 49-2 This ECG tracing shows the pattern of one cardiac cycle in a normal heart. These specific electrical impulses (top) represent the cycle of cardiac contraction and relaxation. The waves and lines (bottom) represent specific parts of the pattern.

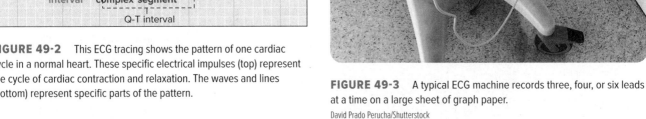

FIGURE 49-3 A typical ECG machine records three, four, or six leads at a time on a large sheet of graph paper.
David Prado Perucha/Shutterstock

term *lead* is used to refer to both the view of the heart on the ECG tracing and the physical location where the electrode is placed on the patient.

Types of Electrocardiographs

Several types of electrocardiographs are in use today. The typical ECG machine sits on a small cart that can be pushed to the patient requiring the ECG. The most common

machine is a 12-lead electrocardiograph, which records the electrical activity of the heart simultaneously from 12 different views. See Figure 49-3. A single-channel electrocardiograph records the electrical activity of one lead and produces a long, thin strip of ECG paper. This strip, or tracing, is sometimes called a **rhythm strip.** When ECG tracings are evaluated, a single lead tracing is either in print or electronic.

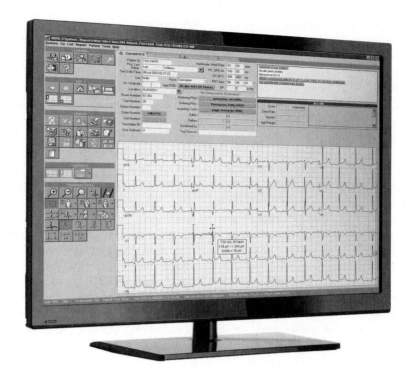

FIGURE 49-4 The electronically stored ECG retrieved by the MUSE Cardiology Information System by GE Healthcare looks just like the printed record.
Courtesy of GE Healthcare Systems

The multichannel ECG produces a 8 ½ by 11 inch sheet of paper containing a printout with all 12 leads. The actual recording time is about 10 seconds. Some models of multichannel ECGs provide a diagnosis or an interpretation of the electrocardiogram. The interpretive option can be turned on or off. Even though the interpretive electrocardiograph can provide a diagnosis, the physician will review the tracing and confirm the diagnosis before treatment is ordered. Many medical facilities use an electronic health records (EHR) software program so that electrocardiograms can be inserted into the patient medical record and transmitted to specialists to interpret. Electrocardiograms can be transmitted electronically or by fax or telephone, depending on the software and model of the electrocardiograph (see Figure 49-4).

Electrodes

Disposable electrodes (electrical sensors) are attached to the patient's skin during electrocardiography (Figure 49-5). Because the skin does not conduct electricity well, an electrolyte (a substance that enhances transmission of electric current) is needed with each electrode. Disposable electrodes come with an electrolyte preparation in place.

When performing routine electrocardiography, you place electrodes on 10 areas of the body: 1 each on the right arm (RA), left arm (LA), right leg (RL), and left leg (LL) and 6 on specific locations on the chest wall. The right leg cable is designated as the ground. These 10 electrodes are used to evaluate 12 different pathways of the heart's electrical activity (leads). This is why it is called a 12-lead ECG. Evaluating different leads—the electrical activity measured through various combinations of electrodes—enables the physician to

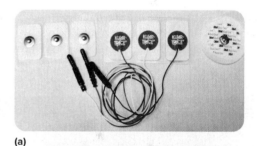

(a)

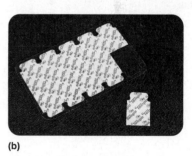

(b)

FIGURE 49-5 (a) Disposable electrodes come in various shapes and sizes. (b) Standard resting tab electrodes are inexpensive, disposable, and easy to use for a routine ECG.
©Total Care Programming, Inc.

pinpoint the origin of certain problems such as dysrhythmias, myocardial infarction (heart attack), and heart block.

Leads

Each lead provides an image, or view, of the heart's electrical activity from a different angle. Together, the images give the doctor a full picture of electrical activity moving up and down, left and right, and forward and backward through the heart. Monitoring the electrodes on the arms and leg in two different ways produces six leads that record electrical impulses that move up and down and left and right. The electrodes placed on the chest provide six more leads, showing electrical activity moving forward and backward (from the front of the body toward the back and vice versa). Each lead is given a specific designation and code. See Table 49-3.

Limb Leads Of the six leads that directly monitor electrodes on the arms and legs, three are standard and three are augmented. Each of the standard leads monitors two limb electrodes, recording electrical activity between them. These leads are also called *bipolar leads* because they monitor two electrodes. The augmented leads monitor one limb electrode and a point midway between two other limb electrodes, recording electrical activity between the monitored electrode and the midway point. Because they directly monitor only one electrode, augmented leads are also called *unipolar leads*. The electrical activity recorded by these leads is very slight, requiring the machine to augment (amplify) the tracings to produce readable waves and lines on the ECG paper. The standard limb leads appear on the ECG as I, II, and III and the augmented limb leads appear as aVF (augmented vector-foot), aVR (augmented vector-right), and aVL (augmented vector-left).

Precordial Leads The six precordial, or chest, leads are unipolar leads. The electrodes are placed across the chest in a precise, specific pattern. Each precordial lead monitors one electrode and a point within the heart. The precordial leads are each designated by a letter and a number: V_1 through V_6.

ECG Paper

ECG paper is provided in a long, continuous roll or pad. It is both heat- and pressure-sensitive and is marked with light and dark lines in a standard pattern. Each small square, or square area delineated by dots, measures 1 mm by 1 mm. Each large square measures 5 mm by 5 mm.

The vertical, or short, axis of the paper records the voltage, or strength of the impulse; the horizontal axis measures time. Normally, the paper moves through the machine at a speed of 25 mm per second. This means the distance across 1 small square represents 0.04 second. The distance across 1 large square represents 0.2 second. The distance across 5 large squares represents 1.0 second. In 1 minute (60 seconds), the paper advances 300 large squares, or 1,500 mm (150 cm).

Each electrocardiograph is standardized before use so that 1 small square represents 0.1 millivolt (mV). One large square represents 0.5 mV and 2 large squares represent 1.0 mV. See Figure 49-6.

Electrocardiograph Controls

The location of knobs and buttons on an electrocardiograph varies from model to model. However, certain features are common to most machines, including the on/off switch, standardization control, speed selector, sensitivity control, lead selector, centering control, and line control.

On/Off Switch The on/off switch turns the machine on and off. Most machines have an indicator light that signals when the power is on.

Standardization and Sensitivity Control Before you obtain an ECG, you must correctly standardize the machine. The standardization control, if present, uses a 1-mV impulse to produce a standardization mark on the ECG paper. Most newer machines standardize automatically and place a standardization mark on the tracing.

The sensitivity control—normally set on 1—adjusts the height of the standardization mark and the tracing. It is important to check the sensitivity prior to running an ECG on the patient to assure the voltages (PQRST waves) are represented as directed by the practitioner. When an ECG tracing's height is too high to fit completely on the paper, adjust this control to ½ (5mm/mV) to reduce the size of both the standardization mark and the tracing by half. For tracings that have very low peaks, set this control on 2 to double (20mm/mV) the standardization mark and the height of the tracing. Note this change on the ECG. Digital machines standardize the wave output height (gain) automatically and an adjustment may not need to be made. Always check the manufacturer's instructions to ensure the standardization is correct.

Speed Selector The paper is normally set to run at 25 mm per second for adults. When you run an ECG on infants and children or on adults with a rapid heartbeat, the deflections may appear too close together. In these cases, you may

TABLE 49-3	ECG Lead Designations
Lead	**Electrodes and Points Monitored**
Standard limb	
I	RA and LA
II	RA and LL
III	LA and LL
Augmented limb	
aVR	heart to right arm (no view). Used for dextrocardia and beneficial in detecting limb lead reversal.
aVL	heart to left arm – lateral wall view of the left ventricle
aVF	heart to left leg – inferior view of the left ventricle
Precordial	
V_1	V_1 and (LA – RA – LL)
V_2	V_2 and (LA – RA – LL)
V_3	V_3 and (LA – RA – LL)
V_4	V_4 and (LA – RA – LL)
V_5	V_5 and (LA – RA – LL)
V_6	V_6 and (LA – RA – LL)

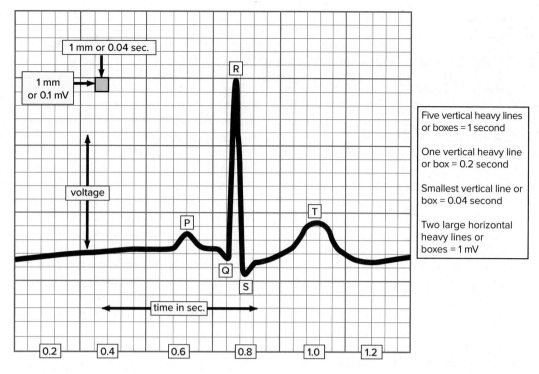

FIGURE 49-6 The ECG paper is standardized and includes heavy lines that allow measurement of both time and voltage. Note that each small box is either 0.1 mV in voltage or 0.04 second in time.

need to adjust the speed to 50 mm per second to separate the peaks and create a tracing that is easier to read. If you must set the speed at 50 mm per second, note it on the strip. Otherwise, a speed of 25 mm per second is assumed. In any case, do not change the speed selection unless the licensed practitioner directs you to do so.

Lead Selector Most electrocardiographs have a setting that enables a standard 12-lead tracing to run automatically. All machines have a lead selector that allows you to run each lead individually, in case you need to repeat a strip containing **artifacts,** which are erroneous marks or defects on the tracking.

▶ Performing an ECG LO 49.4

You must obtain a good-quality tracing when performing electrocardiography. To do so, you must be able to recognize an artifact or a generally defective ECG tracing when you see one. Proper technique is also essential to help you obtain the best-quality tracing. The following sections guide you through the general process; however, you must be familiar with the equipment you will be using. The steps in obtaining a standard 12-lead ECG are listed in Procedure 49-1 at the end of this chapter.

Preparing the Room and Equipment

Be sure the room and equipment are properly set up before you begin to administer an electrocardiogram. The accuracy of an ECG can sometimes be affected by electrical currents emitted from nearby machines. Although some electrocardiographs have filters to minimize outside electrical interference, it is always a good idea to perform electrocardiography in a room

away from all other electrical equipment—air conditioners, refrigerators, fans, and laboratory and diagnostic equipment.

The room should be in a quiet, private location, protected from interruptions. Because the patient must partially disrobe, adjust the room temperature to a comfortable level.

The examining table should be sturdy and comfortable. Make sure the table paper is fresh and the table is disinfected after each patient's use.

Before using the electrocardiograph, check the date of its last inspection. Each machine should be periodically inspected and certified safe to use for a specific period of time. Using a machine only within this time period helps ensure safety for both you and your patient. It is good practice to check the ECG paper and ECG electrodes prior to preparing the patient, restocking these supplies if necessary, as this will save time for you and the physician.

Preparing the Patient

Introduce yourself, identify the patient, explain the procedure, and answer any questions the patient has. Keep in mind, some patients are apprehensive about undergoing electrocardiography. Anxiety often stems from the fear of receiving an electric shock from the machine. See the *Caution: Handle with Care* section for ways to allay a patient's anxiety about having an ECG.

Applying the Electrodes and the Connecting Wires

You must prepare the patient's skin before applying the electrodes. Proper contact between an electrode and the skin allows for proper conduction of the impulses. Depending on your office policy, you may be required to trim chest or leg hair if it is dense

Allaying Patient Anxiety About Having Electrocardiography

The most common reason for a patient's anxiety is not knowing what to expect from electrocardiography. The patient may be fearful of being hooked up to an electrical device and worried about receiving an electric shock.

Calmly and simply explain the procedure in detail, both before you begin and while you prepare the patient for the test. Assure the patient it is a safe procedure that will last less than 10 minutes total and the actual tracing will take much less time. Explain that the machine measures the heart's electrical activity and that no outside electricity will pass through the body. It is also helpful to explain why the doctor has ordered the procedure, without giving any diagnosis or prognosis.

Above all, talk to and listen to the patient. Encourage her to express her concerns and ask questions. Respond to the patient's concerns and questions calmly, fully, and respectfully.

Ensuring Patient Comfort

Ensuring that the patient is comfortable will help her feel more at ease. It also will result in less body movement and a more accurate ECG.

First, make sure the room temperature is right for the patient. If she says the room feels too cool, provide an extra blanket to prevent chills, as this can make a patient shiver and increase her anxiety. Shivering can cause muscle tremor artifacts known as somatic tremor. Next, ensure that the patient is comfortable on the examining table. Placing a small pillow under the head can help, but make sure it does not touch the shoulders or raise them off the table. For most patients, placing a pillow under the knees helps relax the abdomen and lower extremities and prevents lower back pain. Try this arrangement and let the patient decide if this feels comfortable. If the patient has trouble breathing, shift her into a sitting-up (Fowler's or semi-Fowler's) position. Use the position that is most comfortable for the patient. If the patient chooses a position other than on her back (supine), be sure to note the position in her chart.

to ensure proper contact. This should be done with scissors. Shaving is no longer recommended because of the risk of infection or bleeding. However, some facilities still practice shaving, so follow the policies at your facility. If you must shave the patient, remember to clean their skin prior to shaving the patient. Cleaning the skin after shaving can be painful for the patient.

Cleaning is done to remove dead skin, oils, moisturizers, powder and dirt. Rough up the skin a little with a coarse gauze and an approved skin cleansing solution. This will improve adhesion of the sensor to the skin and improve gel to skin contact. This can reduce artifact and improve tracing quality. If you ever have to move an electrode or reattach it, dispose of it and use a new "fresh" electrode.

Electrodes Apply disposable electrodes by simply removing the adhesive backing and pressing the electrode firmly into place on the skin. You must position electrodes at 10 locations on the body (Figure 49-7). This includes 4 limb electrodes and 6 chest electrodes.

Limb Electrodes Limb electrodes are most commonly placed on the inside of the fleshy part of the calf muscle and on the outside of the upper arm. Sometimes they are placed on the thigh, on the abdomen, and above the wrist. Follow office policy on limb placement, but remember, a consistent technique will ensure that all ECGs will be standardized, even with different equipment models. It is generally better to place arm electrodes on the upper arm because this reduces the amount of artifact caused by arm movement. Attach the electrodes to a smooth and fleshy part of each limb to ensure optimal conduction of impulses.

Limb electrodes must always be placed at the same level on both arms and on both legs. If a patient has had a leg amputated, both leg electrodes should be placed on the thighs or abdomen, parallel to each other. If the patient has had an arm amputated, place both electrodes at shoulder level. Note the alternate electrode placement in the patient's chart and the ECG tracing because differences in placement can cause changes in the ECG tracing.

Precordial Electrodes Unlike the limb electrodes, the precordial electrodes must be placed at precise, specific locations on the chest to obtain accurate readings. These locations specify intercostal spaces—the spaces between the ribs—which are numbered from top to bottom. Refer to Figure 49-8 for the exact description of each location.

Determine the position for the first precordial electrode (V_1) by counting to the fourth intercostal space to the right of the sternum (breastbone). The V_1 electrode should be placed over this space, directly adjacent to the sternum. After you have this electrode in place, use it as a guide to position the other electrodes.

Place the V_2 electrode in the fourth intercostal space to the left of the sternum in the same manner. Note that the V_1 and V_2 positions may not line up exactly; one may be higher than the other. Perfect symmetry is rare in the human body.

Next, place the V_4 electrode in the fifth intercostal space where it intersects an imaginary line drawn straight down from the middle of the clavicle (midclavicular line). When the V_4 electrode is in place, place the V_3 electrode midway between V_2 and V_4 in the fifth intercostal space.

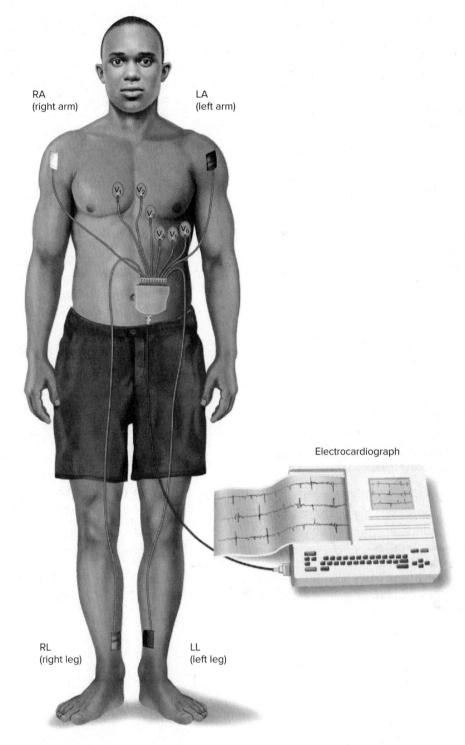

RA
(right arm)

LA
(left arm)

Electrocardiograph

RL
(right leg)

LL
(left leg)

FIGURE 49-7   There are 10 electrode positions for electrocardiography.

Place the V_6 electrode in the fifth intercostal space directly below the middle of the armpit (midaxillary line). Place the last electrode (V_5) in the fifth intercostal space midway between V_4 and V_6.

Attaching the Wires   After placing the electrodes, attach the wires that connect the electrodes to the electrocardiograph. Numbers and letters on the wires correspond to numbers and

letters for the electrodes. For example, RA stands for right arm, LL stands for left leg, and so on. The precordial electrode wires are labeled V_1 through V_6. Connect the limb wires first, then the precordial wires, in the sequence already described. Some wires are also color-coded.

Connect the wires to the electrodes using the clips or snaps on the end of the wires. Wires should follow the patient's body contours and lie flat against the body. Drape the wires over the patient to avoid putting tension on the electrodes, which could cause interference. You also may bundle the wires together to form a single cable.

Operating the Electrocardiograph

Before running the ECG, remind the patient to remain as still as possible and not to talk.

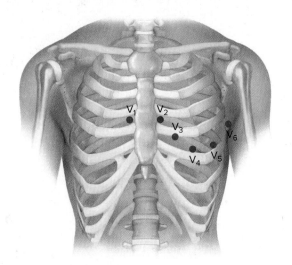

V₁ Fourth intercostal space (between the ribs), to the right of the sternum (breastbone)
V₂ Fourth intercostal space, to the left of the sternum
V₄ Fifth intercostal space, on the left midclavicular line
V₃ Fifth intercostal space, midway between V₂ and V₄
V₆ Fifth intercostal space, on the left midaxillary line
V₅ Fifth intercostal space, midway between V₄ and V₆

FIGURE 49-8 Six precordial electrodes are arranged in specific positions on the chest. Notice that electrode V₄ must be positioned before V₃ and V₆ before V₅.

Preparing the Electrocardiograph Enter patient identifying information into the ECG machine's LCD display. If the machine does not allow data entry, write the information on the tracing report once completed.

Standardization may be necessary; however, digital ECG machines standardize the wave output heights automatically. These calibration marks can be seen at the beginning or end of a 12-lead tracing. See Figure 49-9. For manual standardization, check the manufacturer's instructions.

Running the ECG You can now run the ECG. On most machines, turning the lead selector to the automatic mode produces a standard 12-lead strip. Depending upon the machine you may need to press the run button.

Multiple-Channel Electrocardiographs Some electrocardiographs have multiple channels that can record three, four, or six leads simultaneously (Figure 49-10). Electrode placement is the same as for single-channel electrocardiographs.

Checking the ECG Tracing After running the 12 leads and before disconnecting the patient from the machine, check all tracings to make sure they are clear and free of artifacts. If any of the leads do not appear on a tracing, it may mean a wire has come loose. In this case, reconnect the wire and repeat the tracing. Repeat any unclear tracings.

Also, check that all tracings are contained within the paper's boundaries and that no waves peak above its edges. Increase or decrease the sensitivity setting to adjust the size of the peaks.

If the peaks in a tracing are too close together, increase the paper speed to 50 mm per second. Increasing the speed separates the peaks and makes the tracing easier to read.

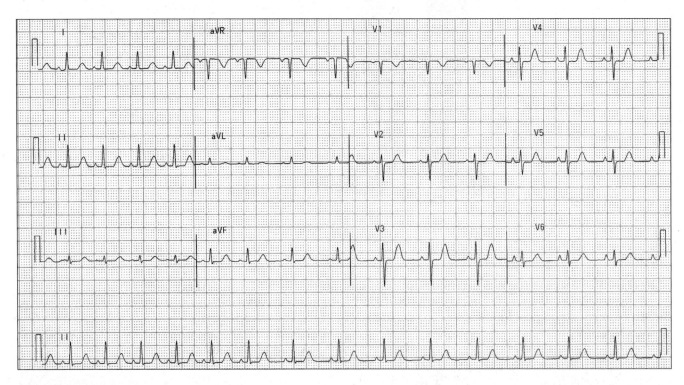

FIGURE 49-9 The tracing from each lead will differ. The long tracing of a single lead along the bottom is the rhythm strip. Notice the calibration marks at the beginning and end of each lead.

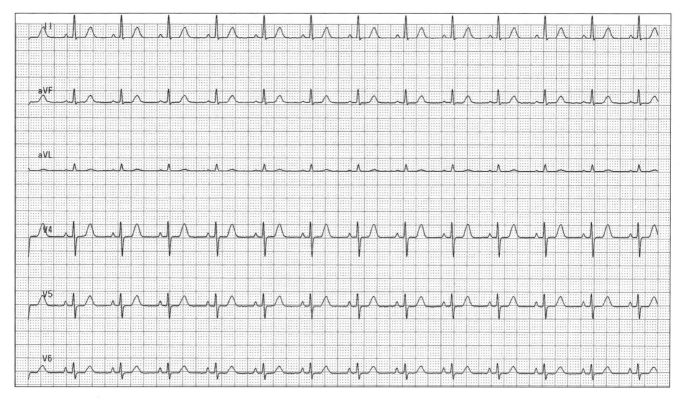

FIGURE 49-10 Some electrocardiographs allow you to run six leads at the same time.

Depending on your facility policy, you may need permission prior to increasing the paper speed.

Make a note on the ECG tracing whenever it is necessary to adjust sensitivity or speed settings. This information is vital to the interpretation of the test.

Troubleshooting: Artifacts and Other Problems

To ensure high-quality tracings, it is essential to recognize artifacts and identify sources of interference. You also must know how to correct them.

Artifacts Improper technique, poor conduction, outside electrical interference, and improper handling of a tracing can cause artifacts. If artifacts are present on an ECG tracing, the licensed practitioner may not be able to make an accurate diagnosis of the patient's condition.

There are several types of artifacts. Among the common ones you may see are a wandering baseline or a flat line. Recognizing the presence of an artifact in the baseline during setup allows you to correct the problem before the tracing is recorded. You also may see marks that are not characteristic of a tracing; large, erratic spikes; or uniform, small spikes. Table 49-4 outlines these artifacts and summarizes possible causes and solutions. Follow these guidelines to correct artifacts when recording an ECG.

Wandering Baseline A wandering baseline, shown in Figure 49-11, is identified by a shift in the baseline from the center position for that lead. Causes include a variety of mechanical problems. Mechanical problems may include

improper application of electrodes (too loose or incorrectly placed), tension on electrodes caused by a dangling wire, inadequate skin preparation, or the presence of creams or lotions on the skin. Proper skin preparation and electrode placement are essential. When the electrocardiography appointment is made, instruct the patient to use no creams or lotions, deodorant, perfume, or powder. Be sure to include specific instructions in patient education materials and ask the patient whether any of these substances were used before the procedure. If so, clean each area of electrode placement thoroughly with alcohol to avoid conduction disturbances.

Flat Line A flat line on one of the lead's tracings (Figure 49-12) is typically caused by a loose or disconnected wire. If flat lines occur on more than one lead, two of the wires may have been switched. If flat lines occur on all leads, the patient cable may be loose or disconnected, or there may be a break (short) somewhere in the unit. On the other hand, a flat line on all leads can indicate cardiac arrest. If a flat line occurs on all leads, always check the patient's pulse and respiration first.

Alternating Current (AC) Interference AC interference occurs when the electrocardiograph picks up a small amount of electric current given off by another piece of electrical equipment. The tracing's line will be jagged, consisting of a series of uniform, small spikes (Figure 49-13). Many newer electrocardiographs have filters to reduce or eliminate most of this interference, and it often can be eliminated by turning off or unplugging other appliances in the room. Keeping the examining table away from the wall also can help, as wiring in the wall can contribute to AC interference.

TABLE 49-4 Correcting ECG Artifacts

Problem	Possible Causes	Solutions
Wandering baseline	Poor skin preparation	Repeat skin preparation and lead placement.
	Loose electrode	Reapply electrode.
	Improper electrode placement	Reapply electrode.
Flat line	Detached/loose wire or cable	Reattach wires or cable.
	Crossed wires	Check/switch wires.
	Short circuit in wires	Check/replace broken equipment.
	Cardiac arrest	Check pulse/respiration; begin CPR.
Marks not part of tracing	Careless handling	Handle carefully.
	Use of paper clips	Use a rubber band.
	Wet hands	Ensure that hands are dry.
Uniform, small spikes	AC interference	Turn off/unplug other electrical equipment; remove patient's watch.
	Improper electrode placement	Reapply electrode.
	Inadequate grounding	Check and apply proper grounding.
	Dirty electrode	Clean and reapply electrode.
Large, erratic spikes	Somatic interference	Help patient relax and be comfortable.
	Loose/dry electrode	Reapply electrode.

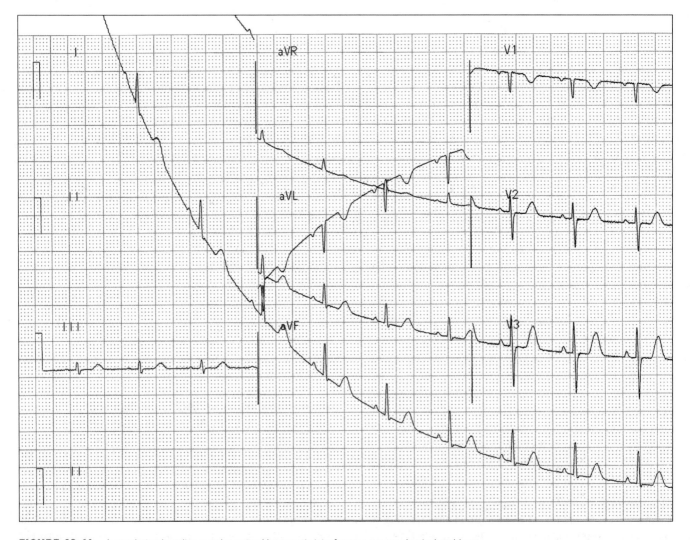

FIGURE 49-11   A wandering baseline may be caused by somatic interference or a mechanical problem.

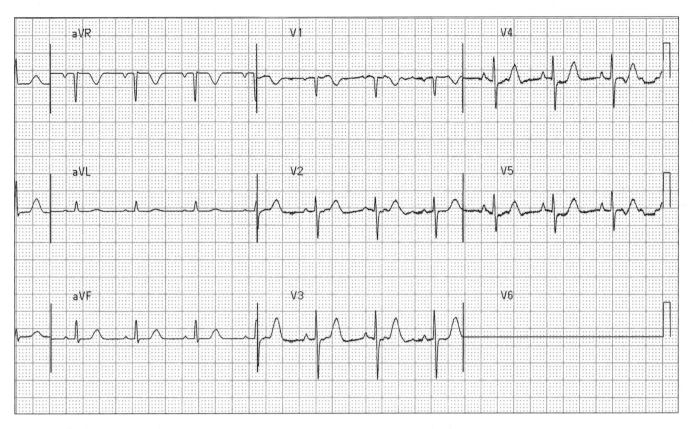

FIGURE 49-12 A flat line on one of the leads is caused by a loose or disconnected wire.

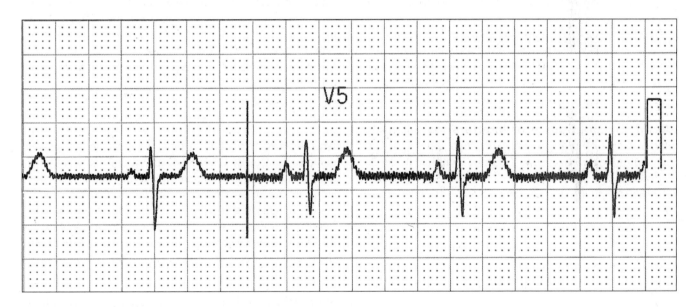

FIGURE 49-13 This type of artifact is caused by AC interference.

If the wires are crossed and the lead wires are not following the patient's body contour, this can cause AC interference. Make sure the ECG cable is not underneath the examination table. If these remedies do not work, check to see whether the electrodes are dirty or attached improperly or whether the machine is incorrectly grounded.

Somatic Interference Muscle movement—tensing of voluntary muscles, shifting of body position, tremors, or even talking (which requires muscular contractions that generate electrical impulses)—causes somatic interference. A sensitive electrocardiograph detects these impulses, possibly resulting in large, erratic spikes and a shifting baseline (Figure 49-14).

Eliminate this type of interference by reminding the patient to remain still and to refrain from talking. To reduce the chance of the patient shivering, shifting, and moving, be sure the room temperature is comfortable for the patient and/or provide a blanket if available.

Placing the limb electrodes closer to the body's trunk—on the upper arms, close to the shoulder, and on the upper

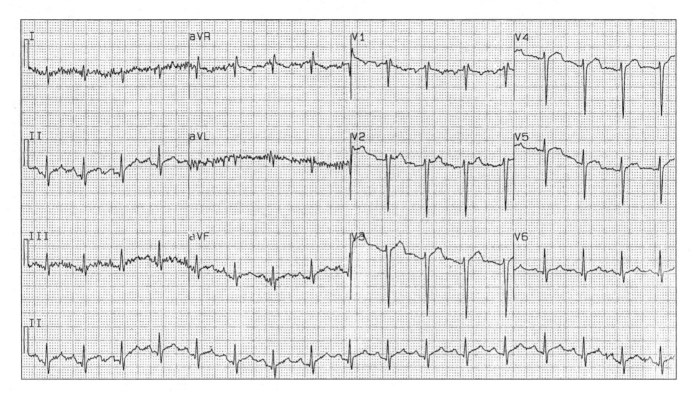

FIGURE 49-14 The somatic interference in this ECG was caused by patient tremors.

thighs—can reduce interference. Reducing patient anxiety by explaining the procedure also can help reduce somatic interference.

Certain nervous system disorders, such as Parkinson's disease, cause patients to experience involuntary movements that can cause interference. So, although placing the limb electrodes closer to the body's trunk is often helpful, it may be necessary to interrupt the tracing until the tremors subside.

Identifying the Source of Interference Frequently, interference is caused by one of the limb electrodes. The source of interference on an ECG can be identified by checking the ECG tracings obtained on leads I, II, and III. If there is a problem with a particular limb electrode, the interference will be prominent in two leads.

Use these guidelines:

- If there is interference in leads I and II on the tracing, check the right arm electrode.
- If there is interference in leads I and III, check the left arm electrode.
- If there is interference in leads II and III, check the left leg electrode.

If the cause of the artifact or the source of interference cannot be determined, stop the machine and notify your supervisor or the physician. Do not disconnect the patient from the electrocardiograph.

Completing the Procedure

When you are sure the quality of all ECG tracings is acceptable, disconnect the patient from the machine. Remove the tracing and label if necessary; then disconnect the wires from

the electrodes and remove the electrodes from the patient. Wipe excess electrolyte from the patient's skin with a moist towel if needed. Assist the patient to a sitting position, allowing a moment's rest before assisting the patient from the table. Help the patient dress, if necessary, or allow the patient privacy to dress. Remove disposable paper covers from the table and pillows, clean surfaces according to OSHA guidelines, and discard all disposable materials in a biohazardous waste container.

Interpreting the ECG Although you are not responsible for interpreting an ECG as a medical assistant, knowing something about how ECGs are interpreted may allow you to recognize an urgent problem. Some of the features assessed by an ECG include heart rhythm, heart rate, the length and position of intervals and segments, and wave changes. A series of ECGs is often taken before a physician makes a diagnosis. The tracings are compared for changes in a patient's condition, progress, or response to a specific medication.

Heart Rhythm The ECG is the best way to assess heart rhythm—the regularity of the heartbeat. A normal heart rhythm is indicated on the ECG by regularly spaced complexes. In regularly spaced complexes, the distance between one P wave and the next P wave—or one R wave and the next R wave—is consistent. The physician assesses the patient's rhythm by viewing the rhythm strip you obtain from lead II.

Heart Rate The heart rate can be determined easily by counting the number of QRS complexes in a 6-second strip of the tracing (30 large squares at 25 mm per second) and multiplying by 10. Heart rate irregularities may result from conduction abnormalities or reactions to certain drugs.

Intervals and Segments Variations in the length and position of the intervals and segments can indicate many heart conditions, including conduction disturbances and myocardial infarction. For example, during a myocardial infarction, the ST segment will be elevated in the tracing for a period of time. Thus, the ECG can be used to determine not only the occurrence of a myocardial infarction but also whether it occurred recently. Electrolyte disturbances in the blood and drug reactions also can affect intervals and segments.

Wave Changes The direction of certain waves may vary, depending on which lead is being viewed. Normally, each wave should have a similar appearance in each of the leads. Changes in the height, width, or direction of a wave may indicate a problem. During the early stages of a myocardial infarction, for example, the T wave forms a large peak. Not long afterward, the T wave inverts and appears below the baseline.

Cardiac Dysrhythmias

Irregularities in heart rhythm are called **dysrhythmias,** also known as *arrhythmias.* Although some dysrhythmias do not cause problems, many of them can be dangerous, so it is important to detect these irregularities with an ECG.

Ventricular Fibrillation (V-fib) Ventricular fibrillation, commonly referred to as *v-fib,* is a life-threatening heart condition in which the ventricles of the heart appear to "quiver" and there is no cardiac output. Electrical activity within the heart is chaotic during fibrillation resulting in a chaotic waveform seen on the tracing. The patient will quickly lose consciousness, and cardioversion (defibrillation) must be used to stop the dysrhythmia. Ventricular fibrillation is seen in patients experiencing a myocardial infarction. (Figure 49-15).

Premature Ventricular Contractions (PVCs) Premature ventricular contractions (PVCs) are premature heartbeats that originate from the heart's ventricles. A PVC is identified as a beat that occurs early in the cycle, followed by a pause before the next cycle (Figure 49-16). PVCs are premature because they occur before the regular heartbeat. These heartbeats are the result of an irritability of the heart muscle in the ventricles and can be caused by myocardial infarctions, electrolyte imbalances, lack of oxygen, or certain medications. A PVC appears on the ECG as having no P wave, a wide QRS complex, and T waves that deflect in the opposite direction from the R wave.

Atrial Fibrillation Atrial dysrhythmias occur because of electrical disturbances in the atria and/or the AV node, which lead to fast heartbeats (tachycardia). Atrial fibrillation is a common atrial dysrhythmia that causes chaotic, rapid, multiple electrical signals that fire from other areas in the atria rather than from the SA node. Causes of atrial fibrillation include myocardial infarction; hypertension; heart failure; mitral valve diseases, such as MVP; overactive thyroid; pulmonary embolisms (blood clots); excessive alcohol consumption; emphysema; and pericarditis. Atrial fibrillation is seen on the ECG as small, irregular, uncoordinated complexes that are difficult to interpret because the P waves cannot be identified (Figure 49-17).

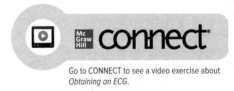

Go to CONNECT to see a video exercise about *Obtaining an ECG.*

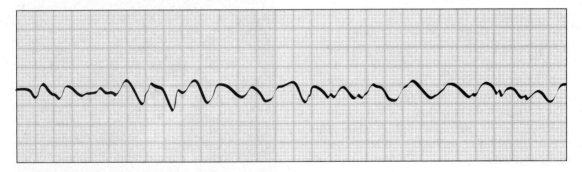

FIGURE 49-15 Ventricular fibrillation is irregular electrical activity with no discernible pattern on the ECG tracing.

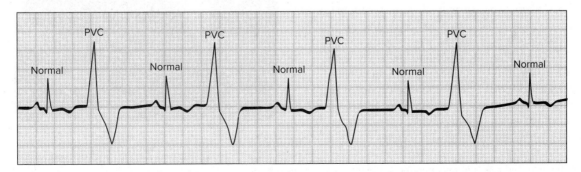

FIGURE 49-16 This rhythm strip compares a normal deflection to a premature ventricular contraction (PVC).

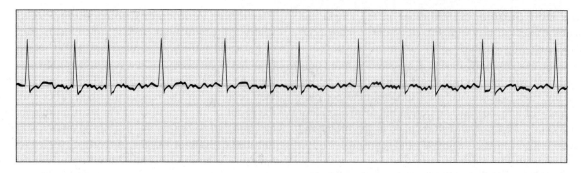

FIGURE 49-17   Atrial fibrillation.

▶ Exercise Electrocardiography (Stress Testing) and Echocardiography   LO 49.5

The resting ECG does not always provide a physician with enough information to diagnose a problem. A licensed practitioner can use several additional tests for diagnosing heart diseases and disorders. Exercise electrocardiography, more commonly known as a **stress test,** assesses the heart's conduction system during exercise, when the demand for oxygen increases. This test measures a patient's response to a constant or increasing workload. **Echocardiography** uses ultrasound to view the heart in motion. This can be done at rest or after strenuous activity such as riding a bike or walking on a treadmill.

Exercise Electrocardiography

A stress test may be performed on a patient who has had surgery or a myocardial infarction to determine how the heart is functioning. It is sometimes used to screen a patient for heart disease and to determine a patient's ability to undertake an exercise program.

During the procedure, the patient is required to walk on a treadmill, pedal a stationary bicycle, or walk on a stair-stepping ergometer while ECG readings are taken (Figure 49-18). An ergonometer measures work performed. You are responsible for preparing the patient for electrocardiography and monitoring blood pressure throughout the procedure. The test continues until the patient reaches a target heart rate, experiences chest pain or fatigue, or develops complications, such as tachycardia or another dysrhythmia.

A patient who undergoes stress testing is often suspected of having a heart problem or is recovering from a myocardial infarction or surgery. Consequently, there may be a risk of cardiac distress, myocardial infarction, or cardiac arrest during testing. Because of the risks, the patient must sign an informed consent form before the procedure and a physician must monitor the patient throughout the test. Emergency medication and equipment, such as a defibrillator, always must be present in the room. Medical assistants and other healthcare professionals should maintain current provider or professional level CPR credentials when working with patients during a stress test.

Because of the potential risk, patients may be apprehensive about the test. As a medical assistant, you can be instrumental in helping them feel comfortable about undergoing the procedure and in making the procedure as safe as possible for them. See the *Caution: Handle with Care* section for ways to help a patient safely undergo stress testing.

Echocardiography

The ability to view the moving heart is essential to understanding how the structures within the heart are functioning. An echocardiogram produces a video image of the working heart valves and chambers and shows how well blood moves through these structures. There are several types of echocardiograms:

- Transthoracic—the ultrasound transducer is moved around on the chest and/or abdomen to produce heart images.

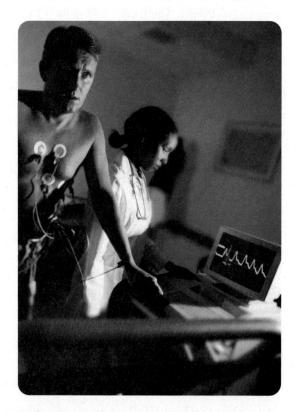

FIGURE 49-18   During a stress test, the patient exercises on special equipment to see how well the heart handles increased physical demands.
©Stockbyte/Getty Images

CAUTION: HANDLE WITH CARE

Ensuring Patient Safety During Stress Testing

Although some risk is involved in exercise electrocardiography, the risk of having a myocardial infarction during a stress test is less than 1 in 500. Patients are sometimes apprehensive about the procedure, especially patients who have recently had a myocardial infarction. You can help educate patients to reduce their apprehension and prepare them for stress tests. Assist before and during the procedure using these techniques:

- Ask patients to wear comfortable shoes and clothes so that they will be more comfortable during the exercise portion of the text.
- Inform the patient of the symptoms he can expect during the test—including fatigue, slight breathlessness, an increased heart rate, and increased perspiration—so that the patient will be better able to cope with the test.
- Explain that advance notice of adjustments or changes during the test, such as an increased workload, will be given.

- Assure the patient that there are few risks associated with the test and that the test can be stopped if he experiences chest pain or extreme fatigue.
- Tell the patient that both you and the physician will be monitoring his vital signs during and after the procedure and that all safety precautions will be taken.
- Explain the presence of the safety equipment—for example, the crash cart with medication, equipment, and supplies in the remote chance that an emergency occurs.
- Encourage the patient to report any symptoms during the test. Even symptoms that are not cardiac-related should be reported.
- Observe the patient for signs of distress and inform the physician immediately if such symptoms appear.

- Transesophageal—the transducer is passed into the esophagus, where it produces clearer images of the heart because it is closer to the heart and the sound waves do not have to penetrate the ribs.
- Doppler—uses a special type of ultrasound to look at blood flow through the heart. The direction and speed of blood flow through the heart are assessed with this type of test, giving the physician information about coronary artery blockage and heart valve damage.
- Stress echo—echocardiography is done before and after exercise or injection of a drug that makes the heart work faster and harder. This is usually done in conjunction with an electrocardiogram to assess how well the heart responds to increased demand.

Pretest Preparation There is usually no special pretest preparation for transthoracic and doppler echocardiography. The patient should not eat a heavy meal prior to a stress echo. Because patients having transesophageal echocardiography receive a sedative and the transducer is passed into the esophagus, they should not eat for at least 6 hours prior to the test. Make sure you carefully explain all pretest instructions verbally and in writing and give the patient an opportunity to ask any questions. Reassure the patient of the limited risk during the procedure. Finally, have the patient sign a consent form prior to having the echocardiogram.

▶ Ambulatory Electrocardiography (Holter Monitoring)   LO 49.6

Patients who experience intermittent chest pain or discomfort may have a normal resting ECG and a normal stress test. When this is the case, the electrical activity of the patient's heart can be monitored over a 24- to 48-hour period of normal

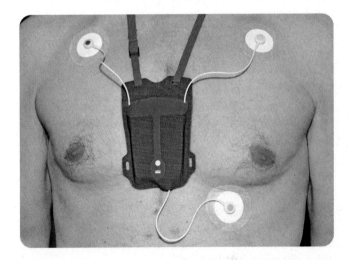

FIGURE 49-19 An ambulatory monitor is used to determine electrical activity of a patient's heart over a 24- to 48-hour period.
©Prisma by Dukas/Getty Images

activity to help diagnose the problem. An ambulatory monitor is used for this purpose.

Functions and Types of Ambulatory Monitors

A common type of ambulatory monitor, often called a **Holter monitor,** is an electrocardiography device that includes a microchip recorder and is worn around a patient's waist or on a shoulder strap to record the heart's electrical activity. The monitor is connected to electrodes on the patient's chest (Figure 49-19). During the testing period, the patient is asked to perform usual daily activities and to keep a log of activities undertaken and of stress or symptoms experienced. Any symptoms or abnormal sensations such as chest pain, indigestion, or dizziness should be recorded. If symptoms do occur, the patient is asked to monitor the symptoms and what he or she was doing prior to and during the symptoms.

To aid in the diagnosis, some monitors allow patients to press a button or apply the monitor device whenever symptoms appear. These symptom event monitors may be worn up to 30 days.

The patient returns to the office at the end of the testing period to turn in their diary, if required, and have the monitor and electrodes removed. The recording is analyzed by a computer in the office or at a reference laboratory and a printout of the results is prepared. When the tracing has been evaluated, the doctor can correlate cardiac irregularities, such as dysrhythmias or ST segment changes, with the activities and symptoms listed in the patient's diary.

In addition to its role as a diagnostic tool, Holter monitoring can be used to evaluate the status of a patient who is recovering from a myocardial infarction. It can indicate progress or the need to change therapy or the rehabilitation plan.

Patient Education

It is essential that the patient continue normal activities during Holter monitoring. Give the patient the following additional instructions:

- Record all activities, emotional upsets, physical symptoms, and medications taken.
- Wear loose-fitting clothing that opens in the front while wearing the monitor.
- Avoid going near magnets, metal detectors, and high-voltage areas and avoid using electric blankets during the monitoring period. These devices and areas can interfere with the recording.
- Avoid getting the monitor wet. Do not take a bath or shower. A sponge bath is permissible.

Show the patient how to check the monitor to make sure it is working properly. This step is particularly important if any of the electrodes seem loose. Instruct the patient to inform the office if there are any problems.

Connecting the Patient

Ambulatory monitors have either three or five electrodes, depending on the unit. As with a resting ECG, correct placement of the electrodes is necessary for accurate readings. Before connecting the patient to the monitor, make sure he has signed an informed consent form and explain that you need to attach electrodes to the patient's skin.

Because the electrodes may stay in place for 24 hours, you may need to clip the hair in the areas where the electrodes are attached to permit optimum adherence. The wires may be connected to the electrodes before they are attached to minimize patient discomfort.

After the electrodes and wires are attached and the monitor is in place, tape the wires to the patient's chest to eliminate tension on the wires or electrodes. Be sure that the unit has a fresh battery, that an SD card or other data storage device has been inserted if necessary, and that the unit is turned on. The steps in performing ambulatory monitoring are outlined in Procedure 49-2 at the end of this chapter.

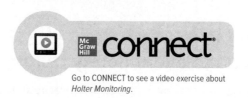

Go to CONNECT to see a video exercise about *Holter Monitoring.*

▶ Pulmonary Function Testing   LO 49.7

Pulmonary function tests (PFTs) help the doctor evaluate ventilatory function of the lungs and chest wall. They evaluate lung volume and capacity and are commonly used to evaluate shortness of breath and to help detect and classify pulmonary disorders. They also may be performed as part of a general examination. PFTs are used to monitor conditions such as asthma, certain allergies, cystic fibrosis, and chronic obstructive pulmonary disease (COPD), a chronic lung disorder. The tests also are used to evaluate the effectiveness of particular treatments on a patient's lung function.

Spirometry

Spirometry is a test used to measure breathing capacity. An instrument called a **spirometer** measures the air taken in by and expelled from the lungs. Several different measurements related to lung volume and capacity can be made with a spirometer. Some of these measurements are made directly by the spirometer; others are calculated. For more information about lung volumes and capacities, see the chapter *The Respiratory System.*

Forced Vital Capacity

The **forced vital capacity (FVC)** is the greatest volume of air that can be expelled when a person performs rapid, forced expiration. To obtain the FVC, ask the patient to take as deep a breath as possible and to exhale into the spirometer as quickly and completely as possible. You can determine the lung's ability to function by taking into account the volume of air expelled and the time it takes to perform this maneuver.

Types of Spirometers

Many models of computerized spirometers are used in physicians' offices. Each consists of a mouthpiece or a mouthpiece and a tube to carry air to the machine, a mechanism to measure the volume or flow of air, and a means of calculating and printing the results.

Computerized spirometers measure air volume and airflow, perform various calculations, and print a graphic representation of the information. Figure 49-20 shows a computerized spirometer.

Performing Spirometry

The technique for performing pulmonary function testing is similar for all types of spirometers. Successful spirometry depends on proper patient preparation and consistent technique in performing the procedure and analyzing the results. The steps involved in measuring forced vital capacity using a spirometer are described in detail here and outlined in Procedure 49-3 at the end of this chapter.

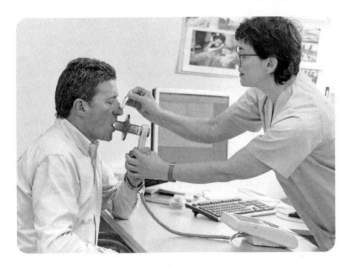

FIGURE 49-20 This computerized spirometer measures air volume and airflow.
©Javier Larrea/Getty Images

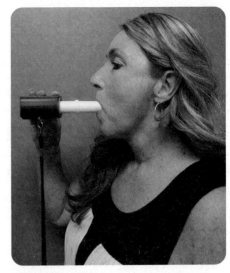

(a) Correct position

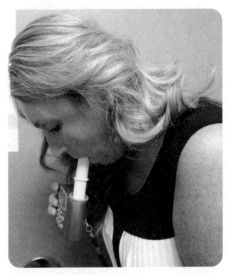

(b) Incorrect position

FIGURE 49-21 During a pulmonary function test, the patient must maintain the proper position. (a) The chin should be slightly elevated and the neck slightly extended. (b) The chin should not approach the chest. Images showing position only, in the correct position the nose should be held or a nose clip should be in place.
©McGraw-Hill Education/David Moyer, photographer

Patient Preparation Certain conditions and activities affect the accuracy of pulmonary function tests. Patients should be made aware of these conditions prior to scheduling to ensure accuracy:

- Viral infection or acute illness within the previous 2 to 3 weeks.
- Serious medical condition, such as a recent myocardial infarction.
- Recent use of a prescribed medication if the test order calls for spirometry before and after prescribed medication.
- Use of a sedative or opioid substance before the test.
- Smoking or eating a heavy meal within 1 hour of taking the test.

Review the conditions and activities with patients again on the day of the test to ensure that none apply. If there are no contraindications, weigh and measure patients. Use simple terms to explain the procedure and its purpose. Have them loosen tight clothing so that they will be comfortable and their breathing will not be restricted in any way. The procedure is performed with patients sitting down. Make sure their legs are not crossed and that both feet are flat on the floor.

Explain that they need to wear a nose clip or hold the nose tightly closed to be sure they will inhale and exhale through the mouth. The mouthpiece of the unit may be a disposable cardboard tube or a reusable rubber one that can be disinfected after use. If disposable mouthpieces are used, instruct patients to avoid biting down on them, as that will obstruct airflow. Be sure patients form a tight seal around the mouthpiece with their lips. Dentures normally help maintain a tight seal; however, they should be removed if they hinder the process.

Proper Positioning Instruct patients to keep their chin and neck in the correct position during the procedure. The chin should be slightly elevated and the neck slightly extended. Bending the chin to the chest tends to restrict airflow and should be avoided (Figure 49-21). Some bending at the waist is acceptable.

Explaining and Demonstrating the Procedure Tell patients to take the deepest breath possible, insert the mouthpiece into the mouth, form a tight seal, and then blow into the mouthpiece as hard and as fast as possible to completely exhale. Tell them to exhale as long as they can to force air from the lungs. Remind them that the initial force of their exhalation must be strong to get a valid reading. Demonstrate the procedure to show how to do the test correctly.

Performing the Maneuver You can improve patients' performance during the maneuver by actively and forcefully coaching them. Urge patients to blow hard and to continue blowing. After a maneuver, give them feedback on their performance and indicate corrective actions they can take to improve the next maneuver.

Some spirometers indicate whether a particular maneuver was of adequate force and duration to be measured. However, adequate force does not indicate that the maneuver was acceptable. An acceptable maneuver must have the following five features:

1. No coughing, particularly during the first second.
2. A quick and forceful start.
3. An adequate length of time (a minimum of 6 seconds).
4. A consistent and fast flow with no variability.
5. Consistency with other maneuvers.

Spirometry tracings plot volume and time. You will need to obtain three acceptable maneuvers, which may require more than three attempts. Observe the patient for signs of breathing difficulty, dizziness, light-headedness, or changes in pulse and blood pressure. If necessary, allow the patient to rest briefly before continuing. Notify the physician immediately if symptoms are severe.

Determining the Effectiveness of Medication
Spirometry is often used to determine the effectiveness of certain medications a patient is taking. You will perform two sets of maneuvers if this determination is required. Instruct the patient to refrain from taking the prescribed medication on the day of the test. Before performing the test, confirm that the patient has followed this instruction. Conduct the first set of maneuvers, ensuring that they are acceptable. After obtaining the results, instruct the patient to take the prescribed medication. Allow the medication to take effect and then perform a second set of maneuvers. Comparing the two sets of readings shows whether the medication has effectively improved the patient's lung function. Some computerized spirometers can graph both sets of readings together to simplify the comparison (Figure 49-22).

Special Considerations On occasion, you may have to deal with an uncooperative patient, one who cannot understand or follow directions, or one who cannot perform the procedure. In these situations, patience and skill are essential for obtaining an acceptable spirometry tracing.

The doctor may be able to convince an uncooperative patient to perform the maneuver. You can help by taking a no-nonsense approach, perhaps stating that the doctor needs these test results to help the patient. Patients who cannot understand or follow directions—the very young, the very old, those who have limited proficiency in English, or those with a hearing impairment—may need extra attention and patience to obtain acceptable results. Explain the procedure in simple terms and repeat instructions as necessary. If, after eight attempts, the patient is unable to perform the procedure, stop and report the situation to the licensed practitioner.

The Importance of Calibration Spirometers should be calibrated each day they are used to ensure accurate readings.

You may be responsible for this procedure, which requires the use of a standardized measuring instrument called a **calibration syringe** (Figure 49-23). When the plunger is pulled back, this syringe contains a fixed volume of air. Connect the syringe to the patient tubing (this tubing runs from the mouthpiece to the machine) and depress the plunger to inject the entire volume of air. The spirometer reading should be within 3% of the stated volume. Keep a calibration logbook for each spirometer.

While calibrating the spirometer, you can detect leaks by checking the volume/time graph. The volume should remain

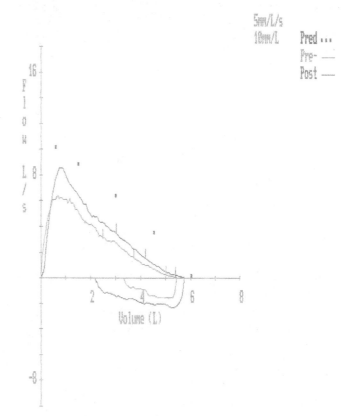

FIGURE 49-22 These spirometry tracings show air volume per second before and after use of a medication.

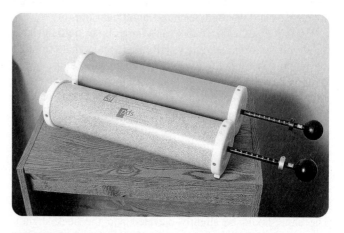

FIGURE 49-23 A calibration syringe delivers a fixed volume of air.
©Cliff Moore

at a steady reading; if it declines with time, a leak exists in the system.

Infection Control After a patient completes the pulmonary function test, you must clean the spirometer and other pulmonary function devices thoroughly to prevent transmission of microorganisms. If disposable mouthpieces, nose clips, and patient tubing are used, discard them in a biohazardous waste container. If reusable mouthpieces, nose clips, and tubing are used, clean and disinfect them between patients. Most importantly, wash your hands thoroughly before and after performing a pulmonary function test.

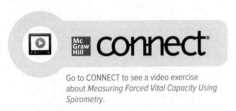

Go to CONNECT to see a video exercise about *Measuring Forced Vital Capacity Using Spirometry*.

Peak Expiratory Flow Rate (PEFR)

A **peak expiratory flow rate (PEFR)** is a measurement taken to determine the amount of air that can be quickly forced from the lungs. A peak flow meter—a small, handheld device that can be used in the medical office or the patient's home (Figure 49-24)—is often used to obtain a PEFR. Patients who suffer from asthma are commonly asked to monitor their asthma by using a peak flow meter and recording their results. During an asthma flare-up, the large airways of the lungs begin to narrow, which slows the speed of air leaving the lungs. A peak flow meter, when used properly, can reveal narrowing of the airways in advance of an asthma attack. Peak flow meters can help determine:

- When to seek emergency medical care.
- The effectiveness of an asthma management treatment plan.
- When to stop or add medication as directed by a physician.
- Asthma triggers, such as stress or exercise.

Procedure 49-4, at the end of this chapter, explains the procedure for obtaining a peak expiratory rate using a peak flow meter.

Peak Flow Zones After obtaining a peak expiratory flow rate, the type of patient care given will be determined based on the individual's results. The physician will instruct the patient about the peak flow zones and how to respond to each zone. Peak flow zones are different for each patient and are determined by the physician. The three peak flow zones are green, yellow, and red. These three color zones can be seen in Figure 49-24.

Green Zone The green zone indicates good control of asthma, with peak flow rates of 80% to 100% of the highest peak flow rate. Measurements in this zone indicate that air

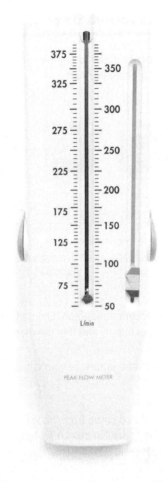

FIGURE 49-24 Peak expiratory flow meter markings determine the patient's treatment based on accurate readings.
©abalcazar/Getty Images

moves well through the large airways and the patient's usual activities can be continued.

Yellow Zone Peak flow rates in the yellow zone range from 50% to 80% of the highest peak flow rate. Measurements in this zone indicate that the large airways are beginning to narrow and medication is needed. Patient symptoms include tiredness and tightening of the chest.

Red Zone Peak flow rates in the red zone are less than 50% of the highest or best personal reading recorded. Narrowing of the largest airways has occurred and is considered a medical emergency. Medical treatment should be sought immediately. Patients are usually directed to take a bronchodilator or other medication that will open the airway and call their physician. Symptoms include wheezing, shortness of breath, and trouble walking and talking.

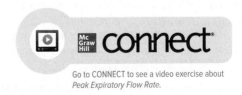

Go to CONNECT to see a video exercise about *Peak Expiratory Flow Rate*.

Procedure Goal: To obtain a graphic representation of the electrical activity of a patient's heart

OSHA Guidelines:

Materials:

Patient chart/progress note, electrocardiograph, ECG paper, electrodes, electrolyte preparation, wires, patient gown, drape, blanket, pillows, gauze pads, alcohol, moist towel, and scissors for trimming hair (if needed)

Method:

1. Turn on the electrocardiograph. Ensure that there is an adequate paper supply and that the machine inspection is up to date.

2. Identify the patient, introduce yourself, and explain the procedure.

3. Wash your hands.

4. Ask the patient to disrobe from the waist up and remove jewelry, socks or stockings, bra, and shoes. If the electrodes will be placed on the patient's legs, have the patient roll up his or her pant legs. Sometimes the electrodes are placed on the sides of the lower abdomen—check the manufacturer's instructions. Provide a gown for female patients and instruct her to wear the gown with the opening in front.
   RATIONALE: *Making sure the patient knows exactly what clothing to remove and the correct way to put on the gown will make the process more efficient.*

5. Assist the patient onto the table and into a supine position. Cover the patient with a drape (and a blanket if the room is cool). If the patient experiences difficulty breathing or cannot tolerate lying flat, use a Fowler's or semi-Fowler's position, adjusting with pillows under the head and knees for comfort if needed.

6. Tell the patient to rest quietly and breathe normally. Explain the importance of lying still to prevent false readings.

7. Wash the patient's skin, using gauze pads moistened with alcohol. If needed, rub it vigorously with dry gauze pads to promote better contact of the electrodes.
   RATIONALE: *If a patient has applied lotion or body powder, or has oily or sweaty skin in the areas where electrodes are placed, it may cause conduction problems.*

8. If the patient's leg or chest hair is dense, use a small pair of scissors to closely trim the hair where you will attach the electrode. (Shaving is generally not allowed because of the risk of bleeding and infection. Follow the procedure specified at your facility.)

9. Apply electrodes to fleshy portions of the limbs, making sure the electrodes on one arm and leg are placed similarly to those on the other arm and leg. Attach electrodes to areas that are not bony or muscular. The arm lead tabs on the electrode point downward and the electrode tabs for the leg leads point upward. Peel off the backings of the disposable electrodes and press them into place.
   RATIONALE: *Using the correct tab position will reduce tension on the limb wires. Artifacts can occur when electrodes are placed on muscles.*

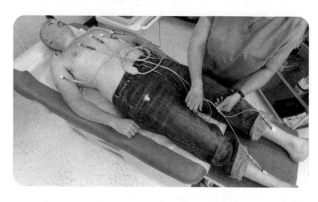

FIGURE Procedure 49-1 Steps 9 and 10 Place electrodes at the specified locations on the chest, arms, and legs.
©McGraw-Hill Education

10. Apply the precordial electrodes at specified locations on the chest. If you are unsure of the placement, check a reliable reference. Precordial electrode tabs point downward.

11. Attach wires and cables, making sure all wire tips follow the patient's body contours.

12. Check all electrodes and wires for proper placement and connection; drape wires over the patient to avoid creating tension on the electrodes, which could result in artifacts.

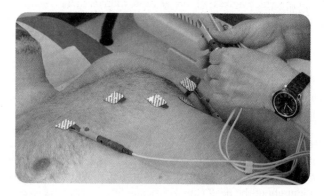

FIGURE Procedure 49-1 Step 12 Attach wires and cables, draping wires over the patient to avoid tension, which can result in artifacts.
©McGraw-Hill Education

13. Enter the patient data into the electrocardiograph. Press the on, run, or record button. If standardization is needed, check the manufacturer's instructions.

14. Remind the patient to lie quietly, and run the ECG.

15. Check tracings for artifacts.

16. Correct problems and repeat any tracings that are not clear.

17. Disconnect the patient from the machine.

18. Remove the tracing from the machine and label it with the patient's name, the date, and your initials if these do not print out with the tracing.

19. Disconnect the wires from the electrodes and remove the electrodes from the patient.

20. Clean the patient's skin with a moist towel.

21. Assist the patient into a sitting position.

22. Allow a moment for rest and then assist the patient from the table.

RATIONALE: *Some patients may experience postural hypotension after lying and may feel dizzy.*

23. Assist the patient in dressing, if necessary, or allow the patient privacy to dress.

24. Wash your hands.

25. Record the procedure in the patient's chart/progress note.

26. Properly dispose of used materials and disposable electrodes.

27. Clean and disinfect the equipment and the room according to OSHA guidelines.

PROCEDURE 49-2 Ambulatory Monitoring

WORK // DOC

Procedure Goal: To monitor the electrical activity of a patient's heart over a period of time to detect cardiac abnormalities that may go undetected during routine electrocardiography or stress testing

OSHA Guidelines:

Materials: Patient chart/progress note; ambulatory monitor; battery; microchip, SD card, or small cassette; patient diary or log, if needed; alcohol; gauze pads; scissors; disposable electrodes; hypoallergenic tape; drape; and electrocardiograph

Method:

1. Identify the patient, introduce yourself, and explain the procedure.

2. Ask the patient to remove clothing from the waist up; provide a drape if necessary.

3. Wash your hands and assemble the equipment.

4. Assist the patient into a comfortable position (sitting or supine).

5. If the patient's body hair is particularly dense, don examination gloves and trim the areas where the electrodes will be attached.
   RATIONALE: *Trimming the area will ensure that the electrodes will stay secure during the 24- to 48-hour period.*

6. Clean the electrode sites with alcohol and gauze.

7. Rub each electrode site vigorously with a dry gauze square.
   RATIONALE: *To help electrodes adhere to the skin.*

8. Attach wires to the electrodes and peel off the paper backing on the electrodes. Apply electrodes at locations as indicated by the manufacturer's instructions. Press firmly to ensure that each electrode is making good contact with the skin.
   RATIONALE: *Good skin contact is essential to obtain an accurate reading.*

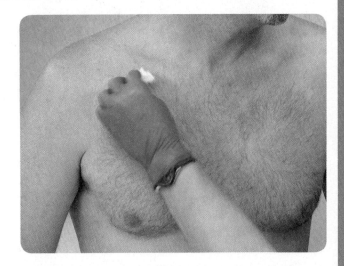

FIGURE Procedure 49-2 Step 7   Rub each electrode site vigorously to ensure that the electrodes adhere and stay in place during the monitoring.
©McGraw-Hill Education

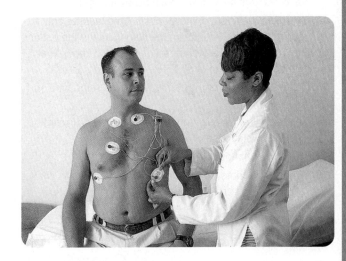

FIGURE Procedure 49-2 Step 8   Correctly connecting the patient to the ambulatory monitor is essential. Check the manufacturer's instructions for the monitor you are using.
©David Kelly Crow

9. Attach the patient cable.

10. Insert a fresh battery and position the unit.

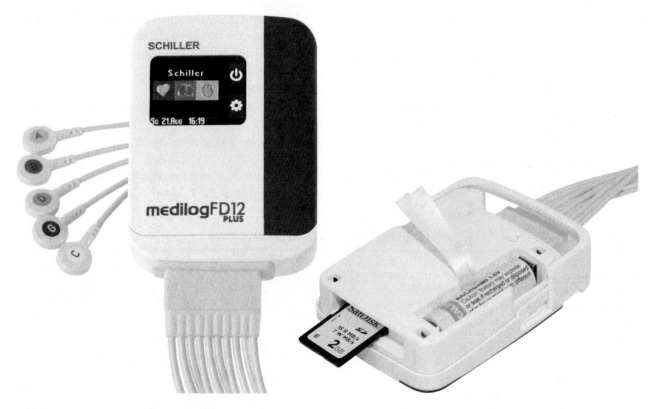

FIGURE Procedure 49-2 Step 10 Make sure that the monitor has a microchip or other type of data storage and a fresh battery.

©2014 SCHILLER AG

11. Tape wires, cable, and electrodes as necessary to avoid tension on the wires as the patient moves.

12. Insert the SD card or other storage device and turn on the unit.

13. Ensure that the unit is on and indicate the start time in the patient's chart.
RATIONALE: *If the unit is not running, results will not be recorded and the test will have to be repeated.*

14. Instruct the patient on proper use of the monitor and how to enter information in the diary. Caution the patient not to alter any diary entries; it is crucial to know what the patient is doing at all times.

15. Schedule the patient's return visit for the same time on the following day.

16. On the following day, remove the electrodes, discard them, and clean the electrode sites.

17. Wash your hands.

18. Transfer the data from the monitor to the patient's chart according to office procedure and the manufacturer's directions.

19. Document the procedure (refer to Progress Note).

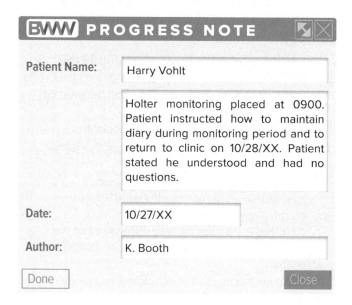

BWW PROGRESS NOTE

Patient Name:

Harry Vohlt

Holter monitoring placed at 0900. Patient instructed how to maintain diary during monitoring period and to return to clinic on 10/28/XX. Patient stated he understood and had no questions.

Date: 10/27/XX

Author: K. Booth

Done   Close

PROCEDURE 49-3 Measuring Forced Vital Capacity Using Spirometry

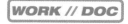

Procedure Goal: To determine a patient's forced vital capacity using a volume-displacing spirometer

OSHA Guidelines:

Materials: Patient chart/progress note, adult scale with height bar, spirometer, patient tubing (tubing that runs from the mouthpiece to the machine), mouthpiece, nose clip, and disinfectant

Method:

1. Prepare the equipment. Ensure that the paper supply in the machine is adequate.

2. Calibrate the machine as necessary.

3. Identify the patient and introduce yourself.

4. Check the patient's chart to see whether there are special instructions to follow.

5. Ask whether the patient has followed instructions.

6. Wash your hands and don examination gloves.

7. Measure and record the patient's height and weight.

8. Explain the proper positioning.

9. Explain the procedure.

10. Demonstrate the procedure.
    RATIONALE: *Explanations and demonstrations are effective patient teaching methods.*

11. Turn on the spirometer and enter applicable patient data and the number of tests to be performed.

12. Ensure that the patient has loosened any tight clothing, is comfortable, and is in the proper position. Apply the nose clip.

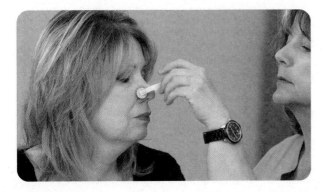

FIGURE Procedure 49-3 Step 12   The nose clip is applied over the fleshy part of the nose.
©McGraw-Hill Education

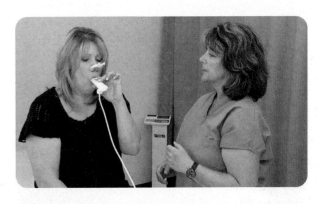

FIGURE Procedure 49-3 Step 13   You may need to coach the patient while performing the maneuver.
©McGraw-Hill Education

13. Have the patient perform the first maneuver, coaching when necessary.

14. Determine whether the maneuver is acceptable.

15. Offer feedback to the patient and recommendations for improvement if necessary.

16. Have the patient perform additional maneuvers until three acceptable maneuvers are obtained.

17. Record the procedure in the patient's chart and place the chart and the test results on the physician's desk for interpretation.

18. Ask the patient to remain until the physician reviews the results.
    RATIONALE: *The physician may want to speak with the patient regarding results or may want to order additional testing.*

19. Properly dispose of used materials and disposable instruments.

20. Sanitize and disinfect patient tubing, reusable mouthpiece, and nose clip.

21. Clean and disinfect the equipment and room according to OSHA guidelines.

PROCEDURE 49-4 Obtaining a Peak Expiratory Flow Rate

Procedure Goal: To determine a patient's peak expiratory flow rate

OSHA Guidelines:

Materials: Patient chart/progress note, peak flow meter, and a disposable mouthpiece

Method:

1. Assemble all necessary equipment and supplies for the test.

2. Wash your hands and identify the patient.

3. Explain and demonstrate the procedure to the patient.
   RATIONALE: *Patient education and understanding are crucial for getting accurate test results.*

4. Position the patient in a sitting or standing position with good posture. Make sure any chewing gum or food is removed from the patient's mouth.

5. Set the indicator to zero.

RATIONALE: *Helps to ensure accurate results.*

6. Ensure that the disposable mouthpiece is securely placed onto the peak flow meter.

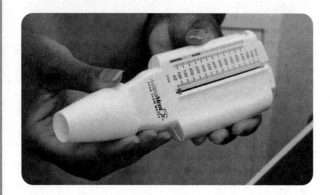

FIGURE Procedure 49-4 Step 6   A disposable mouthpiece is securely fastened to the peak flow meter.
©McGraw-Hill Education

7. Hold the peak flow meter with the gauge uppermost and ensure that your fingers are away from the gauge.

8. Instruct the patient to take as deep a breath as possible.

9. Instruct the patient to place the mouthpiece into his mouth and close his lips tightly around the mouthpiece, sealing his lips around it.

10. Instruct the patient to blow out as fast and as hard as possible.

RATIONALE: *A fast blast is better than a slow blow.*

11. Observe the reading where the arrowhead is on the indicator.

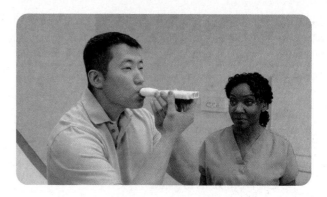

FIGURE Procedure 49-4 Step 9   Have the patient close his lips tightly around the mouthpiece so that no air escapes.
©McGraw-Hill Education

12. Reset the indicator to zero and repeat the procedure two times, for a total of three readings. You will know the technique is correct if the reading results are close. If coughing occurs during the procedure, repeat the step.

13. Document the readings in the patient's chart. The highest reading will be the peak flow rate.

RATIONALE: *The highest reading represents the personal best reading for the patient, and future measurements are based on this result. Do not average the results.*

14. Dispose of the mouthpiece in a biohazardous waste container.

15. Disinfect or dispose of the peak flow meter per office policy.

16. Wash your hands.

SUMMARY OF LEARNING OUTCOMES

OUTCOME	KEY POINTS
49.1 Discuss the medical assistant's role in electrocardiography and pulmonary function testing.	As a medical assistant, you will be responsible for preparing the patient for ECG and pulmonary function tests, maintaining the equipment used for these tests, and performing them.
49.2 Explain the basic principles of electrocardiography and how it relates to the conduction system of the heart.	The heart's conduction system is responsible for the electrical activity that occurs during a heartbeat. The electrical pathway begins with the SA node; travels through the AV node, the bundle of His, and the right and left bundle branches; and ends with the Purkinje fibers. This electrical energy pathway is measured with an electrocardiograph and a tracing of the impulses is produced. The electrical impulses are represented in waveforms or deflections. Deflections are labeled by the letters PQRSTU and represent a part of the pattern.

OUTCOME	KEY POINTS
49.3 Identify the components of an electrocardiograph and what each does.	The electrocardiograph consists of the following components: electrodes, which detect and conduct electrical impulses to the electrocardiograph; amplifier, which increases the signal, making the heartbeat visible; leads, combinations of electrodes that provide different views of the electrical activity of the heart; LCD display and/or ECG paper, where the tracing of the electrical activity is viewed and recorded; and various controls that allow you to input patient information and change things such as the speed of the tracing.
49.4 Carry out the steps necessary to obtain an ECG.	The steps in obtaining an accurate ECG include preparing the room and equipment, identifying the patient, properly placing the limb and chest electrodes, attaching the lead wires, entering the patient data into the ECG machine, running the tracing, checking the tracing for artifacts, disconnecting the patient from the lead wires and removing the electrodes, and assisting the patient as required.
49.5 Summarize exercise electrocardiography and echocardiography.	Exercise electrocardiography is referred to as stress testing. This measures the efficiency of the heart during constant or increasing workload. Echocardiography uses ultrasound to create a picture of the moving heart. This can be done while the patient is resting or after exercise.
49.6 Explain the procedure of ambulatory (Holter) monitoring.	An ambulatory or Holter monitor is used to measure the heart's activity over an extended period, usually 24 hours. This is used when the patient has intermittent chest pain or discomfort and a normal ECG and stress test do not identify the cause.
49.7 Carry out the various types of pulmonary function tests.	Forced vital capacity is the measurement of the greatest volume of air expelled when a patient performs a rapid, forced expiration. The lung's ability to function is measured by the volume of air expelled and the time taken to perform the maneuver. Accurate spirometry testing includes positioning the patient properly, coaching the patient during the procedure, obtaining three acceptable maneuvers, and recording the results in the patient's chart. A peak expiratory flow rate is obtained by having the patient sit or stand using good posture, take in as deep a breath as possible, and blow out through the peak flow meter as fast and as hard as possible three times. The highest reading of the three is the peak flow rate and should be recorded in the patient's chart.

CASE STUDY CRITICAL THINKING

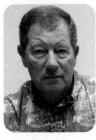

©McGraw-Hill Education

Recall John Miller from the case study at the beginning of the chapter. Now that you have completed the chapter, answer the following questions regarding his case.

1. Explain to John Miller the difference between an ECG and a stress echocardiogram.
2. John Miller expresses concern about having a heart attack during the procedure. How can you alleviate his fear?
3. You must perform an ECG on this patient. Describe the steps in the procedure.

1. (LO 49.2) Which of the following initiates the heartbeat?
   a. AV node
   b. SA node
   c. Bundle of His
   d. Purkinje fibers
   e. Bundle branch

2. (LO 49.4) The ECG tracing is showing somatic interference. What can be done?
   a. Turn off or unplug appliances in the room.
   b. Remove oil from the patient's skin.
   c. Connect a loose wire.
   d. Remind the patient to remain still.
   e. Reschedule the test.

3. (LO 49.5) Which of the following statements best describes echocardiography?
   a. It assesses the heart's conduction system during exercise.
   b. It requires the patient to walk on a stair-stepping ergonometer.
   c. It produces a video image of the working heart valves and chambers.
   d. It is often used to screen patients for heart disease.
   e. It measures a patient's response to an increasing workload.

4. (LO 49.7) When obtaining a peak flow rate, you should _____ the _____ readings.
   a. Average, two
   b. Average, three
   c. Add, two
   d. Document, three
   e. Document, two

5. (LO 49.4) Which of the following irregularities on an ECG would be considered the *most* severe?
   a. PVC
   b. V-fib
   c. A-fib
   d. AC interference
   e. Tachycardia

6. (LO 49.3) The precordial ECG leads are also called
   a. AVR leads
   b. Ground leads
   c. Chest leads
   d. Augmented leads
   e. Limb leads

7. (LO 49.6) Which of the following should a patient do when wearing a Holter monitor?
   a. Avoid normal daily activities and focus on relaxing during the monitoring
   b. Bathe and/or shower as usual because the monitor will not be affected
   c. Wear a tight-fitting shirt to hold the electrodes and monitor in place
   d. Return the Holter monitor through the mail to avoid a return visit
   e. Inform the office if the monitor is not working properly

8. (LO 49.4) Turning off unnecessary electrical equipment in the room when performing an ECG is helpful in reducing which type of artifact?
   a. Extraneous marks
   b. Flatline
   c. Somatic interference
   d. AC interference
   e. Wandering baseline

9. (LO 49.1) An ECG evaluates the _____ and a PFT evaluates the _____.
   a. Heart, lungs
   b. Blood vessels, breathing
   c. Heart, oxygen level
   d. Lungs, blood vessels
   e. Heart, blood vessels

10. (LO 49.7) The greatest volume of air that can be expelled when a person performs rapid, forced expiration is
    a. Peak expiratory flow
    b. Total lung capacity
    c. Maximum voluntary ventilation
    d. Forced vital capacity
    e. Tidal volume

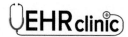

Go to CONNECT to complete the EHRclinic exercises: 49.01 Order an ECG for a Patient and 49.02 Upload an ECG Tracing to a Patient's EHR.

1. Andrea Hochradel arrives to have her Holter monitor removed. She sits down in the exam room, takes the monitor and all the electrodes and wires out of her purse, and plops them on the table. What should you do?

2. John Miller arrives for a pulmonary function test and he has just finished a cigarette. How should you handle this situation?

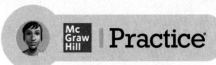

Go to PRACTICE MEDICAL OFFICE and complete the module Clinical: Work Task Proficiencies.

Diagnostic Imaging

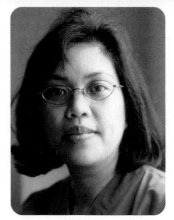
LEARNING OUTCOMES

After completing Chapter 50, you will be able to:

50.1 Explain what X-rays are and how they are used for diagnostic and therapeutic purposes.

50.2 Compare invasive and noninvasive diagnostic procedures.

50.3 Carry out the medical assistant's role in X-ray and diagnostic radiology testing.

50.4 Discuss common diagnostic imaging procedures.

50.5 Describe different types of radiation therapy and how they are used.

50.6 Explain the risks and safety precautions associated with radiology work.

50.7 Relate the advances in medical imaging to EHR.

KEY TERMS

arthrography
barium enema
barium swallow
brachytherapy
cholangiography
contrast medium
diagnostic radiology
dual-energy X-ray absorptiometry (DXA)
intravenous pyelography (IVP)
invasive

KUB radiography
mammography
MUGA scan (nuclear ventriculography)
myelography
noninvasive
nuclear medicine
PET
radiation therapy
retrograde pyelography
SPECT
teletherapy

I.C.9 Analyze pathology for each body system including:
(a) diagnostic measures
(b) treatment modalities

I.P.8 Instruct and prepare a patient for a procedure or a treatment

V.A.4 Explain to a patient the rationale for performance of a procedure

I.A.3 Show awareness of a patient's concerns related to the procedure being performed

2. Anatomy and Physiology
c. Identify diagnostic and treatment modalities as they relate to each body system

7. Administrative Procedures
a. Gather and process documents
f. Maintain inventory of equipment and supplies

8. Clinical Procedures
a. Practice standard precautions and perform disinfection/sterilization techniques

▶ Introduction

Diagnostic radiology has evolved immensely since the discovery of the simple X-ray beam, which has become a valuable screening and clinical diagnostic tool for physicians. In this chapter, you will learn the basics of noninvasive and invasive radiology along with your role as a medical assistant in this testing. Safety issues for the administration of radiologic testing are discussed, as are the proper handling and storage of the films. In addition, you will learn about preparing and instructing patients for the more common radiology procedures.

▶ Brief History of the X-ray   LO 50.1

In 1895, Wilhelm Conrad Roentgen (1845–1923) discovered the X-ray, or roentgen ray, a type of electromagnetic wave. It has a high energy level, traveling at the speed of light (186,000 miles per second), and an extremely short wavelength (one-billionth of an inch) that can penetrate solid objects. X-rays react with photographic film to produce a permanent record (X-ray, or radiograph). The X-ray image is lightest where the film is struck by the least X-ray energy. Differences in tissue densities produce the X-ray image, with the most dense—such as bone—being lightest and the least dense—such as air in the lungs—being darkest on the film.

Today, X-rays and radioactive substances have both diagnostic—such as a wrist X-ray to diagnose a fracture—and therapeutic—such as radiation treatment for cancerous tumors—uses. Radiologic technologists are trained medical personnel, certified to perform certain radiologic procedures upon completion of a 2- to 4-year radiology curriculum. Some radiologic technologists receive further training in radiology subspecialties, such as ultrasound, mammography, magnetic resonance imaging, and nuclear medicine. Radiographers, sonographers, radiation therapists, and nuclear medicine technologists are all radiologic technologists. Invasive radiologic procedures and procedures requiring a high degree of expertise are nearly always performed by a radiologist—a physician who specializes in radiology. A radiologist is also the physician who interprets the films for other physicians. Other specialists who perform radiologic procedures, either alone or with a radiologist's assistance, include cardiologists, orthopedists, obstetricians, and oncologists.

▶ Diagnostic Radiology   LO 50.2

Diagnostic radiology is the use of X-ray technology for diagnostic purposes. Radiologic tests sometimes use contrast media as well as special techniques or instruments for viewing internal body structures and functions. A **contrast medium** is a substance that makes internal organs denser and blocks the passage of X-rays to the photographic film. Introducing contrast media into certain structures or areas of the body can provide a clearer image of organs and tissues and an indication of how well they are functioning. Contrast media include gases (air, oxygen, or carbon dioxide); heavy metal salts (barium sulfate or bismuth carbonate); paramagnetic compounds (substances that are attracted to a magnetic field), which are used for MRI contrast (gadolinium); and iodine compounds. They can be administered orally, parenterally (for example, intravenously), or by routes that introduce them into an organ or a body cavity (for example, by insertion). Types of diagnostic imaging include X-rays, computed tomography (CT), nuclear medicine, magnetic resonance imaging (MRI), and ultrasound.

Invasive Procedures

Diagnostic tests can be invasive or noninvasive. An **invasive** procedure, such as angiography, requires a radiologist to insert a catheter, wire, or other testing device into a patient's blood vessel or organ through the skin or a body orifice. All invasive tests require surgical aseptic technique. Some procedures, including angiography, are performed in a hospital or same-day surgical facility. The patient may need general anesthesia for some procedures. The anesthetist must closely monitor the patient, who is under anesthesia during and after the test, for life-threatening complications such as anaphylaxis.

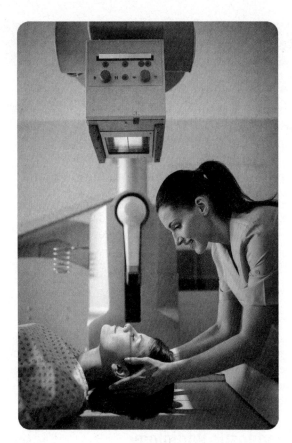

FIGURE 50-1 A standard X-ray is one of the most frequently performed radiologic tests.
©Wavebreakmedia/iStock/Getty Images

Noninvasive Procedures

Noninvasive procedures, such as standard X-rays or ultrasonography, use other technologies to view internal structures. They do not require inserting devices, breaking the skin, or monitoring at the degree needed with invasive procedures.

The most familiar equipment used for diagnostic imaging is the conventional X-ray machine, as shown in Figure 50-1. This machine consists of a table, an X-ray tube, a control panel, and a high-voltage generator. The image produced by a conventional X-ray may be developed on standard X-ray film or captured digitally. Digital radiography is discussed in *section 50.7* of this chapter. Other equipment used for diagnostic radiology includes instruments specifically designed for the test. Examples are a mammography unit, a scanner for CT, and a transducer for ultrasound.

▶ The Medical Assistant's Role in Diagnostic Radiology

LO 50.3

As a medical assistant, you may work with diagnostic radiology in a radiology facility or in a medical office. Your duties in a radiology facility will include assisting a radiologic technologist or a radiologist in performing diagnostic radiologic procedures. Depending on the scope of practice in your state, you may be allowed to learn how to operate certain X-ray equipment. Even if you are not allowed to assist with an X-ray procedure or to operate X-ray equipment, you will probably provide preprocedure and postprocedure patient care. Your duties in an orthopedic office may include assisting a radiologic technologist in performing X-ray procedures. In an obstetric practice, you might assist a physician in performing an ultrasound examination of a pregnant woman. Even if you work in a medical office that does not perform radiologic testing, you still must provide a certain amount of preprocedure care and education. In order to properly explain a test to a patient and to assist a radiologic technologist or radiologist in performing a test, you must have a basic understanding of X-ray technology. You also may need in-service training to ensure accuracy and patient safety for some procedures. See the *Educating the Patient* feature Providing Patient Instruction for Radiologic Procedures.

Preprocedure Care

Preprocedure care varies somewhat, depending on the test. In general, however, you may do the following:

- Schedule the patient's appointment, if necessary. Inform the patient of the location, date, and time of the procedure.

- Provide preparation instructions. Advise the patient about dietary restrictions or requirements (such as fasting or drinking liquids) as well as medication requirements (such as taking a laxative). Always check with the radiology facility for specific requirements and be sure the patient receives this information.

- Explain the procedure to the patient briefly and clearly. Use proper terminology and nontechnical language. Reinforce the doctor's reason for requesting the procedure and provide any available written information about the test. Inform the patient about the length of the examination, possible side effects or safety precautions and warnings, and injections or uncomfortable steps. Check for clarity and understanding by using the mirroring communication technique when communicating with the patient. You must ensure that the patient understands the preprocedure directions.

- Ask pertinent questions. Obtain a medication history from the patient because current medications could interfere with some procedures. If the patient is a woman of childbearing age, ask whether she is pregnant or if there is any chance she could be pregnant. Report the answers to the physician in a medical office or to the radiologic technologist in a radiology facility.

Care During and After the Procedure

If you work in a radiology facility, your responsibilities include preparing and guiding the patient through the procedure. You also may assist the radiologic technologist or the radiologist in performing the procedure by placing, removing, and developing film in the X-ray machine. Procedure 50-1, at the end of this chapter, describes the general process of assisting with a radiologic procedure.

You may care for a patient and assist the radiologic technologist or radiologist during a wide variety of X-ray and other diagnostic imaging tests. While requirements of different procedures vary, you will probably be asked to perform many of the duties described in Procedure 50-1. Although you are unlikely to position the patient, you should know that the position relative to the X-ray source determines the path of the X-rays and the resulting images. Figure 50-2 illustrates common X-ray pathways and the images produced.

Verifying Insurance for Radiologic Procedures

Managed care health insurance plans are the most common type of insurance you will encounter in the office. Patients with HMOs often are required to use the services of certain radiology facilities. Because managed care plans often have facilities with which they are contracted, be sure the patient is sent to a radiology facility that is contracted with his or her health insurance. If needed, verify and complete the necessary referrals for all radiology testing. Make insurance verification a regular step in preprocedure care.

Storing and Filing X-rays

Many X-rays are now stored digitally, but there may be some instances where an actual X-ray film is produced. In this case,

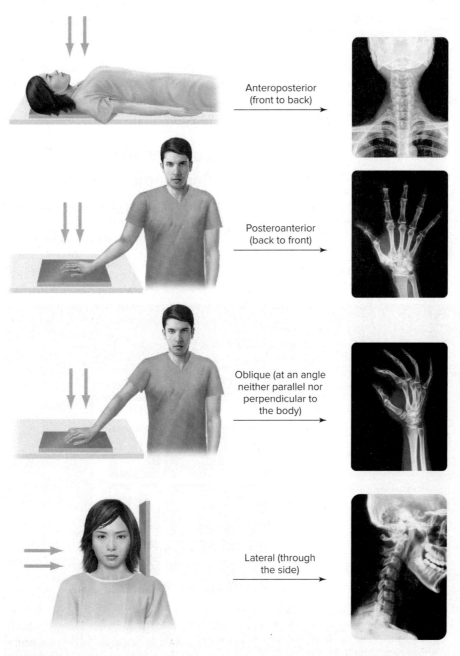

Anteroposterior (front to back)

Posteroanterior (back to front)

Oblique (at an angle neither parallel nor perpendicular to the body)

Lateral (through the side)

FIGURE 50-2 These are X-ray pathways and resulting projections for the most common types of X-rays. (Images are for instruction only. Patients should have protective lead shields during X-ray procedures.)

you may be responsible for storing X-ray films if you work in a radiology facility. Follow these guidelines for proper X-ray storage:

- Keep fresh film on hand at all times.
- Maintain new and exposed films in as good a condition as possible by keeping them at a temperature between 50°F and 70°F (between 10°C and 20°C) and a relative humidity between 30% and 50%. Radiology facilities usually have one or more special rooms for films.

- Prevent pressure marks and keep expiration dates visible by storing packages on end; do not stack them on top of each other.
- Use a first-in, first-out method for using film (that is, use the oldest film first).
- Open film packages or boxes only in the darkroom.
- Do not store film near acid or ammonia vapors.

You also will be responsible for providing accurate record-keeping of X-rays. See Figure 50-3 and Procedure 50-2, at the end of this chapter, for guidelines on documentation and filing techniques.

Remember, X-ray films are the property of the radiology facility or the doctor's office where they are taken. Although the films may be sent (or taken by the patient) to a hospital or another doctor for consultation, they should be returned to the original facility (for example, the radiologist's office). In some facilities, the images are stored on the computer and the patient receives an electronic copy to take to another doctor or medical facility. The information, however, is the patient's property, so the patient need not return reports.

▶ Common Diagnostic Radiologic Tests   LO 50.4

A variety of radiologic imaging tests are available. Table 50-1 identifies some of the most frequently ordered tests and the disorders they are used to diagnose.

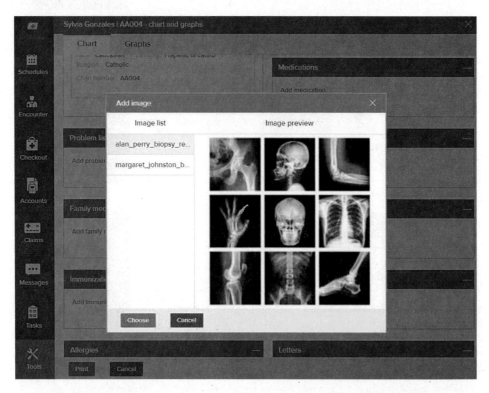

FIGURE 50-3   Patient X-rays are part of the EHR, as shown in this image from ⊍EHRclinic.
©McGraw-Hill Education

TABLE 50-1 Common Radiologic Tests and Disorders Diagnosed

Test	Disorders Diagnosed/Treated
Angiography	
Cardiovascular	Status of blood flow, collateral circulation, malformed vessels, aneurysms, narrowing or blockages of vessels, and presence of hemorrhage
Cerebral	Aneurysm, hemorrhage, evidence of cerebrovascular accident, and arteriosclerosis
Gastrointestinal (GI)	Upper gastrointestinal bleeding
Pulmonary	Pulmonary emboli (especially when lung scan is inconclusive) and evaluation of pulmonary circulation in some heart conditions before surgery
Renal	Abnormalities of blood vessels in urinary system
Arthrography	Joint conditions
Barium enema (lower GI series)	Obstructions, ulcers, polyps, diverticulosis, tumor, and motility problems of colon or rectum
Barium swallow (upper GI series)	Obstructions; ulcers; polyps; diverticulosis; tumor; and motility problems of esophagus, stomach, duodenum, and small intestine
Cholangiography	Gallstones, gallbladder, or common bile duct stones or obstructions and ability of gallbladder to concentrate and store dye
Computed tomography (CT)	Aortic and heart aneurysms, disorders of liver and biliary systems, renal and pulmonary tumors, brain abnormalities (tumors, blood clots, evidence of cerebrovascular accident, outlines of brain ventricles), GI tract lesions, GI disorders (acute pseudocyst of pancreas, abdominal abscesses, biliary obstruction), breast diseases and disorders, spinal disorders, and to guide biopsy procedures
Fluoroscopy	Structure, process, and function of organs in motion to detect abnormalities
HIDA (hepatobiliary) scan	Diagnosis of structural and functional problems with the liver, gallbladder, and bile ducts
Intravenous pyelography (IVP) (excretory urography)	Urinary system abnormalities, including renal pelvis, ureters, and bladder (for example, kidney stones); abnormal size, shape, or structure of kidneys, ureters, or bladder; space-occupying lesions; pyelonephrosis; hydronephrosis; and trauma to the urinary system
KUB (kidneys, ureters, bladder) radiography	Size, shape, and position of urinary organs; urinary system diseases or disorders; and kidney stones
Magnetic resonance imaging (MRI)	Cancerous tissue; atherosclerotic tissue; blood clots; tumors; and deformities, particularly of the heart valves, brain, spine, and joints
Mammography	Breast tumors and lesions
Myelography	Irregularities or compression of spinal cord
Nuclear medicine (radionuclide imaging)	Abnormal function (defects), lesions, or disorders of bone, brain, lungs, kidneys, liver, pancreas, thyroid, and spleen
Radiation therapy	Treatment of cancer
Retrograde pyelogram	Obstruction of ureters, bladder, or urethra (including tumors, stones, strictures, or blood clots) and perinephritic abscess
Ultrasound	Abnormalities of gallbladder, liver, spleen, heart, kidneys, gonads, blood vessels, lymphatic system, and fetal conditions (including number of fetuses; age and sex of fetus; fetal development, position, and deformities)

Contrast Media in Diagnostic Tests

Various procedures involve the use of contrast media to see body structures and observe their function. These procedures include angiography, arthrography, barium enema, barium swallow, cholangiography, cholecystography, cystography, fluoroscopy, hepatobiliary (HIDA) scan, intravenous pyelography, magnetic resonance imaging (sometimes), myelography, nuclear medicine studies, and retrograde pyelography.

As mentioned, contrast media can be administered by mouth, by needle or catheter into a blood vessel, or by a route that introduces the medium into an organ or a body cavity

(for example, into the colon). A contrast medium can cause adverse effects in some patients. Common adverse effects with oral agents include mild and transient abdominal cramping, constipation, nausea, vomiting, diarrhea, skin rashes, itching, heartburn, dizziness, and headache. Intravenous agents cause some of the same adverse effects, as well as localized injection-site reactions and more serious reactions such as anaphylaxis. Because many contrast media contain iodine, a common allergen, patients should be questioned about known allergies to iodine or shellfish, which contain iodine, before procedures involving the use of contrast media. All patients should be observed during such procedures for signs of allergic reaction.

Fluoroscopy

X-rays can cause certain chemicals to fluoresce, or emit visible light. When X-rays penetrate a body structure and are directed onto a fluorescent screen, they produce an image the radiologist can view either directly or through special glasses. Usually, a radiologist, rather than a radiology technician or medical assistant, performs fluoroscopic procedures.

Many diagnostic procedures involve fluoroscopy, which allows viewing of internal organ movement or the movement of a contrast medium, such as barium sulfate, while the contrast medium travels through the alimentary canal. Fluoroscopy also guides the radiologist in locating a precise internal area that needs to be recorded on film or digitally.

Fluoroscopic images are sometimes photographed for further study. Photofluorography is a series of these photographs that records the body's internal movements over time. Cinefluorography is a motion picture of the internal movements of the body.

Hysterosalpingography

Hysterosalpingography, also called uterosalpingography, is a radiologic examination of a woman's uterus and fallopian tubes using fluoroscopy. This procedure is used to examine women who have difficulty becoming pregnant. It is sometimes ordered as part of a fertility exam or when the woman has a history of miscarriages that result from congenital abnormalities of the uterus. It also is used to determine the presence and severity of tumor masses or adhesions, uterine fibroids, and fallopian tube adhesions or obstructions. A hysterosalpingogram (Figure 50-4) assists the radiologist in evaluating the shape and structure of the uterus, the openness (patency) of the fallopian tubes, and any scarring within the fallopian tubes and peritoneal cavity. Hysterosalpingography is usually performed on an outpatient basis.

Angiography

Angiography is a test used to diagnose abnormalities in blood vessels, including the following:

- Aneurysm—a widening or ballooning of an artery.
- Atherosclerotic disease—fatty plaques on the walls of arteries.
- Arteriovenous malformations (AVM)—abnormal connections between arteries and veins.
- Arterial stenosis—narrowing of an artery.

The test is done in one of three ways:

- Catheter angiography with X-rays
- CT angiography
- MRI angiography

Catheter angiography requires a physician (usually a radiologist) to insert a catheter into the patient's vein (venography) or artery (arteriography). The physician first guides the catheter tip to the vessel being examined, then injects a contrast medium through the catheter and takes a series of X-rays to assess the vessel's blood flow and condition (Figure 50-5). The test—used to evaluate the heart vessels (coronary angiography); the brain (cerebral angiography); or the femoral, brachial, or carotid artery—may be performed jointly by a radiologist and a vascular surgeon or other specialist.

Because this procedure requires insertion of a catheter into a blood vessel and the use of local anesthesia, the patient is admitted to a hospital or same-day surgical facility. The physician who performs the examination provides the patient with instructions immediately before the procedure. You, however,

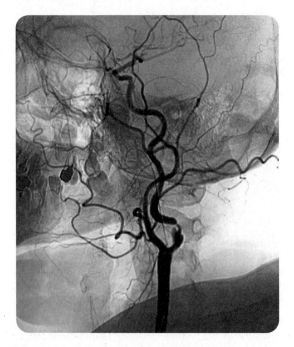

FIGURE 50-5 Carotid angiogram: an intra-arterial catheter is inserted and a contrast medium is injected to create an image of the arteries.

©Science Photo Library/Alamy Stock Photo

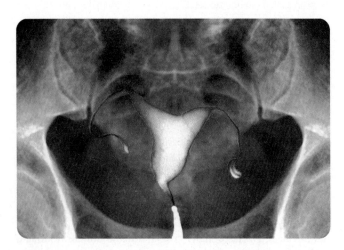

FIGURE 50-4 A hysterosalpingogram of the uterus and fallopian tubes.

©ISM/Phototake

will schedule the procedure, and you can encourage the patient to ask questions. Radiology facilities usually have information sheets for each procedure. If the patient has questions you cannot answer or if you have any doubt about preprocedure instructions, check with your supervisor.

CT and MRI angiography (MRA) may be performed with or without contrast medium. The contrast medium is injected into a vein, usually in the arm, and images are made using computer programs that produce detailed images of blood vessels. Because CT and MRI angiography are less invasive than catheter angiography, they are usually performed on an outpatient basis. CT and MRI are discussed in more detail later in this section.

Arthrography

Arthrography is performed by a radiologist, who uses a contrast medium and fluoroscopy to help diagnose abnormalities or injuries in the cartilage, tendons, or ligaments of the joints—usually the knee or shoulder. Although MRI is used more often to evaluate soft-tissue injuries in joints, arthrography can provide an image while the patient moves the joint. When preparing patients for arthrography or assisting with the procedure, follow these guidelines:

- Describe the procedure to patients and inform them the examination will take about 1 hour. Ask patients about possible allergies to contrast media, iodine, or shellfish. If they have any of these allergies, inform the radiologist immediately.

- Explain to patients that no special preprocedure preparations are necessary.

- Tell patients the doctor will first inject a local anesthetic to numb the area being examined. Then the doctor will inject the contrast medium (dye, air, or both) into the joint and will use a fluoroscope to evaluate the joint's function. Inform patients who are having a knee examined that the doctor may ask them to walk a few steps to spread the contrast medium.

- After the test is completed, advise patients that for 1 or 2 days they may experience some pain or swelling, particularly if the joint is exercised. Tell them to rest and avoid putting strain on the joint.

Barium Enema (Lower GI Series)

A **barium enema** is performed by a radiologist, who instills barium sulfate through the anus into the rectum and then into the colon, to help diagnose and evaluate obstructions, ulcers, polyps, diverticuloses, tumors, or motility problems of the colon or rectum. This procedure is called a *lower GI (gastrointestinal) series*—a series of X-rays of the colon and rectum. The two types of barium enema techniques are single-contrast, in which only barium is instilled into the colon, and double-contrast, in which air is forced into the colon to distend or inflate the tissue. The air may be added while the barium is present, after it has been expelled, or both. The double-contrast technique makes structures more visible by fluoroscopy and allows identification of small lesions. The digestive tract must be totally empty, requiring the patient to thoroughly cleanse the tract with a series of preparatory steps and to have nothing by mouth for 8 hours before the test, except for 1 cup of clear liquid on the morning of the test. In most facilities, a radiologic technologist assists with a barium enema, but you may assist the patient before and after the procedure. If you do assist with a barium enema, you will have various responsibilities before, during, and after the procedure.

Before the Procedure Schedule the patient's appointment in the morning so that he can sleep through most of the period during which his digestive tract must be empty and thus avoid experiencing hunger unnecessarily. Include the following items when you instruct a patient about the preparation for a barium enema:

- Describe the procedure and tell the patient the examination will take 1 to 2 hours.

- Ask about possible allergies to contrast media, iodine, or shellfish and report such allergies to the radiologist.

- Explain the importance of following the preparation instructions so that the colon and rectum are free of residual material. Residual material in the colon or rectum could cause blockages or shadows, resulting in an inaccurate test.

- Preprocedure preparation on the day before the examination includes following a clear liquid diet beginning in the morning (coffee, tea, carbonated beverages, clear gelatin, strained fruit juice, bouillon, or clear broths; milk is not permitted) and taking prescribed amounts of electrolyte solution or other laxative preparations and fluids on a specified schedule.

- Tell the patient he may take his usual medications with a small amount of water on the morning of the examination.

During the Procedure Follow these steps when assisting during a barium enema:

1. Have the patient undress and put on a gown.

2. Tell the patient to expect some discomfort during the examination, as well as frequent side-to-side turning.

3. Have the patient lie on his side. The radiologist inserts the enema tip, designed to help the patient hold the liquid, into the rectum and instills the barium sulfate into the colon. If the patient experiences cramping or the urge to defecate during instillation of the barium, instruct him to relax the abdominal muscles by breathing slowly and deeply through the mouth.

4. Instruct the patient to remain still and hold his breath when X-rays are taken. Using a fluoroscope, the doctor observes the barium as it flows through the lower bowel and periodically takes X-rays while the patient is placed in various positions. You may be asked to assist with placing the patient in these positions.

5. If a double-contrast study is being performed, tell the patient that air will be introduced into the colon to expand the colon tissue. Explain that the combination of air and barium provides a clearer view of structures than only one contrast medium would provide and allows possible identification of small lesions if they are present.

6. When the doctor has completed the barium portion of the examination, including X-rays with both barium and air, tell the patient to use the toilet and expel as much barium as possible. Explain that if enough barium is expelled, the doctor may take a final X-ray of the empty colon.

7. Have the patient wait to dress until the doctor tells you that no additional X-rays are needed.

After the Procedure After the radiologist has completed the barium enema, instruct the patient in postprocedure care. Tell the patient the following:

- He may now have a regular meal.
- The residual barium may make his stools appear whitish or lighter than usual, but this is normal.
- The barium may cause constipation, so he should drink extra water to help relieve constipation and to eliminate the remaining barium sulfate. The physician may order a laxative to be taken if constipation is not relieved within 1 or 2 days.

Barium Swallow (Upper GI Series)

A **barium swallow** involves oral administration of a barium sulfate drink to help diagnose and evaluate obstructions, ulcers, polyps, tumors, or motility problems of the esophagus, stomach, duodenum, and small intestine. This test is called an *upper GI series*. In preparation for this test, the patient can have nothing by mouth for at least 8 hours before the test. You will have various responsibilities before, during, and after the procedure.

Before the Procedure Schedule the patient's appointment in the morning so that she can sleep through most of the period during which her digestive tract is empty and thus avoid experiencing hunger unnecessarily. When instructing a patient about the preparation for an upper GI series, include the following items:

- Describe the procedure and tell the patient the examination will take about 1 hour. If X-rays of the small bowel are needed, the test may take several hours.
- Ask about possible allergies to contrast media, iodine, or shellfish and report such allergies to the radiologist.
- Explain the importance of following the preparation instructions so that the stomach is empty. Preprocedure requirements include having nothing by mouth (food or liquids) after midnight the night before and no breakfast the morning of the examination. If the patient's small bowel is to be evaluated, also tell her to take the prescribed laxative preparation between 2:00 and 4:00 p.m. the day before the examination.
- Instruct the patient not to swallow water when brushing her teeth or rinsing her mouth and, if applicable, to stop smoking because nicotine stimulates gastric secretions and can affect the test results.

During the Procedure When assisting during an upper GI series, take the following steps:

1. Have the patient undress and put on a gown.
2. Explain that she will be drinking a barium sulfate drink that tastes chalky and resembles a milkshake.

3. Have the patient stand and drink part of the barium.
4. The radiologist will use a fluoroscope to observe the flow of the barium and to assess the functioning of the esophagus, stomach, duodenum, and small intestine as the barium passes through the structures. (The doctor will then direct the patient to drink additional barium and continue to observe the function of the various structures.)
5. Place the patient on the X-ray table and move her into different positions (if medical assistants are permitted to do so in your state), as instructed by the doctor, to allow X-rays to be taken of the upper digestive tract. Instruct the patient to remain still and hold her breath when X-rays are taken.

After the Procedure After the physician completes the upper GI series, instruct the patient in postprocedure care. Give the patient the following information:

- She may now have a regular meal.
- Her stools may appear whitish or lighter than usual as the barium is eliminated, but this is normal.
- Sometimes, another examination is required after 24 hours to determine whether the barium has moved into the large intestine. If this test is indicated, tell the patient to follow a clear liquid diet (coffee, tea, carbonated beverages, clear gelatin, strained fruit juices, bouillon, or clear broths; milk is not permitted) and to return in 24 hours.

Cholangiography

Cholangiography is performed by a radiologist to evaluate the function of the bile ducts. It involves injection of the contrast medium directly into the common bile duct (during gallbladder surgery) or through a T tube (after gallbladder surgery or during radiologic testing). X-rays or MRIs are taken immediately after injection. Instruct the patient as follows:

- Describe the procedure to the patient and tell him the examination will take about 2 to 3 hours. Ask the patient about possible allergies to contrast media, iodine, or shellfish and report them to the radiologist.
- Explain the preparation instructions. Tell the patient to eat a light evening meal the night before the examination, to take a laxative (as prescribed by the doctor), and to have no food or liquids after midnight. He also should have no solid food the morning of the examination.

Computed Tomography (CT)

Computed tomography (CT) scans are produced by a specialized X-ray camera that rotates completely around the patient and a computer that compiles one cross-sectional view from each rotation of the camera. The patient is lying on a table that gradually moves through the doughnut-shaped machine containing the rotating camera. Cross-sectional images can be reconfigured by a computer program into different planes (frontal, transverse, and sagittal), creating images that give different views of the same area. The images also can be combined to create three-dimensional images.

CT scans are used to diagnose abnormalities in almost all body structures, including the head, kidneys, heart, chest, liver, biliary tract, pancreas, GI tract, spine, pelvis, bones, and breast. Abnormalities and disorders that can be detected using CT scans include the following:

- Cancer
- Injuries from trauma
- Spinal injury
- Pulmonary embolism (blood clot in the vessels of the lung)
- Aortic aneurysm
- Skeletal injuries and abnormalities

When preparing the patient for a CT scan:

- Ask the patient about possible allergies to contrast media, iodine, or shellfish and report them to the radiologist.
- Tell the patient he will be placed on a table that moves through the scanner but he will be able to see around the room during the test.
- Inform the patient that the procedure will last about 45 to 90 minutes and that he must lie still while the scans are taken.
- If a contrast medium will be used, advise the patient that it will be injected into a vein in the arm or on the back of the hand (except with a CT scan of the spine) to enhance detail of the structure being evaluated.
- If the patient is having a CT scan of the head, chest, abdomen, or pelvis, instruct him not to eat anything for 4 hours or drink any liquids for 2 hours before the examination. Explain that he may experience mild nausea after injection of the contrast medium if the stomach is too full.
- Tell the patient to remove metallic objects that could interfere with the path of the X-rays. Also, ask if the patient has skin staples or metallic prostheses that could interfere.
- Inform the patient that a written report of the results should be available within 24 hours of the test and that a report will be sent to his primary care physician (or the referring physician).

Intravenous Pyelography

Also known as *excretory urography*, **intravenous pyelography (IVP)** is performed by a radiologist who injects a contrast medium into a vein. The doctor then takes a series of X-rays as the contrast medium travels through the kidneys, ureters, and bladder. IVP is used to evaluate urinary system abnormalities or trauma to the urinary system. In most facilities, a radiologic technologist assists with IVP, but you may assist the patient before the procedure. If you assist with IVP, you will have several responsibilities both before and during the procedure.

Before the Procedure Schedule the patient's appointment in the morning so that she can sleep through most of the period during which her digestive tract is empty and thus avoid experiencing hunger unnecessarily. When instructing a patient about the preparation for an IVP, include the following information:

- Describe the procedure and tell the patient the examination will take about 1½ hours.
- Ask the patient about possible allergies to contrast media, iodine, or shellfish and report such allergies to the radiologist.
- Explain the importance of adhering to the preparation instructions so that the bowel is free of any material that could obstruct the view of the urinary organs.
- Tell the patient to follow a liquid diet (coffee, tea, carbonated beverages, clear gelatin, strained fruit juice, bouillon, or clear broths, but no milk) the day before the examination. The patient may be given a laxative preparation to take the night before the examination.
- No food or liquids are allowed after midnight and no breakfast the morning of the examination. Some physicians also order an enema to be taken about 2 hours before the examination.

During and After the Procedure When assisting during an IVP, you will generally proceed in this manner:

1. Have the patient undress and put on a gown.
2. Explain that a contrast medium will be injected into her vein (usually in the arm). Instruct her to inform the physician if she notices shortness of breath or itching after injection of the dye because this can indicate an allergic reaction.
3. Have the patient lie on the X-ray table and move her into different positions, as instructed by the physician, to allow X-rays to be taken of the urinary tract as the contrast medium is excreted. Instruct the patient to remain still and hold her breath when X-rays are taken.
4. Note that some physicians place a compression device on the abdomen, which helps hold the contrast medium in the kidneys and ureters by exerting moderate pressure.
5. After the physician takes the series of X-rays to evaluate urinary system function, ask the patient to urinate, and explain that a final X-ray will be taken.
6. Inform the patient that she may resume a normal diet after the test and that the contrast medium will be eliminated in the urine.

Retrograde Pyelography

Retrograde pyelography is similar to the IVP, except that the doctor injects the contrast medium through a urethral catheter. This procedure, which evaluates function of the ureters, bladder, and urethra, is often used for patients with poor kidney function. Follow the same preparation and assistance instructions as for the IVP.

Kidneys, Ureters, and Bladder (KUB) Radiography

Also called a *flat plate of the abdomen*, **KUB radiography** is an X-ray of the abdomen used to assess the size, shape, and position of the urinary organs; to evaluate urinary system diseases or disorders; and to determine the presence of kidney stones. It also can be helpful in determining the position of an intrauterine device (IUD) or in locating foreign bodies in the digestive tract. No patient preparation is required. A radiologic technologist takes a KUB X-ray; thus, you follow the guidelines you would use for a patient having any type of standard, noninvasive X-ray.

Magnetic Resonance Imaging (MRI)

Magnetic resonance imaging (MRI) uses a strong magnetic field and radio frequency signals in combination with a computer to allow the physician to examine internal structures and soft tissues. The combination of nonionizing (radio frequency) radiation and a magnetic field allows the MRI scanner to produce images based primarily on the water content of tissues, making MRI a useful imaging tool for soft tissues. Because no ionizing radiation (X-ray) is used to produce the image, the risk of harmful effects to the patient is very low. The test may be performed with or without contrast. You will be responsible for preparing the patient for an MRI and assisting with the procedure.

Before the Procedure When instructing a patient about preparing for an MRI, include the following steps:

* If a contrast medium is going to be used, ask the patient and inform the radiologist about possible allergies to contrast media, iodine, or shellfish.

* Screen the patient to determine whether any internal metallic materials are present. (This is especially important because a strong magnetic field is involved in creating the image.) Ask about a pacemaker, brain or aneurysm clips, brain or heart surgery, shunts and heart valves, other surgeries, and shrapnel or metal fragments (particularly in an eye).

* Ask the patient whether he is or has been a metalworker. If so, he may carry metal slivers, chips, or filings under his nails or skin.

* Instruct women not to wear eye makeup the day of the examination, as it often contains metallic ingredients that can cause artifacts on MRI images of the head.

* Describe the procedure to the patient and explain that the examination will take between 45 minutes and 2 hours.

* Inform the patient that he may wear street clothing during the test but to avoid wearing clothing with metallic thread, metal stays or zippers, or thick elastic. Tell the patient that depending upon the location to be examined, he could be asked to undress and put on a gown.

* Tell the patient he does not need to fast before the examination or follow any preprocedure diet, unless he is having an MRI of the pelvis. In that case, instruct him to have no solid food for 6 hours and no liquids for 4 hours before the examination. Inform the patient that he may take prescription medications.

* Explain that he will not be required to drink an oral contrast preparation but should avoid caffeine for 4 hours before the examination. Tell the patient he will probably have no side effects from the examination but that some nausea may occur as a result of the contrast medium.

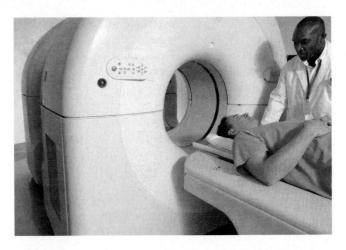

FIGURE 50-6 A patient who is claustrophobic or unable to lie still may require sedation during an MRI.
©UpperCut Images/SuperStock

During and After the Procedure When assisting during an MRI, you will need to follow these specific steps:

1. Have the patient lie on the padded table.

2. Explain that the table will be placed inside a long, narrow tube about 22 inches in diameter and that he will hear a loud knocking noise as the machine scans. Offer the patient hearing protection devices (ear plugs or headphones) during the test. Warn the patient to remain still to avoid blurring the image and the consequent need for a retake. Note that physicians may order sedation for patients who are claustrophobic or cannot lie still for a long period (Figure 50-6).

3. Advise the patient that although the technician will not be in the scanning room during the examination, she will maintain contact with a camera and a microphone. The patient may speak to the technician at any time in case of a problem, but he is encouraged to be still for each series.

4. Inform the patient that his primary care physician or referring doctor should have a preliminary report of test results within about 24 hours.

Mammography

Mammography, the X-ray exam of the internal breast tissues, helps in diagnosing breast abnormalities (Figure 50-7). A specially trained radiologic technologist takes mammograms.

You will have several responsibilities during both setup and patient care before and after mammography. However, a medical assistant does not assist during mammography in most states. Instead, you will prepare the patient for the procedure and ease her fears. For more information regarding patient education before a mammogram, see the *Assisting in Reproductive and Urinary Specialties* chapter.

Stereotactic Breast Biopsy

When a mammogram reveals an abnormality in the breast tissue, the physician may want a biopsy to determine if it is malignant. Because so many abnormalities revealed by mammography are benign and present no health risk, physicians

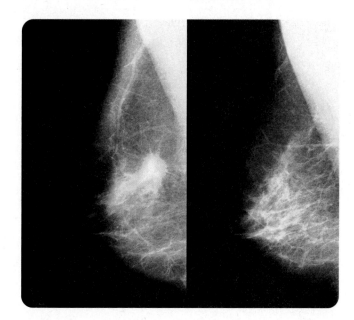

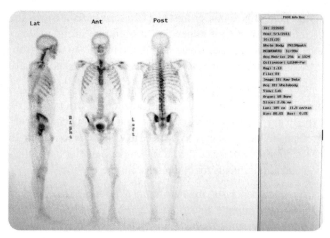

FIGURE 50-7 Mammograms can reveal the presence of tumors that are not detected by other means. The mammogram on the right indicates normal breast tissue, whereas the one on the left suggests a malignancy.
©UHB Trust/Getty Images

now perform *stereotactic breast biopsies,* which are less painful and less invasive than conventional excisional biopsies. The procedure is performed by a physician and a radiologic technologist and is similar to mammography, except that the patient is usually lying face down or sitting rather than standing. The breast is compressed with a compression paddle to confirm that the area of the breast with the lesion is correctly centered in the paddle window. X-rays are taken of the breast from two different angles. A computer is used to help determine the exact positioning of the biopsy needle and the physician uses a needle to take a small sample of tissue for examination by a pathologist. The attending physician later contacts the patient with the test results.

Myelography

Although MRI is used more often to evaluate the spinal cord and spinal nerves, **myelography** is a kind of fluoroscopy of the spinal cord used when MRI is not practical—if a patient has a pacemaker or other medical device that prevents the patient from undergoing MRI. The physician performs a lumbar puncture, removes some cerebrospinal fluid (CSF), and instills a contrast medium to evaluate spinal abnormalities, such as compression of the spinal cord. Sometimes the physician performs pneumoencephalography, which involves instilling air after removal of the CSF to allow viewing of the cerebral cavities.

The physician who performs myelography or pneumoencephalography must be skilled in performing lumbar puncture—most likely a radiologist, neurologist, neurosurgeon, or anesthetist. A radiologic technologist is typically the only other person present for the test. Although myelography is not used as frequently as it was before the invention of CT and MRI, it is still performed when these newer techniques do not provide enough information about the spinal canal. Myelography

may be reserved for cases in which the clinical findings are unusual or the scanning results uncertain.

Nuclear Medicine

Also known as *radionuclide imaging,* **nuclear medicine** involves the use of radionuclides, or radioisotopes (radioactive elements or their compounds). The radionuclides are administered orally, intravenously, or through routes that introduce them into organs or body cavities. The purpose is to evaluate the bone, brain, lungs, kidneys, liver, pancreas, thyroid, or spleen. Sometimes, the entire body is scanned for "hot spots," or places where the radioisotope is concentrated.

For common nuclear medicine scans, the technician uses a scanner called a *gamma camera.* This scanner detects radiation from the radioisotope and converts it into an image (called a *scintiscan* or *scintigram*) to be photographed or displayed on a screen (see Figure 50-8). Some images are produced immediately, whereas others take up to several days. Radionuclide imaging exposes patients to lower doses of radiation than some radiologic techniques because the amount of ionizing radiation in the isotope is less than that emitted from X-ray cameras. Other nuclear medicine procedures include single photon emission computed tomography (SPECT), positron emission tomography (PET), and MUGA (multiple gated acquisition) scan.

- **SPECT** is often used to locate and determine the extent of brain damage from a stroke. The gamma camera detects signals induced by gamma radiation and a computer converts these signals into either two- or three-dimensional images that are displayed on a screen.

- **PET** entails injecting isotopes combined with other substances involved in metabolic activity, such as glucose. These special isotopes emit positrons, which a computer processes and displays on a screen. PET is especially useful for diagnosing brain-related conditions such as epilepsy, mental illnesses, and Parkinson's disease.

- **MUGA scan (nuclear ventriculography)**—evaluates the condition of the heart's myocardium. It can be done while the patient is at rest or in stress (exercise) and involves the injection of radioisotopes that concentrate in the myocardium. The gamma camera allows the physician to measure ventricular contractions to evaluate the patient's heart wall.

When preparing a patient for a nuclear medicine procedure, describe the procedure and explain how long it will take. Also, explain any preparation requirements and other special instructions and tell the patient she will need to wait the required length of time for the uptake of the radioisotope. Length of examination and requirements for common scans are as follows:

- A bone scan lasts about 1 hour; it is done 2 to 3 hours after a 15-minute injection; the patient drinks 1 quart of liquid between the injection and the scan; a normal diet is permitted.

- A liver/spleen or lung scan lasts approximately 1 hour; there are no dietary restrictions.

- A kidney scan lasts about 2 hours; there are no dietary restrictions.

- A thyroid uptake and scan test usually requires 2 days; the patient takes a capsule of contrast medium in the morning and has the scan on the first day; the patient returns 24 hours later for the second scan; there are no dietary restrictions, except the patient must have no fish because of its natural iodine content.

Ultrasound

Ultrasound directs high-frequency sound waves through the skin over the area of the body being examined and produces an image based on the echoes created by the sound waves bouncing off of body structures. A radiologist or an ultrasound sonographer coats the body area with a special gel and passes a transducer (instrument similar to a microphone) over the area. As the transducer passes back and forth, it picks up echoes from the sound waves, which a computer converts into an image—sometimes called a sonogram—on a screen. Ultrasound is used to detect abnormalities in the gallbladder, liver, spleen, heart, and kidneys. It is also safe to use in obstetrics to evaluate the developing fetus or to detect multiple fetuses because it does not expose the patient (or the fetus) to radiation (Figure 50-9). In this case, the obstetrician may perform the test in the office.

One form of ultrasound—Doppler echocardiography— involves sound waves that echo against the flow of blood through vessels. Doppler echocardiography is usually performed by a cardiologist to determine whether blood flow is laminar (normal) or turbulent (disturbed).

Echocardiography, a type of ultrasound test, is used to study the structure and function of the heart. The test is usually performed while the patient is resting and again after exercising on a treadmill or bicycle. Images of the heart before and after exercise help the physician diagnose abnormalities of the structure and function of the heart and heart valves.

When preparing the patient for an ultrasound or assisting with the examination, follow these guidelines:

- Describe the procedure to the patient and inform her that the examination will take about 1½ to 2 hours, depending on the type of ultrasound. For example, a cardiac

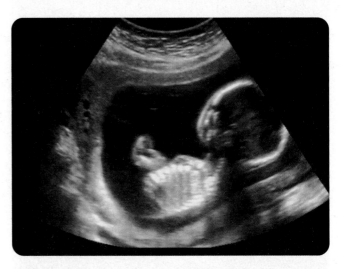

FIGURE 50-9 Ultrasound is commonly used to evaluate the health of a developing fetus.
©GagliardiImages/Shutterstock

ultrasound takes about 1½ hours; pelvic, 1 to 2 hours; and abdominal, ½ to 1 hour.

- Explain the preparation requirements, which vary according to the type of ultrasound. Tell a patient who is having a gallbladder or liver ultrasound not to eat for several hours before the test. Tell a pregnant patient to drink the prescribed amount of water 1 hour before the examination and not to void. Advise a patient having a pelvic ultrasound to take the prescribed laxative (if indicated), drink three to four glasses of water within 1 hour, and not to void within 1 hour of the test. If the patient is having an abdominal ultrasound, instruct her to take a laxative the night before the examination and not to have any food or fluids for 8 hours before the test.

- Advise the patient to wear loose, easy-to-remove clothing.

Dual-Energy X-ray Absorptiometry (DXA)

Dual-energy X-ray absorptiometry (DXA), often called bone densitometry, is a screening test that uses small doses of X-rays to determine the mineral density of a person's bones. The test may be used to diagnose osteoporosis or to monitor treatment of osteoporosis or other conditions that cause bone loss after diagnosis. Patients who take medications known to cause bone loss, such as Dilantin®, corticosteroids, and some barbiturates, should be screened for bone loss using DXA. Bone densitometry is also recommended for people with the following conditions:

- Postmenopausal women
- Smokers
- Hyperthyroidism
- Hyperparathyroidism
- Type 1 diabetes
- Kidney disease
- Recurrent fractures

During the test, the patient will lie on a padded table while very low-dose radiation is generated below the table and detected with a specialized arm that passes over the patient. The patient must lie very still while the test is being performed. DXA is usually completed within 30 minutes.

When instructing patients preparing for a DXA, tell them to wear loose-fitting clothing that does not have zippers, metal buttons, or belts. Patients will be asked to remove wallets, keys, or jewelry in the area being scanned. Tell patients they should avoid taking calcium supplements 24 hours before the test. A patient who has recently had X-rays or CT scans using a contrast medium such as barium may need to wait 2 weeks after the contrast before having a DXA scan.

The test is most often read by a radiologist; however, rheumatologists and endocrinologists also can read DXA scans. The report includes two results: the T score and the Z score. The T score is a measure of the amount of bone the person has compared to that of young adults. This number is used to assess risk of bone fractures. The Z score is the amount of bone the patient has compared to people of the same race, gender, age, and size. If the Z score test is high or low, additional medical tests for other underlying conditions, such as hyperparathyroidism, may be needed.

▶ Common Therapeutic Uses of Radiation   LO 50.5

Used therapeutically, radiology is called **radiation therapy,** which is used to treat cancer by preventing cellular reproduction. The two types of radiation therapy are teletherapy and brachytherapy. **Teletherapy,** also called external beam radiotherapy, is the most common form of radiation therapy and is done on an outpatient basis. It allows deep penetration of tissues and is used primarily for deep tumors. The patient experiences minimal side effects, which may include a "sunburn" effect at the treatment site, mild swelling and tenderness, and sometimes mild fatigue. Generally, the superficial tissues are not permanently damaged.

Stereotactic radiosurgery is a type of teletherapy that uses CT or MRI scanning in conjunction with radiation to treat brain tumors, acoustic neuromas, and arteriovenous malformations—defects in connections between arteries and veins—deep in the brain. In some cases, liver, prostate, and lung tumors also are treated with stereotactic radiosurgery. This method allows for very precise delivery of radiation to areas of the brain or other organs that are normally inaccessible with traditional surgical techniques, helping spare precious healthy tissue while still treating the tumor.

For a patient having stereotactic radiosurgery for brain tumors, first a neurosurgeon temporarily fastens a stereotactic frame to the patient's head using local anesthesia. The frame helps guide the physician to precisely locate the treatment. A CT or MRI scan is then performed to locate the tumor or malformation. Once the frame is in place and the imaging scan is complete, a radiation oncologist and a neurosurgeon plan the patient's treatment. The patient undergoes treatment based on this plan, has the stereotactic frame removed, and, in most cases, can go home the same day.

Localized cancers are treated with **brachytherapy.** In this technique, the radiologist places temporary radioactive implants close to or directly into cancerous tissue. This technique limits radiation exposure to healthy tissue, targeting only the area where the tumor is located. During brachytherapy, both the staff and the patient are subject to radiation exposure, so radiation safety precautions must be closely followed. When preparing the patient for radiation therapy, follow these guidelines:

- Describe the procedure and explain how long it will take, as determined by the radiologist and oncologist according to the patient's diagnosis and condition.
- Encourage patients to tell the physician about all medications, vitamins, or supplements they are taking.
- Inform the patient that the radiologist or oncologist will explain the treatment's possible side effects. Common side effects include nausea, vomiting, hair loss, ulceration of mucous membranes, weakness, and malaise. Other possible effects include localized burns on tissue and damage to organs in the treatment path. Encourage the patient to discuss with the doctor (or the oncology nurse specialist) measures to relieve or minimize stress and discomfort.
- Advise the patient to immediately report any other symptoms to the doctor.
- Encourage the patient to get plenty of rest, eat a balanced diet, and drink plenty of fluids.

▶ Radiation Safety and Dose   LO 50.6

For many years after the X-ray's discovery, the seriousness of radiation hazards was not addressed. In the 1920s, the government of Great Britain took the first steps to limit X-ray exposure. Since World War II, studies have been performed, mostly on the effects of high-dose radiation.

Other studies on the effects of background radiation and nonradiologic versus radiologic (X-ray-related) risks have enabled scientists to assess diagnostic X-ray risks. Results from these studies show the risk of excess radiation from routine X-rays to be minimal.

Reducing Patient Exposure

Advances in diagnostic imaging technology and limits to radiation exposure have helped reduce the dose of radiation to which a patient is exposed during a diagnostic procedure. Another way to reduce excessive radiation exposure risk lies with the physician, who must assess the benefit-to-risk ratio when recommending a diagnostic radiology procedure. Because radiation has a cumulative effect, the physician must have valid medical reasons for ordering the test, particularly if the patient has recently had other X-rays. Some types of X-rays, such as mammograms, should be repeated regularly, however, because of their potential to prevent or promote treatment of life-threatening disorders.

According to a 1993 report by the National Council on Radiation Protection and Measurements (NCRP) titled *Limitation of Exposure to Ionizing Radiation,* one of the earliest pieces of legislation in the United States to limit occupational radiation exposure was enacted in the 1930s. The first legislation to limit public exposure, however, was not enacted until the 1950s.

Safety with X-rays

You are responsible for teaching the patient about X-ray safety. In this role, you will need to obtain pertinent patient history data, answer questions, and provide basic information on X-rays, possible side effects, and other important guidelines. Consider the following points when teaching the patient about X-ray safety.

Patient History

- Ask the patient about X-rays received in the past, including how many and what type, and about the possibility of exposure to radiation in the home, school, or workplace. Explain that the effects of radiation exposure are cumulative; that is, the effects are related to total exposure over the lifetime as well as to exposure from each procedure.

- Ask a female patient about the possibility of pregnancy. Use the 10-day rule—take an X-ray only within 10 days of the last menstrual period to avoid taking an X-ray of a patient who is unknowingly pregnant. If the patient knows she is pregnant, do not schedule an X-ray unless approved by the radiologist.

- Inform the patient about possible radiation exposure side effects, which include fetal abnormality or genetic mutation in a fetus (when a patient is pregnant) and the depression of bone marrow activity, which decreases the production of red blood cells and white blood cells.

Patient Questions

- Always answer questions in simple, easy-to-understand language; make explanations brief and clear. Do not use complex medical terms; however, do include proper terminology. Offer written information about the test, if available.

- Answer fully any questions about examinations, including descriptions of procedures; the doctor's reason for ordering them; their length, side effects, injections, or other uncomfortable aspects; preprocedure requirements; cost and insurance issues; and availability of test results.

- Help reduce the patient's fear or anxiety surrounding the scheduled test and help her feel comfortable and informed about the procedure.

General X-ray Information

- Be aware of the most current guidelines established by the American College of Radiology. Always keep up with new studies on radiation exposure risks.

- Encourage the patient to ask questions about the need for X-rays ordered by the doctor and risks associated with those X-rays.

- If the patient's employer requires annual X-rays or a potential employer asks for preemployment X-rays, advise the patient to question the necessity of these tests.

- Suggest that the patient find out whether the doctor has submittable X-rays on file.

- Advise the patient to discuss testing options with the doctor. For instance, if the doctor orders fluoroscopy, the patient might ask whether standard X-rays can be taken instead, as fluoroscopy, and often mobile X-ray exams, usually carry a higher radiation exposure risk than standard X-rays. Advise the patient to ask questions about X-ray safety standards in the office or hospital in which the tests are to take place.

- Tell the patient to avoid dental X-rays performed with wide-beamed plastic cones; narrow-beamed cones are more exact and less dangerous. In addition, educate the patient about the opinions of the American Dental Association and the National Conference of Dental Radiology, both of which believe X-rays should not be performed solely for insurance claim purposes. Advise the patient to always ask for a lead apron over organs not being studied. Tell the patient to avoid retakes of X-rays because of blurriness or shadows (which are caused by movements or breathing) by remaining still when instructed to do so during X-ray exams.

- Explain the importance of X-rays in proper diagnosis of disorders. Inform the patient about the constant improvements in equipment and X-ray procedures and the much lower doses of radiation now used in these procedures.

- Advise the patient to keep a family record of X-ray exams.

- Educate a female patient without breast disease on the correct schedule for mammography exams. The patient should have a baseline mammogram between ages 35 and 40; a mammogram every 1 to 2 years between ages 40 and 49; and an annual mammogram after age 50.

- Also, tell the patient to see a doctor immediately if she notices a breast mass, lump, or nipple discharge.

The 1993 NCRP report set guidelines for protection from radiation in and out of the workplace. The two primary objectives outlined in the report are to prevent serious general tissue damage from radiation by limiting radiation dose to levels below known thresholds for such damage and to reduce the risk of cancer and genetic effects to a level balanced by potential benefits to the individual and society.

Because radiation exposure always poses some degree of risk, the NCRP recommends that any activity involving radiation exposure be justified, or balanced against the expected benefits to society. Furthermore, the NCRP recommends the cost, or detriment, to society from such activities be kept *as low as reasonably achievable* (ALARA) and that individual dose limits be applied to ensure that justification and ALARA principles do not result in unacceptable risk levels for individuals or groups.

The NCRP has developed detailed lists on radiation doses to achieve the primary objectives stated in the report. Separate specific limits exist for occupational and public exposure.

Safety Precautions

Understanding and following standard safety precautions are crucial for protection from radiation exposure and are essential to the health and safety of both medical personnel and patients.

Personnel Safety If you work in a medical facility that performs radiologic tests, you are at risk for excessive radiation exposure. To protect yourself from exposure, you must adhere to the following guidelines:

- You (and other members of the medical staff) must always wear a radiation exposure badge, or dosimeter. There are several types of exposure badges, the simplest of which is a sensitized piece of film in a holder (Figure 50-10). You must have the badge checked regularly by specially qualified personnel, who measure the degree of radiation uptake on the film to determine the amount of radiation to which you have been exposed.
- Make sure all equipment is in good working order and is checked routinely for radiation leakage and any other problems.
- Be aware that the technician and any other staff members present when equipment is operating should always wear a garment that contains a lead shield.

Patient Safety You must follow all rules governing patient safety from radiation exposure. The *Educating the Patient* feature Safety with X-rays explains safety measures and information that help protect a patient from exposure to unnecessary radiation.

▶ Electronic Medicine LO 50.7

Recent major advances in telemedicine technology, including rapid video and computer-based communications of medical information, enable physicians to "examine" a patient in another city or country, view highly detailed medical images, consult with specialists in other cities, and supervise complex medical procedures. In addition, healthcare personnel, including medical assistants, can participate in interactive teaching conferences by means of closed-circuit television.

In some cities, emergency medical technicians (EMTs) can transmit an electrocardiogram (ECG) electronically to an emergency room physician to obtain life-saving directives from the physician. These directives may involve administration of drugs or other measures the EMTs would not be permitted to perform without a physician's order. Similarly, cardiologists monitor some patients by the transmission of daily ECGs through telephone lines to the cardiologist's office.

Digital Imaging and the EHR

With the emergence of electronic health records (EHR), technology in healthcare is expanding rapidly. However, no department is affected more than radiology because it is the only completely technology-driven specialty. Digital radiology (DR) devices are integrated with the EHR system to provide quality images and rapid access and to eliminate the time and equipment associated with film processing and development (Figure 50-11).

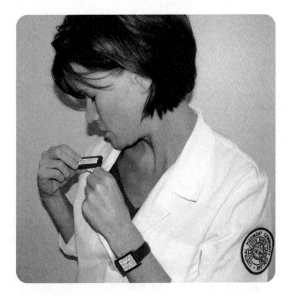

FIGURE 50-10 A radiation exposure badge contains a film that registers the levels of radiation to which a medical staff member is exposed at work.
©Total Care Programming, Inc.

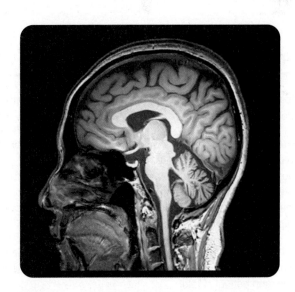

FIGURE 50-11 A digital sagittal MRI image of the brain.
©AkeSak/Shutterstock

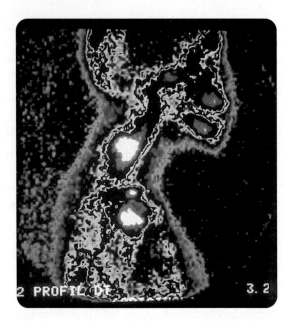

FIGURE 50-12 A digital bone scan of the neck and skull showing malignant tumors.
©SPL/Science Source

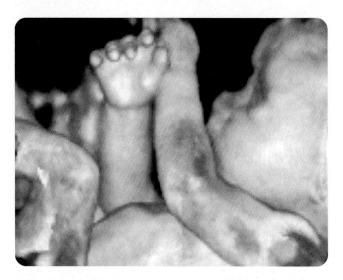

FIGURE 50-13 A 3D ultrasound shows the fetus in great detail.
©GE Medical Systems/Science Source

Digital Radiography

Conventional, film-based radiography is quickly being replaced by digital imaging techniques. Digital radiography uses a digital reader to "capture" or digitize the X-ray image instead of exposing traditional film (Figure 50-12). Using digital radiography has several advantages, including:

- Better image consistency and quality.
- Faster results.
- Decreased radiation to patient.
- Easier X-ray file sharing.
- Simpler storage.
- Environmentally safer (producing the image requires no chemicals).

Digital Imaging and Communications (DICOM) in Medicine Digital Imaging and Communications is a communications protocol or standard for handling, storing, printing, and transmitting information in medical imaging. DICOM was designed as part of the Integrating the Healthcare Enterprise (IHE) initiative that makes it easier for medical systems to share information. A Picture Archive and Communication System (PAC) is the digital storage area where digital images are sent and stored for diagnostic viewing and electronic image storage and distribution.

Advances in Radiology

As radiology continues to experience technological changes, more advances are occurring to enhance digital imaging quality. Some major advances include 3D/4D ultrasound, which provides "live-action" images that allow physicians to observe fetal movement, study body organs, and guide needle biopsies (Figure 50-13).

PROCEDURE 50-1 Assisting with an X-ray Examination ⟦WORK // DOC⟧

Procedure Goal: To assist with a radiologic procedure under the supervision of a radiologic technologist

OSHA Guidelines: This procedure does not involve exposure to blood, body fluids, or tissue. You must wear a radiation exposure badge (dosimeter), however, and will be required to wear a garment containing a lead or approved nonlead shield if you remain in the room during the operation of X-ray equipment.

Materials: Patient chart/progress note, X-ray examination order, X-ray machine, X-ray film and holder, X-ray film developer, drape, and patient shield

Method:

1. Check the X-ray examination order and equipment needed.
2. Identify the patient and introduce yourself.
3. Determine whether the patient has complied with the preprocedure instructions. Do not depend on the patient to inform you, but ask the patient if and how he prepped for the procedure.

   RATIONALE: *If a patient has not been compliant with preprocedural directions, then the test ordered may not be as effective as it should and will need to be rescheduled.*

4. Explain the procedure and the purpose of the examination to the patient.

5. Instruct the patient to remove clothing and all metals (including jewelry) as needed, according to the body area to be examined, and to put on a gown. Explain that metals may interfere with the image. Ask whether the patient has any surgical metal or a pacemaker and report this information to the radiologic technologist. Leave the room to ensure patient privacy.

   Note: Steps 6 through 11 are nearly always performed by a radiologic technologist.

6. Position the patient according to the X-ray view ordered.

7. Drape the patient and place the patient shield appropriately.

8. Instruct the patient about the need to remain still and to hold the breath when requested.

9. Leave the room or stand behind a lead shield during the exposure.

10. Ask the patient to assume a comfortable position while the films are developed. Explain that X-rays sometimes must be repeated.

11. Develop the films.

12. Determine if the X-ray films are satisfactory by allowing the radiologist to review the films.

RATIONALE: *The radiologist may want another film or view.*

13. Instruct the patient to dress and tell the patient when to contact the physician's office for the results.

14. Label the dry, finished X-ray films; place them in a properly labeled envelope; and file them according to your office's policies.

15. Record the X-ray examination, along with the final written findings, in the patient's chart (refer to Progress Note).

BWW PROGRESS NOTE

Patient Name:	Harry Smitts
Date:	AP and lateral chest X-rays completed. Report added to medical record.
Author:	
	11/17/XX
	K. Booth

Done　　Close

PROCEDURE 50-2　Documentation and Filing Techniques for X-rays

WORK // DOC

Procedure Goal: To document X-ray information and file X-ray films properly

OSHA Guidelines: This procedure does not involve exposure to blood, body fluids, or tissues.

Materials: X-ray film(s), patient X-ray record card or book, label, film-filing envelopes, film-filing cabinet, inserts, and a marking pen

Method:

1. Document the patient's X-ray information on the patient record card or in the record book. Include the patient's name, the date, the type of X-ray, and the number of X-rays taken.

2. Verify that the film is properly labeled with the referring doctor's name, the date, and the patient's name. To note corrections or unusual positions or to identify a film that does not include labeling, attach the appropriate label and complete the necessary information. Some facilities also record the name of the radiologist who interpreted the X-ray.
   RATIONALE: *To reduce the likelihood of misidentifying a patient's X-ray.*

X-RAY EXAMINATIONS RECORD

Patient	Date	Type X-Ray	No. Taken	Referring Doctor	Comments
Jill Cabot	2/16	Chest	4	Wapnir	
M. C. Gaines	2/16	Right knee	8	Wright	
J. Hale	2/19	Right wrist	6	McCarthy	
L. Becker	2/23	Left hip	4	Wright	
R. Bell	2/24	Chest	4	Wapnir	
Donna Lin	2/24	Sinuses	6	Harris	
Jon Carey	2/26	Right hand	2	Cohen	

FIGURE Procedure 50-2 Step 1　Keeping accurate records of patient X-ray information is an important duty of the medical assistant.

3. Place the processed film in a film-filing envelope. File the envelope alphabetically or chronologically (or according to your office's protocol) in the filing cabinet.

4. If you remove an envelope for any reason, put an insert or an "out card" in its place until it is returned to the cabinet.
   RATIONALE: *Proper filing techniques save time and prevent litigation.*

OUTCOME	KEY POINTS
50.1 **Explain what X-rays are and how they are used for diagnostic and therapeutic purposes.**	An X-ray is a high-energy electromagnetic wave that travels at the speed of light and can penetrate solid objects. X-rays can be used for diagnosis by producing images of internal body structures. Therapeutically, X-rays are used to treat cancer by preventing cellular reproduction.
50.2 **Compare invasive and noninvasive diagnostic procedures.**	Invasive procedures require a radiologist to insert a catheter, wire, or other testing device into a patient's blood vessel or organ through the skin or a body orifice. Noninvasive diagnostic procedures do not require inserting devices, breaking the skin, or monitoring at the degree needed with invasive procedures.
50.3 **Carry out the medical assistant's role in X-ray and diagnostic radiology testing.**	A medical assistant can work directly with a radiology facility to assist the radiologist or technicians in performing diagnostic procedures. Providing preprocedure and postprocedure care are duties a medical assistant can perform in a medical or radiology facility.
50.4 **Discuss common diagnostic imaging procedures.**	Numerous diagnostic imaging procedures are used in medicine today, including angiography, fluoroscopy, MRI, CT, arthrography, IVP, KUB, mammography, stereotactic breast biopsy, upper and lower GI series, ultrasound, and bone densitometry.
50.5 **Describe different types of radiation therapy and how they are used.**	The two basic types of radiation therapy are teletherapy and brachytherapy. Teletherapy also is called external beam radiotherapy because an external beam of radiation is used to penetrate deep tumors. Brachytherapy uses temporary radioactive implants positioned close to or directly into cancerous tissue to treat the tumor and spare healthy tissue.
50.6 **Explain the risks and safety precautions associated with radiology work.**	The greatest risk associated with a radiology facility is the potential for radiation exposure to patients and healthcare workers. To eliminate this risk, certain safety precautions should be followed. These include careful evaluation by the physician to determine the medical necessity of radiology testing, avoidance of X-rays altogether if a patient is pregnant, and the requirement that all personnel who work in a radiology facility wear a dosimeter.
50.7 **Relate the advances in medical imaging to EHR.**	Major advances in telemedicine technology, including rapid video and computer-based communications of medical information, enable physicians to "examine" a patient in another city or country, view highly detailed medical images, consult with specialists in other cities, and supervise complex medical procedures. Sharing records, including actual radiographic images, between facilities is easier with the advent of digital radiographic procedures and the electronic health record.

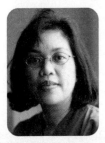

Recall Raja Lautu from the case study at the beginning of the chapter. Now that you have read the chapter, answer the following questions regarding her case.

1. What is the difference between brachytherapy and teletherapy?
2. What should you tell Raja Lautu to help prepare her for her radiation treatment?

©ERproductions Ltd/Blend Images LLC

3. What are the advantages of brachytherapy?
4. What instructions will you give Raja Lautu to prepare for her screening DXA test?
5. Why should the DXA be completed before the brachytherapy?

EXAM PREPARATION QUESTIONS

1. (LO 50.3) Which of the following would the medical assistant *least* likely perform?
   a. Performing stereotactic breast imaging
   b. Filing X-rays
   c. Providing preprocedure instruction for a mammogram
   d. Advising the patient to report symptoms after radiation treatment
   e. Assisting with an ultrasound

2. (LO 50.6) A dosimeter is used to
   a. Prevent radiation exposure
   b. Measure radiation exposure
   c. Measure the dose of medicine given during radiation treatments
   d. Monitor fluctuations in radiation exposure
   e. Determine how much radiation is needed to obtain an image

3. (LO 50.2) Which of the following is considered invasive?
   a. Chest X-ray
   b. Mammogram
   c. MRI
   d. Fluoroscopy
   e. Angiogram

4. (LO 50.4) What organs are evaluated with a KUB?
   a. Kidneys, ureters, bladder
   b. Kidneys, urethra, bladder
   c. Kidneys, ureters, bowels
   d. Kidneys, urethra, bowels
   e. Kidneys and urethra for blood

5. (LO 50.3) Which step in the X-ray procedure would *most* likely be performed by a medical assistant?
   a. Develop the films
   b. Evaluate the films
   c. Label the films
   d. Position the patient
   e. Set up the X-ray machine

6. (LO 50.2) A substance that makes internal organs denser and blocks the passage of X-rays to the photographic film is a
   a. Shielding material
   b. Dosimeter
   c. Radiolucent medication
   d. Digital reader
   e. Contrast medium

7. (LO 50.4) Which of the following is used to detect osteoporosis?
   a. Angiography
   b. DXA
   c. MUGA scan
   d. Lower GI series
   e. IVP

8. (LO 50.4) Hysterosalpingography is used to determine which of the following?
   a. Position of the kidneys
   b. Presence of gallstones
   c. Liver abscess
   d. Patency of the fallopian tubes
   e. Development of the fetus

9. (LO 50.5) Which of the following is used to treat tumors deep in the brain while sparing healthy tissue?
   a. Stereotactic radiosurgery
   b. Chemotherapy
   c. MRI
   d. Cerebral angiography
   e. Paramagnetic contrast

10. (LO 50.1) Wilhelm Conrad Roentgen is credited with discovering
    a. X-rays
    b. Photographic film
    c. Radiation therapy
    d. Magnetic resonance imaging
    e. SPECT scanning

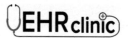

Go to CONNECT to complete the EHRclinic exercises: 50.01 Document Administration of Patient Education - Mammography and 50.02 Upload Mammogram Results to a Patient's EHR.

SOFT SKILLS SUCCESS

Recall Raja Lautu from the case study at the beginning of the chapter. While reviewing the patient preparation information for the DXA scan with Raja Lautu, you notice she is distracted and looks worried. After you complete the instructions, you ask if she has any questions. Raja Lautu tells you that she doesn't understand why she is having the DXA before her brachytherapy and wants to know why she can't wait until they start the treatment for her breast cancer. What should you tell Raja Lautu about the timing of the DXA?

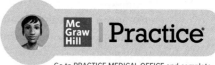

Go to PRACTICE MEDICAL OFFICE and complete the module Clinical: Interactions.

Principles of Pharmacology

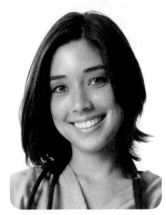
L E A R N I N G O U T C O M E S

After completing Chapter 51, you will be able to:

51.1 Identify the medical assistant's role in pharmacology.

51.2 Recognize the five categories of pharmacology and their importance to medication administration.

51.3 Differentiate the major drug categories, drug names, and their actions.

51.4 Classify over-the-counter (OTC), prescription, and herbal drugs.

51.5 Use credible sources to obtain drug information.

51.6 Carry out the procedure for registering or renewing a physician with the Drug Enforcement Administration (DEA) for permission to administer, dispense, and prescribe controlled drugs.

51.7 Identify the parts of a prescription, including commonly used abbreviations and symbols.

51.8 Discuss nonpharmacologic treatments for pain.

51.9 Describe how vaccines work in the immune system.

K E Y T E R M S

administer	opioid
adverse effects	package insert
controlled substance	pharmacodynamics
dispense	pharmacognosy
efficacy	pharmacokinetics
e-prescribing	pharmacology
generic name	pharmacotherapeutics
indication	prescribe
labeling	side effects
magnetic therapy	toxicology
narcotic	trade name

I.C.11 Identify the classifications of medications including:
(a) indications for use
(b) desired effects
(c) side effects
(d) adverse reactions

II.C.5 Identify abbreviations and symbols used in calculating medication dosages

V.P.3 Use medical terminology correctly and pronounced accurately to communicate information to providers and patients

X.P.5 Perform compliance reporting based on public health statutes

X.P.6 Report an illegal activity in the healthcare setting following proper protocol

3. **Medical Terminology**
   d. Define and use medical abbreviations when appropriate and acceptable

4. **Medical Law and Ethics**
   f. Comply with federal, state, and local health laws and regulations as they relate to healthcare settings

6. **Pharmacology**
   a. Identify drug classification, usual dose, side effects, and contraindications of the top most commonly used medications
   c. Prescriptions
      (1) Identify parts of prescriptions
      (2) Identify appropriate abbreviations that are accepted in prescription writing
      (3) Comply with legal aspects of creating prescriptions, including federal and state laws
   d. Properly utilize the Physician's Desk Reference (PDR), drug handbooks and other drug references to identify a drug's classification, usual dosage, usual side effects, and contraindications

7. **Administrative Procedures**
   a. Gather and process documents

▶ Introduction

Pharmacology—the science of drugs—is a great responsibility of allied health professionals. Medication mistakes can injure or even cause the death of a patient. Before you administer drugs, it is important to begin with a good working knowledge of the foundations of pharmacology, including how medications work, how they should be taken, and what problems can occur when they are taken. This chapter provides an overview of the role of drugs in ambulatory healthcare facilities.

▶ The Medical Assistant's Role in Pharmacology

LO 51.1

As a medical assistant, you will be expected to have a basic knowledge of medications. This includes knowledge of prescription drugs and over-the-counter (OTC) drugs. Prescription drugs require a licensed practitioner's written order to authorize the dispensing (and, sometimes, administering) of drugs to a patient. OTC drugs—available in pharmacies and supermarkets—are purchased by people to treat themselves for ailments ranging from arthritis to colds to stomach ulcers. As a medical assistant, you will need to:

- Ensure that the licensed practitioner is aware of all medications a patient is taking, both prescription and OTC, as well as vitamins and herbal remedies.
- Ask each patient about alcohol and recreational drug use (both past and present).
- Assist in managing and renewing medication prescriptions.
- Educate the patient, using guidelines provided by the licensed practitioner, about the purpose of a drug and how to take the drug for maximum effectiveness and minimum side effects.

As your state and scope of practice permit, you also may be asked to enter medication orders and give drugs to a patient. Safe and effective drug therapy requires additional knowledge and special skills. To handle these important functions, you must understand pharmacologic principles and sources of drug information, be able to read prescriptions accurately, and be prepared to answer basic patient questions (Figure 51-1). You also must adhere to legal requirements and keep accurate records. The Centers for Medicare and Medicaid Services (CMS) ruled in September 2012 that credentialed medical assistants may enter medication orders into a computerized order entry system. This is another excellent reason to become a credentialed medical assistant once you complete your program.

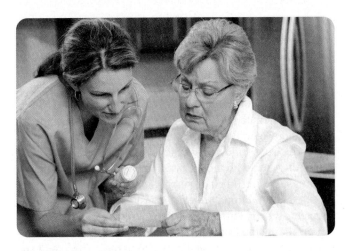

FIGURE 51-1 A medical assistant may need to be prepared to answer the patient's questions about a drug the doctor is prescribing.
©mphillips007/Getty Images

▶ Pharmacology

A drug is a chemical compound used to prevent, diagnose, or treat a disease or other abnormal condition. The study of drugs is called **pharmacology.** A specialist in pharmacology is called a *pharmacologist.* Included in pharmacology are

- **Pharmacognosy** (the study of characteristics of natural drugs and their sources).
- **Pharmacodynamics** (the study of what drugs do to the body).
- **Pharmacokinetics** (the study of what the body does to drugs).
- **Pharmacotherapeutics** (the study of how drugs are used to treat disease).
- **Toxicology** (the study of poisons or poisonous effects of drugs).

According to the Department of Justice's Drug Enforcement Administration (DEA) guidelines, a physician **prescribes,** or orders, a drug either by giving a patient a prescription to be filled by a pharmacy or by sending the order directly to the pharmacy through an electronic system. Electronic prescribing is often called *e-prescribing.* To **administer** a drug is to give it directly by injection, by mouth, or by any other route that introduces the drug into a patient's body. A healthcare professional **dispenses** a drug by distributing it, in a properly labeled container, to a patient who is directed to use it.

There are various types of pharmacies. Traditional pharmacies dispense common prescriptions and also sell other over the counter medications and health care needs. *Compounding pharmacies* compound drugs (mix together two or more ingredients) prescribed by doctors for specific patients with needs that can't be met by commercially available drugs. *Nuclear pharmacies* prepare and dispense patient-specific radiopharmaceutical doses for diagnostic imaging and therapeutic procedures for use in hospital nuclear medicine departments and outpatient clinics.

Sources of Drugs (Pharmacognosy)

Many drugs originate as natural products. Other drugs are developed in the chemical laboratory, as chemists seek to improve existing drugs.

Natural Products Most often, drugs originate as substances from natural products, such as plants, animals, minerals, bacteria, or fungi. For hundreds of years, drugs have been made from seeds, bulbs, roots, stems, buds, leaves, and other parts of plants. Two examples of plant-derived drugs are digitoxin, which comes from the foxglove plant (see Figure 51-2), and quinine, which comes from cinchona tree bark. Digitoxin is used to treat heart failure and abnormal heart rhythms. Quinine is used to treat malaria.

Animals also are used as a source of drugs. Certain animal substances have been shown to be compatible with human physiology. Some examples of animal substances used as drugs are glandular substances, such as thyroid hormones; fats and oils, such as cod-liver oil; enzymes, such as pancreatin and pepsin; and antiserums and antitoxins for vaccines.

Mineral sources yield various substances that can be used as they occur naturally or mixed with other substances. Two drugs derived from mineral sources are potassium chloride and mineral oil. Simple organisms, such as bacteria and fungi, produce substances that are used to make certain antibiotics, such as cephalosporins and penicillins (see Figure 51-3).

Chemical Development A chemist conducts investigations that lead to the synthesis (creation) of drugs based on a natural substance's chemical properties. Some drugs are synthesized by strictly chemical methods. Others are created by manipulating genetic information in a host organism. For example, human insulin is produced by these means, also known as *recombinant deoxyribonucleic acid (rDNA)* techniques.

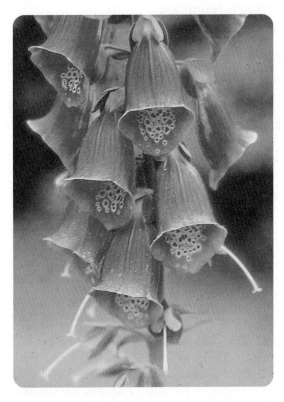

FIGURE 51-2 The foxglove plant, shown here, is the natural source for the medication digitoxin.
©Steven P. Lynch

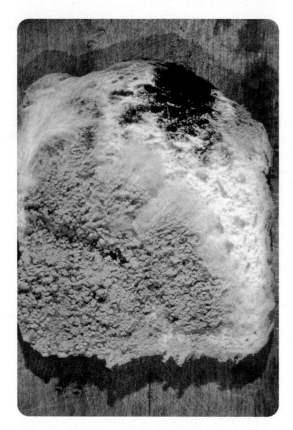

FIGURE 51-3 Bacteria, fungi, and yeasts are natural sources of antibiotics.
©Phototake

Pharmacodynamics

Pharmacodynamics is the study of the mechanism of action, or how the drug works to produce a therapeutic effect. Drugs are placed in categories based on their mechanism of action. Pharmacodynamics includes the interaction between the drug and target cells or tissues and the body's response to that interaction. For example, when a patient with diabetes takes insulin, the drug acts by allowing the movement of glucose across cell membranes. This movement makes the glucose available to cells to use as an energy source. The end result is a decrease in the blood glucose level.

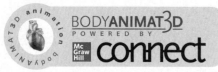

Go to CONNECT to see an animation exercise about *Pharmacokinetics vs. Pharmacodynamics.*

Pharmacokinetics

Pharmacokinetics is what the body does to a drug—that is, how the body absorbs, distributes, metabolizes, and excretes the drug. It is important to understand these processes so that you will be able to explain to patients the reasons for taking a particular drug with food or for drinking plenty of water while taking a drug. These four processes can be remembered by using the acronym ADME: Absorption–Distribution–Metabolism–Excretion.

Absorption Absorption is the process of converting a drug from its dose form, such as a tablet or capsule, into a form the body can use. For example, tablets and capsules are absorbed through the stomach or intestines into the bloodstream. Water or a particular food may either hinder or assist the absorption of a specific drug through the stomach or intestines. Some drugs may irritate the digestive organs if they are taken without food or water. Because of such possible reactions, patients must precisely follow instructions for taking a drug with plenty of water, with food, or without food.

Drugs are absorbed through the skin (intradermally or transdermally), through the tissue just beneath the skin (subcutaneously), or through muscle (intramuscularly), depending on the method of injection. Absorption allows the drug to enter the bloodstream and pass into tissues. The extent and rate of drug absorption depend on several factors, including the route of administration. When the drug is administered by mouth, for example, coatings on tablets or capsules and the amount and type of food consumed with the drug may affect absorption. Drugs administered intravenously do not require absorption; they are directly available to target cells from the bloodstream.

Distribution Distribution is the process of transporting a drug from its administration site, such as the muscle of an injection site, to its site of action. Distribution also pertains to the length of time a drug takes to achieve maximum or peak plasma levels—that is, the length of time between dosing and availability in the bloodstream.

Metabolism Drug metabolism is the process by which drug molecules are transformed into simpler products called *metabolites.* This transformation usually occurs in the liver, where enzymes break down the drug. Some drugs, however, are metabolized in the kidneys. Metabolism can be affected by disease, a patient's age or genetic makeup, a drug's characteristics, and other factors. When drugs metabolized in the liver are prescribed for either children or the elderly, the dose is likely to be lower than that prescribed for young adults. Metabolism in children and the elderly is different from metabolism in other patients; the drugs may remain in the body longer and possibly reach harmful levels. The same concern holds true for any patient with impaired liver or kidney function if prescribed drugs are metabolized in the affected organ.

Excretion *Excretion* describes the manner in which a drug is eliminated from the body. Most drugs are eliminated in urine. Drugs also may be excreted in feces, perspiration, saliva, bile, exhaled air, and breast milk.

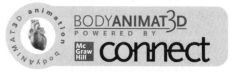

Go to CONNECT to see animation exercises about *Medication Absorption, Medication Distribution, Medication Metabolism,* and *Medication Excretion.*

Pharmacotherapeutics

Pharmacotherapeutics is the study of how drugs are used to treat disease. This area of pharmacology is sometimes called *clinical pharmacology*. Pharmacotherapeutics includes topics such as drug categories, drug indications and labeling, safety, **efficacy** (therapeutic value), and kinds of therapy.

Indications and Labeling An **indication** is a purpose or reason for using a drug. The Food and Drug Administration (FDA) must approve indications before they can become part of a drug's **labeling.** The FDA is an agency of the Department of Health and Human Services. It regulates the manufacture and distribution of every drug approved for use in the United States. Labeling also includes the form of the drug, such as tablet or liquid. Regardless of category, some drugs may be used to treat several different conditions. Multiple uses are possible if the drug affects several body systems or if the drug's primary effect produces significant secondary effects in other body systems.

When a drug is used for multiple indications, one or more indications might not be in its labeling. Off-label prescribing is legal. For example, Benadryl® (diphenhydramine) is an antihistamine used to treat allergic symptoms in both children and adults. Because it tends to make patients sleepy, a physician may use a low dose of Benadryl® as a temporary sedative for an adult. Its use as a sedative, however, is not part of the labeling for Benadryl®.

Another example of a drug with multiple uses is minoxidil. As a trade-name tablet, it is known as the antihypertensive Loniten®; as a trade-name topical solution, it is known as the hair-growth stimulant Rogaine®. In the case of minoxidil, both indications are approved, but the tablet labeling is for hypertension and the topical solution labeling is for hair growth. It is important to be aware of these labeling considerations when dealing with questions from patients. Never assume a drug is appropriate for only one use or administered in only one form. Always consult the licensed practitioner or other approved source of drug information before answering a patient's question.

Safety The safety of a drug is determined by how many and what kinds of adverse reactions are associated with it. Adverse reactions include both side effects and adverse effects. **Side effects** are unintended but fairly mild and common effects of a medication. For example, patients may experience constipation as a side effect of taking codeine for pain. Side effects generally are not severe enough to warrant stopping a medication. Some side effects are common, whereas others are rare. **Adverse effects** are potentially more harmful, but less common, effects. For example, reported adverse effects of Benadryl® include confusion and disturbed coordination. A patient experiencing these effects may be told to stop taking Benadryl® because the adverse effects outweigh the benefit of taking the medication. An adverse effect may require immediate attention.

It is not uncommon for a patient to call the physician's office with complaints of new symptoms soon after beginning therapy with a drug. Be alert for such complaints because they might be signs of an adverse reaction to the drug or an interaction with another medication. These calls should be brought to the attention of the licensed practitioner.

Efficacy A patient may complain that a newly prescribed drug is not doing what the doctor said it would. There are a variety of possible explanations for such a complaint, including:

- The drug is working adequately, but the patient does not understand how it works.
- The dosage (size, frequency, and number of doses) needs to be adjusted.
- The patient is not taking the medication according to the directions.
- The drug has not yet reached a therapeutic level in the bloodstream.
- The wrong drug was prescribed, or the wrong drug was dispensed by the pharmacy (this is rare, but possible).
- Some drugs work better in some patients than in others; not every drug is for everyone (this is particularly true of antihistamines).
- Some forms of a drug work better than others, such as tablets versus injection.
- The generic drug does not work, but the trade-name drug does. A generic drug may not work because it is made with additional or different inert (not active) ingredients. These inert ingredients could interfere with the drug's active ingredient or could change the patient's response to the medication.

Kinds of Therapy Depending on a patient's condition, the licensed practitioner may use drugs for any of the following kinds of therapy:

- Acute: drug is prescribed to improve a life-threatening or serious condition, such as epinephrine for severe allergic reaction.
- Empiric: drug is prescribed according to experience or observation until blood or other tests prove another therapy to be appropriate, such as penicillin for suspected strep throat.
- Maintenance: drug is prescribed to maintain health or protect against exacerbations of a condition, especially in chronic disease, such as an anti-inflammatory medication for inflammatory bowel disease.
- Palliative: drug is prescribed to reduce the severity of symptoms of a condition such as its accompanying pain; for example, morphine is given to reduce the pain caused by cancer.
- Prophylactic: drug is prescribed to prevent a disease or condition, such as immunizations or birth control drugs.
- Replacement: drug is prescribed to provide chemicals otherwise missing in a patient, such as hormone replacement therapy for a woman in menopause.
- Supportive: drug is prescribed for a condition other than the primary disease until that disease resolves, such as a corticosteroid for severe allergic reactions.
- Supplemental: drug or nutrients are prescribed to avoid deficiency, such as iron for a woman who is pregnant.

Toxicology

Toxicology is the study of the poisonous effects, or toxicity, of drugs, including adverse effects and drug interactions. In addition to immediate toxic effects that can occur when drugs are administered, you must be aware of some possible toxic effects that may not be apparent right away:

- An adverse effect on a fetus when the drug crosses the placenta.
- An adverse effect on infants when the drug passes easily into breast milk.
- Adverse reactions reported in clinical trials, such as headache, drowsiness, gastric upset, or other effects.
- An adverse effect in immunocompromised patients who are unable to metabolize a drug normally.
- An adverse effect in pediatric or elderly patients or in patients with hypertension, diabetes mellitus, or other serious chronic conditions.
- An adverse drug interaction when the drug is taken with another drug or food that is incompatible.
- A carcinogenic (cancer-causing) effect in some patients.

Adverse reactions are nearly always encountered during the clinical trials of a drug, and there will be mention of these reactions under that heading in the package insert or in accepted drug reference works. In the reports of clinical trials, the drug company must report all adverse reactions noted during testing. As a result, all of the adverse reactions that, at least theoretically, could be caused by the drug are included.

In dealing with patients who are about to begin drug therapy, use discretion when mentioning specific adverse reactions associated with drugs. The patient must be informed; however, you do not want to cause undue alarm or discourage patients from taking the needed medication. Always ask patients if they have any questions and have the licensed practitioner answer patients' drug-related questions. Because patients will receive lists of possible adverse reactions from the pharmacist, encourage them to discuss concerns with the pharmacist or to call the practitioner's office. Also encourage patients to inform the practitioner of adverse reactions they experience after beginning drug therapy.

▶ Drug Names and Categories LO 51.3

One drug may have several different names, including the drug's **generic name** (official, nonproprietary name), chemical name, and **trade name** (brand, or proprietary, name).

For instance, the trade-name cholesterol-lowering drug prescribed by authorized prescribers as Mevacor® or Altoprev® is also identified by the following names:

- Lovastatin (generic name).
- 2-methyl-1S,2,3R,7S,8S,8aR-hexahydro-3,7-dimethyl-8-[2-[2(2R,4R)-tetrahydro-4-hydroxy-6-oxo-2H-pyran-2-yl]] ethyl-1-naphthalenyl ester, butanoic acid (chemical name).

As a medical assistant, you will probably need to use only generic and trade names. In general, think of the generic name of a drug as a simple form of its chemical name. For each new drug marketed by a manufacturer, the United States Adopted Names (USAN) Council selects a generic name. This name is nonproprietary, meaning it does not belong to any one manufacturer. A generic name also is considered a drug's official name, which is listed in the *United States Pharmacopeia/National Formulary.*

A drug's manufacturer selects the drug's trade name, which is protected by copyright and is the property of the manufacturer. When a new drug enters the market, its manufacturer has a patent on that drug, which means that no other manufacturer can make or sell the drug for 17 years. When the patent runs out, any manufacturer can sell the drug under the generic name or a different trade name. The original manufacturer, however, is the only one allowed to use the drug's original trade name. For example, the antibiotic amoxicillin has two trade names: Amoxil® and Prevpac®. A different manufacturer owns each of these names.

A licensed practitioner may prescribe a drug by its generic or trade name. Because generic drugs are usually less expensive, most practitioners try to prescribe them if possible. Many states allow pharmacists to substitute a generic drug for a trade-name drug unless the practitioner specifies otherwise. In fact, most health insurance prescription plans require the substitution of generic drugs for trade-name drugs (unless otherwise specified by a licensed practitioner). Frequently, they also require the pharmacy to charge a higher copay amount for trade-name drugs than for generic drugs. Some prescription plans offer a mail-in pharmacy, through which a patient can obtain generic drugs with a reduced copayment or without any copayment.

Drugs are categorized by their action on the body, general therapeutic effect, or body system affected. Table 51-1 lists a variety of drug categories, their actions, and common drugs, including drugs from the top 300 drugs most commonly prescribed in the year 2019.

TABLE 51-1 Drug Categories and Actions for Commonly Prescribed Drugs		
Drug Category	**Action of Drug**	**Examples*: Generic Name (Trade Name)**
Analgesic	Relieves mild to severe pain	Acetaminophen (Tylenol®*); acetylsalicylic acid, or aspirin; morphine sulfate (MS Contin®)*; oxycodone HCl (Oxycontin®)*
Anesthetic	Prevents sensation of pain (generally, locally, or topically)	Lidocaine HCl (Xylocaine®, Lidoderm®)*; tetracaine HCl (Pontocaine®)
Antacid/antiulcer	Neutralizes stomach acid	Calcium carbonate (Tums®); esomeprazole (Nexium®)*; lansoprazole (Prevacid®); pantoprazole sodium (Protonix®)*

TABLE 51-1 Drug Categories and Actions for Commonly Prescribed Drugs

Drug Category	Action of Drug	Examples*: Generic Name (Trade Name)
Anthelmintic	Kills, paralyzes, or inhibits the growth of parasitic worms	Mebendazole (Vermox®); pyrantel pamoate (Combantrin®, Antiminth®)
Antidysrythmic (antiarrhythmic)	Normalizes heartbeat in cases of certain cardiac arrhythmias	Disopyramide phosphate (Norpace®); propafenone HCl (Rythmol®); propranolol HCl (Inderal®*)
Antiasthmatic	Treats or prevents asthma attacks	Montelukast (Singulair®)*; fluticasone propionate/salmeterol (Advair Diskus®)*; albuterol (ProAir HFA®)*
Antibiotics (antibacterial)	Kills bacterial microorganisms or inhibits their growth	Amoxicillin (Amoxil®)*; azithromycin (Zithromax®)*; cefprozil (Cefzil®); ciprofloxacin (Cipro®)*; clarithromycin (Biaxin® XL); clindamycin (Cleocin®)*
Anticholinergic	Blocks parasympathetic nerve impulses	Atropine sulfate (Isopto® Atropine); dicyclomine HCl* (Bentyl®); ipratropium (Atrovent®)
Anticoagulant	Prevents blood from clotting	Enoxaparin sodium (Lovenox®); heparin sodium (Hep-Lock®); warfarin sodium (Coumadin®)*
Anticonvulsant	Relieves or controls seizures (convulsions)	Clonazepam (Klonopin®)*; divalproex (Depakote®); phenobarbital sodium (Luminol® Sodium); phenytoin* (Dilantin®)
Antidepressant (four types)	Relieves depression	
Tricyclic		Amitriptyline HCl* (Elavil®); doxepin HCl* (Sinequan®)
Monoamine oxidase inhibitor (MAOI)		Phenelzine sulfate (Nardil®); tranylcypromine sulfate (Parnate®)
Selective serotonin reuptake inhibitor (SSRI)		Escitalopram (Lexapro®)*; fluoxetine HCl (Prozac®); paroxetine (Paxil®)*; sertraline HCl (Zoloft®)*
Serotonin-norepinephrine reuptake inhibitor (SNRI)		Venlafaxine HCl (Effexor XR®)*; duloxetine HCl (Cymbalta®)*
Antidiabetic	Treats diabetes by reducing glucose	Metformin (Glucophage®)*; glipizide (Glucotrol®); pioglitazone HCl (Actos®)*; insulin glargine (Lantus®)*
Antidiarrheal	Relieves diarrhea	Bismuth subsalicylate (Pepto-Bismol®); kaolin and pectin mixtures (Kaopectate®); loperamide HCl* (Imodium®)
Antiemetic	Prevents or relieves nausea and vomiting	Prochlorperazine (Compazine®)*; promethazine (Phenergan®); trimethobenzamide HCl (Tigan®)
Antifungal	Kills or inhibits growth of fungi	Amphotericin B (Fungizone®); fluconazole (Diflucan®)*; nystatin (Mycostatin®); terbinafine (Lamisil®)
Antihistamine	Counteracts effects of histamine and relieves allergic symptoms	Cetirizine HCl (Zyrtec®); diphenhydramine HCl (Benadryl®); fexofenadine (Allegra®); desloratadine (Clarinex®)
Antihypertensive	Reduces blood pressure	Amlodipine (Norvasc®)*; diltiazem HCl (Cartia XL®); quinapril (Prinivil®); metoprolol succinate (Toprol-XL®)*; valsartan (Diovan®)*
Anti-inflammatory (two types)	Reduces inflammation	
Nonsteroidal (NSAIDs)		Naproxen (Aleve)*; colchicine (Colcrys®)*; ibuprofen (Motrin®, Advil®)*; celecoxib (Celebrex®)*
Steroids		Dexamethasone (Decadron®); methylprednisolone (Medrol®)*; prednisone (Deltasone™)*; triamcinolone (Kenalog®)
Antilipemic (antilipidemic)	Lowers blood lipids such as triglycerides	Gemfibrozil (Lopid®); atorvastatin (Lipitor®)*; fenofibrate (TriCor®)*; ezetimibe/simvastatin (Vytorin®)*; ezetimibe (Zetia®)*; rosuvastatin (Crestor®)*
Antineoplastic	Prevents or inhibits the growth of cancer	Bleomycin sulfate (Blenoxane®); dactinomycin (Cosmegen®); paclitaxel (Taxol®); tamoxifen citrate (Nolvadex®)
Antipsychotic	Controls psychotic symptoms	Chlorpromazine HCl (Thorazine®); clozapine (Clozaril®); haloperidol (Haldol®); risperidone (Risperdal®)*; thioridazine HCl (Mellaril®)
Antipyretic	Reduces fever	Acetaminophen (Tylenol®); acetylsalicylic acid, or aspirin

(Continued)

TABLE 51-1 Drug Categories and Actions for Commonly Prescribed Drugs

Drug Category	Action of Drug	Examples*: Generic Name (Trade Name)
Antiseptic	Inhibits growth of microorganisms	Isopropyl alcohol; 70% povidone-iodine (Betadine®); chlorhexidine gluconate (PerioChip®)
Antitussive	Inhibits cough reflex	Codeine; dextromethorphan hydrobromide (component of Robitussin® DM)
Bronchodilator	Dilates bronchi (airways in the lungs)	Albuterol (Proventil®)*; epinephrine (Epinephrine Mist®); salmeterol (Serevent®); tiotropium bromide (Spiriva®)*
Cathartic (laxative)	Induces defecation, alleviates constipation	Bisacodyl (Dulcolax®); casanthranol (Peri-Colace®); magnesium hydroxide (Milk of Magnesia®)
Contraceptive	Reduces risk of pregnancy	Ethinyl estradiol and norgestimate (Ortho Tri-Cyclen®); norethindrone and ethinyl estradiol (Loestrin® 24 Fe)*; norgestrel (Ovrette®)
Decongestant	Relieves nasal swelling and congestion	Oxymetazoline HCl (Afrin®); phenylephrine HCl (Neo-Synephrine®); pseudoephedrine HCl (Sudafed®)
Diuretic	Increases urine output, reduces blood pressure and cardiac output	Bumetanide (Bumex®); furosemide (Lasix®)*; hydrochlorothiazide (HydroDIURIL®)*; mannitol (Osmitrol®); spironolactone (Aldactone®)
Expectorant	Liquefies mucus in bronchi; allows expectoration of sputum, mucus, and phlegm	Guaifenesin* (Mucinex®)
Hemostatic	Controls or stops bleeding by promoting coagulation	Aminocaproic acid (Amicar®); phytonadione or vitamin K_1 (Mephyton®); thrombin (Thrombogen®)
Hormone replacement	Replaces or resolves hormone deficiency	Insulin (Humulin®) for pancreatic deficiency; levothyroxine sodium (Synthroid®)* for thyroid deficiency; conjugated estrogens (Premarin Tabs®)*
Hypnotic (sleep-inducing) or sedative	Induces sleep or relaxation (depending on drug potency and dosage)	Chloral hydrate (Noctec®); secobarbital sodium (Seconal Sodium®); zolpidem* (Ambien®)
Muscle relaxant	Relaxes skeletal muscles	Carisoprodol (Soma®); cyclobenzaprine HCl (Flexeril®)*
Mydriatic	Constricts vessels of eye or nasal passage, raises blood pressure, dilates pupil of eye in ophthalmic preparations	Atropine sulfate (Atropisol®) for ophthalmic use; phenylephrine HCl (Alcon Efrin®) for ophthalmic use or (Neo-Synephrine®) for nasal use
Stimulant (central nervous system)	Increases activity of brain and other organs, decreases appetite	Amphetamine sulfate (Benzedrine®); caffeine (No-Doz®); also a component of many analgesic formulations and coffee
Vasoconstrictor	Constricts blood vessels, increases blood pressure	Dopamine HCl (Intropin®); norepinephrine bitartrate (Levophed®)
Vasodilator	Dilates blood vessels, decreases blood pressure	Enalopril (Vasotec®); lisinopril (Prinivil®)*; nitroglycerin (Nitrostat®, NitroQuick®)

*Indicates top 300 drugs in the year 2019.

Sources: RXList, http://www.rxlist.com, ClinCalc https://clincalc.com/DrugStats/Top300Drugs.aspx

Drug names frequently can be confused because they either look like or sound like other drugs. Pay close attention to the spelling and names of medications. Table 51-2 provides examples of common drugs and their confused equivalents.

TABLE 51-2 Common Drugs and Their Confused Equivalents

Common Drug Name*	Confused Drug Name(s)
ALPRAZolam (Xanax)	LORazepam — clonazePAM
amLODIPine (Norvasc)	aMILoride
ARIPiprazole (Abilify)	RABEprazole
buPROPion (Wellbutrin)	busPIRone

TABLE 51-2 Common Drugs and Their Confused Equivalents

Common Drug Name*	Confused Drug Name(s)
carBAMazepine (Tegretol; Carbatrol; Equetro)	OXcarbazepine
CeleBREX	CeleXA
clonazePAM (Klonopin)	cloNIDine — cloZAPine — cloBAZam — LORazepam
cycloSPORINE (Restasis)	cycloSERINE
diazePAM (Valium)	dilTIAZem
diphenhydrAMINE (Benadryl)	dimenhyDRINATE
DULoxetine (Cymbalta)	FLUoxetine — PARoxetine
EPINEPHrine (EpiPen)	ePHEDrine
fentaNYL (Duragesic and more)	SUFentanil
glipiZIDE (Glucotrol)	glyBURIDE
guaiFENesin (Mucinex and more)	guanFACINE
hydroCHLOROthiazide (HCTZ) (Microzide)	hydrOXYzine — hydrALAZINE
HYDROcodone	oxyCODONE
HYDROmorphone (Dilaudid)	hydrOXYzine — hydralazine — oxyMORphone
inFLIXimab (Remicade)	riTUXimab
ISOtretinoin (Amnesteem, Claravis, Absorica, Accutane)	tretinoin
KlonoPIN	cloNIDine
LaMICtal	LamISIL
lamoTRIgine (Lamictal)	lamiVUDine
levETIRAcetam (Keppra)	levOCARNitine — levoFLOXacin
LORazepam (Ativan)	ALPRAZolam — clonazePAM
metFORMIN (Glucophage)	metroNIDAZOLE
methylPREDNISolone (Medrol)	medroxyPROGESTERone — methylTESTOSTERone
metOLazone (Zaroxolyn)	methIMAzole — methazolAMIDE
NexIUM	NexAVAR
NIFEdipine (Procardia XL and others)	niCARdipine — niMODipine
OLANZapine (Zyprexa)	QUEtiapine
OXcarbazepine (Trileptal)	carBAMazepine
oxyCODONE (OxyContin)	HYDROcodone — OxyCONTIN– oxyMORphone
PARoxetine (Paxil)	FLUoxetine — DULoxetine
predniSONE (Deltasone)	prednisoLONE
PriLOSEC	PROzac
QUEtiapine (Seroquel)	OLANZapine
raNITIdine (Zantac)	riMANTAdine
RisperDAL	rOPINIRole
risperiDONE (Risperdal)	rOPINIRole
SEROquel	SINEquan
SITagliptin (Januvia)	sAXagliptin — SUMAtriptan
SUMAtriptan (Imitrex)	SITagliptin — ZOLMitriptan
TEGretol	TRENtal
traMADol (Rysolt)	traZODone
valACYclovir (Valtrex)	valGANciclovir
ZyPREXA	ZyrTEC

*Tall man letters provided to improve drug name perception and reduce errors. Parentheses ( ) indicate brand name equivalent.

Source: FDA and ISMP Lists of Look-Alike Drug Names with Recommended Tall Man Letters

FDA Regulation and Drugs   LO 51.4

The Food and Drug Administration (FDA) requires that drug manufacturers perform clinical tests on new drugs before humans use the drugs. These tests include toxicity tests in laboratory animals, followed by clinical studies (clinical trials) in controlled groups of volunteers. Some volunteers are patients; others are healthy subjects. Clinical tests are designed to consider the ratio of benefits to the risk of adverse reactions. If the clinical tests prove the drug is safe and effective, the FDA approves it for marketing. The manufacturer must continue to demonstrate the drug's safety and efficacy and must submit reports whenever it discovers unexpected adverse reactions. The FDA can withdraw a drug from the market at any time if evidence suggests it is no longer safe or effective. This is known as a *recall*.

The FDA also regulates drug manufacturing. It ensures that drugs shipped between states have the proper identity, strength, purity, and quality. Each manufacturer must consistently identify each drug by a particular color, form, shape, size, and label. It must produce every dose at the same tested strength, using the exact formula approved by the FDA. The manufacturer also must use high-quality, contaminant-free ingredients. The FDA regulates all drugs, including over-the-counter, prescription, and even complementary and alternative medicine (CAM). See the *Points on Practice* feature The FDA and CAM Therapies. To help regulate the safety of drugs, the FDA has a program called MedWatch for voluntary reporting of adverse events noted during clinical care. An adverse event is any undesirable experience for a patient associated with the use of a medical product. Reporting of these events is done on the FDA site at http://www.fda.gov/Safety/MedWatch/default.htm.

POINTS ON PRACTICE

The FDA and CAM Therapies

Complementary and alternative medicine (CAM) such as dietary supplements, herbal products, and other natural but as yet scientifically unproven therapies are increasing in use. Many licensed practitioners prescribe these therapies and even more patients take them on their own with positive effects.

There is one important difference between dietary supplements and medications. Medications must earn FDA approval prior to being marketed and sold. Drug manufacturers must provide scientific documentation of the effectiveness of a drug before it can be marketed. On the other hand, manufacturers of dietary supplements do not have to provide evidence of effectiveness or safety. Of course, they are not permitted to market or sell a product that is proven unsafe. However, once a supplement is marketed, the FDA must prove that the product is not safe to have it taken from the market. Additionally, dietary supplements are not standardized between batches or among manufacturers. Standardization is a process that ensures the consistency and quality of each batch of supplement produced. Thus, the amount and quality of a dietary supplement may differ between batches produced by one manufacturer or between the same supplement made by two different manufacturers. FDA-approved medications must be standardized and will always be consistent between batches and manufacturers.

The FDA does require that certain information appear on dietary supplement labels. Dietary supplements may include claims on their labels that describe the effect of a substance in maintaining the body's normal structure or function. For example, a label might state "Promotes healthy joints and bones." The FDA does not review or authorize this claim, so the manufacturer also is required to place a disclaimer on the product. This disclaimer is a statement indicating that the claims have not been evaluated by the FDA—for example, "This statement has not been evaluated by the Food and Drug Administration. This product is not intended to diagnose, treat, cure, or prevent disease." Figure 51-4 shows an example of a label that meets the FDA's labeling requirements.

Anatomy of the Requirements for Dietary Supplement Labels (Effective March 1999)

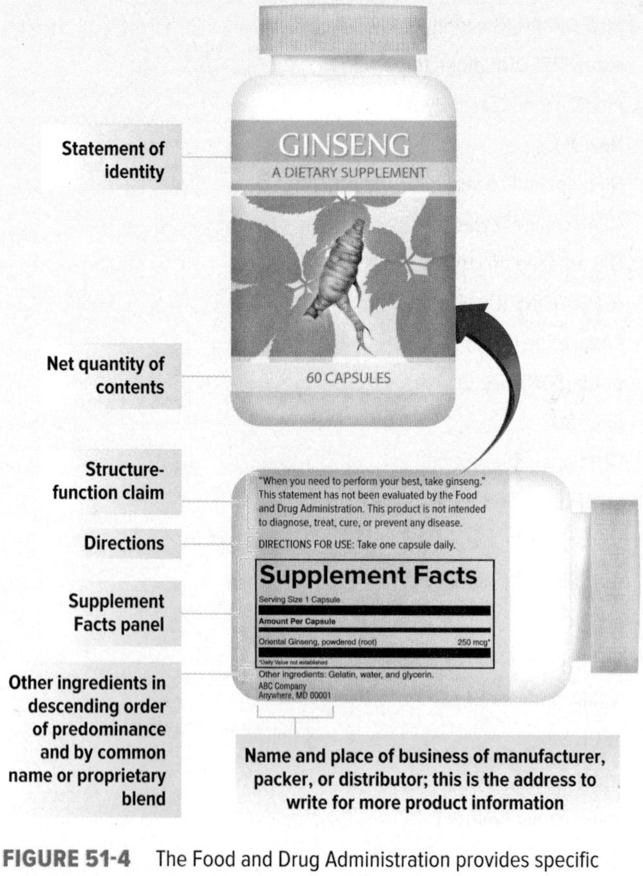

- Statement of identity
- Net quantity of contents
- Structure-function claim
- Directions
- Supplement Facts panel
- Other ingredients in descending order of predominance and by common name or proprietary blend
- Name and place of business of manufacturer, packer, or distributor; this is the address to write for more product information

FIGURE 51-4 The Food and Drug Administration provides specific guidelines for the information to be included on a dietary supplement label.

TABLE 51-3	Pregnancy and Lactation Drug Label Requirements

The FDA requires the following information on prescription drug labels to assist the prescriber and the patient in determining the risks and benefits of each.

Category	Label Requirements
Pregnancy (Includes Labor and Delivery)	• Pregnancy/fetal risk summary • Clinical considerations and data • Inadvertent exposure considerations • Prescribing decisions for pregnant patients • Information for the pregnancy exposure registry when available
Lactation (Includes Nursing Mothers)	• Information about the amount of drug in the breast milk • Information about potential effects of the drug on the breastfed infant
Females and Males of Reproductive Potential	• Need for pregnancy testing when taking the drug • Contraception recommendations • Information about infertility as it relates to the drug

Over-the-Counter Drugs

A nonprescription, or over-the-counter (OTC), drug is one the FDA has approved for use without a licensed healthcare practitioner's supervision. The consumer must follow the manufacturer's directions to use the drug safely. Some drugs, such as aspirin and vitamin supplements, have been OTC drugs for many years. The number of prescription drugs granted OTC status is increasing. Although OTC drugs are safe when used as directed on the package, patient education contributes significantly to their safe use.

Prescription Drugs

A prescription drug is one that can be used only by order of a licensed practitioner. It must be dispensed by a licensed healthcare professional, such as a pharmacist, physician, podiatrist, or licensed midwife. Some prescription drugs are available at much lower strengths as OTC medications. For example, the anti-inflammatory medication ibuprofen is prescribed as 800 mg tablets but is also available as 200 mg tablets over-the-counter.

Pregnancy Categories

Because clinical trials are not typically done on pregnant women, most of the data about the effect of medications on pregnant women are obtained after FDA approval. Drugs can cause defects to the fetus if taken during pregnancy. Prior to June 2015, drugs were labeled as a category A, B, C, D, or X based on the degree to which information has ruled out risk to the fetus. In June 2015, more comprehensive labeling requirements were set for three categories: Pregnancy, Lactation, and Females and Males of Reproductive Potential. The new labels include pregnancy exposure registries that collect and maintain data on the effects of medications used by pregnant women. The new rule dictates what must be included on the drug label based on the three categories. See Table 51-3.

▶ Sources of Drug Information   LO 51.5

Having access to up-to-date and credible sources of drug information in the office is essential. The most up-to-date resources are found online or through smartphone or other electronic applications. Books are available, but resource books are also available online. *Physicians' Desk Reference*® (Figure 51-5), *United States Pharmacopeia/National Formulary, American Hospital Formulary Service* (*AHFS*®), and Epocrates® are

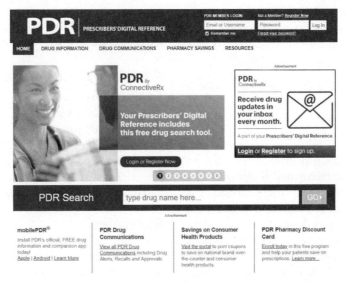

FIGURE 51-5   PDR.net® is a complete and current resource for drug information that includes all the information found in the PDR.
©McGraw-Hill Education

credible sources of drug information. Package inserts and drug labels are also valuable drug information sources. See the *Points on Practice* feature Using Credible Sources.

Physicians' Desk Reference® (PDR)

The *Physicians' Desk Reference*®, or *PDR*, is published annually, along with supplements twice a year. It is sent free to doctors' offices and sold through bookstores. PDR Network, the company that publishes the *PDR*, also publishes separate editions for generic, nonprescription, and ophthalmologic drugs, as well as a guide to drug interactions, adverse effects, and indications. It is also available online. The *PDR* presents information provided by pharmaceutical companies about more than 2,500 prescription drugs. It has the following sections:

- Section 1—manufacturer's index (color-coded white), which includes the pharmaceutical company's name, address, emergency telephone number, and available products.
- Section 2—brand- and generic-name index (color-coded pink).
- Section 3—product category index (color-coded blue).
- Section 4—product identification guide with full-color photos of more than 2,400 medications.
- Section 5—product information.
- Section 6—diagnostic product information.

The product information section is divided according to manufacturer, and the drugs are then grouped alphabetically within each manufacturer's subsection. The information is provided for the *PDR* by the manufacturer and is either the drug package insert or a similar document.

After the large product information section, various smaller other sections are provided, which include diagnostic product information, state drug information centers, ratings for drug use in pregnancy, a state DEA directory, state-aided drug-assistance programs, patient assistance programs, drugs that should not be crushed, dosing instructions in Spanish, and the system for reporting adverse reactions to medications. All of these plus the *PDR* Internet site and *PDR* electronic library that come with the *PDR* are important resources for drug information.

United States Pharmacopeia/National Formulary

The *United States Pharmacopeia/National Formulary,* or *USP-NF*, is the official source of drug standards in the United States, published about every 5 years. It is the official public standards-setting authority for all prescription medications, OTC drugs, dietary supplements, and other healthcare products. By law, every product sold under a name listed in the *USP-NF* must meet the USP's strict standards.

The *USP-NF* describes each product approved by the federal government and lists its standards for purity, composition, and strength as well as its uses, dosages, and storage. The NF portion of the book provides the chemical formulas of the drugs. The *USP-NF* is available online.

American Hospital Formulary Service (AHFS®)

The American Society of Hospital Pharmacists in Bethesda, Maryland, publishes *American Hospital Formulary Service Drug Information*®, or *AHFS DI*. It sells the two-volume set by subscription and provides four to six supplements each year. The *AHFS*® lists generic names and is divided into sections based on drug actions. The *AHFS*® is also available online.

Epocrates®

Epocrates® is available online or can be loaded onto a smartphone or other portable device. Epocrates® includes more than 3,300 brand and generic drugs, alternative medicines, a drug-drug interaction checker, an IV compatibility checker, ICD-10 and CPT codes, and a pill identification.

Package Insert

The **package insert** for each drug describes the drug: its purpose and effects (clinical pharmacology), indications, contraindications (conditions under which the drug should not be administered), warnings, precautions, adverse reactions, drug abuse and dependence, overdosage, and dosage and administration, as well as how the drug is supplied (for example, tablets in different doses, or liquid). The package insert, whether part of the *PDR* or found in the medication package, is a valuable resource for drug information. See Figure 51-6.

Drug Labels

To prepare and administer drugs, you must understand information that appears on drug labels, including the drug name, form, dosage strength, total amount in the container, route of administration, warnings, storage requirements, and manufacturing information. See Figure 51-7. By law, the generic name, as listed in the *USP-NF,* must appear on the drug's label. The drug label also may include the trade (brand) name used to market the drug. The trade name is typically indicated by the registered trademark symbol ®. The form of the drug is included, such as tablet, capsule, or liquid for oral administration. In some cases, a drug may be a combination drug, meaning more than one drug is in each tablet, capsule, or amount of liquid. Drug labels also include information about the amount of the drug present.

On the label, the dosage strength is stated as the amount of drug per dosage unit. In most cases, the amount of the drug is listed in grams (g), milligrams (mg), or micrograms (mcg), or

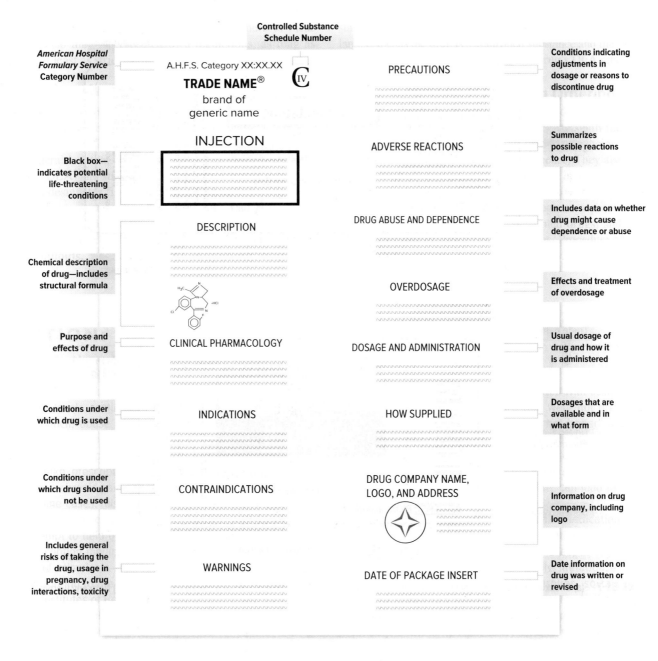

FIGURE 51-6 Use the package insert to become familiar with a drug's indications, contraindications, dosage, and potential adverse reactions.

The basic components of a prescription are

1. *Prescriber information:* Name, address, telephone number, and other information identifying the prescriber.
2. *Patient information:* Patient's full name, date of birth, address, and other information to identify the patient.
3. *Medication prescribed:* Includes generic or brand name, strength, and quantity. This is sometimes called the inscription and is found after the *Rx.*
4. *Subscription:* Instructions to the pharmacist dispensing the medication. This may include generic substitution and refill authorization.
5. *Signa:* Also known as the transcription; refers to patient instructions. These instructions generally follow the abbreviation *Sig,* which means "mark."
6. *Signature:* Prescriber's signature for handwritten prescriptions. The prescriber's signature must be in ink, but it cannot be a stamped signature. A digital signature is used if it is secure; otherwise, the prescription must be printed and then signed or otherwise authorized. The prescriber also must include the date the prescription was generated.
7. *DEA number:* This is required for prescriptions of Schedules II, III, IV, and V medications.

Many terms and abbreviations are used in prescriptions. See Table 51-5 for some examples. Abbreviations for drug names should not be used because there are similar abbreviations for multiple drugs. Recall from the *Patient Interview and History* chapter that there are many abbreviations that should not be used. These are known as the "Do Not Use" abbreviations, as identified by The Joint Commission (http://www.jointcommission.org), and "Error Prone," as identified by the Institute for Safe Medication Practices (http://www.ismp.org).

A medical assistant must be able to interpret a prescription accurately. Refer to Procedure 51-2 at the end of this chapter.

Managing Prescriptions Prescriptions may be printed or handwritten on a prescription blank. They also may be entered electronically and printed, or entered electronically and transmitted directly to a pharmacy. When the information is entered electronically and transmitted directly, this is known as **e-prescribing.** With e-prescribing, the medication information is received at the pharmacy; the actual prescription is never in the patient's hands. This is the most secure and efficient way for prescriptions to be completed. See the *Points on Practice* feature E-Prescribing.

Most frequently, prescriptions are entered into an EHR, then printed and signed for patients to take with them to the pharmacy. In a few cases, preprinted prescription blanks are used that include the licensed practitioner's name, address, telephone number, state license number, and DEA registration number plus blank space for writing the patient's name and address, the date, and other information. To prevent unauthorized use of these prescription blanks, never leave them unattended. If something about a prescription arouses suspicion, the pharmacist who receives a prescription may call the licensed practitioner's office to verify it. You should be able to check the patient's records and tell the pharmacist whether the practitioner wrote a prescription for that patient. If the prescription is a forgery, notify the licensed practitioner and, if she gives you authorization, notify the DEA.

Telephone Prescriptions If requested by the licensed practitioner, you may telephone a new or renewal prescription to the patient's pharmacy. You may not, however, telephone a prescription for a Schedule II drug. In an emergency situation, when a patient needs a drug immediately and no alternative is available, the physician may telephone a prescription for a Schedule II drug. The amount must be limited to the period of emergency and a written prescription must be sent to the pharmacist within 72 hours. The pharmacist must notify the DEA if a written prescription does not arrive within the specified time.

Patient requests for prescription renewals occur daily. The renewal requests may be called in to the receptionist or left on a designated phone or electronic mail system. It is the medical assistant's responsibility, if asked, to handle the prescription renewals/refills in an appropriate manner.

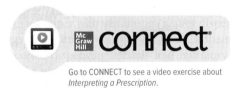

Go to CONNECT to see a video exercise about *Interpreting a Prescription.*

TABLE 51-5	Abbreviations Used in Prescriptions		
Abbreviation	**Meaning**	**Abbreviation**	**Meaning**
ā	Before	min	Minute, minimum
aa	Of each	mL	Milliliters
ac	Before meals	mm	Millimeters
AM	Morning	neb	Nebulizer
amp	Ampule	noct	Night
apl	Applicatorful	NPO	Nothing by mouth
aq	Water	nr	No refills
bid	Twice daily	oz	Ounce

TABLE 51-5   Abbreviations Used in Prescriptions

Abbreviation	Meaning	Abbreviation	Meaning
c̄	With	pc	After meals
cap	Capsule	per	By means of; through
cd	Cycle day (menstrual cycle)	PM	Evening or nighttime
cmpd	Compound	po, PO	By mouth
cr	Cream	PR, pr	Rectally
d	Daily or day	q	Every
DAW	Dispense as written (no generic)	qam	Every morning
disp	Dispense	q4h	Every 4 hours
ds	Double strength	qid	Four times daily
dx	Diagnosis	qs	Sufficient amount
elix	Elixir	r, rec	Rectally
eq	Equivalent	rept	Repeat
g, gm	Gram	rf	Refill(s)
gen	Generic	s̄	Without
gr	Grain (60 to 65 mg)	stat	Immediately
gtt	Drop(s)	subcut, subQ	Subcutaneously
h, hr	Hour	sup	Suppository
H₂O	Water	susp	Suspension
IM	Intramuscularly	sx	Symptoms
inj	Inject, injection	syr	Syrup
IV	Intravenously	tab	Tablet(s)
kg	Kilogram	tbsp	Tablespoon
L	Liter	tsp	Teaspoon
liq	Liquid	tx	Treatment
lot	Lotion	ud, utd	As directed
MDI	Metered dose inhaler	ung	Ointment
mEq	Milliequivalent	vag	Vaginally, into vagina
mg	Milligram(s)	YO	Years old

POINTS ON PRACTICE

E-Prescribing

E-prescribing is intended to bring greater safety to patients by providing for automatic drug and allergy interaction checking and by eliminating medication errors due to poor handwriting. E-prescribing also is designed to bring greater efficiency to the prescribing process for providers, as it dramatically decreases communications from pharmacies, requesting prescription clarifications.

Surescripts is the national clearinghouse for e-prescribing. The company electronically connects authorized prescribers, pharmacists, and payers nationwide, enabling them to exchange health information and prescribe without paper. Surescripts collaborates with national EHR vendors, pharmacies, and health plans to support authorized prescribers using EHR software. With this network in place, healthcare providers can electronically access prescription information from pharmacies, health plans, and other providers to see the patient's total prescription history from all sources. Through e-prescribing, EHRs are providing meaningful improvements in cost, quality, and patient safety. For example, when a medication is taken off the market, a record of all patients who have been prescribed this medication can be queried electronically and the prescribers and patients notified of the change.

Nonpharmacologic Pain Management

Because of drug interactions, adverse reactions, or the risk of dependence, many patients either prefer not to or should not take drugs to relieve chronic pain. The overuse and abuse of pain medications can be a problem. Pain frequently motivates these patients to use complementary and alternative medicine (CAM). The following are some examples:

- Chiropractors use spinal adjustments to treat chronic back or neck pain.
- Massage is used to treat headache or arthritis and to promote healing through relaxation.
- An acupuncture procedure in which very small amounts of electrical current are applied through needles has been used successfully to block the pain of surgery without anesthesia.
- Yoga uses postures to exercise the spine and stimulate the lymphatic system, helping to remove from the body toxins that may cause pain and stiffness in muscles and joints.
- Meditation is said to balance a person's physical, emotional, and mental states and is used as an aid in treating stress, anxiety, and pain.
- Hypnotism may be used to help patients overcome pain caused by stress-induced migraine headaches.
- Glucosamine chondroitin, a dietary supplement, is taken to treat osteoarthritis by reducing pain and slowing down joint cartilage damage.
- **Magnetic therapy** involves the use of magnets of varying sizes and strengths placed on the body to relieve pain or treat disease.
- Biofeedback can help a patient learn to evoke relaxation, which helps block pain perception.

CAM approaches and therapies have become more common in recent years. Some physicians and patients are seeking agents and treatments to manage health problems, such as chronic pain, that are less expensive, have fewer side effects, and are more accessible than traditional medical interventions. Pain clinics that use multiple pain management techniques are common.

Vaccines

LO 51.9

A vaccine is a preparation made from microorganisms and administered to a person to produce reduced sensitivity to, or increased immunity to, an infectious disease. Vaccines are stored with the office supply of drugs and require similar handling. If you work in a pediatrician's office, you will handle the vaccines for childhood diseases. In an adult practice, you can expect to see influenza and pneumonia vaccines and vaccines for diseases to which patients might be exposed in foreign travel.

It is important to know how vaccines work in the immune system. Through the immune system's action, a patient can be protected from—or made not susceptible to—a disease. This immunity results from the formation of antibodies that destroy or alter disease-causing agents. You can review information about immunity discussed in the chapter *The Lymphatic and Immune Systems.*

Antibody Formation

Antigens are foreign substances—bacteria, viruses, and other organisms—that can enter the human body in spite of its natural defenses. In response to an invasion by antigens, the body's specialized white blood cells (lymphocytes) produce antibodies. These antibodies are specific to the invading antigens and combine with the antigens to neutralize them. This action arrests or prevents the reaction or disease that the antigens would otherwise cause. Toxins, pollens, and drugs also can be antigens if the body reacts to them by forming antibodies. (Allergens are antigens that induce an allergic reaction.)

Vaccines contain organisms that have been killed or attenuated (weakened) in a laboratory. Because the organisms have been weakened, they stimulate antibody formation but do not overpower the body and cause disease. They may, however, still be strong enough to cause a fever and slight inflammation at the injection site. Some vaccines, such as those for influenza, may even produce some of the lesser effects of the disease against which they provide protection.

Immunizations made from organisms are called *vaccines.* Those made from the toxins of organisms are called *toxoids.* Some immunizations, such as the polio vaccine, last a lifetime. Others, such as tetanus toxoid, do not. In the latter case, booster immunizations must be used to stimulate the lymphocytes to produce antibodies again.

Immunizations

The Advisory Committee on Immunization Practices, the American Academy of Pediatrics, and the American Academy of Family Physicians jointly publish immunization schedules (see the *Assisting in Pediatrics* chapter). These schedules cover children from infancy through 18 years of age. Just as children receive immunizations before exposure to disease, adults may receive immunizations for influenza, pneumonia, or other diseases, including those to which an adult could be exposed during travel. Figure 51-10 displays the adult immunization schedules based on age. Additional information can be found at https://www.cdc.gov/vaccines/schedules/hcp/imz/adult.html.

Patients are sometimes immunized after exposure. For example, if patients have been exposed to a serious disease and there is too little time for them to produce antibodies, they may receive an antiserum containing antibodies to the disease-carrying organism. These immunizations are made from human or animal serum. If bacterial toxins (rather than bacteria) cause the disease, the patient may receive an antitoxin.

Antiserums and antitoxins must be used cautiously and are usually reserved for life-threatening infectious diseases. Because patients can be allergic to substances in animal antiserums and antitoxins, human serums are usually preferred. An example of a postexposure immunization is one given to a patient who has been exposed to hepatitis B virus (HBV). This patient should be given the antiserum hepatitis B immune globulin (HBV-Ig) within 7 days after exposure and again 28 to 30 days later. Because HBV-Ig is made from human serum, it causes relatively few adverse reactions. Another example is a patient who may have been exposed to tetanus (lockjaw) organisms as the result of an injury such as a puncture wound.

Vaccine	19-21 years	22-26 years	27-49 years	50-64 years	≥65 years
Influenza[1]	1 dose annually				
Tdap[2] or Td[2]	1 dose Tdap, then Td booster every 10 yrs				
MMR [3]	1 or 2 doses depending on indication (if born in 1957 or later)				
VAR[4]	2 doses				
RZV[5] (preferred)				2 doses RZV (preferred)	
or ZVL[5]					or 1 dose ZVL
HPV-Female[6]	2 or 3 doses depending on age at series initiation				
HPV-Male[6]	2 or 3 doses depending on age at series initiation				
PCV13[7]					1 dose
PPSV23[7]	1 or 2 doses depending on indication				1 dose
HepA[8]	2 or 3 doses depending on vaccine				
HepB[9]	3 doses				
MenACWY[10]	1 or 2 doses depending on indication, then booster every 5 yrs if risk remains				
MenB[10]	2 or 3 doses depending on vaccine				
Hib[11]	1 or 3 doses depending on indication				

Recommended for adults who meet the age requirement, lack documentation of vaccination, or lack evidence of past infection | Recommended for adults with other indications | No recommendation

FIGURE 51-10 Adult immunization schedule by age.

Source: https://www.cdc.gov/vaccines/schedules/hcp/imz/adult.html

This patient may receive tetanus immune globulin (T-Ig, a human product) or tetanus antitoxin. Because tetanus antitoxin is made from horse serum, it may cause serious reactions in patients who are allergic to horses or horsehair.

For every vaccine in your medical office, you must be familiar with the indications, contraindications, dosages, administration routes, potential adverse reactions, and methods of storage and handling. You must carefully read the package insert provided with each vaccine and, when necessary, consult drug reference books for further information. Knowledge of correct administration techniques is required and will be discussed in the *Medication Administration* chapter.

PROCEDURE 51-1 Helping the Licensed Practitioner Comply with the Controlled Substances Act of 1970

WORK // DOC

Procedure Goal: To comply with the Controlled Substances Act of 1970

OSHA Guidelines: This procedure does not involve exposure to blood, body fluids, or tissues.

Materials: DEA Form 224, DEA Form 224a, DEA Form 222, DEA Form 41 (available in the workbook that accompanies this textbook or online at the US Department of Justice's website), computer or pen

Method:

1. Use DEA Form 224 to register the licensed practitioner with the Drug Enforcement Administration. Be sure to register each office location at which the practitioner administers or dispenses drugs covered under Schedules II through V. Renew all registrations every 3 years using DEA Form 224a. Form 224 can be printed from the US Department of Justice website. The renewal application (Form 224a) can be completed through registration at this site.

2. Order Schedule II drugs using DEA Form 222, as instructed by the practitioner. (Stocks of these drugs should be kept to a minimum.)

RATIONALE: *Accurate instruction from the practitioner is necessary to ensure safety.*

3. Include the practitioner's DEA registration number on every prescription for a drug in Schedules II through V.
   RATIONALE: *The DEA number is required or prescriptions will not be accepted.*

4. Complete an inventory of all drugs in Schedules II through V every 2 years (as permitted in your state; this task may be reserved for other healthcare professionals).

5. Store all drugs in Schedules II through V in a secure, locked safe or cabinet (as permitted in your state).
   RATIONALE: *To prevent theft.*

6. Keep accurate dispensing and inventory records for at least 2 years.

7. Dispose of expired or unused drugs according to the DEA regulations. Always complete DEA Form 41 when disposing of controlled drugs.

PROCEDURE **51-2** Interpreting a Prescription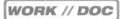

Procedure Goal: To read and accurately interpret a prescription

OSHA Guidelines: This procedure does not involve exposure to blood, body fluids, or tissues.

Materials: Prescription (use Figure 51-9), Table 51-5, and a method of recording (pen or electronic)

Method:

1. Verify the prescriber information. This is especially important in a multiphysician practice or electronic health record.

2. Ensure that patient information is accurate, including correct spelling of name, date of birth, and address. For written prescriptions, check legibility.

3. Confirm the date of the prescription.

4. Check the medication name and double-check spelling.

5. Verify that instructions to the pharmacist are complete and include refill authorization and generic substitution.

6. Interpret the instructions to the patient using abbreviations found in Table 51-5.

7. Make sure that the prescription is signed in ink for handwritten prescriptions and digitally for electronic prescriptions.

SUMMARY OF LEARNING OUTCOMES

OUTCOME	KEY POINTS
51.1 Identify the medical assistant's role in pharmacology.	The role of the medical assistant in pharmacology includes being attentive to ensure that the licensed practitioner is aware of all medications, both prescription and OTC, that a patient is taking; asking each patient about alcohol and recreational drug use (both past and present), as well as herbal remedies; assisting in managing and renewing medication prescriptions; and educating the patient, using guidelines provided by the licensed practitioner, about the purpose of a drug and how to take the drug for maximum effectiveness and minimum adverse reactions.
51.2 Recognize the five categories of pharmacology and their importance to medication administration.	The five categories of pharmacology are pharmacognosy, pharmacokinetics, pharmacodynamics, pharmacotherapeutics, and toxicology. It is important to understand each of these in order to carry out the medical assistant's role in pharmacology.
51.3 Differentiate the major drug categories, drug names, and their actions.	Drug categories are sometimes named based on their action; for example, anticonvulsants are used to treat convulsions (seizures). The major drug categories and their actions are outlined in Table 51-1.
51.4 Classify over-the-counter (OTC), prescription, and herbal drugs.	Nonprescription drugs, including herbal and OTC drugs, can be obtained without a licensed practitioner's order. For prescription drugs, patients must have an authorized prescriber's written (or oral) order.
51.5 Use credible sources to obtain drug information.	Credible sources for drug information are the *Physicians' Desk Reference®(PDR),United States Pharmacopeia/National Formulary,* and *American Hospital Formulary Service (AHFS®).*You also may access medication information from package inserts, drug labels, and reliable Internet sites.
51.6 Carry out the procedure for registering or renewing a physician with the Drug Enforcement Administration (DEA) for permission to administer, dispense, and prescribe controlled drugs.	The medical assistant should assist the licensed practitioner with registration, renewal, and ordering of controlled substances, as outlined in the Controlled Substances Act of 1970 and Procedure 51-1.

OUTCOME	KEY POINTS
51.7 **Identify the parts of a prescription, including commonly used abbreviations and symbols.**	A prescription must be complete to be filled. The medical assistant must be able to interpret a prescription in order to manage new and refilled medications. Procedure 51-2 and Table 51-5 will assist the medical assistant in performing these tasks.
51.8 **Discuss nonpharmacologic treatments for pain.**	Multiple nonpharmacologic methods are used to treat pain, including CAM therapies such as massage, yoga, biofeedback, chiropractic, acupuncture, magnetic therapy, hypnotism, and glucosamine chondroitin.
51.9 **Describe how vaccines work in the immune system.**	Immunizations usually contain killed or weakened organisms. When given, they stimulate the body to build up a resistance to the organism. They are used to provide immunity against specific diseases.

CASE STUDY CRITICAL THINKING

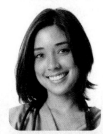

©Rubberball/Getty Images

Recall Kaylyn R. Haddix, RMA (AMT), from the case study at the beginning of the chapter. Now that you have completed the chapter, answer the following questions regarding her case.

1. Detail the steps Kaylyn R. Haddix should take to design and implement an inventory system.
2. What are some credible sources of drug information Kaylyn R. Haddix can use to complete her task?
3. Why is Kaylyn R. Haddix's attention to detail a critical skill for managing the office sample drug inventory and office medications?

EXAM PREPARATION QUESTIONS

1. (LO 51.3) Which drug may prevent an asthma attack?
   a. ProAir HFA®
   b. Elavil®
   c. Lovenox®
   d. Levaquin®
   e. Lipitor®

2. (LO 51.5) Which source of medication information is divided into six major sections?
   a. *American Hospital Formulary Service* (*AHFS®*)
   b. *United States Pharmacopeia/National Formulary*
   c. *Physicians' Desk Reference®* (*PDR*)
   d. Epocrates®
   e. RXList.com

3. (LO 51.6) Which of the following medications has the highest potential for addiction?
   a. Lomotil®
   b. Vicodin®
   c. Valium®
   d. Demerol®
   e. Ambien®

4. (LO 51.6) What method is used for disposing of controlled drugs?
   a. Discard drugs; then complete DEA Form 41.

   b. Use the disposal company that takes your biohazardous waste.
   c. Turn drugs over to a larger healthcare facility.
   d. Complete DEA Form 41 and call the DEA for disposal instructions.
   e. Complete DEA Form 222; then dispose of drugs with biohazardous waste.

5. (LO 51.4) An example of an OTC medication is
   a. Glucophage®
   b. Lasix®
   c. Coumadin®
   d. Lipitor®
   e. Prevacid®

6. (LO 51.7) The *Sig* line of a prescription reads "i tab po bid." What does it mean?
   a. Take 1 tablet by mouth twice a day.
   b. The order is not accurate and cannot be used.
   c. Take 1 tablet by mouth daily.
   d. Take ½ tablet daily.
   e. Take daily 1 tablet.

7. (LO 51.8) A patient would like to know more about nonpharmacologic treatments for pain. Which of the following would you *least* likely discuss with this patient?
   a. Massage therapy
   b. Biofeedback therapy
   c. Acupuncture
   d. Glucosamine chondroitin
   e. Opioids

8. (LO 51.1) Which of the following would *least* likely be the medical assistant's role?
   a. Make sure the licensed practitioner is aware of all medications a patient is taking.
   b. Ask each patient about alcohol and recreational drug use.
   c. Prescribe and dispense certain medications.
   d. Manage and renew medication prescriptions.
   e. Educate the patient according to licensed practitioner guidelines.

9. (LO 51.9) Which of the following is made from micro-organisms and administered to a person to produce reduced sensitivity to an infectious disease?
   a. Controlled substance
   b. Immunity
   c. Vaccine
   d. Antibiotic
   e. Pharmaceutical

10. (LO 51.2) Which of the following is the category of pharmacology that is also called *clinical pharmacology?*
   a. Pharmacodynamics
   b. Pharmacognosy
   c. Pharmacokinetics
   d. Pharmacotherapeutics
   e. Toxicology

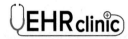

Go to CONNECT to complete the EHRclinic exercises: 51.01 Record Administration of a Vaccine, 51.02 Record Medications in a Patient's EHR, and 51.03 Create a Prescription Refill Request.

SOFT SKILLS SUCCESS

Recall Kaylyn R. Haddix from the case study at the beginning of the chapter. Once Kaylyn R. Haddix finished her organization of the drugs at BWW, she received compliments from Malik, and he even gave her a small raise. She was so excited that at dinner one night with a group of friends, she mentioned how she had organized the drug inventory at work and that she had gotten a raise. Someone at the table jokingly said, "Hey, can you get me some drugs?" Later, the same person, whom Kaylyn R. Haddix did not know very well, asked what kind of drugs she was working with and explained how she had a lot of trouble getting enough medication for her back pain. What should Kaylyn R. Haddix say or do in this situation?

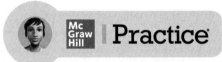

Go to PRACTICE MEDICAL OFFICE and complete the module Clinical: Privacy and Liability.

Dosage Calculations

CASE STUDY

Patient Name	**DOB**	**Allergies**
Christopher Matthews	11/19/2012	NKA
Attending	**MRN**	**Other Information**
Alexis N. Whalen, MD	00-AA-011	Home-schooled

Seven-year-old Christopher Matthews' mother brings him to the clinic today because he has a sore throat and has had a fever since yesterday. Although Chris Matthews is home-schooled, he went to a friend's birthday party last week. According to the friend's mother, her son is displaying similar symptoms. You check and record Chris Matthews' vital signs as follows: BP 110/64, T 101.8, P 96, R 20, Ht. 48 inches,

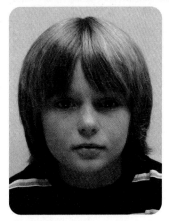

and Wt. 49.5 lb. During the physical exam, the physician notes that Chris Matthews' lymph nodes are swollen and he has some drainage from the tonsillar area. She orders a rapid strep test, which is positive, and diagnoses streptococcal pharyngitis. She writes a prescription for an antibiotic and tells Chris Matthews to take it easy until his symptoms subside.

Keep Chris Matthews in mind as you study this chapter. There will be questions at the end of the chapter based on the case study. The information in the chapter will help you answer these questions.

LEARNING OUTCOMES

After completing Chapter 52, you will be able to:

52.1 Explain the role of the medical assistant to ensure safe dosage calculations.

52.2 Identify systems of measurements and their common uses.

52.3 Convert among systems of measurements.

52.4 Execute dosage calculations accurately.

52.5 Calculate dosages based on body weight and body surface area.

KEY TERMS

amount to administer (A)	metric system
apothecary system	nomogram
body surface area (BSA)	proportion method
desired dose (D)	proportions
dose on hand (H)	quantity (Q)
formula method	volume
household system	weight

CAAHEP

II.C.1	Demonstrate knowledge of basic math computations
II.C.2	Apply mathematical computations to solve equations
II.C.3	Define basic units of measurement in: (a) the metric system (b) the household system
II.C.4	Convert among measurement systems
II.C.5	Identify abbreviations and symbols used in calculating medication dosages
II.P.1	Calculate proper dosages of medication for administration

ABHES

6. Pharmacology
   b. Demonstrate accurate occupational math and metric conversions for proper medication administration

8. Clinical Procedures
   j. Make adaptations for patients with special needs (psychological or physical limitations)

Introduction

Depending on the facility and state where you work as a medical assistant, you may be called on to administer medications. All aspects of this skill require close attention to detail for the safety of the patient. Before you administer a drug, you may need to calculate the dose prescribed by the licensed practitioner. You also should be familiar with the equipment you will be using. You must execute all dosage calculations carefully and accurately in order to prevent medication errors. To do so, you must perform basic math, understand various systems of measurement, and be able to convert from one measurement system to another or within a system. You also may need to know calculations for special patient populations. This chapter will provide the basics of safe dosage calculations. Remember to check the scope of practice in your state and at your place of employment before working with medications and their dosages.

Ensuring Safe Dosage Calculations   LO 52.1

In order to calculate dosages, you must understand and be able to perform basic math accurately. Whether you are using a calculator or doing it by hand, accuracy is key. Remember that a minor mistake in basic math can mean major errors in the patient's medication and consequently the patient's health. When you perform any calculation, think about the answer you obtain and determine if it is reasonable.

Consider this example: While performing a calculation, a medical assistant adds the following numbers: 21¾, 12½, and 1½. He calculates an answer of 49¼. Before he accepts this answer as correct, however, he asks himself, "Is this reasonable?" In order to answer this question, he does a quick estimation. First, he adds the whole numbers from each of the mixed numbers in the problem: 21 + 12 + 1 = 34. Then he rounds each mixed number up to a whole number and

adds them: 22 + 13 + 2 = 37. He recognizes that the correct answer to the problem must be between 34 and 37, so his original answer is incorrect. He probably entered one of the numbers into his calculator incorrectly. When he repeats the original calculation, he now comes up with an answer of 35¾. This is between the values that he expected based on his estimate, so it is a reasonable answer to the problem.

Think about the example. When performing calculations, there are many steps in which an error might be made. In this case, a number had been entered incorrectly into a calculator. While errors like this can happen to anyone, they can usually be detected by performing a quick check to see if the answer

POINTS ON PRACTICE
Math Review

Recall the following math rules while performing dosage calculations.

1. **Order of operations:** When solving a math problem, first divide or multiply from left to right; then add or subtract from left to right. For example, for the equation $\frac{650}{325} \times 3 = x$, you would need to divide 650 by 325 first. This equals 2.

   $x = 2 \times 3$

   Multiply second: $x = 6$

2. **Proportions:** Proportions are two fractions that are equal to each other. When 3 of the 4 values in a proportion are known, the unknown value can be calculated. Proportions using fractions are solved by cross multiplying. For example, to solve for the unknown in $\frac{2}{3} = \frac{x}{12}$, cross multiply ($3 \times x = 2 \times 12$) and then solve for the unknown ($3 \times x = 24$; divide both sides by 3; $x = 8$).

CAUTION: HANDLE WITH CARE

Working with Decimals

Consider the following when working with decimals to prevent errors in dosage calculations.

1. Writing decimals

- Write the whole-number part of the decimal to the left of the decimal point.
- Write the decimal fraction part to the right of the decimal point. Decimal fractions are equivalent to fractions that have denominators of 10, 100, 1,000, and so forth.
- Use zero as a placeholder to the right of the decimal point just as you use zero for whole numbers. The decimal number 4.203 represents 4 ones, 2 tenths, 0 hundredths, and 3 thousandths.

2. Using zeros

- Always write a zero to the left of the decimal point when the decimal number has no whole-number part. Using the zero makes the decimal point more noticeable.

- Never place a zero after the last nonzero digit to the right of the decimal point when working with medication dosages. These "trailing zeros" can be misinterpreted and cause medication errors.

3. Rounding decimals

- Underline the place value to which you want to round.
- Look at the digit to the right of this target place value. If this digit is 4 or less, do not change the digit in the target place value. If this digit is 5 or more, round the digit in the target place value up one unit. For example, to round 2.7384 to the hundredths place, underline the 3, which is in the hundredths place. The digit to the right of the 3 is 8, which is greater than 5, so you round the number up to 2.74.
- Drop all digits to the right of the target place value.

---

is reasonable. You should develop the habit of asking yourself the same question *every time you perform a calculation.* When performing a calculation, analyze the problem and try to estimate a reasonable range for the answer. This critical thinking skill can help you to detect errors and should become a part of every calculation you perform.

Safe dosage calculations depend on your understanding of basic math calculations. Refer to the *Points on Practice* feature Math Review for a quick refresher on some important math concepts.

▶ Measurement Systems LO 52.2

The three systems of measurement used in the United States for pharmacology and drug administration are the metric, apothecary, and household systems. Metric is the most commonly used system. Although apothecary and household systems are rarely used, you may need a basic knowledge of these systems.

To understand drug measurement, focus primarily on remembering the basic units of volume and weight. **Volume** refers to the amount of space a drug occupies. **Weight** refers to its heaviness. Length, which is also a basic unit, is discussed in the *Vital Signs and Measurements* chapter.

Metric System

Like the decimal system, the **metric system** is based on multiples of 10. The greater your confidence working with decimals, the more comfortable you will be working with metric units. See the *Caution: Handle with Care* feature Working with Decimals. The basic units of volume and weight in the decimal-based metric system are liters (L) to measure volume and grams (g) to measure weight. Prefixes are added to these basic units of measurement to indicate multiples, such as kilogram (kg), or fractions, such as milliliter (mL) or microgram (mcg). Common metric units and equivalents are presented in Table 52-1. Note that a cubic centimeter (cc) is the amount of space occupied by 1 mL. Although these two measurements are equal, the accepted medical abbreviation is mL. Do not use the abbreviation "cc," even though you may sometimes see it in practice. Additionally, note that the abbreviation for liters is a capital L instead of a small l. The small l can be confused with the numeral 1.

Apothecary and Household Systems

Although the metric system is preferred for dosage calculations, as a medical assistant you should have basic knowledge of the much older apothecary system, as well as the commonly known **household system**. The **apothecary system** uses units such as fluid ounces, fluid drams, pints, and quarts for volume,

---

TABLE 52-1 Common Metric Units					
Prefix	**Kilo-**	**Base Unit**	**Centi-**	**Milli-**	**Micro-**
Value	× 1000	—	÷ 100	÷ 1,000	÷ 1,000,000
Weight	kilogram (kg) 1,000 g	gram (g) 1 g	centigram (cg) 0.01 g	milligram (mg) 0.001 g	microgram (mcg) 0.000001 g
Volume	kiloliter (kL) 0.01 L	liter (L) 1 L	centiliter (cL) 0.01 L	milliliter (mL) 0.001 L	microliter (mcL) 0.000001 L

TABLE 52-2 Apothecary Units and Equivalents

Apothecary Units	Equivalents
Measures of Volume	
8 fluid drams (fl dr) =	1 fluid ounce (fl oz)
16 fl oz =	1 pint (pt)
2 pt =	1 quart (qt)
4 qt =	1 gallon (gal)
Measures of Weight	
60 gr =	1 dram (dr)
8 dr =	1 ounce (oz)
16 oz =	1 pound (lb)

TABLE 52-3 Household Units and Equivalents

Household Units	Equivalents
Measures of Volume	
60 drops* (gtt) =	1 teaspoon (tsp)
3 tsp =	1 tablespoon (tbsp)
6 tsp =	1 ounce (oz) or 2 tbsp
8 fl oz =	1 cup (c)
2 c =	1 pint (pt)
4 c =	1 quart (qt) or 2 pt

*Droppers may vary.

and drams, ounces, and pounds for weight. The only household units used for measurement are units of volume. They include drops, teaspoons, tablespoons, ounces, cups, pints, quarts, and gallons. Keep in mind that similar units of measurement in both the apothecary and the household systems are equal: An apothecary ounce equals a household ounce. Apothecary and household units and equivalents you may come across in practice are outlined in Tables 52-2 and 52-3.

▶ Conversions Within and Between Measurement Systems LO 52.3

Frequently, you will need to convert units of measure within or between systems of measurement. Most commonly, you will convert within the metric system. For example, you may need to determine how many milligrams of medication to give a patient when the medication only comes in grams. Sometimes you may need to convert from one measurement system to another. For example, a patient may need to take 5 milliliters of medication and the only measuring device she has is a teaspoon.

Converting Within the Metric System

Converting one metric unit of measurement to another is similar to multiplying and dividing decimal numbers. When you convert a quantity from one unit of metric measurement to another, you should follow these rules:

1. Move the decimal point to the right when you convert from a larger to a smaller unit. This is dividing.

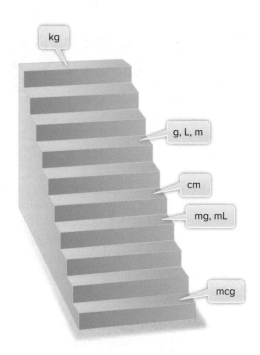

FIGURE 52-1 Use the metric steps to convert between units in the metric system.

2. Move the decimal point to the left when you convert from a smaller to a larger unit. This is multiplying.

Use Table 52-1 and Figure 52-1 to help determine both the direction and the number of places to move the decimal point when you convert between units of metric measurement. For example, milliliter is three decimal places to the right of liter, the basic unit. To convert a quantity from liters (larger) to milliliters (smaller), move the decimal point three places to the right, or three steps down the stairs shown in Figure 52-1. Similarly, to convert a quantity from grams (smaller) to kilograms (larger), move the decimal point three places to the left, or three steps up the stairs.

Let's try these examples.

Example A You need to change the patient's weight from grams to kilograms to determine how much medication should be given based on the patient's weight. An infant weighs 9,600 grams (g). How many kilograms (kg) does she weigh? A gram is smaller than a kilogram, so you need to move the decimal point to the left three steps, or divide by 1,000.

9.600 g ÷ 1,000 = 9.6 kg

Example B The physician orders a patient to have a 1-gram dose of amoxicillin. The medication is supplied in 1,000-mg tablets. You will need to determine how many milligrams are in a gram. A gram is larger than a milligram, so you need to move the decimal point to the right three steps, or multiply by 1,000.

1.000 gram × 1,000 mg

Your Turn A patient takes a daily dose of Synthroid® 100 mcg (micrograms). How many mg (milligrams) does he take?

TABLE 52-4	Common Equivalent Measures for the Metric, Apothecary, and Household Systems*		
1 teaspoon = 5 mL	1 tablespoon = 15 mL	1 fl oz = 30 mL
1 pint = 480 mL	1 kg = 2.2 lb	1 fl oz = 2 tbsp

*Equivalent measures are approximates.

First determine how many mg are in 1 mcg. A microgram is smaller than a milligram, so you need to move the decimal point to the left three steps, or divide by 1,000. The answer is 0.1 mg.

Converting Between Systems of Measurement

When performing dosage calculations, sometimes it will be necessary to convert units from one system to another. In order to do this, you must become familiar with their equivalent measures. Because of the difference in basic units of measure, you must remember that conversions between systems are only approximate equivalents. If you use a conversion chart, read it carefully before administering a drug. Check it several times and place a ruler under the line you are reading to be absolutely sure you are reading the chart properly. Table 52-4 provides equivalent measures for the metric, apothecary, and household systems.

In some cases, you may need to perform a calculation to convert between systems of measurement. You can use the **proportion method** to calculate these conversions. Let's try these examples.

Example A Suppose the licensed practitioner orders 10 milliliters (mL) of Benadryl® elixir. However, there is only a teaspoon (tsp) available to measure the dose. You need to know how many teaspoons are equivalent to 10 mL. To make this conversion, follow these steps.

1. Set up a fraction with the ordered dose on the top and the unknown amount on the bottom:
    $$\frac{10 \text{ mL}}{x \text{ tsp}}$$

2. Next set up a fraction with the standard equivalent. See Table 52-4. Make sure that for this fraction you use units of measure on the top and the bottom that match the units of measure on the top and the bottom of the first fraction:
    $$\frac{5 \text{ mL}}{1 \text{ tsp}}$$

3. Then set up a proportion with both fractions:
    $$\frac{10 \text{ mL}}{x \text{ tsp}} = \frac{5 \text{ mL}}{1 \text{ tsp}}$$

4. Now cross multiply. Multiply the bottom left number by the top right number, and multiply the top left number by the bottom right number:
    $$x \times 5 \text{ mL} = 10 \text{ mL} \times 1 \text{ tsp}$$

5. To solve for x, divide both sides of the equation by 5 mL; then do the arithmetic, canceling out like terms in the top and bottom of each fraction:
    $$\frac{x \times 5 \text{ mL}}{5 \text{ mL}} = \frac{10 \text{ mL} \times 1 \text{ tsp}}{5 \text{ mL}}$$
    $$x = \quad 2 \text{ tsp}$$

Example B Suppose the medication is ordered based on the patient's weight in kilograms. You know the patient's weight is 168 pounds and you need to convert the weight into kilograms To make this conversion, follow these steps:

1. Set up a fraction with the weight in pounds on top and the unknown weight in kilograms on the bottom:
    $$\frac{168 \text{ lb}}{x \text{ kg}}$$

2. Next set up a fraction with the standard equivalent. See Table 52-4. Make sure that for this fraction you use units of measure on the top and the bottom that match the units of measure on the top and the bottom of the first fraction:
    $$\frac{2.2 \text{ lb}}{1 \text{ kg}}$$

3. Then set up a proportion with both fractions:
    $$\frac{168 \text{ lb}}{x \text{ kg}} = \frac{2.2 \text{ lb}}{1 \text{ kg}}$$

4. Now cross multiply. Multiply the bottom left number by the top right number, and multiply the top left number by the bottom right number:
    $$x \times 2.2 \text{ lb} = 168 \text{ lb} \times 1 \text{ kg}$$

5. To solve for x, divide both sides of the equation by 2.2 lb; then do the arithmetic, canceling out like terms in the top and bottom of each fraction and then dividing 168 by 2.2:
    $$\frac{x \times 2.2 \text{ lb}}{2.2 \text{ lb}} = \frac{168 \text{ lb} \times 1 \text{ kg}}{2.2 \text{ lb}}$$
    $$x = 76.36 \text{ kg}$$

6. Follow the rules of rounding. To round to the nearest tenth, the 6 in the hundredth column is greater than 5 so you would round the answer to 76.4 kg. To round to the nearest whole number you would round to the nearest tenth 76.4 kg and since the 4 is less than 4 in the tenths column the nearest whole number would be 76 kg.

Your Turn You need to prepare a solution for the licensed practitioner to clean a wound. He asks for 3½ fluid ounces (fl oz) of saline to be placed in a sterile bowl. Your container of saline is marked in milliliters (mL). Use these steps to make the conversion:

1. Set up a fraction with the ordered dose on the top and the unknown amount on the bottom.

2. Next, set up a fraction with the standard equivalent. See Table 52-4. Make sure that for this fraction you use units of measure on the top and the bottom that match the units of measure on the top and the bottom of the first fraction.

3. Then set up a proportion with both fractions.

4. Now cross multiply. Multiply the bottom left number by the top right number, and multiply the top left number by the bottom right number.

5. To solve for x, cancel out like terms in the top and bottom of each fraction, then do the arithmetic.

6. Round to the nearest whole number.

If you followed each step correctly, you find that you need 105 mL of saline.

▶ Dosage Calculations

As a medical assistant, you may be called on to calculate medication doses. Remember to follow your scope of practice. You may be able to calculate these using either the proportion method or a **formula method**. No matter which method you use, you must be aware that the patient's health or life can depend on your calculations. Always take the time to check and recheck your arithmetic and determine if the answer is reasonable. If you have a question or you are not sure about your calculations, check them again and then have a coworker check. If you are not 100% sure you know how to do dosage calculations correctly, consider buying and using a dosage calculation workbook or searching the Internet for extra practice.

Proportion Method for Dosage Calculations

The proportion method described earlier in the chapter for unit conversion also can be used to perform dosage calculations. Let's try some examples.

Example A Suppose the doctor orders 500 mg of ampicillin, but each tablet contains only 250 mg. To calculate how to provide this dose, follow these steps:

1. Set up a fraction with the amount of the drug ordered over the unknown (in this case, the number of tablets).
$$\frac{500 \text{ mg}}{x \text{ tab}}$$
2. Next, set up a fraction with the amount of drug in a single tablet (dose on hand) over 1 tablet (dosage unit).
$$\frac{250 \text{ mg}}{1 \text{ tab}}$$
3. Now set up the proportion with both fractions, making sure the same units of measure are on the top and bottom of each side of the proportion.
$$\frac{500 \text{ mg}}{x \text{ tab}} = \frac{250 \text{ mg}}{1 \text{ tab}}$$
4. Cross multiply. Multiply the bottom left number by the top right number, and multiply the top left number by the bottom right number:
$$x \text{ tab} \times 250 \text{ mg} = 500 \text{ mg} \times 1 \text{ tab}$$
5. To solve for x, divide both sides of the equation by 250 mg; then do the arithmetic, canceling out like terms in the top and bottom of each fraction:

$$\frac{x \times 250 \text{ mg}}{250 \text{ mg}} = \frac{500 \text{ mg} \times 1 \text{ tab}}{250 \text{ mg}}$$
$$x = \frac{500 \text{ tab}}{250}$$
$$x = 2 \text{ tab}$$

The patient will receive 2 tablets.

Example B The doctor orders 30 mg of Bentyl®, but each capsule (cap) contains only 10 mg. To calculate the prescribed drug dose using the proportion method, you would follow these steps:

1. Set up a fraction with the amount of the drug ordered over the unknown amount (in this case, the number of capsules).
$$\frac{30 \text{ mg}}{x \text{ cap}}$$
2. Next set up a fraction with the amount of drug in a single capsule (dose on hand) over 1 capsule (dosage unit).
$$\frac{10 \text{ mg}}{1 \text{ cap}}$$
3. Now set up the proportion using both fractions, making sure the same units of measure are on the top and bottom of each side of the proportion.
$$\frac{30 \text{ mg}}{x \text{ cap}} = \frac{10 \text{ mg}}{1 \text{ cap}}$$
4. Cross multiply. Multiply the bottom left number by the top right number, and multiply the top left number by the bottom right number:
$$x \text{ cap} \times 10 \text{ mg} = 30 \text{ mg} \times 1 \text{ cap}$$
5. To solve for x, divide both sides of the equation by 10 mg; then do the arithmetic, canceling out like terms in the top and bottom of each fraction:

$$\frac{x \times 10 \text{ mg}}{10 \text{ mg}} = \frac{30 \text{ mg} \times 1 \text{ cap}}{10 \text{ mg}}$$
$$x = \frac{30 \text{ cap}}{10}$$
$$x = 3 \text{ cap}$$

The patient will receive 3 capsules.

Example C Now let's try a liquid medication. The licensed practitioner wants a patient to have 375 mg of valproic acid. You have on hand a bottle of valproic acid oral solution. See the label in Figure 52-2. Follow these steps:

1. Set up a fraction with the amount of the drug ordered over the unknown amount (in this case, the amount of liquid in mL).
$$\frac{375 \text{ mg}}{x \text{ mL}}$$
2. Next set up a fraction with the amount of drug in a single dose (dose on hand) over the number of mL in a single dose (dosage unit).
$$\frac{250 \text{ mg}}{5 \text{ mL}}$$

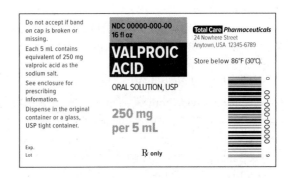

FIGURE 52-2 Valproic acid oral solution.

3. Now set up the proportion using both fractions, making sure the same units of measure are on the top and bottom of each side of the proportion.

$$\frac{375 \text{ mg}}{x \text{ mL}} = \frac{250 \text{ mg}}{5 \text{ mL}}$$

4. Cross multiply. Multiply the bottom left number by the top right number, and multiply the top left number by the bottom right number:

$$x \times 250 \text{ mg} = 375 \text{ mg} \times 5 \text{ mL}$$

5. To solve for x, divide both sides of the equation by 250 mg; then do the arithmetic, canceling out like terms in the top and bottom of each fraction and then multiplying 375 × 5 and dividing by 250:

$$\frac{x \times \cancel{250 \text{ mg}}}{\cancel{250 \text{ mg}}} = \frac{375 \cancel{\text{ mg}} \times 5 \text{ mL}}{250 \cancel{\text{ mg}}}$$
$$x = \frac{375 \times 5 \text{ mL}}{250}$$
$$x = 7.5 \text{ mL}$$

The patient will receive 7.5 mL of medication.

Your Turn The physician has ordered diazepam 4 mg by mouth. You have on hand the bottle of diazepam shown in Figure 52-3. Follow the steps below to determine how much medicine the patient should receive.

1. Set up a fraction with the amount of the drug ordered over the unknown (in this case, the number of tablets).

2. Next, set up a fraction with the amount of drug in a single tablet (dose on hand) over 1 tablet (dosage unit).

3. Now set up the proportion with both fractions, making sure the same units of measure are on the top and bottom of each side of the proportion.

4. Cross multiply. Multiply the bottom left number by the top right number, and multiply the top left number by the bottom right number.

5. To solve for x, cancel out like terms in the top and bottom of each fraction, then do the arithmetic.

If you did the problem correctly, you will discover that the patient needs 2 tablets.

Formula Method for Dosage Calculations

In some instances, you can use a basic formula to calculate drugs that have the same units as the dose ordered—such as milligrams and milligrams—and therefore do not require a conversion. When you use the formula method, you substitute the correct numbers for what each of the letters represents. The basic formula that you would use looks like this:

$$A = \frac{D}{H} \times Q$$

In this formula, A stands for the **amount to administer** (the amount of medication the patient will receive). To use the formula, you will need to know the values of D, H, and Q.

D = **Desired dose** (the amount of medication the licensed practitioner has ordered the patient to take)

H = **Dose on hand** (the amount of medication in each unit of the drug—for example, the number of mcg, mg, or g in each unit dose)

Q = **Quantity** of the dose on hand or dosage unit—for example, a pill or an amount of liquid

Let's try some examples.

Example A Suppose that the licensed practitioner orders acetaminophen 650 milligrams (mg). This is the desired dose (D). However, all that the office has on hand are 325 mg Tylenol® tablets. The dose on hand (H) is 325 mg and the quantity (Q) or dosage unit is 1 tablet because the dose on hand (325 mg) is given per tablet. Follow these steps to perform the calculation:

1. Use the formula, inserting each number, and label all the parts:

$$A = \frac{D}{H} \times Q$$
$$A = \frac{650 \text{ mg}}{325 \text{ mg}} \times 1 \text{ tablet}$$

2. Cancel and solve:

$$A = \frac{650 \cancel{\text{ mg}}}{325 \cancel{\text{ mg}}} \times 1 \text{ tablet}$$
$$A = \frac{650}{325} \times 1 \text{ tablet}$$
$$A = 2 \text{ tablets}$$

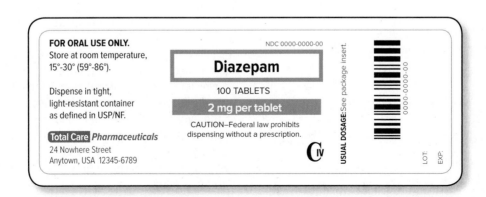

FOR ORAL USE ONLY.
Store at room temperature, 15°-30° (59°-86°).

Dispense in tight, light-resistant container as defined in USP/NF.

Total Care *Pharmaceuticals*
24 Nowhere Street
Anytown, USA 12345-6789

NDC 0000-0000-00

Diazepam

100 TABLETS

2 mg per tablet

CAUTION—Federal law prohibits dispensing without a prescription.

C IV

USUAL DOSAGE: See package insert.

0000-0000-00

LOT: EXP:

FIGURE 52-3 Diazepam tablets.

Two tablets need to be given to the patient. See the *Medication Administration* chapter for the correct procedure for administering a medication.

Example B Now let's say the licensed practitioner asks you to administer 10 mg of Compazine® by injection. The desired dose (*D*) is 10 mg. According to the Compazine® label, the liquid contains 5 mg/mL, which means there are 5 mg of Compazine® in every 1 mL of liquid, so 5 mg is the dose on hand (*H*) and 1 mL is the quantity (*Q*) or dosage unit. Always read the label carefully to determine the dose on hand and the quantity or dosage unit. See the *Caution: Handle with Care* feature Preventing Errors During Dosage Calculations. Follow the same steps to perform the calculation:

1. Use the formula, inserting each number in the correct place, and label all the parts:

$$A = \frac{D}{H} \times Q$$

$$A = \frac{10 \text{ mg}}{5 \text{ mg}} \times 1 \text{ mL}$$

2. Cancel and solve:

$$A = \frac{10 \text{ mg}}{5 \text{ mg}} \times 1 \text{ mL}$$

$$A = \frac{10}{5} \times 1 \text{ mL}$$

$$A = 2 \text{ mL}$$

The amount to administer to the patient is 2 mL. See the *Medication Administration* chapter for the correct procedure for administering a medication.

Example C The licensed practitioner wants a pediatric patient to have 200 mg of clarithromycin. The label of the only bottle you have on hand is pictured in Figure 52-4.

1. Use the formula, inserting each number, and label all the parts:

$$A = \frac{D}{H} \times Q$$

$$A = \frac{200 \text{ mg}}{250 \text{ mg}} \times 5 \text{ mL}$$

2. Cancel and solve:

$$A = \frac{200 \text{ mg}}{250 \text{ mg}} \times 5 \text{ mL}$$

$$A = \frac{200}{250} \times 5 \text{ mL}$$

$$A = 4 \text{ mL}$$

The patient should receive 4 mL of oral suspension. See the *Medication Administration* chapter for the correct procedure for administering an oral medication.

Your Turn The licensed practitioner orders 1.5 mg of granisetron hydrochloride oral solution. You have on hand

CAUTION: HANDLE WITH CARE

Preventing Errors During Dosage Calculations

Medication errors are a serious problem in healthcare. Always pay close attention to the dose and the route of administration (how the medication is given). You must check and recheck the ordered form of the drug as well as the amount of drug per dose of the drug. In the following example, this crucial relationship is illustrated.

Prochlorperazine (Compazine®) is an antiemetic drug for acute nausea and vomiting. It is given to both children and adults. When the vomiting is so severe that a tablet or capsule cannot be swallowed, the drug is administered in injectable or suppository form. This drug is available in multiple forms:

- 10 mL multidose vials with 5 mg of drug per mL, written as 5 mg/mL
- 2 mL single-dose vials with 5 mg/mL
- 4 fl oz bottles of syrup with 5 mg/5 mL (5 mg/1 tsp)
- 5 mg tablets
- 10 mg tablets
- 2 mL prefilled disposable syringes with 5 mg/mL
- 2½ mg suppositories
- 5 mg suppositories
- 25 mg suppositories
- 10 mg extended-release capsules
- 15 mg extended-release capsules

Because so many forms of this drug are available, there is a high risk of error in choosing the correct form. In addition, the route of administration determines how much drug is delivered in one dose. For example, note that suppositories are available in 2½ mg, 5 mg, and 25 mg forms. If the 2½ mg dose were written as 2.5 mg, there could be confusion with the 25 mg dose suppository. Thus, the 2½ mg suppository is always written this way, even in the *PDR*. This clarification helps prevent a child from receiving the adult dose of 25 mg, which could result in serious complications to the central nervous system. This possible confusion is one example of how much difference a decimal point can make. Note also that in the syrup there is a 5 mg dose of drug per 5 mL (1 tsp), whereas in the other liquid forms (vials and prefilled syringes), there is a 5 mg dose of drug per 1 mL. The injectable form is five times more concentrated than the syrup. Therefore, if you were to administer the same amount of injectable liquid as syrup to a patient, you would give the patient five times more drug than in the syrup. Just as a child could be endangered with the 25 mg suppository, an adult could be endangered with the wrong form of liquid. Because elderly patients often receive syrup forms of medication, this instruction could be particularly confusing.

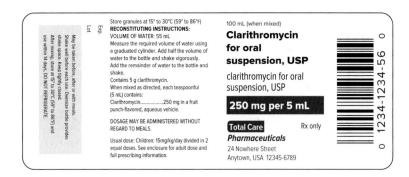

FIGURE 52-4 Clarithromycin for oral suspension.

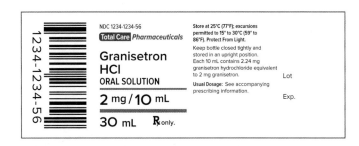

FIGURE 52-5 Granisetron hydrochloride oral solution.

the medication shown in Figure 52-5. How much medication should the patient receive?

1. Use the formula, inserting each number, and label all the parts.
2. Cancel units and solve.

The patient should receive 7.5 mL of medication. See the *Medication Administration* chapter for the correct procedure for administering an oral medication.

▶ Body Weight and Body Surface Area Calculations   LO 52.5

In certain cases, a drug dose is determined based on the patient's weight or the patient's **body surface area (BSA).** This is more common with pediatric and geriatric patients. These patients are at greater risk of harm from medication because of the way they break down and absorb medications. Calculations for these individuals must be precise. Although BSA and weight dosage calculations are usually done by the physician or other licensed healthcare personnel, you may be asked to perform calculations, depending on your area of practice.

Dosages Based on Weight

An order based on weight often states the amount of medication per weight of the patient per unit of time. For example, an order for a 34 lb child may read "Clarithromycin 15 mg/kg/day po q12h." This means that over the course of a day, the patient should receive 15 mg of medication for every kilogram (kg) he or she weighs. A portion of this total amount is to be given every 12 hours, or 2 times during a 24-hour period. You will need to calculate the patient's weight in kilograms, the

total medication to administer in 24 hours, and the amount of medication to administer in each dose. Use these steps:

1. Calculate the weight in kilograms using the proportion method. For accuracy, round the results to the nearest hundredth.
   a. Set up the proportion. Recall from Table 52-4 that 2.2 lb = 1kg.

   $$\frac{34 \text{ lb}}{x \text{ kg}} = \frac{2.2 \text{ lb}}{1 \text{ kg}}$$

   b. Cross multiply. Remember to multiply the bottom left number by the top right number, and multiply the top left number by the bottom right number.

   $$x \text{ kg} \times 2.2 \text{ lb} = 34 \text{ lb} \times 1 \text{ kg}$$

   c. Solve for x (the unknown).

   $$x = \frac{34}{2.2} \text{ kg}$$
   $$x = 15.45 \text{ kg}$$

2. Calculate the desired dose (D) for 24 hours by multiplying the dose ordered by the weight in kilograms. (Round your answer to the nearest milligram.)

   15 mg × 15.45 kg = desired dose (D) for 24 hours

   231.75 mg, rounded to 232 mg = D for 24 hours

3. Calculate the amount of medication to administer in each dose. To do this, divide the amount to be administered in 24 hours by the number of times the medication will be administered in 24 hours. In this case, the medication is to be given two times in 24 hours.

   232 mg ÷ 2 = 116 mg (the desired dose for one dose)

4. Calculate the amount to administer. On hand you have the medication shown in Figure 52-6.

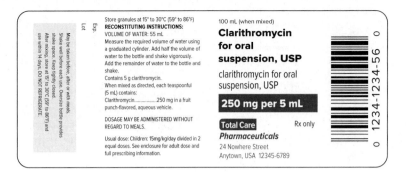

FIGURE 52-6 Clarithromycin for oral suspension.

a. Set up the equation. You want to give 116 mg of medication, and the label shows there are 250 mg in 5 mL of medication.

$$\frac{116 \text{mg}}{x \text{ mL}} = \frac{250 \text{ mg}}{5 \text{ mL}}$$

b. Cross multiply. Remember to multiply the bottom left number by the top right number, and multiply the top left number by the bottom right number.

$$x \text{ mL} \times 250 \text{ mg} = 116 \text{ mg} \times 5 \text{ mL}$$

c. Solve for x to determine the amount of liquid medication to administer to this patient.

$$x \text{ mL} = 116 \times \frac{5}{250} \text{ mL}$$
$$x \text{ mL} = 2.32 \text{ mL}$$
$$x \text{ mL} = 2.3 \text{ mL (rounded to the nearest tenth)}$$

Now that you have determined the amount, refer to the *Medication Administration* chapter before you give the medication to the patient.

Dosages Based on Body Surface Area

The total surface area of the body, or body surface area (BSA), is measured in square meters (m^2). A person's BSA is used to calculate very precise medication dosages. Pediatric patients, as well as burn victims and patients undergoing chemotherapy or radiation therapy, may need BSA dosage calculations. A complex formula or a nomogram, as shown in Figure 52-7, may be used to determine the BSA. A **nomogram** is a set of scales arranged so that a ruler aligned with two of the values shows the corresponding value on the third scale. Aligning the ruler with a person's height and weight shows the body surface area. In this case, the child is 89 cm tall and weighs 13.9 kg. The line drawn between these values in the first and third columns crosses the second column at approximately 0.57, so the child's BSA is 0.57 m^2. For BSA medication ordered as 30 mcg/m^2, this patient would receive 30 mcg × 0.57 = 17.1 mcg of the medication.

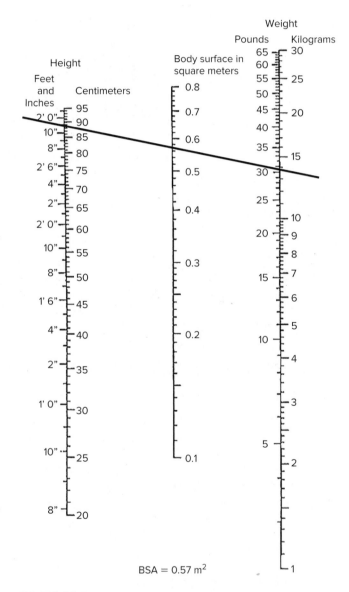

FIGURE 52-7 A nomogram is used to determine the BSA in order to calculate a medication dose.

OUTCOME	KEY POINTS
52.1 Explain the role of the medical assistant to ensure safe dosage calculations.	A medical assistant must be proficient in math and determine whether the answer is reasonable for every calculation he or she performs.
52.2 Identify systems of measurements and their common uses.	The metric system is based on 10 and is the most common system of measurement for dosage calculations. Metric units commonly used for dosage calculations include g, mg, mcg, and mL. The apothecary and household systems have some equal measures, but they are used rarely.
52.3 Convert among systems of measurements.	To convert among systems of measurements, you can refer to a conversion chart or perform a proportion method calculation. Keep in mind that measurements between the metric and the apothecary and household systems are only approximations.
52.4 Execute dosage calculations accurately.	Use the proportion method or formula method to perform dosage calculations. *Proportion Method* 1. Set up a fraction with the amount of the drug ordered over the unknown amount. 2. Set up a fraction with the amount of drug in a single dose (dose on hand) over the dosage unit. 3. Set up the proportion using both fractions, making sure the same units of measure are on the top and bottom of each side of the proportion. 4. Cross multiply. 5. To solve for *x,* do the arithmetic; then cancel out like terms in the top and bottom of each fraction. *Formula Method* $$A = \frac{D}{H} \times Q$$ where A = Amount to administer (the amount of medication the patient will receive). D = Desired dose (the amount of medication the licensed practitioner has ordered the patient to take). H = Dose on hand (the amount of medication in each unit of the drug). Q = Quantity of the dose on hand or dosage unit.
52.5 Calculate dosages based on body weight and body surface area.	Dosages based on body weight and BSA are used when precise amounts of medication must be administered. Body weight calculations are usually ordered in mg/kg/day. BSA calculations use special formulas or a nomogram.

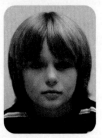

©McGraw-Hill Education

Recall Chris Matthews from the case study at the beginning of the chapter. Now that you have completed the chapter, answer the following questions.

1. The physician ordered amoxicillin 50 mg/kg/day po q8h. What is Chris Matthews' weight in kilograms?

2. The medication on hand is amoxicillin oral suspension 200 mg per 5 mL. How much medication, in milliliters, should Chris Matthews receive for each dose?

3. Name at least three things you can do to ensure that Chris Matthews receives a safe and accurate dose of medication.

There may be more than one correct answer. Circle the *best* answer.

1. (LO 52.1) As a medical assistant, how can you *best* ensure safe dosage calculations?
   a. Use a calculator for every calculation.
   b. Check with a coworker for every calculation you perform.
   c. Do not use the unit of measurement when performing calculations.
   d. Use a trailing zero after the decimal point for whole numbers.
   e. Check your calculation by determining if the results are reasonable.

2. (LO 52.2) What do the following metric prefixes represent in comparison to the base unit: kilo; milli; micro?
   a. × 1,000; ÷ 100; ÷ 1,000,000
   b. × 100; ÷ 1,000; ÷ 1,000,000
   c. ÷ 1,000,000; × 1,000; ÷ 1,000
   d. × 1,000; ÷ 1,000; ÷ 1,000,000
   e. ÷ 1,000; × 1,000; ÷ 1,000,000

3. (LO 52.4) How much medication should be given if the physician ordered Keflex® 500 mg and you have on hand Keflex® 250 mg per 5 mL?
   a. 5 mL
   b. 250 mg
   c. 250 mL
   d. 10 mL
   e. 125 mL

4. (LO 52.4) How much medication would be in the syringe if the physician ordered Decadron® 6 mg IM now and you have on hand Decadron® 4 mg per mL?
   a. 1.5 mg
   b. 1.5 mL
   c. 4 mL
   d. 1 mL
   e. 3 mL

5. (LO 52.4) The doctor orders 5 mg of glyburide, but each tablet contains only 1.25 mg. How many tablets should the patient take?
   a. 3
   b. 1.25
   c. 5
   d. 1
   e. 4

6. (LO 52.5) The physician has ordered gemcitabine 400 mg/m² IV for a patient whose BSA is 0.47m². You have on hand a 200 mg vial of gemcitabine for injection that contains 38 mg per mL. How much medication should this patient receive?
   a. 94 mg
   b. 17.9 mL
   c. 200 mg
   d. 5 mL
   e. 10.5 mL

7. (LO 52.3) The licensed practitioner orders Ceclor® 0.375 g PO bid. You have on hand Ceclor® oral suspension 187 mg per 5 mL. How many mg of Ceclor® are ordered?
   a. 187
   b. 5
   c. 0.375
   d. 375
   e. 0.187

8. (LO 52.4) The licensed practitioner orders Ceclor® 0.375 g PO bid. You have on hand Ceclor® oral suspension 187 mg per 5 mL. How many mL of Ceclor® do you need to administer?
   a. 10
   b. 5
   c. 187
   d. 2.5
   e. 0.375

9. (LO 52.4) The physician wants you to give the patient an IM injection of 135 mg of ceftriaxone. You have on hand the medication pictured here. How many mL of medication would you inject?

a. 2 mL

b. 135 mcg

c. 0.11 mL

d. 1,000 mg

e. 1.35 mL

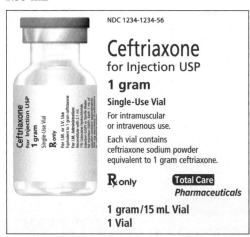

NDC 1234-1234-56

Ceftriaxone
for Injection USP

1 gram

Single-Use Vial

For intramuscular or intravenous use.

Each vial contains ceftriaxone sodium powder equivalent to 1 gram ceftriaxone.

℞ only **Total Care** *Pharmaceuticals*

1 gram/15 mL Vial
1 Vial

10. (LO 52.5) A 5-year-old child weighs 44 lb. The licensed practitioner orders him to receive Zinacef® 50 mg/kg/day IM q6h. How many milligrams of medication should the child receive in one dose?

a. 1,000 mg

b. 167 mg

c. 20 kg

d. 250 mg

e. 50 mg

SOFT SKILLS SUCCESS

1. The patient says she is here for a B$_{12}$ injection and the order reads "Cyanocobalamin 500 mcg IM now." You have never given cyanocobalamin or a B$_{12}$ injection before. What should you do?

2. Using the order in question 1, you find a vial of cyanocobalamin that is 1,000 mcg/mL and give the patient a 1 mL injection in the deltoid muscle of her left arm. When you get ready to chart the medication,

you realize you should have given only 0.5 mL of the medication. What should you do now?

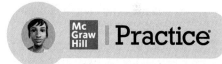

Mc Graw Hill | **Practice**

Go to PRACTICE MEDICAL OFFICE and complete the module Clinical: Privacy and Liability.

Medication Administration

C A S E   S T U D Y

PATIENT INFORMATION	Patient Name	DOB	Allergies
	John Miller	12/05/1954	Bee stings
	Attending	**MRN**	**Other Information**
	Paul F. Buckwalter, MD	00-AA-005	Seeing physical therapist 3X a week for injury.

John Miller has arrived at the clinic for a return-to-work visit. He has a history of hypertension, diabetes Type 2, myocardial infarction (MI) 4 years ago, and congestive heart failure (CHF). He has been taking glyburide 2.5 mg daily, captopril

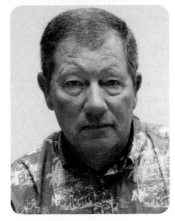

©McGraw-Hill Education

25 mg twice a day, and HCTZ 25 mg daily. He is here for a blood pressure check, and the physician wants to evaluate the medications he just started 3 months ago. He also is scheduled for a pneumococcal immunization. As you read through this chapter, think about what the medical assistant should do next and why.

Keep John Miller in mind as you study this chapter. There will be questions at the end of the chapter based on the case study. The information in the chapter will help you answer these questions.

L E A R N I N G   O U T C O M E S

After completing Chapter 53, you will be able to:

53.1 Describe rules and responsibilities regarding drug administration and the initial preparation for drug administration.

53.2 List the rights of drug administration.

53.3 Recognize the correct equipment to use for administering medications.

53.4 Carry out the procedures for administering oral medications.

53.5 Carry out procedures for administering parenteral medications by injection.

53.6 Carry out procedures for administering parenteral medications by other routes.

53.7 Relate special considerations required for medication administration to pediatric, pregnant, breast-feeding, and geriatric patients.

53.8 Outline patient education information related to medications.

53.9 Implement accurate and complete documentation of medications.

K E Y   T E R M S

buccal
calibrated spoon
diluent
douche
infusion
intradermal (ID)
intramuscular (IM)
intravenous (IV)

ointment
scored
solution
subcutaneous (subcut)
sublingual
transdermal
triple check
Z-track method

I.P.4 Verify the rules of medication administration:
(a) right patient
(b) right medication
(c) right dose
(d) right route
(e) right time
(f) right documentation

I.P.5 Select proper sites for administering parenteral medication

I.P.6 Administer oral medications

I.P.7 Administer parenteral (excluding IV) medications

II.C.5 Identify abbreviations and symbols used in calculating medication dosages

II.P.1 Calculate proper dosages of medication for administration

V.P.4 Coach patients regarding:
(b) health maintenance
(c) disease prevention
(d) treatment plan

X.C.11 Describe the process in compliance reporting:
(a) unsafe activities
(b) errors in patient care
(d) incident reports

X.P.3 Document patient care accurately in the medical record

X.P.6 Report an illegal activity in the healthcare setting following proper protocol

2. Anatomy and Physiology
c. Identify diagnostic and treatment modalities as they relate to each body system

6. Pharmacology
a. Identify drug classification, usual dose, side effects, and contraindications of the top most commonly used medications
d. Properly utilize Physicians' Desk Reference (PDR), drug handbooks and other drug references to identify a drug's classification, usual dosage, usual side effects, and contraindications

8. Clinical Procedures
f. Prepare and administer oral and parenteral medications and monitor intravenous (IV) infusions

▶ Introduction

Drug administration is one of the most important and most dangerous duties for a medical assistant. By following the procedures for proper drug administration, you can help restore patients to health. If you calculate dosages inaccurately, measure drugs incorrectly, or administer drugs improperly, patients' medications may have no therapeutic effect, may worsen their disease or abnormal condition, or may even cause them to die.

To administer drugs safely and effectively to all patient groups, including pediatric, pregnant, and elderly patients, you must know and understand the principles of pharmacology (see the *Principles of Pharmacology* chapter) and how to perform dosage calculations (see the *Dosage Calculations* chapter). This chapter prepares you to understand the fundamentals of drug administration, including:

- Rules and responsibilities of drug administration.
- Rights of drug administration.
- Routes of medication administration.
- Techniques needed to administer drugs.
- Special patient considerations.
- Patient education.

Your role may vary depending on the state and practice where you are employed. Many states have medical practice acts that define the exact duties of medical assistants in drug administration. For example, an act may specify which drugs you are allowed to administer and by which routes. Because state laws vary, you need to research the scope of practice for medical assistants in the state where you will work.

▶ Preparing to Administer a Drug   LO 53.1

To administer drugs, you should know the uses, contraindications, interactions, and adverse effects of common medications. You should be familiar with the medications frequently prescribed in your practice. Furthermore, to be able to assume a role in patient education, you must be comfortable with all aspects of medication administration so that you can instruct patients about the medications prescribed to them.

Although the physician gives the order to administer a medication, the medical assistant has a lot of responsibility before a medication can be administered. As a medical assistant, you often will interview the patient. You must be alert to—and inform the licensed practitioner of—any change in the patient's condition that could affect drug therapy. Some preparation tasks are related to the drugs and drug allergies, administration site, patient condition, and patient consent.

Drugs and Drug Allergies

Before any medication is given, the physician should be aware of the medications the patient is currently taking. As you learned in the *Principles of Pharmacology* chapter, some medications, including herbal medications, can interact in a negative way, so the physician needs to know everything the patient is taking before ordering a medication. The medical assistant is responsible for ensuring that a complete and accurate medication list is maintained on the patient's chart. This medication list must be updated every time the patient comes for an appointment. See Figure 53-1. While asking about medications, you also must ask the patient about any drug allergies. Even though you may see a patient on a regular basis, be in the habit of asking about drugs and drug allergies at every patient visit. Patients often see other physicians or specialists, who may have prescribed different medications. A patient could have had a drug reaction to a medication prescribed by another physician. If applicable, document in the patient chart "NKDA," or "no known drug allergies."

Administration Site

Drugs may be administered for either local or systemic effects. Generally, drugs that have local effects are applied directly to the skin, tissues, or mucous membranes. Drugs that produce systemic effects are administered by routes that allow the drug to be absorbed and distributed in the bloodstream throughout the body. These various routes are discussed in *section 53-3* of this chapter. Before you administer a medication, you must check the site of administration. For example, if you are asked to give an oral medication, you must make sure the patient can take the medication. You may ask if the patient is nauseated, can swallow a pill, or has had anything to eat or drink, depending on the medication.

For an injection, you must locate and inspect the injection site. Find the appropriate injection site by using anatomical landmarks. Inspect the skin by checking for the following conditions, which may eliminate the site:

- Moles
- Scars
- Birthmarks
- Traumatic injury
- Redness
- Rash
- Edema
- Cyanosis
- Burns
- Tattoos
- Site of a mastectomy
- Paralyzed areas
- Warts

If you are unsure about any of these conditions, inform the physician.

Patient Condition

Before administering a medication, observe the patient for any condition that might interfere with the medication you will be administering. For example, a patient who is nauseated or vomiting may not be able to swallow a pill. In addition, review the patient's drug list to ensure that any medications already being taken will not interfere with the ordered drug or route of administration. Double-check the order and ensure that it is appropriate for the patient's age and weight.

Patient Consent Form

Many physicians require that a patient sign a consent form before receiving an injection. A consent is necessary for vaccines, for example. This form provides general information regarding the medication or vaccine and lists the possible side effects or adverse effects. If a consent form is needed, make sure that the patient signs the form and that you have answered any questions prior to giving the injection.

General Rules for Medication Administration

No matter what drug or administration route is ordered, follow these general rules when administering medications.

- Give only the medications the physician has ordered. Written orders are preferable, but oral orders are appropriate for emergencies. If you are unfamiliar with any aspect of a medication the physician orders, consult a credible drug reference.
- Wash your hands before handling the medication. Prepare the medication in a well-lit area, away from distractions. Focus only on the task at hand.
- Perform a **triple check** by checking the medication three times. Check the medication three times even if the dose is prepackaged, labeled, and ready to be administered.

> **1st check**—*when you take it from the storage container and match it to the medication administration record (MAR) or the physician order*
> **2nd check**—*when you prepare it*
> **3rd check**—*before you close the storage container or just before you administer the medication to the patient*

- Calculate the dose if necessary. See the *Dosage Calculations* chapter. Remember, if you are unsure of your computation, ask another medical assistant or a licensed practitioner to check it.
- Avoid leaving a prepared medication unattended, and never administer a medication that someone else has prepared.
- Ask the patient to state his name and date of birth to ensure correct identification. Double-check with the patient about possible drug allergies. Do not rely on documentation in his chart; he may have developed a new allergy that has not yet been added to the record.
- Be sure the physician is in the office when you administer a medication or vaccine. If the patient develops an anaphylactic reaction (sudden, severe allergic reaction) to the medication or vaccine, the physician must administer epinephrine.

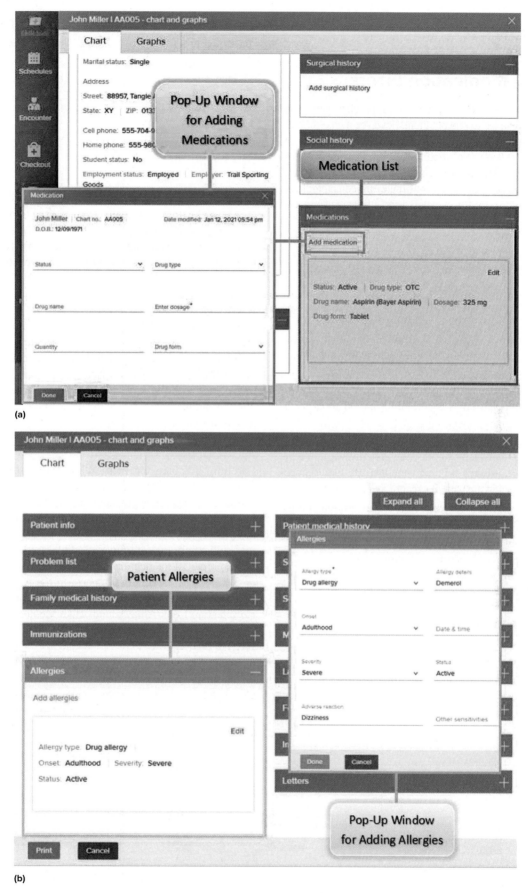

FIGURE 53-1 (a) Each time a patient visits the clinic, update the medication list as needed. (b) Be certain to ask about allergies and record these in the allergy window in the electronic health record.

(a-b) ©McGraw-Hill Education

Handling Medication Errors

Medication errors are a serious yet inevitable problem. Great care always should be taken to prevent them. However, if an error does occur, no matter the cause, it must be reported. Immediately tell the licensed practitioner. Not reporting an error is unethical and in some cases illegal, especially if a serious consequence occurs. Most facilities require that an incident report be completed. This form documents the error. It is completed and then signed by everyone involved, as well as your supervisor. Errors also are reported online through an online program developed by the US Pharmacopeia and the Institute for Safe Medical Practices. Reporting errors at these sites provides information to assist in the prevention of errors.

- After administering the medication, ask the patient to remain in the facility for 10 to 20 minutes so that you can observe the patient for any unexpected effects, such as anaphylaxis. See the *Emergency Preparedness* chapter.

- Give the patient specific instructions about the effects of the medication as well as general information about medication use.

- If the patient refuses to take the medication, discard it according to your facility policy. Do not flush it down the toilet or return it to the original container. Be sure to document the refusal in the patient's record and tell the physician.

- If you make an error in medication administration, tell the physician immediately. See the *Caution: Handle with Care* feature Handling Medication Errors.

- Document the medication and dose immediately after administration; never document administration before giving medicine.

▶ Rights of Medication Administration   LO 53.2

The rights of medication administration are a set of safety checks the medical assistant must follow to prevent errors and ensure patient safety when administering medications (see

TABLE 53-1	The Rights of Medication
Basic Rights	**Additional Rights**
1. Right patient	7. Right reason
2. Right drug	8. Right to know
3. Right dose	9. Right to refuse
4. Right route	10. Right technique
5. Right time	
6. Right documentation	

Table 53-1). The basic rights of medication administration are the following: right patient, right drug, right dose, right route, right time, and right documentation. Additional rights include right reason, right to know, right to refuse, and right technique. A violation of any of the rights constitutes a medication error.

Right Patient

Always check the name and date of birth on the order for a medication or vaccine in the patient's chart, then compare to the name and date of birth that the patient tells you. Do not call the patient by name because a forgetful or confused patient might answer to any name. Have an attending caregiver or family member state the name and date of birth if the patient is unable.

Right Drug

Carefully compare the name of the prescribed medication or vaccine in the patient's chart with the label on the medication container. As you check the medication name on the label, look at the expiration date. Never use a medication that has passed this date (Figure 53-2). If you are unfamiliar with the medication, look it up in a credible drug reference. Also, never prepare a medication from a container with a damaged or handwritten label. Always perform the triple check every time you prepare a medication. See the *Caution: Handle with Care* feature Look-Alike/Sound-Alike Medications.

Right Dose

Compare the dose on the order in the patient's chart with the dose you prepare. To obtain the right dose, read the label closely and calculate accurately. Do not confuse the dose contained in one tablet with the number of tablets in the container.

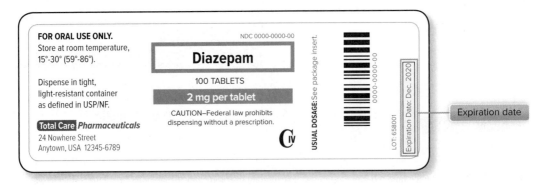

FIGURE 53-2   Check the label for the expiration date before administering a medication.

CAUTION: HANDLE WITH CARE

Look-Alike/Sound-Alike Medications

Recall from the *Principles of Pharmacology* chapter that many medications have very similar names. Although the names may be similar, the drugs often have very different purposes. For example, Cerebyx® is an anti-epileptic drug. The look-alike/sound-alike drug Celebrex® is an anti-inflammatory. It is critical to check the name of each medication carefully. Never assume that the drug is misspelled on the medication order or prescription. If you do not recognize the spelling, *always* look it up in a credible drug reference. (See Table 51-2.)

Right Route

Double-check to make sure the administration route you are preparing to use matches the route the licensed practitioner ordered. Also check that the medication you are using can be administered by the route ordered. For example, do not confuse ear (otic) drops with eye (optic) drops. Check that the patient can receive the medication by this route and that the route seems appropriate. For example, if the patient has an injury at the specified injection site, consult the licensed practitioner for a possible alternative site or a different route.

Right Time

Be sure to give the medication at the right time. If it must be given after meals, make sure the patient has eaten recently. For certain medications, you must ensure that it is the correct time of day and the correct time in a series of doses. For example, timing is crucial with allergy shots because of possible reactions.

Right Documentation

Document the procedure immediately after administering the medication or vaccine to the patient. Do not wait until later and do not document before administration. Be sure to include the date, time, medication or vaccine name, lot number, dose, administration route, patient reaction, and patient education about the medication, as well as your first initial and last name. If the medication is a controlled substance, also document it on the controlled substance inventory record. Always double-check your entry for computer documentation before submitting. Use neat handwriting for written documentation.

Right Reason

The person who administers the medication should know the reason the medication is being given.

Right to Know

All patients have the right to be educated about the medications they are receiving. This should include the reason, the effect, and the side effects of medications.

Right to Refuse

Every patient has the right to refuse a medication. If a patient does refuse a medication or vaccine, you should report this to the physician who ordered the medication. A refusal of medication by a patient should be documented in the patient's medical record.

Right Technique

Always use the proper administration technique. If you have not given a medication or vaccine by the ordered route recently, review the technique before administering the drug.

▸ Drug Routes and Equipment   LO 53.3

The physician may ask you to administer medications by one of the routes outlined in Table 53-2.

TABLE 53-2 Routes and Methods of Drug Administration	
Route and Drug Forms	**Method**
Buccal route Tablets	Place drug between the patient's gum and cheek. To ensure absorption, tell the patient to leave the tablet there until it dissolves and not to chew or swallow it. Tell the patient not to eat, drink, or smoke until the tablet is completely dissolved.

Inhalation therapy (nasal or oral)
   Aerosols
   Sprays
   Mists or steam
	Administer the drug by inhalation to reach the respiratory tract. The drug will be absorbed in 7 to 20 seconds.

Intradermal route
   Solutions
   Powders for reconstitution
	Administer the drug by injection between the upper layers of the patient's skin.

Intramuscular route
   Solutions
   Powders for reconstitution
	Administer the drug by injection into the muscle. The drug will be absorbed in 3 to 5 minutes.

(Continued)

TABLE 53-2   Routes and Methods of Drug Administration   Continued

Route and Drug Forms	Method

Intravenous route
   Solutions (often in bags of 250, 500, or 1,000 mL)
   Powders for reconstitution
   Blood and blood products
	Administer the drug by injection or infusion into a vein. The drug will be absorbed in 15 to 30 seconds.

Ophthalmic (eye) or otic (ear) route
   Solutions
   Ointments
	Apply the drug, usually as drops, in the patient's eye or ear.

Oral route
   Tablets
   Capsules
   Liquids
   Lozenges
	Give the drug to the patient to swallow. The drug will be absorbed in 20 minutes to 3 hours, depending on food and drug ingestion.

Rectal route
   Suppositories
   Solutions
	Insert a suppository into the patient's rectum. Administer a solution as an enema, using a tube and nozzle.

Subcutaneous route
   Solutions
   Powders for reconstitution
	Administer the drug by injection into the subcutaneous layer of skin. The drug will be absorbed in 3 to 5 minutes.

Sublingual route
   Tablets
   Sprays
	Place the drug under the patient's tongue. To ensure absorption, tell the patient to leave the tablet there until it dissolves and not to chew or swallow it. Tell the patient not to eat, drink, or smoke until the tablet is completely dissolved.

Topical route
   Ointments
   Lotions
   Creams
   Tinctures
   Powders
   Sprays
   Solutions
	Apply the drug to the patient's skin or rub it into the skin.

Transdermal route Patches	Apply the drug to a clean, dry, nonhairy area of the patient's skin.
Urethral route Solutions	Administer the drug by instilling it in the patient's bladder, using a catheter.

Vaginal route
   Solutions
   Suppositories
   Ointments
   Foams
   Creams
	Administer a solution as a douche, using a tube and nozzle. Administer other forms by inserting them into the vagina with an applicator.

Most patients take a prescription to a pharmacy to be filled and then take oral medications at home, so you may not need to administer these medications in the office very often. However, you are likely to be asked to:

- Place medications in the patient's mouth between the cheek and gum or under the tongue.
- Administer or teach a parent to administer a medication using a dropper, a medicine cup, an oral syringe, or a calibrated syringe. A **calibrated spoon** has markings (calibrations) that allow you to measure a dose. An oral syringe also has calibrations and a soft, flexible tip. See Figure 53-3.
- Administer a medication by any means other than by mouth (if permitted by your scope of practice and state laws). This would require the use of a syringe and safety-engineered needles, as discussed in *section 53-5* and the *Infection Control Practices* chapter.
- Demonstrate how to use an inhaler.

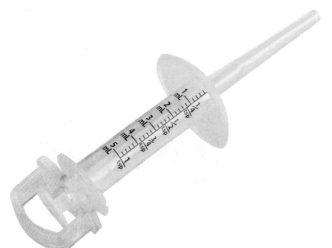

(a) Oral syringe

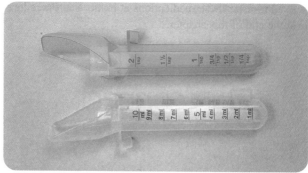

(b) Calibrated spoons

FIGURE 53-3 (a) Oral syringes and (b) calibrated spoons have markings, so that liquid medications given by mouth can be measured accurately.

(a) ©Apothecary Products LLC; (b) ©Total Care Programming, Inc.

- Apply topical medications (those applied to the skin).
- Administer or assist in administering medications into the urethra, vagina, or rectum.
- Administer medications to the eye or ear, as discussed in the *Assisting with Eye and Ear Care* chapter.

These duties require you to master a variety of techniques to give drugs safely by any route.

▶ Medications by Mouth   LO 53.4

Medications that are put in the mouth are usually swallowed. This is called *oral administration.* Some medications that are not meant to be swallowed also may be placed in the mouth. These methods include buccal and sublingual administration.

Oral Administration

Medications that are swallowed are absorbed relatively slowly as they travel along the gastrointestinal (GI) tract. Medications for oral administration include tablets, capsules, lozenges, and liquids. One special type of tablet you should be aware of is a **scored** tablet. See Figure 53-4. This medication can be broken into pieces along a scored (indented) line on the tablet.

Oral administration is contraindicated in patients who have severe nausea, are comatose, or cannot swallow. Certain medications are ineffective when administered orally because the digestive process changes them chemically to an ineffective form or does not deliver them to the bloodstream quickly enough.

Many medications, however, are most effective when given orally. These include antibiotics, vitamins, throat lozenges, and cough syrups. Although these medications are familiar to most people, as a medical assistant, you must follow certain steps to ensure that the patient understands the medication and that the medication is administered safely and effectively. The steps for oral administration are outlined in Procedure 53-1 at the end of this chapter.

Buccal and Sublingual Administration

Although **buccal** and **sublingual** medications are placed in the mouth, they do not continue along the GI tract. Instead, they dissolve and are absorbed in the buccal area (between the cheek and gum) or the sublingual area (under the tongue), where they are placed. The medication is absorbed through tissue that is rich in capillaries and the medication enters the bloodstream directly. Because the medication does not pass into the stomach or intestines before absorption, it produces a therapeutic effect more quickly than do oral medications.

Specially formulated tablets may be given by the buccal or sublingual routes. When you administer buccal or sublingual medications, your role usually includes teaching the patient

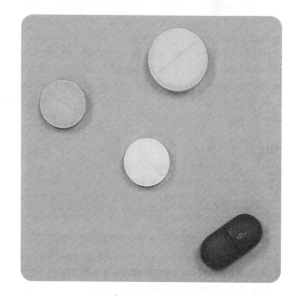

FIGURE 53-4 Unscored tablets should never be broken. Scored tablets, like the ones shown here, can be broken only along the scored line.

©Total Care Programming, Inc.

TABLE 53-3 Suggested Needle Gauge, Length, Injection Amount, and Location

Type	Age	Needle Size*	Needle Length	Maximum Injection Amount	Location
Intradermal (ID)					
ID	All ages	25 to 26 gauge	⅜ to ½ inch	0.1 mL	Interior aspect of forearm (most common)
Subcutaneous (Subcut)					
Subcut	1 to 12 months	23 to 27 gauge	⅝ inch	1 mL	Fatty tissue over anterior lateral thigh muscle
Subcut	>12 months to adult	23 to 27 gauge	½ to ¾ inch; ⅝ is most common	1 mL	Fatty tissue over anterior lateral thigh muscle or over triceps
Intramuscular (IM)					
IM	1 to 28 days	18 to 23 gauge	⅝ inch	1 mL	Anterolateral thigh muscle
IM	1 to 12 months	18 to 23 gauge	1 inch	1 mL	Anterolateral thigh muscle
IM	1 to 2 years	18 to 23 gauge	1 to 1¼ inch; ⅝ to 1 inch	1 mL	Anterolateral thigh muscle / Deltoid muscle of arm
IM	3 to 18 years	18 to 23 gauge	⅝ to 1 inch; 1 to 1¼ inch	2 mL	Deltoid muscle of arm / Anterolateral thigh muscle
IM	All adults ≥19 years <130 lb	18 to 23 gauge	⅝ to 1 inch	3 mL	Deltoid muscle of arm
IM	All adults ≥19 years Female 130 to 200 lb Male 130 to 260 lb	18 to 23 gauge	1 to 1½ inch	3 mL	Deltoid muscle of arm
IM	All adults ≥19 years Female 200+ lb Male 260+ lb	18 to 23 gauge	1½ inch	3 mL	Deltoid muscle of arm

*The needle size varies based upon the viscosity (thickness) of the medicaton.

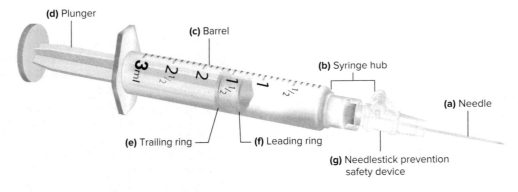

FIGURE 53-9 The parts of a standard syringe include (a) the needle; (b) the syringe hub; (c) the barrel that contains the liquid; (d) the plunger; (e) the trailing ring; (f) the plunger tip, also called the leading ring; and (g) the needlestick prevention safety device.

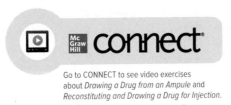

Go to CONNECT to see video exercises about *Drawing a Drug from an Ampule* and *Reconstituting and Drawing a Drug for Injection.*

Methods of Injection

Injections are the most common method of medication administration in a medical office. You need to be knowledgeable about all injection methods: intradermal, subcutaneous, intramuscular, and intravenous.

Intradermal An **intradermal (ID)** injection is administered between the upper layers of skin at an angle almost parallel to the skin, as described in Procedure 53-5 at the end of this chapter. Common sites for intradermal injections are the forearm and back. Intradermal injections are usually used to administer a skin test, such as an allergy test or a TB test. When choosing an injection site on patients, avoid scarred, blemished, or hairy areas because those features interfere with your ability to interpret test results on the skin.

The drug is injected under the top skin layer and a little bubble, or wheal, is raised. If the body reacts to the drug, erythema (redness) and induration (hardening) occur. This

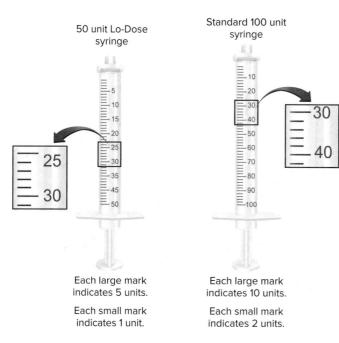

50 unit Lo-Dose syringe

Standard 100 unit syringe

Each large mark indicates 5 units.

Each small mark indicates 1 unit.

Each large mark indicates 10 units.

Each small mark indicates 2 units.

FIGURE 53-10 Always check the calibrations of insulin syringes carefully because the marks on syringes of different sizes use different scales.

reaction generally takes place 15 to 20 minutes after an allergy test and from 48 to 72 hours after a TB test.

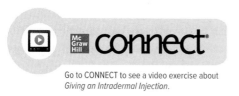

Go to CONNECT to see a video exercise about *Giving an Intradermal Injection.*

Subcutaneous A **subcutaneous (subcut)** injection provides a slow, sustained release of a medication and a relatively long duration of action. Generally, 1 mL or less of a medication can be delivered by a subcut injection (see Procedure 53-6 at the end of this chapter). Various drugs, such as the high-risk drugs insulin and heparin, are commonly administered by a subcut injection. Common subcutaneous injection sites include an area on the back between the shoulder blades, the outer sides of the upper arms and thighs, and the abdomen (except for a 2-inch area around the umbilicus).

To prepare for a subcut injection, select a site away from bones and blood vessels. Do not use an area that is edematous (swollen), scarred, or hardened or one that has a large amount of fat because these areas may not have the capillary network needed for absorption. When patients need regular subcut injections, remember to rotate injection sites systematically. Rotating sites promotes drug absorption and prevents hard subcutaneous lumps from forming. At the injection site, ensure that you can pinch at least a 1-inch skinfold for the injection. If a patient is frail, dehydrated, or thin, you may need to use a site other than the back or abdomen to provide the necessary fold of skin.

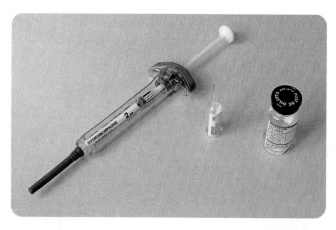

FIGURE 53-11 Injectable medications come in a cartridge (left), an ampule (center), or a vial (right).

©Cliff Moore

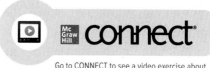

Go to CONNECT to see a video exercise about *Giving a Subcutaneous Injection.*

Intramuscular When a patient requires rapid medication absorption, you may be asked to administer an **intramuscular (IM)** injection, as described in Procedure 53-7 at the end of this chapter. An IM injection usually irritates a patient's tissues less than a subcut injection and allows administration of a larger amount of medication.

Common IM injection sites include the ventrogluteal, vastus lateralis, and deltoid muscles, illustrated in Figure 53-12. The dorsogluteal is used less because of the chance of hitting the sciatic nerve. Before giving an IM injection, identify the site carefully to prevent injury to blood vessels and nerves in the area. As with subcut injections, rotate sites if the patient must receive regular or multiple IM injections.

Take into consideration the patient's layer of fat when choosing an IM injection site. You want the injection to penetrate beyond the fat layer to muscle. If, for example, a patient is heavy in the buttocks and thighs, the deltoid may be the best site for administering an IM injection.

When injecting an IM drug that can irritate subcutaneous tissues, such as iron dextran (Imferon), use the **Z-track method**, illustrated in Figure 53-13. To do this, pull the skin and subcutaneous tissue to the side before inserting the needle at the site. After the drug is injected, release the tissue. This technique creates a zigzag path in the tissue layers, which prevents the drug from leaking into the subcutaneous tissue and causing irritation.

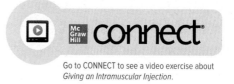

Go to CONNECT to see a video exercise about *Giving an Intramuscular Injection.*

Intravenous Although **intravenous (IV)** injections are not commonly performed in a medical office or by medical

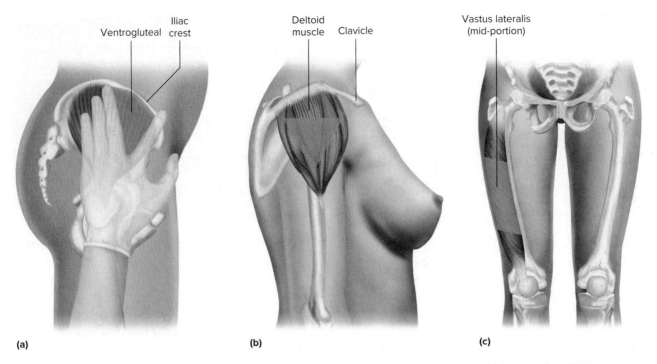

FIGURE 53-12 For intramuscular injection in an adult, use (a) the ventrogluteal site, (b) the deltoid site, or (c) the vastus lateralis site.

assistants, certain drugs may be administered this way. Drugs also may be mixed and dissolved into a **solution** (a homogeneous mixture of a solid, liquid, or gaseous substance in a liquid) and given by IV **infusion** (slow drip) into a vein. Examples of IV drugs include powerful antibiotics, chemotherapeutic drugs, emergency drugs, and electrolytes. Because these drugs are introduced directly into the bloodstream, they produce an almost immediate effect. They also can cause sudden adverse reactions.

Although in most cases a licensed practitioner must administer an IV drug, you may assist by laying out supplies and equipment or monitoring the IV site and flow. When assisting with any intravenous medications, gather the ordered drug and a tourniquet, bedsaver pad, gloves, iodine and alcohol swabs, venipuncture device, tape, and gauze pad, as ordered. Obtain other supplies and equipment depending on the specific type of infusion or injection being administered.

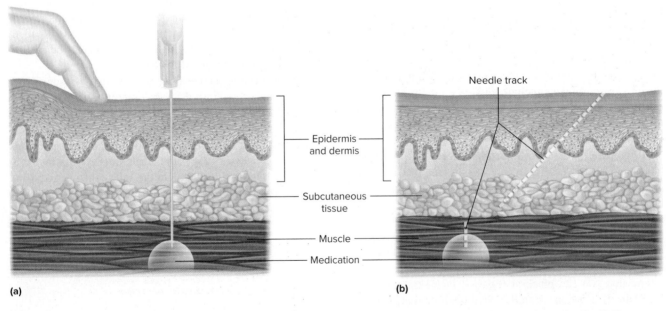

FIGURE 53-13 Use the Z-track method for IM injection of irritating solutions. (a) Pull the skin to one side before inserting the needle. (b) After injecting the drug, release the skin to seal off the needle track.

▶ Other Medication Routes   LO 53.6

Additional parenteral routes of administration include inhalation therapy (sometimes called respiratory therapy); topical application; and urethral, vaginal, and rectal administration.

Inhalation Therapies

Inhalation therapy is medication that is delivered into the respiratory system during inhalation. This medication can be administered through the mouth or nose. There are a number of disorders for which the physician may order an inhaler or aerosol form of medication. For example, an oral inhaler is frequently used by patients with asthma, whereas a nasal inhaler is frequently used for local treatment of nasal congestion. Nasal inhalers also are used to administer medicines for systemic effect, such as a vasopressin derivative for nocturnal bedwetting. Some types of influenza vaccines are now delivered by nasal inhalation. Always read the inserts for inhaled drugs for a detailed description of the exact procedure for the type of inhalation you will be administering. For example, when a corticosteroid medication is delivered by an oral inhaler, the patient should rinse her mouth with water, then spit after the medication is inhaled. This is done to prevent the patient from developing an oral Candida (yeast) infection. Procedure 53-8, at the end of this chapter, provides the basic steps of the procedure, as well as needed patient education.

Topical Application

Topical application is the direct application of a medication on the skin. Topical medications can take the form of creams, lotions, **ointments** (salves), tinctures, powders, sprays, and solutions, which are used for their local effects. They include antibacterial and antifungal drugs, as well as corticosteroids.

To apply a cream, lotion, or ointment, use long, even strokes with a cotton-tipped applicator and/or a gloved finger when rubbing it into the skin. Follow the direction of the hair growth to avoid irritating the hair follicles and skin. To apply a powder, shake it on but do not rub it in.

A specialized type of topical administration that produces a systemic effect is the **transdermal** system (or patch). See Figure 53-14. A medication administered through the transdermal patch is absorbed through the skin directly into the bloodstream. The patch slowly and evenly releases a systemic drug, such as scopolamine, nitroglycerin, estrogen, or fentanyl, through the skin. The patient receives a timed-release dose, usually over a day or several days. See Procedure 53-9 at the end of this chapter.

Urethral Administration

The urethral route is used when antibiotic and antifungal drugs are needed locally—that is, at the site of infection—for some urinary tract infections. Depending on the nature of the infection and the duration of drug action, the physician or a nurse may instill liquid medications only one time or several times a day for a week. Urethral administration is used in both men and women.

Urethral medication administration requires passing a small-diameter urinary catheter into the bladder, instilling a drug through it, and clamping the catheter to let the drug bathe the urinary bladder walls. See Procedure 53-10 at the end of this chapter.

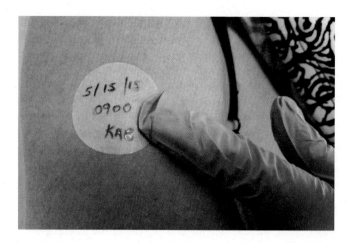

FIGURE 53-14 A medical assistant who applies a transdermal patch should write the date, time, and his or her initials on the patch at the time of application.
©Total Care Programming, Inc.

Vaginal Administration

Physicians usually prescribe vaginal medications to treat local fungal or bacterial infections. They are usually packaged as suppositories (the most common form), solutions, creams, ointments, and foams. The liquid form of vaginal medication is administered by performing a **douche** (vaginal irrigation). This process is similar to giving a urethral medication, but it requires a special irrigating nozzle. Patients frequently ask about administering vaginal medications, and they usually administer such medications at home. Therefore, you must be prepared to provide detailed patient education for this route of administration. The physician may ask you to administer the first dose as a means of teaching a patient the method to use at home, or you may be asked to administer a one-time-only dose. See Procedure 53-11 at the end of this chapter.

Rectal Administration

Certain medications, such as drugs used to treat constipation, nausea, and vomiting, may be administered by the rectal route. These medications may be given in the form of suppositories or enemas and may produce local or systemic effects. See Procedure 53-12 at the end of this chapter.

▶ Special Considerations   LO 53.7

Pediatric, pregnant, breastfeeding, and geriatric patients require special considerations when administering medications. When giving a medication to these patients, you must adjust patient care and technique as needed. Note: Geriatric considerations are discussed in the *Assisting in Geriatrics* chapter.

Pediatric Patients

Children pose special challenges in medication administration and use. Their physiology and immature body systems make medication effects less predictable because drugs are absorbed, distributed, metabolized, and excreted differently in children than in adults. Therefore, plan to observe a pediatric patient closely for adverse effects and interactions.

A child's small size also increases the risk of overdose and toxicity. These factors require dosage adjustments and careful measurement of small doses. To help administer medications safely to pediatric patients, always check your calculations for providing a prescribed dose, and then ask a licensed practitioner to double-check them.

Administration sites and techniques for a child may differ from those for an adult. For example, fewer IM injection sites can be used for a young child. Also, the technique for eardrop administration varies slightly (see the *Assisting with Eye and Ear Care* chapter).

When dealing with an infant or a young child, teach the parents—not the patient—about the medication. With an older child, include parents and patient in the teaching session. Be sure to use age-appropriate language when speaking to children.

Patience and sensitivity are important when working with pediatric patients. The first memorable exposure to an office visit often may determine how the child will react to physician visits for years to come. Infants and children can sense when you are irritated or annoyed. Pay close attention to your nonverbal communication as well as your verbal communication. New mothers are often apprehensive about invasive procedures when it concerns their children, and this apprehension is often reflected in the child. Empathy and compassion are needed to ensure that the office visit is a pleasant one.

Administering medications to a pediatric patient may become a challenge if the child is not cooperative. It is important to ensure that the child receives the full dose as ordered.

Oral Medications When administering oral medications to infants and small children, follow these guidelines:

- Use a pediatric calibrated dropper to measure the ordered dose. See Figure 53-15.
- Administer the medication to the side of the tongue; this method prevents the child from spitting out the medication.
- Hold the child until you are sure the medication has been swallowed. In some cases, you may gently hold the child's mouth closed to ensure that the medication is swallowed.
- If a small amount dribbles from the mouth, do not attempt to give more medication to the child.
- If the child vomits within 5 minutes and you can see the medication in the vomit, you should readminister the medication after the child is calm. If you are unsure of whether to readminister the medication, consult with the physician.
- If the medication comes only in tablet or capsule form and the child is unable to swallow a tablet or capsule, check a creditable drug reference to see if the medication can be crushed and given with food, such as applesauce.

Injections Stress and anxiety will differ from child to child. When giving injections to pediatric patients, the following steps will help ensure a smooth procedure:

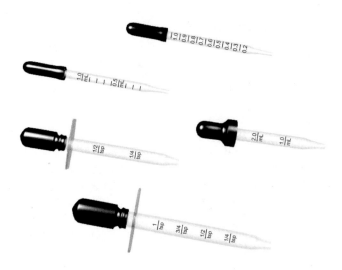

FIGURE 53-15 Pediatric droppers come in various sizes with different calibration marks.

- Distract the patient. Talk to the child while giving the injection. Don't ask permission. Often the injection is performed and over before the child realizes it.
- Use an anesthetic topical agent prior to the injection. This can be applied in the office or at home before the patient arrives in the office.
- Try not to allow the child to see the syringe before giving the injection.
- Be swift. Do not allow a lot of time to pass before giving the injection—the faster the better.
- Praise the child. Say things that promote maturity and self-esteem.

Pediatric Injection Sites Pediatric patients have less muscle development than adults do, which limits the sites for intramuscular injections. The deltoid muscle is not developed enough for an injection and can be painful for the child.

The vastus lateralis and ventrogluteal sites are recommended for infants and children. The vastus lateralis site is good because it is a large and thick muscle that is developed before the child begins to walk. It is also the most desirable site for infants and children because it is not near major nerves and blood vessels. For a child who has been walking for about a year, you can use the ventrogluteal. For an older, well-developed child, use any adult site. The vastus lateralis site is an easier site if you need to incorporate restraining methods.

The most common injections given to pediatric patients are vaccines. Most vaccines are given intramuscularly with a 25-gauge, ⅝-inch needle. The gauge and length vary based on the size of the patient. Use the shortest needle that will allow you to reach muscle, usually ⅝ to 1 inch.

In many cases, pediatric patients require more than one vaccine injection in a single limb (vastus lateralis). When this is the case, the injections should be at least 1 inch apart and the specific location of each vaccine should be documented.

Restraining Methods Sometimes a pediatric patient will need to be restrained in order for you to administer an injection. Two medical assistants may be needed to safely restrain a child while giving an injection. Common restraining methods include the following:

- Have the child "hug the mother." The mother holds the child in front of her, with the child's thighs extended on either side of her torso. As the mother is talking to her child, make the injection in the vastus lateralis.
- Weight-bearing restraining is better than muscular control. Have the child sit on the edge of the examining table and use your weight to immobilize the child's legs against the table.

Pregnant Patients

When dealing with pregnant patients, remember that you are caring for two patients at once: the mother and her fetus. When you give the mother a drug, you also may be giving it to the fetus. Some medications can cause physical defects in the fetus if the mother takes them during pregnancy (especially in the first trimester). It is extremely important to double-check the medication in a credible drug reference for toxicology or pregnancy warnings. After administering the medication, assess the patient carefully for therapeutic and adverse effects of the medication. If the physician orders a medication for a pregnant patient, double-check the order against the pregnancy drug risk categories discussed in the *Principles of Pharmacology* chapter. If it is a high-risk medication, check with the physician before administering the medication.

Patients Who Are Breastfeeding

Some drugs are excreted in breast milk and thus can be ingested by a breastfeeding infant. This ingestion can be dangerous because infants have immature body systems and cannot metabolize and excrete drugs that are safe for the mother. Some medications, such as sedatives, diuretics, and hormones, can reduce the mother's flow of breast milk.

Whenever a medication is ordered for a patient who is breastfeeding, check a drug reference to see whether the medication is contraindicated during lactation. If so, consult the licensed practitioner. If not, teach the mother to recognize signs of adverse drug effects in her infant. If a mother must take a medication that affects lactation, advise her to supplement breast-feeding with infant formula.

▶ Patient Education About Medications
LO 53.8

As a medical assistant, you have an important role in patient instruction about medications. This role may vary depending on your state, training, or place of employment, but the importance of education about medications should not be underestimated. Specific instructions should be given about all the medications a patient is taking, whether prescription or over-the-counter (OTC). Patients also should know how to take and record their medications safely and correctly.

Over-the-Counter Drugs

Even though patients can obtain OTC drugs without a prescription, they need to know several important facts to use them safely. Patients should not treat themselves with OTC drugs as a way to avoid medical care. For example, OTC drugs are available to treat recurrent yeast infections. Nonetheless, a patient should consult a licensed practitioner the first time she develops an infection.

Patients also should know that OTC drugs may not produce enough therapeutic benefit in some cases or be dangerous when used in combination with other substances. For example, a combination of the OTC medication acetaminophen (Tylenol®) and alcohol can cause liver damage. In addition, some OTC drugs even may mask symptoms or aggravate a problem.

Many OTC drugs contain more than one active ingredient. These extra ingredients, such as aspirin, acetaminophen, or caffeine, can cause allergic reactions or other undesirable effects. Excess caffeine can cause elevated heart rates. Too much acetaminophen (Tylenol®)—over 4 grams in 24 hours—can inadvertently be taken, causing severe liver damage.

Prescription Drugs

Before patients begin drug therapy, they should be informed of certain considerations (such as when and how to take the medication) and medication safety precautions. First you must check a credible drug information resource about any medication with which you are not familiar.

As part of your patient education, provide instructions orally and, if possible, in writing. For commonly prescribed medications, you can obtain preprinted information sheets or create one using an electronic health record (EHR) program. Most pharmacies now routinely provide these with each dispensed drug. See Figure 53-16.

An important aspect of this kind of information is teaching the patient how to read a prescription medication label. Instruct the patient to be particularly alert for special instructions and warning labels, such as those shown in Figure 53-17.

Interactions

Interactions may occur between two prescription or nonprescription drugs or between a drug and food and may cause serious effects. The greater the number of drugs the patient takes, including over-the-counter medications or supplements, the greater the chance of a drug interaction.

Drug-Drug Interactions When two drugs are taken at the same time, there are several possible interactions. In some cases, the effects of both drugs are increased, causing either a toxic or beneficial effect. For example, when alcohol is combined with diazepam (Valium®), there is a potential toxic effect of severe central nervous system depression because one drug intensifies the effect of the other. An example of a beneficial effect is the combination of acetaminophen and codeine, which increases the activity of both drugs, allowing the physician to prescribe a lower dose of each. In fact, this combination of drugs is available in one tablet (Tylenol® with codeine).

In other cases, the effects of both drugs are decreased, or one drug cancels out the effect of the other. For example,

BWW Medical Associates, PC
305 Main Street
Port Snead, YZ 12345-9876

Patient Name: Mohammad Nassar

RX#: 711428172

Drug: Albuterol Inhalation Aerosol

COMMON USES:

To treat asthma, bronchitis, and other lung diseases.

HOW SHOULD I USE IT?

Follow your doctor's and/or the package instructions. Shake well before each use. Rinse mouth after each inhalation to avoid dryness. If breathing has not improved in 20 minutes, call the doctor.

ARE THERE ANY SIDE EFFECTS?

Very unlikely, but report: Flushing, trembling, headache, nausea, vomiting, rapid heartbeat, chest pain, weakness, dizziness.

HOW DO I STORE THIS?

Store at room temperature away from moisture and sunlight. Do not puncture. Do not store in the bathroom. Rinse and clean inhaler regularly as described in package instructions.

FIGURE 53-16 Drug information sheets, like this one, are important for consumers to understand the medications they are taking.

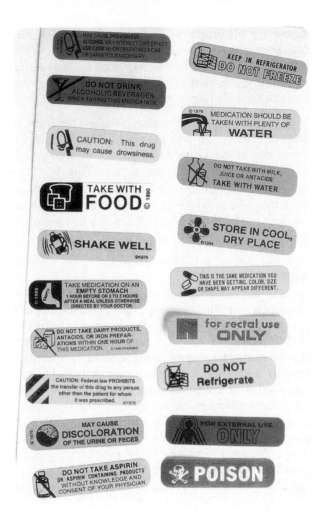

FIGURE 53-17 Teach the patient to heed warning labels and instructions on medication bottles.
©Cliff Moore

combining propranolol (Inderal®) with albuterol (Proventil®) causes each drug to lose its effectiveness.

In still other cases, the effect of one of the drugs is increased by the other. For example, the effect of digoxin (Lanoxin®) is increased by the presence of furosemide (Lasix®), but the furosemide still works at the same degree of effectiveness as when administered alone.

Drug interactions can lead to adverse reactions. For example, a patient who takes the prescription blood modifier (anticoagulant) warfarin (Coumadin®) to prevent blood clots must avoid taking aspirin for pain relief. Taking these drugs together increases the risk of uncontrolled bleeding.

To help prevent unintentional drug interactions, thoroughly check the patient's medication use. Be sure to ask about medications prescribed by specialists as well as OTC drugs and supplements. Question the patient about past and present use of alcohol and recreational drugs as well as herbal remedies. Update the chart as needed. If you detect a potential for drug interactions, notify the physician. Drug interaction checkers are available online.

Also teach patients about possible drug interactions and how to avoid or minimize them. For example, patients may need to take certain drugs at least 4 hours apart. As an example, the hormone replacement drug Synthroid® and calcium should not be taken together. Instruct patients to call the office if they think their drugs are interacting adversely.

Drug-Food Interactions Interactions between a medication and food can alter the medication's therapeutic effect. For example, taking tetracycline with milk can reduce the drug's effectiveness because of decreased absorption from the GI tract. The drug-food interaction between a monoamine oxidase (MAO) inhibitor (such as Parnate®, an antidepressant drug) and aged cheese or meat or other foods containing high levels of tyramine can produce a toxic effect. This interaction can cause a dangerous hypertensive crisis in which the patient's blood pressure rises quickly to dangerous levels, possibly leading to stroke and death.

A food that may interact with drugs is grapefruit and grapefruit juice. Interactions with some heart or blood pressure medications, such as nifedipine, might cause irregularities in heartbeat, called *dysrhythmia*.

Some drug-food interactions can affect the body's use of nutrients. For example, the cholesterol-lowering drugs cholestyramine resin (Locholest®) and colestipol HCl (Colestid®)

may reduce the body's absorption of fat-soluble vitamins (A, D, E, and K) from food.

When teaching a patient about drug-food interactions, specify exactly which foods to avoid and when. For example, a patient should not take tetracycline within 2 hours of consuming milk or milk products, whereas a patient taking an MAO inhibitor must avoid foods that contain high levels of tyramine at all times. Explain what to expect if an interaction occurs and describe how to deal with it.

Adverse Reactions

Reported adverse reactions associated with a drug are somewhat predictable and range from mild side effects, such as stomach upset, to severe or life-threatening allergic responses. For example, certain cholesterol-lowering medications, called statins (e.g., Lipitor®), can increase the likelihood of painful muscle disorders. Unpredictable adverse effects also can occur; they are unique to each patient.

Elderly patients and patients with liver or kidney disease are more susceptible than others to adverse reactions because these conditions affect drug metabolism and excretion. When drugs are not metabolized properly or excreted from the body quickly enough, drugs can reach toxic levels, even with normal doses.

To help prevent adverse reactions, teach the patient to take the drug at the right time, in the right amount, and under the right circumstances. For example, the patient may need to take a cephalosporin with food to avoid nausea and diarrhea. Also teach the patient to recognize significant adverse effects and to call the office if any of them occur. The patient also should report any change in overall health because that change could be drug-related.

Tell patients to inform each of their doctors of any adverse reactions (including allergic reactions) they have had to drugs. Previous adverse reactions may prompt a doctor to adjust a dosage or select a different drug. A history of drug allergies may contraindicate the use of a particular drug.

Complete Medication List

Patients must inform the doctor of all substances they use regularly or periodically. This includes prescription and OTC drugs, plus herbals and supplements. It also includes past and present use of alcohol and recreational drugs. When patients have more than one doctor, tell them to inform each doctor about all medications they are taking. Encourage them to keep up-to-date medication lists with dosages (some patients keep this information on their home computers). This information can help patients and healthcare professionals prevent and monitor for drug interactions. The list should be kept on the patient chart and updated with every visit to the physician's office.

Patient Compliance

To help ensure that patients comply with instructions, confirm that they completely understand the name, dosage, and purpose of each drug prescribed for them. If patients must take more than one drug at a time, be sure they know the correct and relevant information for each one. In addition, cover each of the following points when educating patients about drugs:

- Explain how and when to take each drug to ensure its safety and effectiveness. Some drugs should be taken with food to minimize gastrointestinal irritation. Others should be taken on an empty stomach for proper absorption and metabolism. Some drugs must be taken once a day in the morning; others should be taken three or four times a day. If patients' medication schedules are complex, suggest that they create an alarm, chart, calendar, or diary to remind them of what drug to take and when, or create a schedule for them.

- Tell patients how long to take each drug. In the case of antibiotics, advise them to take the entire course of the drug as scheduled, even if they feel better before finishing it. In the case of medicines prescribed for chronic disease, advise patients that they will need to continue taking the medication unless the doctor tells them to stop. Be aware that some drugs, such as prednisone, must be tapered off slowly to prevent adverse reactions.

- Explain how to identify possible adverse reactions of each drug and safety measures related to adverse reactions. For example, instruct patients to avoid certain activities, such as driving or operating machinery, while taking a drug that causes drowsiness. If appropriate, inform patients that misuse of the drug may lead to dependence, and mention the dangers of drug dependence.

- Tell patients not to save medications that are over 1 year old or share them with anyone else. Old medications and those taken by people other than the patient for whom they were prescribed can cause severe, unexpected adverse effects. Advise patients to check the expiration date on all drugs and to discard them by wrapping in a tightly sealed container and placing in the trash. Flushing is not recommended due to possible water contamination. Some pharmacies will dispose of medications for patients.

- Suggest that patients avoid alcohol when taking certain drugs. Alcohol interacts with some drugs, causing adverse reactions such as lethargy, confusion, or coma.

- Tell patients to ask their pharmacists where to store each medication. Some drugs must be refrigerated. Others should be kept in a dry, cool area. Drugs should not usually be kept in a hot, damp place, such as a bathroom. They must always be kept out of the reach of children.

- Tell patients to take their drugs in a well-lit area so that they can read each drug label carefully before taking each dose. They should never assume that they are taking the right medication without reading the label on the container. If patients have poor vision, print the name of the drug and the dosage schedule clearly on a separate piece of paper or card to attach to the medication container.

- Instruct patients to call the licensed practitioner if they have any questions about their drug therapy.

▶ Charting Medications   LO 53.9

Whenever a patient receives some form of treatment, such as medication, a record is kept of that treatment. Special problems or circumstances also are recorded, such as new symptoms, the patient's own statements, and how the patient tolerated the medications or treatment. Most charting in the physician's office is documented on a progress note or a medication administration record (MAR). These documents are essential to serve as communication tools for all healthcare members who are connected to that patient. The medical record is considered a legal document and is taken as proof that medication or treatment was administered to the patient.

All chart entries must be factual, accurate, complete, current, organized, and confidential. Avoid using words or statements that can be interpreted as your opinion. For example, if a patient gags and spits up cough syrup you have just administered, you would not write that the patient did not like the taste of the medication; you would simply state "patient experienced difficulty in swallowing medication and expelled medication." Avoid terms such as *appear* and *seems,* which can lead you to draw assumptions without objective data to support them. Be specific. Chart what the patient said or did, not what you think. Use abbreviations when appropriate because they allow you to say a great deal in a small space.

Below you can see an EHR medicine charting example or progress note for Valarie Ramirez.

Review your office's medical records to keep consistent with the charting methods used in them. Follow these simple rules:

- Before you begin, make sure you have the right chart and the right location in the chart.
- Chart medications directly from the physician order.
- Be specific. Do not write "Gave Demerol for pain in the evening." Instead, write, "(Date/Time), Demerol 100 mg given IM in right upper outer quadrant of gluteus maximus for c/o sharp pain in left arm, rated 7 on a scale of 10, (lot number, expiration date, initials).
- If using paper charts, do not leave gaps or skip lines. If an entry does not fill a complete line, draw a straight line to fill the gap. Put your signature or first initial and last name and title at the right side directly after the note.
- If you make an error, do not erase it. Draw a line through the mistake. The mistake should still be visible, so do not black it out. Initial it and then rechart the information correctly. Follow the specific procedure for making corrections in an electronic health record.
- Never use ditto marks.
- Write neatly in longhand or carefully enter into the electronic chart and check your note before submitting it. Ensure that your spelling is accurate.
- Use abbreviations and correct symbols. Most facilities have an approved abbreviation list to use as a reference.
- If you are unsure about charting, check with your supervising licensed practitioner.

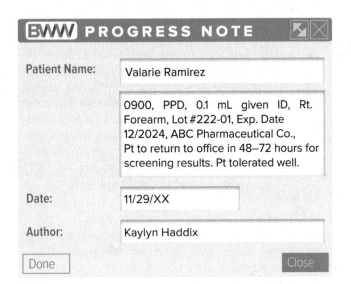

PROGRESS NOTE

Patient Name:	Valarie Ramirez
	0900, PPD, 0.1 mL given ID, Rt. Forearm, Lot #222-01, Exp. Date 12/2024, ABC Pharmaceutical Co., Pt to return to office in 48–72 hours for screening results. Pt tolerated well.
Date:	11/29/XX
Author:	Kaylyn Haddix

Done   Close

PROCEDURE 53-1 Administering Oral Drugs   WORK // DOC

Procedure Goal: To safely administer an oral drug to a patient

OSHA Guidelines: This procedure does not involve exposure to blood, body fluids, or tissues.

Materials: Patient chart/progress note, drug order (in patient chart), container of oral drug, small paper cup (for tablets, capsules, or caplets) or plastic calibrated medicine cup (for liquids), glass of water or juice, straw (optional), package insert or drug information sheet

Method:

1. Identify the patient and wash your hands.
2. Select the ordered drug (tablet, capsule, or liquid).
3. Check the rights, comparing information against the drug order.
   RATIONALE: *To ensure necessary accuracy.*
4. If you are unfamiliar with the drug, check a drug reference, read the package insert, or speak with the physician. Determine whether the drug may be taken with or followed by water or juice.

5. Ask the patient about any drug or food allergies. If the patient is not allergic to the ordered drug or other ingredients used to prepare it, proceed.
   RATIONALE: *To prevent a reaction to the medication.*

6. Perform any calculations needed to provide the prescribed dose. If you are unsure of your calculations, check them with a coworker or the licensed practitioner.

Giving Tablets or Capsules

7. Open the container and tap the correct number into the cap. Do not touch the inside of the cap because it is sterile. If you pour out too many tablets or capsules and you have not touched them, tap the excess back into the container.

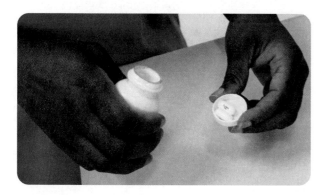

FIGURE Procedure 53-1 Step 7   Tap tablets gently into the cap.
©McGraw-Hill Education

8. Tap the tablets or capsules from the cap into the paper cup.

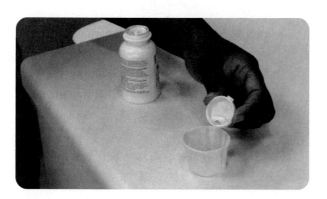

FIGURE Procedure 53-1 Step 8   Tap tablets from the cap into the paper cup.
©McGraw-Hill Education

9. Recap the container immediately.
   RATIONALE: *Recapping immediately protects the medication from exposure to air, which can break down the medication.*

10. Give the patient the cup along with a glass of water or juice. If the patient finds it easier to drink with a straw, unwrap the straw and place it in the fluid. If patients have difficulty swallowing pills, have them drink some water or juice before putting the pills in the mouth.
    RATIONALE: *Additional fluid makes the pills float in the mouth and allows patients to swallow more easily.*

Giving a Liquid Drug

11. If the liquid is a suspension, shake it well.

12. Locate the mark on the medicine cup for the prescribed dose. Keeping your thumbnail on the mark, hold the cup at eye level and pour the correct amount of the drug. Keep the label side of the bottle on top as you pour or put your palm over it.
    RATIONALE: *To prevent liquid drips from obscuring the label.*

13. After pouring the drug, place the cup on a flat surface and check the drug level again. At eye level, the base of the meniscus (the crescent-shaped form at the top of the liquid) should align with the mark that indicates the prescribed dose. If you poured out too much, discard it.
    RATIONALE: *Do not return it to the container because medicine cups are not sterile.*

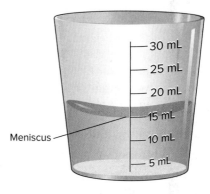

FIGURE Procedure 53-1 Step 13 Looking at eye level, find the base of the meniscus, which is the crescent-shaped form at the top of the liquid, for the correct measure.

14. Give the medicine cup to the patient with instructions to drink the liquid. If indicated, offer a glass of water or juice to wash down the drug.

After You Have Given an Oral Drug

15. Wash your hands.

16. Give the patient an information sheet about the drug. Discuss the information with the patient and answer any questions. If the patient has questions you cannot answer, refer her to the licensed practitioner.

17. Document the drug administration in the patient's chart with date, time, drug name, dosage, expiration date, lot number, manufacturer, route, site, significant patient reactions, and any patient education.

PROCEDURE **53-2** Administering Buccal or Sublingual Drugs

Procedure Goal: To safely administer a buccal or sublingual drug to a patient

OSHA Guidelines: This procedure does not involve exposure to blood, body fluids, or tissues.

Materials: Patient chart/progress note, drug order (in patient chart), container of buccal or sublingual drug, small paper cup, package insert or drug information sheet

Method:

1. Identify the patient and wash your hands.
2. Select the ordered drug.
3. Check the rights, comparing information against the drug order.
   RATIONALE: *To ensure necessary accuracy.*
4. If you are unfamiliar with the drug, check the *PDR* or other credible drug reference, read the package insert, or speak with the licensed practitioner.
5. Ask the patient about any drug or food allergies. If the patient is not allergic to the ordered drug or other ingredients used to prepare it, proceed.
   RATIONALE: *To prevent a reaction to the medication.*
6. Perform any calculations needed to provide the prescribed dose. If you are unsure of your calculations, check them with a coworker or the licensed practitioner.
7. Open the container and tap the correct number into the cap. Do not touch the inside of the cap because it is sterile. If you pour out too many tablets or capsules and you have not touched them, tap the excess back into the container.
8. Tap the tablets or capsules from the cap into the paper cup.
9. Recap the container immediately.
   RATIONALE: *Recapping immediately protects the medication from exposure to air, which can break down the medication.*

Giving Buccal Medication

10. For a *buccal* drug, provide patient instruction, including:
    - Do not chew or swallow the tablet.
    - Place the medication between the cheek and gum until it dissolves.
    RATIONALE: *This area is rich in blood supply to promote rapid absorption of the drug.*
    - Do not eat, drink, or smoke until the tablet is completely dissolved.
    RATIONALE: *Food and fluids wash the drug into the gastrointestinal (GI) tract, slowing absorption or allowing gastric juices to destroy it. Smoking increases salivation, causing impaired absorption of the drug.*

Giving a Sublingual Drug

11. For a *sublingual* drug, provide patient instruction, including:
    - Do not chew or swallow the tablet.

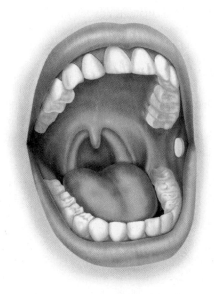

FIGURE Procedure 53-2 Step 10   Place a buccal drug between the cheek and gum.

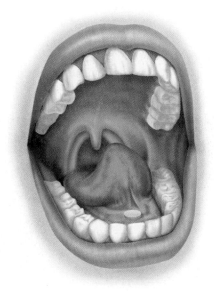

FIGURE Procedure 53-2 Step 11   Place a sublingual drug under the tongue.

- Place the medication under the tongue until it dissolves.
  RATIONALE: *The capillaries in this area promote rapid absorption of the drug.*
- Do not eat, drink, or smoke until the tablet is completely dissolved.
  RATIONALE: *Food and fluids wash the drug into the GI tract, slowing absorption or allowing gastric juices to destroy it. Smoking increases salivation, causing impaired absorption of the drug.*

After You Have Given a Buccal or Sublingual Medication

12. Remain with the patient until the tablet dissolves to monitor for possible adverse reactions and to ensure that the patient has allowed the tablet to dissolve in the mouth instead of chewing or swallowing it.

13. Wash your hands.

14. Give the patient an information sheet about the medication. Discuss the information with the patient and answer any questions. If the patient has questions you cannot answer, refer her to the licensed practitioner.

15. Document the medication administration in the patient's chart with date, time, drug name, dosage, expiration date, lot number, manufacturer, route, site, significant patient reactions, and any patient education.

PROCEDURE 53-3 Drawing a Drug from an Ampule

Procedure Goal: To safely open an ampule and draw a drug, using sterile technique

OSHA Guidelines:

Materials: Ampule of drug, alcohol swab, 2 × 2 gauze square, small file (provided by the drug manufacturer), sterile filtered needle, sterile needle, and a syringe of the appropriate size

Method:

1. Wash your hands and put on exam gloves.
2. Gently tap the top of the ampule with your forefinger to settle the liquid to the bottom of the ampule.
3. Wipe the ampule's neck with an alcohol swab.
4. Wrap the 2 × 2 gauze square around the ampule's neck; then snap the neck away from you. If it does not snap easily, score the neck with the small file and try again.
5. Insert the filtered needle into the ampule without touching the side of the ampule.

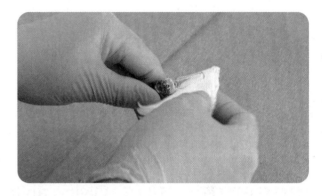

FIGURE Procedure 53-3 Step 4 To prevent possible injury, wrap the neck of the ampule with gauze before snapping.

©McGraw-Hill Education

RATIONALE: *A filtered needle will prevent contamination of the medication.*

6. Pull back on the plunger to aspirate (remove by vacuum or suction) the liquid completely into the syringe.
7. Replace with the regular needle and push the plunger on the syringe until the medication just reaches the tip of the needle. The drug is now ready for injection.

PROCEDURE 53-4 Reconstituting and Drawing a Drug for Injection

Procedure Goal: To reconstitute and draw a drug for injection, using sterile technique

OSHA Guidelines:

Materials: Vial of drug, vial of diluent, alcohol swabs, two disposable sterile needle and syringe sets of appropriate size, sharps container

Method:

1. Wash your hands and put on exam gloves.
2. Place the drug vial and diluent vial on the countertop. Wipe each rubber diaphragm with a fresh alcohol swab.
3. Loosen the cap from the needle and the guard from the syringe. Pull the plunger back to the mark that equals the amount of diluent needed to reconstitute the drug ordered.
   RATIONALE: *This action aspirates air into the syringe.*
4. Puncture the diaphragm of the vial of diluent with the needle and inject the air into the diluent.
   RATIONALE: *This action creates positive pressure that lets you draw the diluent easily. If you do not add air, a vacuum forms, making it difficult to draw the diluent.*

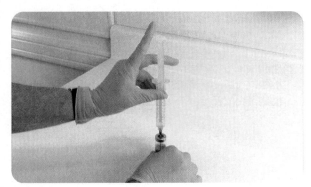

FIGURE Procedure 53-4 Step 4   Injecting air into the diluent.

©McGraw-Hill Education

solution may be clear or cloudy when completely mixed (depending on the drug).

8. Remove the cap and guard from the second needle and syringe.

9. Pull back the plunger to the mark that reflects the amount of drug ordered. Inject the air into the drug vial.

10. Invert the vial and aspirate the proper amount of the drug into the syringe. The drug is now ready for injection.

5. Invert the vial and aspirate the diluent.

6. Remove the needle from the diluent vial, inject the diluent into the drug vial, and withdraw the needle. Properly dispose of this needle and syringe.

7. Roll the vial between your hands to mix the drug and diluent thoroughly. Do not shake the vial unless so directed on the drug label. When completely mixed, the solution in the vial should have no flakes. The

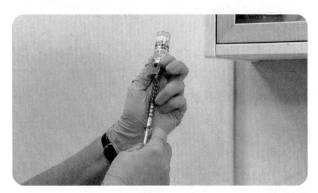

FIGURE Procedure 53-4 Step 10   Aspirating the drug into the syringe.

©McGraw-Hill Education

PROCEDURE 53-5 Giving an Intradermal (ID) Injection   WORK // DOC

Procedure Goal: To administer an intradermal injection safely and effectively, using sterile technique

OSHA Guidelines:

Materials: Patient chart/progress note, drug order (in patient chart), alcohol swab, disposable needle and syringe of the appropriate size filled with the ordered dose of drug, sharps container

Method:

1. Identify the patient. Wash your hands and put on exam gloves.

2. Check the rights, comparing information against the drug order.
   RATIONALE: *To ensure necessary accuracy.*

3. Ask the patient about any drug or food allergies. If the patient is not allergic to the ordered drug or other ingredients used to prepare it, proceed.

4. Identify the injection site on the patient's forearm. To do so, rest the patient's arm on a table with the palm up. Measure two to three finger-widths below the antecubital space and a hand-width above the wrist. The space between is available for the injection.

5. Prepare the skin with the alcohol swab, moving in a circle from the center out.

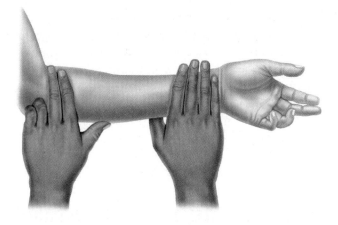

FIGURE Procedure 53-5 Step 4   This space is available for intradermal injection sites.

6. Let the skin dry before giving the injection.
   RATIONALE: *To prevent you from introducing antiseptic under the skin, which could cause irritation and falsify intradermal test results.*

7. Hold the patient's forearm and stretch the skin taut with one hand.

8. With the other hand, place the needle—bevel up—almost flat against the patient's skin. Press the needle against the skin and insert it.

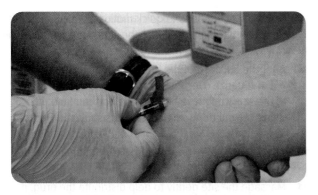

FIGURE Procedure 53-5 Step 8   Inserting the needle for an intradermal injection.

©McGraw-Hill Education

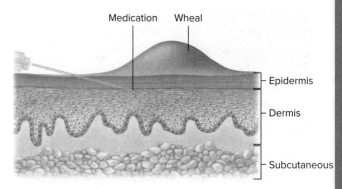

FIGURE Procedure 53-5 Step 9   Medication collects under the skin, forming a wheal, during an intradermal injection.

9. Inject the drug slowly and gently. You should see the needle through the skin and feel resistance. As the drug enters the upper layer of skin, a wheal (raised area of the skin) will form.

10. After the full dose of the drug has been injected, withdraw the needle. Properly dispose of used materials and the needle and syringe immediately.

11. Remove the gloves and wash your hands.

12. Stay with the patient as dictated by the facility to monitor for unexpected reactions.

13. Document the injection in the patient's chart with date, time, drug name, dosage, expiration date, lot number, manufacturer, route, site, significant patient reactions, and any patient education.

PROCEDURE 53-6 Giving a Subcutaneous (Subcut) Injection

WORK // DOC

Procedure Goal: To administer a subcutaneous injection safely and effectively, using sterile technique

OSHA Guidelines:

Materials: Patient chart/progress note, drug order (in patient's chart), alcohol swabs, sterile 2 × 2 gauze or cotton ball, container of the ordered drug, disposable needle and syringe of the appropriate size, sharps container

Method:

1. Identify the patient. Wash your hands and put on exam gloves.

2. Check the rights, comparing information against the drug order.
   RATIONALE: *To ensure necessary accuracy.*

3. Ask the patient about any drug or food allergies. If the patient is not allergic to the ordered drug or other ingredients used to prepare it, proceed.

4. Prepare the drug and draw it up to the mark on the syringe that matches the ordered dose.

5. Choose a site and clean it with an alcohol swab, moving in a circle from the center out. Let the area dry.

6. Pinch the skin firmly to lift the subcutaneous tissue.

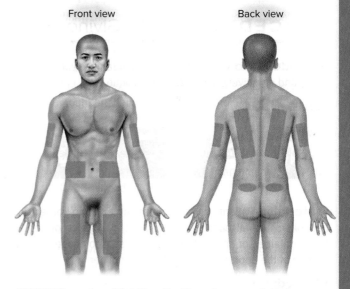

FIGURE Procedure 53-6 Step 5   Many sites are available for subcutaneous injection.

7. Position the needle—bevel up—at a 45- to 90-degree angle to the skin.
   RATIONALE: *The angle of the needle helps ensure that the medication is administered into the correct location. A 90-degree angle is used when you can pinch at least 2 inches. A 45-degree angle is used when you can only pinch 1 inch of skin.*

2. Check the rights, comparing information against the drug order, and explain the procedure and the drug order to the patient.
   RATIONALE: *To ensure necessary accuracy.*

3. Ask the patient about any drug or food allergies. If the patient is not allergic to the ordered drug or other ingredients used to prepare it, proceed.

4. Give the patient the opportunity to empty her bladder before beginning.

5. Assist the patient into the lithotomy position and drape her.
   RATIONALE: *To preserve her modesty while exposing the vulva.*

6. Place a bedsaver pad under the buttocks.

7. Put on gloves.

8. Cleanse the perineum with soap and water, using one cotton ball per stroke, and cleanse the center last, while spreading the labia.

RATIONALE: *This technique prevents contamination of areas already cleaned.*

9. Lubricate the vaginal suppository applicator in lubricant spread on a paper towel. For vaginal drugs in the form of creams, ointments, gels, and tablets, use the appropriate applicator, preparing it according to the package insert.

10. While spreading the labia with one hand, insert the applicator with the other (the applicator should be about 2 inches into the vagina and angled toward the sacrum).

11. Release the labia and push the applicator's plunger to release the suppository into the vagina.

12. Remove the applicator and wipe any excess lubricant off the patient.

13. Help her to a sitting position and assist with dressing if needed.

14. Document the administration with date, time, drug, dose, route, and any significant patient reactions.

PROCEDURE 53-12 Administering a Rectal Medication [WORK // DOC]

Procedure Goal: To safely administer a rectal medication

OSHA Guidelines:

Materials: Patient chart/progress note, prescription or drug order in the patient's chart, a cloth or paper drape, a bedsaver pad, gloves, water-soluble lubricant, and the prescribed drug

Method:

1. Check the rights, comparing information against the drug order.
   RATIONALE: *To ensure necessary accuracy.*

2. Explain the procedure and the drug order to the patient.

3. Ask the patient about any drug or food allergies. If the patient is not allergic to the ordered drug or other ingredients used to prepare it, proceed.

4. Give the patient the opportunity to empty the bladder before beginning.

5. With the patient in a gown, help the patient into the Sims' position and use a drape to prevent exposing the patient. Place a bedsaver pad under the patient.

6. Lift the patient's gown to expose the anus.

7. Wash your hands, put on gloves, and prepare the medication.

Administering a Suppository

8. Lubricate the tapered end of the suppository with about 1 tsp of lubricant.

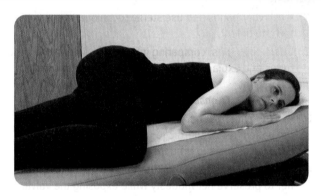

FIGURE Procedure 53-12 Step 5 Place the patient into Sims' position. The patient should be in a gown with a drape in place.

©McGraw-Hill Education

9. While spreading the patient's buttocks with one hand, insert the suppository—tapered end first—into the anus with the other hand.

10. Gently advance the suppository past the sphincter with your index finger. Before it passes the sphincter, the suppository may feel as if it is being pushed back out of the anus. When it passes the sphincter, it seems to disappear.

11. Use tissues to remove excess lubricant from the area.

12. Remove your gloves and ask the patient to lie quietly and retain the suppository for at least 20 minutes. When the treatment is completed, help the patient to a sitting, then standing, position.
    RATIONALE: *To ensure the maximum effectiveness of the medication.*

Administering a Retention Enema

13. Place the tip of a syringe into a rectal tube. Let a little rectal solution flow through the syringe and tube. While holding the tip up, clamp the tubing.

14. Lubricate the end of the tube, spread the patient's buttocks, and slide the tube into the rectum about 4 inches.

15. Slowly pour the rectal solution into the syringe, release the clamp, and let gravity move the solution into the patient. When you have administered the ordered amount of solution, clamp the tube and then remove it.

16. Using tissues, apply pressure over the anus for 20 seconds to stifle the patient's urge to defecate, and then wipe any excess lubricant or solution from the area. Remove your gloves and encourage the patient to retain the enema for the time ordered.

RATIONALE: *To ensure the maximum effectiveness of the medication.*

17. When the time has passed, put on gloves and help the patient use a bedpan or direct the patient to a toilet to expel the solution.

After the Administration Is Complete

18. Remove your gloves and wash your hands.

19. Immediately document the drug administration with date, time, drug, dose, route, and any significant patient reactions.

SUMMARY OF LEARNING OUTCOMES

OUTCOME	KEY POINTS
53.1 Describe the rules and responsibilities regarding drug administration and the initial preparation for drug administration.	Before administering a medication, you should check the patient for allergies and evaluate any drug-drug interactions. You should check all injection sites for abnormalities such as scars, bruises, burns, rash, edema, moles, birthmarks, traumatic injuries, redness, cyanosis, tattoos, warts, site of a mastectomy, and paralyzed areas. Additionally, you should be aware of the patient's condition and have the patient sign a consent form if necessary.
53.2 List the rights of drug administration.	The rights of drug administration include the right patient, right drug, right dose, right route, right time, right documentation, right reason, right to know, right to refuse, and right technique.
53.3 Recognize the correct equipment to use for administering medications.	Drugs may be administered for either local or systemic effects. Generally, drugs that have local effects are applied directly to the skin, tissues, or mucous membranes. Drugs that produce systemic effects are administered by routes that allow the drug to be absorbed and distributed in the bloodstream throughout the body. Table 53-2 outlines the many drug administration routes.
53.4 Carry out the procedures for administering oral medications.	Oral medications typically are swallowed and absorbed through the digestive tract. Sublingual medications go under the tongue, and buccal medications go between the cheek and gum.
53.5 Carry out procedures for administering parenteral medications by injection.	The three most common injection routes are ID, subcut, and IM. IV is less frequently used in a medical office. All injections are given using aseptic technique. Intradermal (ID) injections are administered between the upper layers of skin and create a wheal. Subcutaneous (subcut) injections are administered just under the skin, and intramuscular (IM) injections are administered into a muscle.
53.6 Carry out procedures for administering parenteral medications by other routes.	Other medication routes include inhalants (respiratory), topical (including transdermal), urethral, vaginal, and rectal.

OUTCOME	KEY POINTS
53.7 Relate special considerations required for medication administration to pediatric, pregnant, breast-feeding, and geriatric patients.	Certain special considerations must be made when caring for pediatric, pregnant, and breast-feeding patients. Pediatric patients require extreme care when calculating doses due to the differences in how their bodies absorb, metabolize, eliminate, and distribute the medications. Treat pediatric patients with special care and communication to make the experience as positive as possible. Restraining may be necessary. Checking medications given to pregnant and breast-feeding patients for possible adverse effects is essential. Geriatric considerations are discussed in the *Assisting in Geriatrics* chapter.
53.8 Outline patient education information related to medications.	Patients should be educated about why, when, and how they should take medications. This includes instruction to ensure patient compliance regarding nonprescription and prescription drugs as well as herbal remedies and supplements. Patients also should be instructed about the dangers of medication combinations, and the importance of reporting an adverse effect and maintaining a complete medication list.
53.9 Implement accurate and complete documentation of medications.	Documentation of medication administered should occur immediately after the medication is given and should include name, date, time, medication administered, dose, route, location, lot number, and how the patient tolerated it.

CASE STUDY CRITICAL THINKING

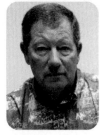

©McGraw-Hill Education

Recall John Miller from the case study at the beginning of the chapter. Now that you have completed this chapter, answer the following questions regarding his case.

1. What questions do you need to ask John Miller during his initial interview regarding his medications?

2. When you get ready to administer the pneumococcal immunization, John Miller states that he had a bad reaction the last time he received a shot. What should you do?

3. If the site of the injection from his last visit was just irritated due to the medication, what could be done to reduce the irritation for his next IM injection?

EXAM PREPARATION QUESTIONS

1. (LO 53.3) Which of the following would you expect to be absorbed in the *least* amount of time?
   a. 200 mL of D5W IV
   b. 5 mL of Compazine® IM
   c. 325 mg of ASA orally
   d. 2 puffs of albuterol by oral inhalation
   e. PPD subcut injection

2. (LO 53.2) Which of the following is *not* a basic right of medication administration?
   a. Right dose
   b. Right drug
   c. Right to refuse
   d. Right patient
   e. Right time

3. (LO 53.8) Which of the following patients has the greatest risk of overdose and toxicity from a medication?
   a. A 35-year-old woman with asthma
   b. A 6-year-old child with the flu
   c. A 50-year-old male with hypertension
   d. A 16-year-old Hispanic girl with mononucleosis
   e. A 25-year-old man with diabetes

4. (LO 53.1) When performing a triple check, which of the following would you *least* likely do?
   a. *1st check*—when you take it from the storage container and match it to the MAR
   b. *2nd check*—when you prepare it
   c. *3rd check*—before you close the storage container
   d. *3rd check*—just after you administer the drug
   e. *3rd check*—just before you administer the drug

5. (LO 53.4) A patient is taking a nitroglycerin tablet under his tongue. What route of administration is this?
   a. Urethral
   b. Topical
   c. Inhalant
   d. Sublingual
   e. Buccal

6. (LO 53.5) You are injecting a medication ID; what would *best* let you know that you have done it correctly?
   a. The patient does not have pain.
   b. There is a wheal on the skin at the site.
   c. The angle of the needle is at 90 degrees.
   d. The medication went into a muscle.
   e. The medication went under the skin.

7. (LO 53.6) You are administering a suppository. What route of administration are you *most* likely performing?
   a. Oral
   b. Vaginal
   c. Respiratory
   d. IV
   e. Topical

8. (LO 53.7) An infant needs an immunization subcut. What site and what needle would be your *best* choice?
   a. Vastus lateralis, 20 gauge, ⅝ inch
   b. Vastus lateralis, 25 gauge, 1½ inch
   c. Ventrogluteal, 25 gauge, ⅝ inch
   d. Dorsogluteal, 23 gauge, 1 inch
   e. Vastus lateralis, 25 gauge, ⅝ inch

9. (LO 53.8) Which of the following would be done to improve patient compliance?
   a. Have patients with multiple meds create an alarm, calendar, or chart.
   b. Remind patients taking antibiotics to stop once they are feeling better.
   c. To avoid waste, encourage patients to share medication if they have too much.
   d. Tell patients to dispose of expired drugs 1 year after the expiration date on the medication.
   e. Encourage anxious patients to have at least three servings of alcohol each day.

10. (LO 53.9) Which of the following is the *most* complete medication documentation?
   a. Gave Demerol® for pain at 2 pm
   b. Demerol® 100 mg IM in deltoid
   c. 4/12/XX Demerol® IM in left deltoid
   d. 4/12/XX Phenergan® 200 mg PO for nausea
   e. Phenergan® PO for nausea—Kaylyn R. Haddix RMA(AMT)

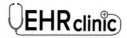

Go to CONNECT to complete the EHRclinic exercises: 53.01 Document Medication Administration, 53.02 Record Medications in a Patient's EHR, and 53.03 Document Allergies in a Patient's EHR.

S O F T   S K I L L S   S U C C E S S

While working at BWW Medical Associates with a medical assisting student from a local school, you enter an examination room with a patient and notice there is a small needle and syringe with medication in it on the tray table. You know that it was the medical assisting student's responsibility to clean the room between patients. What should you do?

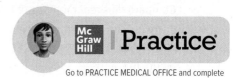

Go to PRACTICE MEDICAL OFFICE and complete the module Clinical: Office Operations.

Physical Therapy and Rehabilitation

CASE STUDY

Patient Name	DOB	Allergies
Christopher Matthews	11/19/2012	NKA

Attending	MRN	Other Information
Alexis N. Whalen, MD	00-AA-011	AP and lateral X-rays right ankle show no signs of fractures.

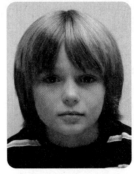
©McGraw-Hill Education

Christopher (Chris) Matthews arrives at the office with a swollen right ankle. Chris Matthews was climbing a tree this morning and jumped from a lower limb to the ground. When he landed, he felt his ankle "turn over" and he could not stand up. Chris Matthews' mother tells you that she thinks it was about 6 feet from the limb to the ground. She also tells you that she put ice on Chris Matthews' ankle after she brought him into the house, but his ankle just kept swelling and Chris Matthews still cannot walk. She says that his ankle is badly bruised. Mrs. Matthews is very distraught and asks that Chris Matthews be seen immediately. You speak with Dr. Whalen, and she asks you to take Chris Matthews to the X-ray department for X-rays. Dr. Whalen examines Chris Matthews and reads the X-rays. She wraps Chris Matthews' ankle and tells you Chris Matthews has a badly sprained ankle and will need crutches for a few weeks using a non-weight-bearing gait.

Keep Chris Matthews in mind as you study this chapter. There will be questions at the end of the chapter based on the case study. The information in the chapter will help you answer these questions.

LEARNING OUTCOMES

After completing Chapter 54, you will be able to:

54.1 Discuss the general principles of physical therapy.

54.2 Relate various cold and heat therapies to their benefits and contraindications.

54.3 Recall hydrotherapy methods.

54.4 Name several methods of exercise therapy.

54.5 Describe the types of massage used in rehabilitation therapy.

54.6 Compare different methods of traction.

54.7 Carry out the procedure for teaching a patient to use a cane, a walker, crutches, and a wheelchair.

54.8 Model the steps you should take when referring a patient to a physical therapist.

KEY TERMS

cryotherapy

diathermy

erythema

fluidotherapy

gait

goniometer

hydrotherapy

mobility aid

physical therapy

posture

range of motion (ROM)

therapeutic team

thermotherapy

traction

I.P.8	Instruct and prepare a patient for a procedure or a treatment	
I.P.9	Assist provider with a patient exam	
I.A.1	Incorporate critical thinking skills when performing patient assessment	
I.A.2	Incorporate critical thinking skills when performing patient care	
I.A.3	Show awareness of a patient's concerns related to the procedure being performed	
V.P.4	Coach patients regarding: (d) treatment plan	
XII.C.7	Identify principles of: (a) body mechanics (b) ergonomics	

2. Anatomy and Physiology

c. Identify diagnostic and treatment modalities as they relate to each body system

8. Clinical Procedures

d. Assist provider with specialty examination including cardiac, respiratory, OB-GYN, neurological, and gastroenterology procedures

e. Perform specialty procedures including but not limited to minor surgery, cardiac, respiratory, OB-GYN, neurological, and gastroenterology

h. Teach self-examination, disease management and health promotion

j. Make adaptations for patients with special needs (psychological or physical limitations)

Introduction

Applying cold and heat therapy and assisting patients with ambulation (walking around) are common responsibilities of a medical assistant. These activities are part of the physical therapy field. For a full program of physical therapy, a physician generally refers a patient to a licensed physical therapist. However, a physician may request that you assist with some forms of physical therapy, including:

- Applying cold and heat.
- Teaching basic exercises.
- Demonstrating how to use a cane, a walker, and crutches.
- Demonstrating how to use a wheelchair.
- Discussing with the patient-specific therapies for use at home.

General Principles of Physical Therapy

LO 54.1

Physical therapy is a medical specialty for the treatment of musculoskeletal, nervous, and cardiopulmonary disorders. A physical therapist uses a variety of treatments, including cold, heat, water, exercise, massage, and traction. Some physical therapy regimens combine two or more treatments. Exercising in a pool, for example, combines the use of water and exercise. In addition, the physical therapist actively promotes patient education and rehabilitation programs.

Physical therapy benefits patients in several ways. It restores and improves muscle function, builds strength, increases joint mobility, relieves pain, and increases circulation. Physical therapy is used to treat various disorders, including arthritis, stroke, lower back pain, muscle spasms, muscle injuries or diseases, pressure sores, skin disorders, and burns.

Assisting Within a Therapeutic Team

Many people who require physical therapy are recovering from traumatic injuries or dealing with chronic illnesses, so they may be receiving therapeutic attention from several specialists. Physicians, nurses, medical assistants, and other specialists who work with patients dealing with chronic illness or recovery from major injuries make up a **therapeutic team.** When you work with such patients, your responsibilities may include:

- Coordinating the patient's schedule of sessions with different specialists.
- Making referrals, as directed by the physician.
- Explaining a specialist's treatment approach to the patient.
- Communicating the physician's findings to the specialist.
- Documenting the specialist's treatments and findings for the physician.
- Reinforcing the specialist's instructions for the patient.
- Answering the patient's questions.

To fulfill these responsibilities, you must have a working knowledge of therapy techniques. If, for example, the physician refers a patient to an art therapist, you would set up an art therapy appointment and explain in general terms what the patient can expect. The *Educating the Patient* feature Specialized Therapies and Their Benefits offers basic information about various specialized therapies.

Besides learning the basic information you need to know about physical therapy, you will want to keep up-to-date on emerging techniques. You may want to become proficient in some of these new techniques. By expanding your knowledge and skills, you increase your value as a member of the therapeutic team.

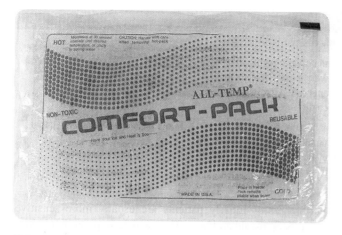

FIGURE 54-3 This chemical pack can be frozen, boiled, or microwaved for cold and heat therapy.
©Total Care Programming, Inc.

60 minutes. Some ice packs come with a soft covering; others must be wrapped in a cloth before they are applied to the skin.

Wet Cold Applications Wet cold applications include cold compresses and ice massage. A cold compress is a cloth or gauze pad moistened with ice water. It may be used to treat the pain associated with a toothache, tooth extraction, eye injury, or headache. The ice used in ice massage may be a cube wrapped in a plastic bag or water frozen in a paper cup. The combination of the cold temperature and the motion of the massage can provide therapeutic relief for the localized pain resulting from a sprain or strain. Although cold causes muscles to contract, the pain-relieving effect can help a patient relax. The procedure for administering cryotherapy is outlined in Procedure 54-1 at the end of this chapter.

Principles of Thermotherapy

The application of thermotherapy causes blood vessels to dilate (expand), which increases the blood supply to the area. Increased blood supply brings about an increased tissue metabolism that carries oxygen and nutrients to the cells of the area being treated. Increased metabolism carries toxins and wastes away from the cells. During thermotherapy, the treated skin becomes warm and develops **erythema** (redness) as the capillaries in the skin's deep layers fill with blood. These physiologic responses can have the following results:

- Relief of pain and congestion.
- Reduction of muscle spasms.
- Muscle relaxation.
- Reduction of inflammation.
- Reduction of swelling by increasing the fluid absorption from the tissues.

Administering Thermotherapy

Thermotherapy is highly effective in relieving pain, congestion, muscle spasms, and inflammation and promoting muscle

relaxation. However, if heat is applied for too long, it may increase skin secretions that soften the skin and lower its resistance to infection. Heat that is too extreme can burn the skin or increase edema. Always monitor patients receiving thermotherapy, particularly children and elderly patients. The three basic types of thermotherapy are dry heat, moist heat, and diathermy. The general principles for administering the following types of thermotherapy are outlined in Procedure 54-2 at the end of this chapter.

Dry Heat Therapies Several types of dry heat therapy are available. They include the use of chemical hot packs, heating pads, hot-water bottles, heat lamps with infrared or ultraviolet bulbs, and fluidotherapy.

Chemical Hot Pack A chemical hot pack is a disposable, flexible pack of chemicals that becomes hot when you activate it by kneading or slapping it. After activating the pack, cover it with a cloth and place it on the patient's skin in the area being treated. Chemical hot packs are pliable and conform to body contours. For best results, follow the manufacturer's directions.

Heating Pad A heating pad is a flat pad with electrical coils between layers of soft fabric. When turned on, the coils provide localized heat. The physician should specify the heating pad temperature (low, medium, or high) and the length of time the pad should be applied.

Before applying a heating pad, cover it with a pillowcase or towel, check to be sure the cord is not frayed, and plug it into an electrical outlet. Make sure the patient's skin is dry. Then turn on the pad and set the temperature selector switch to the specified temperature. The patient should never lie on top of a heating pad, as burns could result.

Hot-Water Bottle A hot-water bottle is a flat, flexible, plastic or rubber bottle with a stopper. Fill the bottle with hot water, using a thermometer to make sure the water temperature does not exceed 125°F. For children under the age of 2 years and for elderly patients, the temperature should range from 105°F to 115°F. For older children, a safe temperature is 115°F to 125°F. Fill the bottle halfway, then compress it to expel air. The half-filled bottle can conform to the area to be treated. A half-filled bottle is also lighter than a full one, so it is more comfortable for the patient. Cover the bottle with a cloth or pillowcase before you apply it.

After you apply the hot-water bottle, check with the patient to make sure the temperature is not too hot. Check the temperature frequently and replace the hot water as needed. Each time you remove the bottle, check the patient's skin to make sure it is merely warm to the touch.

Heat Lamp A heat lamp uses an infrared or ultraviolet bulb to provide heat. When the lamp is turned on, infrared rays heat and penetrate the skin's surface to a depth of 3 to 5 millimeters. To avoid burning the skin, place an infrared heat lamp 2 to 4 feet from the area being treated. Treatment usually lasts for 20 to 30 minutes or as directed by the physician.

Although ultraviolet rays produce little heat, they can burn the skin and damage the eyes. Ultraviolet rays are used to kill bacteria and promote vitamin D formation. They stimulate epithelial cells and cause blood vessels to overfill, increasing the skin's defenses against bacterial infections. Ultraviolet lamps are used to treat psoriasis, pressure sores, and wound infections.

Before recommending the use of an ultraviolet lamp, the healthcare practitioner assesses the patient's sensitivity and determines the treatment duration, which usually ranges from 30 seconds to a few minutes. The duration is usually increased in 10-second intervals. Because ultraviolet rays can burn the skin, monitor the patient closely. Do not leave the room during treatment. Both you and the patient must wear goggles to protect the eyes.

Fluidotherapy **Fluidotherapy** is a technique for stimulating healing, particularly in the hands and feet. The patient places the affected body part in a container of glass beads or other fine, granular particles that are heated and agitated with hot air. Although the therapy is dry, its effect is similar to that of a therapy using water.

Moist Heat Applications Moist heat is often used to increase circulation and decrease pain to specific body areas, especially muscles and tendons. Moist heat applications include hot soak, hot compress, hot pack, and paraffin bath.

Hot Soak With hot-soak therapy, the patient places the affected body part—usually an arm or a leg—in a container of plain or medicated water that has been heated to no more than 110°F. A hot soak should last about 15 minutes.

Hot Compress A compress is a piece of gauze or cloth suitable for covering a small area. After soaking the compress in hot water, wring it out and apply it to the area to be treated. Keep the compress warm either by placing a hot-water bottle on top of it or by frequently rewarming the compress in hot water.

Hot Pack A hot pack is a large canvas bag filled with a heat-retaining gel that is used on a large body area. Like a hot compress, a hot pack retains heat after being placed in hot water.

Paraffin Bath A paraffin bath is a receptacle of heated wax and mineral oil. It is used to reduce pain, muscle spasms, and stiffness in patients with arthritis and similar disorders. The patient's affected area should first be washed. Then it is dipped repeatedly into the mixture until the area is covered with a thick coat of wax. The wax remains on the area for about 30 minutes and then is peeled off. Particularly useful for joints, especially the hands and feet, the paraffin bath has the added benefit of leaving the skin warm, flexible, and soft. Some erythema may result.

Alternating Hot and Cold Packs A physician may order application of a hot pack followed by a cold pack. This increases circulation to the area by dilating and constricting the blood vessels. Be sure to apply the hot pack first. Applying the cold pack first can numb the skin and keep the patient from recognizing a hot pack is too hot. This can result in serious skin burns.

Diathermy **Diathermy** is a type of heat therapy in which a machine produces high-frequency electromagnetic waves that create deep heat penetration in muscle tissue. The heat helps decrease joint stiffness, dilate blood vessels, relieve muscle spasms, and reduce discomfort from sprains and strains. Three types of diathermy are ultrasound, shortwave, and microwave. Equipment for these therapies is continually being improved. Be sure to familiarize yourself with the manufacturer's instructions regarding the specific equipment in your office.

Ultrasound Ultrasound is the most common type of diathermy, used to treat sprains, strains, and other acute ailments. It projects high-frequency sound waves that are converted to heat in muscle tissue.

Ultrasound diathermy may be administered by rubbing a gel-covered transducer over the skin in circular patterns. It also may be administered to a body part under water. Do not use ultrasound in areas where bones are near the skin's surface, as this could cause bone damage.

Shortwave Shortwave diathermy uses radio waves that travel through the body between two condenser plates and are converted to heat in the tissues. This type of diathermy is used to treat acute, subacute, and chronic inflammation. Treatment typically ranges from 20 to 30 minutes. Do not use shortwave diathermy on a patient who has a pacemaker.

Microwave Microwave diathermy uses microwaves to provide heat deep in body tissues. Contraindications include use on patients with pacemakers, use in combination with wet dressings, and use in high dosages on patients with swollen tissue. Also, never use microwave diathermy near metal implants because the reaction between metal and microwaves could cause burns.

▶ Hydrotherapy   LO 54.3

Hydrotherapy is the use of water to treat physical problems. It is typically performed in the physical therapy department of a hospital, in an outpatient clinic, or at home. Common forms of hydrotherapy include the use of whirlpools and contrast baths and underwater exercises.

Whirlpools

Whirlpools are tanks in which water is agitated by jets of air under pressure. Whirlpools vary in size from small (capable of accommodating only one body part) to very large (capable of accommodating a wheelchair or full-body submersion). The agitated water's action in a whirlpool generates a hydromassage, which relaxes muscles and increases circulation. Whirlpools also are used to cleanse and debride (remove foreign matter and dead tissue from) the skin of patients with wounds, ulcers, or burns.

Contrast Baths

Contrast baths are separate baths, one filled with hot water and the other with cold water. The patient alternately moves the treated body part quickly from one bath to the other. This treatment induces relaxation, stimulates improved circulation (which speeds up healing), and results in greater mobility.

Underwater Exercises

Underwater exercises—prescribed for patients with joint injuries, burns, and arthritis—are usually performed in a warm swimming pool. Because the water's buoyancy takes pressure off the joints, these exercises are particularly useful for patients with painful or limited movement. Combined with the movement of the water around the body, the exercises promote relaxation and increased circulation.

▶ Exercise Therapy   LO 54.4

For many patients, exercise is as important as medications or other treatments and offers both preventive and therapeutic benefits. As a patient ages, exercise helps promote flexibility, mobility, muscle tone, and strength. Exercise is a primary treatment for fractures, arthritis, and some respiratory disorders; it can minimize symptoms or help slow disease progression. For patients who have had surgery, stroke, burns, or amputation, regular exercise therapy can help prevent problems caused by inactivity.

A healthcare practitioner orders exercise therapy for many reasons. Exercise improves or restores general health and is especially therapeutic when a patient is weak from illness. Explain to patients that exercise will help them to:

- Improve muscle tone and strength.
- Regain ROM after an injury.
- Prevent ROM from diminishing in chronic conditions.
- Prevent or correct physical deformities.
- Promote neuromuscular coordination.
- Improve circulation.
- Relieve stress.
- Lower cholesterol levels.
- Resume normal daily activities.

Commonly used for treating sports injuries, exercise therapy for injured athletes is described in the *Educating the Patient* feature The Injured Athlete. This type of therapy focuses primarily on regaining muscle strength and flexibility in the injured area.

Role of the Medical Assistant

As a medical assistant, you may have several roles in exercise therapy. As an information resource for the patient and family, you must understand various types of exercise programs and the patient's specific treatment plan. You also may serve as a source of support and encouragement when exercise programs are long and difficult. You may, for example, assist with ROM exercises and teach the patient and family how to perform them at home.

When teaching patients about exercises, give them illustrations of the exercises. Include with each illustration written instructions on the number of times to perform the exercise, as prescribed by the healthcare practitioner.

After demonstrating each exercise, have patients perform it while you watch and give direction. Patients are more likely to perform exercises properly at home if they can perform them correctly in your presence. It is also helpful for patients' caregivers or family members to watch and perform the exercises to become familiar with them.

Types of Exercise

There are various types of exercise in a therapeutic program; however, before a patient begins an exercise program, the healthcare practitioner must evaluate the patient's heart and lung function and overall physical condition. The healthcare practitioner adjusts the level of exercise accordingly and may prescribe other forms of physical therapy, such as cryotherapy, thermotherapy, or hydrotherapy. Careful preparation by the healthcare practitioner and patient before beginning an exercise therapy program helps prevent injuries. Some measures to prevent and treat common exercise therapy problems are outlined in Table 54-2.

Types of exercises in therapeutic programs include active mobility, passive mobility, aided mobility, active resistance, isometric, and ROM.

Active Mobility Exercises Active mobility exercises are exercises the patient performs without assistance to increase muscle strength and function. They often require equipment such as a stationary bicycle or a treadmill.

Passive Mobility Exercises In passive mobility exercises, the physical therapist or a machine moves a patient's body part. The patient does not actively assist in these exercises. Patients who require passive mobility exercises may have neuromuscular disability or weakness. These exercises can help retain patients' ROM and improve their circulation.

TABLE 54-2	Preventing and Treating Common Problems of Exercise Therapy	
Problem	**Prevention Methods**	**Treatment**
Muscle strain	Beginning with gentle warm-up exercises	Rest and application of heat followed by ice
Muscle aches	Keeping track of the number of repetitions and amount of weight (resistance), if used; increasing the number of repetitions or amount of weight slowly	Rest and soaking in hot bath to relieve aches
Impatience with slowness of progress	Discussing expectations with patient; setting realistic goals with patient; stressing necessity of avoiding recurrent injury, which would prolong recovery	Creation of goal sheet, noting small successes as therapy progresses

The Injured Athlete

The risk of injury is associated with most sports, but some sports carry a greater risk of serious injury. Many sports-related injuries affect joints in the neck, shoulders, elbows, wrists, hands, knees, ankles, or feet.

You may be called on to educate injured athletes and to start them on the road to recovery. To do so, you need to understand the mind of the athlete. Why do many athletes get injured in the first place? Here are some reasons:

- The sport they participate in has a high injury rate.
- They return to a sport before their injuries are completely healed.
- They become impatient with a physical therapy regimen.
- They do not work at gradual muscle strengthening.

When does your job begin? After diagnosing the injury, the healthcare practitioner will probably refer the athlete to a sports medicine center or other physical therapy setting, where an individualized program will be set up. As a medical assistant, you will often be responsible for counseling an athlete about the physical therapy program she will be entering. Here are some basic rules you can communicate:

- Follow the physical therapy regimen set up by the physician or physical therapist—even if it is tedious or time-consuming.
- Use only the equipment specified by the therapist: free weights, weight-training equipment, stationary bike, other aerobic equipment, or swimming pool. The physical therapist recommends the designated equipment based

on the type of injury. Using other equipment could cause further injury or interfere with healing.

- Do not rush the therapy in an attempt to recover more quickly.
- Work slowly to strengthen muscles and improve flexibility.
- Continue exercises at home as instructed.
- Be patient.

Explain to the athlete how the physical therapy program will be presented. Knowing what to expect from the physical therapist can improve the athlete's compliance. Here are some explanations you might offer:

- The therapist will demonstrate exercises and then watch you perform them.
- The therapist may increase the number of repetitions or the amount of resistance (weight) but probably not both at the same time.
- The therapist will provide handouts illustrating the exercises, along with instructions on how to perform them.
- The therapist may provide an activity log to help you chart your progress.

An athlete who is impatient with a physical therapy regimen and returns to a sport before an injury has completely healed has an increased risk of repeated injury. Impress on the athlete the importance of the physical therapy process. Emphasize the need for gradual strengthening and healing over a period of time. To help the athlete in the long run, focus on recovery from injury and on the need to prevent recurrent injury.

Aided Mobility Exercises Aided mobility exercises are self-directed exercises. The patient performs them with the aid of a device such as an exercise machine or a therapy pool. Aided mobility exercises help retain or increase patients' ROM.

Active Resistance Exercises In active resistance exercises, the patient works against resistance (counter-pressure) to increase muscle strength. Resistance is provided manually by the therapist or mechanically by an exercise machine.

Isometric Exercises During isometric exercises, the patient relaxes and then contracts the muscles of a body part while in a fixed position. Isometric exercises can maintain the patient's muscle strength when a joint is temporarily or permanently immobilized.

ROM Exercises ROM exercises move each joint through its full range of motion. These exercises should be done slowly and gently. Doing them too quickly or too soon after an injury can cause pain, fracture, or bleeding into the joint. For this reason, a physical therapist assesses the patient and determines a recommended regimen of ROM exercises. You

may be asked to educate the patient and caregiver or family about the regimen.

ROM exercises are typically prescribed after a joint injury. The physical therapist may recommend that the joint be moved in its full range of motion three times, twice a day. ROM exercises also are recommended for elderly people to improve circulation and muscle function. The therapist will prescribe one of three types of ROM exercises for patients:

1. Active range-of-motion exercises: performed by the patient without assistance.
2. Assisted range-of-motion exercises: performed by the patient with the help of another person or a machine.
3. Passive range-of-motion exercises: performed by another person or a machine.

ROM exercises do not build muscle strength but do improve flexibility and mobility. Typical ROM exercises are illustrated in Figure 54-4.

Electrical Stimulation

Electrical stimulation helps prevent atrophy in muscles that cannot move voluntarily by causing the muscles to contract

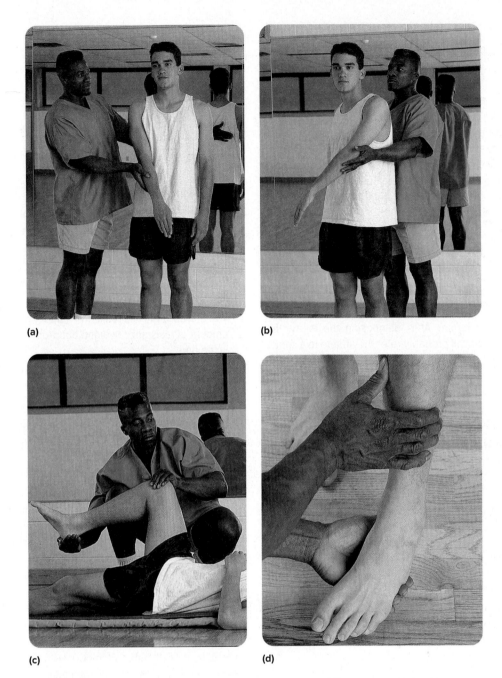

FIGURE 54-4 A medical assistant helps a patient perform typical ROM exercises: (a) shoulder abduction, (b) back rotation, (c) hip flexion, and (d) toe abduction.
©David Kelly Crow

involuntarily (on impulse) and relax. Electrical stimulators deliver controlled amounts of low-voltage electric current to motor and sensory nerves to stimulate muscles. Frequent and regular electrical stimulation also aids in healing injured joints and in revitalizing muscles.

Electrical stimulation can help retrain a patient to use injured muscles by creating a perceivable connection between the stimulus (muscle movement) and the area of the brain that controls those muscles. If a limb does not function because of injury or disease, this therapy can give the patient hope that injured muscles are not dead. Hope often encourages a patient to work harder and to cooperate in the physical therapy regimen, which can be long and arduous.

Wearable electrical stimulation units are being developed for people with spinal cord injuries to help them retrain affected muscles.

▶ Massage   LO 54.5

The practice of massage uses pressure, kneading, stroking, vibration, and tapping to positively affect patients' health and well-being. Massage helps the patient relax and counteracts the effects of stress. During massage, the heart rate and blood pressure are lowered and blood circulation and lymph flow are increased. Massage helps reduce pain caused by tight muscles and helps relax muscle spasms.

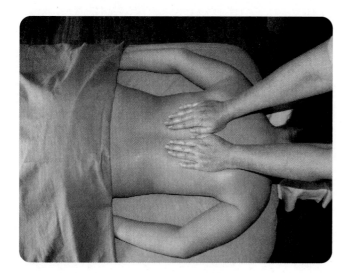

FIGURE 54-5 Swedish massage uses kneading, pressure, stroking, and human touch to alleviate pain and promote healing through relaxation.

©McGraw-Hill Education/Shaana Pritchard, Photographer

Massage benefits the mind as well as the body: It helps improve concentration, promotes restful sleep, and helps the mind relax. Many patients find they handle daily stresses better when they have regular massage. People who get massages on a regular basis find they become ill less often and less severely and they feel less stressed and tense. Some patients notice their muscles beginning to tighten and are aware that if they get a massage, it will decrease muscle tension before it becomes severe.

Swedish Massage

Swedish massage is one of the best known and most frequently taught massage techniques. It stimulates circulation and lymph flow with five basic strokes that manipulate the body's soft tissues. The strokes include pétrissage (kneading), effleurage (stroking), tapotement (percussion), vibration, and friction. Oils and/or lotions are used to reduce friction on the patient's skin. One type of Swedish massage is done on warm muscles immediately after exercise. Another type is a stress-reduction massage that is done with the same basic strokes on patients who have not been exercising (Figure 54-5).

Neuromuscular Massage

Neuromuscular massage is applied to specific muscles and helps release tension and knots, relieve pain and release pressure on nerves, and increase blood flow. Trigger point therapy is one type of neuromuscular massage in which strong finger pressure is applied to trigger points in the muscles.

▶ Traction   LO 54.6

Traction is the pulling of the bones and joints to create a mechanical force that is used to treat fractured bones and dislocated, arthritic, or other diseased joints. It is often performed by a physical therapist using special equipment. The therapist may set up traction in the patient's home and visit regularly to ensure that the equipment is used and maintained properly.

Traction is used to:

- Create and maintain proper bone alignment after a fracture or other injury.
- Reduce or prevent joint stiffening and abnormal muscle shortening.
- Correct deformities.
- Relieve compression of vertebral joints.
- Reduce or relieve muscle spasms.

Although you will not be setting up or performing traction, you should know about its types and uses. This information will prepare you to answer basic questions from patients and family members.

Manual Traction

The physical therapist performs manual traction by using his hands to pull a patient's limb or head gently. Pulling stretches the muscles and separates the joints, allowing for greater motion and less stiffening. Manual traction is used with patients who have muscle spasms, stiffness, and arthritis.

Static Traction

To perform static traction, or weight traction, the therapist places a patient's limb, pelvis, or chin in a harness. The harness is then attached to weights through a pulley system. This type of traction is commonly used to relieve muscle spasms.

Skeletal Traction

Skeletal traction is performed in inpatient facilities on patients whose injuries require long traction time and heavy weights. During surgery, a surgeon inserts pins, wires, or tongs into bones. After surgery, the pins, wires, or tongs are attached to pulleys and weights to provide continuous traction.

Mechanical Traction

Mechanical traction uses a device that intermittently pulls and relaxes a prescribed body part, such as the neck. The therapist sets the time intervals between contractions and relaxations. Mechanical traction is used to promote relaxation.

▶ Mobility Aids   LO 54.7

Mobility aids (also called *mobility assistive devices*) are designed to improve patients' ability to ambulate, or move from one place to another. These include canes, walkers, crutches, and wheelchairs.

The appropriate aid depends on the patient's disability, muscle coordination, strength, and age. The patient may need a device temporarily—perhaps crutches after a sprain—or permanently—such as a wheelchair in the case of permanent paralysis.

Canes

Canes provide support and help patients maintain balance. They come in several styles, including standard, tripod, and quad-base (Figure 54-6), which are all lightweight, are made of wood or aluminum, and have a rubber tip or tips at the bottom. Canes are especially useful for patients with weaknesses

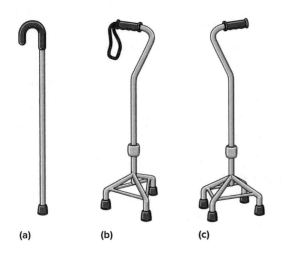

(a) **(b)** **(c)**

FIGURE 54-6 Shown here are three styles of canes: (a) standard, (b) tripod, and (c) quad-base.

on one side of the body (possibly due to a stroke), joint disability, or neuromuscular defects.

A standard cane is best for a patient who needs only a small amount of support. Its curved handle is convenient, allowing the patient to hang it from a pocket or a doorknob. When the patient uses a standard cane, however, the curved handle concentrates most of the patient's weight in one small area of the hand. To avoid stressing the hand in this way, some standard canes have a T-shaped handle, which distributes pressure on the hand more evenly. Tripod canes have three legs, and quad-base canes have four. The multiple legs create a wide base of support, making them more stable than a standard cane. Tripod and quad-base canes can stand alone, freeing up the patient's hands when she sits down. These canes are bulkier and more difficult to pick up and put down than a standard cane, however. Both styles have T-shaped handles.

After determining the most suitable cane for the patient, the physical therapist adjusts the cane's height. When the cane is the correct height, the patient's elbow is flexed at 20 to 25 degrees and the patient stands tall while using the cane (instead of leaning on it for support). The therapist makes sure the handle is the right size for the patient's hand and instructs the patient on how to use the cane. If directed, you may do the teaching or reinforce it, as discussed in Procedure 54-3 at the end of this chapter.

Walkers

A walker is a lightweight, easy-to-use aluminum frame that is open on one side and has four widely placed, adjustable, rubber-tipped legs that can be adjusted to various heights (Figure 54-7). Some models are designed to fold up for storage. To use a walker, the patient stands within the frame and leans on the upper bar, which has a handgrip on each side.

Typically, older patients who are too weak to walk unassisted or who have balance problems use a walker. The walker is designed to give these patients a sense of stability as they ambulate. In tight spaces or in areas with throw rugs, however, a walker may be difficult to manage. A patient who is too weak to pick up the walker may use a walker on wheels. Wheeled walkers have brakes for safety. Patients should never

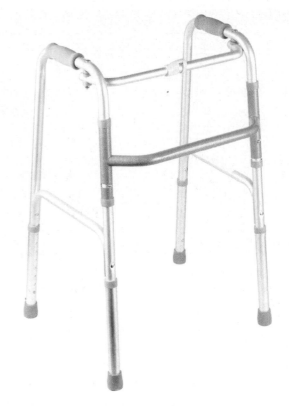

FIGURE 54-7 A standard walker.
©Ingram Publishing/SuperStock

slide a walker that does not have wheels because the movement could easily result in a fall.

A physical therapist selects a walker that suits the patient's abilities and height. A walker should reach the patient's hipbone. See Table 54-3 for more information about different types of walkers. Although the physical therapist usually trains the patient in the use of a walker, you may be asked to do this, or you may need to reinforce the information presented in Procedure 54-4 at the end of this chapter.

Crutches

Crutches allow a patient to walk without putting weight on the feet or legs by transferring that weight to the arms. Crutches are made of aluminum or wood. Aluminum crutches are lighter and usually more expensive than those made of wood. Pediatric crutches are available for children. The two basic types of crutches are axillary and Lofstrand®. Procedure 54-5, at the end of this chapter, provides the steps for teaching patients how to use crutches.

Axillary crutches reach from the ground to the armpit. Each crutch has a rubber tip on the bottom to prevent slipping. This type of crutch is designed for short-term use by patients with injuries such as a sprained ankle.

Lofstrand®, or Canadian, crutches reach from the ground to the forearm, and each one has a rubber tip on the bottom to prevent slipping. For additional support, this type has a handgrip extension attached at a 90-degree angle and a metal cuff that fits securely around the patient's forearm. Lofstrand® crutches are geared for long-term use by patients with disorders such as paraplegia (Figure 54-8).

TABLE 54-3 Types of Walkers

Walker	Features	Advantages	Disadvantages
Standard	No wheels, adjustable legs	Very stable on flat surfaces; easier to use than crutches	Requires upper-body strength to use
Standard folding	No wheels, sides fold in	Easy to transport and store	Requires upper-body strength to use, requires pressing a tab to release and fold
Rolling	Front wheels	Requires less upper-body strength to use	Not as stable as a standard walker
Rolling with brakes	Front wheels and brakes	Disengages wheels when weight from upper body is applied	Not as stable as a standard walker
Three-wheel rolling with brakes	Bicycle-style hand brakes	Better maneuverability; folds for transport and storage	Requires better balance than other walkers
Reciprocal	Each side of walker moves alternately	Allows for more natural gait	Requires better balance and coordination than other walkers; catches on some floor surfaces

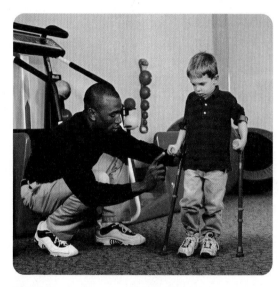

FIGURE 54-8   A child using Lofstrand® crutches.
©Guy Cali/Getty Images

Measuring the Patient for Crutches To prevent back pain and nerve injury to the armpits and palms, crutches must be measured to fit each patient. Axillary crutches that are too long can put pressure on nerves in the armpit, causing a condition called crutch palsy (muscle weakness in the forearm, wrist, and hand). They also can force the patient's shoulders forward, causing strain on the back and making ambulation difficult. Crutches that are too short force the patient to bend forward during ambulation, causing back pain or imbalance, which can lead to falls.

Before a patient who uses crutches leaves the office, make sure the crutches fit properly and that the patient is comfortable walking with them. To confirm a correct fit, check for the following conditions (see Figure 54-9):

- The patient is wearing the type of shoes he will wear when walking.
- The patient is standing erect with feet slightly apart.
- The crutch tips are positioned 4 to 6 inches in front of the patient's feet and 4 to 6 inches to the side of each foot.
- The axillary supports allow two to three finger-widths between supports and armpits. (Use wing nuts and bolts to adjust crutches.)

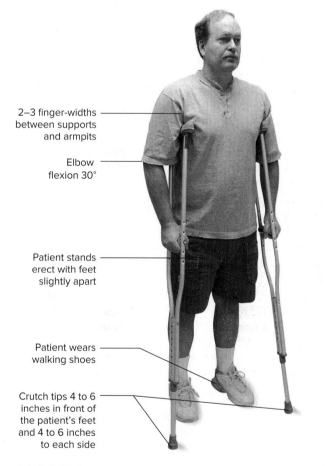

2–3 finger-widths between supports and armpits

Elbow flexion 30°

Patient stands erect with feet slightly apart

Patient wears walking shoes

Crutch tips 4 to 6 inches in front of the patient's feet and 4 to 6 inches to each side

FIGURE 54-9   Use these guidelines when measuring a patient for crutches.
©Total Care Programming, Inc.

- The handgrips are positioned to create 30-degree flexion at the elbows. (Use wing nuts and bolts to adjust; use a goniometer to check flexion.)

Crutch Gaits To teach a patient how to stand and walk with crutches, you must learn the crutch gaits, or walks. First, show the patient the standing, or tripod, position. To do this, have the patient stand erect and look straight ahead. The

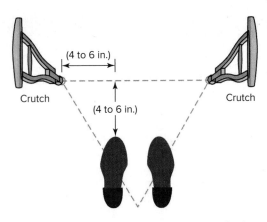

FIGURE 54-10 This is the correct beginning position for the patient's feet and crutches when you are teaching a patient to walk with crutches.

patient should place the crutch tips 4 to 6 inches in front of her feet and 4 to 6 inches away from the side of each foot. See Figure 54-10.

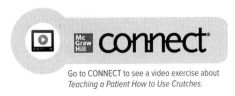

Go to CONNECT to see a video exercise about *Teaching a Patient How to Use Crutches.*

To determine the proper gait for a patient, you will make a preteaching assessment of the patient's muscle coordination and physical condition. In general, instruct a patient to use a slow gait in crowded areas or when feeling tired. The patient can use a faster gait in open places or when feeling more energetic. Using various gaits and speeds enables the patient to exercise different muscle groups and improve overall conditioning.

Four-Point Gait The four-point gait is a slow gait used only when a patient can bear weight on both legs. Because this gait has three points of contact with the ground at all times, it is stable and safe. It is especially useful for patients with leg muscle weakness, spasticity, or poor balance or coordination. To teach this gait, see Figure 54-11a, have the patient start in the tripod position, and give the following instructions.

1. Move the right crutch forward.
2. Move the left foot forward to the level of the left crutch.
3. Move the left crutch forward.
4. Move the right foot forward to level of the right crutch.

See Figure 54-11a.

Three-Point Gait The three-point gait is used when a patient cannot bear weight on one leg but can bear full weight on the unaffected leg. This gait allows the patient's weight to be carried alternately by the crutches and by the unaffected leg. It is appropriate for amputees, patients with tissue or musculoskeletal trauma (such as a fractured or sprained leg), and those recovering from leg surgery. The patient must have good muscle coordination and arm strength, however. To teach this gait, have the patient start in the tripod position. Then give the patient the following instructions, as illustrated in Figure 54-11b:

1. Move both crutches and the affected leg forward.
2. Move the unaffected leg forward while weight is balanced on both crutches.

Two-Point Gait The two-point gait is faster than the four-point gait and is used by patients who can bear some weight on both feet and have good muscle coordination and balance. To teach this gait, have the patient start in the tripod position. Then outline the following steps, as illustrated in Figure 54-11c:

1. Move the left crutch and the right foot forward at the same time.
2. Move the right crutch and the left foot forward at the same time.

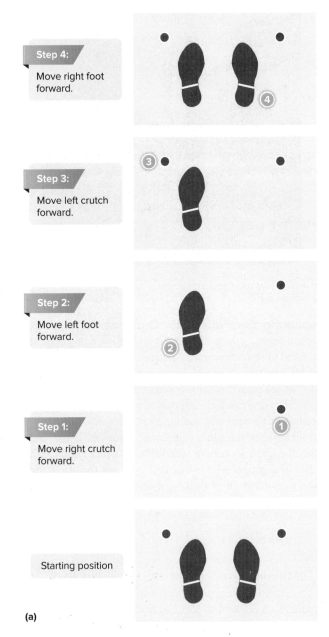

Step 4: Move right foot forward.

Step 3: Move left crutch forward.

Step 2: Move left foot forward.

Step 1: Move right crutch forward.

Starting position

(a)

FIGURE 54-11 Crutch gaits include (a) a four-point gait, (b) a three-point gait, and (c) a two-point gait.

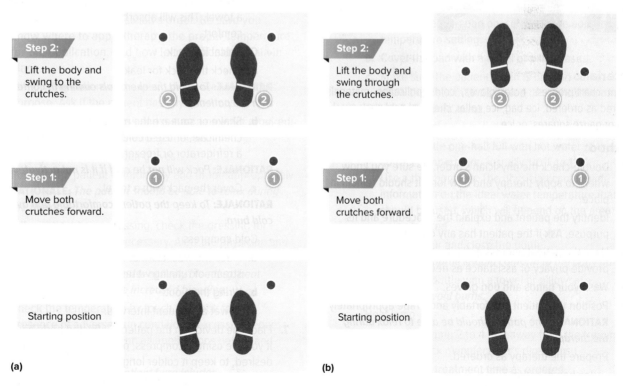

FIGURE 54-11 Crutch gaits include (a) a four-point gait, (b) a three-point gait, and (c) a two-point gait.

Swing Gaits Patients with severe disabilities, such as leg paralysis or deformity, may use one of two swing gaits: the swing-to gait or the swing-through gait (Figure 54-12). To teach the swing-to gait, have the patient start in the tripod position. Then outline the following steps:

1. Move both crutches forward at the same time.

2. Lift the body and swing to the crutches.

3. End with the tripod position again.

To teach the swing-through gait, have the patient start in the tripod position. Then review the following steps:

1. Move both crutches forward.

2. Move the body and swing past the crutches.

FIGURE 54-12 Patients with severe disabilities may walk with crutches using (a) the swing-to gait or (b) the swing-through gait.

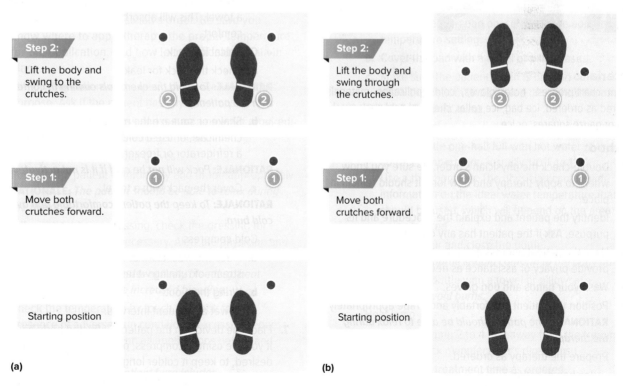

1. (LO 54.1) Which of the following is an example of inversion?
   a. Flexing the foot
   b. Pointing the foot upward
   c. Turning the sole of the foot inward
   d. Rotating the foot back and forth
   e. Turning the sole of the foot downward

2. (LO 54.1) Body position and alignment are known as
   a. Posture
   b. Gait
   c. Range of motion
   d. Flexion
   e. Extension

3. (LO 54.4) Which of the following is a type of exercise whereby the patient relaxes and contracts the muscles of a specific body part without moving the body part?
   a. ROM
   b. Passive mobility
   c. Active resistance
   d. Isometric
   e. Aided mobility

4. (LO 54.6) Another name for weight traction is
   a. Static
   b. Skeletal
   c. Mechanical
   d. Manual
   e. Harness

5. (LO 54.7) Which of the following crutch gaits is the best for someone with leg paralysis?
   a. Two-point
   b. Three-point
   c. Swing-to
   d. Four-point
   e. Crutches are never used by people with leg paralysis.

6. (LO 54.2) Which of the following therapies causes blood vessels to constrict?
   a. Neuromuscular massage
   b. Thermotherapy
   c. ROM
   d. Active resistance exercise
   e. Cryotherapy

7. (LO 54.5) In Swedish massage, which of the following strokes is a percussive stroke?
   a. Pétrissage
   b. Effleurage
   c. Vibration
   d. Tapotement
   e. Friction

8. (LO 54.4) Riding a stationary bicycle is an example of a(n)
   a. Active mobility exercise
   b. Isometric exercise
   c. Passive mobility exercise
   d. Active range-of-motion exercise
   e. Aided mobility exercise

9. (LO 54.7) Which of the following crutch gaits is considered the slowest?
   a. Two-point
   b. Swing-through
   c. Three-point
   d. Swing-to
   e. Four-point

10. (LO 54.1) A goniometer is used to measure
    a. Pain
    b. The effectiveness of cold therapy
    c. Range of motion
    d. Muscle contraction
    e. The type of traction needed

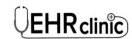

Go to CONNECT to complete the EHRclinic exercise: 54.01 Refer a Patient to Physical Therapy.

Recall Chris Matthews from the case study at the beginning of the chapter. Dr. Whalen asks you to assist with wrapping Chris Matthews' ankle. She wants you to hold and stabilize his leg while she applies the elastic wrap. Chris Matthews' mom asks you if she will need any help rewrapping Chris Matthews' ankle. What should you tell Mrs. Matthews about taking care of Chris Matthews' bandage?

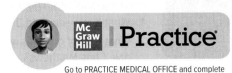

Go to PRACTICE MEDICAL OFFICE and complete the module Clinical: Work Task Proficiencies.

Nutrition and Health

CASE STUDY

Patient Name	DOB	Allergies
Mohammad Nassar	05/17/2005	Animal dander

Attending	MRN	Other Information
Elizabeth H. Williams, MD	00-AA-007	Current medications: Albuterol 4 mg bid

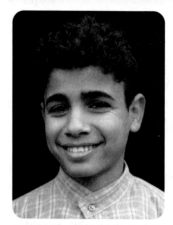

©David Sacks/Getty Images

Mohammad Nassar, is brought to BWW Medical Associates by his parents. As the medical assistant, you take his history and physical, noting that he has a past history of mild asthma. The patient mentions that he is avoiding food because he is being "careful not to eat too many calories" so that he can keep his weight down and have a chance to fight in the lightest weight class. He tells you he hopes to get a scholarship for wrestling so that he can attend college next fall. You note that his vital signs are blood pressure 100/60, height 5'10", weight 131 lb., pulse rate 50. He appears dehydrated and exhibits signs of muscle weakness.

Keep Mohammad Nassar in mind as you study the chapter. There will be questions at the end of the chapter based on the case study. The information in the chapter will help you answer these questions.

LEARNING OUTCOMES

After completing Chapter 55, you will be able to:

55.1 Relate daily energy requirements to the role of calories.

55.2 Identify nutrients and their role in health.

55.3 Implement a plan for a nutritious, well-balanced diet and healthy lifestyle using the USDA's guidelines.

55.4 Describe methods used to assess a patient's nutritional status.

55.5 Explain reasons why a diet may be modified.

55.6 Identify types of patients who require special diets and the modifications required for each.

55.7 Describe the warning signs, symptoms, and treatments for eating disorders.

55.8 Educate patients about nutritional requirements.

KEY TERMS

amino acid

anabolism

anorexia nervosa

antioxidant

behavior modification

body dysmorphic disorder (BDD)

bulimia nervosa

calorie

catabolism

celiac disease

cholesterol

complex carbohydrate

dehydration

fiber

food exchange

gluten

lipid

mineral

parenteral nutrition

protein

saturated fat

unsaturated fat

vitamin

TABLE 55-7 Diabetic Food Exchange Table

Food Exchange	US Unit	Comments
Starches		
15 g Carb, 3 g Protein, 1 g Fat		• Most starches are a good source of B vitamins.
• English muffin	½	• Choose whole-grain foods such as 100% whole-wheat bread and flour, brown rice, and tortillas for nutrients and fiber.
• Graham crackers (2½-inch squares)	3	
• Bagel, large (4 ounces)	¼ (1 oz)	• Combine beans (starch and meat) with grains (starch) for their complementary proteins and fiber.
• Bread: pumpernickel, rye, white, whole-grain	1 slice (1 oz)	
• Bread, reduced calorie	2 slices (1½ oz)	• Combine grains (starch) with milk (milk exchange) or cheese (meat exchange) to complement proteins.
• Cereal: bran, oats, spoon-size shredded wheat, frosted cereals	¼ cup	• Add 1 fat exchange for starchy foods prepared with fat.
• Cereal, unsweetened	¾ cup	
• Grits, cooked	½ cup	
• Tabbouleh, prepared	½ cup	
• Pasta, cooked	⅓ cup	
• Wild rice, cooked	½ cup	
• Corn	½ cup	
• Popcorn, popped	3 cups	
• Potato (large, baked with skin)	¼ (3 oz)	
• Potato, mashed	½ cup	
• Sweet potato	½ cup	
• Squash: acorn, butternut	1 cup	
Add 1 meat exchange for the following starches:		
• Baked beans	⅓ cup	
• Beans, cooked: black, garbanzo, kidney, lima, pinto, navy, white	½ cup	
• Peas, cooked: black-eyed, green	½ cup	
• Refried beans, canned	½ cup	
Vegetables (3–5 exchanges)		
5 g Carb, 2 g Protein		• Choose more dark green leafy and deep yellow vegetables such as spinach, broccoli, carrots, and peppers.
• Raw vegetables	1 cup	
• Cooked vegetables	½ cup	
Fruit (2–4 exchanges)		
15 g Carb		• Choose whole fruits for fiber.
Fresh fruit:		• Choose citrus fruits such as oranges, grapefruits, or tangerines.
• Apple, small (2 inches across)	1 (4 oz)	
• Berries: blackberries, blueberries	¾ cup	
• Grapefruit, large	½	
• Mango, cubed	½ cup	
• Orange, small	1 (6 oz)	
• Strawberries	¼ cup (13½ oz)	
Dried fruit:		
• Apple	4 rings	
• Prunes	3	
• Raisins	2 tbsp	

TABLE 55-7 Diabetic Food Exchange Table

Food Exchange	US Unit	Comments
Canned fruit, unsweetened:		
• Applesauce, apricots, cherries, peaches, pears, pineapple, plums	½ cup	
• Grapefruit	¾ cup	
• Mandarin oranges	¾ cup	
Fruit juice, unsweetened:		
• Apple, grapefruit, orange, pineapple	½ cup (4 fl oz)	
Meat & Substitutes (5–7 exchanges)		
7 g Protein, 0–13 g Fat		• Choose leaner meats such as chicken, fish, and lean cuts of meat; add fat exchange for higher-fat meats and substitutes.
• Beef	1 oz	• Remove skin from poultry.
• Cheese	1 oz	• Limit frying or adding fat.
• Cottage cheese	¼ cup	• Have 2 servings of fish per week for omega-3 fatty acid.
• Egg whites	2	
• Egg substitutes	¼ cup	
• Fish, fresh or frozen	1 oz	
• Pork	1 oz	
• Bacon	2 slices	
• Poultry	1 oz	
• Peanut butter	1 tbsp	
• Tofu	½ cup	
Milk (2–3 exchanges)		
12 g Carb, 8 g Protein, 0–8 g Fat		• Choose lower-fat milks; add fat exchange for higher-fat milk.
• Milk	1 cup	
• Soy milk	1 cup	
• Rice drink, low-fat, flavored	1 cup (8 fl oz)	
• Yogurt, low-fat with fruit	⅔ cup (6 oz)	
Fat (use sparingly)		
5 g Fat		• Eat less fat.
• Almonds	6	• Eat less saturated fat, such as animal fat found in fattier meat, cheese, and butter; also eat less hydrogenated fat.
• Coconut, shredded	2 tbsp	
• Oil: canola, olive, peanut, corn, safflower, soybean, sunflower	1 tsp	• Check Nutrition Facts on food labels; 5 g Fat = 1 Fat exchange.
• Mayonnaise	1 tsp (1 tbsp if reduced-fat)	
• Cream cheese	1 tbsp (1½ tbsp if reduced-fat)	
• Salad dressing	1 tbsp (2 tbsp if reduced-fat)	
• Peanuts	10	
• Avocado	2 tbsp (1 oz)	
• Butter or margarine	1 tsp	

Sources: Diet.com. http://www.diet.com/g/exchange-system, USDA National Agricultural Library. http://fnic.nal.usda.gov/diet-and-disease/diabetes/carbohydrate-counting-and-exchange-lists, and American Diabetes Association. http://www.diabetes.org/food-and-fitness/food/planning-meals/diabetes-meal-plans-and-a-healthy-diet.html. National Heart, Lung, and Blood Institute https://www.nhlbi.nih.gov/health/educational/lose_wt/eat/fd_exch.htm Accessed March 11, 2018.

instructed to remove the tampon immediately and replace it with a sanitary napkin.

TSS is treated with intravenous antibiotics and fluids. The patient will require hospitalization.

Viral Encephalitis

Viral encephalitis is a severe brain inflammation caused directly by a virus or secondary to a complication resulting from a viral infection. Viral encephalitis may result from an epidemic or may arise sporadically. This condition requires accurate identification and prompt treatment. Symptoms develop suddenly, beginning with fever, headache, and vomiting. They quickly progress to stiff neck and back, decreased level of consciousness (from drowsiness to coma), and paralysis and seizures.

The level of consciousness must be monitored frequently in a patient with viral encephalitis. Prepare the patient for treatment with antiviral drugs and arrange for transport to a hospital for a lumbar puncture and other diagnostic tests.

▶ Common Psychosocial Emergencies

LO 57.6

You will probably encounter psychosocial emergencies in the medical office at some point. These may result from drug or alcohol abuse, spousal abuse, child abuse, or elder abuse. Handle these situations as directed in the *Patient Interview and History* chapter. If you encounter patients who have overdosed on drugs, exhibit violent behavior, mention suicide, or have been raped, follow the specific clinical responsibilities described in this section.

You also may be responsible for referring patients with psychosocial emergencies to resources in the community. Some of these resources are listed in Table 57-5.

A patient who is overdosing on drugs can suffer serious medical problems and can even die. If a patient who has taken an overdose is brought to the medical office, call the EMS system immediately and arrange for transport to the hospital.

Patients on drugs may become violent during withdrawal from the substance or while under the influence. If, at any time, a patient becomes aggressive or threatening, follow office protocol for handling violent behavior. The protocol should state when to call the police, how to document the incident, and when to notify the insurance carrier.

During a psychosocial emergency, a patient may tell you he is so depressed that he has thought about killing himself. Allow the patient to talk freely. Listen carefully without interrupting. Whenever a patient mentions suicide or talks about life in ways that make you suspect suicidal tendencies, discuss your suspicions with the physician. Take comments on suicide seriously, no matter how casual they may seem.

Victims of rape may be of any age and either gender, but more than 90% are women. If a patient says she has been raped, provide privacy. Limit the number of people who ask her questions. She may feel traumatized, embarrassed, and fearful. Do not make her go through the office routine at this time.

TABLE 57-5	Resources for Patient Assistance
Resource	
Al-Anon Family Groups	
Alcoholics Anonymous	
Mothers Against Drunk Driving (MADD)	
Narcotics Anonymous	
National Child Abuse Hotline (Childhelp)	
National Coalition Against Domestic Violence	
National Council on Child Abuse and Family Violence	
National Domestic Violence Hotline	
National Institute for Alcohol Abuse and Alcoholism (NIAAA)	
National Institute on Drug Abuse	
National Organization for Victim Assistance (NOVA)	
Students Against Destructive Decisions (SADD)	

If the physician asks you to speak to the patient, explain to her that you are legally required to contact the police so that they can file a report. The patient can decide later whether she wishes to press charges.

Contact the local rape hotline and request that a rape counselor come to the office to stay with the patient during the exam and police report procedures. The physician should be familiar with state laws for collecting specimens and the protocol for caring for a rape victim.

The procedure of ensuring that a specimen is obtained from the victim and is correctly identified, that the specimen is under the uninterrupted control of authorized personnel, and that the specimen has not been altered or replaced is called *establishing chain of custody*. This procedure is required for medicolegal issues such as evidence of rape and for tests for illicit drug use. If the chain between the victim and the specimen cannot be proved to have remained unbroken, the specimen must be considered invalid. The steps for establishing a chain of custody are outlined in the *Collecting, Processing, and Testing Urine and Stool Specimens* chapter and are essentially the same for any specimen with a medicolegal purpose. These general steps help maintain an intact chain of custody. Always refer to your office's procedures to make sure you are meeting all relevant requirements.

▶ The Patient Under Stress

LO 57.7

In emergency situations, patients and family members are under a great deal of stress. You must realize that people react differently to emergency situations. You can learn how to detect signs of extreme stress by being alert for patients whose behavior varies from that previously observed or who cannot focus or follow directions.

Your role during many emergency situations may be to keep victims and their families and friends calm. You can promote calmness by listening carefully and giving your full attention. Your first priority, at all times, is the victim's well-being. If he is very distraught, for example, hold his hand while the doctor examines him. If one of his relatives is crying and causing him to become emotional, suggest that the relative do something to help—for example, fill out paperwork in another room.

You may face special challenges when communicating with victims during emergencies. Victims may not speak your language or may have a visual or hearing impairment. In such instances, follow these guidelines:

- Use gestures throughout the process for non-English-speaking victims. Continue to speak, however, because they may be able to understand some English.
- Tell patients who have visual impairments what you are going to do before you do it and maintain voice and touch contact while caring for them.
- Ask patients who have hearing impairments whether they can read lips. If they can, speak slowly to them and never turn away while you are speaking. If they cannot read lips, communicate by writing and using gestures. At all times, try to remain face to face and keep direct physical contact.

▶ Educating the Patient   LO 57.8

During minor medical emergencies, after major emergencies have been resolved, and during routine office visits, you can educate patients about ways to prevent and handle various medical emergencies. For example, you might tell them how to contact the local American Red Cross office, post notices of upcoming classes the Red Cross offers, and encourage patients and family members to learn basic first aid. You also might develop a first-aid kit checklist and make it available to patients and families.

Make sure all family members, including children, are familiar with the local EMS system and know how to contact it in an emergency. Suggest that families keep emergency numbers by the telephone. In addition, teach parents how to childproof their home for children of various ages. Remember, childproofing differs for different children—for example, for children who can crawl as opposed to children who can walk.

Provide brief, easy-to-read handouts to reinforce the information you present to patients. Prepare handouts in multiple languages if you provide care for non-English-speaking patients. Find and use patient education resources for the types of patients seen by the practice. For example, if you work in an obstetric office, obtain educational materials for pregnant and postpartum patients from companies that provide pregnancy-related products. Ask company representatives what materials are available. Many companies provide free videos and booklets.

▶ Disasters and Pandemics   LO 57.9

Your skills in dealing with emergencies, including first-aid and CPR training, will be an enormous help to your community in the event of a disaster or pandemic illness. To be fully effective, you also must be familiar with standard protocols for responding to disasters and pandemic illness. Table 57-6 shows ways you can help in certain types of disasters. You

may even want to participate in fire or other disaster drills to familiarize yourself with emergency procedures.

Evacuation and Shelter-in-Place Plans

Every office should have evacuation and shelter-in-place plans in the event of an emergency. **Shelter-in-place** refers to an interior room or rooms within your medical facility that have few or no windows and are places to take refuge. Plans should include means of communication for employees during and after the emergency. Maps of the facility with escape routes clearly marked should be posted. These plans should be in writing and there should be periodic practice drills. Employees should be trained in shelter-in-place procedures and their roles in implementing them. If a shelter-in-place option is a part of your emergency plan, be sure to implement a means of alerting your employees to shelter-in-place that is easy to distinguish from alerts used to signal an evacuation.

Pandemic Illness

A rapidly spreading influenza outbreak can overwhelm your office's resources very quickly. The influenza virus is capable of mutating, creating novel strains. Because the population has never been exposed to a novel influenza strain, no one has immunity to the new strain and the virus can spread quickly throughout the world. You must plan for pandemic illness before it occurs. Your office should have a written plan that includes:

- Identification and isolation of patients with potential influenza.
- Communication and reporting.
- Occupational health.
- Education and training of patients and staff.
- Respiratory hygiene.

In the most serious scenario, a worldwide influenza outbreak may last 12 to 24 months. There may be waves of illness that come and go every 6 to 8 weeks. Vaccines may be unavailable at first and antivirals will likely be in short supply. To reduce confusion, essential personnel and their roles should be clearly defined. The practice's plan should be flexible, as it is likely the situation will rapidly change. Having a flexible plan will more easily accommodate an evolving pandemic. For more information, see the *Caution: Handle with Care* feature Planning and Implementing a Preparedness Plan for Pandemic Illness.

Chemical Release Disasters

Whether a chemical release is the result of an industrial or transportation accident or an intentional release during a terrorist event, the results can quickly overwhelm emergency services and medical facilities. As a medical assistant, you may be asked to assist in treating and decontaminating patients exposed to chemicals released into the atmosphere. There are numerous chemicals that, when released into the atmosphere, can cause serious health concerns. Initial decontamination and assessment will most likely occur at the site of the release. Ambulatory patients who may need further decontamination and supportive

OUTCOME	KEY POINTS
57.1 Discuss the importance of first aid during a medical emergency.	Prompt and appropriate first aid can save a life, reduce pain, prevent further injury, reduce the risk of permanent disability, and increase the chance of early recovery.
57.2 Identify items found on a crash cart.	The crash cart should include all appropriate drugs, supplies, and equipment needed for emergencies. These include but are not limited to activated charcoal, atropine, dextrose 50%, epinephrine, lactated Ringer's solution, nitroglycerin tablets, and sodium bicarbonate.
57.3 Recognize various accidental emergencies and how to deal with them.	Accidental injuries you may encounter include bites and stings; burns; choking; ear trauma; eye trauma; falls; fractures, dislocations, sprains, and strains; head injuries; hemorrhaging; multiple injuries; poisoning; weather-related injuries; and wounds.
57.4 List common illnesses that can result in medical emergencies.	Common illnesses that may cause a medical emergency include abdominal pain, asthma, dehydration, diarrhea, fainting, fever, hyperventilation, nosebleed, tachycardia, and vomiting.
57.5 Identify less common illnesses that can result in medical emergencies.	Less common illnesses you may encounter in a medical office include anaphylaxis, bacterial meningitis, diabetic emergencies, gallbladder attack, myocardial infarction, hematemesis, obstetric emergencies, respiratory arrest, seizures, shock, stroke, toxic shock syndrome, and viral encephalitis.
57.6 Discuss your role in caring for people with psychosocial emergencies.	Psychosocial emergencies in the medical office include drug or alcohol abuse, spousal abuse, child abuse, elder abuse, and rape. As a medical assistant, you may be involved in the direct care of someone suffering a psychosocial emergency or may arrange for his or her care at an outside agency.
57.7 Carry out the procedure for calming a patient who is under extreme stress.	A medical assistant can help calm a patient under stress by listening carefully and giving her or his full attention.
57.8 Discuss ways to educate patients about how to prevent and respond to emergencies.	Medical assistants should educate patients about ways to prevent and handle various medical emergencies by providing brief, easy-to-read handouts containing local emergency contact numbers and a first-aid kit checklist. The handouts should be prepared in multiple languages if the practice provides care for non-English-speaking patients.
57.9 Illustrate your role in responding to natural disasters and pandemic illness.	During a disaster, a medical assistant's first-aid and CPR training will be of enormous help. A medical assistant also must be familiar with standard protocols for responding to disasters and pandemic illness.
57.10 Discuss your role in responding to acts of bioterrorism.	Physicians' offices will be on the front lines if a biologic agent is intentionally released as an act of terror. You should be aware of unusual patterns of disease in patients being seen at your office. Indications of a bioterrorist attack might include many patients having been in the same place at the same time or an unusual distribution for common illnesses, such as an increase in chickenpox-like illness in adults that might be smallpox.

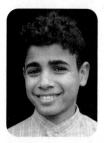

©David Sacks/Getty Images

Recall Mohammad Nassar from the case study at the beginning of the chapter. Now that you have completed the chapter, answer the following questions regarding his case.

1. What action should you take to keep Mohammad Nassar from exposing the other patients in the reception area?

2. What precautions should his mother take?

3. Mohammad Nassar tells you he feels like he is going to vomit. How should you care for Mohammad Nassar?

4. Dr. Williams tells you the office needs to implement the preparedness plan for pandemic illness. What steps should you take?

EXAM PREPARATION QUESTIONS

1. (LO 57.3) What is the first action you should take when administering first aid for an animal bite?
   a. Check to see if the animal has had a rabies vaccination.
   b. Clean the wound with soap and water.
   c. Call animal control.
   d. Administer tetanus toxoid.
   e. Put antibiotic ointment on the wound.

2. (LO 57.3) A displacement of a bone end from the joint is a(n)
   a. Fracture
   b. Sprain
   c. Dislocation
   d. Impaction
   e. Greenstick

3. (LO 57.3) Which of the following is a jarring injury to the brain?
   a. Concussion
   b. Stroke
   c. Seizure
   d. TIA
   e. Aneurysm

4. (LO 57.3) When should you apply a tourniquet to a wound?
   a. To save the limb
   b. If medical help is less than an hour away
   c. Only if the patient is alert
   d. If extremity bleeding cannot be stopped
   e. Before putting pressure on a wound

5. (LO 57.5) Severe hypoglycemia is known as
   a. Insulin shock
   b. Diabetic coma
   c. High blood sugar
   d. Diabetes mellitus
   e. Diabetes insipidus

6. (LO 57.4) The medical term for fainting is
   a. Hypoglycemia
   b. Epistaxis
   c. Shock
   d. Stroke
   e. Syncope

7. (LO 57.5) A severe, often life-threatening allergic reaction is known as
   a. Anaphylaxis
   b. Bee sting
   c. Hives
   d. Toxic shock syndrome
   e. CVA

8. (LO 57.10) The intentional release of a biologic agent with the intent to harm individuals is known as
   a. Pandemic illness
   b. Natural disaster
   c. Mass casualties
   d. Bioterrorism
   e. Radiation contamination

9. (LO 57.6) Drug abuse, attempted suicide, rape, child abuse, and alcohol abuse are examples of
   a. Common illnesses
   b. Psychosocial emergencies
   c. Stress-related diseases
   d. Psychiatric diseases
   e. Medical emergencies

10. (LO 57.3) An injury characterized by a clean, smooth cut through the skin is a(n)
    a. Puncture
    b. Contusion
    c. Laceration
    d. Abrasion
    e. Incision

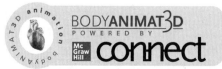

Go to CONNECT to see an animation exercise about *Burns*.

You arrive at the office the morning after a large accidental chemical release at the local fertilizer plant. Your office was utilized by emergency personnel as a decontamination station for victims with mild to moderate exposure. As you are checking the exam rooms, you notice that one of the rooms still has contaminated clothing from a victim of the chemical accident. The clothes are in the corner of the room and are not contained. What should you do?

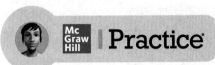

Go to PRACTICE MEDICAL OFFICE and complete the module Clinical: Privacy and Liability.

CASE STUDY

EMPLOYEE INFORMATION

Employee Name	Position	Credentials
Reagan Patrick	Student	In training

Supervisor	DOB	Other Information
Malik Katahri, CMM	09/07/1988	Applying for a position that is opening where she is finishing her applied training.

Reagan Patrick is just finishing her applied training and is beginning her job search. Her applied training included venipuncture, ECG, urinalysis, assisting with exams and procedures, patient reception, insurance claim form completion, patient scheduling, and many other clinical and administrative skills. She lives in a small town but is willing to relocate. She is excited about her new career in healthcare because it is so different from her current job working as a teller at a bank.

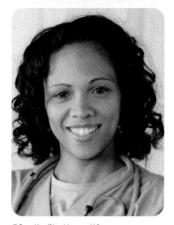

©Terry Vine/Blend Images LLC

Keep Reagan Patrick in mind as you study this chapter. There will be questions at the end of the chapter based on the case study. The information in the chapter will help you answer these questions.

LEARNING OUTCOMES

After completing Chapter 58, you will be able to:

58.1 Carry out professionalism in all applied training scenarios.

58.2 Summarize the steps necessary for obtaining professional certification.

58.3 Describe an appropriate strategy for finding a position.

58.4 Explain key factors for a successful interview.

58.5 Describe ways of becoming a successful employee.

KEY TERMS

affiliation agreement

applied training

applied training coordinator

chronological résumé

clinical preceptor

constructive criticism

functional résumé

networking

portfolio

professional objective

reference

targeted résumé

V.P.8 Compose professional correspondence utilizing electronic technology

1. General Orientation

  c. Describe and comprehend medical assistant credentialing requirements, the process to obtain the credential and the importance of credentialing

4. Medical Law and Ethics

  f. Comply with federal, state, and local health laws and regulations as they relate to healthcare settings

10. Career Development

  a. Perform the essential requirements for employment, such as résumé writing, effective interviewing, dressing professionally, time management, and following up appropriately

  b. Demonstrate professional behavior

  c. Explain what continuing education is and how it is acquired

▶ Introduction

After completing a medical assisting program, you may be both excited and apprehensive about beginning your new career. Such a reaction is perfectly normal. In this chapter, you will learn how to maximize your applied training experience and gain the hands-on experience you need for securing a position in medical assisting. Your applied training is an opportunity for you to explore the different responsibilities required of a medical assistant. After completing this chapter, you will understand the process for becoming a nationally certified medical assistant. You also will know how to effectively begin searching for a position in medical assisting—which includes completing a résumé, cover letter, and thank-you letter—and how to form a strategic plan to secure this position. And as you explore this chapter, you will gain valuable interviewing techniques for successfully competing in the modern healthcare world.

▶ Training in Action

LO 58.1

An **applied training** experience is an opportunity to work in a medical facility to gain essential on-the-job experience for beginning your new career. Some schools call this training an externship, whereas others call it a practicum. Whether it is called an externship or a practicum, it is an opportunity to apply—in an actual medical environment—the knowledge and skills you have learned.

Most applied training is measured by hours attended, usually a minimum of 160 hours. Applied training is a mandatory requirement of fulfilling a medical assisting program in educational institutions that are accredited by the Accrediting Bureau of Health Education Schools (ABHES) and the Commission on Accreditation of Allied Health Education

Programs (CAAHEP). Some of the applied training is completed after the didactic, or academic, portion of the curriculum (for example, during the last module or semester), and some is completed during the academic or didactic last semester. Medical assisting applied training may be performed at physician offices, laboratories, hospitals, administrative billing offices, and clinics.

The Applied Training Process

To make the applied training process possible, the educational institution where the medical assisting student is enrolled partners with local medical facilities throughout the area. Most schools have an **applied training coordinator** who is familiar with medical assisting and the medical community. The applied training coordinator procures applied training sites and qualifies, or assesses, them to make certain that they provide a thorough educational experience. The applied training coordinator is the liaison between the applied training site and the educational institution. A checklist is often designed to ensure that students are given a well-rounded, safe experience (Figure 58-1). Although student applied training experiences are unpaid, the student should be positive about the experience and appreciate the opportunity to train with the facility.

Applied Training Requirements Applied training sites are required to review and sign an **affiliation agreement**. The affiliation agreement states the expectations of the facility and the expectations of the student. Some examples of the expectations of the applied training site include:

- Providing reasonable opportunities for clinical instruction by qualified facility personnel for students participating in the program.

CLINICAL SITE ASSESSMENT

Name of Site _____

Address _____

Specialty _____ Supervisor _____

Telephone # _____ Fax # _____

Number of Staff _____

Administrative/clinical experience available to students
(check all that apply)

_____ Front office skills

_____ Word processing skills

_____ Measurement/recording of vital signs

_____ Blood drawing (venipuncture, fingersticks)

_____ Injections

_____ Electrocardiograms

_____ Specimen collection/diagnostic procedures
(urinalysis, blood sugar, cholesterol, etc.)

_____ Assisting with minor surgical procedures

I have determined that this site meets the needs of the students in the medical assisting program.

Print name of evaluator _____

Signature of evaluator _____ Date _____

FIGURE 58-1 A form such as this clinical site assessment often is used by the applied training coordinator to determine if a clinical site will be appropriate for medical assisting applied training.

- Supervising students in a manner that will provide safe practice and meaningful clinical education.

In addition, the expectations of the educational institution include:

- Reinforcing patient confidentiality by having the student sign a statement of confidentiality.
- Providing professional liability insurance for the student, the educational institution, and the faculty.
- Ensuring that the student is medically able to perform the assigned duties of the applied training facility by providing proof of immunizations and health physicals.

Screening The applied training coordinator places students in applied training clinical sites. It is not uncommon for the clinical site to screen students prior to their applied training. This screening can include:

- Interviewing students.
- Asking students to provide a urine or hair sample for drug screening.

- Asking students to consent to a criminal background check. Some medical facilities check only for felony convictions, and others check for misdemeanors and felonies. Honesty is the best policy for criminal background checks. Some institutions will waive some convictions as long as the student is honest and truthful about the conviction early in the process.

Time Sheets Students receive time sheets to be completed on a daily basis and faxed to the educational facility at the end of every week. The **clinical preceptor** (person at the clinical site who serves as an instructor but is an employee of the site) and the student both sign the time sheet (Figure 58-2). Weekly telephone calls and site visits may be performed by the clinical coordinator or a medical assisting instructor for each student. Some schools require weekly progress reports from each student outlining the procedures and duties the student performed during the week. Figure 58-3 provides an example of this report. When students finish their applied training, the preceptors will complete a final evaluation and the students will be graded on their performance.

Donna Turner-Smith
18 Kingsley Road
Olmsted Falls, OH 44138
(440) 555-4279

PUBLIC HEALTH EDUCATION:

Instructed community groups on HIV awareness
Instructed volunteers on how to set up community programs on domestic violence
Facilitated workshops for parents of teenagers
Provided in-services for public school teachers on signs and symptoms of
substance abuse

COUNSELING:

Consulted with social workers on individual cases for suspected child abuse
Worked with parents from abused homes
Counseled individual abused children

ORGANIZATIONAL:

Wrote grants for federal funds for HIV awareness programs
Served as a liaison for transitional shelters for victims of domestic violence
Served as a liaison between community health agencies and public schools

PROFESSIONAL WORK HISTORY:

2011–2016   Project SAFE, Plymouth, Michigan
                     HIV Public Health Instructor

2016–2019   Department of Child Health and Safety, Cleveland, Ohio
                     Public Health Educator

EDUCATION:

2011 BS Sociology, Eastern Michigan University, Ypsilanti, Michigan

References available upon request

FIGURE 58-4   A functional résumé is often used by people who are reentering the job market.

Example #2 WORK EXPERIENCE

Medical Assistant

Managed eight medical assistants from three different offices. Oversaw three offices in the Greater Cleveland area. Directed the daily operations of the medical offices. Coordinated events and served as secretary for the Cuyahoga County Chapter of the American Association of Medical Assistants. Increased daily patient census by 25% due to the success of a customer service model, "Patient First," which improved patient-facility relations during my tenure.

Résumé Writing Tips

Pay close attention to detail as you create your résumé:

- Organize your information by using a worksheet (Figure 58-7). List all the addresses, dates, phone numbers, and supervisors of previous positions you have held. Write down brief descriptions of all the responsibilities and duties of your positions.

- List your educational institutions and their addresses, your dates of attendance, and the type of diploma or degree, including your major.

Anthony Dalton
1234 West 25th Street
Park Ridge, NJ 07656
(201) 555-8311

WORK EXPERIENCE:

September 2015–Present   NORTH BERGEN CLINIC FOUNDATION

Lead medical assistant for cardiology practice
Patient preparation
EKG and Holter monitor
Assist with stress testing
Patient follow-up

June 2007–August 2015   ST. JOSEPH HOSPITAL

Phlebotomist—inpatient and outpatient

March 2007–June 2007   ST. JOSEPH HOSPITAL

Medical assisting externship
Administrative and clinical responsibilities utilizing all
medical assisting skills in the emergency department

- Patient triage
- Foley catheters
- ECG
- Specimen collection
- Patient intake
- Insurance verification

EDUCATION AND CERTIFICATIONS:

Associate of Applied Science Degree, June 2013, Bergen Community College,
Paramus, New Jersey, 07645

Certified Medical Assistant, August 2007

References available upon request

FIGURE 58-5   A chronological résumé lists a person's job history in chronological order.

- Choose a résumé format that best describes your experience, education, and achievements.
- Use a word processing program and save your résumé so that you can update it as needed.
- Proofread all spelling and grammar. Your completed résumé should be perfect. Do not rely on the spell-checking feature of your computer. Proofread your résumé line by line and ask someone else to also proofread your résumé.
- Choose a clean, easy-to-read font that is 11–12 points. This makes the résumé easier to read.
- Select a high-quality, standard-size (8½ × 11) résumé paper with a weight between 20 and 25 pounds. Use ivory or white paper with matching envelopes.
- Use clear and concise statements and sentences. Your writing should reflect a positive and confident tone. For example, if you are describing your duties as a food service worker, use sentences that focus on customer service, cash management, and the training and development of new food service workers. Avoid using the word "I" because the reader already knows that the résumé is referring to you.

Infectious Diseases Caused by Fungi

NAME	DESCRIPTION
Candidiasis	Commonly called a "yeast infection," this disease can be caused by one of several bacteria in the Candida family but is most commonly caused by *Candida albicans*. It may be oropharyngeal (thrush), vaginal, or invasive.
Pneumocystis pneumonia (PCP)	Infection that causes fever, dry cough, shortness of breath, and fatigue. Caused by *Pneumocystis jirovecii*
Tinea (ringworm)	Fungal skin infection that gets its name because it appears serpentine, like a worm. *Tinea corporis* means the location is on the trunk or body, *tinea capitis* affects the scalp, and *tinea pedis* refers to the feet and is commonly known as athlete's foot.

Infectious Diseases Caused by Parasites and Protozoans

NAME	DESCRIPTION
Amebic dysentery	Condition characterized by loose stools; causes inflammation of the intestines
Giardiasis	Disease transmitted by the oral-fecal route and through untreated water; causes diarrhea
Lice	Can affect the head or the pubic area. Transmitted by contact with personal items used by someone who is infected. Lice and their eggs cause itching in the affected area.
Malaria	Disease transmitted to humans from the bite of an infected Anopheles mosquito. Protozoan parasites invade the red blood cells and create symptoms such as high fever and chills.
Pinworm	Transmitted by the oral-fecal route. This disease is common in children and causes anal itching and nighttime restlessness from eggs that are deposited around the anus.
Scabies	A highly contagious skin condition that results from a mite that burrows beneath the skin, leaving its feces behind. The feces leave red lines of inflammation on the skin.
Trichomoniasis	Condition that affects the reproductive organs and can be transmitted through sexual intercourse

Infectious Diseases Caused by Viruses

NAME	DESCRIPTION
Acquired immune deficiency syndrome (AIDS)	Syndrome caused by HIV (human immunodeficiency virus), resulting in decreased resistance to infections. Transmitted by blood and body fluids
Chickenpox	Highly contagious disease caused by the varicella-zoster virus. Also called varicella, it is characterized by the presence of skin lesions. Shingles is also caused by varicella and is seen in patients who have previously had chickenpox.
Hepatitis	Hepatitis types A, B, C, D, and E are all caused by a virus. This disease affects the liver and can cause mild to moderate symptoms or chronic illness and possibly death. Healthcare workers are encouraged to be vaccinated for hepatitis B because they are at risk for contact with client blood and body fluids.
Herpes simplex virus types 1 and 2 (HSV-1, HSV-2)	Typically, HSV-1 causes cold sores, is very contagious, and is spread through contact with infected saliva. HSV-2, known as genital herpes, is sexually transmitted. However, it should be noted that there can be crossing over, with HSV-1 infecting the genitals and HSV-2 infecting the mouth.
Human immunodeficiency virus (HIV)	Virus that destroys the immune system and can result in AIDS (acquired immune deficiency syndrome)
Human papillomavirus (HPV)	The most common sexually transmitted infection. Some strains of HPV cause harmless verrucae (warts); other strains are the greatest single risk factor for cervical cancer and may cause other, less common cancers such as cancer of the vagina, penis, and oropharynx.
Influenza	Commonly called "the flu"; an infection of both the upper and lower respiratory tracts
Mononucleosis	Highly contagious viral infection spread through the saliva of the infected person. Caused by either the Epstein-Barr virus or the cytomegalovirus (CMV)

Infectious Diseases Caused by Viruses *(concluded)*

NAME	DESCRIPTION
Norovirus	Most common cause of foodborne illness in the United States. Causes diarrhea, nausea, stomach pain, vomiting, fever, headache, and body aches
Respiratory syncytial virus (RSV)	Infection that causes cough, sneezing, runny nose, fever, loss of appetite, wheezing, and dyspnea
Severe acute respiratory syndrome (SARS)	Highly contagious disease that causes severe flu-like symptoms
Upper respiratory (tract) infection (URI)	The common cold, including pharyngitis (sore throat). Caused by the rhinovirus

Genetic Diseases

DISEASE	DESCRIPTION
Albinism	Genetic condition in which a person is born with little or no pigmentation in the skin, eyes, or hair
Cystic fibrosis	Life-threatening disease that affects the lungs and pancreas. It is one of the most common inherited life-threatening disorders among Caucasians in the United States.
Down syndrome	Abnormal cell division involving chromosome 21 that results in physical abnormalities and some form of mental disability. It is the single most common type of birth defect.
Fragile X syndrome	Most common inherited cause of learning disability, caused by a defect on one of the genes on the X chromosome. It affects boys more severely than girls.
Hemophilia	Inheritable bleeding disorder in which an essential clotting factor is low or missing, primarily affecting males
Klinefelter's syndrome	Disorder in which males have an extra X chromosome, resulting in tall stature, pear-shaped fat distribution, small testes, sparse body hair, infertility, and slightly lower intelligence
Muscular dystrophy	Group of genetic disorders that affect the muscular and nervous systems, most often affecting males
Phenylketonuria (PKU)	Genetic disorder in which the body is unable to properly eliminate phenylalanine, which is an essential amino acid. Organ damage, mental disability, and even death are possible.
Turner's syndrome	Disorder that results when females have a single X chromosome. Symptoms include a webbed neck, broad chest, short stature, and infertility. Intelligence is normal.

Common Diseases and Disorders in the United States*

DISEASE	EXAMPLES	SCREENING AND PREVENTION
Heart disease	Coronary artery disease, atherosclerosis, congestive heart failure	Monitor blood pressure and cholesterol and triglyceride levels, and have routine electrocardiograms (ECG).
Cancer	Skin, lung, breast, prostate, blood, colorectal, gynecologic, HPV-related	Have routine breast or prostate exam, Pap smear, and colonoscopy. Monitor size and shape of skin lesions. Maintain healthy eating habits and a good body weight, exercise, do not use tobacco products, and limit alcohol consumption.
Cerebrovascular diseases	Stroke, deep vein thrombosis, aneurysm, embolism	Maintain healthy eating habits and a good body weight, exercise, do not use tobacco products, and limit alcohol consumption. Have routine screening tests and physical exams.
Chronic lower respiratory diseases	Asthma, COPD, bronchitis	Do not use tobacco products, avoid irritants and allergens, and monitor air quality. Have routine screening tests (TB skin test) and vaccinations.

*Entries ordered from most to least common.

Common Diseases and Disorders in the United States* *(concluded)*

DISEASE	EXAMPLES	SCREENING AND PREVENTION
Diabetes mellitus	Type 1, Type 2, gestational	Have blood glucose tests, including fasting blood sugar, and hemoglobin A1c blood test. Maintain healthy eating habits and a good body weight, exercise, and limit alcohol and sugar consumption.
Alzheimer's disease ·		Maintain a healthy lifestyle and have a regular physical examination.
Influenza, pneumonia		Maintain a healthy lifestyle and obtain yearly flu and pneumonia vaccinations.
Nephritis/nephrosis	Chronic renal disease (CRD), end-stage renal disease (ESRD)	Have routine urinalysis. Maintain healthy eating habits and a good body weight, exercise, do not use tobacco products, and limit alcohol consumption.

*Entries ordered from most to least common.

Skin Lesions

NAME AND EXAMPLE	DESCRIPTION
Bulla	A large blister or cluster of blisters
Cherry angioma	A common, noncancerous skin growth made up of blood
Crust	Dried blood or pus on the skin
Ecchymosis	A black-and-blue mark, or bruise
Erosion	A shallow area of skin worn away by friction or pressure

NAME AND EXAMPLE	DESCRIPTION
Excoriation	A scratch; may be covered with dried blood
Fissure	A crack in the skin's surface
Keloid	An overgrowth of scar tissue
Macule	A flat skin discoloration, such as a freckle or a flat mole
Nodule	A large pimple or small node (larger than 1 cm)
Papule	An elevated mass similar to but smaller than a nodule
Patch color	A spot on the skin that is lighter or darker than regular skin
Petechiae	Pinpoint skin hemorrhages that result from bleeding disorders

NAME AND EXAMPLE	DESCRIPTION
Plaque	A small, flat, scaly area of the skin
Purpura	Purple-red bruises; usually the result of clotting abnormalities
Pustule	An elevated (infected) lesion containing pus
Scale	A thin plaque of epithelial tissue on the skin's surface
Telangiesctasia	Widely open (dilated) blood vessels in the outer layer of the skin
Tumor	A swelling of abnormal tissue growth
Ulcer	A wound that results from tissue loss
Vesicle	A blister
Wheal	A hive

Classifications of Fractures

NAME AND EXAMPLE	DESCRIPTION
Closed fracture (simple fracture)	Fracture in which the skin remains intact
Comminuted fracture	Fracture in which the bone has broken into several fragments
Complete fracture	Fracture that goes across the entire bone

NAME AND EXAMPLE	DESCRIPTION
Greenstick fracture	Fracture commonly seen in children; occurs in bones that are not completely ossified, so there is a bending and only one side of the bone is fractured, rather than a complete breaking of bone
Impacted fracture	Fracture in which one end of the fractured bone is driven into the interior of the other
Incomplete fracture	Fracture that goes through only part of the bone

Classifications of Fractures *(concluded)*

NAME AND EXAMPLE	DESCRIPTION
Open fracture (compound fracture)	Fracture in which the skin is broken

Bone Disorders

NAME	DESCRIPTION
Bursitis	Inflammation of a bursa, which is the fluid-filled sac that cushions tendons. (Tendons attach muscles to bone.)
Carpal tunnel syndrome (CTS)	Occurs when the median nerve in the wrist is excessively compressed by an inflamed tendon (the flexor retinaculum)
Fractures	Cracks, breaks, or splintering of a bone
Gout (gouty arthritis)	A type of arthritis associated with high uric acid levels in the blood with crystalline deposits in the joints, kidneys, and various soft tissues
Kyphosis	An abnormal, exaggerated curvature of the spine, most often at the thoracic level. This condition is often referred to as humpback.
Lordosis	An exaggerated inward (convex) curvature of the lumbar spine. The condition is sometimes called swayback.
Osteoarthritis (OA)	Also known as degenerative joint disease (DJD) or wear-and-tear arthritis
Osteogenesis imperfecta (brittle bone disease)	People with brittle bone disease have decreased amounts of collagen in their bones, which leads to very fragile bones.
Osteoporosis	A condition in which bones become thin (more porous) over time
Osteosarcoma	A type of bone cancer that originates from osteoblasts, the cells that make bone tissue. It is most often seen in children, teens, and young adults and occurs more often in males than females.
Paget's disease	Causes bones to enlarge and become deformed and weak. It usually affects people older than 40 years of age.
Rheumatoid arthritis (RA)	A chronic, systemic inflammatory disease that attacks the smaller joints such as those in the hands and feet
Scoliosis	An abnormal, S-shaped lateral curvature of the thoracic or lumbar spine

Classifications of Burns

NAME	DESCRIPTION
First-degree ©Sheila Terry/Science Source	A superficial burn that causes pain and makes the surrounding skin turn red
Second-degree ©Dr. P. Marazzi/Science Source	A partial-thickness burn that extends deeper into the skin than first-degree burns; causes blistering along with pain and redness
Third-degree ©John Radcliffe Hospital/Science Source	A full-thickness burn that involves all layers of the skin and requires immediate medical assistance

Diseases and Disorders of the Integumentary System

NAME	DESCRIPTION
Acne vulgaris	An inflammatory condition of the skin follicles and sebaceous glands
Alopecia	The absence or loss of hair, especially of the head (baldness)
Basal cell carcinoma	Skin cancer that originates from the basal layer of the epidermis and rarely metastasizes (spreads)
Cellulitis	An inflammation of the connective tissue in skin that is most often seen on the face and legs. A bacterial infection by *Staphylococcus aureus* or *Streptococcus* is the most common cause.
Comedos	Commonly known as blackheads; collections of bacteria, dead epithelial cells, and dried sebum
Dermatitis	A general term describing any inflammation of the skin; can be caused by a wide range of disorders
Eczema	A common chronic dermatitis that often has acute phases or flareups followed by periods of remission. The rash of eczema can appear anywhere on the body and appears as a red, scaly, pruritic (itchy) rash that may be painful.

Diseases and Disorders of the Integumentary System *(concluded)*

NAME	DESCRIPTION
Folliculitis	Inflammation of hair follicles. When it involves a single hair follicle, the condition is called a furuncle. When more than one hair follicle is involved, it is a carbuncle.
Herpes simplex types 1 and 2	Type 1 causes cold sores and is very contagious. Type 2, which is genital herpes, is sexually transmitted.
Jaundice	A yellow cast to the skin that often occurs with liver disease
Lentigos	Commonly called liver spots or age spots; these are not caused by the liver but are the result of excessive melanin production due to overexposure to sunlight (UV rays)
Malignant melanoma	Skin cancer that arises from melanocytes and often metastasizes (spreads)
Psoriasis	A common chronic inflammatory skin condition that has an autoimmune basis
Rosacea	A skin disorder that commonly appears as facial redness, predominantly over the cheeks and nose
Squamous cell carcinoma	Skin cancer that arises from the upper cells of the epidermis and often metastasizes (spreads)

Diseases and Disorders of the Muscular System

NAME	DESCRIPTION
Fibromyalgia	A fairly common condition that results in chronic pain primarily in joints, muscles, and tendons. It most commonly affects women between the ages of 20 and 50.
Muscular dystrophy (MD)	A group of inherited disorders characterized by muscle weakness and a loss of muscle tissue
Myasthenia gravis	A condition in which affected persons experience muscle weakness. In this autoimmune condition, a person produces antibodies that prevent muscles from receiving neurotransmitters from neurons.
Sprains	Injuries that excessively stretch or tear ligaments at a joint
Strains	Caused by stretching or tearing of muscles or tendons
Tendonitis	Painful inflammation of a tendon as well as of the tendon–muscle attachment to a bone
Tetanus	A condition caused by a toxin produced by the bacterium *Clostridium tetani*. It has a high mortality rate but is completely preventable through regular vaccinations.
Torticollis	Also known as wry neck. This condition is due to abnormally contracted neck muscles. The head typically bends toward the side of the contracted muscle, and the chin rotates to the opposite side.

Diseases and Disorders of the Blood and Circulatory System

NAME	DESCRIPTION
Anemia	A symptom of an underlying disease process. Anemia occurs when the blood has less than its normal oxygen-carrying capacity. Anemia is the most common blood disorder in the United States and occurs more often in women than in men.
Aneurysm	A ballooned, weakened arterial wall. The most common locations of aneurysms are the aorta and the arteries in the brain, legs, intestines, and spleen. An aortic aneurysm is a bulge in the wall of the aorta.
Leukemia	A neoplastic condition in which the bone marrow produces a large number of WBCs that are not normal
Thrombocythemia	A condition in which there is an increase in the platelet count. This condition is the opposite of thrombocytopenia.
Thrombocytopenia	A condition in which there are too few platelets, causing abnormal bleeding. This can be caused by a variety of situations, such as leukemia, certain medications, or idiopathic (unknown) reasons. The bleeding may be mild or life-threatening.
Thrombophlebitis	A condition in which a thrombus and inflammation develop in a vein. It most commonly occurs in the deeper veins of the legs.
Varicose veins (varices or varicosities)	Tortuous or twisted, dilated veins that are usually seen in the legs. They affect women more often than men.

Diseases and Disorders of the Cardiovascular System

NAME	DESCRIPTION
Congenital heart disease	A problem with the heart's structure and function due to abnormal heart development before birth
Congestive heart failure (CHF)	Failure of the heart to pump effectively. The heart weakens over time and loses its ability to supply blood to the body.
Coronary artery disease (CAD), atherosclerosis	A condition involving partial or complete blockage of major coronary arteries that supply blood to the heart
Dysrhythmias	Also known as arrhythmias; abnormal heart rhythms and/or rates
Endocarditis	An inflammation of the innermost lining of the heart and heart valves, usually caused by bacterial infections
Murmurs	Abnormal heart sounds. Not all murmurs indicate a heart disorder. Murmurs are graded from 1 to 6, with 6 being quite loud and the most serious.
Myocardial infarction (MI, heart attack)	Death of heart tissue due to deprivation of oxygen. The cardiac muscle sustains damage because of ischemia.
Myocarditis	An inflammation of the muscular layer of the heart caused by a viral infection. It leads to weakening of the heart wall.
Pericarditis	An inflammation of the pericardium, usually caused by complications of viral or bacterial infections, MIs, or chest injuries

Diseases and Disorders of the Lymphatic and Immune Systems

NAME	DESCRIPTION
Allergies	Excessive immune responses to stimuli that would not ordinarily cause a reaction
Autoimmune disease	A disease in which the immune system targets itself
Chronic fatigue syndrome (CFS)	Causes a person to feel severe tiredness; possibly caused by the Epstein-Barr virus (EBV)
HIV/AIDS	A viral disease spread through blood and body fluids. AIDS is caused by the human immunodeficiency virus (HIV). HIV attacks T lymphocytes.
Lymphadenitis	Inflammation of lymph nodes; can be viral or bacterial
Lymphadenopathy	Any disease involving the lymph nodes; causes can be autoimmune disease or malignancy.
Lymphedema	Blockage of lymphatic vessels; can be caused by genetics, parasitic infections, trauma to the vessels, tumors, radiation therapy, cellulitis, and surgeries
Systemic lupus erythematosus (SLE)	An autoimmune disorder that affects women more often than men. Affects many organ systems of the body and has numerous symptoms, usually including joint pain and swelling

Diseases and Disorders of the Respiratory System

NAME	DESCRIPTION
Allergic rhinitis	A hypersensitivity reaction to various airborne allergens
Asthma	Hyperactivity of the bronchioles; an inflammatory response with excess mucus production
Atelectasis	Commonly called collapsed lung; may occur after surgery or due to pleural effusion
Bronchitis	Inflammation of the bronchi; can be acute or chronic. Often follows a cold. One common cause of chronic bronchitis is cigarette smoking.
Chronic obstructive pulmonary disease (COPD)	A group of lung disorders in which obstruction limits airflow to the lungs. COPD includes chronic bronchitis and emphysema.

Diseases and Disorders of the Respiratory System *(concluded)*

NAME	DESCRIPTION
Emphysema	A lung disease in which the alveolar walls are destroyed; often caused by cigarette smoking
Laryngitis	An acute inflammation of the larynx; caused by viruses, bacteria, polyp formation, excessive use due to talking and singing, allergies, smoking, heartburn, alcohol use, nerve damage, or stroke
Lung cancer	The leading cancer-related cause of death in the United States. Caused by smoking or exposure to radon, asbestos, and industrial carcinogens. The three types are small cell lung cancer, squamous cell lung cancer, and adenocarcinoma.
Mesothelioma	A type of cancer that affects the pleura and is a result of asbestos exposure
Pleuritis or pleurisy	A condition in which the pleura become inflamed
Pneumonia (pneumonitis)	An inflammation of the lungs caused by a bacterial, viral, or fungal infection
Pneumonoconiosis	Lung diseases that result from years of exposure to different environmental or occupational types of dust
Pulmonary edema	A condition in which fluids fill the alveoli of the lungs, most commonly occurring with left heart failure
Pulmonary embolism	A blocked artery in the lungs, usually caused by a blood clot
Respiratory distress syndrome (RDS)	Kills apparently healthy infants; cause is unknown
Severe acute respiratory syndrome (SARS)	A viral disease that is highly contagious and sometimes fatal
Sinusitis	An inflammation of the membranes lining the sinuses. It can be acute or chronic.
Sudden infant death syndrome (SIDS)	The sudden and unexpected death of an infant under 1 year of age. There is no explainable cause of death.

Diseases and Disorders of the Nervous System

NAME	DESCRIPTION
Alzheimer's disease	A progressive, degenerative disease of the gray matter of the brain that causes dementia
Amyotrophic lateral sclerosis (ALS)	Commonly known as Lou Gehrig's disease; a fatal disorder characterized by the degeneration of neurons in the spinal cord and brain
Bell's palsy	A disorder in which facial muscles are very weak or temporarily totally paralyzed. Results from damage to the facial nerve; causes are unknown
Brain tumors and cancers	Abnormal growths in the brain. Malignant tumors that start in brain tissue are called primary brain cancers. Those that start elsewhere and metastasize to the brain are classified as secondary brain cancers.
Epilepsy	A condition in which the brain experiences repeated spontaneous seizures due to abnormal electrical activity of the brain
Guillain-Barré syndrome	A disorder in which the body's immune system attacks part of the peripheral nervous system. It has a sudden and unexpected onset.
Headaches	Caused by a variety of factors. Include episodic tension headaches, chronic tension headaches, migraines, and cluster headaches
Meningitis	An inflammation of the meninges
Multiple sclerosis (MS)	A chronic disease of the central nervous system in which myelin is destroyed. Some known causes are viruses, genetic factors, and immune system abnormalities.

Diseases and Disorders of the Nervous System *(concluded)*

NAME	DESCRIPTION
Neuralgia	A group of disorders commonly referred to as nerve pain; most frequently occur in the nerves of the face
Parkinson's disease	A nervous system disorder that is slowly progressive and degenerative
Sciatica	A condition in which the sciatic nerve is damaged, commonly due to excessive pressure on the nerve from prolonged sitting
Stroke or cerebrovascular accident (CVA)	Occurs when brain cells die because of inadequate blood perfusion of the brain

Diseases and Disorders of the Urinary System

NAME	DESCRIPTION
Acute kidney (renal) failure (ARF)	A sudden loss of kidney function due to burns, dehydration, low blood pressure, hemorrhage, allergic reactions, obstructions, poisons, alcohol abuse, or trauma
Chronic kidney (renal) failure (CRF)	A condition in which the kidneys slowly lose their ability to function due to diabetes, hypertension, kidney disease, or heart failure
Cystitis	A urinary bladder infection caused by different types of bacteria
Glomerulonephritis	An inflammation of the glomeruli of the kidney, caused by bacterial infections, renal diseases, and immune disorders.
Incontinence	A condition in which an adult cannot control urination. Can be temporary or long lasting; caused by various medications, UTIs, nervous system disorders, cancers, surgery, trauma, or pregnancy
Polycystic kidney disease (PKD)	A disorder in which the kidneys enlarge because of the presence of many cysts within them. The cause is hereditary.
Pyelonephritis	A type of complicated UTI that begins as a bladder infection and spreads up one or both ureters into the kidneys
Renal calculi (kidney stones)	Solid masses of crystals that obstruct the ducts within the kidneys or ureters. Painful condition caused by gouty arthritis, ureter defects, overly concentrated urine, or UTIs

Diseases and Disorders of the Male Reproductive System

NAME	DESCRIPTION
Benign prostatic hypertrophy (BPH)	The nonmalignant enlargement of the prostate gland
Epididymitis	An inflammation of the epididymis. Most cases start as an infection of the urinary tract.
Impotence, or erectile dysfunction (ED)	A disorder in which a male cannot achieve or maintain an erection to complete sexual intercourse. Can be caused by many physical or psychological conditions
Prostate cancer	One of the most common cancers in men older than 40. A high-fat diet, increased age, and genetic predisposition all increase the risk.
Prostatitis	An inflammation of the prostate gland; can be acute or chronic. May be caused by bacterial infections, catheterization, trauma, excessive alcohol consumption, or scarring
Testicular cancer	A malignant growth in one or both testicles. Occurs more commonly in males 15 to 30 years of age and is very aggressive

Diseases and Disorders of the Female Reproductive System

NAME	DESCRIPTION
Breast cancer	One of the most common cancers in females. Evaluated and graded based on tumor size and how far cells have traveled from the site of origin
Cervical cancer	This type of cancer usually develops slowly, and with early detection by a yearly Pap smear, treatment is often successful.
Cervicitis	Inflammation of the cervix caused by an infection
Dysmenorrhea	Condition of experiencing severe menstrual cramps that limit normal daily activities
Endometriosis	A condition in which tissues that make up the lining of the uterus grow outside the uterus
Fibrocystic breast change	A common condition consisting of abnormal but usually benign cysts in the breasts that vary in size related to the menstrual cycle
Fibroids	Benign tumors that grow in the uterine wall
Infertility	The inability to conceive a child due to scarring of the fallopian tubes, STIs, PID, endometriosis, or hormone imbalance
Ovarian cancer	Considered more deadly than the other types of gynecologic cancers because its symptoms are mild and indistinct.
Pelvic inflammatory disease (PID)	An acute or chronic infection of the reproductive tract caused by untreated STIs or bacteria
Premenstrual syndrome (PMS)	A collection of symptoms that occur just before the menstrual period. Symptoms include anxiety, depression, irritability, bloating, and diarrhea.
Uterine (endometrial) cancer	Most common in postmenopausal women. It may be related to increased levels of estrogen.
Vaginitis	An inflammation of the vagina, associated with abnormal vaginal discharge
Vulvovaginitis	An inflammation of the vulva and vagina

Diseases and Disorders of the Digestive System

NAME	DESCRIPTION
Appendicitis	An inflammation of the appendix. If not treated promptly, it can be life-threatening.
Cholelithiasis (gallstones)	Hardened deposits of bile that can form in the gallbladder. Two types of calculi are cholesterol and pigment stones.
Cirrhosis	A chronic liver disease in which normal liver tissue is replaced with nonfunctional scar tissue
Colitis	An inflammation of the large intestine. This condition can be chronic or short-lived, depending on the cause.
Colorectal cancer	Usually arises from the lining of the rectum or colon. This type of cancer is curable if diagnosed and treated early. It is the third most common cause of death due to cancer in both men and women.
Constipation	The condition of difficult defecation or elimination of feces
Crohn's disease	A type of inflammatory bowel disease. It can affect any region of the digestive tract from the mouth to the anus, but most often affects the ileum (lower part of the small intestine).
Diarrhea	The condition of watery and frequent feces. Many cases of diarrhea do not require treatment because they are usually self-limiting and stop within a day or two.
Diverticulitis	An inflammation of diverticuli in the intestine. Diverticuli are abnormal dilations or pouches in the intestinal wall. When the diverticuli are not inflamed, the condition is known as *diverticulosis*.
Gastric, or stomach, ulcers	Occur when the lining of the stomach breaks down

Diseases and Disorders of the Digestive System *(concluded)*

NAME	DESCRIPTION
Gastritis	An inflammation of the stomach lining; often referred to as an upset stomach
Gastroesophageal reflux disorder (GERD)	This occurs when stomach acids are pushed into the esophagus (also called heartburn). If not treated, GERD can cause erosion of the esophagus and even esophageal cancer.
Helicobacter pylori (H. pylori)	Organism implicated as being responsible for many diseases and disorders, including gastric ulcers
Hemorrhoids	Varicosities (varicose veins) of the rectum or anus
Hepatitis	An inflammation of the liver. There are many different types of hepatitis, but they all involve inflammation of the liver. Many signs and symptoms are shared, regardless of the cause of the inflammation.
Hiatal hernias	Occur when a portion of the stomach protrudes into the thoracic cavity through an opening (esophageal hiatus) in the diaphragm
Inguinal hernias	Occur when a portion of the large intestine protrudes into the inguinal canal, which is located where the thigh and the body trunk meet. In males, the hernia can also protrude into the scrotum.
Oral cancer	Usually involves the lips or tongue but can occur anywhere in the mouth. This type of cancer tends to spread rapidly to other organs because of the high vascularity of this area.
Pancreatic cancer	The fourth leading cause of cancer death in the United States. The poor prognosis and 5-year survival rate of only 5% are due to the late diagnosis in many cases.
Stomach cancer	Most commonly occurs in the uppermost (cardiac) portion of the stomach. It appears to occur more frequently in Japan, Chile, and Iceland than in the United States. This may be due to diets high in nitrates that are known to be carcinogenic.
Stomach ulcer	A condition in which the lining of the stomach breaks down

Diseases and Disorders of Metabolism and Nutrition

NAME	DESCRIPTION
Anorexia nervosa	An eating disorder in which individuals have a perception of being overweight regardless of their actual weight
Bulimia nervosa	An eating disorder in which the person may be of normal weight and may eat normal or even excessive amounts of food but then vomits to rid himself or herself of the calories. Also called binge-and-purge eating
Celiac disease	An immune reaction to eating gluten that causes the individual's body to attack the small intestinal mucosa. In a similar disorder, known as non-celiac gluten sensitivity, patients cannot tolerate gluten and have similar symptoms, with the addition of headache, joint pain, and numbness in the extremities.
Hypercholesterolemia	An excess of cholesterol in the blood
Kwashiorkor	A type of starvation in which there is too little protein in the diet
Malnutrition	Inadequate or excessive caloric intake
Marasmus	A type of starvation that entails both protein and calorie insufficiency
Metabolic syndrome	A group of symptoms such as hypertension, hyperinsulinism, excess body fat around the waist, and hypercholesterolemia. Lifestyle changes, medication, and regular appointments with a healthcare provider are essential.
Obesity	A body weight greater than 20% above the standard is considered obesity, and 50% over the standard is considered morbid obesity.
Starvation	A type of malnutrition resulting from inadequate caloric intake, inadequate resources, dietary imbalances, illness, or self-imposed starvation

Diseases and Disorders of the Endocrine System

NAME	DESCRIPTION
Acromegaly	A condition caused by the secretion of too much growth hormone after puberty that causes the hands, feet, and face to take on unusual enlargement
Addison's syndrome	Hyposecretion of ACTH in which patients experience anorexia, fatigue, weight loss, GI problems, and bronzing of the skin
Diabetes insipidus	Hyposecretion of ADH. Symptoms include excessive urination, thirst, and dehydration.
Diabetes mellitus	Hyposecretion of insulin, categorized into Type 1 (insulin dependent) and Type 2 (non-insulin dependent)
Dwarfism	Abnormal underdevelopment of the body due to hyposecretion of growth hormone (GH). Adult height is 4 feet 10 inches or less.
Epinephrine and norepinephrine imbalances	Cause increase in blood pressure, tachycardia, and tachypnea
Estrogen imbalances	Hyposecretion before or during menopause results in hot flashes, vaginal dryness, mood changes, depression, and loss of bone density.
Gigantism	An abnormal increase in the length of long bones due to hypersecretion of growth hormone during childhood
Hypercalcemia	An increase in blood calcium levels, resulting in more calcium going into bone
Hyperthyroidism	Excess secretion of thyroid hormone (TSH). Also called Grave's disease, it causes an overall increase in metabolism.
Hypocalcemia	A condition in which there is too little calcium in the blood
Hypoglycemia	A low level of glucose in the blood
Hypothyroidism	Too little TSH is secreted, resulting in slowing of metabolism.
Melatonin imbalances	Hyposecretion disturbs the sleep cycle and contributes to depression.
Pancreatic tumors	Malignant tumors have a poor prognosis due to difficulty in diagnosing.
Pheochromocytoma	A benign tumor of the adrenal medulla that can cause an increase in blood pressure.
Thymosin imbalances	Hyposecretion results in lack of mature T lymphocytes and a decrease in immunity.
Thyroid tumor	An abnormal growth on the thyroid gland. May be benign or malignant

Diseases and Disorders of the Special Senses—the Eye

NAME	DESCRIPTION
Amblyopia	Commonly called lazy eye; occurs when a child does not use one eye regularly
Astigmatism	Occurs when the cornea or lens has an abnormal shape, which causes blurred images in near or distant vision
Blepharitis	An inflammation of the eyelid, as well as corneal abrasions (scratching of the cornea)
Cataracts	Opaque structures within the lens that prevent light from going through the lens. Over time, images begin to look fuzzy; if left untreated, cataracts may cause blindness.
Color blindness	The inability to see certain colors. May be inherited; occurs more commonly in males
Dry eye syndrome (xerophthalmia)	One of the most common eye problems treated by physicians. This syndrome results from a decreased production of the oil within tears, which normally occurs with age.
Ectropion	Eversion of the lower eyelid
Entropion	Inversion of the lower eyelid

Diseases and Disorders of the Special Senses—the Eye *(concluded)*

NAME	DESCRIPTION
Glaucoma	Indicated by an increase in intraocular pressure, caused by a buildup of aqueous humor in the anterior chamber. If untreated, this excess pressure can lead to permanent damage of the optic nerve that can result in blindness.
Hyperopia	Farsightedness
Macular degeneration	A progressive disease that usually affects people over the age of 50. It occurs when the retina no longer receives an adequate blood supply. It is the most common cause of vision loss in the United States.
Myopia	Nearsightedness
Nystagmus	Rapid, involuntary eye movements. The movements may be horizontal or vertical.
Presbyopia	A common eye disorder that results in the loss of lens elasticity. It develops with age and causes a person to have difficulty seeing objects that are close up.
Retinal detachment	Occurs when the layers of the retina separate. It is considered a medical emergency and if not treated right away leads to permanent vision loss.
Strabismus	A misalignment of the eyes. Convergent strabismus is commonly referred to as crossed eyes.

Diseases and Disorders of the Special Senses—the Ear

NAME	DESCRIPTION
Cerumen impaction	A buildup of ear wax within the external auditory canal.
Menière's disease	A disturbance in the equilibrium characterized by *vertigo* (dizziness), ringing in the ears, nausea, and progressive hearing loss
Otitis externa	An inflammation of the outer ear
Otitis media	An inflammation of the middle ear
Otosclerosis	The immobilization of the stapes within the middle ear; a common cause of conductive hearing loss
Presbycusis	Hearing loss because of the aging process
Tinnitus	Ringing in the ears
Vertigo	Dizziness

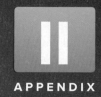
NOTE: When referencing this appendix, note that some word parts are used in more than one way. For example, "cyt" serves as a word root in "cytology" but as a suffix in "astrocyte." If you do not initially find the word part you are looking for, check the other sections of this appendix to see if it is listed as another type of word part.

Prefixes

a-, an- without, not
ab- from, away
acr-, acro- extremity, topmost
ad- to, toward
ambi-, amph-, amphi- both, on both sides, around
ante- before
antero- in front of
anti- against, opposing
aque- water
astro- star-like
auto- self
bi- twice, double
brachy- short
brady- slow
carboxy- containing carbon and oxygen or a carboxyl group
cata- down, lower, under
centi- hundred
cephal- head
chol-, chole-, cholo- gall
chromo- color
circum- around
co-, com-, con- together, with
contra- against
cryo- cold
crypt-, crypto- hidden
cyan-, cyano- blue
de- down, from
deca- ten
deci- tenth
demi- half
dextro- to the right
di- double, twice
dia- through, apart, between
dipla-, diplo- double, twin
dis- apart, away from
dys- difficult, painful, bad, abnormal
e-, ec-, ecto- away, from, without, outside
echo- sound, sound wave
electro- electric
em-, en- in, into, inside
endo- within, inside
ento- within, inner
epi- on, above
erythro- red
eu- good
ex-, exo- outside of, beyond, without
excori- scratch or abrasion, loss of skin

extra- outside of, beyond, in addition
fore- before, in front of
glauc-, glauco- gray
gyn-, gyne-, gyneco-, gyno- woman, female
hemi- half
hetero- other, unlike
homeo-, homo- same, like
hyper- above, over, increased, excessive
hypo- below, under, decreased
idio- personal, self-produced
im-, in-, ir- not
in- in, into
inferi- below
infra- beneath
inter- between, among
intra-, intro- into, within, during
juxta- near, nearby
kata-, kath- down, lower, under
kineto- motion
leuco-, leuko- white
levo- to the left
macro- large, long
mal- bad
mega-, megalo- large, great
meio- contraction
melan-, melano- black
membran- pertaining to a membrane
mes-, meso- middle
metr-, metro- pertaining to the uterus
meta- beyond
micro- small
mid- middle
mio- smaller, less
mono- single, one
multi- many
neo- new
non-, not- no
nulli- none
ob- against
olig-, oligo- few, less than normal
ortho- straight
oxy- sharp, acid
pachy- thick
pan- all, every
par-, para- alongside of, with; woman who has given birth
per- through, excessive
peri- around
pes- foot

pluri- more, several
pneo- breathing
poly- many, much
post-, posteri- after, behind
pre-, pro- before, in front of
presby-, presbyo- old age
primi- first
pseudo- false
quadri- four
re- back, again
retro- backward, behind
semi- half
steno- contracted, narrow
stereo- firm, solid, three-dimensional
sub- under
super-, supra- above, upon, excess
sym-, syn- with, together
tachy- fast
tele- distant, far
tetra- four
tomo- incision, section
trans- across
tri- three
tropho- nutrition, growth
ultra- beyond, excess
uni- one
veni- vein
xanth-, xantho- yellow

Suffixes

-ad to, toward
-aesthesia, -esthesia sensation
-al characterized by, pertaining to
-algia pain
-ase enzyme
-asthenia weakness
-cele swelling, tumor
-centesis puncture, tapping
-ceps heads
-cidal killing
-cide causing death
-cise cut
-clast to break
-coele cavity
-crine to excrete
-cyst bladder, bag
-cyte cell, cellular
-duction to pull or move
-dynia pain
-ectomy cutting out, surgical removal

-edema fluid buildup
-emesis vomiting
-emia blood
-esthesia sensation
-extension increasing the angle of a joint
-flexion bending
-form shape
-fuge driving away
-gen, -genesis, -gon born, produced
-gene, -genesis, -genetic, -genic, -genous arising from, origin, formation
-glia pertaining to glial cells
-globin, -globulin protein
-gram recorded information
-graph instrument for recording
-graphy the process of recording
-ia condition
-iasis condition of
-ic, -ical pertaining to
-ician specialist in a field
-id having the characteristics of
-ism condition, process, theory
-itis inflammation of
-ium membrane
-ive with the properties of
-ize to cause to be, to become, to treat by special method
-kinesis, -kinetic motion
-lepsis, -lepsy seizure, convulsion
-lith stone
-logy science of, study of
-lysis setting free, disintegration, decomposition
-malacia abnormal softening
-mania abnormal desire or compulsion
-megaly enlargement
-meter measure
-metrist one who measures
-metry process of measuring
-motor movement
-odynia pain
-oid resembling
-ole small, little
-oma tumor
-opia vision
-opsy to view
-osis disease, condition of
-or relating to
-ostomy to make a mouth, opening
-otomy incision, surgical cutting
-ous having
-pathy disease, suffering
-pelvic pelvis
-penia too few, lack, decreased
-pexy surgical fixation
-phage, -phagia eating, consuming, swallowing
-phobia fear, abnormal fear
-phylaxis protection
-plasia formation or development
-plastic molded
-plasty operation to reconstruct, surgical repair

-plegia paralysis
-pnea breathing
-poiesis to make or produce
-ptysis spitting
-receptor cell that can send a signal to the brain
-rrhage, -rrhagia abnormal or excessive discharge, hemorrhage, flow
-rrhaphy suture of
-rrhea flow, discharge
-sarcoma malignant tumor
-sclerosis hardening
-scope instrument used to examine
-scopy examining
-sepsis poisoning, infection
-spasm cramp or twitching
-stalsis contraction
-stasis stoppage
-stomy opening
-thalamus pertaining to the thalamus
-therapy treatment
-thermy heat
-thorax chest
-tome cutting instrument
-tomy incision, section
-tory pertaining to
-toxic poison
-tripsy surgical crushing
-trophy turning, tendency
-tropic in response to a stimulus
-tropy turning, tendency
-ula, -ule little
-uretic pertaining to urine
-uria urine
-verse, -version turned or directed

Word Roots/Combining Forms

abdomino- abdomen
adeno- gland, glandular
adipo- fat
adreno- adrenal glands
aero- air
andr-, andro- man, male
ambly- dull, dim
angio- blood vessel
ano- anus
anthrac-, anthraco- coal, carbon
arterio- artery
arthro- joint
athero- soft, fatty deposit
atrio- pertaining to the atria of the heart
audi- hearing
baro- weight, pressure
bili- bile
bio- life
blast-, blasto- developing stage, bud, immature
bracheo- arm
broncho- bronchial (windpipe)
burs- bursa
carcino- cancer
cardio- heart
caud- tail

cellul- cells
cephalo- head
cerebr-, cerebro- brain
cervico- neck
chondro- cartilage
chromo- color
colo- colon
colp-, colpo- vagina
conjunctiv- conjunctiva
coro- body
cortico- cortex
cost-, costo- rib
cox- hip
crani-, cranio- skull
cusp- projection
cysto- bladder, bag
cyto- cell, cellular
dacry-, dacryo- tears, lacrimal apparatus
dactyl-, dactylo- finger, toe
dent-, denti-, dento- teeth
derma-, dermat-, dermato- skin
dist- farthest from the point of attachment
diverticul- diverticula
dorsi-, dorso- back
dur-, dura- pertaining to the dura mater of the brain
encephalo- brain
entero- intestine
episi-, episio pertaining to the pubic region
esophag- esophagus
esthesio- sensation
femor- femur
fibro- connective tissue
follicul- follicle
front- forehead
galact-, galacto- milk
gastr-, gastro- stomach
gingiv- gums
glomerulo- glomerulus
glosso- tongue
gluco-, glyco- sugar, sweet
granulo- granules
gravid- pregnant
haemo-, hem-, hemato-, hemo- blood
hepa-, hepar-, hepato- liver
herni- rupture
hidro- sweat (perspiration)
histo- tissue
hydra-, hydro- water
hyster-, hystero- uterus
ictero- jaundice
ileo- ileum
immuno- pertaining to the immune system
interstit- interstices
karyo- nucleus, nut
kera-, kerato- horn, hardness, cornea
keratino- keratin
labyrinth- pertaining to the labyrinth of the ears
lacrim-, lacrimo- tears
lact-, lactifer- milk

laparo- abdomen
laryngo- pertaining to the larynx
later-, latero- side
linguo- tongue
lipo- fat
lith- stone
lobo- lobe
lun-, luna- moon
lymph-, lympho- lymphatic, spring water
mast-, masto- breast
med-, medi- middle
mening- meninges (covers the brain)
metacarpo- pertaining to the metacarpal bones
metatarso- pertaining to the metatarsal bones
metra-, metro- uterus
my-, myo- muscle
myel-, myelo- marrow
narco- sleep
nas-, naso- nose
nat-, nato- born
natri- sodium
necro- dead
nephr-, nephro- kidney
neu-, neuro- nerve
niter-, nitro- nitrogen
nucleo- nucleus
oculo- eye
odont- tooth
omphalo- navel, umbilicus
onco- tumor
onych-, onycho- pertaining to the nail of a finger or toe
oo- ovum, egg
oophor- ovary
ophthalmo- eye
opt-, opto- vision
or-, oro- pertaining to the mouth

orchid- testicle
os- mouth, opening
oste-, osteo- bone
oto- ear
ov-, ovi-, ovo- pertaining to an ovum or egg
paedo-, pedo- child
palpebro- eyelid
pancrea- pancreas
path-, patho- disease, suffering
pedicul- lice
pepso- digestion
peptid- pertaining to a peptide
phag-, phago- eating, consuming, swallowing
phalang- pertaining to the phalanges
pharyng-, pharyngo- throat, pharynx
phlebo- vein
photo- pertaining to light
pleuro- side, rib
pneumo- air, lungs
pod- foot
procto- rectum
proxim- close to the point of attachment
psych- the mind
pulmon-, pulmono- lung
pus-, pyo- pus
pyelo- pelvis (renal)
pylor- pylorus (part of the stomach)
pyro- fever, heat
refract- refraction, refractive
reni-, reno- kidney
retino- retina
rhabdo- rod-shaped
rhino- nose
sacchar- sugar
sacro- sacrum
sagitt- dividing into left and right
salpingo- tube, fallopian tube
sarco- flesh

sclero- hard, sclera
scolio- lateral curvature
sebace- oil
sensori- the senses
septi-, septic-, septico- poison, infection
sigmo- S-shaped
som-, soma- body
sperma-, spermato- semen, spermatozoa
spleno- spleen
steroid- steroid (lipid-soluble substance)
stomato- mouth
sudorifer- sweat
superfic- near the surface
superi- above
synapt- pertaining to a synapse
synov- synovium
tempor- pertaining to the temple
tendon-, teno-, tenoto- tendon
thermo- heat
thio- sulfa
thoraco- chest
thrombo- blood clot
thymo- thymus
thyro- thyroid gland
tricho- hair
tubulo- tube, tubule
tympan- eardrum
ureth- urethra
urino-, uro- urine, urinary organs
utero- uterus, uterine
uvulo- uvula
vagin- vagina
vasculo-, vaso- vessel
ventr- front
ventricul-, ventriculo- pertaining to the ventricles of the heart
ventri-, ventro- abdomen
vesico- blister
vulvo- pertaining to the vulva

Abbreviations

a before
a̅a̅, A̅A̅ of each
ABGs arterial blood gases
a.c. before meals
ADD attention deficit disorder
ADL activities of daily living
ad lib as desired
ADT admission, discharge, transfer
AED automated external defibrillator
AIDS acquired immunodeficiency syndrome
AKA above-knee amputation
a.m.a., AMA against medical advice
AMA American Medical Association
amp. ampule
amt amount
AND allow natural death
aq., AQ water; aqueous
ASHD atherosclerotic heart disease
ausc. auscultation
ax axis
B both
Bib, bib drink
b.i.d., bid, BID twice a day
BKA below-knee amputation
BM bowel movement
BP, B/P blood pressure
BPC blood pressure check
BPH benign prostatic hypertrophy
bpm beats per minute
BSA body surface area
Bx biopsy
c̄ with
Ca, CA calcium; cancer
CABG coronary artery bypass graft
cap, caps capsules
CBC complete blood (cell) count
C.C., CC chief complaint
CCU coronary care unit
CDC Centers for Disease Control and Prevention
CHF congestive heart failure
chr chronic
cm centimeter
CNS central nervous system
Comp, comp compound
COPD chronic obstructive pulmonary disease
CP chest pain
CPE complete physical examination
CPR cardiopulmonary resuscitation
CSF cerebrospinal fluid
CT computed tomography

CV cardiovascular
CVA cerebrovascular accident
CXR chest X-ray
d day
D&C dilation and curettage
DEA Drug Enforcement Administration
Dil, dil dilute
DM diabetes mellitus
DNAR do not attempt resuscitation
DNR do not resuscitate
DOB date of birth
DOC date of conception
Dr. doctor
DRE digital rectal exam
DTaP diphtheria-tetanus-acellular pertussis vaccine
DTs delirium tremens
DVT deep venous thrombosis
D/W dextrose in water
Dx, dx diagnosis
ECG, EKG electrocardiogram
ED emergency department
EDD estimated delivery date
EEG electroencephalogram
EENT eyes, ears, nose, and throat
EHR electronic health record
EMR electronic medical record
EP established patient
ER emergency room
ESR erythrocyte sedimentation rate
FBS fasting blood sugar
FDA Food and Drug Administration
FH family history
Fl, fl, fld fluid
fl oz fluid ounce
F/u, F/U, f/u follow-up
FUO fever of unknown origin
Fx, FX fracture
g gram
GBS gallbladder series
G&D growth and development
GI gastrointestinal
Gm, gm gram
gr grain
gt, gtt drop, drops
GTT glucose tolerance test
GU genitourinary
GYN gynecology
HA headache
HB, Hgb hemoglobin
hct hematocrit
HEENT head, eyes, ears, nose, throat
HIV human immunodeficiency virus
HO, H/O history of

H&P history and physical
HPI history of present illness
HPV human papillomavirus
HTN hypertension
Hx history
ICU intensive care unit
I&D incision and drainage
IDDM insulin-dependent diabetes mellitus
IIHI individually identifiable health information
IM intramuscular
inf. infusion; inferior
inj injection
I&O intake and output
IT inhalation therapy
IUD intrauterine device
IV intravenous
KUB kidneys, ureters, bladder
L liter or left
L1, L2, etc. lumbar vertebrae
lab laboratory
lb pound
LBP low back pain
LBW low birth weight
liq liquid
LLE left lower extremity (left leg)
LLL left lower lobe
LLQ left lower quadrant
LMP last menstrual period
LUE left upper extremity (left arm)
LUQ left upper quadrant
m meter
M mix (Latin *misce*)
mcg microgram
mg milligram
MI myocardial infarction
mL milliliter
mm millimeter
MM mucous membrane
mmHg millimeters of mercury
MOLST medical orders for life-sustaining treatment
MOST medical orders for scope of treatment
MRI magnetic resonance imaging
MS multiple sclerosis
NB newborn
NED no evidence of disease
NIDDM noninsulin-dependent diabetes mellitus
NKA no known allergies
no, # number
noc, noct night
npo, NPO nothing by mouth

NP new patient
NS normal saline
NSAID nonsteroidal anti-inflammatory drug
NTP normal temperature and pressure
N&V, N/V nausea and vomiting
NYD not yet diagnosed
OB obstetrics
OC oral contraceptive
oint ointment
OOB out of bed
OPD outpatient department
OPS outpatient services
OR operating room
OT occupational therapy
OTC over-the-counter
oz ounce
p̄ after
P&P Pap smear (Papanicolaou smear) and pelvic exam
PA posteroanterior
Pap Pap smear
Path pathology
p.c., pc after meals
PE physical examination
per by, with
PET positron emission tomography
PH past history
PHI protected health information
PID pelvic inflammatory disease
PMFSH past medical, family, social history
PMS premenstrual syndrome
po by mouth
p/o postoperative
POCT point of care tests
POL physician's office laboratory
POLST physician orders for scope of treatment
POMR problem-oriented medical record
POST physician orders for scope of treatment
PPD packs per day
PPE personal protective equipment
p.r.n., prn, PRN whenever necessary
pt pint
Pt patient
PT physical therapy
PTA prior to admission
pulv powder
PVC premature ventricular contraction
q. every
q2, q2h every 2 hours
q.a.m., qam every morning
q.h., qh every hour
qns, QNS quantity not sufficient
qs, QS quantity sufficient
qt quart
R right
RA rheumatoid arthritis; right atrium
RBC red blood cells; red blood (cell) count
RDA recommended dietary allowance; recommended daily allowance
REM rapid eye movement

RF rheumatoid factor
RLE right lower extremity (right leg)
RLL right lower lobe
RLQ right lower quadrant
R/O rule out
ROM range of motion
ROS/SR review of systems/systems review
RUE right upper extremity (right arm)
RUQ right upper quadrant
RV right ventricle
Rx prescription; take
s̄ without
SAD seasonal affective disorder
SIDS sudden infant death syndrome
sig sigmoidoscopy
Sig directions
SL sublingual
SOAP subjective, objective, assessment, plan
SOB shortness of breath
sol solution
SOMR source-oriented medical record
S/R suture removal
SSI surgical site infection
Staph staphylococcus
stat, STAT immediately
STI sexually transmitted infection
Strep streptococcus
subcu, subcut, subQ subcutaneous
subling sublingual
surg surgery
S/W saline in water
SX symptoms
T1, T2, etc. thoracic vertebrae
T&A tonsillectomy and adenoidectomy
tab tablet
TB tuberculosis
tbs, tbsp tablespoon
TIA transient ischemic attack
t.i.d., tid, TID three times a day
tinc, tinct, tr tincture
TMJ temporomandibular joint
top topically
TPR temperature, pulse, and respiration
TSH thyroid-stimulating hormone
tsp teaspoon
Tx treatment
U unit
UA urinalysis
UCHD usual childhood diseases
UGI upper gastrointestinal
ung, ungt ointment
URI upper respiratory infection
US ultrasound
UTI urinary tract infection
VA visual acuity
VD venereal disease
VF visual field
VS vital signs
WBC white blood cells; white blood (cell) count
WNL within normal limits
wt weight

y/o, Y/O year(s) old

Symbols
Weights and Measures
\# pounds
° degrees
′ foot; minute
″ inch; second
mEq milliequivalent
mL milliliter
dL deciliter
mg% milligrams percent; milligrams per 100 mL

Mathematical Functions and Terms
\# number
+ plus; positive; acid reaction
− minus; negative; alkaline reaction
± plus or minus; either positive or negative; indefinite
× multiply; magnification; crossed with, hybrid
÷ , / divided by
= equal to
≈ approximately equal to
> greater than; from which is derived
< less than; derived from
≮ not less than
≯ not greater than
≤ less than or equal to
≥ greater than or equal to
≠ not equal to
$\sqrt{\ }$ square root
$\sqrt[3]{\ }$ cube root
∞ infinity
: ratio; "is to"
∴ therefore
% percent
π pi (3.14159)—the ratio of circumference of a circle to its diameter

Chemical Notations
Δ change; heat
⇌ reversible reaction
↑ increase
↓ decrease

Warnings
Ⓒ Schedule I controlled substance
Ⓒ Schedule II controlled substance
Ⓒ Schedule III controlled substance
Ⓒ Schedule IV controlled substance
Ⓒ Schedule V controlled substance
☠ poison
☢ radiation
☣ biohazard

Others
℞ prescription; take
□, ♂ male
○, ♀ female
† one
†† two
††† three

10× lens (ten x lenz) A magnifying lens in the ocular of a microscope that magnifies an image ten times.

24-hour urine specimen (twen'tē for owr yūr'in spes'i-měn) A urine specimen collected over a 24-hour period and used to complete a quantitative and qualitative analysis of one or more substances, such as sodium, chloride, and calcium.

ABA number (nŭm'běr) A fraction appearing in the upper-right corner of all printed checks that identifies the geographic area and specific bank on which the check is drawn.

abandonment (ă-ban'dŏn-měnt) A situation in which a healthcare professional stops caring for a patient without arranging for care by an equally qualified substitute.

abscess (ab'ses) A collection of pus (white blood cells, bacteria, and dead skin cells) that forms as a result of infection.

accessibility (ak-ses'ă-bil'i-tē) The ease with which people can move into and out of a space.

accommodation (ă-kom'ŏ-dā'shŭn) The ability of the lens to change shape, allowing the eye to focus images of objects that are near or far away.

accounting (ă-kownt'ing) The process of communicating the income and expenses of a business and its financial health.

accounts payable (A/P) (ă-kownts' pā'ă-běl) Money owed by a business; the practice's expenses.

accounts receivable (A/R) (ă-kownts' rě-sē'vă-běl) Income or money owed to a business.

accreditation (ă-kred'i-tā'shŭn) The documentation of official authorization or approval of a program.

Accrediting Bureau of Health Education Schools (ABHES) (ă-kre'dăt-ing byoor'-oh helth ed´yū-kā´shŭn skulz) An accrediting body that accredits private postsecondary institutions and programs that prepare individuals for entry into the medical assisting profession.

acetylcholine (as'ě-til-kō'lēn) A neurotransmitter released by the parasympathetic nerves onto organs and glands for resting and digesting.

acetylcholinesterase (as'ě-til-kō'lin-es'těr-ās) An enzyme within the nervous system that hydrolyzes acetylcholine to acetate and choline.

acid-fast stain (as'id-fast stān) A staining procedure for identifying bacteria that have a waxy cell wall.

active file (ăk'tĭv fīl) A file used on a consistent basis.

active listening (ak'tiv lis'ĕn-ing) Part of two-way communication, such as offering feedback or asking questions; contrast with **passive listening.**

ADA Amendments Act of 2008 (ADAAA) (ă-mend'měnts akt) A 2008 amendment to the ADA that broadens the definition of disability, making it easier for individuals who seek ADA protection to establish that they have a disability.

add-on code (ad'on' kōd) A code indicating procedures that are usually carried out in addition to another procedure. Add-on codes are used together with the primary code.

add-on safety features (ad'on sāf'tē fē'chūrz) Features on injection, phlebotomy, and winged steel needles that provide protection from needlestick injury. They consist of a hinged or sliding sheath attached to the needle that can be activated with one hand, keeping the user's hands behind the needle.

addiction (ă-dik'shŭn) A physical or psychological dependence on a substance, usually involving a pattern of behavior that includes obsessive or compulsive preoccupation with the substance and the security of its supply, as well as a high rate of relapse after withdrawal.

administer (ad-min'i-stir) To give a drug directly by injection, by mouth, or by any other route that introduces the drug into the body.

advance scheduling (ad-vans' sked'jūl-ing) Booking an appointment several weeks or even months in advance.

adverse effect (ad-věrs' e-fekt') An unintended negative reaction to a medication or treatment. Adverse effects are potentially more harmful than side effects, but are less common.

aerobes (ār'ōbz) Bacteria that grow best in the presence of oxygen.

afebrile (ā-feb'ril) Having a body temperature within one's normal range.

afferent nerves (af'ĕr-ĕnt něrvz) Sensory nerves that are responsible for detecting sensory information from the environment or from inside the body and taking it to the CNS for interpretation.

affiliation agreement (ă-fi'lē-ā'shŭn ă-grē'měnt) An agreement that applied training participants must sign that states the expectations of the facility and the expectations of the student.

agar (ā'gar) A gelatin-like substance derived from seaweed that gives a culture medium its semisolid consistency.

age analysis (āj ă-nal'i-sis) The process of clarifying and reviewing past-due accounts by age from the first date of billing.

agenda (ă-jěn'dă) The list of topics discussed or presented at a meeting, in order of presentation.

agglutination (ă-glū-ti-nā'shŭn) The clumping of red blood cells following a blood transfusion.

aggressive (ă-gres'iv) Imposing one's position on others or trying to manipulate them.

agonist (ag'ŏn-ist) The muscle responsible for most of the movement when a body movement is produced by a group of muscles. Also called a *prime mover.*

agranulocyte (ā-grăn'ŭ-lō-sīt) A type of leukocyte (white blood cell) with a solid nucleus and clear cytoplasm; includes lymphocytes and monocytes. Also called **agranular leukocyte.**

albumins (al-bū'minz) The smallest of the plasma proteins. Albumins are important for pulling water into the bloodstream to help maintain blood pressure.

alcohol-based hand disinfectants (AHD) (al'kŏ-hol bāsd hand disinfek'tănts) Gels, foams, or liquids with an alcohol content of 60% to 95% that are used for hand disinfection.

alimentary canal (al'i-men'tăr-ē kă-nal') The organs of the digestive system that extend from the mouth to the anus.

allowed charge (ă-lowd' chahrj) The amount that is the most the payer will pay any provider for each procedure or service.

alopecia (al-ō-pē'shē-ă) The clinical term for baldness.

alphabetic filing system (āl'fə-bĕt'ĭk fī'lĭng sis'təm) A filing system in which the files are arranged in alphabetical order, with the patient's last name first, followed by the first name and middle initial.

Alphabetic Index (al'fă'bet-ik in'deks) One of two ways diagnoses are listed in the ICD manual. They appear in alphabetical order with their corresponding diagnosis codes.

alveoli (al-vē'ō-lī) Clusters of air sacs in which the exchange of gases between air and blood takes place; located in the lungs.

amenorrhea (ā-men-ŏ-rē'ă) Absence or abnormal cessation of the menses.

American Association of Medical Assistants (AAMA) (ă-mer'i-kăn ă-sō'sē-ā'shŭn med'i-kăl ă-sis'tănts) The professional organization that certifies medical assistants and works to maintain professional standards in the medical assisting profession.

American Medical Technologists (AMT) (ă-mer'i-kăn med'i-kăl tek-nol'ŏ-jists) The registering organization for medical assistants that provides online continuing education, certification information, and member news.

Americans with Disabilities Act (ADA) (ă-mer'i-kănz dis'ă-bil'i-tēz akt) A US civil rights act forbidding discrimination against people because of a physical or mental disability.

amino acid (ă-mē'nō as'id) Natural organic compound found in plant and animal foods and used by the body to create protein.

amnion (am'nē-on) The innermost membrane enveloping the embryo and containing amniotic fluid.

amount to administer (A) (ă-mownt' ad-min'ĭ-stĭr') The amount of medication the patient will receive.

anabolism (ă-nab'ŏ-lizm) The stage of metabolism in which substances such as nutrients are changed into more complex substances and used to build body tissues.

anaerobe (an'ār-ōb) A bacterium that grows best in the absence of oxygen.

anaphylactic shock (an'ă-fi-lak'tik shok) A severe, often fatal form of shock characterized by smooth muscle contraction and capillary dilation initiated by cytotropic (IgE class) antibodies.

anaphylaxis (an'ă-fi-lak'sis) A severe allergic reaction with symptoms that include respiratory distress, difficulty in swallowing, pallor, and a drastic drop in blood pressure that can lead to circulatory collapse.

anatomical position (an-ă-tom'i-kăl pŏ-zish'ŏn) When the body is standing upright and facing forward with the arms at the side and the palms of the hands facing forward.

anatomy (ă-nat'ŏ-mē) The scientific term for the study of body structure.

anesthesia (an'es-thē'zē-ă) A loss of sensation, particularly the feeling of pain.

anesthetic (an'es-thet'ik) A medication that causes anesthesia.

angiography (an-jē-og'ră-fē) An X-ray examination of a blood vessel, performed after the injection of a contrast medium, that evaluates the function and structure of one or more arteries or veins.

annotate (an'ō-tāt') To underline or highlight key points of a document or to write reminders, make comments, and suggest actions in the margins.

anorexia nervosa (an'ŏ-rek'sē-ă nĕr-vō'să) An eating disorder in which people starve themselves because they fear that if they lose control of eating, they will become grossly overweight.

anoscope (ā'nō-skōp) An instrument used to open the anus (rectal opening) for an exam.

anoxia (ă'nox sē ă) An absense of oxygen.

antagonist (an-tag'ŏ-nist) A muscle that produces the opposite movement of the prime mover.

antibodies (ăn'ti-bod'ēz) Highly specific proteins that attach themselves to foreign substances in an initial step in destroying such substances, as part of the body's defenses.

antibody-mediated response (an'ti-bod'ē mē'dē-āt-ed rĕ-spons') The part of our body's immune response that occurs when B cells respond to antigens by becoming plasma cells, which make antibodies that attach to antigens.

anticoagulants (an'tē-kō-ag'yŭ-lăntz) Substances that prevent clotting.

antigens (an'ti-jenz) Foreign substances that stimulate white blood cells to create antibodies when they enter the body.

antioxidant (an'tē-ok'si-dănt) Chemical agent that fights cell-destroying chemical substances called free radicals.

anuria (an-yū'rē-ă) The absence of urine production.

APGAR (ap'gar) A test performed 1 minute and 5 minutes after a baby is born to determine how well the baby is breathing and how well the heart is working. Its five categories are respiratory effort, heart rate, skin color, reflexes, and muscle tone.

apnea (ap'nē-ă) The absence of respiration.

apocrine gland (ap'ō-krin glănd) A type of sweat gland. It produces a thicker type of sweat than other sweat glands and contains more proteins.

aponeurosis (ap'ō-nū-rō'sis) A tough, sheet-like structure that is made of fibrous connective tissue. It typically attaches muscles to other muscles.

apothecary system (ă-poth'ĕ-kăr-ē sis'tĕm) An older system of measurement that includes units such as fluid ounces, fluid drams, pints, and quarts.

appendicular (ap'en-dik'yū-lăr) The division of the skeletal system that consists of the bones of the arms, legs, pectoral girdle, and pelvic girdle.

applied training (ă-plīd' trān'ing) An opportunity to work in a medical facility to gain the essential on-the-job experience for beginning your new career, sometimes known as an externship or practicum.

applied training coordinator (ă-plīd' trān'ing kō-ōr'di-nā-tŏr) A professional who procures applied training sites and qualifies, or assesses, them to make certain that they provide a thorough educational experience. Also may be known as a clinical coordinator.

approximate (a-prŏk'si-māt) To bring the edges of a wound together so that the tissue surfaces are close in order to protect the area from further contamination and to minimize scar and scab formation.

arrector pili (ă-rek'tōr pī'lī) Muscles attached to most hair follicles and found in the dermis.

arthrography (ahr-throg'ră-fē) A radiologic procedure performed by a radiologist, who uses a contrast medium and fluoroscopy to help diagnose abnormalities or injuries in the cartilage, tendons, or ligaments of the joints—usually the knee or shoulder.

arthroscopy (ahr-thros'kŏ-pē) A procedure in which an orthopedist examines a joint, usually the knee or shoulder, with a tubular instrument called an arthroscope; also used to guide surgical procedures.

articulations (ahr-tik'yū-lā'shŭnz) The areas where bones are joined together; joints.

artifact (ahr'ti-fakt) Any irrelevant object or mark observed when examining specimens or graphic records that is not related to the object being examined—for example, a foreign object visible through a microscope or an erroneous mark on an ECG strip.

asepsis (ā-sep'sis) The condition in which pathogens are absent or controlled.

assault (ă-sawlt') The open threat of bodily harm to another.

assertive (ă-sĕr'tiv) Being firm and standing up for oneself while showing respect for others.

astigmatism (ă-stig'mă-tizm) A condition in which the cornea has an abnormal shape, which causes blurred images during near or distant vision.

atrioventricular node (AV node) (ā'trē-ō-ven-trik'yū-lar nōd) A node that is located between the atria of the heart. After the electrical impulse reaches the atrioventricular node, the atria contract and the impulse is sent to the ventricles.

attitude (at'i-tūd) A disposition to act in a certain way.

audiologist (aw-dē-ol'ō-jist) A healthcare specialist who focuses on evaluating and correcting hearing problems.

audiometer (aw-dē-om'ĕ-ter) An electronic device that measures hearing acuity by producing sounds in specific frequencies and intensities.

audit (aw'dit) To examine and review a group of patient records for completeness and accuracy—particularly as related to their ability to back up the charges sent to health insurance carriers for reimbursement.

auricle (awr'i-kĕl) The outside part of the ear, made of cartilage and covered with skin.

auscultated blood pressure (aws'kŭl-tāt-ĕd blŭd presh'ŭr) Blood pressure as measured by listening with a stethoscope.

auscultation (aws'kŭl-tā'shŭn) The process of listening to body sounds.

autoclave (aw'tō-klāv) A device that uses pressurized steam to sterilize instruments and equipment.

autoimmune disease (aw'tō-i-myūn' di-zēz') Any condition in which the body attacks its own antigens, causing illness to the patient.

automated external defibrillator (AED) (aw'tō-mā-tĕd eks-tĕr'năl dē-fib'ri-lā-tŏr) A computerized defibrillator programmed to recognize lethal heart rhythms and deliver an electric shock to restore a normal rhythm.

automated voice response unit (aw'tō-mā'tĕd voys rĕ-spons' yū'nit) Automated answering unit with a recorded voice that offers the caller various options for routing the call.

automatic puncturing device (aw'tō-mat'ik pungk'shŭr-ing dĕ-vīs') A type of lancet that is spring loaded, is self-contained, and has a mechanically controlled skin puncture depth.

autonomic nervous system (aw'tō-nom'ik nĕr'vŭs sis'tĕm) A system that is in charge of the body's automatic functions, such as the respiratory and gastrointestinal systems.

autopsy (aw'top-sē) The examination of a cadaver to determine or confirm the cause of death.

axial (ak'sē-ăl) The division of the skeletal system that consists of the skull, vertebral column, and rib cage.

axon (ak'son) A type of nerve fiber that is typically long and branches far from the cell body of a neuron. Its function is to send information away from the cell body.

bacillus (bă-sil'ŭs) A rod-shaped bacterium.

balloon angioplasty (bă-lūn' an'jē-ō-plas-tē) A procedure using a slender, hollow tube passed through a coronary artery to compress a blockage in the artery.

barium enema (bar'ē-ŭm en'ĕ-mă) A radiologic procedure performed by a radiologist who administers barium sulfate through the anus, into the rectum, and then into the colon to help diagnose and evaluate obstructions, ulcers, polyps, diverticuloses, tumors, or motility problems of the colon or rectum; also called a lower GI (gastrointestinal) series.

barium swallow (bar'ē-ŭm swahl'ō) A radiologic procedure that involves oral administration of a barium sulfate drink to help diagnose and evaluate obstructions, ulcers, polyps, tumors, or motility problems of the esophagus, stomach, duodenum, and small intestine; also called an upper GI (gastrointestinal) series.

Bartholin's glands (bahr'tō-lĭnz glandz) Glands lateral to the vagina that produce mucus for lubrication of the vagina.

basophil (bā'sō-fil) A type of granular leukocyte that produces the chemical histamine, which aids the body in controlling allergic reactions and other exaggerated immunologic responses.

battery (bat'ĕr-ē) An action that causes bodily harm to another.

behavior modification (bē-hāv'yŏr mod'i-fi-kā'shŭn) The altering of personal habits to promote a healthier lifestyle.

benefits (ben'ĕ-fits) Payments for medical services.

benign (bē-nīn') A noncancerous or nonmalignant growth or condition.

bile (bīl) A substance created in the liver and stored in the gallbladder. Bile is a bitter, yellow-green fluid that is used in the digestion of fats.

bilirubin (bil'i-rū'bin) A bile pigment formed by the breakdown of hemoglobin in the liver.

bioethics (bī-ō-ĕth'ĭks) Principles of right and wrong in issues that arise from medical advances.

biological indicator (bī'ŏ-loj'i-kăl in'di-kā-tŏr) An indicator consisting of bacterial spores that is used as a quality control method in autoclaves to confirm that sterilization has occurred.

biopsy (bī'op-sē) The removal and examination of a sample of tissue from a living body for diagnostic purposes.

bioterrorism (bī'o-ter'ŏr-izm) The intentional release of a biologic agent with the intent to harm individuals.

birthday rule (bĭrth'dā rūl) A rule that states that the insurance policy of a policyholder whose birthday comes first in the year is the primary payer for all dependents.

blastocyst (blas'tō-sist) A morula that has traveled down the uterine tube to the uterus and is invaded with fluid. It then implants into the wall of the uterus.

board-certified physician (bōrd sĕr'ti-fīd fi-zish'ŭn) A licensed practitioner who has obtained education and licensing for 9 to 12 years and taken multiple tests known as board tests.

body (bod'ē) Single-spaced lines of text that are the content of a business letter.

body dysmorphic disorder (BDD) (bod'ē dis-mōr'fic dis-ōr'der) Disorder in which a person cannot stop worrying about and trying to correct a perceived physical flaw, whether or not the flaw actually exists. Examples include facial blemishes, appearance of veins, and breast size. In some cases, people who have anorexia nervosa also may have BDD.

body language (bod'ē lang'gwăj) Non-verbal communication, including facial expressions, eye contact, posture, touch, and attention to personal space.

body mass index (BMI) (bod'ē mas in'deks) A reliable indicator of healthy weight that is calculated based on height and weight.

body mechanics (bod'ē mĕ-kan'iks) The application of physical principles to achieve maximum efficiency and to limit risk of physical stress or injury to the practitioner of physical therapy, massage therapy, or chiropractic or osteopathic manipulation.

body surface area (BSA) (bod'ē sŭr'făs ār'ē-ă) The area of the external surface of the body, expressed in square meters (m²); used to calculate metabolic, electrolyte, and nutritional requirements; drug dosage; and expected pulmonary function measurements.

bolus (bō'lŭs) The mass created when food is combined with saliva and mucus.

bookkeeping (buk'kēp'ing) The systematic recording of business transactions.

boundaries (bown'dăr-ēz) A physical or psychological space that indicates the limit of appropriate versus inappropriate behavior.

Bowman's capsule (bō'mănz kap'sŭl) A capsule that surrounds the **glomerulus** of the kidney.

brachytherapy (brak-ē-thār'ă-pe') A radiation therapy technique in which a radiologist places temporary radioactive implants close to or directly into cancerous tissue; used for treating localized cancers.

bradycardia (brad'ē-kahr'dē-ă) A slow heart rate; usually less than 60 beats per minute.

breach of contract (brēch kon'trakt) The violation of or failure to live up to a contract's terms.

bronchi (brong'kī) The two branches of the trachea that enter the lungs.

bronchioles (brong'kē-ōlz) A part of the respiratory tract that branches from the tertiary bronchi.

buccal (bŭk'ăl) Between the cheek and gum.

budget (bŭj'ĕt) The total sum of money allocated for a particular purpose or period of time.

buffy coat (buf'ē kōt) The layer between the packed red blood cells and plasma in a centrifuged blood sample; this layer contains the white blood cells and platelets.

bulbourethral glands (bŭl'bō-yū-re'thrăl glăndz) Glands that lie beneath the prostate and empty their fluid into the urethra. Their fluid aids in sperm movement.

bulimia nervosa (bŭ-lĭm'ē-ă nĕr-vō'să) An eating disorder in which people eat a large quantity of food in a short period of time (bingeing) and then attempt to counter the effects of bingeing by self-induced vomiting, use of laxatives or diuretics, and/or excessive exercise.

bundle of His (bŭn'dĕl hiss) Also known as the AV bundle, this is the node located between the ventricles of the heart that carries the electrical impulse from the AV node to the bundle branches.

bundled codes (bŭn'dĕld kōds) When healthcare services that are usually separate are considered as a single entity for purposes of classification and payment.

butterfly system (bŭt'ĕr-flī sis'tĕm) A type of needle used to draw blood from patients with small or fragile veins. Sometimes called a winged infusion set, it has flexible wings attached to the needle and a length of flexible tubing.

calibrate (kal'i-brāt) To determine the caliber of; to standardize a measuring instrument.

calibrated spoon (kal'i-brā-tĕd spūn) A spoon that has special markings, or calibrations, that allow you to measure a dose of liquid medication.

calibration syringe (kal'i-brā'shŭn sir-inj') A standardized measuring instrument used to check and adjust the volume indicator on a spirometer.

calorie (kal'ŏr-ē) A unit used to measure the amount of energy food produces; the amount of energy needed to raise the temperature of 1 kg of water by 1°C.

capillary puncture (kap'i-lār-ē pungk'shŭr) A blood-drawing technique that requires a superficial puncture of the skin with a sharp point.

capitation (kap'i-tā'shŭn) A payment structure in which a health maintenance organization prepays an annual set fee per patient to a physician.

cardiac catheterization (kahr'dē-ak kath'ĕ-tĕr-ī-zā'shŭn) A diagnostic method in which a catheter is inserted into a vein or an artery in the arm or leg and passed through blood vessels into the heart.

cardiac cycle (kahr'dē-ak sī'kĕl) The sequence of contraction and relaxation that makes up a complete heartbeat.

cardiac output (kahr'dē-ak owt'put) The product of heart rate and stroke volume, measured in liters per minute; the amount of blood that is pumped by the heart in 1 minute.

cardiac sphincter (kahr'dē-ak sfingk'tĕr) The valve-like structure composed of a circular band of muscle at the juncture of the esophagus and stomach. Also known as the esophageal sphincter.

carrier (kar'ē-ĕr) A reservoir host who is unaware of the presence of a pathogen and so spreads the disease while exhibiting no symptoms of infection.

cash flow statement (kash flō stāt'mĕnt) A statement that shows the cash on hand at the beginning of a period, the income and disbursements made during the period, and the new amount of cash on hand at the end of the period.

cashier's check (ka-shērz' chĕk) A bank check issued by a bank on bank paper and signed by a bank representative; usually purchased by individuals who do not have checking accounts.

cast (kast) (1) Cylinder-shaped elements with flat or rounded ends, differing in composition and size, that form when protein from the breakdown of cells accumulates and precipitates in the kidney tubules and is washed into the urine. (2) A rigid, external dressing, usually made of plaster or fiber-glass, that is molded to the contours of the body part to which it is applied; used to immobilize a fractured or dislocated bone.

catabolism (kă-tab'ō-lizm) The stage of metabolism in which complex substances, including nutrients and body tissues, are broken down into simpler substances and converted into energy.

cataracts (kat'ăr-akts) Cloudy areas that form in the lens of the eye that prevent light from reaching visual receptors.

category (kat'ĕ-gōr'ē) In ICD-10, the first three digits of the diagnosis code.

catheter-associated urinary tract infection (CAUTI) (kath'ĕ-tĕr ă-sō'sē-āt-ĕd yūr'i-nar-ē trakt in-fek'shŭn) A urinary tract infection that may be caused by long-term use of urinary catheters; the longer the catheter is in place, the greater the chance of infection.

catheterization (kath'ĕ-ter-ī-zā'shun) The procedure during which a catheter is inserted into a vessel, an organ, or a body cavity.

celiac disease (sē'lē-ak di-zēz') An intolerance to gluten that causes an immune response in the body and reduces the absorption of nutrients in the small intestine.

cell body (sel bŏd'ē) The portion of the neuron that contains the nucleus and organelles.

cell-mediated response (sel mē'dē-āt-ed rĕ-spons') The part of our body's immune response that occurs when T cells bind to antigens on cells and attack the antigens directly.

cells (selz) The smallest living units of structure and function.

central line (sen'trăl līn) A catheter placed in a large vein, usually in the neck, chest, or groin, that is used to give fluids or medications.

central line–associated bloodstream infections (CLABSI) (sen'trăl līn ă-sō'sē-āt-ĕd blŭd'strēm in-fek'shŭnz) Bloodstream infections caused by the entry of infectious microorganisms into the bloodstream through a central line.

central nervous system (CNS) (sen'trăl nĕr'vŭs sis'tĕm) A system that consists of the brain and the spinal cord.

central processing unit (CPU) (sen'trăl pros'es-ing yū'nit) A microprocessor, the primary computer chip responsible for interpreting and executing programs.

centrifuge (sen'tri-fyūzh) A device used to spin a specimen at high speed until it separates into its component parts.

cerebrospinal fluid (CSF) (ser-ē'brō-spī'năl flū'ĭd) The fluid in the subarachnoid space of the meninges and the central canal of the spinal cord.

cerebrovascular accident (CVA) (ser'ĕ-brō-vas'kyū-lăr ak'si-dĕnt) A stroke; caused by a hemorrhage in the brain or more often by a clot lodged in a cerebral artery.

Certificate of Waiver tests (sĕr-ti'fi-kŭt wāv'ĕr tests) Laboratory tests that pose an insignificant risk to the patient if they are performed or interpreted incorrectly, are simple and accurate to such a degree that the risk of obtaining incorrect results is minimal, and have been approved by the Food and Drug Administration for use by patients at home; laboratories performing only Certificate of Waiver tests must meet less stringent standards than laboratories that perform tests in other categories.

certification (sĕr'ti-fi-kā'shŭn) The attainment of board approval and credentialing in a specialty.

certified check (sĕr'ti-fīd chĕk) A payer's check written and signed by the payer that is stamped "certified" by the bank. The bank has already drawn money from the payer's account to guarantee that the check will be paid.

Certified Medical Assistant (CMA) (sĕr'ti-fīd med'i-kăl ă-sis'tănt) A medical assistant whose knowledge about the skills of medical assistants, as summarized by the 2003 AAMA Role Delineation Study areas of competence, has been certified by the Certifying Board of the American Association of Medical Assistants (AAMA).

cerumen (sĕ-rū'mĕn) A wax-like substance produced by glands in the ear canal; also called earwax.

chain of command (chān kŏ-mand') A command hierarchy where a group of people are committed to carrying out orders from the highest authority.

chapters (chap'tĕrz) The breakdown of diagnosis codes by body system or disease. There are 21 chapters in ICD-10.

check (chĕk) A bank draft or order written by a payer that directs the bank to pay a sum of money on demand to the payee.

CHEDDAR (ched'er) C: Chief complaint. H: History. E: Examination. D: Details of problem and complaints. D: Drugs and dosage. A: Assessment. R: Return visit information or referral, if applicable.

chemical digestion (kem'i-kăl dī-jes'chŭn) The breaking down of food for use by the body caused by enzymes in the body such as amylase.

chemistry (kem'is-trē) The study of the composition of matter and how matter changes.

chief complaint (CC) (chēf kŏm-plānt') The patient's main issue of pain or ailment.

cholangiography (kō-lan-jē-og'ră-fē) A test that evaluates the function of the bile ducts by injection of a contrast medium directly into the common bile duct (during gallbladder surgery) or through a T-tube (after gallbladder surgery or during radiologic testing) and taking an X-ray.

cholesterol (kŏ-les'tĕr-ol) A fat-related substance that the body produces in the liver and obtains from dietary sources; needed in small amounts to carry out several vital functions. High levels of cholesterol in the blood increase the risk of heart and artery disease.

chordae tendineae (kōr'dē ten-din'ē-ē) Cord-like structures that attach the cusps of the heart valves to the papillary muscles in the ventricles.

choroid (kōr'oyd) The middle layer of the eye, which contains the iris, the ciliary body, and most of the eye's blood vessels.

chromosome (krō'mə-sōm') Thread-like structure composed of DNA.

chronological résumé (kron'ŏ-lo'ji-kĕl rez'ŭm-ā) The type of résumé used by individuals who have job experience. Jobs are listed according to date, with the most recent listed first.

chyme (kīm) The mixture of food and gastric juice.

civil law (si'vĭl law) Involves crimes against persons. A person can sue another person, business, or the government. Judgments often require a payment of money.

clarification (klar'i-fi-kā'shŭn) Asking questions that provide an increased understanding of a problem.

clarity (klār'i-tē) Clearness in writing or stating a message.

clavicle (klav'i-kĕl) A slender, curved long bone that connects the sternum and the scapula; also called the collar bone.

clean-catch midstream urine specimen (klēn kach mid-strēm yūr'in spes'i-mĕn) A type of urine specimen that requires special cleansing of the external genitalia to avoid contamination by organisms residing near the external opening of the urethra and is used to identify the number and types of pathogens present in urine; sometimes referred to as midvoid.

clearinghouse (klēr'ing-hows) A group that takes nonstandard medical billing software formats and translates them into the standard EDI formats.

clinical diagnosis (klin'i-kăl dī-ăg-nō'sis) A diagnosis based on the signs and symptoms of a disease or condition, and on the results of any laboratory tests that have been ordered.

Clinical Laboratory Improvement Amendments of 1988 (CLIA '88) (klin'i-kăl la'bōr-ă-tōr'ē im-prūv'ment ă-mend'ments) A law enacted by Congress in 1988 that placed all laboratory facilities that conduct tests for diagnosing, preventing, or treating human disease or for assessing human health under federal regulations administered by the Health Care Financing Administration (HCFA) and the Centers for Disease Control and Prevention (CDC).

clinical preceptor (klin'i-kăl prē'sep-tŏr) The person at the clinical site who serves as an instructor but is an employee of the site.

closed file (klōzd fīl) A file for a patient who has died, has moved away, or for some other reason no longer consults the office for medical expertise.

closed posture (klōzd pŏs'chŭr) A position that conveys the feeling of not being totally receptive to what is being said; arms are often rigid or folded across the chest.

cluster scheduling (klŭs'tĕr sked'jūl-ing) The scheduling of similar appointments together at a certain time of the day or week.

coagulation (kō-ag'yū-lā'shŭn) The process by which a clot forms in blood.

coccus (kŏk'ŭs) A spherical, round, or ovoid bacterium.

cochlea (kok'lē-ă) A spiral-shaped canal in the inner ear that contains the hearing receptors.

cochlear implant (kok'lē-ăr im'plant) Amplification device surgically implanted with its stimulating electrodes inserted directly into the nonfunctioning cochlea.

coding (kōd'ing) Putting an identifying mark or phrase on a document to ensure that it is placed in the correct file folder.

coinsurance (kō-in-shŭr'ăns) A fixed percentage of covered charges paid by the insured person after a deductible has been met.

colonoscopy (kō-lon-os'kŏ-pē) A procedure used to determine the cause of diarrhea, constipation, bleeding, or lower abdominal pain by inserting a scope through the anus to provide direct visualization of the large intestine.

colony (kol'ŏ-nē) A distinct group of microorganisms, visible with the naked eye, on the surface of a culture medium.

color family (kŭl'ŏr fam'i-lē) A group of colors that share certain characteristics, such as warmth or coolness, allowing them to blend well together.

combination code (kom'bi-nā'shŭn kōd) An ICD code in which two diagnoses are included in one code.

Commission on Accreditation of Allied Health Education Programs (CAAHEP) (kŏ-mish'ŭn ă-kred'i-tā'shŭn al'īd helth) A voluntary organization that accredits allied health education programs.

compactible file (kŏm-pakt'ăbl fīl) File kept on rolling shelves that slide along permanent tracks in the floor and stored close together or stacked when not in use.

complements (kom'plē-mĕnts) Proteins, present in serum, that are involved in specific defenses.

complete blood (cell) count (CBC) (kŏmplēt' blŭd kownt) A combination of the following determinations: red blood cell indices and count, white blood cell count, hematocrit, hemoglobin, platelets, and differential blood count.

complex carbohydrate (kom'pleks kahr-bō-hī'drāt) A long chain of sugar units; also known as a polysaccharide.

complimentary closing (kom'plē-mĕnt-ă-rē klōz-ing) The closing remark of a business letter found two lines below the last line of the body of the letter.

compound microscope (kom'pownd mī'krŏ-skōp) A microscope that uses two lenses to magnify the image created by condensed light focused through the object being examined.

comprehension (kom'prē-hen'shŭn) Knowledge or understanding of an object, a situation, an event, or a verbal statement.

computed tomography (kŏm-pyū'tĕd tŏ-mog'ră-fē) A radiographic examination that produces a three-dimensional, cross-sectional view of an area of the body; may be performed with or without a contrast medium.

concise (kon-sīs') Brief; using no unnecessary words

concurrent care (kŏn-kŭr'ĕnt kār) Care being provided by more than one physician, such as with specialists.

concussion (kŏn-kŭsh'ŭn) A jarring injury to the brain; the most common type of head injury.

conductive hearing loss (kon-dŭk'tiv hēr'ing laws) A type of hearing loss that occurs when sound waves cannot be conducted through the ear. Most types are temporary.

conflict (kŏn'flikt) An opposition of opinions or ideas.

conjunctiva (kŏn'jŭngk-tī'vă) The protective membrane that lines the eyelid and covers the anterior of the sclera, or the white of the eye.

conjunctivitis (kon-jŭngk'ti-vī'tis) An infection of the conjunctiva caused by bacteria, viruses, and allergies. The symptoms may include discharge, red eyes, itching, and swollen eyelids; also commonly called pinkeye. Both bacterial and viral conjunctivitis are highly contagious.

consent (kŏn-sent') A voluntary agreement that a patient gives to allow a medically trained person the permission to touch, examine, and perform a treatment.

constructive criticism (kon-strŭk'tiv krit'ĭ-siz'ŭm) A type of critique aimed at giving an individual feedback about his or her performance in order to improve that performance.

consultation (kon'sŭl-tā'shŭn) Meeting of two or more physicians or surgeons to evaluate the nature and progress of disease in a particular patient and to establish diagnosis, prognosis, and/or therapy.

consumable (kŏn-sūm'ă-bĕl) Able to be emptied or used up, as with supplies.

consumer education (kŏn-sum'ĕr ed'yū-kā'shŭn) The process by which the average person learns to make informed decisions about goods and services, including healthcare.

contagious (kŏn-tā'jŭs) Having a disease that can be transmitted easily to others.

continuing education (kŏn-tin'yū-ing ed'yū-kā'shŭn) Systematic professional learning experiences designed to augment knowledge and skills of healthcare professionals; education completed after the initial educational program; required for relicensure in some fields.

contract (kon'trakt) A voluntary agreement between two parties in which specific promises are made.

contraindication (kon'tră-in-di-kā'shŭn) A symptom that renders use of a remedy or procedure inadvisable, usually because of risk.

contrast medium (kon'trast mē'dē-ŭm) A substance that makes internal organs denser and blocks the passage of X-rays to photographic film. Introducing a contrast medium into certain structures or areas of the body can provide a clear image of organs and tissues and highlight indications of how well they are functioning.

control sample (kŏn-trŏl' sam'pĕl) A specimen that has a known value; used as a comparison for test results on a patient sample.

controlled substance (kŏn-trōld' sŭb'stăns) A drug or drug product that is categorized as potentially dangerous and addictive and is strictly regulated by federal laws.

contusion (kŏn-tū'zhŭn) A closed wound, or bruise.

conventions (kŏn-vĕn'shŭnz) A list of abbreviations, punctuation, symbols, typefaces, and instructional notes appearing in the beginning of the ICD-10. The items provide guidelines for using the code set.

copayment (kō'pā'mĕnt) A fixed or set amount paid for each healthcare or medical service; the remainder is paid by the health insurance plan. Also called a copay.

cornea (kōr'nē-ă) A transparent area on the front of the outer layer of the eye that acts as a window to let light into the eye.

coronary artery bypass graft (CABG) (kŏr'ŏ-nār-ē ahr'tĕr-ē bī'pās graft) A surgery performed to bypass a blockage within a coronary artery with a vessel taken from another area.

coronary circulation (kōr'ŏ-nār-ē sĭr'kyū-lā'shŭn) The part of systemic circulation that provides the heart muscle with oxygen and nutrients and carries away waste products.

counseling (kown'sĕl-ing) Provision of advice and instruction by a healthcare professional to patients.

counter check (kown'tĕr chĕk) A special bank check that allows a depositor to draw funds from his own account only, as when he has forgotten his checkbook.

covered entity (kŭv'ĕrd en'ti-tē) Any organization that transmits health information in an electronic form that is related in any way with a HIPAA-covered business.

Cowper's glands (kow'pĕrz glandz) Bulbourethral glands.

CPT See *Current Procedural Terminology.*

crash cart (krăsh kärt) A rolling cart of emergency supplies and equipment.

creatine phosphate (krē'ă-tēn fos'fāt) A protein that stores extra phosphate groups.

credit (krĕd'ĭt) An extension of time to pay for services, which are provided on trust.

credit bureau (krĕd'ĭt būr-ō) A company that provides information about the credit-worthiness of a person seeking credit.

criminal law (krim'i-năl lô) Involves crimes against the state. When a state or federal law is violated, the government brings criminal charges against the alleged offender.

critical care (krit'i-kăl kār) Care provided to unstable, critically ill patients. Constant bedside attention is needed in order to code critical care.

critical thinking (krit'i-kăl thingk'ing) The practice of considering all aspects of a situation when deciding what to believe or what to do.

cross-reference (kraws ref'rĕns) The notation within the ICD-10 of the word *see* after a main term in the index. The *see* reference means that the main term first checked is not correct. Another category must then be used.

cross-referenced (kraws ref'rĕnsd') Filed in two or more places, with each place noted in each file; the exact contents of the file may be duplicated, or a cross-reference form can be created, listing all the places to find the file.

cross-training (kraws trān'ing) The acquisition of training in a variety of tasks and skills.

cryosurgery (krī'ō-sŭr'jĕr-ē) The use of extreme cold to destroy unwanted tissue, such as skin lesions.

cryotherapy (krī'ō-thār'ă-pē) The application of cold to a patient's body for therapeutic reasons.

crystal (kris'tăl) Naturally produced solid of definite form; commonly seen in urine specimens, especially those permitted to cool.

cultural competence (kŭl'chŭr-ăl kom'pĕ-tens) The ability to react appropriately in situations that may arise due to a patient's (or coworker's) cultural background.

cultural diversity (kŭl'chŭr-ăl di-vĕr'si-tē) The inevitable variety in customs, attitudes, practices, and behavior that exists among groups of people from different ethnic, racial, or national backgrounds who come into contact.

culture (kŭl'chŭr) (1) In the sociologic sense, a pattern of assumptions, beliefs, and practices that shape the way people think and act. (2) To place a sample of a specimen in or on a substance that allows microorganisms to grow in order to identify the microorganisms present.

culture and sensitivity (C&S) (kŭl'chŭr sen'si-tiv'i-tē) A procedure that involves culturing a specimen and then testing the isolated bacteria's susceptibility (sensitivity) to certain antibiotics to determine which antibiotics would be most effective in treating an infection.

***Current Procedural Terminology* (CPT) (kŭr'rĕnt prō-sē'jŭr-ăl tĕr-mi-nol'ŏ-jē)** A book with the most commonly used system of procedure codes. It is the HIPAA-required code set for physicians' procedures.

customized (kŭs'tŏm-īzd) Altering something to meet individual specifications such as when creating unique settings within an EHR software program to meet the needs of a specialty physician or medical office.

cycle billing (sī'kĕl bil'ing) A system that sends invoices to groups of patients every few days, spreading the work of billing all patients over the month while billing each patient only once.

cytokines (sī'tō-kīnz) Chemicals secreted by T lymphocytes in response to an antigen. Cytokines increase T- and B-cell production, kill cells that have antigens, and stimulate red bone marrow to produce more white blood cells.

cytokinesis (sī'tō-ki-nē'sis) Splitting of the cytoplasm during cell division.

database (dā'tă-bās) A collection of records created and stored on a computer.

debridement (dā-brēd-mon') The removal of debris or dead tissue from a wound to expose healthy tissue.

decibels (des'i-bĕlz) Units for measuring the relative intensity of sounds on a scale from 0 to 130.

deductible (dĕ-dŭk'ti-bĕl) A fixed dollar amount that must be paid by the insured before additional expenses are covered by an insurer.

defamation (def'ĕ-mā'shŭn) Damaging a person's reputation by making public statements that are both false and malicious.

deflection (dĕ-flek'shŭn) A peak or valley on an electrocardiogram.

dehydration (dē-hī-drā'shŭn) The condition that results from a lack of adequate water in the body.

demographic (dĕ-mŏ-gră'-fik) Statistical data relating to the population and particular groups within it.

dendrite (dĕn'drīt) A type of nerve fiber that is short and branches near the cell body. Its function is to receive information from the neuron.

dependent (dĕ-pen'dĕnt) A person who depends on another person for financial support.

depolarization (dē-pō'lăr-i-zā'shŭn) The loss of polarity, or opposite charges inside and outside; the electrical impulse that initiates a chain reaction resulting in contraction.

deposition (de-pə-zi'shən) A sworn statement regarding the facts of a case that is used to prepare a case for trial.

dermatome (děr'mă-tōm) An area of skin innervated by a spinal nerve.

dermis (děr'mis) The middle layer of the skin, which contains connective tissue, nerve endings, hair follicles, sweat glands, and oil glands.

desired dose (D) (di-zīrd' dōs) The amount of medication the licensed practitioner has ordered the patient to take.

detrusor muscle (dě-trū'sŏr mŭs'ĕl) A smooth muscle that contracts to push urine from the bladder into the urethra.

diagnosis (Dx) (dī-ăg-nō'sis) The primary condition for which a patient is receiving care.

diagnosis code (dī-ăg-nō'sis kōd) The way a diagnosis is communicated to the third-party payer on the healthcare claim.

diagnostic radiology (dī-ăg-nōs'tik rā'dē-ol'ŏ-jē) The use of X-ray technology to determine the cause of a patient's symptoms.

diaphysis (dī-af'i-sis) The shaft of a long bone.

diastolic pressure (dī'ă-stol'ik presh'ŭr) The blood pressure measured when the heart relaxes.

diathermy (dī'ă-thěr-mē) A type of heat therapy in which a machine produces high-frequency electromagnetic waves that achieve deep heat penetration in muscle tissue.

differential diagnosis (dif'ĕr-en'shăl dī-ăg-nō'sis) The process of determining the correct diagnosis when two or more diagnoses are possible.

digital examination (dij'i-tăl eg-zam'in-ā'shŭn) Part of a physical examination in which the physician inserts one or two gloved fingers of one hand into the opening of a body canal such as the vagina or the rectum; used to palpate the canal and related structures.

digital subscriber line (DSL) (dij'i-tăl sŭb-skrīb'ĕr līn) A type of modem that operates over telephone lines but uses a different frequency than a telephone, allowing a computer to access the Internet at the same time that a telephone is being used.

diluent (dil'yū-ĕnt) A liquid used to dissolve and dilute another substance, such as a drug.

disbursement (dis-běrs'mĕnt) Any payment of funds made by the physician's office for goods and services.

disclaimer (dis-clām'ĕr) A statement of denial of legal liability or that refutes the authenticity of a claim.

disclosure statement (dis-klō'zhŭr stāt'mĕnt) A written description of agreed terms of payment; also called a federal Truth in Lending Statement.

disinfection (dis-in-fek'shŭn) Destruction of pathogenic microorganisms or their toxins or vectors by direct exposure to chemical or physical agents.

dislocation (dis'lō-kā'shŭn) The displacement of a bone end from a joint.

dispense (dis-pens') To distribute a drug, in a properly labeled container, to a patient who is to use it.

distal convoluted tubule (dis'tăl kon'vŏ-lūt'ed tū'byūl) The last twisted section of the renal tubule; it is located after the loop of Henle. Several of these tubules merge together to form collecting ducts.

diversity (di-věr'si-tē) Differences among people in terms of identity, age, sex, race, physical ability, ethnicity, religious beliefs, values and mores, sexual orientation, and personality.

diverticula (dī'věr-tik'yū-lă) Pouches or sacs opening from a tubular or saccular organ, such as the gut or bladder. Plural of *diverticulum*.

documentation (dok'yū-měn-tā'shŭn) The recording of information in a patient's medical record; includes detailed notes about each contact with the patient and about the treatment plan, patient progress, and treatment outcomes.

dose on hand (H) (dōs hand) The amount of medication in each unit of the drug.

double-booking system (dŭb'ĕl buk'ing sis'těm) A system of scheduling in which two or more patients are booked for the same appointment slot, with the assumption that both patients will be seen by the doctor within the scheduled period.

douche (dūsh) Vaginal irrigation, which can be used to administer vaginal medication in liquid form.

downcoding (down'kōd-ing) The insurance carrier bases reimbursement on a code level lower than the one submitted by the provider.

dual coverage (dyū'ăl kŭv'ĕr-ăj) Term used when a patient is covered by Medicare and Medicaid.

dual-energy X-ray absorptiometry (DXA) (dū'ăl en'ĕr-jē eks'rā ăb-sōrp'shē-om'ĕ-trē) A screening test that uses small doses of X-rays to determine the mineral density of a person's bones; also called *bone densitometry*.

ductus arteriosus (dŭk'tŭs ar-tēr'ē-ō'sus) The connection in the fetus between the pulmonary trunk and the aorta.

ductus venosus (duk'tŭs vē-nō'sŭs) A blood vessel that allows most of the blood to bypass the liver in the fetus.

durable power of attorney (dūr'ă-bĕl pow'ĕr ă-tŏr'nē) A document naming the person who will make decisions regarding medical care on behalf of another person if that person becomes unable to do so.

dysmenorrhea (dis-men-ōr-ē'ă) Severe menstrual cramps that limit daily activity.

dyspnea (disp'nē-ă) Difficult or painful breathing (*dys* = difficult, painful, bad, abnormal; *pneo* = breathing).

dysrhythmia (dis-rith'mē-ă) An irregularity in heart rhythm; also called *arrhythmia*.

e-prescribing (ē-prě-skrīb'ing) Prescriptions are entered electronically and transmitted directly to the pharmacy.

E/M codes (ē/ĕm kōds) Evaluation and management codes that are often considered the most important of all CPT codes. The E/M section guidelines explain how to code different levels of services.

eccrine gland (ek'rin glănd) The most numerous type of sweat gland. Eccrine sweat glands produce a watery type of sweat and are activated primarily by heat.

ECG See **electrocardiogram**.

echocardiography (ek'ō-kahr-dē-og'ră-fē) A procedure that tests the structure and function of the heart through the use of reflected sound waves, or echoes.

editing (ed'i-ting) The process of ensuring that a document is accurate, clear, and complete; free of grammatical errors; organized logically; and written in the appropriate style.

efferent nerves (ef'ĕr-ĕnt něrvz) Motor nerves that take information or impulses from the central nervous system to the peripheral nervous system to control the movement or action of a muscle or gland.

efficacy (ef'i-kă-sē) The therapeutic value of a procedure or therapy, such as a drug.

elderly (el'dĕr-lē) Individuals over the age of 65.

elective procedure (ĕ-lek'tiv prŏ-sē'jŭr) A medical procedure that is not required to sustain life but is requested for payment to the third-party payer by the patient or physician. Some elective procedures are paid for by third-party payers, whereas others are not.

electrocardiogram (ECG) (ĕ-lek'trō-kahr'dē-ō-gram) The tracing made by an electrocardiograph.

electrocardiograph (ĕ-lek'trō-kahr'dē-ō-graf) An instrument that measures and displays the waves of electrical impulses responsible for the cardiac cycle.

electrocardiography (ĕ-lek'trō-kahr-dē-og'ră-fē) The process by which a graphic pattern is created to reflect the electrical impulses generated by the heart as it pumps.

electrocauterization (ĕ-lek'trō-kaw'tĕr-ī-zā'shŭn) The use of a needle, probe, or loop heated by electric current to remove growths such as warts, to stop bleeding, and to control nosebleeds that either will not subside or continually recur.

electrode (ĕ-lek'trōd) Sensor that detects electrical activity.

electroencephalography (ĕ-lek'trō-en-sef'ă-log'ră-fē) A procedure that records the electrical activity of the brain as a tracing called an electroencephalogram, or EEG, on a strip of graph paper.

electrolytes (ĕ-lek'trō-līts) Substances that carry electrical current through the movement of ions.

electromyography (ĕ-lek'trō-mī-og'ră-fē) A procedure in which needle electrodes are inserted into some of the skeletal muscles and a monitor records the nerve impulses and measures conduction time; used to detect neuromuscular disorders or nerve damage.

electronic health records (EHR) (ĕ-lek-tron'ik helth rek'ōrdz) Patient health records created and stored on a computer or other electronic storage device. Also known as *electronic medical records.*

electronic medical record (EMR) (ĕ-lek-tron'ik med'i-kăl rek'ōrd) Patient medical record created and stored on a computer or other electronic storage device.

embolus (em'bŏ-lŭs) A portion of a thrombus that breaks off and moves through the bloodstream.

embryo (em'brē-ō) A group of cells, called the *inner cell mass,* that develops from the blastocyst during the embryonic prenatal period to become the fetus.

empathy (ĕm'pă-thē) Identification with or sensitivity to another person's feelings and problems.

employee handbook (em-ploy'ē hand'buk) A synopsis of human resources policies and procedures.

endocardium (en'dō-kahr'dē-ŭm) The innermost layer of the heart.

endocrine gland (en'dō-krin gland) A gland that secretes its products directly into tissue, fluid, or blood.

endogenous infection (en-doj'ĕ-nŭs in-fek'shŭn) An infection in which an abnormality or a malfunction in routine body processes causes normally beneficial or harmless microorganisms to become pathogenic.

endorsement (en-dōrs'mĕnt) Signature on the back of a check with the terms for accepting the check as payment.

endoscopy (en-dos'kŏ-pē) Any procedure in which a scope is used to visually inspect a canal or cavity within the body.

engineered safety devices (en'jin-ērd sāf'tē dĕ-vīs') Devices specifically designed to isolate or remove a hazard. These include needles with safety shields and self-shielding needles.

enunciation (ē-nŭn-sē-ā'shŭn) Clear and distinct speaking.

enuresis (en-yūr-ē'sis) Bed-wetting.

eosinophil (ē-ō-sin'ō-fil) A type of granular leukocyte that captures invading bacteria and antigen-antibody complexes through phagocytosis.

epicardium (ep-i-kar'dē-ŭm) The outermost layer of the wall of the heart. Also known as the **visceral pericardium.**

epidermis (ep'i-dĕr'mis) The most superficial layer of the skin.

epiglottis (ep-i-glot'is) The flap-like structure that closes off the larynx during swallowing.

epiphysis (e-pif'i-sis) The expanded end of a long bone.

epistaxis (ĕp'i-stak'sis) Nosebleed.

ergonomics (ĕr'gŏ-nom'iks) The science of workplace, tools, and equipment designed to reduce worker discomfort, strain, and fatigue and to prevent work-related injuries.

erythema (er-i-thē'mă) Redness of the skin.

erythrocyte (ĕ-rith'rŏ-sīt) Red blood cell.

erythrocyte sedimentation rate (ESR) (ĕ-rith'rŏ-sīt sed'i-mĕn-tā'shŭn rāt) The rate at which red blood cells, the heaviest blood component, settle to the bottom of a blood sample.

erythropoietin (ĕ-rith'rō-poy'ĕ-tin) A hormone secreted by the kidney and responsible for regulating the production of red blood cells.

esophageal hiatus (ĕ-sof'ă-jē'ăl hī-ā'tŭs) Hole in the diaphragm through which the esophagus passes.

established patient (es-tab'lisht pā'shĕnt) A patient who has seen the physician within the past 3 years. This determination is important when using E/M codes.

ethics (ĕth'īks) General principles of right and wrong, as opposed to requirements of law.

ethylenediaminetetraacetic acid (EDTA) (eth'i-lēn-dī'ă-mēn-tet'ră-ă-sē'tik as'id) A chelating agent and anticoagulant; added to blood specimens for hematologic and other tests.

etiologic agent (ē'tē-e-lŏj'ĭk ā'jent) A living microorganism or its toxin that may cause human disease.

etiology (ē'tē-ol'ŏ-jē) The science and study of the causes of disease and their mode of operation.

etiquette (ĕt'ĭ-ket') Good manners.

eustachian tube (yū-stā'-shē-an tūb) An opening in the middle ear, leading to the back of the throat, that helps equalize air pressure on both sides of the eardrum.

examination light (eg-zam'i-nā'shŭn līt) A flexible arm light source used for better visualization of a patient during an examination.

exocrine gland (ek'sō-krin gland) A gland that secretes its product into a duct.

exogenous infection (eks-oj'ĕ-nŭs in-fek'shŭn) An infection that is caused by the introduction of a pathogen from outside the body.

expiration (eks'pir-ā'shŭn) The process of breathing out; also called exhalation.

explanation of benefits (EOB) (eks'plă-nā'shŭn ben'ĕ-fits) Information that explains the medical claim in detail; also called **remittance advice (RA).**

explanation of payment (EOP) (eks'plă-nā'shŭn pā'mĕnt) Document sent by an insurance carrier when payment is made describing the terms of the payments. Also known as **explanation of benefits (EOB)** or **remittance advice (RA).**

expressed contract (eks-prest' kon'trakt) A contract clearly stated in written or spoken words.

external auditory canal (eks-tĕr'năl aw'di-tōr-ē kă-nal') Canal that carries sound waves to the tympanic membrane; commonly called the ear canal.

face page (fās pāj) A screen that provides an overview or "snapshot" of the patient demographic information in an EHR system.

face sheet (fās shēt) A screen that provides an overview or "snapshot" of the patient demographic information in an EHR system.

factual teaching (fak'chū-ăl tēch'ing) Method of teaching that provides the patient with details of the information that is being taught.

facultative (fak'ŭl-tā-tiv) Able to adapt to different conditions; in microbiology, able to grow in environments either with or without oxygen.

fascicle (fas'i-kĕl) Sections of a muscle divided by connective tissue called perimysium.

febrile (feb'ril) Having a body temperature above one's normal range.

fecal occult blood test (FOBT) (fē'kăl ŏ-kŭlt' blŭd test) A test to find hidden blood in the stool.

feces (fē'sēz) Material found in the large intestine and made from leftover chyme. Feces are eventually eliminated through the anus.

Federal Insurance Contributions Act (FICA) (fed'ĕr-ăl in-shŭr'ăns kon'tri-byū'shunz akt) A law that requires employers to deduct a certain amount from each employee's paycheck to fund Social Security and Medicare.

Federal Unemployment Tax Act (FUTA) (fĕd'ĕr-al em-ploy'mĕnt taks akt) This act requires employers to pay a percentage of each employee's income up to a certain dollar amount.

fee schedule (fē sked'jūl) A list of the costs of common services and procedures performed by a physician.

fee-for-service (fē sĕr'vis) A major type of health plan. It repays policyholders for the costs of healthcare that are due to illness and accidents.

feedback (fēd'băk) Verbal and nonverbal evidence that a message was received and understood.

feedback loop (fēd'băk lūp) A mechanism to control hormone levels. The two types are positive and negative feedback loops.

felony (fel'ŏ-nē) A serious crime, such as murder or rape, that is punishable by imprisonment. In certain crimes, a felony is punishable by death.

femur (fē'mŭr) The bone in the upper leg; commonly called the thigh bone.

fenestrated drape (fen'ĕs-trāt-ĕd drāp) A drape that has a round or slit-like opening that provides access to the surgical site.

fetus (fē'tŭs) The product of conception from the end of the eighth week to the moment of birth.

fiber (fī'bĕr) The tough, stringy part of vegetables and grains, which is not absorbed by the body but aids in a variety of bodily functions.

fibrinogen (fī-brin'ō-jen) A protein found in plasma that is important for blood clotting.

fibula (fib'yū-lă) The lateral bone of the lower leg.

file guide (fīl gīd) A heavy cardboard or plastic insert used to identify a group of file folders in a file drawer.

first morning urine specimen (first mōr'ning yūr'in spes'i-mĕn) A urine specimen that is collected after a night's sleep; contains greater concentrations of substances that collect over time than specimens taken during the day.

fixative (fik'să-tiv) A solution sprayed on a slide immediately after the specimen is applied. It is used to preserve and hold the cells in place until a microscopic examination is performed.

fluidotherapy (flū'id-ō-thăr'ă-pē) A technique for stimulating healing, particularly in the hands and feet, by placing the affected body part in a container of glass beads that are heated and agitated with hot air.

follicle (fol'i-kĕl) An accessory organ of the skin that is found in the dermis and the sites at which hairs emerge.

fomite (fō'mīt) An inanimate object, such as clothing, body fluids, water, or food, that may be contaminated with infectious organisms and thus transmit disease.

fontanels (fon'tă-nelz') Soft spots in an infant's skull that consist of tough membranes that connect to incompletely developed bone.

food exchange (fūd eks-chānj') A unit of food in a particular food category that provides the same amounts of protein, fat, and carbohydrates as all other units of food in that category.

foramen ovale (fōr-ā'mĕn ō-va'lē) A hole in the fetal heart between the right atrium and the left atrium.

forced vital capacity (FVC) (fōrst vī'tăl kă-pas'i-tē) The greatest volume of air that a person is able to expel when performing rapid, forced expiration.

Form I-9 A federal form for verifying that an employee is a US citizen, a legally admitted alien, or an alien authorized to work in the United States.

Form W-2 The tax form that an employer must send to an employee and the IRS at the end of the year. It reports an employee's annual wages and the amount of taxes withheld from his or her paycheck.

Form W-4 A tax form completed by an employee to indicate his or her tax situation, such as exemptions and status, to the employer.

formalin (fōr'mă-lin) A dilute solution of formaldehyde used to preserve biological specimens.

formed elements (fōrmd el'ĕ-mĕnts) Red blood cells, white blood cells, and platelets; compose 45% of blood volume.

formula method (fōrm'yū-lă meth'ŏd) A basic formula to calculate dosage. $D/H \times Q$, where D = desired dose, H = dose on hand, and Q = quantity of the dose.

fraud (frawd) An act of deception that is used to take advantage of another person or entity.

frequency (frē'kwĕn-sē) The number of complete fluctuations of energy per second in the form of waves.

full-block letter style (ful' blok let'ĕr stīl) A letter format in which all lines begin flush left; also called block style.

functional résumé (fŭngk'shŭn-ăl rez'ŭm-ā) A résumé that highlights specialty areas of a person's accomplishments and strengths.

G-protein (jē-prō'tēn) A substance that causes enzymes in the cell to activate following the activation of the hormone-receptor complex in the cell membrane.

gait (gāt) The way a person walks, consisting of two phases: stance and swing.

ganglia (gang'glē-ă) Collections of neuron cell bodies outside the central nervous system.

gene (jēn) A segment of DNA that determines a body trait.

general duty clause (jen'ĕr-ăl dū'tē klawz) An OSHA clause that requires an employer to maintain a workplace free from hazards that are recognized as likely to cause death or serious injury.

general physical examination (jen'ĕr-ăl fiz'i-kăl eg-zam'i-nā'shŭn) An examination performed by a physician to confirm a patient's health or to diagnose a medical problem.

generic name (jĕ-ner'ik nām) A drug's official name.

geriatrician (jer'ē-ă-trish'ăn) A specialist who cares for elderly individuals, usually those over the age of 65.

glaucoma (glaw-kō'mă) A condition in which too much pressure is created in the eye by excessive aqueous humor. This excess pressure can lead to permanent damage of the optic nerves, resulting in blindness.

global period (glō'băl pēr'ē-ŏd) The period of time that is covered for follow-up care of a procedure or surgical service.

Globally Harmonized System of Classification and Labeling of Chemicals (GHS) (glō'băl-lē har'mōn-izd sis'tĕm klas'i-fi-kā'shŭn lā'bĕl-ing kem'i-kălz) A system for standardizing the classification and labeling of chemicals developed by the United Nations as a guide for regulatory systems around the world. In the United States, OSHA's Hazard Communication Standard is now aligned with the GHS.

globulins (glob'yū-linz) Plasma proteins that transport lipids and some vitamins.

glomerulus (glō-mer'yū-lŭs) A group of capillaries in the renal corpuscle.

glottis (glot'is) The opening between the vocal cords.

gluten (glū'tĕn) The insoluble protein (prolamines) constituent of wheat and other grains; a mixture of gliadin, glutenin, and other proteins; believed to be an agent in celiac disease.

glycogen (glī'kō-jen) An excess of glucose that is stored in the liver and in skeletal muscle.

glycosuria (glī'kō-syūr'ē-ă) The presence of significant levels of glucose in the urine.

gonads (gō'nădz) The reproductive organs: namely, in women the ovaries and in men the testes.

goniometer (gō'nē-om'ĕ-tĕr) A protractor device that measures range of motion.

Gram stain (gram stān) A method of staining that differentiates bacteria according to the chemical composition of their cell walls.

Gram-negative (gram nĕg'ă-tĭv) Referring to bacteria that lose their purple color when a decolorizer has been added during a Gram stain.

Gram-positive (gram pŏz'ĭ-tĭv) Referring to bacteria that retain their purple color after a decolorizer has been added during a Gram stain.

granulocyte (gran'yū-lō-sīt) A type of leukocyte (white blood cell) with a segmented nucleus and granulated cytoplasm; also known as a polymorphonuclear leukocyte or **granular leukocyte.**

grievance process (grē'văns pros'es) A mediation process through the human resources department utilized when an employee or employees feel they are treated unjustly.

gross earnings (grōs ĕrn'ingz) The total amount an employee earns before deductions.

growth chart (grōth chahrt) A chart consisting of percentile curves that are used to determine a child's growth in relation to average rates.

guarantor (gar'ăn-tōr) The patient, caregiver, or entity responsible for payment of the healthcare bill.

gustatory cortex (gŭs'tă-tōr-ē kōr'teks) An area of the brain that is responsible for interpreting taste sensations by integrating information from the taste cells with other information to provide a more complete interpretation.

hapten (hap'tĕn) Foreign substances in the body too small to start an immune response by themselves.

hard skills (hahrd skilz) Specific technical and operational proficiencies.

hardware (hahrd'wār) The physical components of a computer system, including the monitor, keyboard, and printer.

Hazard Communication Standard (HCS) (haz'ărd kŏ-myūn'i-kā'shŭn stan'dărd) OSHA's standard for worker safety when working with hazardous chemicals. In 2012, the standard was updated to align with the Globally Harmonized System of Classification and Labeling of Chemicals (GHS).

hazard label (haz'ărd lā'bĕl) A shortened version of the Safety Data Sheet; permanently affixed to a hazardous substance container.

HCPCS See **Healthcare Common Procedure Coding System.**

HCPCS Level II codes (hik'piks lĕv'ĕl tū kōdz) Codes that cover many supplies such as sterile trays, drugs, and durable medical equipment; also referred to as national codes. They also cover services and procedures not included in the CPT.

health maintenance organization (HMO) (helth mān'tĕn-ăns ōr'găn-ī-zā'shŭn) A healthcare organization that provides specific services to individuals and their dependents who are enrolled in the plan. Doctors who enroll in an HMO agree to provide certain services in exchange for a prepaid fee.

Healthcare Common Procedure Coding System (HCPCS) (helth'kār kom'ŏn prŏ-sē'jŭr kōd'ing sis'tĕm) A coding system developed by the Centers for Medicare and Medicaid Services that is used in coding services for Medicare patients.

healthcare-associated infections (HAI) (helth'kār ă-sō'sē-āt-ed in-fek'shŭns) Infections acquired by a patient in a healthcare facility.

hematemesis (hē'mă-tem'ĕ-sis) The vomiting of blood.

hematocrit (Hct) (hē-mat'ō-krit) The percentage of the volume of a sample made up of red blood cells after the sample has been spun in a centrifuge.

hematoma (hē'mă-tō'mă) A swelling caused by blood under the skin.

hematuria (hē'mă-tyūr'ē-ă) The presence of blood in the urine.

hemoglobin (Hgb) (hē'mō-glō'bin) A protein that contains iron and bonds with and carries oxygen to cells; the main component of erythrocytes.

hemolysis (hē-mol'ĭ-sis) The rupturing of red blood cells, which releases hemoglobin.

hemostasis (hē'mō-stā'sis) The stoppage of bleeding.

hepatic portal system (hĕ-pat'ik pōr'tăl sis'tĕm) The collection of veins carrying blood to the liver.

hierarchy (hī'ĕr-ahr-kē) A term that pertains to Abraham Maslow's hierarchy of needs. This hierarchy states that human beings are motivated by unsatisfied needs and that certain lower needs must be satisfied before higher needs can be met.

hilum (hī'lŭm) The indented side of a lymph node. Also, the part of the renal sinus of the kidney through which the renal artery, renal vein, and ureter enter the kidney.

HIPAA (Health Insurance Portability and Accountability Act) (hĭp-uh) A set of regulations whose goals include the following: (1) improving the portability and continuity of healthcare coverage in group and individual markets; (2) combating waste, fraud, and abuse in healthcare insurance and healthcare delivery; (3) promoting the use of a medical savings account; (4) improving access to long-term care services and coverage; and (5) simplifying the administration of health insurance.

HITECH (Health Information Technology for Economics and Clinical Health) Act (hī-tek' akt) The expansion of HIPAA coverage through increased regulations and enforcement penalties related to EHR and practice management systems.

Holter monitor (hōl'tĕr mon'i-tŏr) An electrocardiography device that includes a microchip or a small cassette recorder worn around a patient's waist or on a shoulder strap to record the heart's electrical activity.

homeostasis (hō'mē-ō-stā'sĭs) A balanced, stable state within the body.

hormone (hōr'mōn) A chemical secreted by a cell that affects the functions of other cells.

hospice (hŏs'pĭs) Healthcare professionals and volunteers who work with terminally ill patients and their families.

household system (hows'hōld sis'tĕm) A system of measurement that includes drops, teaspoons, tablespoons, ounces, cups, pints, quarts, and gallons.

hydrotherapy (hī'drō-thār'ă-pē) The therapeutic use of water to treat physical problems.

hyperglycemia (hī'pĕr-glī-sē'mē-ă) High blood sugar.

hyperopia (hī'pĕr-ō'pē-ă) A condition that occurs when light entering the eye is focused behind the retina; commonly called farsightedness.

hyperpnea (hī-pĕr-nē'ă, hī-pĕrp'nē-ă) Abnormally deep, rapid breathing.

hyperpyrexia (hī'pĕr-pī-rek'sē-ă) An exceptionally high fever.

hypertension (hī'pĕr-ten'shŭn) High blood pressure.

hyperventilation (hī'pĕr-ven'ti-lā'shŭn) The condition of breathing rapidly and deeply. Hyperventilating decreases the amount of carbon dioxide in the blood.

hypodermis (hī'pō-dĕr'mis) The subcutaneous layer of the skin that is largely made of adipose tissue.

hypoglycemia (hī'pō-glī-sē'mē-ă) Low blood sugar.

hypotension (hī'pō-tĕn'shŭn) Low blood pressure.

hypovolemic shock (hī'pō-vŏ-lē'mik shŏk) A state of shock resulting from insufficient blood volume in the circulatory system.

hypoxemia (hī'pok-sē'mē-ă) Subnormal oxygenation (low oxygen) of arterial blood, short of anoxia.

icons (ī'konz') Pictorial images; on a computer screen, graphic symbols that identify menu choices.

immunization (im'yū-nī-zā'shŭn) Administration of a vaccine to protect susceptible individuals from communicable diseases.

immunoglobulins (im'yū-nō-glob'yū-linz) A class of structurally related proteins that include IgG, IgA, IgM, and IgE; also called **antibodies.**

implied contract (ĭm-plīd' kon'trakt) A contract that is created by the acceptance or conduct of the parties rather than the written word.

inactive file (in-ak'tiv fīl) A file used infrequently.

incident report (in'si-dĕnt rē-pōrt') A report required by a facility when an adverse incident with risk of liability occurs.

incision (in-sizh'ŭn) A surgical wound made by cutting into body tissue.

incontinence (in-kon'ti-nens) The involuntary leakage of urine.

indexing (in'dĕks'ing) The naming of a file.

indexing rules (in'dĕks'ing rūlz) Rules used as guidelines for the sequencing of files based on current business practice.

indication (in'di-kā'shŭn) The purpose or reason for using a drug, as approved by the FDA.

indirect filing system (in'dir-ekt' fīl'ing sis'tĕm) A numeric filing system, which organizes files by numbers instead of by names.

induction (in-dŭk'shŭn) The pregnant patient is admitted to the delivering healthcare facility, then given medication to start uterine contractions.

infectious waste (in-fek'shŭs wāst) Waste that can be dangerous to those who handle it or to the environment; includes human waste, human tissue, and body fluids as well as potentially hazardous waste, such as used needles, scalpels, and dressings, and cultures of human cells.

infertility (in'fĕr-til'i-tē) Diminished ability to produce offspring; does not imply sterility.

inflammatory phase (in-flam'ă-tōr-ē fāz) The initial phase of wound healing in which bleeding is reduced as blood vessels in the affected area constrict.

infundibulum (in-fŭn-dib'yū-lŭm) The funnel-like end of the uterine tube near an ovary. It catches the secondary oocyte as it leaves the ovary.

infusion (in-fyū'zhŭn) A slow drip, as of an intravenous solution into a vein.

innate immunity (i-nāt' i-myū'ni-tē) The body's mechanisms to protect itself against pathogens in general; also called nonspecific defenses.

insertion (in-sĕr'shŭn) An attachment site of a skeletal muscle that moves when a muscle contracts.

inside address (ĭn-sīd' ă-dres') The name and address of the person to whom the letter is being sent. It appears on a business letter two to four lines down from the date. It should be two, three, or four lines in length.

inspecting (conditioning) (in-spek'ting; kuhn-dih'shun-ing) The process of making sure an item is ready for filing, including removing paper clips and stapling related documents together.

inspection (ĭn-spĕk'shŭn) The visual examination of the patient's entire body and overall appearance.

inspiration (in'spir-ā'shŭn) The act of breathing in; also called inhalation.

integrity (in-teg'ri-tē) Adhering to the appropriate code of law and ethics and being honest and trustworthy.

interactive pager (in'tĕr-ak'tiv pāj'ĕr) A pager designed for two-way communication. The pager screen displays a printed message and allows the physician to respond by way of a mini-keyboard.

International Classification of Diseases (in'tĕr-nash'ŭn-ăl klas'i-fi-kā'shŭn di-zēz'ĕz) Code set that is based on a system maintained by the World Health Organization of the United Nations. The use of the ICD-10 codes in the healthcare industry is mandated by HIPAA for reporting patients' diseases, conditions, and signs and symptoms. ICD-10 codes, adopted October 1, 2015, allow for more specificity and accuracy when coding.

interneurons (in'tĕr-nū'ronz) Structures found only in the central nervous system that link sensory and motor neurons together.

interpersonal skills (in′tĕr-pĕr′sŏn-ăl skĭlz) Attitudes, qualities, and abilities that influence the level of success and satisfaction achieved in interacting with other people.

interstitial fluid (in′tĕr-stish′ăl flū′id) Fluid found between tissue cells that is absorbed by lymphatic capillaries to become lymph.

intradermal (ID) (in′tră-der′măl) Within the upper layers of the skin.

intradermal test (in′tră-dĕr′măl tĕst) An allergy test in which dilute solutions of allergens are introduced into the skin of the inner forearm or upper back with a fine-gauge needle.

intramuscular (IM) (in′tră-mŭs′kyū-lăr) Within muscle; an IM injection allows administration of a larger amount of a drug than a subcutaneous injection allows.

intraoperative (in′tră-op′ĕr-ă-tiv) Taking place during surgery.

intravenous (IV) (in′tră-vē′nŭs) Injected directly into a vein.

intravenous pyelography (IVP) (in′tră-vē′nŭs pī′ĕ-log′ră-fē) A radiologic procedure in which the doctor injects a contrast medium into a vein and takes a series of X-rays of the kidneys, ureters, and bladder to evaluate urinary system abnormalities or trauma to the urinary system; also known as excretory urography.

invasive (ĭn-vā′sĭv) Referring to a procedure in which a catheter, wire, or other foreign object is introduced into a blood vessel or organ through the skin or a body orifice. Surgical asepsis is required during all invasive tests.

invasive procedure (in-vā′siv prŏ-sē′jur) Any procedure that requires entry into a body cavity or cutting into skin or mucous membranes.

invoice (ĭn′vois) A listing of products or services rendered that is used when billing for that product or service..

ions (ī′onz) Positively or negatively charged particles.

islets of Langerhans (ī′lĕts lahng′er-hahnz) Structures in the pancreas that secrete insulin and glucagon into the bloodstream.

itinerary (ī-tĭn′ĕ-rar′ē) A detailed travel plan listing dates and times for specific transportation arrangements and events, the location of meetings and lodgings, and phone numbers.

jaundice (jawn′dis) A condition characterized by yellowness of the skin, eyes, mucous membranes, and excretions; occurs in newborns due to an inability to break down bilirubin and in people of all ages during the second stage of hepatitis infection.

journalizing (jûr′nă-līz′ĭng) The process of logging charges and receipts in a chronological list each day; used in the single-entry system of bookkeeping.

keratin (kĕr′ă-tĭn) A tough, hard protein contained in skin, hair, and nails.

keratinocyte (kĕ-rat′i-nō-sīt) The most common cell type in the epidermis of the skin.

KOH mount (kā′ō-āch mownt) A type of mount used when a physician suspects a patient has a fungal infection of the skin, nails, or hair and to which potassium hydroxide is added to dissolve the keratin in cell walls.

KUB radiography (kā′yoo-bē rā′dē-og′ră-fē) The process of X-raying the abdomen to help assess the size, shape, and position of the urinary organs; evaluate urinary system diseases or disorders; or determine the presence of kidney stones. It also can be helpful in determining the position of an intrauterine device (IUD) or in locating foreign bodies in the digestive tract; also called a flat plate of the abdomen.

kyphosis (kī-fō′sis) A deformity of the spine characterized by a bent-over position; more commonly called humpback.

labeling (lā′bĕl-ing) Information provided with a drug, including FDA-approved indications and the form of the drug.

labor relations (lā′bŏr rĕ-lā′shŭnz) An HR role that refers to issues that arise between employees and management.

labyrinth (lab′i-rinth) The inner ear.

laceration (las′ĕr-ā′shŭn) A jagged, open wound in the skin that can extend down into the underlying tissue.

lacrimal apparatus (lak′ri-măl ap′ă-rat′ŭs) A structure that consists of the lacrimal glands and nasolacrimal ducts.

lactic acid (lăk′tĭk ăs′ĭd) A waste product that must be released from the cell. It is produced when a cell is low on oxygen and converts pyruvic acid.

lancet (lăn′sĭt) A small, disposable instrument with a sharp point used to puncture the skin and make a shallow incision; used for capillary puncture.

laryngeal mirror (lă-rĭn′jē-al mir′or) A small mirrored instrument used to examine the inside of the mouth and throat.

laryngopharynx (lă-ring′gō-făr′ingks) The portion of the pharynx behind the larynx.

larynx (lăr′ingks) The part of the respiratory tract between the pharynx and the trachea that is responsible for voice production; also called the voice box.

last menstrual period (LMP) (lăst men′strū-ăl pēr′ē-ŏd) The date of the first day of the last menstruation; used to determine an estimated expected delivery date for a pregnant patient.

lateral file (lat′ĕr-ăl fīl) A horizontal filing cabinet that features doors that flip up and a pull-out drawer, where files are arranged with sides facing out.

laterality (lat′ĕr-al′i-tē) In ICD-10, the side of the body affected by the diagnosis.

law (lô) A rule of conduct established and enforced by an authority or governing body, such as the federal government.

lead (lēd) A view of a specific area of the heart on an electrocardiogram.

lentigos (len-tī′gōz) Brown macules resembling a freckle except that the border is usually regular and microscopic proliferation of rete ridges is present; scattered melanocytes are seen in the basal cell layer. They are usually caused by sun exposure in someone of middle age or older.

leukocyte (lū′kō-sīt) White blood cell.

licensed practitioner (lī′sĕnst prak-ti′shŭn-ĕr) A healthcare provider who has obtained the necessary education and skills and is licensed to provide specified healthcare to patients.

ligature (lig′ă-chŭr) Suture material.

limited check (lĭm′ĭ-ted chĕk) A check that is void after a certain time limit; commonly used for payroll.

lipid (lip′id) Fats, oils, and waxy substances that are not soluble in water. Lipids can be used by the body as a source of energy. They are also a major component of cell membranes.

lithotripsy (lith′ō-trip-sē) The crushing of a stone in the renal pelvis, ureter, or bladder by mechanical force or sound waves.

local area network (LAN) (lō′kăl ār′ē-ă net′wŏrk) A network that connects computers in one building or a group of buildings.

locum tenens **(lō′kum ten′enz)** A substitute physician hired to see patients while the regular physician is away from the office.

loop electrosurgical excision procedure (LEEP) (lūp ĕ-lek'trō-sŭr'jik-ăl ek-sizh'ŭn prŏ-sē'jŭr) A diagnostic and therapeutic gynecologic surgical technique for removing dysplastic cells from the cervix with a small wire loop.

loop of Henle (lūp hen'lē) The portion of the renal tubule that curves back toward the renal corpuscle and twists again to become the distal convoluted tubule.

lubricant (lū'bri-kănt) A water-soluble gel used during examination of the rectum or vaginal cavity.

lymph (limf) The fluid inside lymphatic vessels.

lymph nodes (limf nōdz) Very small, glandular structures that filter pathogens from lymph and generate lymphocytes.

lymphocytes (lĭm'fō-sīts) Granular leukocytes formed in lymphoid tissue. Lymphocytes are generally small and include T lymphocytes and B lymphocytes.

lymphokines (lĭm'fō-kīnz) A type of cytokine secreted by T cells that increases T-cell production and directly kills cells with antigens.

macrophages (mak'rō-fāj-ez) A type of phagocytic cell found in the liver, spleen, lungs, bone marrow, and connective tissue. Macrophages play several roles in humoral and cell-mediated immunity, including presenting the antigens to the lymphocytes involved in these defenses; also known as monocytes while in the bloodstream.

magnetic resonance imaging (MRI) (mag-net'ik rez'ō-năns im'ăj-ing) A viewing technique that uses a powerful magnetic field to produce an image of internal body structures.

magnetic therapy (măg-nĕt'ĭk thār'ă-pē) A type of therapy in which magnets are placed on the body to penetrate and correct the body's energy fields.

major histocompatibility complex (MHC) (mā'jŏr his'tō-kŏm-pat'i-bil'i-tē kom'pleks) A large protein complex that plays a role in T-cell activation.

malignant (mă-lig'nănt) A type of tumor or neoplasm that is invasive and destructive and that tends to metastasize; it is commonly known as cancerous.

mammography (mă-mog'ră-fē) X-ray examination of the breasts.

manipulation (mă-nip'yū-lā'shŭn) The systematic movement of a patient's body parts.

matrix (mā'trĭks) The basic format of an appointment book, established by

blocking off times on the schedule during which the doctor is able to see patients. Also, the material between the cells of connective tissue.

matter (măt'er) Anything that takes up space and has weight. Liquids, solids, and gases are matter.

maturation phase (mach'ūr-ā'shŭn fāz) The third phase of wound healing, in which scar tissue forms.

meaningful use (mēn'ing-ful yüs) The use of certified electronic health record technology to improve quality, safety, and efficiency, and reduce health disparities; to engage patients and family; to improve care coordination, and population and public health; and to maintain privacy and security of patient health information.

mechanical digestion (mĕ-kan'i-kăl dī-jes'chŭn) The breaking down of food for use by the body by a physical method such as chewing.

mediation (mē'dē-ā'shun) Intervention in a dispute in order to resolve it.

medical asepsis (med'i-kăl ā-sep'sis) Measures taken to reduce the number of microorganisms, such as handwashing and wearing examination gloves, that do not necessarily eliminate microorganisms; also called clean technique.

meiosis (mī-ō'sis) A type of cell division in which each new cell contains only one member of each chromosome pair.

melanin (mel'ă-nĭn) A pigment that is deposited throughout the layers of the epidermis.

melanocyte (mel'ă-nō-sīt) A cell type within the epidermis that makes the pigment **melanin.**

menarche (men'ahr-kē) A woman's first menstrual period.

Ménière's disease (men-yerz' di-zēz') An inner-ear disease characterized by attacks of vertigo, tinnitus, and nausea. Permanent hearing loss may result.

meninges (mĕ-nin'jēz) Membranes that protect the brain and spinal cord.

menopause (men'ō-pawz) The termination of the menstrual cycle due to the normal aging of the ovaries.

menorrhagia (men-ŏ-rā'jē-ă) Excessively prolonged or profuse menses.

menstruation (men'strū-ā'shŭn) Cyclic endometrial shedding and discharge of a bloody fluid from the uterus during the menstrual cycle.

mensuration (men'sŭr-ā'shŭn) The process of measuring.

meridians (mĕr-id'ē-anz) Pathways of energetic flow that are distributed symmetrically throughout the body. These pathways are used in acupuncture, traditional Chinese medicine, and Ayurveda.

metabolic wastes (met'ă-bol'ik wāsts) Waste substances produced by normal body processes, such as respiration and digestion, that are filtered out of the blood by the kidneys and excreted through the urine.

metabolism (mĕ-tab'ĕ-lizm) The overall chemical functioning of the body, including all body processes that build small molecules into large ones (anabolism) and break down large molecules into small ones (catabolism).

metacarpal (met'ă-kahr'păl) One of the bones that form the palms of the hand.

metatarsal (met'ă-tahr'săl) One of the bones that form the front of the foot.

metric system (met'rik sis'tĕm) A system of measurement based on multiples of 10.

metrorrhagia (mē-trō-rā'jē-ă) Any irregular, acyclic bleeding from the uterus between periods.

micropipette (mī'krō-pĭ-pet') A small pipette that holds a small, precise volume of fluid; used to collect capillary blood.

micturition (mik-chŭr-ish'ŭn) The process of urination.

middle digit (mid'ĕl dij'it) A small group of two to three numbers in the middle of a patient number that is used as an identifying unit in a filing system.

midlevel provider (mid-lev'ĕl prō-vī'dĕr) Physician assistant or nurse practitioner who provides patient care under the supervision of a physician.

mineral (min'ĕr-ăl) Natural, inorganic substance the body needs to help build and maintain body tissues and carry on life functions.

minor (mī'nŏr) Anyone under the age of majority—18 in most states, 21 in some jurisdictions.

minutes (min'ŭtz) A report of what happened and what was discussed and decided at a meeting.

mirroring (mir'ŏr-ing) Restating in your own words what a person is saying.

misdemeanor (mis'di-mēn'ŏr) A less serious crime such as theft under a certain dollar amount or disturbing the peace. A misdemeanor is punishable by fines or imprisonment.

mitosis (mī-tō'sĭs) A type of cell division that produces ordinary body, or somatic, cells; each new cell receives a complete set of paired chromosomes.

mobility aid (mō-bil'i-tē ād) Device that improves one's ability to move from one place to another; also called mobility assistive device.

modeling (mod'ĕl-ing) The process of teaching the patient a new skill by having the patient observe and imitate it.

modified-block letter style (mod'i-fīd blok let'ĕr stīl) A letter format similar to full-block style, except that the dateline, complimentary closing, signature block, and notations are aligned and begin at the center of the page or slightly to the right of center.

modified-wave scheduling (mod'i-fīd wāv sked'jūl-ing) A scheduling system similar to the wave system, with patients arriving at planned intervals during the hour, allowing time to catch up before the next hour begins.

modifier (mod'i-fī'ĕr) One or more 2-digit codes assigned to the 5-digit main code to show that some special circumstance applied to the service or procedure that the physician performed.

molecule (mol'ĕ-kyūl) The smallest unit into which an element can be divided and still retain its properties; it is formed when atoms bond together.

money order (mŭn'ē ôr'dĕr) A certificate of guaranteed payment, which may be purchased from a bank, a post office, or some convenience stores.

monocyte (mon'o-sīt) A type of phagocyte that is formed in bone marrow and circulates throughout the blood for a very short period of time. It then migrates to specific tissues and is called a macrophage.

monokines (mon'ō-kīnz) A type of cytokine secreted by lymphocytes and macrophages that assists in regulating the immune response by increasing B-cell production and stimulating red bone marrow to produce more white blood cells.

morbidity (mōr-bid'i-tē) The frequency of the appearance of complications following a surgical procedure or other treatment; a disease state.

mordant (mōr'dănt) A substance, such as iodine, that can intensify or deepen the response a specimen has to a stain.

moro reflex (mō'rō rē'fleks) A reflex in which an infant's arms spread out and then back in, often with crying, because the infant feels as if she is falling. The

moro reflex is a result of the infant's immature nervous system.

morphology (mōr-fol'ŏ-jē) The study of the shape or form of objects.

mortality (mōr-tal'i-tē) A fatal outcome.

mucous membranes (myū'kus mem'brānz) Specialized tissue that lines the body openings and cavities. Mucous membranes are found inside the mouth, digestive system, and lungs.

MUGA scan (nuclear ventriculography) (mŭg'ă skan [noo'klē-ĕr ven-trĭk-ū-log'ră-fē]) A radiologic procedure that evaluates the condition of the heart's myocardium; it involves injection of radioisotopes that concentrate in the myocardium, followed by the use of a gamma camera to measure ventricular contractions to evaluate the patient's heart wall.

multi-unit smooth muscle (mŭl'tē yū'nit smūth mŭs'ĕl) A type of smooth muscle that is found in the iris of the eye and in the walls of blood vessels.

multiskilled healthcare professional (MSHP) (mŭl'tē-skild helth'kār prŏ-fesh'i-năl) A healthcare team member who has been cross-trained to handle many different duties.

myelin sheath (mī'ĕ-lin shēth) Insulation around some nerve cell axons that allows nerve impulses to move more quickly through the axons.

myelography (mī'ĕ-log'ră-fē) An X-ray visualization of the spinal cord after the injection of a radioactive contrast medium or air into the spinal subarachnoid space (between the second and innermost of three membranes that cover the spinal cord). This test can reveal tumors, cysts, spinal stenosis, or herniated disks.

myocardium (mī'ō-kahr'dē-ŭm) The middle and thickest layer of the heart. It is made primarily of cardiac muscle.

myofibrils (mī-ō-fī'brilz) Long structures that fill the sarcoplasm of a muscle fiber.

myopia (mī-ō'pē-ă) A condition that occurs when light entering the eye is focused in front of the retina; commonly called nearsightedness.

nail bed (nāl bĕd) The layer beneath each nail.

narcotic (nahr-kot'ik) A popular term for an opioid and term of choice in government agencies; see **opioid.**

nares (nā'rēz) The openings of the nose, or nostrils.

nasal conchae (nā'zăl kon'kē) Structures that extend from the lateral walls of the nasal cavity.

nasal mucosa (nā'zăl myū-kō'să) The lining of the nose.

nasal speculum (nā'zăl spek'yŭ-lŭm) An instrument used to enlarge the nasal opening to permit viewing inside the nose.

nasopharynx (nā'zō-făr'ingks) The portion of the pharynx behind the nasal cavity.

natural killer (NK) cells (na'chŭr-ăl kil'ĕr selz) Non-B and non-T lymphocytes. NK cells kill cancer cells and virus-infected cells without previous exposure to the antigen.

needle biopsy (nē'dĕl bī'op-sē) A procedure in which a needle and syringe are used to aspirate (withdraw by suction) fluid or tissue cells.

negligence (nĕg'lĭ-jĕns) A medical professional's failure to perform an essential action or performance of an improper action that directly results in the harm of a patient.

negotiable (nĭ-gō'shē-ă-bel) Legally transferable from one person to another.

nephrons (nef'ronz) Microscopic structures in the kidneys that filter waste products from the blood and form urine.

net earnings (net ûr'nĭngz) Take-home pay, calculated by subtracting total deductions from gross earnings.

networking (nĕt'wŏrk-ĭng) Making contacts with relatives, friends, and acquaintances who may have information about how to find a job in your field.

neuroglia (nūr-ŏg'lē-ă) Structures that function as support cells for other neurons, including astrocytes, microglia, and oligodendrocytes; also called *neuroglial cells.*

neurotransmitter (nūr'ō-trans'mit-ĕr) A chemical within the vesicles of the synaptic knob that is released into the postsynaptic structures when a nerve impulse reaches the synaptic knob.

neutrophil (nū'trō-fil) A type of granular leukocyte that aids in phagocytosis by attacking bacterial invaders; also responsible for the release of pyrogens.

new patient (nū pā'shĕnt) Patient that, for CPT reporting purposes, has not received professional services from the physician within the past 3 years.

no-show (nō shō) A patient who does not call to cancel and does not come to an appointment.

nocturia (nok-tyūr'ē-ă) Excessive nighttime urination.

nomogram (nō'mō-gram) A form of line chart showing scales for the variables

with other substances involved in metabolic activity, such as glucose. These isotopes emit positrons, which a computer processes and displays on a screen.

phagocytosis (fag'ŏ-sī-tō'sis) The process by which white blood cells defend the body against infection by engulfing invading pathogens.

pharmacodynamics (far'mă-kō-dī-nam'iks) The study of what drugs do to the body: the mechanism of action, or how they work to produce a therapeutic effect.

pharmacognosy (far-mă-kog'nō-sē) The study of characteristics of natural drugs and their sources.

pharmacokinetics (far'mă-kō-ki-net'iks) The study of what the body does to drugs: how the body absorbs, metabolizes, distributes, and excretes the drugs.

pharmacology (far'ma-kŏl'ŏ-jē) The study of drugs.

pharmacotherapeutics (far'mă-kō-thār'ă-pyū'tiks) The study of how drugs are used to treat disease; also called clinical pharmacology.

pharynx (făr'ĭngks) Structure below the mouth and nasal cavities that is an organ of the respiratory system as well as the digestive system.

phenylketonuria (PKU) (fen'il-kē'tō-nyūr'ē-ă) A genetically inherited disorder in which the body cannot properly metabolize the nutrient phenylalanine, resulting in the buildup of phenylketones in the blood and their presence in the urine. The accumulation of phenylketones results in mental retardation.

philosophy (fĭ-lŏs'ĕ-fē) The system of values and principles an office has adopted in its everyday practice.

phlebotomy (fle-bot'ŏ-mē) The insertion of a needle or cannula (small tube) into a vein for the purpose of withdrawing blood.

photometer (fō-tom'ĕ-tĕr) An instrument that measures light intensity.

physical therapy (fiz'i-kăl thār'ă-pē) A medical specialty that uses cold, heat, water, exercise, massage, traction, and other physical means to treat musculoskeletal, nervous, and cardiopulmonary disorders.

physician assistant (PA) (fi-zish'ŭn ă-sis'tănt) A healthcare provider who practices medicine under the supervision of a physician.

physician's office laboratory (POL) (fi-zish'ŭnz aw'fis lă'brūh-tō-rē) A laboratory contained in a physician's office; processing tests in the POL produces quick turnaround and eliminates the need for patients to travel to other test locations.

physiology (fĭz'ē-ŏl'ŏ-jē) The science of the study of the body's functions.

pineal body (pin'ē-ăl bŏd'ē) A small gland located between the cerebral hemispheres that secretes melatonin.

pitch (pĭch) The high or low quality in the sound of a person's speaking voice.

placenta (plă-sen'tă) An organ located between the mother and the fetus that envelops the fetus during development. The placenta permits the absorption of nutrients and oxygen. In some cases, harmful substances such as viruses are absorbed through the placenta.

platelets (plăt'lĕts) Fragments of cytoplasm in the blood that are crucial to clot formation; also called thrombocytes.

pleura (plūr'ă) The membranes that surround the lungs.

plexus (plĕk'sŭs) A structure that is formed when spinal nerves fuse together. It includes the cervical, brachial, and lumbosacral nerves.

point of care tests (POCT) (poynt of kār tests) Tests performed at or near the patient, normally where the patient is being treated.

polarity (pō-lăr'ĭ-tē) The condition of having two separate poles, one of which is positive and the other negative.

policies and procedures (P&P) manual (pol'i-sēz prŏ-sē'jŭrz) A key written communication tool in the medical office that covers all office policies for administrative and clinical procedures.

POLST (Physician Orders for Life-Sustaining Treatment) form A set of medical orders completed by a healthcare provider after a discussion with the patient regarding his or her desires for treatment; it serves as a set of portable treatment orders.

polypharmacy (pol'ē-fahr'mă-sē) The administration of many drugs at the same time.

POMR The problem-oriented medical record system for keeping patients' charts. Information in a POMR includes the database of information about the patient and the patient's condition, the problem list, the diagnostic and treatment plan, and progress notes.

portfolio (pôrt-fō'lē-ō') A collection of an applicant's résumé, reference letters, and other documents of interest to a potential employer.

positive tilt test (pŏz'ĭ-tĭv tĭlt tĕst) When the pulse rate increases more than 10 beats per minute (bpm) and the blood pressure drops more than 20 points while taking vital signs in the lying, sitting, and standing positions.

positron emission tomography (PET) (poz'ĭ-tron ĕ-mish'ŭn tŏ-mog'ră-fē) A radiologic procedure that entails injecting isotopes combined with other substances involved in metabolic activity, such as glucose. These isotopes emit positrons, which a computer processes and displays on a screen.

postcoital (pōst-kō'i-tăl) After sexual union.

postoperative (pōst-op'ĕr-ă-tiv) Taking place after a surgical procedure.

postural hypotension (pŏs'chŭr-ăl hī'pō-tĕn'shŭn) A situation in which blood pressure becomes low and the pulse increases when a patient is moved from a lying to a standing position; also known as orthostatic hypotension.

posture (pŏs'chŭr) Body position and alignment.

power of attorney (pow'ĕr ă-tŏr'nē) The legal right to act as the attorney or agent of another person, including handling that person's financial matters.

PPE See **personal protective equipment.**

practice management system (prak'tis man'ăj-mĕnt sis'tĕm) Multifunctional electronic health system programs that, in addition to medical records management, provide other functionalities including, but not limited to, electronic scheduler, billing and accounts receivable capability, report writer, insurance eligibility and referral management system, and billing and coding software.

preauthorization (prē'awth'ŏr-ī-zā'shun) Authorization or approval for payment from a third-party payer requested in advance of a specific procedure.

precertification (prē'sĕr-ti-fi-kā'shŭn) A determination of the amount of money that will be paid by a third-party payer for a specific procedure before the procedure is conducted.

preferred provider organization (PPO) (prĕ-fĕrd' prŏ-vī'dĕr ŏr'gă-nī-zā'shŭn) A managed care plan that establishes a network of providers to perform services for plan members.

prefix (prē'fĭks) A word part that comes at the beginning of a medical term that alters the meaning of the term.

premium (prē'mē-ŭm) The basic annual cost of healthcare insurance.

preoperative (prē-op'ĕr-ă-tiv) Taking place prior to surgery.

presbyopia (prez-bē-ō'pē-ă) A common eye disorder that results in the loss of lens elasticity. Presbyopia develops with age and causes a person to have difficulty seeing objects close up.

prescribe (prĕ-skrīb') To order a medication for a patient from a pharmacy. A licensed practitioner can prescribe medications by giving the patient a prescription to take to a pharmacy or by sending the prescription directly to the pharmacy electronically (known as *e-prescribing*).

preventive care (prĕ-ven'tiv kār) Screening tests and drugs to prevent disease.

preventive medicine (prĕ-ven'tiv med'i-sin) The branch of medical science concerned with the prevention of disease and with promotion of physical and mental health, through study of the etiology and epidemiology of disease processes.

primary care physician (PCP) (prī'mar-ē kār fi-zish'ŭn) A physician who provides routine medical care and referrals to specialists.

primary diagnosis (prī'mar-ē dī'ăg-nō'sis) The diagnosis given as the primary reason for the patient seeking care.

primary germ layers (prī'mar-ē jĕrm lā'ĕrz) The layers of an inner cell mass: the ectoderm, mesoderm, and endoderm.

prime mover (prīm mū'vĕr) The muscle responsible for most of the movement when a body movement is produced by a group of muscles. Also called an *agonist*.

principal diagnosis (prin'si-păl dī'ăg-nō'sis) The diagnosis that is found, after testing and study, to be the main reason for the patient's need for healthcare services.

prioritizing (prī-ôr'i-tīz-ing) Sorting and dealing with matters in the order of urgency and importance.

probationary period (prō-bā'shŭn-ār'ē pēr'ē-ŏd) A trial period during which the employer may terminate the new employee without cause.

problem solving (prob'lĕm sŏlv-ing) A step-by-step approach that uses critical thinking and good judgment to deal with situations or occurrences that need resolution.

procedure code (prŏ-sē'jĕr kōd) Code that represents a medical procedure, such as surgery and diagnostic tests, and medical services, such as an examination to evaluate a patient's condition.

professional development (prŏ-fesh'ŭn-ăl dĕ-vel'ŏp-mĕnt) The skills and knowledge attained for both personal development and career advancement.

professional objective (prŏ-fesh'un-ăl ŏb-jek'tiv) A brief, general statement that demonstrates a career goal.

proficiency testing program (prō-fish'ĕn-sē test'ing prō'grăm) A required set of tests for clinical laboratories; the tests measure the accuracy of the laboratory's test results and adherence to standard operating procedures.

prognosis (prŏg-nō'sĭs) A prediction of the probable course of a disease in an individual and the chances of recovery.

prolapse (prō'laps) A sinking of an organ or other part, especially its appearance at a natural or artificial orifice.

proliferation phase (prō-lif'ĕr-ā'shŭn fāz) The second phase of wound healing, in which new tissue forms, closing off the wound.

pronunciation (prō-nun'sē-ā'shŭn) The sounding out of words.

proofreading (prūf'rēd-ing) Checking a document for formatting, data, and mechanical errors.

proportion (prŏ-pōr'shŭn) Two fractions that are equal to each other. When three of the four values are known, the fourth value can be calculated by cross-multiplying and solving for the unknown value.

proportion method (prō-pōr'shŭn meth'ŏd) A fraction formula based on ratios and proportions that is used to calculate dosage.

prostaglandins (pros-tă-glan'dinz) Local hormones derived from lipid molecules. Prostaglandins typically do not travel in the bloodstream to find their target cells because their targets are close by. These hormones have numerous effects, including uterine stimulation during childbirth.

protein (prō'tēn) Macromolecules consisting of long sequences of a-amino acids [H_2N-CHR-COOH] in peptide (amide) linkage (elimination of H_2O between the a-NH_2 and a-COOH of successive residues). Protein is three-fourths of the dry weight of most cell matter and is involved in structures, hormones, enzymes, muscle contraction, immunologic response, and essential life functions. The amino acids involved are generally the 20 a-amino acids (glycine, l-alanine) recognized by the genetic code. Cross-links yielding globular forms of protein are often effected through the 2SH groups of two sulfur-containing l-cysteinyl residues, as well as by noncovalent forces (such as hydrogen bonds, lipophilic attractions).

proteinuria (prō'tē-nyūr'ē-ă) An excess of protein in the urine.

proximal convoluted tubule (prok'si-măl kon'vō-lūt'ed tū'byŭl) The portion of the renal tubule that is directly attached to the glomerular capsule and becomes the loop of Henle.

puberty (pyu'bĕr-tē) The period of adolescence when a person begins to develop secondary sexual traits and reproductive functions.

pulmonary circulation (pul'mŏ-nar-ē sĭr'kyū-lā'shŭn) The passage of blood from the right ventricle through the pulmonary artery to the lungs and back through the pulmonary veins to the left atrium.

pulmonary function test (pul'mŏ-nār-ē fŭngk'shŭn test) A test that evaluates a patient's lung volume and capacity; used to detect and diagnose pulmonary problems or to monitor certain respiratory disorders and evaluate the effectiveness of treatment.

punctuality (pŭngk'chū-ăl'i-tē) Showing up on appointed dates and at appointed times.

puncture wound (pungk'shŭr wūnd) A deep wound caused by a sharp, pointed object.

purchase order (pŭr'chăs ōr'dĕr) A form that authorizes a purchase for the practice.

Purkinje fibers (pŭr-kin'jē fī'bĕrz) Cardiac fibers located in the lateral walls of the ventricles.

quadrant (kwahd'rănt) One of four equal sections, such as those into which the abdomen is figuratively divided during an examination.

qualitative test response (kwahl'i-tā'tiv test rĕ-spons') A test result that indicates the substance tested for is either present or absent.

quality assurance (kwahl'i-tē ă-shŭr'ăns) Procedures that ensure that the services provided in the medical practice meet or exceed requirements and standards.

quality assurance program (kwahl'i-tē ă-shŭr'ăns prō'gram) A required program for clinical laboratories designed to monitor the quality of patient care, including quality control, instrument and equipment maintenance, proficiency testing, training and continuing education, and standard operating procedures documentation.

quality control program (kwahl'i-tē kŏn-trōl' prō'gram) A component of a quality assurance program that focuses on ensuring accuracy in laboratory test results through careful monitoring of test procedures.

quantitative test results (kwahn'ti-tā'tiv test rē-sŭlt) The concentration of a test substance in a specimen.

quantity (Q) (kwahn'ti-tē) Amount of a medication on hand; for example, a pill or an amount of liquid.

radiation therapy (rā'dē-ā'shŭn thăr'ă-pē) The use of X-rays and radioactive substances to treat cancer.

radius (rā'dē-ŭs) The lateral bone of the forearm.

rales (rahlz) Noisy respirations usually due to blockage of the bronchial tubes.

random-access memory (RAM) (ran'dŏm ak'ses mem'ŏ-rē) The temporary, or programmable, memory in a computer.

range of motion (ROM) (rānj mō'shŭn) The degree to which a joint is able to move.

rapport (ră-pôr') A harmonious, positive relationship.

re-sheathing scalpel (rē-shēth'ing skalp'ĕl) A single-use, disposable scalpel that has a sheath that can be slid over the blade and locked in position after use.

read-only memory (ROM) (rēd ōn'lē mem'ŏ-rē) A computer's permanent memory, which can be read by the computer but not changed. It provides the computer with the basic operating instructions it needs to function.

reagent (rē-ā'jĕnt) A chemical or chemically treated substance used in test procedures and formulated to react in specific ways when exposed under specific conditions.

reception (rī-sep'shŭn) The place or event where one is greeted, usually where a patient is first greeted and checks in at a healthcare facility.

reconciliation (rĕ-kon-sil'ē-ā'shŭn) A comparison of the office's financial records with bank records to ensure that they are consistent and accurate; usually done when the monthly checking account statement is received from the bank.

records management system (rĕ'kôrdz man'ăj-mĕnt sis'tĕm) How patient records are created, filed, and maintained.

reference (ref'er-rĕns) A recommendation for employment from a facility or a preceptor.

reference laboratory (ref'er-rĕns lă'brŭh-tō-rē) A laboratory owned and operated by an organization outside the physician's practice.

reflection (rĕ-flek'shŭn) When a thought, an idea, or an opinion is formed as a result of deeper thought.

reflex hammer (rē'fleks ha'mer) An instrument with a hard triangular head used to check a patient's reflexes.

refraction (rē-frak'shŭn) The bending of light by the cornea, lens, and eye fluids to focus light onto the retina.

refraction examination (rē-frak'shŭn eg-zam'i-nā'shŭn) An eye examination in which the patient looks through a succession of different lenses to find out which ones create the clearest image.

refractometer (rē-frak-tom'ĕ-ter) An optical instrument that measures the refraction, or bending, of light as it passes through a liquid.

Registered Medical Assistant (RMA) (rej'i-stĕrd med'i-kăl ă-sis'tănt) A medical assistant who has met the educational requirements and taken and passed the certification examination for medical assisting given by the American Medical Technologists (AMT).

registration (rej'is-trā'shŭn) The recording of information (e.g., licensure, birth or death date).

releasing (rĕ-lēs'ing) Placing a mark or stamp on an item that indicates that the responsible licensed practitioner has seen the document and is giving permission to file it in the patient's medical record.

remittance advice (RA) (rē-mit'ăns ad-vīs') A form that the patient and the practice receive for each encounter that outlines the amount billed by the practice, the amount allowed, the amount of subscriber liability, the amount paid, and notations of any service not covered, including an explanation of why that service is not covered; also called an explanation of benefits.

renal column (rē'năl kol'ŭm) The portion of the renal cortex that extends down between the renal pyramids.

renal corpuscle (rē'năl kŏr'pŭs-ĕl) Corpuscle that is composed of the glomerulus and the glomerular capsule. The filtration of blood occurs here.

renal cortex (rē'năl kŏr'teks) The outermost layer of the kidney.

renal medulla (rē'năl mĕ-dŭl'ă) The middle portion of the kidney.

renal pelvis (rē'năl pel'vis) The internal structure of the renal sinus in the kidney. Urine flows from the renal pelvis down the ureter.

renal pyramids (rē'năl pir'ă-midz) Triangular-shaped areas in the medulla of the kidney.

renal sinus (rē'năl sī'nŭs) The medial depression of a kidney.

renal tubule (rē'năl tū'byūl) Structure that extends from the glomerular capsule of a nephron and is composed of the proximal convoluted tubule, the loop of Henle, and the distal convoluted tubule.

repolarization (rē-pō'lăr-i-zā'shŭn) The process of returning to the original polar (resting) state.

requisition (rĕk'wĭ-zĭsh'ŭn) A formal request from a staff member or physician for the purchase of equipment or supplies. Also a physician's order for laboratory tests.

reservoir host (rĕz'er-vwahr' hōst) An animal, insect, or human whose body is susceptible to growth of a pathogen.

resource-based relative value scale (RBRVS) (rē'sōrs-băst rel'ă-tiv val'yū skāl) The payment system used by Medicare. It establishes the relative value units for services, replacing the providers' consensus on usual fees.

respiratory capacity (res'pir-ă-tōr-ē kă-pas'i-tē) The amount of air the lungs can hold; calculated by adding certain respiratory volumes together.

respiratory hygiene/cough etiquette (res'pir-ă-tōr-ē hī'jĕn kawf e'ti-ket) Infection control guideline that includes teaching the patient to cover his or her mouth/nose when coughing and dispose of tissues in the proper receptacle.

respiratory volume (res'pir-ă-tōr-ē vol'yūm) The different volumes of air that move into and out of the lungs during different breathing intensities. These volumes can be measured to assess the healthiness of the respiratory system.

restatement (rē-stāt'ment) Repeating what a patient says in your own words back to the patient.

résumé (re-zūm-ā') A document summarizing one's employment and educational history.

retention schedule (rĭ-ten'shŭn sked'jūl) A schedule that details how long to keep different types of patient records in the office after they have become inactive or closed and how long the records should be stored.

retina (ret'i-nă) The inner layer of the eye; contains light-sensing nerve cells.

retractable needle (rē-trak'tă-běl nē'děl) A needle that retracts inside the barrel of a syringe after it is activated.

retrograde pyelography (ret'rō-grād pī'ě-log'ră-fē) A radiologic procedure in which the doctor injects a contrast medium through a urethral catheter and takes a series of X-rays to evaluate function of the ureters, bladder, and urethra.

return demonstration (rē-tŭrn' dem'on-strā'shŭn) Participatory teaching method in which the technique is first described to the patient and then demonstrated to the patient; the patient is then asked to repeat the demonstration.

reverse chronological order (rě-věrs' kron'ŏ-loj'ik-ěl ōr'děr) A filing system in which the most recent files (by date) are inserted so they are on top of documents with earlier dates in the file folder.

review of systems (rē-vū' sis'těm) A process of gathering information about a patient's health history regardless of apparent relevance to the chief complaint.

rhonchi (rong'kī) Deep snoring or rattling sounds during breathing; associated with asthma, acute bronchitis, or any condition involving partial obstruction of the lung's airway.

rhythm strip (rith'ŭm strip) An ECG tracing obtained using an electrocardiograph machine.

risk management (RM) (risk man'ăj-měnt) Plans and processes that continually identify, assess, correct, and monitor functions of the medical office to prevent negative outcomes and minimize exposure to risk and consequent liability.

rubrics (rū'briks) Three-character ICD categories used to specify diseases, injuries, and symptoms.

Safety Data Sheet (SDS) (sāf'tē dā'tă shēt) A form that is required for all hazardous chemicals or other substances used in the laboratory and that contains information about the product's name,

ingredients, chemical characteristics, physical and health hazards, guidelines for safe handling, and procedures to be followed in the event of exposure.

salutation (sal'yū-tā'shŭn) A written greeting, such as "Dear," used at the beginning of a letter.

sanitization (san'i-ti-zā'shŭn) A reduction of the number of microorganisms on an object or a surface to a fairly safe level.

sarcolemma (sahr'kō-lem'ă) The cell membrane of a muscle fiber.

sarcoplasm (sahr'kō-plazm) The cytoplasm of a muscle fiber.

sarcoplasmic reticulum (sahr'kō-plaz'mik rě-tik'yū-lŭm) The endoplasmic reticulum of a muscle fiber.

saturated fat (sach'ūr-āt-ěd fat) Fat, derived primarily from animal sources, that is usually solid at room temperature and that tends to raise blood cholesterol levels.

scapula (skap'yū-lă) Thin, triangular-shaped flat bone located on the dorsal surface of the rib cage; also called shoulder blade.

Schwann cells (shwahn sělz) Cells whose cell membrane coats the axons of some neurons in the peripheral nervous system.

scoliosis (skō'lē-ō'sis) A lateral curvature of the spine, which is normally straight when viewed from behind.

scope of practice (skōp prak'tis) The procedures, processes, and actions a healthcare worker is allowed to perform under the terms of his or her career or professional license.

scored (skōrd) An indented line on a tablet where the medication can be broken into equal pieces.

scratch test (skrăch těst) An allergy test in which extracts of suspected allergens are applied to the patient's skin and the skin is then scratched to allow the extracts to penetrate.

screening (skrēn'ĭng) Performing a diagnostic test on a person who is typically free of symptoms.

sebaceous (sě-bā'shŭs) A type of oil gland found in the dermis.

sebum (sē'bŭm) An oily substance produced by sebaceous glands.

secondary diagnosis (sek'ŏn-dār-ē dī'ăg-nō'sis) Diagnosis other than the primary diagnosis for other conditions that are also affecting the patient at the time of the visit.

self-blunting/blunt tip, blood-drawing needle (self blŭnt'ing) A blood-drawing needle that has a blunt tip that slides forward through the needle past the sharp point to protect the user from needlestick injury.

self-confidence (self-kŏn'fĭ-děns) Believing in oneself; assured.

self-sheathing needle (self-shēth'ing) A needle that has a sheath over the barrel of the syringe. After injecting the medication, the user slides the sheath forward over the needle and locks it in place to prevent needlestick injuries.

semicircular canals (sem'ē-sĭr'kyū-lăr kă-nalz') Structures in the inner ear that help a person maintain balance; each of the three canals is positioned at right angles to the other two.

seminiferous tubules (sem'i-nif'er-ŭs tū'byūlz) Tubes located in the lobules of the testes that contain spermatogenic cells.

sensorineural hearing loss (sen'sěr-ē-nūr'ăl hēr'ing laws) Hearing loss that occurs when neural structures associated with the ear are damaged. Neural structures include hearing receptors and the auditory nerve.

sensory adaptation (sen'sŏr-ē ad'ap-tā' shŭn) A process in which the same chemical can stimulate receptors only for a limited amount of time until the receptors eventually no longer respond to the chemical.

sensory teaching (sen'sŏr-ē tēch'ing) Method of teaching that provides a patient with a description of the physical sensations he or she may have as part of the learning or the procedure involved.

septic shock (sěp'tĭk shŏk) A state of shock resulting from massive, widespread infection that affects the blood vessels' ability to circulate blood.

sequential order (sē-kwen'shăl ōr'děr) One after another in a predictable pattern or sequence.

serum (sēr'ŭm) The liquid portion of blood (plasma) when all of the clotting factors have been removed.

serum separators (sēr'ŭm sep'ăr-ā'tŏrz) A type of blood collection tube with an additive that, when centrifuged, forms a gel-like barrier between serum and the clot in a coagulated blood sample.

sexual harassment (sek'shū-ăl hăr-ăs'ment) Unwelcome verbal, visual, or physical conduct of a sexual nature that is severe or pervasive and affects working conditions or creates a hostile work environment.

shelter-in-place (shel'tĕr in plās) An interior room or rooms with few or no windows that form a place to take refuge in case of an emergency or a disaster.

side effects (sīd e-fekts') Unintended but fairly mild and common effects of a medication.

sigmoidoscopy (sig'moy-dos'kŏ-pē) A procedure in which the interior of the sigmoid area of the large intestine, between the descending colon and the rectum, is examined with a sigmoidoscope, a lighted instrument with a magnifying lens.

sign (sīn) An objective, or external, factor, such as blood pressure, rash, or swelling, that can be seen or felt by the physician or measured by an instrument.

signature block (sig'nă-chŭr blok) The writer's name and business title found four lines below the complimentary closing in a business letter.

simplified letter style (sim'pli-fīd let'ĕr stīl) A modification of the full-block style in which the salutation and complimentary closing are omitted and a subject line typed in all capital letters is placed between the address and the body of the letter.

single-entry account (sing'gĕl en'trē ă-kownt') An account that has only one charge, usually for a small amount, for a patient who does not come in regularly.

sinoatrial node (SA node) (sī'nō-ā'trē-ăl nōd) A small bundle of heart muscle tissue in the superior wall of the right atrium that sets the rhythm (pattern) of the heart's contractions; also called sinus node or pacemaker.

skip (skĭp) A patient who has moved without leaving a forwarding address and his bill is unpaid.

sleep apnea (slēp ap'nē-ă) A condition characterized by pauses in breathing during sleep.

slit lamp (slit lămp) An instrument composed of a magnifying lens combined with a light source; used to provide a minute examination of the eye's anatomy.

SOAP (sōp) An approach to medical records documentation that documents information in the following order: S (subjective data), O (objective data), A (assessment), P (plan of action).

soft skills (sawft skilz) Personal attributes that enhance an individual's interactions, job performance, and career prospects.

software (soft'wār) A program, or set of instructions, that tells a computer what to do.

solution (sŏ-lū'shŭn) A homogeneous mixture of a solid, liquid, or gaseous substance in a liquid, such as a dissolved drug in liquid form.

somatic nervous system (sō-măt'ik nĕr'vŭs sis'tĕm) A system that governs the body's skeletal, or voluntary, muscles.

SOMR Source-oriented medical record. The information in this type of medical record is arranged according to the provider type supplying the data.

SPECT (spĕkt) Single photon emission computed tomography; a radiologic procedure in which a gamma camera detects signals induced by gamma radiation and a computer converts these signals into two- or three-dimensional images that are displayed on a screen.

speculum (spek'yū-lŭm) An instrument that expands the vaginal opening to permit viewing of the vagina and cervix.

spermatogenesis (sper-măt'ō-jen'ĕ-sis) The process of sperm cell formation.

sphincter (sfĭngk'tĕr) A valve-like structure formed from circular bands of muscle. Sphincters are located around various body openings and passages.

sphygmomanometer (sfig'mō-mă-nom'ĕ-ter) An instrument for measuring blood pressure; consists of an inflatable cuff, a pressure bulb used to inflate the cuff, and a device to read the pressure.

spirillum (spī-ril'ŭm) A spiral-shaped bacterium.

spirometer (spī-rom'ĕ-ter) An instrument that measures the air taken in and expelled from the lungs.

spirometry (spī-rom'ĕ-trē) A test used to measure breathing capacity.

spleen (splēn) An abdominal organ that assists in the production and removal of blood cells.

splint (splĭnt) A device used to immobilize and protect a body part.

spores (spōrz) A resistant form of certain species of bacteria.

sprain (sprān) An injury characterized by partial tearing of a ligament that supports a joint, such as the ankle. A sprain also may involve injuries to tendons, muscles, and local blood vessels and contusions of the surrounding soft tissue.

stain (stān) In microbiology, a solution of a dye or group of dyes that imparts a color to microorganisms.

standard (stan'dărd) A specimen for which test values are already known; used to calibrate test equipment.

standard of care (stan'dărd kār) A legal term that refers to the care that would ordinarily be provided by an average, prudent healthcare provider in a given situation.

standard precautions (stan'dărd prē-kaw'shŭnz) A combination of universal precautions and Body Substance Isolation guidelines; used in hospitals for the care of all patients.

statement (stāt'mĕnt) Similar to an invoice; a summary of total amounts owed, including outstanding charges as well as payments received for services provided by the office.

statute of limitations (sta'chyūt lim'i-tā'shŭnz) A state law that sets a time limit on when a collection suit on a past-due account can legally be filed.

stenosis (stĕ-nō'sis) An abnormal narrowing of a body passage.

stent (stĕnt) A metal mesh tube used to hold a vessel open.

stereotyping (ster'ē-ō-tī'ping) A negative statement about the specific traits of a group that is applied unfairly to an entire population.

sterile field (ster'il fēld) An area free of microorganisms used as a work area during a surgical procedure.

sterilization (ster'i-li-zā'shŭn) The destruction of all microorganisms, including bacterial spores, by specific means.

sterilization indicator (ster'i-li-zā'shŭn in'di-kā-tŏr) A tag, insert, tape, tube, or strip that confirms that the items in an autoclave have been exposed to the correct volume of steam at the correct temperature for the correct amount of time.

sternum (stĕr'nŭm) A bone that forms the front and middle portion of the rib cage; also called the breastbone or breast plate.

steroidal hormone (ster-oy'dăl hōr'mōn) A hormone derived from steroids that are soluble in lipids and can cross cell membranes very easily.

stethoscope (stĕth'ĕ-skōp) An instrument that amplifies body sounds.

strain (strān) A muscle injury that results from overexertion or overstretching.

stratum basale (strat'ŭm bā-sā'lē) The deepest layer of the epidermis of the skin.

stratum corneum (strat'ŭm kōr'nē-ŭm) The most superficial layer of the epidermis of the skin.

stress test (stres tĕst) A procedure that involves recording an electrocardiogram while the patient is exercising on a stationary bicycle, treadmill, or stair-stepping ergometer, which measures work performed.

stressor (stres'or) Any stimulus that produces stress.

striations (strī-ā'shŭnz) Bands produced from the arrangement of filaments in myofibrils in skeletal and cardiac muscle cells.

subcategory (sŭb-kăt'ĭ-gôr'ē) The fourth digit added to many ICD-10 codes giving further specificity to the diagnosis.

subcutaneous (subcut) (sŭb'kyŭ-tā'nē-ŭs) Under the skin.

subject line (sŭb'jekt līn) Optional line of two to three words that appears three lines below the inside address of a business letter.

subjective (sŭb-jĕk'tĭv) Pertaining to data that are obtained from conversation with a person or patient.

subjective data (sŭb-jĕk'tĭv dā'tă) Information about the patient's condition that includes thoughts, feelings, and perceptions.

sublingual (sŭb-ling'gwăl) Under the tongue.

substance abuse (sŭb'stăns ă-byūs') The use of a substance in a way that is not medically approved, such as using diet pills to stay awake or consuming large quantities of cough syrup that contains codeine. Substance abusers are not necessarily addicts.

sudoriferous (sŭ'dŏr-if'ĕr-ŭs) The sweat glands.

suffix (sŭ'fiks) A word part that comes at the end of a medical term that alters the meaning of the term.

supernatant (sū-per-nā'tănt) The liquid portion of a substance from which solids have settled to the bottom, as with a urine specimen after centrifugation.

surfactant (sŭr-fak'tănt) Fatty substance secreted by some alveolar cells that helps maintain the inflation of the alveoli so that they do not collapse in on themselves between inspirations.

surgical asepsis (sŭr'ji-kăl ā-sep'sis) The elimination of all microorganisms from objects or working areas; also called sterile technique.

surgical site infection (SSI) (sŭr'ji-kăl sīt in-fek'shŭn) An infection that occurs after a surgical procedure at the site of surgery.

susceptible host (sŭ-sep'ti-bĕl hōst) An individual who has little or no immunity to infection by a particular organism.

suture (sū'chŭr) Fibrous joint in the skull. Also, a surgical stitch made to close a wound.

swaged needle (swājd nē'dĕl) A suturing needle that has the suture material permanently attached to the needle.

symmetry (sim'ĕ-trē) The degree to which one side of the body is the same as the other.

sympathetic branch (sim'pă-thet'ik branch) A branch of the autonomic nervous system that prepares organs for fight-or-flight (stressful) situations.

symptom (simp'tŏm) A subjective, or internal, condition felt by a patient, such as pain, headache, or nausea, or another indication that generally cannot be seen or felt by the doctor or measured by instruments.

synaptic knob (si-nap'tik nŏb) An enlargement at the end of an axon branch that produces and releases neurotransmitters.

synergist (sĭn'er-jist) Muscle that helps the prime mover by stabilizing joints.

systemic circulation (sis-tem'ik sĭr'kyū-lā'shŭn) The circulation of blood through the arteries, capillaries, and veins of the general system, from the left ventricle to the right atrium.

systolic pressure (sis-tol'ik presh'ŭr) The blood pressure measured when the left ventricle of the heart contracts.

Tabular List (tab'yŭ-lăr list) One of two ways that diagnoses are listed in the ICD-10. In the Tabular List, the diagnosis codes are listed in numeric order with additional instructions.

tachycardia (tak'i-kahr'dē-ă) Rapid heart rate, generally in excess of 100 beats per minute.

tachypnea (tăk-ip-nē'ă) Abnormally rapid breathing.

targeted résumé (tahr'gĕt-ed rez'ŭm-ā) A résumé that is focused on a specific job target.

tax liability account (taks lī'ă-bil'ĭ-tē ă-kownt') Money withheld from employees' paychecks and held in a separate account that must be used to pay taxes to appropriate government agencies.

teamwork (tēm'wŏrk) Working with others in the best interest of completing the job.

telecommunications device for the deaf (TDD) (tel'ĕ-kŏ-myū'ni-kā'shŭnz dĕ-vīs' def) Telephone accessory that transmits and receives text over standard telephone lines.

telephone triage (tĕl'ĕ-fōn' trē'ahzh) A process of determining the level of urgency of each incoming telephone call and how it should be handled.

teletherapy (tel-ĕ-thăr'ă-pē) A radiation therapy technique that allows deeper penetration than brachytherapy; used primarily for deep tumors.

template (tem'plăt) A guide that ensures consistency and accuracy.

temporal mandibular joint (TMJ) (tem'pŏr-ăl man-dib'yū-lăr joynt) The location where the mandible attaches to the temporal bone.

terminal digit (tĕr'mi-năl dij'it) A small group of two to three numbers at the end of a patient number that is used as an identifying unit in a filing system.

testes (tĕs'tēz) The primary organs of the male reproductive system. Testes produce the hormone **testosterone.**

therapeutic team (thăr'ă-pyū'tik tēm) A group of physicians, nurses, medical assistants, and other specialists who work with patients dealing with chronic illness or recovery from major injuries.

thermometer (ther-mom'ĕ-ter) An instrument, either electronic or disposable, that is used to measure body temperature.

thermotherapy (ther'mō-thăr'ă-pē) The application of heat to the body to treat a disorder or injury.

third-party check (thĭrd-pahr'tē chĕk) A check made out to one recipient and given in payment to another, as with one made out to a patient rather than the medical practice.

third-party payer (thĭrd-pahr'tē pā'ĕr) A health plan that agrees to carry the risk of paying for patient services.

thoracocentesis (thōr'ă-kō-sen-tē'sis) Medical procedure in which a sterile needle is introduced into the chest to remove fluid and pus.

thoracostomy (thōr'ă-kos'tŏ-mē) The surgical insertion of a chest tube to provide continuous drainage of the thoracic (chest) cavity. (thoraco- = chest; -stomy = opening)

thorax (thō'raks) The chest cavity.

thrombocytes (throm'bō-sīts) Fragments of cytoplasm in the blood that are crucial to clot formation; also called **platelets.**

thrombus (thrŏm′bŭs)   A blood clot that forms on the inside of an injured blood vessel wall.

thymus (thī′mŭs)   A gland that lies between the lungs. It secretes a hormone called thymosin.

thyroid gland (thī′royd gland)   An endocrine gland, consisting of irregularly spheroid follicles, lying in front and to the sides of the upper part of the trachea, in a horseshoe shape, with two lateral lobes connected by a narrow central portion, the isthmus; occasionally an elongated offshoot, the pyramidal lobe, passes upward from the isthmus in front of the trachea. It is supplied by branches from the external carotid and subclavian arteries, and its nerves are derived from the middle cervical and cervicothoracic ganglia of the sympathetic system. It secretes thyroid hormone and calcitonin.

tibia (ti′bē-ă)   The medial bone of the lower leg; commonly called the shin bone.

tickler file (tĭk′lĕr fīl)   A reminder file for keeping track of time-sensitive obligations.

time management (tīm man′ăj-mĕnt)   Utilizing time in an effective manner to accomplish the desired results.

time-specified scheduling (tīm spĕs′i-fīd sked′jūl-ing)   A system of scheduling where patients arrive at regular, specified intervals, ensuring the practice a steady stream of patients throughout the day.

tinnitus (tin′i-tŭs)   An abnormal ringing in the ear.

tissue (tish′ū)   A structure that is formed when cells of the same type organize together.

tonometer (tō-nom′ĕ-tĕr)   An instrument for determining pressure or tension, especially determining ocular tension.

tonsils (ton′silz)   Sets of lymphoid tissue in and around the oral cavity. The three sets are the pharyngeal tonsils (adenoids), palatine tonsils, and lingual tonsils.

tort (tōrt)   In civil law, a breach of some obligation that causes harm or injury to someone.

tourniquet (tŭr′ni-kĕt)   An instrument for temporarily arresting the flow of blood to or from a distal part by pressure applied with an encircling device.

toxicology (tŏk′sĭ-kŏl′ŏ-jē)   The study of poisons or poisonous effects of drugs.

trachea (trā′kē-ă)   The part of the respiratory tract between the larynx and the bronchial tree that is tubular and made of rings of cartilage and smooth muscle; also called the windpipe.

tracking (trăk′ĭng)   Watching for changes in spending so as to help control expenses.

traction (trak′shŭn)   The pulling or stretching of the musculoskeletal system to treat dislocated joints, joints afflicted by arthritis or other diseases, and fractured bones.

trade name (trād nām)   A drug's brand, or proprietary, name.

transcription (trăn-skrĭp′shŭn)   The transforming of spoken notes into accurate written form.

transdermal (trans-der′măl)   A type of topical drug administration that slowly and evenly releases a systemic drug through the skin directly into the bloodstream; a transdermal unit is also called a patch.

transmission-based precautions (tranz-mish′ŭn-bāsd prē-kaw′shŭnz)   CDC guidelines that supplement standard precautions when caring for patients with suspected or confirmed infection. The three types of transmission-based precautions are contact, droplet, and airborne precautions.

traveler's check (trăv′ĕl-rz chĕk)   A check purchased and signed at a bank and later signed over to a payee.

triage (trē′ahzh)   To assess the urgency and types of conditions patients present as well as their immediate medical needs.

triglycerides (trī-glis′ĕr-īdz)   Simple lipids consisting of glycerol (an alcohol) and three fatty acids.

trigone (trī′gōn)   The triangle formed by the openings of the two ureters and the urethra in the internal floor of the bladder.

triple check (trip′ĕl chek)   The process of checking a medication three times before administering it. First check is when you take it from the storage container and match it to the MAR or physician order; second check is when you prepare the medication; third check is before you close the container or just before you administer the medication.

Truth in Lending Statement (trūth lend′ing stāt′mĕnt)   A written description of the agreed terms of payment between the patient and medical practice when payment will be made in more than four installments.

turbidity (ter-bid′i-tē)   Cloudiness, often due to small particles present in a liquid.

tympanic membrane (tim-păn′ik mĕm′brān)   A fibrous partition located at the inner end of the ear canal and separating the outer ear from the middle ear; also called the eardrum.

ulna (ŭl′nă)   The medial bone of the lower arm.

unbundling (ŭn-bŭnd′ling)   Use of several *Current Procedural Terminology* codes for a service when one inclusive code is available.

underbooking (ŭn′dĕr-buk′ing)   Leaving large, unused gaps in the doctor's schedule; this approach does not make the best use of the doctor's time.

unit (yū′nit)   A part of an individual's name or title, described in indexing rules.

unsaturated fats (ŭn-săch′ŭr-āt-ĕd fats)   Fats, including most vegetable oils, that are usually liquid at room temperature and tend to lower blood cholesterol.

upcoding (ŭp′kōd-ing)   Coding to a higher level of service than that provided to obtain higher reimbursements.

ureters (yūr′ĕ-tĕrz)   Long, slender, muscular tubes that carry urine from the kidneys to the urinary bladder.

urethra (yūr-ē′thră)   The tube that conveys urine from the bladder during urination.

urinalysis (yūr′in-al′i-sis)   The physical, chemical, and microscopic evaluation of urine to obtain information about body health and disease.

urinary pH (yūr′i-nar-ē)   A measure of the degree of acidity or alkalinity of urine.

urine culture (yūr′in kŭl′chŭr)   A laboratory test in which urine is placed on a growth medium and bacteria are allowed to grow for 24 to 48 hours. Any large growths of bacteria are then identified. Urine cultures are often followed by a sensitivity or susceptibility test to determine which antibiotic will be most effective against the bacteria.

urine specific gravity (yūr′in spĕ-sif′ik grav′i-tē)   A measure of the concentration or amount (total weight) of substances dissolved in urine.

urobilinogen (yūr-ō-bī-lin′ō-jen)   A colorless compound formed by the breakdown of hemoglobin in the intestines. Elevated levels in urine may indicate increased red blood cell destruction or liver disease, whereas lack of urobilinogen in the urine may suggest total bile duct obstruction.

utilization review (UR) (yū'ti-li-zā'shŭn rē-vyū') The process of reviewing medical care in individual cases to be sure that all services provided were medically necessary and that there was appropriate use of medical resources; performed by medical peers and used as a cost control measure by managed care organizations.

uvula (ū'vyū-lă) The part of the soft palate that hangs down in the back of the throat.

vasectomy (vas-ek'tō-mē) A male sterilization procedure in which a section of each vas deferens is removed.

vasoconstriction (vā'sō-kŏn-strik'shŭn) The constriction of the muscular wall of an artery to increase blood pressure.

vasodilation (vā-sō-dī-lā'shŭn) The widening of the muscular wall of an artery to decrease blood pressure.

vector (vek'tŏr) A living organism, such as an insect, that carries microorganisms from an infected person to another person.

venipuncture (ven'i-pŭngk'shŭr) The puncture of a vein, usually with a needle, for the purpose of drawing blood.

venoscope (vē'no-skōp) An instrument that helps visualize a vein; LED lights illuminate the subcutaneous tissue to highlight the veins.

ventricular fibrillation (VF) (ven-trik'yū-lăr fib'ri-lā'shŭn) An abnormal heart rhythm that is the most common cause of cardiac arrest.

verbalizing (vûr'bă-līz'ĭng) Stating what you believe the patient is suggesting or implying.

vertical file (věr'ti-kăl fīl) A filing cabinet featuring pull-out drawers that usually contain a metal frame or bar equipped to handle letter- or legal-sized documents in hanging file folders.

vestibule (ves'ti-byūl) The area in the inner ear between the semicircular canals and the cochlea.

vibrio (vib'rē-ō) A comma-shaped bacterium.

video relay services (VRS) (vĭ'dē-ō rē'lā ser'vĭ-sěz) A type of telecommunication that allows persons with hearing disabilities to use American Sign Language to communicate with voice telephone users through video equipment, rather than through typed text.

virtual private network (VPN) (vir'chū-ăl prī'văt net'wŏrk) These are used to connect two or more computer systems.

visceral smooth muscle (vis'ĕr-ăl smūth mŭs'ĕl) A type of smooth muscle containing sheets of muscle that closely contact each other. It is found in the walls of hollow organs such as the stomach, intestines, bladder, and uterus.

viscosity (vis-kos'i-tē) Thickness.

vitamin (vīt'ă-min) Organic substance that is essential for normal body growth and maintenance and resistance to infection.

volume (vol'yūm) The amount of space an object, such as a drug, occupies.

voucher check (vow'chĕr chĕk) A business check with an attached stub, which is kept as a receipt.

walk-in (wôk'in) A patient who arrives without an appointment.

wave scheduling (wāv sked'jūl-ing) A system of scheduling in which the number of patients seen each hour is determined by dividing the hour by the length of the average visit and then giving that number of patients appointments with the doctor at the beginning of each hour.

weight (wāt) The product of the force of gravity, defined internationally as 9.81 (m/sec)/sec, × the mass of the body.

wellness (wěl'něs) A philosophy of life and personal hygiene that views health as not merely the absence of illness but the fullest realization of one's physical and mental potential, as achieved through positive attitudes, fitness training, a diet low in fat and high in fiber, and the avoidance of unhealthful practices.

wet mount (wět mount) A preparation of a specimen in a liquid that allows the organisms to remain alive and mobile while they are being identified.

whole blood (hōl blŭd) The total volume of plasma and formed elements, or blood in which the elements have not been separated by coagulation or centrifugation.

whole foods (hōl fūdz) Foods that have little or no processing before they are eaten.

wide-area network (WAN) (wīd ār'ē-ă net'wŏrk) A computer network in which the computers connected may be far apart, generally having a radius of half a mile or more.

Wood's light examination (wudz līt eg-zam'i-nā'shŭn) A type of dermatologic examination in which a physician inspects the patient's skin under an ultraviolet lamp in a darkened room.

word root (wŏrd rūt) The base meaning of a medical term.

work ethic (wŏrk eth'ik) A set of values of hard work held by employees.

work practice controls (wŏrk prak'tis kŏn-trōlz') Controlling workplace injuries by altering the way a task is performed.

work quality (wŏrk kwahl'i-tē) Striving for excellence in doing the job; pride in one's performance.

World Health Organization (WHO) (wŏrld helth ŏr'găn-ĭ-zā'shŭn) A unit of the United Nations devoted to international health problems.

write-it-once (pegboard) system (rīt it wŭns pĕg'bōrd sis'tĕm) A manual bookkeeping system where the daily log has prepunched holes on the right or left side of the log. Prepunched charge sheets (of NCR paper) are placed in designated areas on top of the day sheet, which has been placed on the pegboard. The patient ledger card is placed between the day sheet and the charge sheet and an entry is made; it appears on all three documents at the same time.

written-contract account (rě'ten kŏn'trăkt ă-kownt') An agreement between the physician and patient stating that the patient will pay a bill in more than four installments.

Z-track method (zē'trăk měth'ŏd) A technique used when injecting an intramuscular (IM) drug that can irritate subcutaneous tissue; involves pulling the skin and subcutaneous tissue to the side before inserting the needle at the site and creating a zigzag path in the tissue layers that prevents the drug from leaking into the subcutaneous tissue and causing irritation.

zygote (zī'gōt) The cell that is formed from the union of the egg and sperm.

Page numbers in **boldface** indicate figures. Page numbers followed by b indicate box features, p procedures, and t tables, respectively.

POLST forms, 61–62, 63t
preoperative duties and, 661
standard of care, 55
statute of limitations, 58
terminating care of patients, **54,** 54–55
uniform donor cards, 62–63
withdrawing from a case, **54,** 54–55, 59–60
Lawyers, telephone calls from, 171
Laxatives, 850t
Lazy eye, 625
LDLs (low-density lipoproteins), 304, 775t, 940
Leading questions, 469t
Leads, in ECGs, 795–798, 798t
Lead selector, on electrocardiographs, 799
Learning, domains of, 186, **186**
Learning disabilities, 572
LEEP (loop electrosurgical excision procedure), 540
Left atrioventricular valve, 284
Legal documents
advance medical directives, 62, 63t
durable power of attorney, 62
living wills, 39, 61
POLST forms, 61–62, 63t
uniform donor cards, 62–63
Legal issues. *See* Laws and legal issues
Legionella pneumophila, 705t
Legionnaire's disease, 335b, 705t, A–1
Legislation. *See* Laws and legal issues; *specific legislation*
Legs
bones of, 256, **256**
muscles of, **271,** 273
Leiomyomas, 542t
Lens, **429,** 430, 432t
Lentigos, 585, **585,** A–11
Leprosy, 704, 706t
Lesbian, gay, bisexual, transsexual, queer (LGBTQ) persons, 41
Letters
cover letters, 1006–1007, **1009**
thank-you letters, 1010
withdrawing from a case, **54,** 54–55, 60
Leukemia, 309b, 603t, A–11
Leukocytes. *See* White blood cells (WBCs)
Leukocytosis, 302
Leukopenia, 304
LGBTQ (lesbian, gay, bisexual, transsexual, queer) persons, 41
LH (luteinizing hormone), 377, 382, **414,** 415t, 416
Liability, 52, 57
Liability insurance, 58
Libel, 51
Libraries, as patient education resource, 191
Lice, 241b, 392–393b, 571t, 708t, 711, A–2
Licensed practitioners, 2
Lidocaine, 663
LifeSign Status Mono, 781

Lifespan development model, 31, **31**
Lifting objects, guidelines for, 105
Ligaments, 209, 256
Ligatures, 652, 658
Lighting, 111, 135, 680, **680**
Limb electrodes, 800, **801**
Limb leads, 798, 798t
Limbus, **429,** 430
Limitation of Exposure to Ionizing Radiation (NCRP), 835
Lingual frenulum, 398
Lingual tonsils, 315, 398, **400**
Linoleic acid, 405
Lipids, 219, 405, **939,** 939–940, 940t
Lipoproteins, 304
Listening skills, 34, **34,** 468
Listeria monocytogenes, 706t
Literacy, 39, 511b
Lithotomy position, 512–513, **513,** 521p
Lithotripsy, 369b, 406–407b
Liver. *See also* Hepatitis
cancer of, 603t
cirrhosis of, 406b
structure and function of, **398,** 403, **403**
Liver, cirrhosis of, A–15
Liver spots, 585, **585**
Living wills, 39, 61
LMP (last menstrual period), 530
Lobes
of brain, 347, **348**
of lungs, 330
Local anesthetics, 651, **663,** 663–664
Lockjaw, 277b
Locum tenens, 56
Lofstrand® crutches, 924
Long bones, 247, **248, 250**
Longitudinal fissure, 347
Loniten, 847
Look-alike/sound-alike medications, 850, 850–851t, 885b
Loop electrosurgical excision procedure (LEEP), 540
Loop of Henle, 363, **364**
Lordosis, 259b, A–9
Lou Gehrig's disease, 354b, A–13
Love/belonging needs, 32, **32**
Low-cholesterol diets, 947
Low-density lipoproteins (LDLs), 304, 775t, 940
Lower esophageal sphincter, 401, **401**
Lower GI series. *See* Barium enema
Low-sodium diets, 947
Low-tyramine diets, 947
LSD, 472t, 858t
Lubricants, 132, 138
Lubrication, 382
Lumbar enlargement, 346, **346**
Lumbar puncture, 352–353, 615
Lumbar trunk, 313
Lumbar vertebrae, 252, 252t, **253**
Lumbosacral plexus, 351
Lung cancer, 335–336b, **336,** 603t, A–13
Lung flukes, 708t

Lungs
anatomy and structure of, **328,** 330
cancer of, 335–336b, **336,** 603t
collapsed, 333–334b
diseases and disorders of, 333–339b
examination of, 517
mechanisms of breathing and, **330,** 330–331
pulmonary circulation and, 289–290, **290**
systemic circulation and, 290, **290**
Lunula, 234, **234**
Lupus, 322–323b, A–12
Luteinizing hormone (LH), 377, 382, **414,** 415t, 416
Lyme disease, 85, 703, 705t, 711, A–1
Lymph, 313, 314, **314**
Lymphadenitis, 315, A–12
Lymphadenopathy, 315, A–12
Lymphatic capillaries, 313, **314**
Lymphatic ducts, 313–314, **314**
Lymphatic system, 313–319. *See also* Immune system
defenses against disease, 316–318, 317t, **319**
interstitial fluid and lymph, 313, **314**
lymph nodes, 314, 315, **315**
organs and tissues of, 315–316, **315–316,** 316t
structure and function of, **212,** 313–316, **314**
thymus and spleen in, 315, **316**
vessels and circulation in, 313–314, **314**
Lymphatic trunks, 313–314, **314**
Lymphatic vessels, 313–314, **314**
Lymphedema, 322b, A–12
Lymph nodes, 314, 315, **315,** 316t
Lymph nodules, 315–316
Lymphocytes
B cells, 318, **319–320**
function of, 303t, 304, 315
normal ranges for, 773t
specific defense and, 317–318
staining characteristics of, 776, 777t
T cells, 304, 318, **319**
Lymphokines, 318
Lysosomes, 220, **220**
Lysozymes, 317, 430

M

MAC (*Mycobacterium avium* complex) infection, 702
Macrophages, 209, 302, 315, 317, 318
Macular degeneration, 624–625, A–18
Macules, **232,** 233, 233t, A–5
Mad cow disease, 699t
MADD (Mothers Against Drunk Driving), 982t
Magazines, for reception areas, **111,** 111–112
Magnesium, 406, 943
Magnetic resonance imaging (MRI)
in cardiology, 612
disorders diagnosed with, 827t

in neurologic testing, 353, 615, **615**
in oncology, 615
in orthopedics, 616
procedure for, 832, **832**
Magnetic therapy, 862
Mail. *See also* Letters
e-mail, 17
specimens sent by, 715–716, **716**
U.S. Postal Service, 715
Maintenance
of examination instruments, 136–137
quality control and, 686–688, **688–689**
of testing equipment, 688, **689**
Maintenance drug therapy, 847
Major histocompatibility complex (MHC), 318
Malaria, 85, 707, 708t, 711, A–2
Male reproductive system, 373–379. *See also* Testes
contraception and, 389–390, **390**
diseases and disorders of, 378–379b, 542–545, 603t, A–14
erection, orgasm and ejaculation, 377
examination of, 518
external accessory organs of, 376–377
hormones of, 377
infertility, 390–391
internal accessory organs of, 374, 376
sexually transmitted infections and, 544–545, 544b
structure and function of, **213,** 373, **374**
testicular self-exams, 541, 541b
Malfeasance, 56
Malignant hypertension, 495
Malignant tumors, 321b, 602
Malleus, 435, **435**
Malnutrition, A–16
Malpractice, 55–59
civil law and, 57
courtroom conduct in, 57–58
defined, 51
examples of, 55–56
four Cs of prevention, 58–59
insurance for, 57, 58
laws of agency and, 57
negligence and, 55–58
proving, 56–57
reasons patients sue, 58
risk management and, 55
settling suits of, 57
statute of limitations and, 58
Maltase, 402
MALT (mucosa-associated lymphoid tissue), 315
Mammary glands, 381, **381**
Mammography/mammograms
disorders diagnosed with, 827t, **833**
medical assistant's role in, 832
patient education on, 537b
procedure for, 536, **536**
recommendations for, 530–531